2000 Edition

Questionable Doctors

Sidney Wolfe, M.D.
Phyllis McCarthy
Alana Bame
Benita Marcus Adler

Disciplined by State and Federal Governments

Arizona, Colorado, Nevada, New Mexico, Utah

Public Citizen
Health Research Group

Public Citizen is a nonprofit membership organization in Washington, D.C., dedicate to advancing consumer rights through lobbying, litigation, research, publications an information services.

Since its founding by Ralph Nader in 1971, Public Citizen has fought for consumer right in the marketplace, for safe and secure health care, for fair trade, for clean and safe energ sources, and for corporate and government accountability

First printing

Region 3: Arizona, Colorado, Nevada, New Mexico, Utah ISBN 1-58231-004-1

Acknowledgments

The authors would like to acknowledge the important efforts of many people and institutions which made this study possible.

First, we are grateful to the state licensing or disciplinary boards which cooperated with our requests for doctor-specific information by sending us lists which, in many cases, required them to reorganize data in a form which would be more useful to us. Similarly, the Inspector General's Office of the Department of Health and Human Services (HHS) has been extremely cooperative with our requests for information on those physicians who were sanctioned by the Peer Review Organizations and those who were the subject of other HHS sanctions. The Drug Enforcement Administration (DEA), initially, belatedly, incompletely and only in the face of a lawsuit from Public Citizen, gave us the data on doctors with uncontested restrictions or revocations of their narcotics licenses. Several consumer groups, including the New York Public Interest Research Group (NYPIRG) have also provided us with valuable information.

But the lion's share of time spent on this report was in the time-consuming process of data entry, checking, rechecking and *rechecking* for accuracy and editing of information. A group of Public Citizen employees and former Public Citizen employees assisted in this enormous task including Kimberly Ferlauto, Luisa Hegedus, Salwa Nassar, Demian Larry and Ragin Jennings.

Jason Stele, Public Citizen's Manager of Information Systems, spent many long hours desiging our programs and providing computer assistance. Sean R. Witte, our computer consultant offered valuable assistance.

David Vladeck, an attorney with and Director of the Public Citizen Litigation Group, spent many long hours going over our summaries of the legal actions taken by state boards to ensure that they correctly interpreted the lengthier statements we received from the states.

Previous authors of the first four editions were Nicole Simmons, Ingrid VanTuinen, Durrie McKnew, Mary Gabay and Katie Franklin. Other Public Citizen employees who worked on earlier editions include Toufic Rahman, Dana Hull, Lynn Soffer, Joan Stieber, Joanne Mott, Stephen Moore, Beverly Wellman, Kate Moore, Lauren Kanee, Kathy Cashel. Elizabeth Hanson, Edith T. Burpee, Christine E. Dehlendorf, Lauren Dame, and Elizabeth Schramm.

Table of Contents

Executive Summary

Information in the one federal repository of disciplinary actions by state medical boards and federal agencies--the National Practitioner Data Bank--is kept secret from both patients and from almost all physicians thanks to the American Medical Association's successful lobbying for secrecy when the legislation concerning the Data Bank was being considered. It is partially in protest to this congressionally-mandated secrecy that Public Citizen's Health Research Group has established our own publicly-available data bank of doctors who have been disciplined. What follows are just a few of the main findings from our study of the data as reported in the national version of *20,125 Questionable Doctors* and in the regional versions:

* 20,125 doctors disciplined by either state medical boards or federal agencies are listed in the national books. This represents an increase of 6,185 new physicians since the last version of this report.

* These 20,125 doctors had a total of 38,589 disciplinary actions taken against them, the most common of which were probation (7,431 times), license suspension (3,704 times), fine (3,708 times) and license revocation (3,045 times). (See other types of disciplinary actions in Table D, Findings, pg. 21.) Although these and other serious actions made up 70% of all actions, far too many physicians received slaps on the wrist in the form of fines or reprimands despite having committed serious offenses. (see Tables F through J, pages 24-28.)

* For those doctors with disciplinary actions for which the states or federal agencies supplied specific information on the offenses they had committed, the following numbers of doctors committed the five most serious offenses (see other types of offenses in Table E, Findings, pg. 23):

1. Sexual abuse of or sexual misconduct with a patient: 547 doctors
2. Substandard care, incompetence or negligence: 3,215 doctors
3. Criminal Conviction (includes plea of guilty or no contest): 2,963 doctors
4. Misprescribing or overprescribing of drugs: 1,318 doctors
5. Substance abuse: 1,715 doctors

Of the 24,042 disciplinary actions for which offenses were listed (See Table E, pg. 23) for

7,132, the reason listed was "disciplinary action taken by another state or agency," leaving 16,910 offenses with specific details as to the nature of the offense. For 15,310 of these offenses or 90.6% of them, the offense was one of the five listed above or another serious offense such as providing false information, loss of hospital privileges or insurance fraud.

An analysis of the 2,366 doctors who were the subjects of DEA disciplinary actions revealed that hundreds were not the subject of any state disciplinary action even though their federal narcotics license had been revoked or restricted.

Similarly, of the 3,232 Medicare doctors who were the subjects of Medicare disciplinary actions, hundreds were not disciplined by their state boards even though most had involved exclusion from Medicare.

Thus, many states are not acting promptly, if at all, against physicians about whom a federal agency has already compiled sufficient information to discipline them for very serious offenses. Even for those states which do discipline these doctors, for most of the serious offenses involved in DEA or Medicare actions, some states frequently do little more than slap physicians on the wrist, leaving the majority free to practice with few if any restrictions.

Overall, the majority of physicians who were disciplined for the five most serious offenses--sexual abuse or sexual misconduct, substandard care, incompetence, or negligence, criminal conviction, misprescribing or overprescribing of drugs, or substance abuse were not required to stop practicing even temporarily. The most common disciplinary action for each of these five offenses was probation, the severity of which varies widely from state to state. Following are the percentages and numbers of physicians for each offense who did not have to stop practicing despite the offenses which they had committed:

* Sexual abuse of or sexual misconduct with a patient: 547 doctors.
  Only 52.3% of these physicians had to stop practicing, even temporarily. 47.7% or 261 doctors were not required to stop.
* Substandard care, incompetence or negligence: 3,215 doctors.
  Only 29.3% of these physicians had to stop practicing, even temporarily. 70.7% or 2,273 were not required to stop.
* Criminal conviction (includes plea of guilty or no contest): 2,963 doctors.
  Only 39.2% of these doctors had to stop practicing, even temporarily. 60.8% or 1,802 were not required to stop.
* Misprescribing or overprescribing of drugs: 1,318 doctors.
  Only 27.9% of these physicians had to stop practicing, even temporarily. 72.1% or 950

were not required to stop.

* Substance abuse: 1,715 doctors.

  Only 32.4% of these doctors had to stop practicing, even temporarily. 67.6% or 1,159 were not required to stop.

(See Tables F through J pages 24-28.)

Thus, it is likely that most of the doctors in these above five categories of very serious offenses are currently practicing medicine, with few if any of their patients aware of these offenses.

Precisely because regulators provide so many protections for these health care practitioners, in 1988 the Congressional Office of Technology Assessment concluded that a formal disciplinary action against a doctor provides a good reason to question his or her care.

Our study of the nation's medical quality control system led us to conclude that:

* Too little discipline is still being done. The rate of serious disciplinary actions by state medical boards was only 3.50 serious actions per 1,000 doctors or 2,696 serious actions in 1999. Therefore only an extremely small fraction of the nation's doctors face any serious state sanctions each year despite the fact that at least 80,000 patients are killed and 234,000 injured as a result of negligence in hospitals, most cases involving doctors.
* Far too few state medical board disciplinary actions are for medical negligence or incompetence. Of the 16,910 disciplinary actions in which we knew the basis (the offense) for which the action was taken and for which the basis of the action was not an action by another state, only 3,184 of those cases (18.8%) were for substandard care, incompetence or negligence.

This country's system for ensuring medical quality needs to be made much stronger. We suggest several avenues towards improvement. Most states need to strengthen their medical practice statutes, restructure their medical boards, and dramatically increase both funding and staffing. Most states should also establish programs to audit and weed out bad doctors so that patient injuries can be prevented rather than simply reacted to.

The total number of serious state disciplinary actions against physicians decreased from 2,803 reported for 1995 to 2,696 in 1999 for a nationwide rate of 3.50 serious actions per 1,000 physicians. A difference greater than 10-fold exists between Alaska, the state with the highest rate (10.34 per 1,000), and Delaware, with the lowest rate, (0.96). (See Table A, pg. 14.)

It is clear that state-by-state performance is spotty. Only one of the nation's 15 largest states, Ohio, is represented among those 10 states with the highest disciplinary rates, as it also was in

1996, 1997 and 1998. Other large states such as, New York, Michigan and California (14th, 19th and 20th respectively in 1999) have shown improvement from 40th, 49th and 37th in 1991. But other large states such as Texas, Pennsylvania, Massachusetts and Illinois (34th, 36th, 39th and 43rd in 1999) have not done very much doctor discipline for many of the last 10 years. It is not unreasonable to estimate that a nationwide average rate of at least 10 serious disciplinary actions per 1,000 doctors can be attained (the number was 3.50 in 1999) since, in most years, one or more states (Alaska, in 1999) actually takes this many actions. This would amount to 7,703 serious disciplinary actions a year, far in excess of the 2,696 serious disciplinary actions in 1999. If this had occurred, there would have been 5,007 more serious disciplinary actions that year--almost three times the number of actions which actually were taken.

Recommendations

Congress should require cooperation and routine data-sharing between state medical boards, Medicare Peer Review Organizations, state Medicaid agencies, the Drug Enforcement Administration and hospitals in catching and sanctioning malfeasant physicians.

The National Practitioner Data Bank, which began collecting information on questionable doctors in September 1990, should be opened to the public. This change will require legislation. Although there have been Congressional hearings on this topic in 2000, there is not any evidence that Congress has enough guts to take on the A.M.A.

The Drug Enforcement Administration should routinely tell the public and pharmacists which doctors' controlled substances prescription licenses it has pulled or restricted.

State medical boards should be required to promptly make public all their disciplinary actions and the offenses for which their actions were taken, and to regularly distribute lists of actions to consumers, the press, and other health care consumer organizations. In addition, boards should publicly disclose information they have concerning final hospital disciplinary actions and malpractice payouts against doctors.

In the past two years, many medical boards have started putting varying degrees of disciplinary information on their web sites. (for a report on the status of these sites--with grades A to X for completeness--visit our web site at http://www.citizen.org/hrg/publications/1506.htm) Unfortunately, most states either have no web site with disciplinary information or an inadequate amount of information about this important topic. Combined with the fact that only slightly more than half of the people in this country have access to the internet, this means that probably 75% of the people in this country do not have internet access to an adequate amount of this information. It is inexcusable that all states do not have detailed information about actions and offenses about every doctor who has been disciplined, including a copy of the board's order spelling out the details as to why the action was taken.

How to Use This Report

Questionable Doctors was designed to assist consumers in making better informed health care choices. The individual doctor listings aid patients in understanding the quality of care they would potentially receive or have already received from a particular practitioner. The general discussion of disciplinary actions and offenses within a state and the nation help to interpret the information we received.

Please Note...

Names sound alike. Just because a doctor whose name resembles your doctor's is listed in this report doesn't mean your doctor has been sanctioned. Some states failed to give us much identifying information on each doctor, and of the half a million doctors in this country, at least two are bound to have the same name.

Many things change with time. While your doctor's license may be listed as having been revoked, suspended or restricted in this edition of the report, this doesn't necessarily mean those restrictions are still in effect. The information contained in this edition is information we received from the state medical boards by January 31, 2000. We also included information received through May 31, 2000 regarding previous actions which were either overturned or terminated, leaving the physician with an unrestricted license. However, the state may have fully reinstated a doctor's license or lifted their probation or other restrictions in materials received after our deadlines.

Boards don't always have the final say. Your doctor may have appealed his or her disciplinary action and had it overturned by a court. Although we strive to provide the most current information, we are unable to obtain information on many appeals.

If you are selecting a doctor...

* Call the medical board in the state where the doctor practices or used to practice. The board can frequently provide information on the physician's educational and specialty background, and whether the doctor has been disciplined or formally charged with misconduct. (Contact information for each state board is listed at the end of each state's introductory section

in this book.)

* Check to see if your local consumer group has published a guide to local doctors.

* Look your doctor up in the American Medical Association's American Medical Directory or the Directory of Medical Specialists, which can be found in all medical libraries and many large public libraries. These directories list the physician's educational background and whether or not he or she is board-certified in a specialty. You should not select a self-designated specialist who has not been trained in the specialty field.

* Ask the doctor for the names of hospitals where he or she has admitting privileges. Your local university teaching hospital will probably be the most selective about the physicians it admits to its staff. Also, should you need to be hospitalized, you will want a doctor who can admit you to the best hospital.

If your current doctor is on this list...

* Check which state(s) or federal agency has disciplined him or her.

* Request a copy of the doctor's disciplinary file from the state or federal agency. State agency addresses are listed in the "Addresses" section of each state section. Federal addresses are in Appendix 3, pg. 50.

* Read the file before making a decision about whether to switch doctors. Some of the information contained in our report is sketchy and may not include a full explanation of the reason for the disciplinary action because states may not have sent these details to us. Some of the actions taken involve offenses that were administrative in nature and do not necessarily reflect on the physician's ability to practice.

* Ask your doctor why he or she was disciplined. If your doctor can convince you that any problem that resulted in the disciplinary action has been resolved or is irrelevant to your future care, fine. Otherwise, you should consider switching.

If you have a complaint about a doctor...

Some examples of reportable actions are:

* if a doctor over-charged you or charged for treatment that was not delivered;
* if a physician failed to order or properly administer appropriate tests or treatment;
* if you suspect that a doctor may be abusing drugs or alcohol;
* if a physician inappropriately touched you in a sexual manner or conducted a sexual relationship with you while you were a patient;

* if you suspect a physician is unable to function mentally or physically.

* Find out what degree your doctor has, whether a medical doctor (M.D.), osteopathic physician (D.O.), chiropractor (D.C.), podiatrist (D.P.M.), or dentist (D.D.S. or D.M.D.). Different state agencies often regulate these different professionals.

* File your complaint with the state medical disciplinary agency. This agency is the only one that can remove dangerous or incompetent doctors from practice, impose limitations on a physician's license to practice, and truly protect other patients from being harmed. Your complaint could lead to the suspension or revocation of a doctor's license directly, or it could aid the medical board in detecting a pattern of poor medical care.

* File the complaint in the state where the doctor is licensed--i.e., where his or her office is located. Turn to that state's section under our "State by State Listings." Find the "Address" heading. Look for the address of the agency that regulates that type of doctor.

* If your care was within a hospital, you should also file a complaint with the hospital's peer review committee, which has the power to revoke or limit a doctor's privileges to practice there.

* You may also want to file a complaint with Medicare (Addresses, Appendix 3, pg. 50).

* Call the agency you have found to inquire about how to file a formal complaint. Some agencies have toll-free hotlines for complaints. Others require complaints to be filed on a specific form.

* Ask whether your complaint will remain confidential. State laws vary. If the agency intends to reveal your name to your doctor, you may want to consider switching to another physician before pursuing any action.

* File a written complaint containing as much information as possible. Make sure to include the doctor's full name, correctly spelled, office address, and the exact date when the conduct you are complaining of occurred. The state may also ask you to release your medical records for review.

* Ask the agency to notify you of the outcome of your complaint.

If you want to improve medical quality assurance in the state or the nation...

* Write your state representatives, your congressional representative, and your senators. Ask them to pass the legislation we recommend on pg. 32.

Introduction

For more than a quarter of a century, Public Citizen's Health Research Group has been providing consumers with information they can use to make educated choices about their doctors. It has not been an easy road. Doctors generally don't like comparative information on quality to be released.

In the nation's first consumer's directory of local physicians, which we published in 1974 for Prince Georges County, Maryland, we wrote, "Most people can find out more about a car they plan to buy than they can about a doctor who may hold their life in his or her hands."[1] Unfortunately, that statement is still largely true today. In the process of collecting information from doctors for that directory, the Maryland State Medical Association threatened doctors who cooperated with loss of their license, arguing that "information that would point out differences between doctors" is illegal.

Another example of the barriers to public access to information on specific doctors: the federal government began collecting information on state disciplinary actions, malpractice payments, and revocations and restrictions of hospital privileges for its National Practitioner Data Bank (NPDB) in September 1990. The problem is that consumers (and even doctors--except for information on themselves) are forbidden by law to have access to the data. This information is available only to hospitals, Health Maintenance Organizations, and state and federal government agencies that regulate the quality of medical care.[2,3,4]

In the wake of efforts to pass legislation to open up the NPDB, the American Medical Association, whose earlier efforts had succeeded in a prohibition against public disclosure when the law creating the NPDB was passed in 1986, passed a resolution at its 1993 annual convention stating: "Resolved, that the American Medical Association...call for the dissolution of the National Practitioner Data Bank." Now, as then, the AMA seems to want to protect the minority of American physicians about whom there is data in the NPDB from the scrutiny of their own patients and other physicians.

It should be noted that a number of states have been increasingly using their disciplinary power to address administrative issues. Illinois and Medicare are sanctioning many physicians for defaulting on student loans; the District of Columbia targets physicians who failed to renew their license before the expiration date; and Pennsylvania suspends doctors for not paying a liability insurance surcharge. Although we do not advocate physicians shirking financial responsibilities, we feel that the public would be better served if boards focused more of their resources on exposing and preventing more serious patient abuses. We include such actions in our book because the agencies supplying this information have labeled them "disciplinary;" consumers, however, can and should differentiate between physicians sanctioned for true quality of care issues and administrative violations. These administrative actions, however, make up only a small fraction of cases listed in *20,125 Questionable Doctors.*

There has been some progress in the area of informing the public about poorly practicing physicians. Much information on state and federal government discipline of physicians is now public, although often difficult to obtain, and we have used that data to compile this report. State medical boards, licensing bureaus, and medical societies have increased public access to physician sanctions and license status via toll-free numbers and Internet postings (See our report on State Medical Board Web Sites at www.citizen.org/hrg/1506.htm); New York and California have made concerted efforts to enhance the exchange of information with other medical boards.

The United States has approximately 770,320 licensed medical doctors, most of them competent and dedicated. *20,125 Questionable Doctors* includes only that 2.6% of physicians whose care or conduct was substandard enough to be cited by a state medical disciplinary board, Medicare, or the federal Drug Enforcement Administration, or whose eligibility to participate in Food and Drug Administration (FDA) experiments was rescinded.

In a 1988 study on medical care quality assessment, the Congressional Office of Technology Assessment concluded that "a sanction imposed on a physician by a state or a Medicare Peer Review Organization is good reason to question the quality of his or her care.[5] The rigorous due process followed by state medical boards lends credibility to the validity of their formal disciplinary actions against physicians," stated the report. "State boards are reluctant to censure physicians and accord accused physicians extensive opportunities for appeal."

But until the day that consumers can have access to as much information about their health care providers as they can about buying a car Public Citizen will continue to battle the shroud of secrecy in which the medical community envelops itself.

The U.S. "System" of Medical Quality Control

The United States has a patchwork system for protecting the public from poor quality health care that is still largely uncoordinated and ineffective.

The first lines of defense are the state medical boards, the state government agencies charged with licensing physicians who meet certain standards. These boards are also responsible for catching already-licensed doctors who fall below standards of conduct or competence in any of a number of areas. They are legally empowered to discipline these doctors: to reprimand them, require them to take course work, impose fines, place them on probation, and, in the worst cases, to suspend them from practice or revoke their licenses altogether.

These licensing and disciplinary systems vary from state to state. In some states the medical board is an independent state agency. In others, it is contained within the state department of licensing, of health, or of consumer affairs. In some states there is one board or agency for medical licensing and another for medical discipline. In a few states, one board or agency regulates all the health care professions--doctors, nurses, dentists, and so forth. In others, there are separate licensing and disciplinary boards for medical (allopathic) physicians, for osteopathic physicians, for dentists, and so on.[6]

In all states, the licensing boards are required to provide consumers with some disciplinary information about a specific doctor. The state agencies' addresses, including their website address if applicable, and phone numbers are listed in the "Addresses" section of each state's listing in this report.

The U.S. Department of Health and Human Services, through its Medicare and Medicaid programs, also disciplines health practitioners. It excludes doctors from participation in Medicare or Medicaid for specified periods of time, and may fine them for violations as well.

The Department's Inspector General must exclude a doctor for at least five years for a criminal conviction related to the Medicare or Medicaid programs and for patient abuse or neglect.[7] It may also impose sanctions based on other types of convictions, on license revocation or suspension by a state agency, or on a sanction by any state Medicaid program. The Inspector General may also sanction a doctor for fraud, for accepting kickbacks, for failing to cooperate with investigators, for failing to pay loans, and, based on a recommendation by the Medicare Peer Review Organizations for each state, for providing substandard or unnecessary care. The Inspector General's office accepts consumer complaints at the phone numbers and addresses listed in Appendix 3, pg. 50.

The Drug Enforcement Administration (DEA), which is part of the U.S. Department of

Justice, tracks down doctors who overprescribe or abuse the so-called "scheduled drugs"--drugs such as narcotics, tranquilizers, and amphetamines that may be addictive or otherwise abused. The DEA issues licenses to doctors and dentists that allow them to prescribe these "controlled dangerous substances." No doctor may legally prescribe drugs listed as controlled substances without a valid DEA license. Some states require a separate state controlled substance license as well.

The DEA may deny a license to prescribe these drugs, restrict a doctor's prescription privileges, or revoke his or her privileges to prescribe controlled substances. It publishes notices of such disciplinary actions in the *Federal Register* when the actions have been contested. The address to direct complaints to the DEA is listed in Appendix 3, pg. 50.

The Food and Drug Administration (FDA) sanctions physicians who violated FDA laws, regulations, or policies regarding clinical research on patients. In addition, the FDA permanently debars from ever working for an FDA-regulated company any one--including physicians--who was convicted of a felony related to FDA regulation of drugs.

State medical societies and specialty societies, both of which are unofficial trade associations for doctors, not government agencies, have peer review committees and have a role to play in medical discipline. However, they cannot prevent a doctor from continuing to practice, and their vested interest, in most cases, is in protecting their members, not the public.

Hospitals are required to have peer review committees to review the quality of medical care in their institutions. Consumers who have complaints about the quality of care in a hospital should file them with these committees. The committees may throw doctors off their staffs or restrict doctors' privileges to practice there. Unfortunately, most hospitals regard their peer review activities and disciplinary actions as confidential and will not inform patients about them. The National Practitioner Data Bank (NPDB), as of December 31, 1997, contained information on 6,793 clinical privilege actions against doctors[8] but, as mentioned above, these data are kept secret. There is also serious concern that hospitals are not reporting all of the hospital disciplinary actions against doctors as required by law. During the first three years and four months of operation of the NPDB, 75 percent of U.S. hospitals had not reported even one physician to the NPDB.[9] By 1996, according to NPDB staff, the situation had improved and "only" two-thirds of hospitals had not reported a single physician to the NPDB.By early 2000, almost 10 years after the NPDB had started its operations, 59% of U.S. hospitals, over 4000 hospitals, had still never reported any physicians to the data bank. One of the ways hospitals are said to be gaming the system and avoiding reporting doctors is related to the requirement that only those hospital disciplinary actions against doctors which are more than 30 days in duration need to be reported. Many hospitals are apparently taking a plethora of 27, 28 or 29-day actions so they will not have to report doctors whose cash flow of patient referrals they do not want to jeopardize.

Malpractice insurers can also play a role in quality control: they can cancel the policy of a physician who presents a bad risk, raise his or her rates, or offer coverage only if his or her practice is restricted.[10] Unfortunately, many states guarantee every doctor access to malpractice insurance, no matter how poor his or her record. Without an insurance policy, few doctors could afford to continue practicing and, in many states, would not be legally allowed to. Some state medical boards are informed when a doctor has had malpractice insurance canceled and will tell consumers.

The Magnitude of the Problem of Inadequate Doctor Discipline

Though it has improved during the past 15 years, the nation's system for protecting the public from medical incompetence and malfeasance is still far from adequate.

Gaps and breakdowns in communication still exist, although the National Practitioner Data Bank is helping to prevent doctors from being able to indiscriminately cross state lines to evade disciplinary boards. Those dangerous doctors who do fall through the cracks continue to kill, maim, defraud, and otherwise injure their unknowing patients.

Too many state medical boards, despite a clear duty to protect the public,[11] still believe their first responsibility is to rehabilitate "impaired physicians" and to protect them from the public's prying eyes. And the definition of "impaired" has expanded: it now covers doctors who may be drunk on the job, strung out on drugs, mentally ill, or habitual sex offenders.

Arizona, unlike any of the other state medical boards, states in its orders about doctors that it interprets the Americans with Disabilities Act as a reason for not "disciplining" physicians for substance abuse simply because they are already in or will be required to be in a rehabilitation program. Therefore, these actions are viewed as a "voluntary agreement" between the Board and the doctors, not as a disciplinary action.

While it is important for doctors who suffer from emotional problems or drug or alcohol addiction to receive appropriate treatment, this must be balanced with the state's responsibility to protect the public from doctors who are not able to deliver good medical care. Some states show a dangerous pattern of letting chemically dependent doctors return to practice after numerous failed attempts at rehabilitation. And while behavior that is sexually abusive may result from a mental illness, it is also a crime and is never acceptable in the context of patient care.

Although medical boards are now able to communicate with each other, at least indirectly, about doctors they have disciplined, the boards are often far too slow to act on what they have learned. And many state medical boards seldom communicate with the other agencies that guard against medical incompetence, fraud, and abuse--the federal Department of Health and Human Services, the Medicare Peer Review Organizations, the federal Drug Enforcement Administration, and the agencies that run state Medicaid programs.[12] Many of our recommendations to the states and federal government call for improved and regular communication between these groups.

Only a few of the country's medical boards, for example those in Utah, West Virginia, Georgia, Oregon, and a few others attempt to proactively sleuth out highly questionable physicians before receiving complaints, in order to prevent misconduct and poor care.

The College of Physicians and Surgeons in the Canadian province of Ontario, by contrast, visits physicians' offices and performs random audits of their care in order to "be assured that licensed physicians meet minimal requirements for safe practice."[13,14] Physicians who fail to meet those standards, as many as 12% of family doctors and 2% of specialists, must undergo intensive educational retraining and in rare cases face disciplinary action. To our knowledge, no American state has yet attempted such a far-reaching quality control program.

Most importantly, most state medical boards have not refined the art of speaking to their primary constituency: the public.

Because of a commendable increase in requirements to report malpractice information to them, states are now repositories of masses of information on the quality of individual doctors, but most states have not begun effective ways of disseminating all of it.

Many consumers when selecting a doctor still feel that they are floundering in the dark. They are unfamiliar with the role or the existence of medical boards. They are unaware that they can request disciplinary information, or that they can file complaints. Unwarned, too many of these people are treated by doctors guilty of previous acts of malpractice. And unwarned, too many of them are harmed.

Too little discipline is still being done. Fewer than one-half of 1% of the nation's doctors face any serious state sanctions each year. 2,696 total serious disciplinary actions a year, the number state medical boards took in 1999,[15] (see Table A, pg. 14) is a pittance compared to the volume of injury and death of patients caused by negligence of doctors. A recent study by the Institute of Medicine of the National Academy of Sciences estimated that as many as 98,000 patients may be killed each year in hospitals alone as a result of medical errors.[16] Earlier studies also found that this was a serious national problem.

* Harvard researchers found that 1% of a representative sample of patients treated in New York state hospitals in 1984 were injured, and one-quarter of those died, because of medical negligence.[17] Nationwide, that would have translated into 234,000 injuries and 80,000 deaths in 1988 from negligence in American hospitals. Most of this involves physicians. There is no clear evidence that there has been significant improvement since then.
* A similar study conducted in California in 1974 found that 0.8% of hospital patients had either been injured by negligence in the hospital or had been hospitalized because of negligent care.[18] Extrapolation of those findings would have yielded an estimate of 249,000 injuries and deaths from negligent medical practice in 1988.
* In 1976 the HEW Malpractice Commission estimated similarly that one-half of 1% of all patients entering hospitals are injured there due to negligence. That estimate would have indicated 156,000 injuries and deaths resulting from doctor negligence in 1988.[19]

Expanding these estimates to include general medical practice outside of a hospital, the potential abuse by physicians is even greater. An in-depth interview with 53 family physicians revealed that 47% of the doctors recalled a case in which the patient died due to physician error. Only four of the total reported errors led to malpractice suits, and none of these errors resulted in an action by a peer review organization.[20]

Medical students at SUNY-Buffalo were asked to recall incidents during their clinical training that raised ethical concerns. More than 200 students responded (40% of total sample); the majority of instances they reported (60%) did not in the researchers' opinions threaten the patient's life, health or welfare. This, however, implies that potentially 40% did.[21]

Systemic changes over time may also suggest a rise in physician malpractice. In a journal commentary, Dr. Alvan R. Feinstein reflects that in his 40 years of experience the manner in which medicine is now conducted may be sufficiently more complex as to contribute to an "epidemic of negligent medical errors."[22] A review of 43 malpractice insurance claims also indicates that systemic causes significantly contribute to pediatrician error; 91% of these claims, however, were also attributed to alleged errors of physician judgment involving diagnosis and treatment.[23] Even medical students and residents are now being held legally accountable for their mistakes,[24] thus broadening the pool of recognized physician error.

Given that many state medical boards now have the same information on claims and payments, they should be able to discipline at least as many doctors as malpractice carriers do. A 1989 Tufts University study found that physician-owned malpractice insurers sanctioned 13.6 of every 1,000 doctors they covered. The insurers terminated policies of 6.6 of every 1,000 policyholders in 1985 because of negligence-prone behavior, and they restricted the practice or imposed other sanctions on another 7 of every 1,000 doctors whose care was found to be substandard.[25] In an estimated population of 770,320 nonfederal doctors, this would translate to 10,476 doctors being disciplined a year.

The Impact of Substance Abuse

Specific physician attributes also contribute to this rate. Two studies surveyed residents to determine the incidence of substance use. Recent alcohol use was extremely high in both groups (87% within the last year for emergency medicine residents; 74% within the past 30 days for surgery residents).[26,27] Additional findings proved extremely disturbing; although the emergency medicine program directors accurately determined the incidence of alcohol use amongst residents, they dramatically underestimated the percent who were actually impaired by the substance as indicated by diagnostic tests (1% estimate impaired vs. 13% diagnosed.)[28]

This does not bode well for creating a medical system that prevents mishaps before they occur. And although the surgery residents reported negligible recent cocaine use, when employed, the drug was typically obtained from the hospital supply,[29] indicating a greater ease of access than for the general population.

Hughes reported that approximately 1-3% of physicians are disciplined or treated for substance abuse with an AMA estimated lifetime prevalence of 6-8% for alcoholism and 1-2% for drug dependency.[30] In 1985, Smith proposed that 17,000 doctors suffered from substance abuse.[31] Six percent of physicians indicated lifetime alcohol abuse and 1.6% reported either alcohol dependency or abuse within the last year alone.[32] If only 1% of physicians needed disciplining for chemical dependency, that alone would translate to 6,891 doctors.

Sexual Abuse or Misconduct

Sexual abuse of or sexual misconduct with a patient is also a serious issue. Six to ten percent of psychiatrists surveyed confessed to having engaged in sexual contact with a patient[33,34] and in a longitudinal study, Garfinkel at al. noted that of the original 70 psychiatrists they tracked, 2 (2.9%) had lost their medical licenses due to repeated violations of sexual boundaries with patients.[35] In reviewing their own rate of disciplinary actions for the years 1991-1995, the Oregon Board of Medical Examiners determined that of 100 open complaints investigated against 80 doctors during this time period, 5.9% were alleged to be sexual misconduct. More than one-third (39%) of these were classified as sexual impropriety, 31% were categorized as sexual transgression and 30% sexual violation. Disciplinary action was reported in 5%, 27%, and 54% of the instances, respectively. Twenty-five percent of the closed complaints also resulted in reportable disciplinary action.[36]

In light of these findings, it is not unreasonable to estimate that at least 1 percent of doctors in this country deserve some serious disciplinary action each year. This would amount to 7,703 physicians being disciplined each year, a number that, unfortunately far exceeds the actual number of physicians disciplined.

Findings

Public Citizen National Ranking of State Disciplinary Actions

Based on the Federation of State Medical Boards' (FSMB) data released annually on the number of disciplinary actions taken against doctors, Public Citizen calculated the rate of serious disciplinary actions per 1,000 doctors in each state and compiled a national report ranking state boards by the extent to which they are taking serious disciplinary actions against doctors in 1999 (See Table A, Findings, pg. 14).

Public Citizen has had and continues to have, two disputes with the FSMB over these data. First, we choose to look only at the most serious actions taken by state medical boards as a way of evaluating them, whereas the FSMB looks at "prejudicial" actions, a broader category which includes relative slaps on the wrist such as fines and reprimands as well as what we deem "serious" disciplinary actions. This category, in our view, should include only license revocations, suspensions or surrenders, plus probations, restrictions or other limitations on license (categories A & B in the FSMB data).

Second, the Federation states "it is virtually impossible to make sound comparisons of one medical board to another," and thereby avoids doing a ranking of state boards. We strongly disagree, and the Federation admits that the structure and funding of medical boards may have a direct impact on their effectiveness. Public Citizen believes that a valid uniform measure of board effectiveness is the rate of serious disciplinary actions per 1,000 doctors per year--a belief shared by Richard Kusserow, formerly Inspector General of the federal Department of Health and Human Services.

According to James R. Winn, M.D., the Federation's executive vice-president, "Boards that are independent or semi-autonomous, adopting their own budgets and allocating revenues to their operations, appear to perform their role of public protectors more effectively than those boards that are classified as subordinate or advisory." So, although the FSMB disagrees with the idea of our rankings based on their data, it admits to differences in structure and funding between boards which are amongst the probable causes of the differences in rates of serious disciplinary action.

Table A Ranking of Serious Doctor Disciplinary Actions by State Medical Licensing Boards 1999

1999 Rank	State	Number Of Serious Actions 1999	Total Number of Nonfederal Doctors 1998	Serious Actions Per 1,000 Doctors
1	Alaska	12	1160	10.34
2	North Dakota	14	1596	8.77
3	Wyoming	8	981	8.15
4	Idaho	16	2278	7.02
5	Oklahoma	37	6216	5.95
6	Kentucky	54	9115	5.92
7	Ohio	190	32220	5.90
8	Mississippi	30	5107	5.87
9	Vermont	11	2061	5.34
10	Colorado	59	11253	5.24
11	Iowa	33	6602	5.00
12	Arkansas	27	5486	4.92
13	Alabama	45	9559	4.71
14	New York	366	77781	4.71
15	Georgia	82	17961	4.57
16	Indiana	60	13267	4.52
17	West Virginia	19	4249	4.47
18	New Hampshire	14	3309	4.23
19	Michigan	101	24001	4.21
20	California	367	90940	4.04
21	Arizona	42	11025	3.81
22	Virginia	70	18441	3.80
23	Louisiana	43	11581	3.71
24	Maine	11	3195	3.44
25	Nevada	11	3373	3.26
26	North Carolina	62	19615	3.16
27	New Mexico	13	4138	3.14
28	New Jersey	89	28432	3.13
29	South Carolina	27	8923	3.03
30	Oregon	27	8984	3.01
31	Missouri	45	15211	2.96
32	Montana	6	2036	2.95
33	Utah	13	4770	2.73
34	Texas	124	45707	2.71
35	Rhode Island	10	3784	2.64
36	Pennsylvania	97	38080	2.55
37	Washington	38	15254	2.49
38	Florida	105	42169	2.49
39	Massachusetts	67	27622	2.43
40	Maryland	51	21116	2.42
41	District of Columbia	9	4121	2.18
42	Wisconsin	28	13567	2.06
43	Illinois	73	35581	2.05
44	South Dakota	3	1562	1.92
45	Kansas	12	6577	1.82
46	Connecticut	23	12910	1.78
47	Hawaii	6	3555	1.69
48	Minnesota	21	13275	1.58
49	Tennessee	18	14412	1.25
50	Nebraska	5	4070	1.23
51	Delaware	2	2092	0.96
	Total	**2696**	**770320**	**3.50**

Our calculation of rates of serious disciplinary actions per 1,000 doctors by state is created by taking the number of such actions (as defined above) and dividing it by the American Medical Association data on non-federal M.D.s, and then multiplying the result by 1,000 to get state disciplinary rates. Nationwide, there were 2,696 serious disciplinary actions in 1999 out of 770,320 nonfederal M.D.s, which is a rate of 3.50 serious disciplinary actions per 1,000 physicians. State rates ranged from 10.34 (Alaska) to 0.96 (Delaware).

Best States. The top 10 states, or those with the highest rate of serious disciplinary actions per 1,000 physicians are (in order): Alaska (10.34/1,000 physicians), North Dakota (8.77), Wyoming (8.15), Idaho (7.02), Oklahoma (5.95), Kentucky (5.92), Ohio (5.90), Mississippi (5.87), Vermont (5.34), and Colorado (5.24). Five of these 10 states (Alaska, Oklahoma, Mississippi, Wyoming, and Ohio) were also in the top 10 in 1997 and 1998 and two, (Mississippi and Alaska) have been in the top 10 for nine straight years. Oklahoma, 5th this year, has been in the top 10 states for eight of the last nine years. Wyoming, 3rd this year, has been in the top 10 for seven of the last nine years and Vermont, 9th this year and Ohio, 7th this year, have been in the top ten for five of the last nine years.

It is clear that state-by-state performance is spotty. Only one of the nation's 15 largest states, Ohio, is represented among those 10 states with the highest disciplinary rates, as it also was in 1996, 1997 and 1998. Other large states such as, New York, Michigan and California (14th, 19th and 20th respectively in 1999) have shown improvement from 40th, 49th and 37th in 1991. But other large states such as Texas, Pennsylvania, Massachusetts and Illinois (34th, 36th, 39th and 43rd in 1999) have not done very much doctor discipline for many of the last 10 years.

Worst States. The bottom 15 states, those with the lowest serious disciplinary rates in 1998, were, starting with the lowest: Delaware 0.96 per 1,000 physicians), Nebraska (1.23), Tennessee (1.25), Minnesota (1.58), Hawaii (1.69), Connecticut (1.78), Kansas (1.82), South Dakota (1.92), Illinois (2.05), Wisconsin (2.06), D.C. (2.18), Maryland (2.42), Massachusetts (2.43), Florida (2.49), and Washington (2.49). Massachusetts, Tennessee, Minnesota, Wisconsin, Kansas, Hawaii, and Delaware were also in the bottom 15 states in 1997 and 1998. In 1999, the bottom 20 states all had rates of serious disciplinary action that were one-half or less than the rate of all of the top five states.

Table B Ranking of States 1991-1999: Serious Disciplinary Actions

Rank 1999	Rank 1998	Rank 1997	Rank 1996	Rank 1995	Rank 1994	Rank 1993	Rank 1992	Rank 1992	State
1	1	2	6	8	2	8	7	6	Alaska
2	11	9	2	34	10	3	5	13	N. Dakota
3	7	3	31	3	1	21	4	9	Wyoming
4	25	30	21	36	30	37/38	23	34/35	Idaho
5	2	5	7	12	5	2	1	2	Oklahoma
6	14	7/8	14	14	4	4	16	5	Kentucky
7	10	7/8	8	9	24	22/23	19	23	Ohio
8	3	1	1	1	9	9	6	6	Mississippi
9	6	25/26	10	6	39	17	15	10	Vermont
10	18	6	4	5	12	6	8	17	Colorado
11	23	4	3	2	7	5	2	3	Iowa
12	4	13	15	23	28	26	18	29	Arkansas
13	17	23/24	38	30	43/44	29	30	31	Alabama
14	16	16	18	17	29	34	39	49	New York
15	12	23/24	19	4	8	10	9	4	Georgia
16	21	19/20	33	28	16	7	14	15	Indiana
17	5	12	11	7	6	1	3	8	W. Virginia
18	30	46	51	49	49	47	47	44	New Hampshire
19	13	15	28	21	34/35	35	40	40	Michigan
20	27	18	27	20	34/35	32	42	37	California
21	38	19/20	5	10	17	16	22	22	Arizona
22	40	34/35	50	41/42	32	30	37	32	Virginia
23	15	34/35	44	13	18	11	12	7	Louisiana
24	9	22	17	32	33	41	44	46	Maine
25	26	32	9	11	31	20	25	26	Nevada
26	43	33	48/49	35	36	40	34	42/43	N. Carolina
27	8	50	23	15	43/44	49	33	33	New Mexico
28	35	42	20	25	19	18	28	20	New Jersey
29	22	40	45	44	14	15	11	11	S. Carolina
30	31	28/29	29	16	20	22/23	24	14	Oregon
31	48	17	30	37	13	12	13	12	Missouri
32	34	11	13	18	3	14	10	19	Montana
33	20	25/26	16	38	46	39	43	18	Utah
34	28/29	37	35	19	23	28	29	21	Texas
35	24	10	25	26	26	42	41	50/51	Rhode Island
36	45	27	32	43	47	48	48	47	Pennsylvania
37	36/37	28/29	40	24	27	24	17	24	Washington
38	49	36	22	22	25	25	21	27	Florida
39	47	45	43	40	37	45	46	48	Massachusetts
40	36/37	38	41	29	21	19	27	42/43	Maryland
41	33	44	36	50	51	51	45	45	D. Columbia
42	46	39	34	47	41	27	26	34/35	Wisconsin
43	41	21	46	45	40	31	36	36	Illinois
44	19	14	42	33	11	13	32	50/51	S. Dakota
45	44	41	12	46	22	37/38	20	25	Kansas
46	32	31	37	27	42	36	35	30	Connecticut
47	39	49	39	51	50	46	50	41	Hawaii
48	42	51	47	39	45	33	31	28	Minnesota
49	51	48	48/49	31	38	44	49	38	Tennessee
50	28/29	43	24	41/42	15	50	38	39	Nebraska
51	50	47	26	48	48	43	51	16	Delaware

Table B, on pg. 16, shows the ranking of state boards for the last nine years. It can be seen that there are some states which have consistently been among the highest-ranking ones, others which have stayed consistently toward the bottom and yet others which have gone from better to worse or vice versa.

This analysis raises serious questions about the extent to which patients in many states with poorer records of serious doctor discipline are being protected from physicians who might well be barred from practice in states with boards that are doing a better job of disciplining physicians. It is likely, if not certain that patients are being injured or killed more often in states with poor doctor disciplinary records than in states with consistent top 10 performances. It is not unreasonable to estimate that at least 1 percent of doctors in this country deserve some serious disciplinary action each year, a number comparable to Alaska's rate of 10.32 actions per 1,000 doctors or 1.032 percent. In fact, each year one or more states achieves a rate of serious disciplinary actions of approximately 10 per 10,000 doctors. This would amount to 7,703 (1% of 770,320 non-federal doctors) serious actions a year, which cover only a small fraction of the 98,000 patient deaths thought to occur each year in American hospitals as a result of errors, almost all of it involving physicians. The current overall national rate of serious disciplinary actions, 3.50 per 1,000 or .350 percent is far short of the rate of 1.034 percent in Alaska. If the rate of serious disciplinary actions had been 10 per 1,000 (1 percent), the national total would have been 7,703 actions or 5,007 more actions in 1999 (2.8 times more) than the 2,696 that actually occurred in 1999.

Considering what is known about substandard doctoring, not even Alaska's disciplinary rate seems adequate. Most states have a long way to go before they even begin to offer serious protection for citizens from doctors who are incompetent, who sexually abuse patients or who otherwise have serious problems that interfere with delivery of high-quality medical care in a compassionate way. All states, even those with best records, need to strengthen the structure and functions of their licensing boards. The statement by the Federation that you cannot compare the disciplinary rates of boards with each other because they are set-up, structured and funded differently is preposterous.

Disciplinary Actions from Public Citizen's Database

As shown in Table C, pg. 19, of the 38,589 disciplinary actions reported by state boards or the federal government to Public Citizen (representing actions against 20,125 doctors), the majority (32,868 or 85.2%) of these were imposed by state medical boards. A description and statistical breakdown of the actions provided to Public Citizen by each state is provided in the "State by State Listings" section. These counts represent the two most serious disciplinary actions for each sanction reported. Some sanctions included more than two actions against the doctors. These less serious actions are not included in these counts. (For a more detailed discussion of how disciplinary actions are reported, refer to "How We Compiled This Report," Appendix 2, pg. 40.)

Please note that the period of years covered in the database varies from state to state. However, of the 50 states and the District of Columbia, for 44 of these jurisdictions, (86%), we have 10 years of data, from the beginning of 1990 through 1999. For the remaining 7 states, we have between 6 and 3/4 years of data (Arkansas) and 9 and 1/2 years of disciplinary data (Florida).

The federal agencies account for the remaining 5721 disciplinary actions imposed; 6.4% (2,462) were DEA sanctions in contested and uncontested cases, 8.3% (3,234) were fines and exclusions from the Medicare program, and 25 were restrictions placed on a physician's eligibility to participate as investigators in FDA experiments or to work for FDA-regulated companies.

An analysis of the 2,366 doctors who were the subject of DEA disciplinary actions revealed that hundreds were not the subject of any state disciplinary action even though their federal narcotics license had been revoked, surrendered, or restricted.

Similarly, of the 3,232 Medicare doctors who were the subjects of the 3,234 Medicare disciplinary actions, hundreds were not disciplined by their state boards even though most had involved exclusion from Medicare.

Table C Disciplinary Actions by State and Federal Agencies

State/Federal Agency	Number of Actions	State/Federal Agency	Number of Actions
Alabama	366	Mississippi	298
Alaska	161	Missouri	630
Arizona	942	Montana	97
Arkansas	168	Nebraska	114
California	2670	Nevada	151
Colorado	884	New Hampshire	117
Connecticut	440	New Jersey	1472
Delaware	44	New Mexico	145
District of Columbia	242	New York	2993
DEA	***2462***	North Carolina	523
Florida	2746	North Dakota	131
FDA	***25***	Ohio	1484
Georgia	855	Oklahoma	592
Hawaii	119	Oregon	344
Idaho	51	Pennsylvania	1230
Illinois	1390	Rhode Island	176
Indiana	556	South Carolina	389
Iowa	526	South Dakota	75
Kansas	250	Tennessee	409
Kentucky	595	Texas	2035
Louisiana	505	Utah	218
Maine	177	Vermont	132
Maryland	803	Virginia	567
Massachusetts	586	Washington	596
Medicare	***3234***	West Virginia	419
Michigan	1341	Wisconsin	501
Minnesota	493	Wyoming	68
		TOTAL	**38,589**

Thus, many states are not acting promptly, if at all, against physicians about whom a federal agency has already compiled sufficient information to discipline them for very serious offenses.

Types of Disciplinary Actions and Offenses

The following tables provide a statistical national look at the types of disciplinary actions and the offenses for which they were taken.

Table D, Types of Disciplinary Actions Reported to Public Citizen (pg. 21) shows that the most common type of state disciplinary action of those submitted to us was probation. States imposed probation 19.3% of the times (7,431 times) when practitioners were disciplined. They revoked licenses 7.9% of the time (3,045 times), suspended licenses 9.6% of the time (3,704 times), and accepted a doctor's surrender of his or her license 7.9% of the time (3,063 times). Cumulatively, only 9,812 or 25.4% of the actions against doctors listed in this report were ones which resulted in at least a temporary loss of ability to practice medicine (revocation, suspension and surrender). Most of the doctors who are listed in this book never had to stop practicing medicine and many more who had suspensions may once again be practicing. It is not likely that many of their patients are aware of these actions. **A total of 20,125 different physicians were the subject of the 38,589 disciplinary actions taken by state and federal agencies.**

Table D Disciplinary Actions Reported to Public Citizen: A Breakdown of the Types of Disciplinary Actions Contained in This Report

Disciplinary Action	Number	Percent
Probation	7431	19.3%
Suspension	3704	9.6%
Revocation	3045	7.9%
Fine	3708	9.6%
Surrender	3063	7.9%
Reprimand	3094	8.0%
Exclusion from the Medicare Program	3220	8.3%
Practice Restriction	2243	5.8%
Revocation, Surrender, Suspension of Controlled Substance License	2275	5.9%
Restriction of Controlled Substance License	1317	3.4%
Emergency Suspension	1231	3.2%
Education	1357	3.5%
Physician Monitoring	1251	3.2%
License Denial, Reinstatement or Nonrenewal	803	2.1%
Required to Enter an Impaired Physicians Program or Substance Abuse Treatment	266	0.7%
Other Actions	581	1.5%
Total Actions	**38589**	**100.0%**

Table E, Offenses for which Disciplinary Action was Taken (pg. 23). The reason an action was taken--the offense--was provided by state and federal authorities for 24,042 of the records in our database. For a number of offenses, more than one action was taken. In 7,132 cases, the stated reason for the listed actions was "disciplinary action taken by another state agency," leaving 16,910 offenses with specific details as to the nature of the offense. For 15,310 of these offenses or 90.6% of them, the offense was one of the five discussed previoiusly--substandard care, incompetence or negligence, criminal conviction, substance abuse, misprescribing or over prescribing of drugs or sex-related offenses--or another serious offense such as providing false information, loss of hospital privileges or fraud. Among those 16,910 actions for which specific reasons other than discipline by another state or agency were reported, the five most serious offenses were as follows.

Sexual abuse of or sexual misconduct with a patient accounted for 3.2% of the total known offenses for which doctors were disciplined. A total of 547 different doctors were disciplined for these offenses.

Substandard care, incompetence or negligence: The most common single reason for which states disciplined doctors was for offenses involving substandard care, incompetence or negligence. which accounted for 18.8% of all the 16,910 actions for which a specific offense was stated. A total of 3,215 different doctors were disciplined for this offense.

Criminal conviction, the second largest category, accounted for 17.2% of known offenses other than those listed as disciplinary action by another state. A total of 2,963 different doctors were disciplined for criminal conviction (plea of guilty or nolo contendere--no contest).

Disciplinary actions taken because of *misprescribing or overprescribing drugs* accounted for an additional 7.7% of known offenses. A total of 1,318 different doctors were disciplined for these offenses.

Substance abuse accounted for an additional 10.0% of known offenses for which doctors were disciplined. A total of 1,715 different doctors were disciplined for these offenses.

The five offenses listed above, all extremely serious, accounted for 56.9% or more than half of all of those disciplinary actions in which a specific offense other than discipline by another state or agency was listed.

Table E	Offenses for which Disciplinary Action was Taken*	
Offense	**Number**	**Percent**
Criminal Conviction	2901	12.1%
Disciplinary Action Taken by Another State or Agency	7132	29.7%
Substandard Care, Incompetence, or Negligence	3184	13.2%
Misprescribing or Overprescribing Drugs	1302	5.4%
Substance Abuse	1683	7.0%
Professional Misconduct	2182	9.1%
Noncompliance with a Board Order	1274	5.3%
Noncompliance with a Professional Rule	2075	8.6%
Practicing without a License	420	1.7%
Practicing without a Controlled Substance License	70	0.3%
Providing False Information to Medical Board or Other Health Agency	417	1.7%
Sexual Abuse of or Sexual Misconduct with a Patient	536	2.2%
Physical or Mental Impairment	472	2.0%
Hospital Privilege Loss or Restriction	236	1.0%
Insurance or Medicare/Medicaid Fraud	72	0.3%
Falsifying/Altering Medical Records	38	0.2%
Overcharging	34	0.1%
Exceeding Professional Limitations	14	0.1%
Total Records With Offense Cited	**24042**	**100.0%**

* Frequencies and types of violations cited by states or federal government for disciplinary actions. Includes only those actions for which an offense was reported and for which we had a corresponding term in our database. This table does not include the 5,371 cases in which the stated reason was action by another state.

Table F, Disciplinary Actions Taken Against Doctors Cited for Sexual Abuse of or Sexual Misconduct with a Patient, below, shows that of the 547 different doctors who were disciplined for sexual abuse of or sexual misconduct with a patient, there were 302 actions (81 revocations, 46 surrenders, 130 suspensions plus 45 emergency suspensions) which required those doctors, at least temporarily, to stop practicing medicine. Switching from actions to doctors, there were 286 doctors (52.3%) who were, at least temporarily, removed from practice by license suspension, surrender or revocation. But this means that at least 47.7% of doctors (261 doctors) were allowed to continue practicing, their behavior probably unknown to most if not all of their patients. It is likely that other doctors, especially those whose licenses were only suspended temporarily, are once again practicing medicine.

Table F Disciplinary Actions Taken Against Doctors Cited for Sexual Abuse of or Sexual Misconduct with a Patient

Action	Number	Percent
Revocation	81	10.3%
Surrender	46	5.9%
Suspension	130	16.6%
Emergency Suspension	45	5.7%
Probation	189	24.1%
Fine	77	9.8%
Other Actions	217	27.6%
Total Actions	**785**	**100.0%**

Table G, Disciplinary Actions Taken Against Doctors Cited for Substandard Care, Incompetence or Negligence, below, shows that of the 3,215 different doctors who were disciplined for substandard care, incompetence or negligence, there were 987 actions (315 revocations, 244 surrenders, 338 suspensions plus 90 emergency suspensions) which required those doctors, at least temporarily, to stop practicing medicine. Switching from actions to doctors, there were 942 doctors (29.3%) who were, at least temporarily, removed from practice by license suspension, surrender or revocation. But this means that at least 70.7% of doctors (2,273 doctors) were allowed to continue practicing, their behavior probably unknown to most if not all of their patients. It is likely that other doctors, especially those whose licenses were only suspended temporarily, are once again practicing medicine.

Table G Disciplinary Actions Taken Against Doctors Cited for Substandard Care, Incompetence or Negligence

Action	Number	Percent
Revocation	315	6.8%
Surrender	244	5.3%
Suspension	338	7.3%
Emergency Suspension	90	2.0%
Probation	1181	25.6%
Practice Restriction	359	7.8%
Fine	809	17.6%
Reprimand	491	10.7%
Other Actions	779	16.9%
Total Actions	**4606**	**100.0%**

Table H, Disciplinary Actions Taken Against Doctors Cited for Criminal Convictions, below, shows that of the 2,963 different doctors who were disciplined because of a criminal conviction, there were 1,363 actions (563 revocations, 159 surrenders, 491 suspensions plus 150 emergency suspensions) which required those doctors, at least temporarily, to stop practicing medicine. Switching from actions to doctors, there were 1,162 doctors (39.2%) who were, at least temporarily, removed from practice by license suspension, surrender or revocation. But this means that at least 60.8% of doctors (1,801 doctors) were allowed to continue practicing, their behavior probably unknown to most if not all of their patients. It is likely that other doctors, especially those whose licenses were only suspended temporarily, are once again practicing medicine.

Table H Disciplinary Actions Taken Against Doctors Cited for Criminal Convictions

Action	Number	Percent
Revocation	563	16.2%
Surrender	159	4.6%
Suspension	491	14.1%
Emergency Suspension	150	4.3%
Probation	587	16.9%
Fine	203	5.8%
Other Actions	1319	38.0%
Total Actions	**3472**	**100.0%**

Table I, Disciplinary Actions Taken Against Doctors Cited for Misprescribing or Overprescribing Drugs, below, shows that of the 1,318 different doctors who were disciplined because of misprescribing or overprescribing drugs, there were 378 actions (96 revocations, 85 surrenders, 155 suspensions plus 42 emergency suspensions) which required those doctors, at least temporarily, to stop practicing medicine. Switching from actions to doctors, there were 368 doctors (27.9%) who were, at least temporarily, removed from practice by license suspension, surrender or revocation. But this means that at least 72.1% of doctors (950 doctors) were allowed to continue practicing, their behavior probably unknown to most if not all of their patients. It is likely that other doctors, especially those whose licenses were only suspended temporarily, are once again practicing medicine.

Table I Disciplinary Actions Taken Against Doctors Cited for Misprescribing or Overprescribing Drugs

Action	Number	Percent
Revocation	96	5.0%
Surrender	85	4.4%
Revocation, Surrender, or Suspension of Controlled Substance License	171	8.9%
Suspension	155	8.1%
Emergency Suspension	42	2.2%
Probation	486	25.2%
Restriction of Controlled Substance License	211	11.0%
Fine	200	10.4%
Education	141	7.3%
Other Actions	338	17.6%
Total Actions	**1925**	**100.0%**

Table J, Disciplinary Actions Taken Against Doctors Cited for Substance Abuse, below, shows that of the 1,715 different doctors who were disciplined because of substance abuse, there were 611 actions (71 revocations, 111 surrenders, 293 suspensions plus 136 emergency suspensions) which required those doctors, at least temporarily, to stop practicing medicine. Switching from actions to doctors, there were 556 doctors (32.4%) who were, at least temporarily, removed from practice by license suspension, surrender or revocation. But this means that at least 67.6% of doctors (1,159 doctors) were allowed to continue practicing, their behavior probably unknown to most if not all of their patients. It is likely that other doctors, especially those whose licenses were only suspended temporarily, are once again practicing medicine.

Table J Disciplinary Actions Taken Against Doctors Cited for Substance Abuse

Action	Number	Percent
Revocation	71	2.9%
Surrender	111	4.5%
Revocation, Surrender, or Suspension of Controlled Substance License	116	4.7%
Suspension	293	11.8%
Emergency Suspension	136	5.5%
Probation	741	29.9%
Restriction of Controlled Substance License	143	5.8%
Fine	43	1.7%
Required to Enter an Impaired Physician Program or Substance Abuse Treatment	161	6.5%
Other Actions	665	26.8%
Total Actions	**2480**	**100.0%**

Conclusions

1. The current rate of serious disciplinary actions is a dangerously small drop in the bucket of adequate, consumer-protective doctor discipline.
2. All states, especially those with the worst records, need to strengthen the structure and functions of their licensing boards.
3. The increase in the total number of disciplinary actions in a given state may not indicate that more doctors are being caught. Much of the disciplinary activity, in states such as New York, involves insuring that doctors, once caught by one state, are disciplined when they move to another. There has also been a noticeable increase in sanctioning doctors for administrative purposes.
4. Questionable doctors can still cross state borders, though with less impunity than before. The extent to which one board shares information with another still varies widely by state.

   * In many instances discipline is still too slow although the case backlogs in some states have been greatly reduced. Wisconsin sanctioned a number of doctors only after they had already retired from practice.

   * The vast majority of states continue to require reporting of hospital disciplinary actions and malpractice claims or payments to the medical board, but few check whether the required reports have actually been filed. And some still fail to act promptly, if at all, on the information they receive.

   * Medical boards are much too forgiving. Many still see their priority as "rehabilitation," and their disciplinary actions are too light. Probation is the most common sanction against doctors for all of the five most serious offenses: sexual abuse or misconduct; substandard care; conviction; prescription violations, or substance abuse. Arizona, for example, interprets the Americans with Disabilities Act to indicate that action for substance abuse is a "voluntary agreement" between the physician and the Board, not a disciplinary action.

   * Far too few board actions, only 18.8% of the 16,910 identified offenses (other than those listed as action by another state), were for medical negligence or incompetence. Instead boards focus on more easily documentable offenses such as

prescription violations and fraud convictions or disciplinary action in another state as potential indicators of substandard care. Other instances of incompetence may be overlooked because the investigations soak up resources like a sponge.

To date, legislation--mainly at the state level--on medical malpractice, the injury and death of patients caused by doctor negligence, has been to punish the victim instead of disciplining the perpetrator. Legislative attention must be given to requiring states to significantly improve the discipline of physicians in order to prevent future death and injury.

Recommendations for Action

Complain. As discussed in *How To Use This Report*, pg. 1, file your complaints about poor medical care or medical misconduct with your state medical board and with the federal Department of Health and Human Services. If the offense occurred in a hospital, also file a complaint with the hospital peer review committee. Your complaints are needed to protect others!

Organize. Form citizens' action or victims' rights groups to improve medical quality assurance in your area. The American Association of Retired Persons publishes a guide that can help you mobilize a group for reform.[37] Try to get a representative of your group appointed to the state medical board or the Medicare Peer Review Organization for your state.

Write to your Congresspersons, at both state and federal levels urging actions as listed below.

Recommendations for the Federal Government

Create grants and standards. Congress should create a small program of grants-in-aid to state medical boards. The grants should be tied to the boards' agreements to meet certain performance standards, which should be developed by the Public Health Service, as the Department of Health and Human Services Office of Inspector General recommended in 1990.[38]

In developing these standards, the Public Health Service should work with the Federation of State Medical Boards' Assessment Task Force. In September 1990 the FSMB received a federal contract for $200,000 to undertake the development of a self-assessment instrument for state medical boards. The goal of the task force was to produce a sound and objective means by which boards could assess their performance over time and in comparison with other boards.[39] In April 1992 the Federation released its "Self-Assessment Instrument for State Medical Boards" and the accompanying handbook. The Instrument is a survey that each board can fill out regarding its own activities, enabling boards to eventually share information with each other and compare resources and performance. The standards should include (but not be limited to) the following: processing complaints within a certain limited period of time; maintaining a certain level of staffing and having staff meet certain qualifications; disseminating disciplinary information to the public; having at least 30% of board members be consumer members; regularly publishing a newsletter that includes names of disciplined physicians and descriptions of the disciplinary actions taken against them; issuing an annual report that includes meaningful disciplinary statistics; and other standards.

The Medicare Peer Review Organizations (PRO), which have been practically moribund in disciplining physicians for substandard care, should become more aggressive. The PROs should hire investigators and advisers trained in law enforcement so that fewer of their sanctions will be overturned.

As a 1990 Institute of Medicine report noted, the PROs are not evaluated on their ability to detect and correct poor quality care.[40] The Department of Health and Human Services should change its evaluation procedures to place more emphasis on quality.

Open the National Practitioner Data Bank (NPDB). In 1986 Congress passed the Health Care Quality Improvement Act. This act mandated the establishment of a data bank containing information on adverse professional review actions taken against doctors, and on doctors who had been sued for malpractice and on whose behalf settlement or adjudicated payments had been made. Unfortunately, the law establishing the data bank also required that it be closed to the general public. Congress should pass legislation opening the data bank to consumers and loudly rebuke the American Medical Association's resolution to destroy the data bank. Although there have been Congressional hearings in 2000 on the topic of opening up the NPDB, as this report goes to press, there is no significant likelihood that such legislation is likely to become law.

The Drug Enforcement Administration should release a monthly list of all practitioners whose controlled substance prescription licenses have been revoked, surrendered, restricted, or denied. The list should be widely distributed to pharmacies, state pharmacy and medical boards, and the general public. Far too many doctors continue to prescribe controlled substances after their DEA licenses have expired or have been revoked. The DEA should consider requiring pharmacies to subscribe to an on-line service with which they could check the validity of these DEA license numbers.

Require doctor recertification. Congress should consider legislation proposed by Rep. Pete Stark, D-California, to require physicians who accept Medicare patients to be periodically recertified for competency.

Recommendations for States

Strengthen the statutes. States that have not already done so should adopt legislation at least as strong as that in the Model Medical Practice Act developed by the Federation of State Medical

Boards,[41] or, preferably, stronger laws.

Restructure the boards. States should sever any remaining formal, debilitating links between state licensing boards and state medical societies. Members of medical boards (and separate disciplinary boards, where present) should be appointed by the governor, and the governor's choice of appointees should not be limited to a medical society's nominees. At least 50% of the members of each state medical board and disciplinary board should be well-informed and well-trained public members who have no ties to health care providers and who, preferably, have a history of advocacy on behalf of patients. The governor should appoint members to the Medical Board whose top priority is protecting the public's health, not providing assistance to physicians who are trying to evade disciplinary actions.

Inform the public. Each state's Open Records Law and its Medical Practice Act should state that all formal disciplinary actions against licensed professionals are fully public records. Each legislature should require widespread dissemination of final disciplinary orders. Lists of those disciplined and full disciplinary orders should be promptly available by mail to all requesting them.

Notices of disciplinary actions should be sent to the local news media and to all hospitals, health maintenance organizations (HMOs), and other health care providers in the state, as well as to other state agencies, the federal Department of Health and Human Services, and the federal Drug Enforcement Administration. Federal law already requires that such information be reported to the National Practitioner Data Bank, which began operating on September 1, 1990.

As has already begun to happen in many states, all states should make disciplinary actions they take against physicians promptly available on their web sites and it should include all details such as the full text of the board order against the physician.

Strengthen board authority. Every medical board should have the authority to impose emergency suspensions pending formal hearing in cases where a doctor poses a potential danger to the public health. Boards should aggressively use this authority when they learn of a potentially dangerous doctor. The legal standard for disciplining physicians should be a preponderance of the evidence, not more difficult to accomplish standards.

Medical boards should have the authority to rapidly, after confirmation, accept the findings of other state boards and of the federal Department of Health and Human Services and the Drug Enforcement Administration. If a physician has been disciplined by another state, any subsequent state's medical board should be required to impose sanctions at least as stringent as those imposed by the first state. Each state should require physicians who have been licensed in other states and who seek licensure in a new state to submit affidavits that they are not under investigation elsewhere before being granted a new license. Physicians who are under investigation should not be permitted to practice until the board has heard the details of their case and can evaluate their competency. Each legislature should grant its state medical licensing board the authority to examine physicians for physical, mental and professional competence and to test them for alcohol and drug use upon reason to believe that a problem exists in one of these areas.

Encourage complaints. Each legislature should provide for the protection of confidentiality and immunity to those who report violations of the Medical Practice Act to a board. Such protections should also be extended to board members, their staff, and consultants.

Each legislature should require all licensed health care practitioners to report Medical Practice Act violations by other practitioners to the medical board, with large civil penalties for failure to do so. Boards should aggressively use their authority to enforce the requirement that all health care providers report such violations. Each legislature should also require hospitals to report all revocations, restrictions, or voluntary surrenders of privileges.

Courts should be required to report all indictments and convictions of physicians to the medical disciplinary board. In addition, each legislature should require liability insurers to report all claims, payments, and policy cancellations to state medical disciplinary boards. It should request reports from other state agencies, Medicare, the DEA and other federal agencies. It should also require impaired physicians' programs to report the names of doctors who fail to successfully complete their programs. Medical boards should conduct random audits of institutions to check compliance with these reporting requirements, and should fine those who fail to comply. After a doctor is disciplined, a board should fine any other practitioners who knew of that doctor's offense, but failed to report it.

Keep the courts in check. Each legislature should pass laws that make clear their intent that the judgements of the medical board be given extreme deference, and that, barring extraordinary circumstances, disciplinary actions should take immediate effect pending appeal.

Each legislature should adopt the 'preponderance of the evidence' standard of proof in medical disciplinary cases, replacing the tougher-to-meet 'clear and convincing evidence' standard now in effect in most states. According to the August 1990 report on state medical boards issued by the Office of the Inspector General, "The 'clear and convincing evidence' standard of proof is more rigorous than the 'preponderance of evidence' standard that is typically required to justify tort damages for negligence in civil cases. The more rigorous standard provides greater protection for physicians, but adds complexity to the investigative process and appears to make it less likely that a board will persevere on a case through a full evidentiary hearing."[42]

Furthermore, the Project Work Panel of the Federation of State Medical Boards, in its August 1989 report "Elements of a Modern State Medical Board: A Proposal," recommended that each state medical board "use preponderance of evidence as the standard of proof" and that they each have the power "to issue final decisions when acting as trier of fact in the performance of [their] adjudicatory duties."[43]

Beef up funding and staffing. Each legislature should permit the medical board to spend all the revenue from medical licensing fees, rather than being forced to give part to the state Treasury. The medical boards should raise their fees to $500 a year. All boards could benefit from hiring new investigators and legal staff. Boards should employ adequate staff to process and investigate all complaints within 30 days, to review all malpractice claims filed with the board, to monitor and regularly visit doctors who have been disciplined to ensure their compliance with the sanctions imposed, and to ensure compliance with reporting requirements. They should hire investigators to seek out errant doctors, through review of pharmacy records, consultation with medical examiners, and targeted office audits of those doctors practicing alone and suspected of poor care.

Require risk prevention. States should adopt a law, similar to one in Massachusetts, that requires all hospitals and other health care providers to have a meaningful, functioning risk prevention program designed to prevent injury to patients. Massachusetts also requires all adverse incidents occurring in hospitals or in doctors' offices to be reported to the medical board.

Require periodic recertification of doctors based on a written exam and audit of their patients' medical care records.

Appendix 1
Glossary

Controlled substances, controlled dangerous substances: drugs which are regulated under the federal Controlled Substances Act because of their potential for addiction or abuse.

D.O.: the academic degree awarded to osteopathic physicians.

DEA: the federal Drug Enforcement Administration, an agency of the U.S. Justice Department. Its mission is to enforce controlled substances laws.

DEA license, DEA registration, or DEA certificate: every person who handles or prescribes controlled substances, including physicians and dentists, must legally have a registration number issued by the Drug Enforcement Administration.

Disciplinary action: any of a number of ways a regulatory agency can limit or forbid a doctor's practice or formally indicate its displeasure. Includes license revocations, suspensions, and probations, consent agreements placing conditions on a doctor's continuing practice, monetary fines, and letters of reprimand.

Disciplinary action rate: total state disciplinary actions per 1,000 M.D.s practicing in a state.

Emergency suspension: a disciplinary action in which a medical board may remove a doctor from practice temporarily, without a formal disciplinary hearing, if it finds the doctor's continued practice could endanger the public health. Generally, boards are required to then hold a formal hearing on the case within a specified time period.

Impaired physicians program: a program to rehabilitate physicians suffering from an illness. Impaired physicians programs generally serve alcohol and drug abusers, but they have also been used to aid the mentally or physically ill, as well as habitual sex offenders.

Liability insurer: a company that insures doctors against malpractice lawsuits.

M.D.: the academic degree awarded to U.S. medical doctors, or allopathic physicians.

Medical Board: used generically, any state regulatory agency that licenses and/or disciplines M.D.s. Medical boards may also license other practitioners and health care paraprofessionals.

Osteopath: a physician who graduated from a school of osteopathic medicine. Osteopaths have training in skeletal manipulation in addition to their medical training.

Peer Review Committee: a hospital committee that reviews the quality of care in the institution. The committee may admit physicians to the hospital staff or revoke or limit their privileges.

Peer Review Organization: a state-based group under contract to the federal Medicare program to audit the necessity and quality of Medicare patients' care.

Probation: a disciplinary action or agreement wherein a doctor must abide by certain conditions for a definite or indefinite period of time, or face a more severe penalty. Probationary conditions are generally tailored to the individual.

Reinstatement: issuance of a new medical license to a doctor who previously surrendered his or her license or had it revoked.

Reprimand: a formal letter to a doctor criticizing a particular episode of misconduct or poor care. Sometimes called an admonition or letter of censure.

Restriction: a disciplinary action which limits the type of medicine a doctor may practice. For instance, a doctor's license may be restricted to prevent him or her from practicing surgery, or to limit practice to a certain clinic.

Revocation: the cancellation of a doctor's state or DEA license. State laws regarding revocations vary. In some states, revocations are permanent; in others, doctors may reapply for a new license immediately; in others, doctors must wait for a certain time period before reapplying.

Sanction: a formal disciplinary action.

Schedule I: controlled substances such as marijuana and heroin, which are usually held to have no approved medical purpose.

Schedule II: controlled substances with approved medical uses, but with high potential for addiction or abuse. This category includes raw opium, codeine, amphetamines, and some barbiturates.

Schedule III: controlled substances whose use may lead to low-moderate physical dependence or high psychological dependence and are therefore considered to have some potential for abuse. This category includes many barbiturates and other depressant drugs, and narcotics which include moderate amounts of codeine.

Schedule IV: controlled substances whose use may lead to limited physical and psychological dependence. This category includes Valium, Xanax, and other benzodiazepine tranquilizers, sleeping pills such as Halcion and anorectic stimulants, which are frequently used for weight loss.

Schedule V: controlled substances whose abuse potential is low. This category includes many non-prescription narcotic antidiarrheal drugs and cough suppressants.

Scheduled drugs: see Controlled Substances.

Serious disciplinary actions: Public Citizen's term for revocations, suspensions, surrenders, and probations, as they are reported by the Federation of State Medical Boards.

Serious disciplinary action rate: the number of revocations, suspensions, surrenders and probations per 1,000 M.D.s practicing in a state.

Summary suspension: see emergency suspension.

Surrender: a voluntary agreement by a doctor to give up his or her license to practice. Some surrender agreements permit a doctor to reapply for a new license; others are permanent.

State medical society: a local trade association of physicians. It serves no governmental function.

Stay: a stayed disciplinary action is like a suspended sentence: it does not take effect unless the doctor who has been disciplined disobeys the board or commits some further offense.

Suspension: the temporary removal of a doctor from practice. Some suspensions run for a definite period of time; others are indefinite, and a doctor must apply for the suspension to be lifted.

Triplicate prescription program: a program, now in effect in nine states, that requires copies of prescriptions for certain scheduled drugs to be sent to the state regulatory authority. Intended to prevent drug dealing and overprescribing of drugs that can easily be abused.

Appendix 2
How We Compiled This Report

Sources of Information

In the fall of 1989, using a list published by the Federation of State Medical Boards, Public Citizen contacted all the medical boards from the 50 states and the District of Columbia and requested the name of every physician the boards had disciplined since the beginning of 1985. We also asked at that time to be placed on the boards' mailing lists to receive notification of future disciplinary orders. Since that initial request, Public Citizen has periodically contacted these boards to obtain additional information on disciplinary actions. Most recently, we sent a letter to each state in March 2000 requesting updated information for this edition of *Questionable Doctors.*

This edition reflects disciplinary actions taken against doctors from all 50 states, the District of Columbia, the U.S. Department of Health and Human Services, the Drug Enforcement Administration, and the Food and Drug Administration. The extent of information each medical board provides regarding disciplinary actions varies by state; some boards enclose a detailed synopsis of the case history and findings, whereas others simply supply the physician's name and resulting action within a quarterly newsletter. A description of the information we received from each state is included in the "State by State Listing" section of this report

The time period reflected in this edition of *Questionable Doctors* spans from 1990 through 1999. Public Citizen made every effort to include information from every state for each of these years, but due to either periodic board inactivity or inoperation, data was not always available. The cutoff date for receipt of disciplinary materials in this report was January 31, 2000. Although the earliest editions of *Questionable Doctors* included disciplinary actions against dentists, chiropractors, and podiatrists if the state Board provided that information, because we did not consistently receive information on such health care providers from all medical boards, we decided to eliminate these entries on such professionals from our database.

Public Citizen obtained from the Inspector General's office of the U.S. Department of Health and Human Services a list of all health care providers excluded from the Medicare program for disciplinary purposes through December 1999. The list is called the

Medicare/Medicaid Sanction--Reinstatement Report. It includes the doctor's name, degree and/or specialty, address, date of the sanction notice, period of exclusion from the program, and section of the Social Security Act violated. We included all physicians (both M.D.s and D.O.s) listed in these reports in our database. Previously, from January 1990 through October 1990, the Inspector General's office also provided Public Citizen with copies of the notices of all sanctions, both fines and exclusions, imposed by the Department of Health and Human Services as a result of recommendations from Medicare Peer Review Organizations (PROs), which may sanction doctors for substandard or unnecessary care. The sanction notices included the physician's name, address, the PRO that recommended disciplinary action, the number of cases of substandard or unnecessary care for which the doctor was cited, sometimes the Department's findings about that care, the type of disciplinary action being taken, the length of an exclusion or the amount of a fine, and any information on appeals then available.

Public Citizen obtained from the *Federal Register* notices about doctors whose Drug Enforcement Administration registrations to prescribe controlled substances were revoked, restricted or denied following contested cases dated from 1990 through 1999. The *Federal Register* notices include the doctor's name, address, and DEA certificate number, a description of the conduct that led to the agency's action, the type of action taken, and the effective date. *20,125 Questionable Doctors* also includes most of the physicians who did not contest the DEA's decision and agreed to surrender or restrict their prescribing privilege. This information was obtained directly from the DEA.

From the Food and Drug Administration, Public Citizen obtained information on physicians who were sanctioned because they had violated FDA laws, regulations, or policies regarding clinical research on patients or were convicted of a crime regarding their contract. These physicians are ineligible to receive investigational products for research purposes. Our database includes actions taken through December 1999.

Generating the Database

From the information received from the states, the Drug Enforcement Administration, the Food and Drug Administration, and the Department of Health and Human Services, we created database entries on individual practitioners. Each entry included (when available) the doctor's full name, degree, license number, date of birth, and location (street address, city and state), the disciplinary state or agency, and the date of the disciplinary action. When it was unclear whether a physician was an M.D. or D.O., we listed the physician's degree as "DR".

We included up to two types of disciplinary actions taken on a given action date, and one violation or offense that served as the basis for that action (see below). Any additional actions were described in the "Notes" heading of items on individual doctors. Details and information on appeals, when available, are also included in this section. Information regarding appeals was not generally available, and hence it is possible that some doctors have had their sanctions stayed or overturned on appeal. Public Citizen made a special effort to obtain information on court actions/decisions that overrule or change previous disciplinary actions taken by state boards. In March 2000, we sent a letter to all boards requesting this information. Not all boards were able to fulfill this request, but of the information received, any actions that were overturned by the courts on appeal or for which litigation in the matter had ended in the physician's favor were deleted from the database.

Each disciplinary action was classified into one of 27 categories. For each disciplinary order, we chose what we viewed as the two most "severe" actions. These were included under the heading "Disciplinary Action:" on the individual doctor listings.

Following is a listing of our categories of disciplinary actions, in order of "severity."

* license revocation
* surrender of license
* nonrenewal of license
* revocation of license to prescribe controlled substances
* surrender of license to prescribe controlled substances
* nonrenewal of license to prescribe controlled substances
* denial of new license
* denial of license reinstatement (following surrender or revocation)
* license reinstatement (following surrender or revocation)
* license suspension
* suspension of authority to prescribe controlled substances
* emergency suspension (pending a formal disciplinary hearing)
* probation
* controlled substance license placed on probation
* fine
* restriction placed on license to practice
* restriction placed on license to prescribe controlled substances

* public reprimand
* required to take additional medical education
* required to enter an impaired physician program or substance abuse treatment
* required to enter an impaired physician program or treatment
* cease and desist order
* monitoring of physician performance
* community service

Medicare program sanctions and actions taken against physicians by the Food and Drug Administration were classified in the following three categories respectively:

* exclusion from the Medicare program
* investigator ineligible to receive investigational new drugs for experimental purposes
* debarment from the FDA's contract program

We placed any further details about disciplinary actions under the heading "Notes." Any disciplinary actions that do not fall into the above categories are detailed in the notes sections and classified as "Other Actions" in our charts and statistical summaries.

When a state provided information on the legal violation or offense that led them to discipline a doctor, we classified that violation into one of 18 categories. If several violations were listed by the Board, we chose the one that appeared to contribute the most to the disciplinary decision. If that choice was unclear, we selected the offense that ranked highest on our hierarchy of offenses as listed below. We included the violation under the heading "Offense" in the listings of individual doctors.

Following are the lists of our categories of offenses, and definitions as needed, in order of presumed importance:

* disciplinary action by another state or agency
* criminal conviction or plea of guilty, nolo contendere, or no contest to a crime
* practicing without a valid license
* practicing without a valid controlled substance license
* loss or restriction of hospital privileges
* failure to comply with a previous board order
* providing false information to the medical board or other health agency
* substandard care, incompetence or negligence
* sexual abuse of or sexual misconduct with a patient
* substance abuse

* overprescribing or misprescribing drugs
* physical or mental illness inhibiting the ability to practice with skill and safety
* insurance, Medicare or Medicaid fraud
* falsifying or altering patient records or medical reports
* overcharging
* exceeding professional limitations
* professional misconduct (see below)
* failure to comply with a professional rule (see below)

The category "professional misconduct" includes a variety of offenses that are more serious than the violation of a professional rule but do not fit into any of the other categories listed above. Some examples of offenses classified as professional misconduct are:

* "unprofessional conduct"
* a criminal offense of which the physician has not been actually convicted
* ordering or performing unnecessary or inappropriate procedures for a patient deliberately, rather than because of incompetence
* failing to supervise a physician's assistant, or other non-medical personnel
* permitting an unlicensed person to practice medicine
* tax violations
* intimidating a patient in an attempt to convince them not to seek a second opinion
* terminating a patient's medical care without transferring the patient to another's care
* abandonment of a patient
* making fraudulent representations in medical practice
* assuring a cure for an incurable disease
* offering to treat by a "secret method"
* accepting payments from laboratories for sending them patients' tests
* procuring a criminal abortion
* performing medical services that the board has declared to be of no value (frequently chelation therapy)
* soliciting patients in a deceitful manner
* disruption of residency program
* improperly transferring a patient from a treatment center to a hospital
* engaging in lewd conduct
* clearly excessive use of diagnostic procedures

* unlawful possession of a controlled substance outside the practice of medicine
* fraud in medical research
* operating an illegal drug lab
* unspecified perjury
* diversion of drugs (not specifically prescription drugs) or drug use
* presigning blank prescription pads so that an unlicensed person may practice medicine
* breaching physician-patient confidentiality
* charging for services as supervising physician even though not present during the course of treatment
* selling drugs and devices for financial gain
* sending out letters to request payment using an attorney's name without the attorney's knowledge or consent
* use of disposable syringes on multiple patients
* rendering a psychiatric evaluation without properly examining and treating the subject of said evaluation
* sexual abuse of a person other than a patient, or of an unspecified person
* not getting a consent form signed
* failing to provide information on license applications, renewals, etc., rather than actually giving false information
* unspecified malpractice settlement
* patient abuse

Examples of the types of violations included in the category "Failure to comply with a professional rule" are:

* violation of restrictions on advertising
* failure to respond to the board
* failure to maintain sanitary practice conditions
* violation of medical records laws (except for falsifying records) including failure to provide copies of records when requested or excessive charges for providing records
* requiring patients to purchase drugs or devices from physician
* failure to keep required documents on file
* employing an agent to solicit patients
* making excessive claims of expertise
* violating AMA ethics standards

* failure to report a disciplinary action in another state
* failure to report child abuse
* failure to pay fees
* failure to display a valid license
* endorsing a product
* keeping outdated or misbranded drugs
* failure to keep proper controlled substance records
* failure to report other medical personnel who are violating the Medical Practice Act to the medical board
* fee-splitting
* failure to report a suspicious death to the police
* failure to meet continuing medical education requirements
* allowing someone not in the doctor's employ and not under direct supervision to demonstrate a medical device to patients
* two-tiered billing
* failure to have liability insurance
* practicing under a name other than the one on his or her physician's license
* violating patient dumping regulations
* nonpayment of student loan

Counting Physicians and Actions

Counting physicians: It is impossible for us to know exactly how many physicians are in our database. There are two main reasons for this:

Many states are not consistent in how they list the names of physicians who have been disciplined, i.e. they may have reported only a first and last name in one newsletter, but included a middle initial and suffix (such as Jr. or Sr.) in another. We made numerous phone calls to try and resolve questions about multiple actions taken against what appeared to be a single physician by a single state and in some cases made calls regarding multiple actions taken against what appeared to be the same person by different states. We also used board web sites to try and verify middle initials, license numbers, etc. These attempts were not always successful.

Many states do not include license numbers or birth dates in their listings of disciplined doctors, which can quickly clarify situations in which names appear similar but are not exactly alike.

After entering the corrected information obtained through phone calls, we counted all the physicians in the database. This is done by using a computer program that compared physician identifying information. The program used six database fields to "match" entries: last name, first name, middle name, the suffix (Jr., Sr., etc.), license number, and birth date. It compared two entries with the same first and last name and "matched" them if one or more of the following was true:

* they had the same birth date;
* they were sanctioned by the same state and had the same license number;
* a middle name in one matched the middle name in the other;
* a middle name in one matched the middle initial in the other; or
* a suffix in one matched the suffix in the other.

Entries within the same state with the same first and last name were not matched if they had differing birth dates or license numbers. When one record included a middle name and the other did not, the records were not considered a match unless the birth dates or license numbers matched. The same is true if one record had a suffix (Jr., Sr., etc.) and another did not.

Counting actions: Although each sanction may consist of several disciplinary actions, we entered only the two most serious disciplinary actions in each case. Both of these disciplinary actions were included when generating counts of actions taken by the state boards or federal agencies. Because we calculated only the two most serious actions, the counts of the less serious actions (such as fines, restrictions, education, and monitoring) will not reveal the frequency with which these less serious actions were imposed. Rather, they will only demonstrate how often these actions were among the two most serious actions levied.

Generation of the State-by-State Lists

In the "Disciplinary Actions" sections of each state listing, we attempted to include all doctors who had any connection with the state. For example, the New York "Disciplinary Actions" section includes:

* All disciplinary actions taken by the New York State Board of Regents;
* All disciplinary actions by other states, the Drug Enforcement Administration, the Food and Drug Administration or Medicare/Medicaid against doctors for whom a New York state address is given;

* All other disciplinary actions against doctors with names like those included above, i.e., actions taken by another state or agency that the computer program described above "matched" to doctors disciplined by New York or located in New York.

Any time a doctor's license number is listed in an action, it is the license number of the state that is sanctioning the doctor.

Some state listings may include doctors with similar names who are not, in fact, the same doctor.

When we were informed by state medical boards or other sources that a physician listed in the book had died, we deleted all records for the deceased doctor from the database. Using the matching program we ensured that all records that matched to the physician's identifying information were also deleted.

Although we have made every effort to match physicians' names correctly, some materials we received did not include complete information on middle names, license numbers, or birth dates. Therefore, consumers should remember that non-disciplined physicians and physicians with different disciplinary actions may have similar names to those physicians listed in the state listing of disciplinary actions. Consumers should also remember that if they want the most current information on the status of a physician's license, they should contact the medical board of the state in which the physician practices or has practiced in the past.

Appeals, Reinstatements

While we attempted to acquire as much up-to-date information as possible on doctors whose disciplinary actions have been appealed to and/or overturned by the courts, we do not have information on all appellate actions. Therefore, we cannot guarantee that a doctor listed here as being disciplined has not had that action overturned or stayed by a court. We entered into our database all disciplinary actions we received by January 31, 2000 and all reinstatements to an unrestricted license and court appeals we received by May 31, 2000. Again, the medical board should be contacted for more detailed and up-to-date information.

> Some states did not supply us with information on license reinstatements or the lifting of license restrictions. We cannot guarantee that a physician listed as being suspended or restricted has not had that suspension or restriction lifted, or that a physician whose license was revoked has not obtained a new license.

Charts, Tables, Statistics

This report uses data on disciplinary actions from two general sources: Public Citizen's analysis of information on disciplinary actions provided by each state; and, the 1999 statistical summaries of state serious disciplinary actions released by the Federation of State Medical Boards. This latter source is only used to generate Tables A and B (pgs. 14 and 16) in the national and regional reports.

These two data sources are not always comparable. States may not have published or sent Public Citizen all the disciplinary actions they counted in their statistical summaries or reported to the Federation of State Medical Boards. Furthermore, our categorization of disciplinary actions may differ from the Federation's.

In our rankings of the numbers of serious state disciplinary actions, we use the Federation statistics because they are the only statistics that are relatively uniform from state to state. However, the Federation is dependent on the states to supply it with disciplinary information, and the types of actions reported may be different from state to state. This may lead to inconsistencies in the rankings. In this report we have ranked states based on the total number of serious disciplinary actions reported to the Federation in 1999 (see Table A, pg. 14) and, in Table B, pg. 16, show the rankings of states for the past nine years as far as the rate of serious disciplinary actions per 1,000 physicians.

For the tables summarizing the disciplinary actions taken by a state over a period of several years, we used our own method of counting only those actions in our database. Therefore, the numbers in these tables may look different from the numbers the Federation has released.

Appendix 3
Addresses of Federal Agencies

Drug Enforcement Administration (DEA)

Drug Enforcement Administration
U.S. Department of Justice
1405 I Street, NW
Washington, D.C. 20005

For questions regarding Physician Registration of the Controlled Substances Act (CSA):

Drug Enforcement Administration

Office of Diversion Control
600 Army Navy Drive
Arlington, VA 22202

Information Services Section (CPI)
700 Army Navy Drive
Arlington, VA 22202

U.S. Department of Health and Human Services

Use these addresses and phone numbers for information on the Medicare/Medicaid sanctions program:

June Gibbs Brown
Inspector General
Department of Health and Human Services
330 Independence Ave. SW
Room 5246 Cohen Bldg.
Washington, DC 20201
(202) 619-3148

Judy Holtz
Public Affairs Office
Office of Inspector General
Department of Health and Human Services
330 Independence Ave. SW
Room 5246 Cohen Building
Washington DC 20201
(202) 619-1343

To get a current list of those sanctioned, contact:

William M. Libercci
Deputy Director
Health Care Administrative Sanctions
Office of Investigations
Office of Inspector General
Department of Health and Human Services
Room N2-01-26
7500 Security Boulevard
Baltimore MD 21244-1850
(410) 786-9603

Use these numbers and addresses to file complaints about health care providers with the Medicare sanctions program:

Nationwide, 24-hour complaints hotline
Toll free 1-800-447-8477

Region I - Boston
(Connecticut, Maine, Massachusetts, New Hampshire, Rhode Island, Vermont,)
Regional Inspector General
Room 2425, JFK Federal Bldg.
Boston, MA 02203
(617) 565-2689

Region II - New York
(New York, New Jersey, Puerto Rico, Virgin Islands)
Regional Inspector General
Room 3900B, Federal Bldg.
26 Federal Plaza
New York, NY 10278
(212) 264-1691

Region III - Philadelphia
(Pennsylvania, Delaware, Maryland, Virginia, West Virginia, District of Columbia)
Regional Inspector General
P.O. Box 13716
Mailstop #9
Philadelphia, PA 19101
(215) 861-4587

Region IV - Atlanta
(Alabama, Florida, Georgia, Kentucky, Mississippi, North Carolina, South Carolina, Tennessee)
Regional Inspector General
Atlanta Federal Center
61 Forsyth Street, SW
Suite 5T18
Atlanta, GA 30303-8909
(404) 562-7603

Region V - Chicago
(Illinois, Indiana, Michigan, Minnesota, Ohio, Wisconsin)
Regional Inspector General
233 North Michigan, Suite 1330
Chicago, IL 60601
(312) 353-2740

Region VI - Dallas
(Arkansas, Louisiana, Montana, New Mexico, Oklahoma, Texas)
Regional Inspector General
Room 6B-13, Federal Bldg.
1100 Commerce Street
Dallas, TX 75242
(214) 767-8406

Region VII - Kansas City
(Kansas, Nebraska, Missouri, Iowa)
Regional Inspector General
Room 284B Richard Bolling Federal Bldg.
601 E. 12th Street
Kansas City, MO 64106
(816) 426-5959

Region VIII - Denver
(Colorado, Montana, North Dakota, South Dakota, Utah, Wyoming)
Division of Health Standards and Quality
Federal Building 1961 Stout Street
Denver, CO 80294
(303) 844-2121

Region IX - San Francisco
(Arizona, California, Hawaii, Nevada, Guam, American Samoa)
Regional Inspector General
DHHS, OIG, OI
Room 174, Federal Office Bldg.
50 United Nations Plaza
San Francisco, CA 94102
(415) 437-7961

Region X - Seattle
Regional Inspector General
(Alaska, Washington, Oregon, Idaho)
2201 Sixth Avenue, MS/RX-40
Seattle, WA 98121-2500
(206) 615-2306

References

1. Public Citizen's Health Research Group. A Consumer's Directory of Prince George's County Doctors 1974.

2. Public Health Service, Department of Health and Human Services. National Practitioner Data Bank for Adverse Information on Physicians and Other Health Care Providers. 45 CFR Part 60, *Federal Register*, October 17, 1989.

3. The Health Care Quality Improvement Act of 1986. *New Jersey Medicine* June 1987;84 (6): 401-403.

4. Iglehart John K. Congress Moves to Bolster Peer Review: The Health Care Quality Improvement Act of 1986. *New England Journal of Medicine* 1987;316 (15):960-964.

5. Office of Technology Assessment. The Quality of Medical Care: Information for Consumers. OTA-H-386. Washington, DC: U.S. Government Printing Office June 1988.

6. Federation of State Medical Boards. Exchange. Section 3: Physician Licensing Boards and Physician Discipline 1989/1990 edition.

Federation of State Medical Boards. Exchange. Section 3: Physician Licensing Boards and Physician Discipline 1988 edition.

7. Title II of the Social Security Act in Compilation of Social Security Laws including Social Security Act as amended and related enactments through January 1, 1989, Vol. 1, U.S. Government Printing Office 1989.

8. Health Resources and Services Administration. National Practitioner Data Bank Statistical Summary, As of Month Ending December 31, 1997.

9. Office of the Inspector General, Department of Health and Human Services. Hospital Reporting to the National Practitioner Data Bank. OEI-01-94-00050 February 1995.

10. Quality-of-Care Data Bank for Patients Coming Soon. *Internal Medicine News* April 15-30, 1989; 22 (8):9.

11. *Dent v. West Virginia*, 127 U.S. 114 (1889); see also *Klafter v. State Board of Examiners of Architects*, 259 Ill. 15, 102 N.E. 193 (1913); *In re Polk License Revocation*, 90 N.J. 550, 449 A.2nd 7 (1982).

12. Office of Evaluation and Inspections, Office of the Inspector General, U.S. Department of Health and Human Services. State Medical Boards and Medical Discipline, draft report April 1990.

13. McAuley R.G. Letter to the Editor, *New England Journal of Medicine* August 8, 1985.

14. Kusserow Richard, Inspector General, U.S. Department of Health and Human Services. Testimony before the U.S. House of Representatives Committee on Small Business, Subcommittee on Regulation, Business Opportunities and Energy June 8, 1990.

15. Federation of State Medical Boards. 1999 Summary of Board Actions Reported by State Licensing and Disciplinary Boards April 2000.

16. To Err is Human: Institute of Medicine, Washington, D.C., 1999.

17. Harvard Medical Practice Study Group. Patients, Doctors and Lawyers: Medical Injury, Malpractice Litigation and Patient Compensation in New York 1990.

18. Mills, D.H. ed. California Medical Association and California Hospital Association Report on the Medical Insurance Feasibility Study. San Francisco: Sutter Publications 1977.

19. *Journal of Legal Medicine* February 1976.

20. Ely John W, Levinson Wendy, Elder Nancy C, Mainous Arch G III, Vinson Daniel C. Perceived Causes of Family Physicians' Errors. *The Journal of Family Practice* 1995;40(4):337-344.

21. Bissonette Raymond, O'Shea Robert M, Horwitz Mary, Route Cynde F. A Data-Generated Basis for Medical Ethics Education: Categorizing Issues Experienced by Students During Clinical Training. *Academic Medicine* 1995;70(11):1035-1037.

22. Feinstein Alvan R. System, Supervision, Standards, and the 'Epidemic' of Negligent Medical Errors. *Archives of Internal Medicine* 1997;157:1285-1289.

23. Pichert James W, Hickson Gerald B, Bledsoe Sandy, Trotter Tinsla, Quinn Doris. Understanding the Etiology of Serious Medical Events Involving Children: Implications for Pediatricians and Their Risk Managers. *Pediatric Annal* 1997;26(3):160-172.

24. Butters Janice M, Strope John L. Legal Standards of Conduct for Students and Residents: Implications for Health Profession Educators. *Academic Medicine* 1996;1(6):583-590.

25. Schwartz William B, Mendelson Daniel N. The Role of Physician-Owned Insurance Companies in the Detection and Deterrence of Negligence. *Journal of the American Medical Association* 1989;260(10):1342-1346.

26. McNamara Robert M, Margulies Jeffrey L. Chemical Dependency in Emergency Medicine Residency Programs: Perspective of the Program Directors. *Annals of Emergency Medicine* 1994;23(5):1072-1076.

27. Hyde Gordon L, Wolfe James. Alcohol and Drug Use by Surgery Residents. *Journal of the American College of Surgeons* 1995;181(1):1-5.

28. McNamara, op. cit.

29. Hyde, op. cit.

30. Hughes Patrick H, Brandenburg Nancy, Baldwin DeWitt C Jr, Storr Carla L, Williams Kristine M, Anthony James C, Sheehan David V. Prevalence of Substance Use Among US Physicians. *Journal of the American Medical Association* 1992;267(17):2333-2339.

31. Smith DE, Seymour R. A Clinical Approach to the Impaired Health Professional. *The International Journal of the Addictions* 1985;20(5):713-722, as cited in Centrella Michael. Physician Addiction and Impairment--Current Thinking: A Review. *Journal of Addictive Diseases* 1994;13:91-105.

32. Hughes, op. cit.

33. Gartrell N, Herman J, Olarte S, Feldsteing M, Localio R. Prevalence of Psychiatrist-Patient Sexual Contact. Sexual Exploitation in Professional Relationships. Washington, DC: American Psychiatric Press 1989:3-13, as cited in Garfinkel Paul E, Bagby RM, Waring EM, and Dorian Barbara. Boundary Violations and Personality Traits among Psychiatrists. *Canadian Journal of Psychiatry* 1997;42:758-763.

34. Kardener SH, Fuller M, Mensh IN. A Survey of Physician's Attitudes and Practices Regarding Erotic and Nonerotic Contact with Patients. *American Journal of Psychiatry* 1973;139:1077-81, as cited in Garfinkel, op. cit.

35. Garfinkel, op. cit.

36. Enbom John A, Thomas Claire D. Evaluation of Sexual Misconduct Complaints: The Oregon Board of Medical Examiners, 1991 to 1995. *American Journal of Obstetrics and Gynecology* 1997;176(6):1340-1348.

37. American Association of Retired Persons. Effective Physician Oversight: Prescription for Medical Licensing Board Reform 1987.

38. Lohr Kathleen N, Schroeder Steven A, Institute of Medicine. A Strategy for Quality Assurance in Medicare. *New England Journal of Medicine* 1990;322(10):707-712.

39. Federation Receives Federal Contract to Develop Self-Assessment Instrument for State Medical Boards. *FSMB Newsletter* September 1990;36.

40. Lohr, op. cit.

41. Federation of State Medical Boards. Elements of a Modern State Medical Board: A Proposal August 1989.

42. Office of Evaluation and Inspections, Office of the Inspector General, U.S. Department of Health and Human Services. State Medical Boards and Medical Discipline August 1990:9.

43. Federation of State Medical Boards August 1989, op. cit.

ARIZONA

1999 serious action rate: 3.81/1000

1999 ranking: 21st

The Arizona State Board of Medical Examiners sent copies of disciplinary orders for 1990 and minutes of the Arizona Board meetings from 1991 through 1999. The orders include the physician's name, degree, license number, the date and type of action taken and the reason for the action. The meeting minutes list the physician's name, degree, license number, the date and type of action taken, and the reason for the action. The reports contain information on modifications and terminations of board actions and some minimal information on court decisions affecting board actions. Arizona also sent separate information on these actions.

One hundred and ten doctors in Arizona were placed on rehabilitation contracts. The Board designated this as not a disciplinary action based on their interpretation of the Americans With Disabilities Act. Public Citizen felt that it was important to include this information for Arizona consumers. Therefore, these doctors are listed separately at the end of the Arizona physicians' listing.

The Arizona Board of Osteopathic Examiners sent copies of disciplinary orders for 1990 through 1999. The orders include the physician's name, degree, license number, addresses (for orders after April 1993), date and type of action taken and the reason for the action. The orders contain information on modifications and terminations of board actions but not on court decisions affecting board actions. Arizona sent separate information on these actions.

The information provided covers disciplinary actions taken against allopathic physicians (MDs) and osteopathic physicians (DOs).

Besides disciplinary actions taken by the State Medical Boards, this listing also includes actions taken by the Medicare/Medicaid programs, the FDA, and the DEA against physicians located in this state. Disciplinary actions taken by other states against physicians located in Arizona or that match a physician disciplined by Arizona (see Appendix 2 for an explanation of the matching protocol) are also included.

Although we have made every effort to match physicians' names correctly, some materials we received did not include complete information on middle names, license numbers, birth dates or addresses. Therefore, consumers should remember that non-disciplined physicians and physicians with different disciplinary actions may have similar names to those disciplined physicians listed in this state. Consumers should also remember that if they want the most current information on the status on a physician's license, they should contact the medical board of the state in which the physician practices or had practiced. (See board address below.) Internet address: *http://www.docboard.org/bomex/index.htm.* This state has a web site which we have graded B on a scale of A (best) to X (worst). This is a measure of the completeness of the information on disciplined doctors. Those state licensing boards with web sites make independent choices about the type of information to be included on their site and how often it is updated.

According to the Federation of State Medical Boards, Arizona took 42 serious disciplinary actions against MDs in 1999. Compared to the 11,025 MDs licensed in the state, the Board had a serious disciplinary action rate of 3.81 serious actions per 1,000 MDs and ranked 21st on that list (see Table A, Findings, pg. 14).

The tables below summarize the data Public Citizen received from Arizona.

Table 1. Disciplinary Actions Against MDs and DOs 1990 through 1999*

Action	Number	Percent**
Revocation	65	6.9%
Surrender	8	0.9%
Suspension	89	9.4%
Probation	177	18.8%
Practice Restriction	114	12.1%
Action Taken Against Controlled Substance License	36	3.8%
Other Actions	453	48.1%
Total Actions	**942**	**100.0%**

* This table lists only the two most serious disciplinary actions taken against a physician.
** Percentages may not total 100% due to rounding.

Table 2. Offenses for which MDs and DOs were Disciplined 1990 through 1999*

Offense	Number	Percent
Criminal Conviction	13	2.3%
Sexual Abuse of or Sexual Misconduct with a Patient	12	2.1%
Substandard Care, Incompetence or Negligence	82	14.7%
Misprescribing or Overprescribing Drugs	43	7.7%
Substance Abuse	96	17.2%
Disciplinary Action Taken Against License by Another State or Agency	66	11.8%
Other Offenses	247	44.2%
Total Records With Offense Listed	**559**	**100.0%**

* Includes only those actions for which an offense was listed and for which we had a corresponding term in our database.

Table 3. Disciplinary Actions Taken for Sexual Abuse of or Sexual Misconduct with a Patient

Action	Number	Percent
Revocation	3	20.0%
Emergency Suspension	3	20.0%
Probation	2	13.3%
Other Actions	7	46.7%
Total Actions	**15**	**100.0%**

Table 4. Disciplinary Actions Taken for Substandard Care, Incompetence or Negligence

Action	Number	Percent
Revocation	3	3.7%
Suspension	1	1.2%
Probation	21	25.9%
Practice Restriction	13	16.0%
Fine	3	3.7%
Reprimand	12	14.8%
Other Actions	28	34.6%
Total Actions	**81**	**100.0%**

Table 5. Disciplinary Actions Taken for Criminal Conviction

Action	Number	Percent
Revocation	6	35.3%
Suspension	2	11.8%
Emergency Suspension	1	5.9%
Probation	4	23.5%
Fine	3	17.6%
Other Actions	1	5.9%
Total Actions	**17**	**100.0%**

Table 6. Disciplinary Actions Taken for Misprescribing or Overprescribing Drugs

Action	Number	Percent
Revocation	2	3.3%
Revocation, Surrender, or Suspension of Controlled Substance License	1	1.6%
Suspension	3	4.9%
Emergency Suspension	2	3.3%
Probation	12	19.7%
Restriction of Controlled Substance License	8	13.1%
Fine	2	3.3%
Education	17	27.9%
Other Actions	14	23.0%
Total Actions	**61**	**100.0%**

Table 7. Disciplinary Actions Taken for Substance Abuse		
Action	**Number**	**Percent**
Revocation	2	1.2%
Suspension	12	7.1%
Emergency Suspension	2	1.2%
Probation	37	22.0%
Restriction of Controlled Substance License	8	4.8%
Fine	1	0.6%
Required to Enter an Impaired Physician Program or Substance Abuse Treatment	55	32.7%
Other Actions	51	30.4%
Total Actions	**168**	**100.0%**

If you feel that your doctor has not given you proper medical care or has mistreated you in any way--whether or not he or she is listed in this report--it is important that you let your state medical board know. Even if they do not immediately act on your complaint, it is important that the information be recorded in their files because it is possible that other people may have filed or will file complaints about the same doctor. Send a brief written description of what occurred to the addresses below or call the phone numbers listed for more information on how to file a complaint.

Addresses

Arizona State Board of Medical Examiners
Mark R. Speicher, Executive Director
9545 East Doubletree Ranch Road
Scottsdale, AZ 85258-5539
(480) 551-2700
Fax: (480) 551-2704

Arizona Board of Osteopathic Examiners in Medicine and Surgery
Anne Marie Berger, Executive Secretary
9545 East Doubletree Ranch Road
Scottsdale, AZ 85258
(480) 657-7703

Listing of Doctors Sanctioned by Offense

Sexual Abuse of or Sexual Misconduct with a Patient

CLOUSE, RICHARD G
COPPELLI, LUIS A
GERSTENBERGER, DEAN L
GERTZ, EDWARD W
HERMAN, RICHARD M
KRAMOLC, NICHOLAS I
MILLER, KEITH E
RODELAS, RAUL M
SHARP, JEFFREY A
WESTMAN, LINCOLN H
YEE, DENNIS W

Substandard Care, Incompetence, or Negligence

AGBEBIYI, JONATHAN A
ANDREWS, CYNTHIA C
AQUILERA, RUBIN
ASLAM, KHALID S
BENCE, LAWRENCE W
BERMAN, ROBERT L
BISKIND, JOHN I
BLATTSTEIN, DEBORAH
BODNAR, THOMAS
BOTTNER, MELVIN
BRENNAN, MICHAEL JAMES
BURNETT, DAVID W
CARTER, H EUGENE
CASTRO, RONALD J
CAZARES, CARLOS
CURTIS, BRUCE NELSON
DAVIS, ROGER
ELTOUKHY, MOHAMED SAMY
EMBRY, THOMAS L
FLEISCHER, ALAN S
FORD, ARTHUR
FORD, LAVELL
FOSDICK, WILLIAM M
FRASER, KENNETH R
GALLAGHER, WILLIAM B
GARLAND, DONALD J
GHAZI-ASKAR, MEHDI
GLADHART, RODNEY
GOODMAN, HERBERT D
GROVES, THOMAS J
HAYASHI, JOE T
HIGUERA, JOSE A
HILL, RICHARD J
HOPWOOD, DON M
HURM, RAYMOND A
HYDE, ROBERT L
KHAN, MUHAMMED AZAM
KLIEWER, PAUL
LAORR, ANAN K
LAPRADE, PAUL W
LEAVITT, J ALLEN
LEIBSOHN, STEVEN
LUTHRA, ADARSH
MARQUEZ, ALBERTO B
MCCRACKEN, JOHN
MCGAREY, WILLIAM C
MILLER, JAMES I
MOSHREFZADEH, MASHALLA
OH, RICHARD D
PAYNE, DAVID L
PINERES, EFRAIM
POWELL, TOM
PREISER, FRANKLIN M
QUIROZ, EDWARD E
RAIKHELKAR, KRANTINATH V
RATH, JOGESWAR
REGER, HARRY L
RUBIN, MARTIN H
SACKS, ALAN CHASBY
SAULTS, CHARLES J
SAVAJIYANI, RAJENDRAKUMAR D
SCHULER, CALVIN
SHAMOS, RAYMOND F
SHAUT, CHRISTOPHER ALDERSON
SHAW, GERALD P
SWENSON, EUGENE J
THORPE, DAVID
VALEROS, QUIRINO
WEBB, DALE F
WESTERVELT, MARK
WESTERVELT, MARK JUSTIN
WILLIAMS, HARVEY E
WILSON, JACK HERBERT
WOO, FRANCIS J
ZIMMERMAN, MARC H

Caution: This list is designed to be used only in conjunction with the rest of this book which includes additional information on each physician such as license number, date of action and more complete descriptions of the offenses.

Criminal Conviction or Plea of Guilty, Nolo Contendere, or No Contest to a Crime

BALMES, RUBEN A
BERTSCH, DALE ROGER
BIGELSEN, HARVEY
BROWNE, ALLEN
CALKINS, GREGORY PAUL
COY, JOHN R
FINLEY, LIEUTENANT WAYNE
KOGIANES, MICHAEL G
KROFT, VADEE
MORGAN, JEROLD
SIEGEL, BERTON
WILLIAMS, KIRK G
ZUERLEIN, KEVIN

Misprescribing or Overprescribing Drugs

AGARWAL, SUDHIR P
BIDWELL, GEORGETTA
BISCOE, MICHAEL
BODNAR, THOMAS
BREWER, EDWARD A
BROWN, RICHARD C
CARIDEO, CAROL
CHAVES, JESUS V
CLARK, ROBERT W
COMPTON, SAMUEL P
GABROY, JAMES B
GOTTESMAN, JOSEPH R
GREEN, JAMES C
HEARTER, WILLIAM R
HUBBARD, JOHN R
HUGHES, THOMAS J
HUNTER, WILLARD S
HURLEY, JAMES M
INFORZATO, NANCY M
KAHLE, JOHN F
LANSING, CORNELIUS
LEBEIS, KERWIN J
LINGENFELTER, JOHN
LUKE, WILLIAM J
MCBRIDE, CRIS D
MEYER, KARL L
MINOR, DAVID
O'DONNELL, ROBERT
PORTER, JOHN C
RUTZ, VIRGINIA
SAYEGH, ABRAHAM J
SCHROEDER, WALTER G
SETTLES, RICHARD
SIMONS, MORTON
SMITH, DIANA J
SMITH, RICHARD L
SMITH, SUSAN M
STEVENS, ROBERT E
TEAGUE, ROBERT C
TEKELL, GORDON SILAS
WADE, MICHAEL G
WALDRIP, ROBERT C
WHITLOW, FRANCIS

Substance Abuse

ADAMS, RICHARD A
AUSTEIN, MARK ROBERT
BLASS, GARY S
BOLES, STEVEN C
BRAZIE, ROBERT WILLARD
BROWN, RICHARD C
BRYANT, GEORGE
BUBIEN, JOHN F
BURKS, JAMES R
CHERISH, LAWRENCE
CLARKE, GEORGE
CLEMENTS, MARK
CUNNIEN, ALAN J
DEMARSE, CORWIN F
DENICOLE, MICHAEL A
DENOVELLIS, ANNA
DENSON, MARK L
DIEHL, CRAIG
DISNEY, THOMAS F
DOLORES, MICHAEL A
DORN, JANICE B
FELLENS, THOMAS E
FLYNN, STEPHEN E
GEAR, PHILLIP E
GILLETTE, WARREN
GRADE, THOMAS J
GRIGGS, JAMES A
HARGIS, THOMAS C
HICKS, WILLIAM R
HOFFERT, KEVIN G
HORSLEY, WILLIAM W
HOWARD, MILES WAYNE
INFORZATO, NANCY M
JANIKOWSKI, MARY DARIN
JOHNSON, PATRICIA
KINCAID, JOSEPH P

Caution: This list is designed to be used only in conjunction with the rest of this book which includes additional information on each physician such as license number, date of action and more complete descriptions of the offenses.

Substance Abuse (cont'd)

KOPPULA, SAMPURNARAO
KREUZER, FREDERICK A
LARSON, DEBORAH J
LEPPERD, FLOYD CHARLES
LEWIS, LEO
LOCNIKAR, STEVEN
MACLACHLAN, ROBERT T
MADRID, EDWARD J
MARQUEZ, ALBERTO B
MARSH, PATRICK J
MAUK, JOHN D
MCRAE, BART L
MERI, BASEM
MICHALAK, PETER
MORITZ, TERRELL CONWAY
NEVIUS, FRED L
ONGLEY, GLENN M
PARDI, EUGENE HANNIBAL
PENA, FRANCISCO
PETERSEN, RICHARD J
PIMIENTA, GILBERT
PUMA, LILLIAN D
RAPPAPORT, WILLIAM DAVID
RICHARDSON, ROBERT ALAN
ROBERTS, BERNICE
RYAN, MARGARET A
SAYEGH, ABRAHAM J
SCHOENHALS, MICHAEL R
SCOTT, MICHAEL E
SHERMAN, SCOTT J
SMITH, SUSAN M
SORGEN, ROBERT WILLIAM
SPINAZZOLA, VICTORIA
SUFFECOOL, STEVEN L
SWEENEY, MICHAEL W
TENORIO, PAUL A
TINSLEY, MARK S
TOUR, ROBERT LOUIS
TUTT, MICHAEL L
URUCHURTU, RICHARD
WELLS, MARILYN
WILCOX, MELINDA J
WILLIAMS, ROBERT A
WRY, ORLIN V
ZALES, MICHAEL R
ZUERLEIN, KEVIN

Caution: This list is designed to be used only in conjunction with the rest of this book which includes additional information on each physician such as license number, date of action and more complete descriptions of the offenses.

ADAMS, RICHARD A MD, LICENSE NUMBER 0016375, WAS DISCIPLINED BY ARIZONA ON JULY 15, 1994
DISCIPLINARY ACTION: LICENSE SUSPENSION; REQUIRED TO ENTER AN IMPAIRED PHYSICIAN PROGRAM OR SUBSTANCE ABUSE TREATMENT
OFFENSE: SUBSTANCE ABUSE

NOTES: DRANK ALCOHOL IN VIOLATION OF ARIZONA BOARD STATUTE AND WAS ADMITTED TO RECOVERY CENTER; AGREES TO ENTER LONG-TERM RESIDENTIAL/IN-PATIENT TREATMENT FOR CHEMICAL DEPENDENCY AND ALCOHOLISM AND TO SUCCESSFULLY COMPLETE ALL TREATMENT RECOMMENDED BY THE TREATMENT FACILITY; CANNOT REACTIVATE HIS LICENSE UNTIL HE MEETS WITH BOARD AND COMPLIES WITH THEIR REQUESTS.

ADAMS, RICHARD A MD OF 6553 E. BAYWOOD AVE PO BOX 11000, MESA, AZ, WAS DISCIPLINED BY DEA ON SEPTEMBER 8, 1994
DISCIPLINARY ACTION: SURRENDER OF CONTROLLED SUBSTANCE LICENSE

NOTES: IN LIEU OF PUBLIC INTEREST REVOCATION.

ADAMS, RICHARD A MD, LICENSE NUMBER 0016375, WAS DISCIPLINED BY ARIZONA ON NOVEMBER 14, 1994
DISCIPLINARY ACTION: 120-MONTH PROBATION; REQUIRED TO ENTER AN IMPAIRED PHYSICIAN PROGRAM OR SUBSTANCE ABUSE TREATMENT
OFFENSE: SUBSTANCE ABUSE

NOTES: LICENSE PLACED ON INACTIVE STATUS 4/15/94 AFTER HE WAS ARRESTED FOR DRIVING WHILE IMPAIRED BY INTOXICATING LIQUOR; DISCHARGED FROM INPATIENT RECOVERY 9/94. LICENSE REACTIVATED ON PROBATION. PROBATION HAS FOLLOWING TERMS AND CONDITIONS: MUST IMMEDIATELY PARTICIPATE IN A BOARD-APPROVED MONITORED AFTERCARE TREATMENT PROGRAM WHOSE THERAPIST MUST SUBMIT QUARTERLY REPORTS; MUST PARTICIPATE IN 90 12-STEP MEETINGS FOR SUBSTANCE ABUSE WITHIN 90 DAYS; MUST THEN PARTICIPATE IN A 12-STEP RECOVERY PROGRAM AS DETERMINED BY HIS TREATING THERAPIST AND ATTEND AT LEAST THREE WEEKLY MEETINGS; SHALL OBTAIN A BOARD-APPROVED TREATING PHYSICIAN; SHALL ABSTAIN COMPLETELY FROM THE CONSUMPTION OF ALCOHOLIC BEVERAGES AND DRUGS EXCEPT WHEN PRESCRIBED BY HIS TREATING PHYSICIAN; MUST SUBMIT TO WITNESSED RANDOM BIOLOGICAL FLUID COLLECTION; KEEP A LOG OF ANY AND ALL MEDICATIONS PRESCRIBED FOR HIM; SHALL SUBMIT TO ANY EXAMINATIONS OR THERAPY ORDERED BY BOARD; SHALL APPEAR BEFORE BOARD FOR INTERVIEWS UPON REQUEST; SHALL INFORM BOARD OF CHANGE OF ADDRESS OR IF AWAY FOR MORE THAN FIVE DAYS. ON 3/15/97 PROBATION TERMINATED AND HE ENTERED INTO A NONDISCIPLINARY REHABILITATION CONTRACT; SHALL MEET WITH MONITORED AFTERCARE COMMITTEE IN 3/98.

AGAHI, FARSHAD MD, DATE OF BIRTH SEPTEMBER 28, 1943, LICENSE NUMBER 0022389 OF 515 W. BUCKEYE ROAD #201, PHOENIX, AZ, WAS DISCIPLINED BY IOWA ON NOVEMBER 2, 1990
DISCIPLINARY ACTION: PROBATION

NOTES: INDEFINITE PROBATION. ON 7/23/92 PROBATION TERMINATED. LICENSE RETURNED TO FULL PRIVILEGES.

AGARWAL, SUDHIR P DR, LICENSE NUMBER 0028660, WAS DISCIPLINED BY MINNESOTA ON JANUARY 9, 1993

NOTES: STAYED SUSPENSION. ON 1/21/95 GRANTED UNCONDITIONAL LICENSE.

AGARWAL, SUDHIR P MD, LICENSE NUMBER 0017587, WAS DISCIPLINED BY ARIZONA ON APRIL 6, 1995
OFFENSE: OVERPRESCRIBING OR MISPRESCRIBING DRUGS

NOTES: INTERVIEWED BY BOARD MEMBERS RELATIVE TO MALPRACTICE CLAIM ALLEGING THAT HE INAPPROPRIATELY PRESCRIBED A CONTROLLED SUBSTANCE TO A PATIENT; FELL BELOW THE STANDARD OF CARE IN HIS TREATMENT BETWEEN 7/89 AND 7/90 OF A PATIENT WITH A HISTORY OF DRUG ABUSE: FAILED TO REQUIRE PATIENT TO COME INTO HIS OFFICE FOR EVALUATION AND/OR EXAMINATION BEFORE PRESCRIBING DIAZEPAM (VALIUM); CONTINUED TO PRESCRIBE VALIUM WITHOUT SEEING THE PATIENT; FAILED TO TAKE AN APPROPRIATE HISTORY, WHICH WOULD HAVE REVEALED THAT THE PATIENT HAD BEEN TO TWO TREATMENT FACILITIES AND THAT PHYSICIANS AT THE SECOND FACILITY PRESCRIBED IMIPRAMINE FOR HIM, WHICH HE WAS TAKING AT THE SAME TIME THAT HE WAS REQUESTING VALIUM PRESCRIPTIONS; ONCE DR. AGARWAL PRESCRIBED THE VALIUM, HE FAILED TO WARN PATIENT OF THE SIDE EFFECTS OF VALIUM AND IMIPRAMINE AND/OR TO WARN HIM THAT HE SHOULD NOT DRIVE AN AUTOMOBILE WHILE TAKING THESE DRUGS BECAUSE OF THE DRASTIC EFFECTS THAT THE COMBINATION OF THE DRUGS COULD HAVE UPON A PERSON'S ABILITY TO DRIVE A MOTOR VEHICLE SAFELY: ON 7/26/90, SIX DAYS AFTER THE FINAL REFILL OF VALIUM, A CAR DRIVEN BY THE PATIENT CROSSED OVER THE CENTER LINE AND COLLIDED HEAD-ON WITH A CAR IN WHICH TWO POLICE OFFICERS WERE KILLED. AT THE TIME, PATIENT'S ABILITY TO DRIVE WAS IMPAIRED DUE TO THE USE OF VALIUM, IMIPRAMINE AND COCAINE. PHYSICIAN STATED AT HIS INFORMAL INTERVIEW WITH THE BOARD THAT, PRIOR TO 1991, HE ALSO PRESCRIBED MEDICATION TO OTHER PATIENTS ON A SOCIAL BASIS WITHOUT SEEING THEM IN THE OFFICE. CENSURED.

AGARWAL, SUDHIR P DR, LICENSE NUMBER 0028660, WAS DISCIPLINED BY MINNESOTA ON NOVEMBER 18, 1995
DISCIPLINARY ACTION: REPRIMAND

AGBEBIYI, JONATHAN MD OF 6707 NORTH 19TH STREET #103, PHOENIX, AZ, WAS DISCIPLINED BY MEDICARE ON SEPTEMBER 1, 1994
DISCIPLINARY ACTION: EXCLUSION FROM THE MEDICARE AND/OR MEDICAID PROGRAM
OFFENSE: DISCIPLINARY ACTION BY ANOTHER STATE OR AGENCY

NOTES: LICENSE REVOKED FOR REASONS BEARING ON PROFESSIONAL PERFORMANCE.

AGBEBIYI, JONATHAN A MD, LICENSE NUMBER 0013271, WAS DISCIPLINED BY ARIZONA ON JANUARY 24, 1991
OFFENSE: SUBSTANDARD CARE, INCOMPETENCE OR NEGLIGENCE

NOTES: CHARGED WITH UNPROFESSIONAL CONDUCT: GROSS MALPRACTICE, REPEATED MALPRACTICE, OR ANY MALPRACTICE RESULTING IN THE DEATH OF A PATIENT; KNOWINGLY MAKING ANY FALSE OR FRAUDULENT STATEMENT IN CONNECTION WITH THE PRACTICE OF MEDICINE; AND FAILING TO FURNISH INFORMATION IN A TIMELY MANNER FOR THE BOARD. ISSUED A DECREE OF CENSURE AND MUST REPORT BACK TO THE BOARD WITHIN 30 DAYS THAT HE HAS CORRECTED MATTERS; SHALL NOT UTILIZE VITAMIN

B12 INJECTIONS, EXCEPT FOR MEDICALLY INDICATED REASONS.

AGBEBIYI, JONATHAN A MD, LICENSE NUMBER 0013271, WAS DISCIPLINED BY ARIZONA ON JUNE 19, 1991
DISCIPLINARY ACTION: 60-MONTH PROBATION; FINE
OFFENSE: OVERCHARGING

NOTES: BOARD INVESTIGATED POSSIBLE OVERCHARGING OF THREE PATIENTS. ORDERED TO PAY RESTITUTION TO TWO PATIENTS DESCRIBED. DURING PROBATION THE BOARD WILL CONDUCT A REEVALUATION OF HIS BILLING PROCEDURES. $2,500 FINE. ORDER MODIFIED ON 10/11/91: ORDER OF PROBATION AND FINE CANCELED; ONLY ONE CASE OF OVERCHARGING WAS CONSIDERED. SHALL PAY RESTITUTION; SURVEY WILL BE CONDUCTED OF PRACTICE WITHIN ONE YEAR.

AGBEBIYI, JONATHAN A MD, LICENSE NUMBER 0013271 OF PHOENIX, AZ, WAS DISCIPLINED BY ARIZONA ON JANUARY 26, 1994
DISCIPLINARY ACTION: LICENSE REVOCATION
OFFENSE: SUBSTANDARD CARE, INCOMPETENCE OR NEGLIGENCE

NOTES: IN 3/91 PERFORMED A HYSTERECTOMY DURING WHICH HE SHOULD HAVE BEEN MORE AGGRESSIVE IN STOPPING BLOOD LOSS WHICH WAS A HEALTH-THREATENING SITUATION. IN 7/91 MEDICAL MANAGEMENT AND CLINICAL JUDGMENT IN HANDLING A PATIENT WERE INADEQUATE AND PATIENT WAS PLACED IN SERIOUS JEOPARDY DUE TO THE UNEXPLAINED DELAY BETWEEN DIAGNOSIS AND SURGERY. IN BOTH CASES OPERATIVE REPORTS AND DISCHARGE SUMMARIES WERE NOT FILLED OUT IN A TIMELY MANNER. HOSPITAL PRIVILEGES WERE SUSPENDED ON 12/20/91 PARTIALLY BECAUSE OF UNWILLINGNESS TO ACCEPT RESPONSIBILITY FOR ACTIONS OR MAINTAIN MALPRACTICE INSURANCE; ENTERED INTO AGREEMENT WITH HOSPITAL ON 2/19/92. DID NOT PROPERLY HANDLE HIS OFFICE CLOSURE WITH REGARD TO ONE PATIENT WHO HAD PAID HIM IN ADVANCE FOR A DELIVERY AND WHOM HE DID NOT INFORM HE WAS CLOSING HIS PRACTICE NOR HAD HE REFERRED HER TO ANOTHER PHYSICIAN; ONLY ABOUT 1/2 OF PATIENT RECORDS WERE RETRIEVED AFTER HIS OFFICE CLOSED. AS OF DATE OF ORDER WAS WORKING IN CORPUS CHRISTI, TEXAS. ORDER OF REVOCATION AFFIRMED BY COURT ON 4/28/95; TIME TO APPEAL HAS RUN.

AGBEBIYI, JONATHAN A MD, LICENSE NUMBER 0G46725 OF CORPUS CHRISTI, TX, WAS DISCIPLINED BY CALIFORNIA ON JUNE 30, 1995
DISCIPLINARY ACTION: 60-MONTH PROBATION
OFFENSE: DISCIPLINARY ACTION BY ANOTHER STATE OR AGENCY

NOTES: DISCIPLINE BY ARIZONA BOARD FOR OB-GYN PRACTICE THAT WAS HARMFUL OR DANGEROUS TO PATIENTS. REVOCATION STAYED.

AGBEBIYI, JONATHAN ADESHINA MD, DATE OF BIRTH SEPTEMBER 7, 1949, LICENSE NUMBER 1041053 OF PO BOX 181135, CORPUS CHRISTI, TX, WAS DISCIPLINED BY MICHIGAN ON AUGUST 7, 1995
DISCIPLINARY ACTION: EMERGENCY SUSPENSION
OFFENSE: SUBSTANDARD CARE, INCOMPETENCE OR NEGLIGENCE

NOTES: NEGLIGENCE; INCOMPETENCE.

AGBEBIYI, JONATHAN ADESHINA MD, DATE OF BIRTH SEPTEMBER 7, 1949, LICENSE NUMBER 1041053 OF PO BOX 181135, CORPUS CHRISTI, TX, WAS DISCIPLINED BY MICHIGAN ON JANUARY 12, 1996
DISCIPLINARY ACTION: LICENSE REVOCATION; FINE
OFFENSE: SUBSTANDARD CARE, INCOMPETENCE OR NEGLIGENCE

NOTES: NEGLIGENCE; INCOMPETENCE. $1,000 FINE.

AGBEBIYI, JONATHAN ADESHINA MD, DATE OF BIRTH SEPTEMBER 7, 1949 OF PO BOX 181298, CORPUS CHRISTI, TX, WAS DISCIPLINED BY MEDICARE ON APRIL 23, 1996
DISCIPLINARY ACTION: EXCLUSION FROM THE MEDICARE AND/OR MEDICAID PROGRAM
OFFENSE: DISCIPLINARY ACTION BY ANOTHER STATE OR AGENCY

NOTES: LICENSE REVOKED FOR REASONS BEARING ON PROFESSIONAL PERFORMANCE.

ALEXANDER, CLIFTON J MD, LICENSE NUMBER 0002715, WAS DISCIPLINED BY ARIZONA ON DECEMBER 17, 1990

NOTES: BOARD GRANTED INACTIVE STATUS FOR CAUSE ON HIS LICENSE BECAUSE HE FAILED THE SPECIAL PURPOSE LICENSING EXAM TWICE; HE SHALL NOT PRACTICE ANYWHERE WHILE HIS LICENSE IS IN INACTIVE STATUS; WILL NOT HOLD DEA REGISTRATION WHILE LICENSE IS INACTIVE.

AMBER, SAUL MD, LICENSE NUMBER 0010916, WAS DISCIPLINED BY ARIZONA ON SEPTEMBER 23, 1996
DISCIPLINARY ACTION: MONITORING OF PHYSICIAN PERFORMANCE

NOTES: WITHIN THREE MONTHS SHALL OBTAIN PSYCHOLOGICAL COUNSELING FROM A BOARD-APPROVED THERAPIST; REMAIN IN THERAPY FOR THE DURATION OF THIS STIPULATION; AND AUTHORIZE AND REQUIRE THE THERAPIST TO PROVIDE QUARTERLY REPORTS TO THE BOARD. ON 9/26/97 ORDER TERMINATED.

ANDREWS, BRIAN C MD, WAS DISCIPLINED BY ARIZONA ON JULY 30, 1999
DISCIPLINARY ACTION: RESTRICTION PLACED ON LICENSE

NOTES: LICENSE GRANTED WITH PRACTICE RESTRICTION.

ANDREWS, CYNTHIA C MD, LICENSE NUMBER 17902, WAS DISCIPLINED BY ARIZONA ON SEPTEMBER 26, 1997
DISCIPLINARY ACTION: REPRIMAND
OFFENSE: SUBSTANDARD CARE, INCOMPETENCE OR NEGLIGENCE

NOTES: DURING 1995 IN CONNECTION WITH LITIGATION FILED BY A DECEASED PATIENT'S ESTATE, IT WAS FOUND THAT DR. ANDREWS DESTROYED THE ORIGINAL OFFICE VISIT FORM OF THIS PATIENT FROM 3/22/95 SINCE SHE WAS CONCERNED THAT ANYONE REVIEWING THE RECORD WOULD FIND IT ILLEGIBLE OR SUSPECT ADDED INFORMATION TO THE ORIGINAL NOTES; SHE ALSO ASKED A NURSE TO REWRITE HER NOTES ON A NEW, BLANK OFFICE VISIT FORM WHICH WAS THEN SUBSTITUTED IN THE FILE FOR THE ORIGINAL; ALTHOUGH THE CORRECT DIAGNOSES FOR THE PATIENT WAS NOT READILY APPARENT NOR DID THE PATIENT HAVE AN OBVIOUS UNDERLYING PNEUMONIA, PNEUMOCOCCAL INFECTION SHOULD BE SUSPECTED. DR. ANDREWS WAS ISSUED A DECREE OF CENSURE.

ANDREWS, JANIS L MD, LICENSE NUMBER 0019667, WAS DISCIPLINED BY ARIZONA ON AUGUST 31, 1990
DISCIPLINARY ACTION: RESTRICTION PLACED ON LICENSE; MONITORING OF PHYSICIAN PERFORMANCE

NOTES: SHALL CONTINUE TO PARTICIPATE IN BOARD-APPROVED COUNSELING WITH MONTHLY REPORTS SUBMITTED TO THE BOARD; SHALL PRACTICE IN A SETTING WHICH WILL PROVIDE FOR ONGOING PEER REVIEW AND IMMEDIATE ACCESS TO A LICENSED PHYSICIAN; SHALL PROVIDE A COPY OF THE ORDER

TO HER EMPLOYER WHO SHALL PROVIDE MONTHLY STATUS REPORTS TO THE BOARD; SHALL NOT SEEK TO MODIFY ORDER PRIOR TO 4/1/92. ON 10/11/91 ORDER MODIFIED SUCH THAT SHE BE ALLOWED TO PRACTICE IN AN UNSUPERVISED SETTING WHERE SHE IS NOT RESPONSIBLE FOR PATIENT CARE AND TREATMENT IN WHICH RECORDS SHALL BE AVAILABLE FOR REVIEW. ON 4/11/92 BOARD AMENDED PREVIOUS ORDER (WHICH IS NOT DISCIPLINARY IN NATURE AND DOES NOT RELATE TO THE QUALITY OF CARE AFFORDED HER PATIENTS, BUT RATHER IS DESIGNED FOR PERSONAL REHABILITATIVE PURPOSES ONLY): SHALL IMMEDIATELY PARTICIPATE IN ONGOING PSYCHIATRIC THERAPY WITH A BOARD-APPROVED PSYCHIATRIST WHO SHALL PROVIDE MONTHLY REPORTS TO BOARD; SHALL PRACTICE IN A SUPERVISED SETTING EXCEPT INSOFAR AS SHE MAY PRACTICE IN A SETTING WHERE SHE IS NOT RESPONSIBLE FOR PATIENT CARE AND TREATMENT, IN WHICH CASE SHE WILL MAKE HER PATIENT RECORDS AVAILABLE TO BOARD; SHALL PROVIDE COPY OF ORDER TO EMPLOYER WHO SHALL PROVIDE MONTHLY STATUS REPORTS TO BOARD. ORDER MODIFIED ON 10/11/95: SHALL CONTINUE TO PARTICIPATE IN ONGOING PSYCHOLOGICAL COUNSELING AND THERAPY WITH A BOARD APPROVED THERAPIST WHO SHALL PROVIDE REPORTS MONTHLY TO THE BOARD; SHALL PRACTICE MEDICINE IN A SUPERVISED SETTING WHERE SHE IS NOT RESPONSIBLE FOR PATIENT CARE AND TREATMENT AND SHALL MAKE HER PATIENT RECORDS AVAILABLE UPON BOARD REQUEST; SHALL PROVIDE A COPY OF THIS ORDER TO HER EMPLOYER WHO SHALL PROVIDE THE BOARD WITH MONTHLY STATUS REPORTS CONCERNING HER PERFORMANCE AND PATIENT CARE.

AQUILERA, RUBIN MD, WAS DISCIPLINED BY ARIZONA ON SEPTEMBER 24, 1998
DISCIPLINARY ACTION: REQUIRED TO TAKE ADDITIONAL MEDICAL EDUCATION
OFFENSE: SUBSTANDARD CARE, INCOMPETENCE OR NEGLIGENCE

NOTES: PRESCRIBED MEDICATION FOR A PATIENT'S HEADACHES WITHOUT ADEQUATE WORKUP. MUST OBTAIN 10 HOURS OF CONTINUING MEDICAL EDUCATION IN OBESITY TREATMENT AND RECORD KEEPING WITHIN SIX MONTHS.

AREBALO, RONALD E MD, LICENSE NUMBER 0020144, WAS DISCIPLINED BY ARIZONA ON FEBRUARY 15, 1996
DISCIPLINARY ACTION: LICENSE SUSPENSION
OFFENSE: FAILURE TO COMPLY WITH PREVIOUS BOARD ORDER

NOTES: IN VIOLATION OF HIS REHABILITATION STIPULATION AND ORDER DUE TO CHEMICAL RELAPSE. SHALL UNDERGO TREATMENT AT TALBOTT RECOVERY CENTER. LICENSE PLACED IN INACTIVE STATUS WITH CAUSE.

AREBALO, RONALD E MD OF 130 S. COCHISE #790, SPRINGERVILLE, AZ, WAS DISCIPLINED BY DEA ON JULY 25, 1997
DISCIPLINARY ACTION: SURRENDER OF CONTROLLED SUBSTANCE LICENSE

NOTES: IN LIEU OF PUBLIC INTEREST REVOCATION.

ASHBY, RALPH R MD OF PHOENIX, AZ, WAS DISCIPLINED BY IOWA ON MARCH 28, 1997
DISCIPLINARY ACTION: PROBATION
OFFENSE: DISCIPLINARY ACTION BY ANOTHER STATE OR AGENCY

NOTES: ACTION FILED IN CONNECTION WITH HIS ENTRY INTO A VOLUNTARY AGREEMENT WITH THE ARIZONA MEDICAL BOARD WHICH PLACED CERTAIN RESTRICTIONS ON HIS ARIZONA LICENSE. AS A CONDITION OF PROBATION HE MUST COMPLY WITH THE TERMS OF THE ARIZONA AGREEMENT.

ASLAM, KHALID S MD, LICENSE NUMBER 0013474, WAS DISCIPLINED BY ARIZONA ON DECEMBER 30, 1996
DISCIPLINARY ACTION: PROBATION; REQUIRED TO TAKE ADDITIONAL MEDICAL EDUCATION
OFFENSE: SUBSTANDARD CARE, INCOMPETENCE OR NEGLIGENCE

NOTES: PRACTICED GROSS AND REPEATED NEGLIGENCE WHICH RESULTED IN HARM TO PATIENTS WITH REGARD TO SIX PATIENTS HE TREATED BETWEEN 10/90 AND 8/91 WHICH INCLUDED: FAILING TO NOTE AT FIRST PAST HISTORY, FAMILY HISTORY, REVIEW OF SYSTEMS OR THAT THE PATIENT WAS AN INSULIN DEPENDENT DIABETIC; FAILING TO PROMPTLY RESPOND TO A NURSE'S CALL ABOUT A PATIENT HAVING POST-OPERATIVE COMPLICATIONS; FAILING TO ESTABLISH A DIAGNOSIS BEFORE HE PERFORMED AN ARTHRODESIS ON ONE PATIENT AND NOTED THAT THE CARTILAGE APPEARED TO BE DISEASED ALTHOUGH HE SUBMITTED NO PATHOLOGY SPECIMEN; DELAYED SURGICAL INTERVENTION IN ONE CASE; AND OTHER RELEVANT INFORMATION ON OTHER PATIENT'S RECORDS. INDEFINITE PROBATION INCLUDES: SHALL NOT PRACTICE UNTIL HE SUCCESSFULLY COMPLETES ONE YEAR OF POST-GRADUATE TRAINING IN ORTHOPEDIC SURGERY IN AN APPROVED PROGRAM AND TAKES AND PASSES THE AMERICAN BOARD OF ORTHOPEDIC SURGERY CERTIFICATION EXAM. UPON COMPLETION OF THE FIRST CONDITION ABOVE, HE MAY BE SUBJECT TO THE FOLLOWING: SHALL IMMEDIATELY PROVIDE NOTIFICATION IN WRITING OF HIS PRACTICE LOCATION UPON RETURN TO ARIZONA; SHALL MAKE HIS RECORDS AND PRACTICE AVAILABLE TO BOARD TO REVIEW AT ANY TIME; AND SHALL UNDERGO A PRACTICE SURVEY BY THE BOARD WITHIN ONE YEAR OF HIS RETURN TO ARIZONA.

ASLAM, KHALID S MD, LICENSE NUMBER 13474, WAS DISCIPLINED BY ARIZONA ON JANUARY 24, 1997
DISCIPLINARY ACTION: PROBATION; REQUIRED TO TAKE ADDITIONAL MEDICAL EDUCATION
OFFENSE: SUBSTANDARD CARE, INCOMPETENCE OR NEGLIGENCE

NOTES: IN SIX PATIENTS DR. ASLAM TREATED BETWEEN 10/90 AND 9/93 THE BOARD DETERMINED THERE TO BE GROSS NEGLIGENCE, REPEATED NEGLIGENCE OR NEGLIGENCE RESULTING IN HARM OR DEATH TO THE PATIENT. THESE CASES INCLUDED: ONE PATIENT FOR WHICH HE INITIALLY FAILED TO NOTE PAST HISTORY, FAMILY HISTORY, REVIEW OF SYSTEMS OR THAT THE PATIENT WAS AN INSULIN DEPENDENT DIABETIC; IN ANOTHER PATIENT LEFT DETAILS OUT OF REPORT AND DID NOT ARRIVE AT HOSPITAL UNTIL AT LEAST 3 1/2 HOURS AFTER NURSES NOTIFIED HIM OF COMPLICATIONS; IN A THIRD PATIENT, HE FAILED TO ESTABLISH A DIAGNOSIS, DID NOT CONSIDER ASPIRATING A SWOLLEN JOINT AND DESPITE NO INDICATION OF ARTHRITIS IN THE JOINT, RECOMMENDED A JOINT PROCEDURE WHICH HE PERFORMED AND WAS DETERMINED EXCESSIVE BY ANOTHER DOCTOR; ON ANOTHER PATIENT, HE DELAYED PERFORMING SURGICAL INTERVENTION AND FAILED TO DOCUMENT THE NATURE AND EXTENT OF A ULNAR NEUROPATHY WHICH LATER DEVELOPED POST-OPERATIVELY. PLACED ON INDEFINITE PROBATION WITH THE FOLLOWING TERMS AND CONDITIONS: SHALL SUCCESSFULLY COMPLETE ONE

YEAR OF POST-GRADUATE TRAINING IN ORTHOPEDIC SURGERY IN AN APPROVED PROGRAM; SHALL TAKE AND PASS THE AMERICAN BOARD OF ORTHOPEDIC SURGERY CERTIFICATION EXAM. ONCE HE COMPLETES HIS TRAINING HE MAY PRACTICE IN ARIZONA UNDER THE FOLLOWING CONDITIONS: SHALL IMMEDIATELY PROVIDE NOTIFICATION TO THE BOARD IN WRITING OF HIS PRACTICE LOCATION UPON RETURN TO ARIZONA; SHALL MAKE HIS RECORDS AND PRACTICE AVAILABLE TO THE BOARD ANY TIME FOR REVIEW; SHALL UNDERGO A PRACTICE SURVEY WITHIN ONE YEAR OF HIS RETURN TO ARIZONA.

ASLAM, KHALID S MD, DATE OF BIRTH AUGUST 18, 1949 OF 48 HOUSE 150 F10/4, ISLAMABAD PAKISTAN, WAS DISCIPLINED BY MEDICARE ON JANUARY 20, 1999
DISCIPLINARY ACTION: EXCLUSION FROM THE MEDICARE AND/OR MEDICAID PROGRAM
OFFENSE: DISCIPLINARY ACTION BY ANOTHER STATE OR AGENCY

NOTES: LICENSE REVOKED, SUSPENDED, SURRENDERED OR OTHERWISE LOST FOR REASONS BEARING ON PROFESSIONAL PERFORMANCE, PROFESSIONAL COMPETENCE OR FINANCIAL INTEGRITY.

ASLAM, KHALID SALEEM MD, LICENSE NUMBER A39443 OF ISLAMABAD PAKISTAN, WAS DISCIPLINED BY CALIFORNIA ON MAY 8, 1998
DISCIPLINARY ACTION: LICENSE REVOCATION
OFFENSE: DISCIPLINARY ACTION BY ANOTHER STATE OR AGENCY

NOTES: DISCIPLINED BY ARIZONA FOR GROSS NEGLIGENCE OR NEGLIGENCE RESULTING IN HARM TO OR DEATH OF A PATIENT.

ATHANS, JOHN DO OF 13020 N SURREY CIRCLE, PHOENIX, AZ, WAS DISCIPLINED BY DEA ON MAY 21, 1999
DISCIPLINARY ACTION: SURRENDER OF CONTROLLED SUBSTANCE LICENSE

ATHANS, JOHN J DO, LICENSE NUMBER 2118 OF 13020 N SURREY CIRCLE, PHOENIX, AZ, WAS DISCIPLINED BY ARIZONA ON MARCH 28, 1998
DISCIPLINARY ACTION: EMERGENCY SUSPENSION
OFFENSE: LOSS OR RESTRICTION OF HOSPITAL PRIVILEGES

NOTES: ON 3/25/98 HIS HOSPITAL PRIVILEGES WERE SUSPENDED DUE TO ALLEGATIONS OF SUBSTANCE ABUSE AND NARCOTICS WHICH WERE UNACCOUNTED FOR; ON 3/25/98 HE TESTED POSITIVE FOR BENZODIAZEPINES AND ADMITTED TO SELF-MEDICATING WITH VALIUM, PROZAC AND TAGAMET.

ATHANS, JOHN J DO, LICENSE NUMBER 2118 OF 13020 N SURREY CIRCLE, PHOENIX, AZ, WAS DISCIPLINED BY ARIZONA ON MAY 16, 1998
DISCIPLINARY ACTION: LICENSE SUSPENSION; 60-MONTH PROBATION
OFFENSE: LOSS OR RESTRICTION OF HOSPITAL PRIVILEGES

NOTES: ON 3/25/98 HOSPITAL PRIVILEGES WERE SUMMARILY SUSPENDED DUE TO ALLEGATIONS OF SUBSTANCE ABUSE AND NARCOTICS WHICH WERE UNACCOUNTED FOR; HE REFUSED TO TAKE A URINE SCREEN AS REQUIRED BY THE HOSPITAL; TESTED POSITIVE FOR BENZODIAZEPINES; ON 3/27/98 ADMITTED HE WAS SELF-MEDICATING WITH VALIUM, PROZAC AND TAGAMET. HE SHALL REFRAIN FROM PRACTICING OSTEOPATHIC MEDICINE AND SURGERY UNTIL HE HAS COMPLIED WITH THE FOLLOWING TERMS AND CONDITIONS: SHALL SUCCESSFULLY COMPLETE AN INPATIENT EVALUATION FOR POSSIBLE CHEMICAL DEPENDENCY; WILL PROVIDE COPIES OF ANY AND ALL RECORDS PERTINENT TO HIS DIAGNOSIS AND TREATMENT WHILE A PATIENT AT A TREATMENT FACILITY; SHALL DEVELOP A PLAN FOR AFTERCARE TREATMENT WHICH SHALL INCLUDE COUNSELING, RANDOM BODY FLUID TESTING, PROHIBITION FROM USE OF ALCOHOL AND CONTROLLED SUBSTANCES AND MEETINGS WITH THE BOARD. CONDITIONS OF PROBATION: SHALL PARTICIPATE IN A MINI-RESIDENCY REGARDING PRESCRIPTION HABITS WITHIN SIX MONTHS AND SHALL OBTAIN AT LEAST 20 CONTINUING MEDICAL EDUCATION CREDITS IN PRESCRIBING OF NARCOTICS AND CONTROLLED SUBSTANCES AND SUBSTANCE ADDICTION IN THE FIRST TWO YEARS OF PROBATION; SHALL NOT CONSUME ILLICIT DRUGS OR TAKE ANY CONTROLLED SUBSTANCES UNLESS PRESCRIBED BY THE TREATING PHYSICIAN AND SHALL MAINTAIN A MONTHLY LOG OF ALL PRESCRIPTION DRUGS TAKEN BY HIM AND PROVIDE A COPY TO THE BOARD; SHALL SUBMIT TO ANY INDEPENDENT MEDICAL OR PSYCHOLOGICAL EVALUATION ORDERED; SHALL SUBMIT TO RANDOM BIOLOGICAL FLUID TESTING; SHALL PROVIDE A COPY OF THE ORDER TO ANY HEALTH CARE ENTITY WHERE HE IS EMPLOYED; SHALL INFORM BOARD IF HE LEAVES ARIZONA; SHALL PAY COSTS.

ATHANS, JOHN J DO, LICENSE NUMBER 2118 OF 13020 N. SURREY CIRCLE, PHOENIX, AZ, WAS DISCIPLINED BY ARIZONA ON MARCH 6, 1999
DISCIPLINARY ACTION: LICENSE REVOCATION
OFFENSE: FAILURE TO COMPLY WITH PREVIOUS BOARD ORDER

NOTES: VIOLATED 5/16/98 BOARD ORDER BY ADMITTING THAT HE WAS PURCHASING AND SELF-MEDICATING WITH THE DRUG KETAMINE SINCE 5/98; ON 1/11/99 WHEN HE WAS REQUESTED TO HAVE AN EVALUATION REGARDING THE ALLEGATION OF A POSSIBLE DRUG RELAPSE, HE REFUSED TO GO INTO TREATMENT AND STATED HE NEVER WANTED TO PRACTICE MEDICINE AGAIN.

ATHANS, JOHN J DO, DATE OF BIRTH DECEMBER 21, 1953, LICENSE NUMBER 1009476 OF 13020 N SURREY CIRCLE, PHOENIX, AZ, WAS DISCIPLINED BY MICHIGAN ON MAY 19, 1999
DISCIPLINARY ACTION: LICENSE SUSPENSION; FINE
OFFENSE: DISCIPLINARY ACTION BY ANOTHER STATE OR AGENCY

NOTES: FAILURE TO REPORT/COMPLY. LICENSE SUSPENDED FOR A MINIMUM OF SIX MONTHS AND ONE DAY. $1000 FINE.

AUSTEIN, MARK ROBERT MD, LICENSE NUMBER 0014196, WAS DISCIPLINED BY ARIZONA ON OCTOBER 15, 1993
DISCIPLINARY ACTION: LICENSE SUSPENSION
OFFENSE: SUBSTANCE ABUSE

NOTES: TREATED FOR CHEMICAL DEPENDENCY AND LEFT TREATMENT AGAINST STAFF ADVICE; AN INPATIENT EVALUATION AT PARKSIDE HOSPITAL ALSO INDICATED A NEED FOR FURTHER LONG-TERM RESIDENTIAL TREATMENT. PRIOR TO APPLYING FOR REACTIVATION OF LICENSURE, MUST FIRST DEMONSTRATE TO THE SATISFACTION OF THE BOARD THAT HE IS PHYSICALLY, MENTALLY AND MEDICALLY COMPETENT TO SAFELY ENGAGE IN THE PRACTICE OF MEDICINE, AND PROVIDE PROOF THAT HE HAS NOT MISUSED ALCOHOL AND/OR LICIT OR ILLICIT DRUGS OR SUBSTANCES. RETROACTIVE TO 8/18/93.

AUSTEIN, MARK ROBERT MD OF 1925 W ORANGE GROVE RD SUITE 204, TUCSON, AZ, WAS DISCIPLINED BY DEA ON MARCH 4, 1994

DISCIPLINARY ACTION: SURRENDER OF CONTROLLED SUBSTANCE LICENSE

NOTES: IN LIEU OF PUBLIC INTEREST REVOCATION.

AUSTEIN, MARK ROBERT MD, LICENSE NUMBER 0014196, WAS DISCIPLINED BY ARIZONA ON APRIL 8, 1995
DISCIPLINARY ACTION: 60-MONTH PROBATION; REQUIRED TO TAKE ADDITIONAL MEDICAL EDUCATION
OFFENSE: SUBSTANCE ABUSE

NOTES: REINSTATEMENT TO PROBATION WITH CONDITIONS: MUST IMMEDIATELY PARTICIPATE IN A BOARD-APPROVED MONITORED AFTERCARE TREATMENT PROGRAM WHOSE THERAPIST MUST SUBMIT QUARTERLY REPORTS; HAS PREVIOUSLY PARTICIPATED IN 90 12-STEP MEETINGS FOR SUBSTANCE ABUSE; MUST PARTICIPATE IN A 12-STEP RECOVERY PROGRAM AS DETERMINED BY HIS TREATING THERAPIST AND ATTEND AT LEAST THREE WEEKLY MEETINGS; SHALL OBTAIN A BOARD-APPROVED TREATING PHYSICIAN; SHALL ABSTAIN COMPLETELY FROM THE CONSUMPTION OF ALCOHOLIC BEVERAGES AND DRUGS EXCEPT WHEN PRESCRIBED BY HIS TREATING PHYSICIAN; MUST SUBMIT TO WITNESSED RANDOM BIOLOGICAL FLUID COLLECTION; MUST KEEP A LOG OF ANY AND ALL MEDICATIONS PRESCRIBED FOR HIM; SHALL SUBMIT TO ANY EXAMINATIONS OR THERAPY ORDERED BY BOARD; SHALL APPEAR BEFORE BOARD FOR INTERVIEWS UPON REQUEST; SHALL INFORM THE BOARD OF CHANGE OF ADDRESS OR IF AWAY FOR MORE THAN FIVE DAYS. WITHIN 90 DAYS, SHALL OBTAIN 16 HOURS OF CONTINUING MEDICAL EDUCATION IN INTERNAL MEDICINE REVIEW APPROVED BY BOARD STAFF.

BAKER, DUANE MD, LICENSE NUMBER 0005290, WAS DISCIPLINED BY ARIZONA ON OCTOBER 15, 1993
OFFENSE: DISCIPLINARY ACTION BY ANOTHER STATE OR AGENCY

NOTES: ORDER OF SUSPENSION ISSUED IN NEBRASKA; CHEMICAL DEPENDENCY RELAPSE. SHALL NOT ENGAGE IN THE PRACTICE OF MEDICINE IN ARIZONA UNTIL HE HAS FIRST ADVISED THE BOARD OF MEDICAL EXAMINERS OF ARIZONA IN WRITING OF HIS INTENTION TO DO SO; AGREES TO RELEASE ANY AND ALL INFORMATION GATHERED BY NEBRASKA, THE AFTERCARE PROGRAM AND OTHER INDIVIDUALS OR ENTITIES AS NECESSARY TO REVIEW HIS COMPLIANCE WITH THE NEBRASKA ORDER OF PROBATION.

BALDWIN, STEVEN MD, WAS DISCIPLINED BY ARIZONA ON JULY 17, 1996
DISCIPLINARY ACTION: REQUIRED TO TAKE ADDITIONAL MEDICAL EDUCATION; MONITORING OF PHYSICIAN PERFORMANCE

NOTES: INTERVIEWED BY THE BOARD REGARDING HIS PRESCRIBING OF CONTROLLED SUBSTANCES. SHALL COMPLETE 30 HOURS OF CONTINUING MEDICAL EDUCATION IN THE PHARMACOLOGY OF CHRONIC PAIN MANAGEMENT; AND THAT STAFF PERFORM A FOLLOW-UP OFFICE SURVEY IN ONE YEAR. ON 8/8/98 ORDER TERMINATED.

BALIZADO, ALFREDO DIVINA MD, LICENSE NUMBER 0006702, WAS DISCIPLINED BY ARIZONA ON NOVEMBER 26, 1990
OFFENSE: LOSS OR RESTRICTION OF HOSPITAL PRIVILEGES

NOTES: PRACTICE PRIVILEGES WERE SUSPENDED OR RESTRICTED AT SEVERAL HOSPITALS. IN SEVERAL CASES HE WAS INVOLVED WITH HIS CARE AS AN ANESTHESIOLOGIST MANIFESTED THE FOLLOWING INADEQUACIES: INADEQUATE INTRAOPERATIVE MONITORING AND FLUID AND BLOOD REPLACEMENT; INAPPROPRIATE DRUG DOSAGES; INADEQUATE EXTUBATION CRITERIA; ABANDONED AN UNRESPONSIVE CYANOTIC PATIENT IN POST-OP WHO LATER DIED; TAMPERED WITH RECORDS; NONCOMPLIANCE WITH DEMANDS FROM ANESTHESIA COMMITTEE. CENSURED FOR UNPROFESSIONAL CONDUCT.

BALIZADO, ALFREDO DIVINA MD, LICENSE NUMBER 0006702, WAS DISCIPLINED BY ARIZONA ON JANUARY 25, 1991
DISCIPLINARY ACTION: REQUIRED TO TAKE ADDITIONAL MEDICAL EDUCATION

NOTES: MUST COMPLETE 70 HOURS OF ANESTHESIA EDUCATION PROGRAMS DURING EACH OF THE THREE YEARS FROM THE DATE OF THIS ORDER, TO BE REPORTED WITH RENEWAL OF HIS LICENSE FOR 1992, 1993, AND 1994; MUST PROVIDE BOARD DOCUMENTED PROOF OF COMPLETION OF THESE EDUCATIONAL REQUIREMENTS.

BALMES, RUBEN A MD, WAS DISCIPLINED BY ARIZONA ON OCTOBER 11, 1991
DISCIPLINARY ACTION: LICENSE SUSPENSION
OFFENSE: CRIMINAL CONVICTION OR PLEA OF GUILTY, NOLO CONTENDERE, OR NO CONTEST TO A CRIME

NOTES: FOUND GUILTY OF A MISDEMEANOR INVOLVING MORAL TURPITUDE ISSUES. REQUEST THAT BOARD ACCEPT HIS SIGNED STIPULATED AGREEMENT FOR SUSPENSION OF HIS LICENSE WITH CAUSE WAS ACCEPTED.

BALMES, RUBEN A MD, LICENSE NUMBER 0C41700 OF SAN DIEGO, CA, WAS DISCIPLINED BY CALIFORNIA ON JULY 25, 1992
DISCIPLINARY ACTION: LICENSE REVOCATION

BALMES, RUBEN ALONZO MD, LICENSE NUMBER 032009L OF TEMPE, AZ, WAS DISCIPLINED BY PENNSYLVANIA ON JANUARY 19, 1995
DISCIPLINARY ACTION: LICENSE REVOCATION
OFFENSE: DISCIPLINARY ACTION BY ANOTHER STATE OR AGENCY

NOTES: RECIPROCAL ACTION TAKEN IN CALIFORNIA; BOARD UPHELD REVOCATION.

BALMES, RUBEN ALONZO MD, DATE OF BIRTH FEBRUARY 22, 1932 OF 1644 N EL CAMINO DRIVE, TEMPE, AZ, WAS DISCIPLINED BY MEDICARE ON SEPTEMBER 11, 1995
DISCIPLINARY ACTION: EXCLUSION FROM THE MEDICARE AND/OR MEDICAID PROGRAM
OFFENSE: DISCIPLINARY ACTION BY ANOTHER STATE OR AGENCY

NOTES: LICENSE REVOKED FOR REASONS BEARING ON PROFESSIONAL PERFORMANCE.

BARNET, EMMANUEL MD, WAS DISCIPLINED BY ARIZONA ON JANUARY 18, 1996

NOTES: DID NOT RESPOND TO BOARD REQUEST OF 9/95 THAT HE UNDERGO PHYSICAL AND PSYCHOLOGICAL EVALUATIONS AND A PERIOD OF URINE DRUG TESTING; WHEN CONTACTED BY TELEPHONE ABOUT REQUEST, HE INDICATED THAT HE WOULD NOT COMPLY WITH RECOMMENDATIONS FOR EVALUATION OR URINE DRUG TESTING. ORDERED BY THE BOARD TO UNDERGO PSYCHOLOGICAL, PSYCHIATRIC AND PSYCHOMETRIC EVALUATIONS WITHIN 30 DAYS.

BARNET, EMMANUEL MD, LICENSE NUMBER 2227, WAS DISCIPLINED BY ARIZONA ON MAY 19, 1999
DISCIPLINARY ACTION: SURRENDER OF LICENSE

NOTES: HIS SON OBTAINED A GUARDIANSHIP ORDER AND STATED THAT HE WOULD BE WILLING TO ENTER INTO A STIPULATED ORDER TO VOLUNTARILY SURRENDER HIS FATHER'S LICENSE WITH CAUSE.

BARNET, EMMANUEL MD, WAS DISCIPLINED BY ARIZONA ON JULY 30, 1999
DISCIPLINARY ACTION: LICENSE REVOCATION

NOTES: CANCELLATION OF LICENSE WITH CAUSE.

BARNETT, HARVEY A MD, LICENSE NUMBER 0015269, WAS DISCIPLINED BY ARIZONA ON MARCH 29, 1996
DISCIPLINARY ACTION: MONITORING OF PHYSICIAN PERFORMANCE

NOTES: WITHIN SIX MONTHS SHALL OBTAIN THE SERVICES OF AN OFFICE PRACTICE CONSULTANT WHO SHALL BE APPROVED BY THE BOARD.

BARRICKMAN, LES L DO, DATE OF BIRTH NOVEMBER 2, 1953, LICENSE NUMBER 0001988 OF 938 TALWRN COURT, IOWA CITY, IA, WAS DISCIPLINED BY IOWA ON JUNE 3, 1993
DISCIPLINARY ACTION: 48-MONTH PROBATION; FINE
OFFENSE: CRIMINAL CONVICTION OR PLEA OF GUILTY, NOLO CONTENDERE, OR NO CONTEST TO A CRIME

NOTES: ALLEGATIONS OF CRIMINAL CONVICTIONS RELATED TO ILLEGAL POSSESSION OF CONTROLLED DRUGS. $5,000 CIVIL PENALTY.

BARRICKMAN, LES L DO, DATE OF BIRTH NOVEMBER 2, 1953, LICENSE NUMBER 0099794, WAS DISCIPLINED BY NEW MEXICO ON FEBRUARY 12, 1994
DISCIPLINARY ACTION: PROBATION
OFFENSE: DISCIPLINARY ACTION BY ANOTHER STATE OR AGENCY

NOTES: ACTION IN ANOTHER STATE. ON 10/21/95 A PERMANENT LICENSE WITH FULL PRIVILEGES ISSUED.

BARRICKMAN, LES L DO, DATE OF BIRTH NOVEMBER 2, 1953, LICENSE NUMBER 0002676 OF 2316 CAMIO DE LOS ARTESANOS NW, ALBUQUERQUE, NM, WAS DISCIPLINED BY ARIZONA ON MAY 13, 1994
DISCIPLINARY ACTION: MONITORING OF PHYSICIAN PERFORMANCE
OFFENSE: DISCIPLINARY ACTION BY ANOTHER STATE OR AGENCY

NOTES: ACTION IN NEW MEXICO ON 2/12/94 BASED ON TWO GUILTY PLEAS TO POSSESSION OF A CONTROLLED SUBSTANCE ON 1/15/93 IN IOWA; ON 6/3/93 IOWA LICENSE PLACED ON PROBATION BASED ON THESE ACTIONS. AGREEMENT WITH ARIZONA: SHALL COMPLY WITH THE NEW MEXICO BOARD ORDER; SHALL MEET WITH THE BOARD UPON REQUEST; SHALL AUTHORIZE NEW MEXICO TO RELEASE TO THE BOARD UPON REQUEST A RECORD OF COMPLIANCE WITH THE TERMS AND CONDITIONS IN NEW MEXICO; IF HE CHOOSES TO PRACTICE IN ARIZONA BOARD RESERVES THE RIGHT TO REVIEW THE COMPLIANCE WITH THIS ORDER.

BARRICKMAN, LES L DO, DATE OF BIRTH NOVEMBER 2, 1953, LICENSE NUMBER 0025600 OF IOWA CITY, IA, WAS DISCIPLINED BY COLORADO ON MAY 20, 1994
DISCIPLINARY ACTION: SURRENDER OF LICENSE
OFFENSE: DISCIPLINARY ACTION BY ANOTHER STATE OR AGENCY

NOTES: BASED ON IOWA DISCIPLINE. NO UNPROFESSIONAL CONDUCT IDENTIFIED. PERMANENT LICENSE SURRENDER.

BARRICKMAN, LES L DO OF HI, WAS DISCIPLINED BY IOWA ON MAY 22, 1997
DISCIPLINARY ACTION: SURRENDER OF LICENSE
OFFENSE: DISCIPLINARY ACTION BY ANOTHER STATE OR AGENCY

NOTES: CHARGED WITH VIOLATING THE TERMS OF A PREVIOUS AGREEMENT WITH THE BOARD AS WELL AS IN CONNECTION WITH DISCIPLINE TAKEN BY ARIZONA.

BARRICKMAN, LES L DO, LICENSE NUMBER 782 OF 509 UNIVERSITY AVENUE, #104, HONOLULU, HI, WAS DISCIPLINED BY HAWAII ON DECEMBER 11, 1998
DISCIPLINARY ACTION: FINE
OFFENSE: DISCIPLINARY ACTION BY ANOTHER STATE OR AGENCY

NOTES: FAILED TO TIMELY INFORM THE HAWAII BOARD OF DISCIPLINARY ACTIONS AGAINST HIS LICENSE IN ARIZONA AND IOWA; ACTION ALSO TAKEN IN NEW MEXICO. $500 FINE

BARTON, LOUIS A MD, DATE OF BIRTH NOVEMBER 1, 1956, LICENSE NUMBER 0033024 OF 61022 SHORTER AVE #149, ROME, GA, WAS DISCIPLINED BY GEORGIA ON NOVEMBER 10, 1992
DISCIPLINARY ACTION: 4-MONTH LICENSE SUSPENSION; 60-MONTH PROBATION
OFFENSE: PROFESSIONAL MISCONDUCT

BARTON, LOUIS A MD, LICENSE NUMBER 0019125, WAS DISCIPLINED BY ARIZONA ON JULY 14, 1994
DISCIPLINARY ACTION: LICENSE REVOCATION
OFFENSE: DISCIPLINARY ACTION BY ANOTHER STATE OR AGENCY

NOTES: GEORGIA BOARD TOOK ACTION AGAINST HIM FOR ENGAGING IN INAPPROPRIATE SEXUAL CONTACT WITH TWO PATIENTS, INCLUDING SEXUAL INTERCOURSE WITH ONE PATIENT DURING A TIME WHEN HE HAD ESTABLISHED A PSYCHIATRIST/PATIENT RELATIONSHIP WITH THEM.

BARTON, LOUIS ANTHONY MD, LICENSE NUMBER 0051293 OF ROME, GA, WAS DISCIPLINED BY OHIO ON MARCH 9, 1995
DISCIPLINARY ACTION: LICENSE SUSPENSION; PROBATION
OFFENSE: DISCIPLINARY ACTION BY ANOTHER STATE OR AGENCY

NOTES: ACTION BY GEORGIA BOARD FOR ENGAGING IN INAPPROPRIATE SEXUAL CONTACT WITH TWO PATIENTS WHO WERE UNDER HIS PSYCHIATRIC CARE AND TREATMENT, INCLUDING SEXUAL INTERCOURSE WITH ONE PATIENT. HE HAD SUBSEQUENT TREATMENT AND AFTERCARE; REVOCATION STAYED; INDEFINITE SUSPENSION MINIMUM ONE YEAR; CONDITIONS FOR REINSTATEMENT. AGREEMENT TO REMAIN IN EFFECT FOR A MINIMUM OF TWO YEARS SUBSEQUENT TO REINSTATEMENT PRIOR TO ANY REQUEST FOR RELEASE FROM PROBATION.

BATES, MARVIN L MD, LICENSE NUMBER 0013114, WAS DISCIPLINED BY ARIZONA ON OCTOBER 21, 1994
DISCIPLINARY ACTION: LICENSE SUSPENSION
OFFENSE: NONCOMPLIANCE WITH A PROFESSIONAL RULE

NOTES: FAILED THE SPECIAL PURPOSE EXAMINATION TWICE. CONDITIONS OF LICENSE ON INACTIVE LICENSE STATUS INCLUDE: HE SHALL NOT ENGAGE IN THE PRACTICE OF MEDICINE IN ARIZONA OR ANY OTHER STATE OR A FOREIGN COUNTRY OR CONTINUE TO HOLD OR MAINTAIN A DRUG ENFORCEMENT ADMINISTRATION CONTROLLED SUBSTANCES REGISTRATION CERTIFICATE; WILL DEVOTE HIS VERY BEST EFFORTS TO ARRANGING FOR SOMEONE TO COVER HIS PRACTICE WHILE HIS LICENSE IS

INACTIVE; HIS LICENSE SHALL REMAIN INACTIVE UNTIL HE PASSES THE SPEX EXAM AND MEETS WITH THE BOARD AT THE NEXT REGULARLY SCHEDULED MEETING.

BATES, MARVIN L MD, LICENSE NUMBER 0013114, WAS DISCIPLINED BY ARIZONA ON JULY 22, 1995
DISCIPLINARY ACTION: 60-MONTH PROBATION; RESTRICTION PLACED ON LICENSE
OFFENSE: NONCOMPLIANCE WITH A PROFESSIONAL RULE

NOTES: INTERVIEWED BY THE BOARD ON 1/26/94 TO DISCUSS ALLEGATIONS OF EXCESSIVE PRESCRIBING OF CONTROLLED SUBSTANCES. PRIOR TO INTERVIEW, BOARD REVIEWED THE CHARTS OF 11 OF HIS PATIENTS, WHOM HE HAD SEEN BETWEEN 8/85 AND 6/92 WHICH REVEALED FREQUENT COMPLAINTS AND/OR PRESCRIPTION OF CONTROLLED SUBSTANCES FOR THESE COMPLAINTS WITHOUT RECORDED PHYSICAL EXAMINATIONS OR ELABORATION OF HISTORY. ON 1/26/94, BOARD ORDERED HIM TO TAKE AND PASS THE SPECIAL PURPOSE EXAMINATION WITHIN SIX MONTHS; FAILED THE EXAMINATION TWICE WITHIN THE DESIGNATED TIME PERIOD; RETOOK THE SPECIAL PURPOSE EXAMINATION IN 1995 AND PASSED WITH A SCORE OF 76. PROBATION WITH CONDITIONS: SHALL NOT PRACTICE MEDICINE IN A SOLO PRACTICE SETTING; SHALL NOT PRESCRIBE CONTROLLED SUBSTANCES; WITHIN SIX MONTHS, SHALL COMPLETE 40 HOURS OF CONTINUING MEDICAL EDUCATION, 30 HOURS IN PRESCRIBING CONTROLLED SUBSTANCES AND 10 HOURS IN MAINTAINING ADEQUATE MEDICAL RECORDS; BOARD SHALL CONDUCT A REVIEW OF 30 CHARTS IN HIS OFFICE AT THE END OF SIX MONTHS. ON 1/19/96 ORDER TERMINATED.

BATES, MARVIN LYLE MD OF 220 WEST GRANT, WILLIAMS, AZ, WAS DISCIPLINED BY DEA ON MARCH 20, 1995
DISCIPLINARY ACTION: SURRENDER OF CONTROLLED SUBSTANCE LICENSE
OFFENSE: DISCIPLINARY ACTION BY ANOTHER STATE OR AGENCY

NOTES: STATE BOARD.

BAUDER, MARC A MD, LICENSE NUMBER 15235, WAS DISCIPLINED BY ARIZONA ON JANUARY 22, 1998
DISCIPLINARY ACTION: RESTRICTION PLACED ON LICENSE; REQUIRED TO ENTER AN IMPAIRED PHYSICIAN PROGRAM OR SUBSTANCE ABUSE TREATMENT

NOTES: CONDITIONS ARE AS FOLLOWS: SHALL HAVE A FEMALE CHAPERONE PRESENT DURING ALL PHYSICAL EXAMINATIONS OF FEMALE PATIENTS WHEN THE PATIENT DISROBES, WHETHER IN HIS OFFICE OR AT ANY OTHER LOCATION; SHALL NOT TREAT OR OTHERWISE HAVE ANY PROFESSIONAL INVOLVEMENT WITH WOMEN, OR FAMILY MEMBERS OF WOMEN, WITH WHOM HE HAD SEXUAL CONTACT OR A SOCIAL RELATIONSHIP; SHALL RETAIN AN INDIVIDUAL THERAPIST IN THE AREA OF SEXUAL ADDICTION APPROVED BY BOARD STAFF AND SHALL REMAIN IN THERAPY UNTIL FURTHER ORDER OF THE BOARD WITH QUARTERLY REPORTS; IT WAS ALSO AGREED THAT HE ENTER INTO A NONDISCIPLINARY MONITORING AGREEMENT WHICH INCLUDED THE FOLLOWING CONDITIONS: MUST IMMEDIATELY PARTICIPATE IN A BOARD-APPROVED MONITORED AFTERCARE TREATMENT PROGRAM WHOSE THERAPIST MUST SUBMIT MONTHLY REPORTS; MUST PARTICIPATE IN 90 12-STEP MEETINGS FOR SUBSTANCE ABUSE WITHIN 90 DAYS; MUST THEN PARTICIPATE IN A 12-STEP RECOVERY PROGRAM AS DETERMINED BY HIS TREATING THERAPIST AND ATTEND AT LEAST THREE WEEKLY MEETINGS; SHALL OBTAIN A BOARD-APPROVED TREATING PHYSICIAN; SHALL ABSTAIN COMPLETELY FROM THE CONSUMPTION OF ALCOHOLIC BEVERAGES AND DRUGS EXCEPT WHEN PRESCRIBED BY HIS TREATING PHYSICIAN; SHALL NOT CONSUME FOOD OR SUBSTANCES CONTAINING POPPYSEEDS; MUST SUBMIT TO WITNESSED RANDOM BIOLOGICAL FLUID COLLECTION; MUST KEEP A LOG OF ANY AND ALL MEDICATIONS PRESCRIBED FOR HIM; SHALL SUBMIT TO ANY EXAMINATIONS OR THERAPY ORDERED BY BOARD; SHALL APPEAR BEFORE BOARD FOR INTERVIEWS UPON REQUEST; SHALL INFORM BOARD OF CHANGE OF ADDRESS OR IF AWAY FOR MORE THAN FIVE DAYS; ARIZONA, IN COMPLIANCE WITH THE AMERICANS WITH DISABILITIES ACT, PROCLAIMS THIS IS NOT A DISCIPLINARY ACTION BUT MERELY A MONITORING PROCEDURE WHICH HE VOLUNTARILY ENTERED INTO; SHALL IMMEDIATELY OBTAIN A TREATING PSYCHIATRIST APPROVED BY THE BOARD AND SHALL REMAIN IN TREATMENT WITH THE PSYCHIATRIST UNTIL FURTHER ORDER OF THE BOARD WITH QUARTERLY REPORTS.

BELENYESSY, LASZLO I MD, LICENSE NUMBER 0A32670 OF LOS ANGELES, CA, WAS DISCIPLINED BY CALIFORNIA ON AUGUST 30, 1993
DISCIPLINARY ACTION: SURRENDER OF LICENSE

NOTES: VOLUNTARY SURRENDER WHILE CHARGES PENDING.

BELENYESSY, LASZLO I MD, LICENSE NUMBER 0133807 OF 4002 NORTH 40TH STREET, PHOENIX, AZ, WAS DISCIPLINED BY NEW YORK ON AUGUST 21, 1995
DISCIPLINARY ACTION: LICENSE REVOCATION
OFFENSE: DISCIPLINARY ACTION BY ANOTHER STATE OR AGENCY

NOTES: ACTION IN CALIFORNIA FOR HIS NEGLIGENT TREATMENT OF TWO PATIENTS DURING THE PRACTICE OF GENERAL MEDICINE.

BENCE, LAWRENCE W MD, LICENSE NUMBER 0015956 OF FLORENCE, AZ, WAS DISCIPLINED BY ARIZONA ON APRIL 14, 1994
OFFENSE: SUBSTANDARD CARE, INCOMPETENCE OR NEGLIGENCE

NOTES: MANAGEMENT OF PATIENT IN OCTOBER 1991 TO WHOM HE PRESCRIBED COUMADIN ON A DAILY BASIS WITH NO CLEAR CUT PLANS TO OBTAIN DAILY PROTHROMBIN TIMES; PATIENT EXPIRED ON 10/21/91 OF AN INTERCEREBRAL HEMATOMA. CENSURED.

BENDING, GLENVILLE C DR, LICENSE NUMBER 0015819, WAS DISCIPLINED BY MINNESOTA ON SEPTEMBER 11, 1993

NOTES: STAYED SUSPENSION.

BENDING, GLENVILLE C MD, LICENSE NUMBER 0005453 OF TUCSON, AZ, WAS DISCIPLINED BY ARIZONA ON APRIL 14, 1994

NOTES: SHALL NOT PRACTICE IN ARIZONA PRIOR TO MEETING WITH THE BOARD.

BENDING, GLENVILLE CHARLES MD, LICENSE NUMBER MD07773 OF NEWPORT, OR, WAS DISCIPLINED BY OREGON ON JULY 9, 1992
DISCIPLINARY ACTION: RESTRICTION PLACED ON LICENSE

BENDING, GLENVILLE CHARLES MD, LICENSE NUMBER 0013279, WAS DISCIPLINED BY WASHINGTON ON MARCH 19, 1993
DISCIPLINARY ACTION: RESTRICTION PLACED ON LICENSE; MONITORING OF PHYSICIAN PERFORMANCE

OFFENSE: DISCIPLINARY ACTION BY ANOTHER STATE OR AGENCY

NOTES: ON 7/8/92 OREGON LICENSE LIMITED IN THAT HE WILL OBTAIN A SECOND OPINION FOR PATIENTS FOR WHOM HE RECOMMENDS CATARACT SURGERY. LICENSE LIMITED INDEFINITELY AND HE SHALL COMPLY WITH THE TERMS OF THE VOLUNTARY LIMITATION OF HIS MEDICAL PRACTICE INTO WHICH HE ENTERED WITH THE OREGON BOARD SO LONG AS THAT VOLUNTARY LIMITATION IS IN EFFECT; IF HE ESTABLISHES A PRACTICE IN WASHINGTON THE BOARD MAY MAKE ANNOUNCED VISITS TO INSPECT OFFICE AND/OR MEDICAL RECORDS; INTERVIEW OFFICE STAFF OR SUPERVISORS; AND REVIEW OTHER ASPECTS OF HIS PRACTICE; SHALL ASSUME ALL COSTS; SHALL INFORM THE BOARD IN WRITING OF CHANGES IN HIS PRACTICE AND RESIDENCE ADDRESS.

BERG, GARY L MD, DATE OF BIRTH AUGUST 6, 1945, LICENSE NUMBER 0025607 OF 11777 E BELLA VISTA, SCOTTSDALE, AZ, WAS DISCIPLINED BY IOWA ON JUNE 29, 1992
DISCIPLINARY ACTION: FINE
OFFENSE: PROFESSIONAL MISCONDUCT

NOTES: $250 CIVIL PENALTY AS SETTLEMENT TO CHARGES OF UNETHICAL CONDUCT.

BERG, GARY L MD, DATE OF BIRTH AUGUST 6, 1945, WAS DISCIPLINED BY ARIZONA ON OCTOBER 23, 1992
DISCIPLINARY ACTION: MONITORING OF PHYSICIAN PERFORMANCE

NOTES: LICENSE GRANTED WITH STIPULATION: SHALL OBTAIN A BOARD APPROVED MENTAL HEALTH THERAPIST, WHO SHALL SUBMIT QUARTERLY REPORTS TO BOARD. ON 1/27/94 BOARD DENIED HIS REQUEST TO TERMINATE ORDER.

BERG, GARY L MD, DATE OF BIRTH AUGUST 6, 1945, LICENSE NUMBER 0008646 OF NEWPORT, VT, WAS DISCIPLINED BY VERMONT ON DECEMBER 7, 1992

NOTES: CONDITIONED LICENSE. ORDER MODIFIED ON 1/11/94.

BERG, GARY L DR, LICENSE NUMBER 0036005, WAS DISCIPLINED BY MINNESOTA ON MARCH 11, 1995
DISCIPLINARY ACTION: RESTRICTION PLACED ON LICENSE

NOTES: ON 5/17/97 GRANTED UNCONDITIONAL LICENSE.

BERG, GARY L MD, DATE OF BIRTH AUGUST 6, 1945, LICENSE NUMBER 0027435 OF 11777 EAST BELLA VISTA, SCOTTSDALE, AZ, WAS DISCIPLINED BY WISCONSIN ON AUGUST 23, 1995
DISCIPLINARY ACTION: REPRIMAND
OFFENSE: DISCIPLINARY ACTION BY ANOTHER STATE OR AGENCY

NOTES: DISCIPLINARY ACTION IN IOWA ON 6/29/92. ON 8/05/91 WAS CONVICTED OF TWO COUNTS OF MISDEMEANOR ASSAULT FOR INCIDENTS WHICH OCCURRED WITH ANOTHER PHYSICIAN IN A HOSPITAL SETTING WHILE HE WAS ENGAGED IN DUTIES RELATED TO THE PRACTICE OF MEDICINE. SENTENCED BY THE COURT TO PAY FINES TOTALING $150 AND TO MAKE RESTITUTION TO THE VICTIM OF THE ASSAULT. PAID A $250.00 CIVIL FINE TO THE IOWA BOARD. ON 11/13/92 THE ARIZONA BOARD ISSUED HIM A LIMITED LICENSE WHICH REQUIRED HIM TO ENTER AND REMAIN IN THERAPY FOR AS LONG AS THE THERAPIST DEEMED IT NECESSARY. ON 12/07/92 THE VERMONT BOARD LIMITED HIS LICENSE AND REQUIRED HIM TO ENTER AND REMAIN IN THERAPY FOR AS LONG AS NECESSARY. $200 COSTS IN WISCONSIN.

BERGESON, PAUL S MD OF PHOENIX, AZ, WAS DISCIPLINED BY UTAH ON MAY 17, 1991
OFFENSE: DISCIPLINARY ACTION BY ANOTHER STATE OR AGENCY

NOTES: ABUSED ALCOHOL OR CONTROLLED SUBSTANCES IN ANOTHER JURISDICTION RESULTING IN SANCTIONS UPON HIS LICENSE IN THAT JURISDICTION. THE ORDER ENTERED INTO IN ARIZONA IS ADOPTED AS FULLY BINDING IN UTAH; IF HE WISHES TO PRACTICE IN UTAH, HE IS TO MEET WITH THE DIVISION TO DETERMINE IF ANY FURTHER CONDITIONS SHOULD APPLY TO HIS LICENSE. LICENSE REINSTATED WITH FULL PRIVILEGES EFFECTIVE 6/8/92.

BERMAN, ROBERT L MD, LICENSE NUMBER 0014040, WAS DISCIPLINED BY ARIZONA ON OCTOBER 18, 1996
OFFENSE: SUBSTANDARD CARE, INCOMPETENCE OR NEGLIGENCE

NOTES: NEGLIGENCE RESULTING IN HARM TO OR DEATH; IN 11/95, HE DID NOT APPROPRIATELY AND ADEQUATELY OXYGENATE THE PATIENT OR MANAGE THE AIRWAY IN A CRITICALLY ILL PATIENT AND THEN INAPPROPRIATELY ANESTHETIZED THE PATIENT UNDERGOING AN ARREST; ALSO IN 11/95, A PATIENT DIED IN PART AS A RESULT OF HIS POOR WATCHFULNESS; HIS DOCUMENTATION WAS SUBSTANDARD IN BOTH OF THESE CASES. CENSURED.

BERNHARD, JEROME J DO OF PHOENIX, AZ, WAS DISCIPLINED BY MISSOURI ON AUGUST 2, 1990
DISCIPLINARY ACTION: REPRIMAND
OFFENSE: DISCIPLINARY ACTION BY ANOTHER STATE OR AGENCY

BERTSCH, DALE R MD, DATE OF BIRTH MAY 17, 1931 OF PO BOX 3500, DLC#113443, FLORENCE, AZ, WAS DISCIPLINED BY MEDICARE ON OCTOBER 20, 1998
DISCIPLINARY ACTION: EXCLUSION FROM THE MEDICARE AND/OR MEDICAID PROGRAM
OFFENSE: DISCIPLINARY ACTION BY ANOTHER STATE OR AGENCY

NOTES: LICENSE REVOKED, SUSPENDED, SURRENDERED OR OTHERWISE LOST FOR REASONS BEARING ON PROFESSIONAL PERFORMANCE, PROFESSIONAL COMPETENCE OR FINANCIAL INTEGRITY.

BERTSCH, DALE ROGER DR, LICENSE NUMBER 0009406, WAS DISCIPLINED BY ARIZONA ON JULY 15, 1994
DISCIPLINARY ACTION: LICENSE SUSPENSION
OFFENSE: NONCOMPLIANCE WITH A PROFESSIONAL RULE

NOTES: FAILURE TO PAY RENEWAL FEE DURING PENDING INVESTIGATION.

BERTSCH, DALE ROGER MD, LICENSE NUMBER 0009406, WAS DISCIPLINED BY ARIZONA ON JANUARY 19, 1996
DISCIPLINARY ACTION: LICENSE REVOCATION
OFFENSE: CRIMINAL CONVICTION OR PLEA OF GUILTY, NOLO CONTENDERE, OR NO CONTEST TO A CRIME

NOTES: CONVICTED IN 8/94 OF ONE COUNT OF FIRST DEGREE MURDER; ON 5/24/95, SENTENCED TO LIFE IN PRISON, REQUIRING HIM TO SERVE AT LEAST 25 YEARS BEFORE BEING ELIGIBLE FOR PAROLE. PERMANENTLY REVOKED; FINAL BOARD DECISION WITH NO OPPORTUNITY FOR REHEARING OR REVIEW.

BERTSCH, DALE ROGER MD, LICENSE NUMBER G7956 OF PHOENIX, AZ, WAS DISCIPLINED BY CALIFORNIA ON JUNE 9, 1997
DISCIPLINARY ACTION: LICENSE REVOCATION
OFFENSE: DISCIPLINARY ACTION BY ANOTHER STATE OR AGENCY

NOTES: REVOKED BY ARIZONA FOLLOWING HIS CONVICTION

FOR MURDER. DEFAULT DECISION.

BEYER, E CAROLYN THOMAS D0, LICENSE NUMBER 0001480 OF 419 SOUTH JACKSON, CHESTERTON, IN, WAS DISCIPLINED BY ARIZONA ON JANUARY 10, 1996
DISCIPLINARY ACTION: 60-MONTH PROBATION; MONITORING OF PHYSICIAN PERFORMANCE
OFFENSE: DISCIPLINARY ACTION BY ANOTHER STATE OR AGENCY

NOTES: ON 4/29/93 INDIANA PLACED LICENSE ON INDEFINITE PROBATION. THIS ACTION WAS BASED ON THE FACT THAT SHE FAILED TO PRESCRIBE THE PROPER DOSAGE OF OXSORALEN-ULTRA BASED ON HER PATIENT'S WEIGHT; FAILED TO ADEQUATELY WARN HER PATIENT IN WRITING OF THE DANGERS OF OVEREXPOSURE TO UV RADIATION WHEN USING OXSORALEN-ULTRA; DID NOT UNDERSTAND HOW ULTRA-VIOLET RADIATION IS TO BE ADMINISTERED; SHOULD NOT HAVE SENT HER PATIENT TO A TANNING SALON TO RECEIVE UV RADIATION WITHOUT MEDICAL SUPERVISION. ARIZONA PROBATION UNDER TERMS AND CONDITIONS: SHALL COMPLY WITH THE INDIANA ORDERS; SHALL PROVIDE A COPY OF THIS ORDER TO ALL FACILITIES IN ARIZONA WHERE SHE IS CURRENTLY EMPLOYED AS A PHYSICIAN OR HAS PRIVILEGES TO ENGAGE IN THE PRACTICE OF MEDICINE; SHALL COMPLY WITH ANY CONDITION PLACED ON HOSPITAL PRIVILEGES; SHALL AUTHORIZE INDIANA TO RELEASE REPORTS; SHALL MEET WITH THE BOARD TO DISCUSS HER COMPLIANCE WHILE RESIDING OR PRACTICING IN ARIZONA.

BIDWELL, GEORGETTA MD, LICENSE NUMBER 0007104, WAS DISCIPLINED BY ARIZONA ON MARCH 19, 1996
DISCIPLINARY ACTION: REPRIMAND
OFFENSE: OVERPRESCRIBING OR MISPRESCRIBING DRUGS

NOTES: FAILED TO RECORD CONTROLLED SUBSTANCE PRESCRIPTIONS IN THE MEDICAL RECORDS OF TWO PATIENTS.

BIGELSEN, HARVEY MD, LICENSE NUMBER 0009667, WAS DISCIPLINED BY ARIZONA ON APRIL 14, 1994
DISCIPLINARY ACTION: LICENSE REVOCATION
OFFENSE: CRIMINAL CONVICTION OR PLEA OF GUILTY, NOLO CONTENDERE, OR NO CONTEST TO A CRIME

NOTES: ON 10/21/93 PLED GUILTY TO FILING FALSE, FICTITIOUS, OR FRAUDULENT CLAIMS, MAIL FRAUD AND CONSPIRACY TO OBSTRUCT JUSTICE. ONE OF THE CONDITIONS OF THE PLEA AGREEMENT IS THAT HE WILL RELINQUISH ALL MEDICAL AND HOMEOPATHIC LICENSES SO THAT HE WILL BE UNABLE TO PRACTICE HOMEOPATHIC OR ALLOPATHIC MEDICINE.

BIGELSEN, HARVEY MD OF SCOTTSDALE, AZ, WAS DISCIPLINED BY DEA ON APRIL 17, 1997
DISCIPLINARY ACTION: REVOCATION OF CONTROLLED SUBSTANCE LICENSE
OFFENSE: DISCIPLINARY ACTION BY ANOTHER STATE OR AGENCY

NOTES: ON 5/2/94 THE ARIZONA BOARD ENTERED INTO A CONSENT ORDER WHEREBY HIS LICENSE WAS CANCELED AS A RESULT OF A PLEA AGREEMENT HE ENTERED ON 10/21/93 ON CHARGES OF FILING FALSE, FICTITIOUS OR FRAUDULENT CLAIMS, MAIL FRAUD, AND CONSPIRING TO OBSTRUCT JUSTICE; PART OF THIS PLEA AGREEMENT IS THAT HE AGREED TO VOLUNTARILY RELINQUISH HIS LICENSES IN ARIZONA, NEW YORK AND NEW JERSEY.

BINDELGLAS, PAUL M MD, LICENSE NUMBER 0003579, WAS DISCIPLINED BY ARIZONA ON JANUARY 17, 1996
DISCIPLINARY ACTION: REQUIRED TO TAKE ADDITIONAL MEDICAL EDUCATION

NOTES: INTERVIEWED REGARDING INFORMATION RECEIVED BY THE BOARD QUESTIONING HIS CARE AND TREATMENT OF TWO PATIENTS AND THE RESULTS OF AN OFFICE RECORD REVIEW. WITHIN SIX MONTHS, SHALL SUCCESSFULLY COMPLETE AN 80-HOUR BOARD-APPROVED MINI-RESIDENCY IN PSYCHOTHERAPY WITH PSYCHOPHARMACOLOGY AND RECORD KEEPING COMPONENTS AND SUBMIT TO THE BOARD EVIDENCE OF HIS SUCCESSFUL COMPLETION. ON 4/16/96 BOARD APPROVED HIS LISTING OF SUBMITTED COURSES. ON 10/18/96 ORDER TERMINATED.

BINETTE, MARK MD OF MESA, AZ, WAS DISCIPLINED BY DEA ON SEPTEMBER 7, 1999
DISCIPLINARY ACTION: REQUIRED TO ENTER AN IMPAIRED PHYSICIAN PROGRAM OR SUBSTANCE ABUSE TREATMENT; MONITORING OF PHYSICIAN PERFORMANCE
OFFENSE: DISCIPLINARY ACTION BY ANOTHER STATE OR AGENCY

NOTES: PREVIOUS DEA REGISTRATION EXPIRED ON 1/31/95; STARTED SMOKING MARIJUANA IN COLLEGE IN THE 1970S AND OCCASIONALLY USED IT BETWEEN 1977 AND 1992 BUT DID NOT BELIEVE HE HAD AN ADDICTION PROBLEM; IN 1992 BEGAN TO USE METHAMPHETAMINE TO KEEP HIMSELF AWAKE WHEN WORKING EXTRA JOBS DURING HIS RESIDENCY; BEGAN OBTAINING STREET METHAMPHETAMINE AND SMOKED IT SEVERAL TIMES A DAY; ON 4/1/0/93 CHARGED WITH POSSESSION OF A CONTROLLED SUBSTANCE AND RELEASED ON HIS OWN RECOGNIZANCE; BETWEEN 8/93 AND 1/94 THIS RELEASE WAS REVERSED; STARTED TREATMENT BUT DID NOT FINISH BECAUSE HE COULD NOT AFFORD IT; ON 5/13/94 THE ARIZONA BOARD PROHIBITED HIM FROM USING CONTROLLED SUBSTANCES AND SAID HE COULD NOT PRACTICE UNTIL HE FINISHED TREATMENT; A PERSON WHO RECEIVED A PACKAGE OF METHAMPHETAMINE WITH A STREET VALUE OF $2,800 STREET VALUE CLAIMED DR. BINETTE HAD SENT IT ; CLAIMED HE MAILED TWO PACKAGES IN 4/94 AND 5/94; ON 10/31/94 PLED GUILTY TO ONE FELONY COUNT OF USING A COMMUNICATION FACILITY TO FACILITATE THE DISTRIBUTION OF A CONTROLLED SUBSTANCE AND ONE MISDEMEANOR COUNT OF SIMPLE POSSESSION OF A CONTROLLED SUBSTANCE; ARIZONA LICENSE PLACED ON INACTIVE STATUS ON 10/20/94; PARTICIPATED IN TREATMENT AND ARIZONA BOARD ON 2/13/96 ISSUED A REHABILITATION STIPULATION ORDER; ORDER MODIFIED ON 3/23/97 TERMINATING THE PROBATION BUT WITH MUCH THE SAME CONDITIONS; CLAIMED HIS LAST ILLEGAL DRUG USE WAS 6/94 AND HE IS PARTICIPATING IN TREATMENT AND MONITORING PROGRAMS. DEA REGISTRATION GRANTED WITH THE FOLLOWING CONDITIONS: MUST CONTINUE WITH MONITORED AFTERCARE PROGRAM; SHALL CONSENT TO PERIODIC INSPECTIONS BY DEA.

BINETTE, MARK J MD, LICENSE NUMBER 0020392, WAS DISCIPLINED BY ARIZONA ON SEPTEMBER 19, 1994
DISCIPLINARY ACTION: LICENSE SUSPENSION
OFFENSE: FAILURE TO COMPLY WITH PREVIOUS BOARD ORDER

NOTES: VIOLATED PREVIOUS BOARD ORDER BY USING METHAMPHETAMINES AND WAS INDICTED IN THE U.S. DISTRICT COURT ON CHARGES OF CONSPIRACY TO DISTRIBUTE A CONTROLLED SUBSTANCE; DISTRIBUTION AND POSSESSION WITH INTENT TO

DISTRIBUTE A CONTROLLED SUBSTANCE; AND USE OF A COMMUNICATION FACILITY TO FACILITATE SUCH DISTRIBUTION. REQUESTED THAT HIS ARIZONA MEDICAL LICENSE BE PLACED ON INACTIVE STATUS WITH CAUSE. CONDITIONS OF SUSPENSION INCLUDE: HE AGREES NOT TO PRACTICE MEDICINE IN ARIZONA OR ANY OTHER STATE WHILE ARIZONA LICENSE IS CLASSIFIED AS INACTIVE; MAY NOT HOLD REGISTRATION WITH THE DRUG ENFORCEMENT ADMINISTRATION OR WRITE PRESCRIPTIONS AS LONG AS LICENSE INACTIVE; SHALL NOT REQUEST REACTIVATION OF LICENSE TO PRACTICE MEDICINE UNTIL HE MEETS WITH THE BOARD AT A REGULARLY SCHEDULED MEETING AND COMPLIES WITH ANY REQUESTS OF THE BOARD.

BISCOE, MICHAEL MD, LICENSE NUMBER 0020915, WAS DISCIPLINED BY ARIZONA ON APRIL 6, 1995
DISCIPLINARY ACTION: MONITORING OF PHYSICIAN PERFORMANCE
OFFENSE: OVERPRESCRIBING OR MISPRESCRIBING DRUGS

NOTES: IMPROPER MONITORING OF METHOTREXATE IN A PATIENT; INAPPROPRIATE PRESCRIBING OF TESTOSTERONE; EXCESSIVE LABORATORY STUDIES. SHALL PROMPTLY OBTAIN A BOARD-APPROVED TREATING PSYCHOLOGIST OR PSYCHIATRIST TO SUBMIT QUARTERLY REPORTS TO THE BOARD REGARDING HIS DIAGNOSIS, PROGNOSIS AND RECOMMENDATION FOR HIS CONTINUING CARE AND TREATMENT. ON 1/24/97 ORDER TERMINATED. ON 7/30/99 ORDER AMENDED.

BISCOE, MICHAEL S MD OF 1818 EAST SOUTHERN, MESA, AZ, WAS DISCIPLINED BY DEA ON APRIL 16, 1996
DISCIPLINARY ACTION: SURRENDER OF CONTROLLED SUBSTANCE LICENSE
OFFENSE: DISCIPLINARY ACTION BY ANOTHER STATE OR AGENCY

NOTES: STATE BOARD.

BISKIND, JOHN I MD, LICENSE NUMBER 0012642, WAS DISCIPLINED BY ARIZONA ON JANUARY 18, 1996
OFFENSE: SUBSTANDARD CARE, INCOMPETENCE OR NEGLIGENCE

NOTES: ENGAGED IN CONDUCT THAT THE BOARD DETERMINES IS GROSS NEGLIGENCE, REPEATED NEGLIGENCE OR NEGLIGENCE RESULTING IN DEATH OF A PATIENT IN THAT IN 2/95 HE PERFORMED AN ABORTION ON A 26 YEAR OLD WOMAN WHO WAS 20.6 WEEKS PREGNANT, WHO DIED SHORTLY AFTER OF MASSIVE INTRA-ABDOMINAL HEMORRHAGE RESULTING FROM PERFORATION OF THE UTERUS DURING THE SURGERY; PATIENT SIGNED CONSENT FORM, ON WHICH WAS PRINTED BENEATH HER SIGNATURE THAT SHE WOULD STAY WITHIN 15 MINUTES FROM THE FACILITY AND SHE LEFT THE OPERATING ROOM IN GOOD CONDITION; HER BLOOD PRESSURE AND PULSE WERE TAKEN AT 11:05 AND 11:20 AND SHE WAS NOTED TO BE ALERT AND ORIENTED; SHE WAS DISCHARGED AT 11:30 AM; WHEN SHE EXPERIENCED DIFFICULTY BREATHING, EMERGENCY MEDICAL SERVICE PERSONNEL WERE CALLED AND SHE WAS TRANSPORTED TO A HOSPITAL WHERE SHE WAS PRONOUNCED DEAD AT 4:55 PM; THE NEXT DAY AUTOPSY REPORT INDICATED THE PRESENCE OF APPROXIMATELY 2000 CC'S OF BLOOD IN THE ABDOMEN AND AN 8 CENTIMETER LACERATION OF THE UTERUS. CENSURED.

BISKIND, JOHN I MD, WAS DISCIPLINED BY ARIZONA ON JULY 20, 1998
DISCIPLINARY ACTION: EMERGENCY SUSPENSION
OFFENSE: PROFESSIONAL MISCONDUCT

BISKIND, JOHN ISRAEL MD, LICENSE NUMBER 19703 OF CLEVELAND, OH, WAS DISCIPLINED BY OHIO ON SEPTEMBER 8, 1998
DISCIPLINARY ACTION: LICENSE REVOCATION
OFFENSE: DISCIPLINARY ACTION BY ANOTHER STATE OR AGENCY

NOTES: ACTION BASED ON REVOCATION BY ARIZONA'S MEDICAL BOARD FOLLOWING ITS CONCLUSION THAT HE ENGAGED IN UNPROFESSIONAL CONDUCT. PERMANENT REVOCATION AUTHORIZED BY DOCTOR IN LIEU OF FORMAL DISCIPLINARY PROCEEDINGS.

BISLA, RANJIT S MD, WAS DISCIPLINED BY ARIZONA ON JANUARY 21, 1992

NOTES: PETITION FOR REINSTATEMENT OF PRIVILEGES FOR BACK AND NECK SURGERY DENIED. ORDERED TO EITHER TAKE AND PASS THE SPEX EXAM OR PART I OF THE ORTHOPAEDIC BOARD'S WRITTEN EXAM BY 8/1/92.

BISLA, RANJIT S MD, DATE OF BIRTH JUNE 18, 1944 OF 1415 N 7TH, PHOENIX, AZ, WAS DISCIPLINED BY MEDICARE ON DECEMBER 4, 1994
DISCIPLINARY ACTION: EXCLUSION FROM THE MEDICARE AND/OR MEDICAID PROGRAM
OFFENSE: DISCIPLINARY ACTION BY ANOTHER STATE OR AGENCY

NOTES: LICENSE SURRENDERED FOR REASONS BEARING ON PROFESSIONAL COMPETENCE.

BISLA, RANJIT SINGH MD, LICENSE NUMBER 0122015 OF 3002 EAST PALO VERDE DRIVE, PHOENIX, AZ, WAS DISCIPLINED BY NEW YORK ON MARCH 21, 1994
DISCIPLINARY ACTION: SURRENDER OF LICENSE
OFFENSE: DISCIPLINARY ACTION BY ANOTHER STATE OR AGENCY

NOTES: DISCIPLINARY ACTION TAKEN BY THE ARIZONA BOARD

BLANKSTEIN, EDWARD MD, LICENSE NUMBER 10529, WAS DISCIPLINED BY ARIZONA ON JULY 28, 1999
DISCIPLINARY ACTION: 36-MONTH PROBATION; REQUIRED TO TAKE ADDITIONAL MEDICAL EDUCATION
OFFENSE: NONCOMPLIANCE WITH A PROFESSIONAL RULE

NOTES: PROBATION WITH THE FOLLOWING TERMS: THAT HE OBTAIN A PRACTICE MANAGEMENT CONSULTANT WITHIN SIX MONTHS, AT HIS OWN EXPENSE, FOR RECORD KEEPING, BILLING PRACTICES AND CODING, THAT HE OBTAIN 20 HOURS OF BOARD APPROVED CONTINUING MEDICAL EDUCATION IN CHILD AND ADULT PSYCHIATRY, IN ADDITION TO THE 20 HOURS REQUIRED FOR LICENSE RENEWAL, AND THAT STAFF PERFORM RANDOM YEARLY CHART REVIEWS FOR THE NEXT THREE YEARS.

BLASS, GARY S MD, WAS DISCIPLINED BY ARIZONA ON JANUARY 25, 1994
DISCIPLINARY ACTION: 60-MONTH PROBATION; REQUIRED TO ENTER AN IMPAIRED PHYSICIAN PROGRAM OR SUBSTANCE ABUSE TREATMENT
OFFENSE: SUBSTANCE ABUSE

NOTES: IN 1981 PLED GUILTY IN U.S. DISTRICT COURT IN MARYLAND OF POSSESSION OF A SCHEDULE III NON-NARCOTIC CONTROLLED SUBSTANCE; PLACED ON PROBATION AND ENTERED DRUG REHABILITATION WHICH HE COMPLETED IN 3/83; GRADUATED MEDICAL SCHOOL IN 3/89; ENTERED PENNSYLVANIA'S IMPAIRED PHYSICIAN PROGRAM; HAD A RELAPSE IN 1990 AND WAS TERMINATED FROM HIS RESIDENCY; CONTINUED OUTPATIENT TREATMENT IN PENNSYLVANIA

THROUGH 1/93 AND HAS BEEN MONITORED BY NEW JERSEY BOARD THROUGH THE PRESENT. CONDITIONS OF PROBATION: MUST IMMEDIATELY PARTICIPATE IN A BOARD-APPROVED MONITORED AFTERCARE TREATMENT PROGRAM WHOSE THERAPIST MUST SUBMIT QUARTERLY REPORTS; MUST PARTICIPATE IN A 12-STEP RECOVERY PROGRAM AS DETERMINED BY HIS TREATING THERAPIST AND ATTEND AT LEAST THREE WEEKLY MEETINGS; SHALL OBTAIN A BOARD-APPROVED TREATING PHYSICIAN; SHALL ABSTAIN COMPLETELY FROM THE CONSUMPTION OF ALCOHOLIC BEVERAGES AND DRUGS EXCEPT WHEN PRESCRIBED BY HIS TREATING PHYSICIAN; MUST SUBMIT TO WITNESSED RANDOM BIOLOGICAL FLUID COLLECTION; KEEP A LOG OF ANY AND ALL MEDICATIONS PRESCRIBED FOR HIM; SHALL SUBMIT TO ANY EXAMINATIONS OR THERAPY ORDERED BY BOARD; SHALL APPEAR BEFORE BOARD FOR INTERVIEWS UPON REQUEST; SHALL INFORM BOARD OF CHANGE OF ADDRESS OF IF AWAY FOR MORE THAN FIVE DAYS. ON 1/25/97 THIS ORDER TERMINATED.

BLATTSTEIN, DEBORAH MD, LICENSE NUMBER 15649, WAS DISCIPLINED BY ARIZONA ON MAY 20, 1999

NOTES: INTERIM ORDER TO UNDERGO PHYSICAL, PSYCHIATRIC AND PSYCHOMETRIC EVALUATIONS BY EVALUATORS CHOSEN BY BOARD STAFF WITHIN 60 DAYS. ON 9/21/99 IT WAS ORDERED THAT SHE COMPLY WITH THIS ORDER WITHIN 30 DAYS, AND IF SHE DOES NOT COMPLY, THAT THE MATTER BE REFERRED TO A FORMAL HEARING.

BLATTSTEIN, DEBORAH MD, LICENSE NUMBER 15649, WAS DISCIPLINED BY ARIZONA ON JULY 28, 1999
DISCIPLINARY ACTION: PROBATION; RESTRICTION PLACED ON LICENSE
OFFENSE: SUBSTANDARD CARE, INCOMPETENCE OR NEGLIGENCE

NOTES: INAPPROPRIATE TREATMENT FOR A PATIENT'S SCAR. RESTRICTED FROM PRACTICING ANY COSMETIC LASER SURGERY, WITH THE EXCEPTION OF FACIAL RESURFACING; SHALL RETAIN, AT HER EXPENSE, THE SERVICES OF A BOARD APPROVED MEDICAL OFFICE PRACTICE CONSULTANT; CONSULTANT IS TO PROVIDE THE BOARD A WRITTEN REPORT ON APPROPRIATE BUSINESS AND PATIENT RECORDING PRACTICES AND PROCEDURES WITH THE RECOMMENDED PROVISIONS TO CURRENT PROCEDURES. ON 11/19/99 THE BOARD DENIED A MOTION FOR REHEARING.

BLEAK, EARL MD, LICENSE NUMBER 6019, WAS DISCIPLINED BY ARIZONA ON MARCH 24, 1999

NOTES: INTERIM STIPULATION THAT HE NOT PRACTICE MEDICINE IN ARIZONA.

BLUM, JACK MD, DATE OF BIRTH JANUARY 9, 1934, LICENSE NUMBER 0C28144 OF FAIR OAKS, CA, WAS DISCIPLINED BY CALIFORNIA ON JUNE 22, 1990
DISCIPLINARY ACTION: SURRENDER OF LICENSE

NOTES: VOLUNTARY SURRENDER ACCEPTED WHILE CHARGES PENDING.

BLUM, JACK MD, DATE OF BIRTH JANUARY 9, 1934, LICENSE NUMBER 0005293, WAS DISCIPLINED BY ARIZONA ON JANUARY 23, 1992
DISCIPLINARY ACTION: PROBATION
OFFENSE: DISCIPLINARY ACTION BY ANOTHER STATE OR AGENCY

NOTES: CALIFORNIA LICENSE SURRENDERED EFFECTIVE 6/22/90 IN CONJUNCTION WITH DISCIPLINARY PROCEEDINGS PENDING AGAINST HIM IN CALIFORNIA. ADMITTED THAT HE USED OR ADMINISTERED TO HIMSELF CONTROLLED SUBSTANCES AND DANGEROUS DRUGS WHICH CAUSED URINE SAMPLES TO TEST POSITIVE ON SIX TESTS DURING THE PERIOD FROM 4/18/88 THROUGH 6/22/89. DR. BLUM IS GUILTY OF UNPROFESSIONAL CONDUCT FOR USE OF CONTROLLED SUBSTANCES EXCEPT IF PRESCRIBED BY ANOTHER PHYSICIAN FOR USE DURING A PRESCRIBED COURSE OF TREATMENT. SHALL MEET WITH THE ARIZONA BOARD PRIOR TO PRACTICING MEDICINE IN ARIZONA AND SHALL BE SUBJECT TO ANY PSYCHIATRIC, PSYCHOMETRIC AND PHYSICAL EVALUATION OR COMPETENCY TESTS THAT THE BOARD MAY DEEM NECESSARY PRIOR TO PERMITTING HIM TO PRACTICE MEDICINE.

BLUM, JACK MD, DATE OF BIRTH JANUARY 9, 1934, LICENSE NUMBER 0003057 OF DALLAS, TX, WAS DISCIPLINED BY VERMONT ON OCTOBER 15, 1992
OFFENSE: DISCIPLINARY ACTION BY ANOTHER STATE OR AGENCY

NOTES: SURRENDERED LICENSE IN CALIFORNIA ON 3/29/90. DISCIPLINED FOR UNPROFESSIONAL CONDUCT, IN THAT HE ADMITTED HE USED OR ADMINISTERED TO HIMSELF CONTROLLED SUBSTANCES AND DANGEROUS DRUGS WHICH CAUSED URINE SAMPLES TO TEST POSITIVE BETWEEN 1/19/89 AND 6/22/89. IF HE SHOULD REAPPLY FOR LICENSURE IN CALIFORNIA, HIS APPLICATION SHALL BE TREATED AS AN ORIGINAL APPLICATION AND HE SHALL BE REQUIRED TO MEET ALL THE REQUIREMENTS OF A NEW APPLICANT. BEFORE PRACTICING IN VERMONT, WILL APPEAR BEFORE THE BOARD AND BE SUBJECT TO ANY COMPETENCY TESTS THEY DEEM NECESSARY.

BLUM, JACK MD, DATE OF BIRTH JANUARY 9, 1934, LICENSE NUMBER 00D2660 OF 10044 INWOOD ROAD, DALLAS, TX, WAS DISCIPLINED BY TEXAS ON JANUARY 29, 1993
DISCIPLINARY ACTION: 60-MONTH PROBATION; RESTRICTION PLACED ON CONTROLLED SUBSTANCE LICENSE
OFFENSE: DISCIPLINARY ACTION BY ANOTHER STATE OR AGENCY

NOTES: DISCIPLINED BY CALIFORNIA BOARD FOR SELF-ADMINISTRATION OF DANGEROUS OR CONTROLLED SUBSTANCES LEADING TO SURRENDER OF HIS LICENSE; MISSISSIPPI LICENSE ALSO SURRENDERED ALTHOUGH HE HAD NEVER PRACTICED THERE; DISCIPLINED BY ARIZONA BOARD ALTHOUGH HE NEVER PRACTICED THERE; SELF-ADMINISTERED DIAZEPAM, CODEINE, PHENERGAN, AND PROCARDIA; CURRENTLY PRACTICING IN GEORGIA. 5 YEAR SUSPENSION STAYED. CONDITIONS OF PROBATION: SHALL PARTICIPATE IN ACTIVITIES OF A PHYSICIAN HEALTH AND REHABILITATION COMMITTEE AND ATTEND WEEKLY MEETINGS WITH QUARTERLY REPORTS; SHALL PARTICIPATE IN AA'S 12 STEP PROGRAM NOT LESS THAN 2 TIMES A WEEK WITH QUARTERLY REPORTS; SHALL FURNISH THE BOARD WITH WRITTEN REPORTS ON HIS MEDICAL CONDITION AND COMPLIANCE WITH THIS ORDER WHEN REQUESTED; SHALL ABSTAIN FROM THE CONSUMPTION OF ALCOHOL/CONTROLLED SUBSTANCES IN ANY FORM; SHALL SUBMIT HIMSELF FOR APPROPRIATE EXAMS INCLUDING DRUG OR ALCOHOL SCREENS; SHALL NOT TREAT OR OTHERWISE SERVE AS THE PHYSICIAN, PRESCRIBE, DISPENSE OR ADMINISTER DRUGS THAT MAY BE SUBJECT TO ABUSE TO HIMSELF OR ANY MEMBER OF HIS FAMILY; SHALL NOT POSSESS, ADMINISTER,

DISPENSE OR PRESCRIBE SCHEDULE II OR IIN CONTROLLED SUBSTANCES OUTSIDE OF A HOSPITAL SETTING; SHALL MAINTAIN A SEPARATE LOG OF ALL PRESCRIPTIONS WRITTEN FOR CONTROLLED SUBSTANCES WHICH SHALL BE AVAILABLE FOR INSPECTION; SHALL OBTAIN THE SERVICES OF A PRIMARY CARE PHYSICIAN WHO SHALL RELEASE INFORMATION TO THE BOARD; BOARD WILL BE INFORMED IF ANY DRUG HAVING ADDICTION-FORMING OR ADDICTION-SUSTAINING LIABILITY IS PRESCRIBED; SHALL OBTAIN NO PRESCRIPTIONS FROM ANY OTHER PHYSICIAN UNLESS IT IS APPROVED IN WRITING WITHIN 24 HOURS; ANY PRESCRIPTIONS WRITTEN CAN BE FILLED ONLY AT BOARD-APPROVED PHARMACIES; SHALL BE EVALUATED BY A BOARD-APPROVED PSYCHIATRIST TO WHOM HE WILL PROVIDE A COPY OF THE ORDER; SHALL COOPERATE WITH THE BOARD IN VERIFYING COMPLIANCE; SHALL INFORM BOARD OF CHANGE OF ADDRESS WITHIN 10 DAYS; TIME SPENT OUT OF TEXAS OR GEORGIA DOES NOT COUNT TOWARD PROBATION; SHALL APPEAR BEFORE THE BOARD ONCE A YEAR; SHALL APPEAR BEFORE THE BOARD PRIOR TO PRACTICING IN TEXAS. SHALL NOT SEEK MODIFICATION UNTIL FEBRUARY 6, 1994.

BLUM, JACK MD, DATE OF BIRTH JANUARY 9, 1934, LICENSE NUMBER 0016004 OF 101 BOWENS MILL ROAD, DOUGLAS, GA, WAS DISCIPLINED BY GEORGIA ON JUNE 28, 1993
DISCIPLINARY ACTION: EMERGENCY SUSPENSION

NOTES: IMPAIRMENT.

BLUM, JACK MD, DATE OF BIRTH JANUARY 9, 1934, LICENSE NUMBER 0016004 OF 10044 INWOOD ROAD, DALLAS, TX, WAS DISCIPLINED BY GEORGIA ON OCTOBER 7, 1993
DISCIPLINARY ACTION: LICENSE SUSPENSION

NOTES: IMPAIRMENT; SHALL NOT ENGAGE IN OR RETURN TO PRACTICE OF MEDICINE IN GEORGIA UNTIL FURTHER ORDER OF THE BOARD.

BLUM, JACK MD, DATE OF BIRTH JANUARY 9, 1934, LICENSE NUMBER 00D2660 OF DALLAS, TX, WAS DISCIPLINED BY TEXAS ON OCTOBER 14, 1993
DISCIPLINARY ACTION: EMERGENCY SUSPENSION
OFFENSE: FAILURE TO COMPLY WITH PREVIOUS BOARD ORDER

NOTES: VIOLATED 1/29/93 ORDER IN THAT HE REFUSED TO SUPPLY A URINE SAMPLE IN 8/93 AND INGESTED CONTROLLED SUBSTANCES IN 9/93.

BLUM, JACK MD, DATE OF BIRTH JANUARY 9, 1934, LICENSE NUMBER 00D2660 OF DALLAS, TX, WAS DISCIPLINED BY TEXAS ON JUNE 22, 1994
DISCIPLINARY ACTION: PROBATION
OFFENSE: FAILURE TO COMPLY WITH PREVIOUS BOARD ORDER

NOTES: VIOLATED 1/29/93 TEXAS ORDER IN THAT HE REFUSED TO SUPPLY A URINE SAMPLE ON 8/26/93, INGESTED CONTROLLED SUBSTANCES THREE TIMES IN 9/93; SURRENDERED HIS DEA CONTROLLED SUBSTANCES REGISTRATION ON 11/22/93. SUSPENSION STAYED. CONDITIONS OF INDEFINITE PROBATION: SHALL NOT PRACTICE MEDICINE UNTIL HE HAS UNDERGONE A 72 HOUR INPATIENT EVALUATION FOR CHEMICAL DEPENDENCY, HAS OBTAINED A COMPLETE NEUROLOGIC EXAM FROM A BOARD APPROVED PSYCHIATRIST, CAN DEMONSTRATE COMPLIANCE WITH THIS PSYCHIATRIST'S RECOMMENDATIONS AND APPEARS BEFORE THE BOARD TO REQUEST PERMISSION TO PRACTICE. UPON AN ADEQUATE SHOWING BEFORE THE BOARD THAT HE IS ABLE TO SAFELY PRACTICE MEDICINE, HE SHALL BE ALLOWED TO RESUME THE PRACTICE OF MEDICINE UNDER VARIOUS TERMS AND CONDITIONS.

BLUM, JACK MD, DATE OF BIRTH JANUARY 9, 1934, LICENSE NUMBER 00D2660, WAS DISCIPLINED BY TEXAS ON JANUARY 5, 1995
DISCIPLINARY ACTION: 120-MONTH PROBATION; RESTRICTION PLACED ON CONTROLLED SUBSTANCE LICENSE
OFFENSE: FAILURE TO COMPLY WITH PREVIOUS BOARD ORDER

NOTES: SUSPENSION STAYED. CONDITIONS OF PROBATION: SHALL ABSTAIN FROM THE CONSUMPTION OR ALCOHOL OR CONTROLLED SUBSTANCES IN ANY FORM UNLESS PRESCRIBED BY ANOTHER PHYSICIAN FOR A LEGITIMATE AND THERAPEUTIC PURPOSE; SHALL SUBMIT HIMSELF FOR APPROPRIATE EXAMS INCLUDING DRUG OR ALCOHOL SCREENS; SHALL NOT TREAT OR OTHERWISE SERVE AS PHYSICIAN FOR HIMSELF OR ANY MEMBER OF HIS FAMILY AND SHALL NOT PRESCRIBE, DISPENSE OR ADMINISTER ANY DRUGS THAT MAY BE SUBJECT TO ABUSE TO HIMSELF OR ANY MEMBER OF HIS FAMILY; SHALL ONLY ORDER AND ADMINISTER CONTROLLED SUBSTANCES FOR PERSONS UNDERGOING INPATIENT PROCEDURES AND/OR TREATMENTS AT A HOSPITAL FOR PURPOSES OF INPATIENT CARE; SHALL SURRENDER ALL UNUSED TRIPLICATE PRESCRIPTION FORMS AND CONTROLLED SUBSTANCES IN HIS POSSESSION INCLUDING SAMPLES; SHALL BE MONITORED BY A BOARD-APPROVED PHYSICIAN WITH QUARTERLY REPORTS TO THE BOARD; SEPARATE FROM PATIENT RECORDS SHALL MAINTAIN A FILE OF EVERY PRESCRIPTION WRITTEN FOR DANGEROUS DRUGS WHICH SHALL BE AVAILABLE FOR REVIEW; SHALL NOT TELEPHONE ANY PRESCRIPTION TO A PHARMACY FOR DANGEROUS DRUGS THAT MAY BE HABIT-FORMING; SHALL PARTICIPATE IN THE ACTIVITIES OF A PHYSICIANS' HEALTH AND REHABILITATION COMMITTEE AND ABIDE BY TERMS OF AN AFTERCARE PROGRAM CONTRACT WITH QUARTERLY REPORTS; SHALL PARTICIPATE IN AA'S PROGRAMS NOT LESS THAN THREE TIMES A WEEK WITH QUARTERLY REPORTS TO THE BOARD; SHALL SUBMIT HIMSELF FOR EVALUATION AND TREATMENT TO A BOARD-APPROVED PSYCHIATRIST WITH QUARTERLY REPORTS; SHALL ATTEND AT LEAST 40 HOURS OF CONTINUING MEDICAL EDUCATION PER YEAR; SHALL APPEAR BEFORE THE BOARD TWICE A YEAR; SHALL GIVE A COPY OF THIS ORDER TO ANY HEALTH CARE ENTITY WHERE HE HAS PRIVILEGES; SHALL COOPERATE WITH THE BOARD IN VERIFYING COMPLIANCE; SHALL INFORM BOARD OF CHANGE OF ADDRESS WITHIN 10 DAYS OR IF HE LEAVES THE STATE; TIME SPENT OUT OF TEXAS DOES NOT COUNT TOWARD PROBATION. SHALL NOT SEEK MODIFICATION FOR ONE YEAR.

BLUM, JACK MD, DATE OF BIRTH JANUARY 9, 1934, LICENSE NUMBER 00D2660, WAS DISCIPLINED BY TEXAS ON JUNE 28, 1995
DISCIPLINARY ACTION: LICENSE REVOCATION
OFFENSE: FAILURE TO COMPLY WITH PREVIOUS BOARD ORDER

NOTES: BETWEEN 10/6/94 AND 1/5/95 DIAGNOSED, TREATED, AND PRESCRIBED TO PATIENTS IN VIOLATION OF ORDER; NONCOMPLIANCE TO 1/05/95 ORDER IN THAT HE FAILED TO CAUSE HIS TREATING PHYSICIAN TO REPORT THE INGESTION OF FIORCET AND DIRECTED A MEDICAL ASSISTANT OF HIS MONITORING PHYSICIAN TO PREPARE PRESCRIPTIONS OF CHLORAL HYDRATE AND DIAZEPAM IN HIS WIFE'S NAME WHICH HE TRIED TO FILL, NEITHER OF WHICH WERE AUTHORIZED OR DIRECTED BY HIS MONITORING PHYSICIAN. ON 1/29/99 PETITION TO

REINSTATE LICENSE DENIED.

BLUM, JACK MD, DATE OF BIRTH JANUARY 9, 1934, LICENSE NUMBER 0003057 OF DALLAS, TX, WAS DISCIPLINED BY VERMONT ON NOVEMBER 3, 1995
DISCIPLINARY ACTION: LICENSE REVOCATION
OFFENSE: DISCIPLINARY ACTION BY ANOTHER STATE OR AGENCY

NOTES: TEXAS BOARD TOOK DISCIPLINARY ACTION AGAINST HIS MEDICAL LICENSE; ON HIS 1994-1996 LICENSE RENEWAL APPLICATION HE FALSELY ANSWERED "NO" TO A QUESTION REGARDING DISCIPLINARY ACTION TAKEN BY ANOTHER STATE WHEN HE HAD ACTIONS TAKEN BY SEVERAL STATES BETWEEN 1990 AND 1993; ALSO ANSWERED "NO" TO A QUESTION REGARDING REDUCTION, SUSPENSION OR REVOCATION OF STAFF PRIVILEGES, EMPLOYMENT OR APPOINTMENT IN A HOSPITAL OR OTHER HEALTH CARE INSTITUTION WHEN HE HAD RESIGNED FROM A HOSPITAL IN GEORGIA IN 4/93.

BLUM, JACK MD, DATE OF BIRTH JANUARY 9, 1934, LICENSE NUMBER 0005293, WAS DISCIPLINED BY ARIZONA ON JANUARY 19, 1996
DISCIPLINARY ACTION: LICENSE REVOCATION
OFFENSE: DISCIPLINARY ACTION BY ANOTHER STATE OR AGENCY

NOTES: VIOLATED TERMS OF TEXAS PROBATION OF 1/93 IN THAT HE REFUSED TO SUPPLY A URINE SAMPLE AT THE REQUEST OF A COMPLIANCE OFFICER IN 8/93; IN 9/93, INGESTED CHLORAL HYDRATE, CODEINE, AND XANAX WITHOUT A PRESCRIPTION FROM HIS PRIMARY PHYSICIAN AS REQUIRED BY PROBATION TERMS; SURRENDERED HIS DEA CONTROLLED SUBSTANCES REGISTRATION ON 11/22/93; PLACED ON 10 YEAR PROBATION IN TEXAS IN 1/95 BASED ON NONCOMPLIANCE. IN 1993,1994 AND 1995 APPLICATIONS FOR LICENSE RENEWAL IN ARIZONA, HE DENIED ANY DISCIPLINARY ACTION TAKEN AGAINST HIS LICENSE DURING THE REGISTRATION PERIODS AND DENIED ANY DENIAL, RESTRICTION, SUSPENSION, OR LOSS/REVOCATION OF DEA OR PRESCRIPTION PERMIT, DESPITE ACTIONS BY ARIZONA, TEXAS AND SURRENDER OF HIS DEA REGISTRATION DURING THOSE PERIODS. PERMANENT REVOCATION; FINAL DECISION WITH NO OPPORTUNITY FOR REHEARING OR REVIEW.

BLUM, JACK MD, DATE OF BIRTH JANUARY 9, 1934, LICENSE NUMBER 18306, WAS DISCIPLINED BY COLORADO ON APRIL 10, 1997
DISCIPLINARY ACTION: SURRENDER OF LICENSE

NOTES: NO UNPROFESSIONAL CONDUCT IDENTIFIED.

BLUME, HORST G MD, DATE OF BIRTH MARCH 12, 1926, LICENSE NUMBER 0017208 OF SIOUX CITY, IA, WAS DISCIPLINED BY IOWA ON FEBRUARY 22, 1990
DISCIPLINARY ACTION: 60-MONTH PROBATION; 3-MONTH RESTRICTION PLACED ON CONTROLLED SUBSTANCE LICENSE

NOTES: MAY NOT PRESCRIBE ADMINISTER OR DISPENSE CONTROLLED SUBSTANCES EXCEPT IN HOSPITAL

BLUME, HORST G MD, WAS DISCIPLINED BY ARIZONA ON JUNE 21, 1991
OFFENSE: DISCIPLINARY ACTION BY ANOTHER STATE OR AGENCY

NOTES: PLACED ON PROBATION FOR 5 YEARS BY IOWA. BOARD ACCEPTED THE SIGNED STIPULATION AND ORDER SAYING THAT HE WILL NOT PRACTICE MEDICINE IN ARIZONA UNTIL HE HAS FIRST MET WITH THE BOARD.

BLUME, HORST G MD, WAS DISCIPLINED BY NEBRASKA ON NOVEMBER 21, 1991
DISCIPLINARY ACTION: PROBATION
OFFENSE: DISCIPLINARY ACTION BY ANOTHER STATE OR AGENCY

BLUME, HORST G MD OF SIOUX CITY, IA, WAS DISCIPLINED BY MISSOURI ON OCTOBER 1, 1992
DISCIPLINARY ACTION: 60-MONTH PROBATION
OFFENSE: DISCIPLINARY ACTION BY ANOTHER STATE OR AGENCY

NOTES: ALSO PRESCRIPTION VIOLATIONS.

BLUME, HORST GUNTHER MD, LICENSE NUMBER 00D1551 OF SIOUX CITY, IA, WAS DISCIPLINED BY TEXAS ON OCTOBER 26, 1990

NOTES: MUST COMPLY WITH IOWA RESTRICTIONS AND AUTHORIZE IOWA BOARD TO RELEASE INFORMATION AS TO STATUS AND PROBATIONARY COMPLIANCE; MUST RECEIVE APPROVAL FROM TEXAS BOARD PRIOR TO PRACTICING MEDICINE IN TEXAS.

BLUME, HORST GUNTHER MD, LICENSE NUMBER D1551 OF SIOUX CITY, IA, WAS DISCIPLINED BY TEXAS ON OCTOBER 24, 1998
DISCIPLINARY ACTION: FINE
OFFENSE: PROFESSIONAL MISCONDUCT

NOTES: IN 4/96 HE TESTIFIED AS AN EXPERT WITNESS IN A LAWSUIT IN ST. LOUIS, MISSOURI; IN A DEPOSITION HE TESTIFIED CONCERNING THE STATUS OF HIS TEXAS LICENSE; SINCE THE 1990 TEXAS ORDER HAD BEEN BASED UPON THE IOWA ORDER, HE BELIEVED THAT TERMINATION OF AN IOWA ORDER SIMILARLY SATISFIED THE TERM OF THE TEXAS ORDER; HE CONTENDS THAT HE DID NOT UNDERSTAND HIS TEXAS LICENSE TO BE IN A PROBATIONARY OR RESTRICTED STATUS, SINCE HE WAS NOT AND HAD NOT BEEN PRACTICING IN TEXAS; HE DENIES INTENTIONALLY OR KNOWINGLY TESTIFYING IN A FALSE OR MISLEADING MANNER; THE 1990 TEXAS ORDER REQUIRING HIM TO APPEAR BEFORE BOARD BEFORE PRACTICING REMAINS IN EFFECT TO DATE. $7,500 FINE.

BOBER, ARTHUR P MD, LICENSE NUMBER 0015442, WAS DISCIPLINED BY ARIZONA ON APRIL 15, 1994
DISCIPLINARY ACTION: LICENSE SUSPENSION; REQUIRED TO ENTER AN IMPAIRED PHYSICIAN PROGRAM OR SUBSTANCE ABUSE TREATMENT
OFFENSE: FAILURE TO COMPLY WITH PREVIOUS BOARD ORDER

NOTES: ENTERED INTO AGREEMENT WITH BOARD ON 12/21/93 THAT HE WOULD ABSTAIN FROM THE CONSUMPTION OF ALCOHOL AND IF THERE WAS A RELAPSE WOULD GO TO A RECOVERY CENTER. WAS ARRESTED ON 2/18/94 FOR "DOMESTIC VIOLENCE" RELATED TO DRINKING; AS OF THE DATE OF THE ORDER HE HAD NOT ENTERED A RECOVERY PROGRAM. SHALL IMMEDIATELY PROCEED TO TALBOTT RECOVERY CENTERS FOR EVALUATION AND TREATMENT FOR CHEMICAL DEPENDENCY.

BOBER, ARTHUR P MD, DATE OF BIRTH FEBRUARY 5, 1949, LICENSE NUMBER 1046534 OF 25545 TWEED, FRANKLIN, MI, WAS DISCIPLINED BY MICHIGAN ON MARCH 25, 1996
DISCIPLINARY ACTION: EMERGENCY SUSPENSION
OFFENSE: SUBSTANCE ABUSE

BOBER, ARTHUR P MD, DATE OF BIRTH FEBRUARY 5, 1949, LICENSE NUMBER 1046534 OF 25545 TWEED, FRANKLIN, MI, WAS DISCIPLINED BY MICHIGAN ON JULY 13, 1997

DISCIPLINARY ACTION: 6-MONTH LICENSE SUSPENSION
OFFENSE: SUBSTANCE ABUSE

NOTES: ON 9/27/99 REINSTATEMENT DENIED.

BODNAR, THOMAS MD, LICENSE NUMBER 0007036, WAS DISCIPLINED BY ARIZONA ON OCTOBER 11, 1990
DISCIPLINARY ACTION: RESTRICTION PLACED ON CONTROLLED SUBSTANCE LICENSE; REQUIRED TO TAKE ADDITIONAL MEDICAL EDUCATION

NOTES: SHALL ONLY ADMINISTER SCHEDULE II CONTROLLED SUBSTANCES FOR HOSPITAL INPATIENTS AND OUTPATIENT SURGERY CENTER PATIENTS. SHALL NOT OTHERWISE PRESCRIBE OR DISPENSE CONTROLLED SUBSTANCES TO PATIENTS. SHALL COMPLETE 40 HOURS OF CONTINUING MEDICAL EDUCATION IN PHARMACOLOGY AND PAIN CONTROL DURING 1991. HE COMPLETED ALL REQUIREMENTS OF HIS STIPULATION AND THIS ORDER WAS TERMINATED ON 1/21/93.

BODNAR, THOMAS MD, LICENSE NUMBER 0007036, WAS DISCIPLINED BY ARIZONA ON JULY 20, 1995
DISCIPLINARY ACTION: RESTRICTION PLACED ON LICENSE
OFFENSE: SUBSTANDARD CARE, INCOMPETENCE OR NEGLIGENCE

NOTES: INTERVIEWED BY BOARD RELATIVE TO ALLEGING NEGLIGENT SURGERY IN REVISION OF A TOTAL HIP ARTHROPLASTY. SHALL NO LONGER PERFORM REVISION HIP REPLACEMENT SURGERY. ON 10/19/95 HIS REQUEST THAT THE BOARD RECONSIDER THIS STIPULATION WAS DENIED.

BODNAR, THOMAS MD, WAS DISCIPLINED BY ARIZONA ON APRIL 19, 1996
DISCIPLINARY ACTION: REQUIRED TO TAKE ADDITIONAL MEDICAL EDUCATION
OFFENSE: SUBSTANDARD CARE, INCOMPETENCE OR NEGLIGENCE

NOTES: INTERVIEWED BY THE BOARD REGARDING MALPRACTICE CLAIM ALLEGING NEGLIGENT CARE OF A FINGER SURGERY. SHALL TAKE AND PASS THE NEXT ADMINISTRATION OF THE ORTHOPEDIC RECERTIFICATION EXAMINATION; SHALL PARTICIPATE IN A TWO-WEEK MINI-RESIDENCY IN ORTHOPEDICS TO BE COMPLETED IN SIX MONTHS. ON 10/15/96 ORDERED THAT IF HE IS INELIGIBLE OR UNABLE TO REGISTER FOR THE RECERTIFICATION EXAMINATION OF THE AMERICAN BOARD OF ORTHOPEDIC SURGERY IN 1997 HE SHALL TAKE AND PASS THE SPEX WITH A SCALED SCORE OF 75 OR GREATER PRIOR TO 2/28/97.

BODNAR, THOMAS MD, LICENSE NUMBER 7036, WAS DISCIPLINED BY ARIZONA ON JULY 25, 1997
DISCIPLINARY ACTION: REPRIMAND
OFFENSE: OVERPRESCRIBING OR MISPRESCRIBING DRUGS

NOTES: IN 12/95 A PHYSICIAN WHO SHARED OFFICE SPACE WITH DR. BODNAR, DISCOVERED THAT DR. BODNAR HAD INSTRUCTED OFFICE STAFF TO USE HIS ASSOCIATE'S NAME WHEN PHONING IN PRESCRIPTIONS TO A PHARMACY FOR A PATIENT WHO WAS A MEMBER OF DR. BODNAR'S FAMILY; THE ASSOCIATE DID NOT CONSENT TO THE USE OF HIS NAME ON THESE PRESCRIPTIONS; DR. BODNAR OVERPRESCRIBED BARBITURATES TO THIS PATIENT.

BODNAR, THOMAS MD OF PHOENIX, AZ, WAS DISCIPLINED BY IOWA ON OCTOBER 2, 1997
DISCIPLINARY ACTION: DENIAL OF NEW LICENSE
OFFENSE: DISCIPLINARY ACTION BY ANOTHER STATE OR AGENCY

NOTES: ACTION TAKEN BY ARIZONA. FAILED TO COMPLY WITH THE ARIZONA ORDER WHICH REQUIRED HIM TO COMPLETE A TWO WEEK MINI-RESIDENCY AND PASS THE SPEX EXAM.

BODNAR, THOMAS MD, LICENSE NUMBER 7036, WAS DISCIPLINED BY ARIZONA ON JANUARY 22, 1998
DISCIPLINARY ACTION: RESTRICTION PLACED ON LICENSE; MONITORING OF PHYSICIAN PERFORMANCE

NOTES: INTERIM ORDER. CONDITIONS OF THE ORDER INCLUDE: HE MUST TAKE AND PASS THE SPEX EXAM; HE MAY NOT PERFORM MAJOR SURGERY; HE MUST LIMIT HIS PRACTICE TO A GROUP SETTING (A MINIMUM OF ONE OTHER PHYSICIAN); THE CHARTS OF THE PATIENTS HE SEES IN A SOLO SETTING MUST BE REVIEWED BY THE OTHER PHYSICIANS IN THE DOCTOR'S PRACTICE AND THAT REVIEW MUST BE DOCUMENTED BY THE REVIEWER'S SIGNATURE IN THE CHART. ORDER TERMINATED ON 3/27/98.

BODNAR, THOMAS MD, WAS DISCIPLINED BY ARIZONA ON MARCH 27, 1998
DISCIPLINARY ACTION: REQUIRED TO TAKE ADDITIONAL MEDICAL EDUCATION

NOTES: HE SHALL SUCCESSFULLY COMPLETE 40 HOURS OF BOARD-APPROVED CONTINUING MEDICAL EDUCATION COURSES IN BOTH FRACTURE CARE AND MAJOR POINT REVISION AND REPLACEMENT WITHIN NINE MONTHS. AFTER COMPLETION OF THE COURSES, HE SHALL MEET WITH THE BOARD PRIOR TO RESUMING PRACTICE.

BODNAR, THOMAS MD, LICENSE NUMBER 7036, WAS DISCIPLINED BY ARIZONA ON NOVEMBER 17, 1999
DISCIPLINARY ACTION: REPRIMAND
OFFENSE: NONCOMPLIANCE WITH A PROFESSIONAL RULE

NOTES: FAILURE TO PROVIDE MATERIALS TO THE BOARD IN A TIMELY MANNER, WHEN LEGALLY REQUESTED.

BOLES, STEVEN C DO, LICENSE NUMBER 1869 OF 702 E BELL B119, PHOENIX, AZ, WAS DISCIPLINED BY ARIZONA ON JUNE 24, 1997
DISCIPLINARY ACTION: EMERGENCY SUSPENSION
OFFENSE: SUBSTANCE ABUSE

NOTES: IN 6/97 OBTAINED NARCOTIC AND PRESCRIPTION ONLY DRUGS BY FRAUD FOR PERSONAL USE; WAS USING THREE SEPARATE ALIASES AT FOUR SEPARATE LOCATIONS; CHARGED WITH FELONY COUNTS OF OBTAINING THESE DRUGS BY FRAUD; ADMITTED THAT HE WAS CONTINUING TO PRACTICE WHILE CONTEMPLATING ENTERING A SUBSTANCE ABUSE PROGRAM. SHALL SUBMIT HIMSELF FOR MENTAL, PHYSICAL AND/OR ORAL WRITTEN MEDICAL COMPETENCY EXAMINATIONS AS DESIGNATED BY THE BOARD.

BOLES, STEVEN C DO, LICENSE NUMBER 1869 OF 702 E BELL ROAD, B119, PHOENIX, AZ, WAS DISCIPLINED BY ARIZONA ON AUGUST 23, 1997
DISCIPLINARY ACTION: 60-MONTH PROBATION; RESTRICTION PLACED ON LICENSE
OFFENSE: SUBSTANCE ABUSE

NOTES: HAVING COMPLETED INPATIENT AND NOW CONTINUING OUTPATIENT TREATMENT FOR REHABILITATION OF HIS ADDICTION, HE REQUESTED THAT THE BOARD RELEASE HIS LICENSE FROM SUSPENSION AND ENTER INTO A STIPULATED CONSENT ORDER. TERMS AND CONDITIONS ARE AS FOLLOWS: SHALL IMMEDIATELY OBTAIN A TREATING PSYCHIATRIST APPROVED BY THE BOARD AND SHALL

REMAIN IN TREATMENT WITH THE PSYCHIATRIST UNTIL FURTHER ORDER OF THE BOARD WITH MONTHLY REPORTS FOR SIX MONTHS THEN QUARTERLY; SHALL PROVIDE A COPY OF THIS ORDER TO ANY HEALTH CARE ENTITY WHERE SHE HAS PRIVILEGES; SHALL ABSTAIN COMPLETELY FROM THE CONSUMPTION OF ALCOHOLIC BEVERAGES AND DRUGS EXCEPT WHEN PRESCRIBED BY HIS TREATING PHYSICIAN; MUST SUBMIT TO WITNESSED RANDOM BIOLOGICAL FLUID COLLECTION; MUST KEEP A LOG OF ANY AND ALL MEDICATIONS PRESCRIBED FOR HIM; SHALL SUBMIT TO ANY EVALUATIONS ORDERED BY BOARD; SHALL PARTICIPATE IN A MINIMUM OF THREE SELF-HELP MEETINGS PER WEEK THROUGH ORGANIZATIONS SUCH AS AA, NARCOTICS ANONYMOUS, AND DOCTOR'S CADUCEUS GROUPS; SHALL APPEAR BEFORE BOARD FOR INTERVIEWS UPON REQUEST; SHALL INFORM BOARD OF CHANGE OF ADDRESS OR IF HE LEAVES ARIZONA; SHALL NOT PRESCRIBE ANY CONTROLLED SUBSTANCES EXCEPT FOR THE FOLLOWING AND UNDER THESE CONDITIONS: SCHEDULE IV AND V, IN A DOSAGE AMOUNT FOR NOT MORE THAN SEVEN DAYS AND THE PRESCRIPTION MAY NOT BE RENEWED TELEPHONICALLY; SHALL LIMIT HIS WORK HOURS TO AN AVERAGE OF 40 PER WEEK. ON 11/19/97, ORDER AMENDED, DELETING RESTRICTION PRESCRIBING SCHEDULES IV AND V DRUGS.

BORJESON, ROBBI MD, LICENSE NUMBER 0024093, WAS DISCIPLINED BY ARIZONA ON APRIL 20, 1996
DISCIPLINARY ACTION: RESTRICTION PLACED ON LICENSE; MONITORING OF PHYSICIAN PERFORMANCE

NOTES: INTERVIEWED BY BOARD REGARDING APPLICATION FOR ARIZONA LICENSE. SHALL CONTINUE PSYCHOLOGICAL TREATMENT WITH A BOARD-APPROVED PSYCHOLOGIST WHO SHALL SUBMIT QUARTERLY REPORTS TO THE BOARD; SHALL PRACTICE MEDICINE ONLY IN A STRUCTURED SETTING; FOR SIX MONTHS, SHALL SUBMIT TO WITNESSED RANDOM BIOLOGICAL FLUID TESTING BY BOARD OR ITS DESIGNEES WITHIN TWO HOURS OF REQUEST.

BORJESON, ROBBI MD, LICENSE NUMBER 24093, WAS DISCIPLINED BY ARIZONA ON JULY 25, 1997
DISCIPLINARY ACTION: REPRIMAND
OFFENSE: FAILURE TO COMPLY WITH PREVIOUS BOARD ORDER

NOTES: ADMITTED THAT SHE HAD NOT BEEN IN COMPLIANCE WITH 5/24/96 ORDER THAT INCLUDED A REQUIREMENT THAT SHE WOULD CONTINUE PSYCHOLOGICAL TREATMENT WITH A BOARD-APPROVED PSYCHOLOGIST WITH QUARTERLY REPORTS; STATED HER WILLINGNESS TO IMMEDIATELY COMPLY AND SUBMITTED THE NAME OF A PSYCHOLOGIST FOR APPROVAL.

BORJESON, ROBBI LIN MD, DATE OF BIRTH MARCH 28, 1956 OF 3644 E. ROSEMONTE DRIVE, PHOENIX, AZ, WAS DISCIPLINED BY MEDICARE ON APRIL 20, 1999
DISCIPLINARY ACTION: EXCLUSION FROM THE MEDICARE AND/OR MEDICAID PROGRAM
OFFENSE: NONCOMPLIANCE WITH A PROFESSIONAL RULE

NOTES: DEFAULTED ON PUBLIC HEALTH SERVICE EDUCATION LOAN.

BOTNIK, EDWARD L MD, LICENSE NUMBER 0011688, WAS DISCIPLINED BY ARIZONA ON AUGUST 5, 1996
DISCIPLINARY ACTION: REPRIMAND
OFFENSE: PROFESSIONAL MISCONDUCT

NOTES: IN 10/92, BOARD RECEIVED AN EXCESSIVE PURCHASES REPORT FROM THE DRUG ENFORCEMENT ADMINISTRATION WHICH STATED THAT HE HAD ORDERED CONTROLLED SUBSTANCES TO BE SENT TO HIS HOME ADDRESS; AT THE TIME, HE WAS NOT REGISTERED WITH THE BOARD AS A DISPENSING PHYSICIAN; IN 1/93, ADMITTED TO THE BOARD THAT HE HAD ORDERED THE CONTROLLED SUBSTANCES FOR HIS OWN PERSONAL USE; IN 10/93, AGREED TO BE EVALUATED PSYCHIATRICALLY AND UNDERGO RANDOM URINE TESTING FOR APPROXIMATELY FOUR MONTHS; ON 1/19/94, A RANDOM BIOLOGICAL FLUID SPECIMEN OBTAINED FROM HIM TESTED POSITIVE FOR DARVON; FAILED TO RESPOND TO FOUR REQUESTS FOR RANDOM URINE DRUG SCREENS IN 3/94 AND 4/94.

BOTNIK, EDWARD L MD, LICENSE NUMBER C26065 OF SUN LAKES, AZ, WAS DISCIPLINED BY CALIFORNIA ON JANUARY 8, 1998
DISCIPLINARY ACTION: REPRIMAND
OFFENSE: DISCIPLINARY ACTION BY ANOTHER STATE OR AGENCY

NOTES: DISCIPLINED BY ARIZONA FOR ORDERING CONTROLLED SUBSTANCES THAT WERE SENT TO HIS HOME FOR HIS OWN USE.

BOTNIK, EDWARD L MD, LICENSE NUMBER 25280 OF SUN LAKES, AZ, WAS DISCIPLINED BY OHIO ON AUGUST 5, 1998
DISCIPLINARY ACTION: LICENSE SUSPENSION; PROBATION
OFFENSE: DISCIPLINARY ACTION BY ANOTHER STATE OR AGENCY

NOTES: ACTION BY ARIZONA'S MEDICAL BOARD WHICH DETERMINED THAT HE ORDERED BOTTLES OF FIVE SPECIFIED CONTROLLED SUBSTANCES FOR HIS OWN USE, HIS BIOLOGICAL FLUID SPECIMEN TESTED POSITIVE FOR DARVON NOT PRESCRIBED BY HIS TREATING PHYSICIAN, AND HE FAILED TO RESPOND TO REQUESTS FOR RANDOM DRUG SCREENS ON FOUR SPECIFIED DATES.

BOTTNER, MELVIN MD, WAS DISCIPLINED BY ARIZONA ON JANUARY 23, 1997
DISCIPLINARY ACTION: REQUIRED TO TAKE ADDITIONAL MEDICAL EDUCATION
OFFENSE: SUBSTANDARD CARE, INCOMPETENCE OR NEGLIGENCE

NOTES: ADMINISTERED ASPIRIN TO A PATIENT WITH A KNOWN ALLERGY TO ASPIRIN. MUST OBTAIN THE SERVICES OF AN OFFICE MANAGEMENT CONSULTANT AND COMPLETE 20 HOURS OF CONTINUING MEDICAL EDUCATION IN PHARMACOLOGY, SPECIFICALLY, MEDICATION PRESCRIBING AND MEDICINE ALLERGIES.

BOUCHER, VICTOR MD, WAS DISCIPLINED BY ARIZONA ON NOVEMBER 20, 1998
DISCIPLINARY ACTION: LICENSE SUSPENSION

NOTES: BOARD ACCEPTED HIS SIGNED REQUEST FOR AND ORDER GRANTING INACTIVE STATUS WITH CAUSE.

BRANDT, PAMELA MD OF 1501 N CAMPBELL AVENUE #7415, TUCSON, AZ, WAS DISCIPLINED BY DEA ON AUGUST 31, 1999
DISCIPLINARY ACTION: SURRENDER OF CONTROLLED SUBSTANCE LICENSE

NOTES: INAPPROPRIATE PRESCRIBING.

BRAVERMAN, ERIC R MD, DATE OF BIRTH DECEMBER 28, 1957, LICENSE NUMBER 0045071 OF 212 COMMONS WAY BLDG. #2, PRINCETON, NJ, WAS DISCIPLINED BY NEW JERSEY ON JULY 11, 1996
DISCIPLINARY ACTION: EMERGENCY SUSPENSION

OFFENSE: SUBSTANDARD CARE, INCOMPETENCE OR NEGLIGENCE

NOTES: BASED ON MALPRACTICE/NEGLIGENCE. DURING THE PERIOD OF 7/11/96 TO 7/18/96 SHALL SEE NO NEW PATIENTS; SHALL ARRANGE FOR THE TRANSFER OF CURRENT PATIENTS TO THE CARE OF OTHER PHYSICIANS; SHALL CEASE AND DESIST FROM ANY PRACTICE IN NEW JERSEY AS OF 7/18/96.

BRAVERMAN, ERIC R MD, DATE OF BIRTH DECEMBER 28, 1957, LICENSE NUMBER 042712E OF 212 COMMONS WAY, PRINCETON, NJ, WAS DISCIPLINED BY PENNSYLVANIA ON JULY 24, 1996
DISCIPLINARY ACTION: EMERGENCY SUSPENSION
OFFENSE: DISCIPLINARY ACTION BY ANOTHER STATE OR AGENCY

NOTES: ACTION IN NEW JERSEY. CLEAR AND IMMEDIATE DANGER TO PUBLIC HEALTH AND SAFETY. IMMEDIATE SUSPENSION UNTIL VACATED BY THE BOARD, BUT NO LONGER THAN 180 DAYS, PLUS ANY DAYS WAIVED.

BRAVERMAN, ERIC R MD, WAS DISCIPLINED BY ALABAMA ON AUGUST 28, 1996
DISCIPLINARY ACTION: EMERGENCY SUSPENSION
OFFENSE: DISCIPLINARY ACTION BY ANOTHER STATE OR AGENCY

NOTES: DISCIPLINARY ACTION TAKEN BY NEW JERSEY.

BRAVERMAN, ERIC R MD, LICENSE NUMBER 0159238 OF 212 COMMONS WAY BUILDING 2, PRINCETON, NJ, WAS DISCIPLINED BY NEW YORK ON DECEMBER 11, 1996
DISCIPLINARY ACTION: EMERGENCY SUSPENSION

BRAVERMAN, ERIC R MD, LICENSE NUMBER 16127 OF 777 CHERRY HILL ROAD, PRINCETON, NJ, WAS DISCIPLINED BY ARIZONA ON FEBRUARY 3, 1997

NOTES: SHALL NOT PRACTICE MEDICINE UNTIL HE MEETS WITH THE BOARD AND RECEIVES ITS AFFIRMATIVE APPROVAL TO DO SO. INTERIM ORDER. ON 7/28/99, THIS STIPULATION WAS TERMINATED AS HE WAS IN COMPLIANCE WITH THE 5/97 NEW JERSEY CONSENT ORDER.

BRAVERMAN, ERIC R MD, DATE OF BIRTH DECEMBER 28, 1957, LICENSE NUMBER 45071 OF 664 ROUTE 518, SKILLMAN, NJ, WAS DISCIPLINED BY NEW JERSEY ON MAY 28, 1997
DISCIPLINARY ACTION: REPRIMAND; REQUIRED TO TAKE ADDITIONAL MEDICAL EDUCATION
OFFENSE: PRACTICING WITHOUT A VALID LICENSE

NOTES: INADEQUATE RECORD KEEPING, INCOMPLETE EXAMINATION OF ONE PATIENT, AND PRACTICING WHILE UNDER TEMPORARY SUSPENSION. MUST TAKE COURSE IN CONTROLLED DANGEROUS SUBSTANCES AND AN ETHICS COURSE; AGREES TO CHART REVIEW FOR ONE YEAR BEGINNING THE DAY HE OPENS OR BECOMES EMPLOYED BY A MEDICAL PRACTICE IN NEW JERSEY; CHART REVIEW TO BE PERFORMED BY A BOARD APPROVED PHYSICIAN WITH MONTHLY REPORTS; ASSESSED COSTS OF $20,000. LICENSE REINSTATED PROVIDED HE WILL NOT RESUME PRACTICE IN NEW JERSEY UNTIL HE HAS NOTIFIED THE BOARD IN WRITING.

BRAVERMAN, ERIC R MD, DATE OF BIRTH DECEMBER 28, 1957, LICENSE NUMBER 042712E OF 142 BELLEVUE AVENUE, PENNDEL, PA, WAS DISCIPLINED BY PENNSYLVANIA ON MARCH 24, 1998
DISCIPLINARY ACTION: REPRIMAND; REQUIRED TO TAKE ADDITIONAL MEDICAL EDUCATION
OFFENSE: DISCIPLINARY ACTION BY ANOTHER STATE OR AGENCY

NOTES: DISCIPLINARY ACTION TAKEN BY NEW JERSEY. REQUIRED TO SUBMIT PROOF OF COMPLETION OF THE 2 CONTINUING MEDICAL EDUCATION COURSES REQUIRED BY NEW JERSEY AND COPIES OF ALL REPORTS SUBMITTED TO NEW JERSEY.

BRAVERMAN, ERIC RANDALL MD, LICENSE NUMBER 14896, WAS DISCIPLINED BY ALABAMA ON NOVEMBER 26, 1997

NOTES: UNSPECIFIED CONSENT ORDER.

BRAZIE, ROBERT WILLARD MD, LICENSE NUMBER 0003293, WAS DISCIPLINED BY ARIZONA ON OCTOBER 15, 1993
DISCIPLINARY ACTION: 12-MONTH RESTRICTION PLACED ON CONTROLLED SUBSTANCE LICENSE; REQUIRED TO ENTER AN IMPAIRED PHYSICIAN PROGRAM OR SUBSTANCE ABUSE TREATMENT
OFFENSE: SUBSTANCE ABUSE

NOTES: CHEMICAL SUBSTANCE MISUSE RELAPSE. SHALL SURRENDER HIS SCHEDULE II PROVIDER CERTIFICATE (DEA REGISTRATION) FOR ONE YEAR; SHALL NOT RECEIVE, STORE OR DISPENSE SAMPLES OF CONTROLLED SUBSTANCES IN ANY PRACTICE LOCATION; MUST IMMEDIATELY PARTICIPATE IN A BOARD-APPROVED MONITORED AFTERCARE TREATMENT PROGRAM WHOSE THERAPIST MUST SUBMIT QUARTERLY REPORTS; MUST PARTICIPATE IN 90 12-STEP MEETINGS FOR SUBSTANCE ABUSE WITHIN 90 DAYS; MUST THEN PARTICIPATE IN A 12-STEP RECOVERY PROGRAM AS DETERMINED BY HIS TREATING THERAPIST AND ATTEND AT LEAST THREE WEEKLY MEETINGS; SHALL OBTAIN A BOARD-APPROVED TREATING PHYSICIAN; SHALL ABSTAIN COMPLETELY FROM THE CONSUMPTION OF ALCOHOLIC BEVERAGES AND DRUGS EXCEPT WHEN PRESCRIBED BY HIS TREATING PHYSICIAN; MUST SUBMIT TO WITNESSED RANDOM BIOLOGICAL FLUID COLLECTION; KEEP A LOG OF ANY AND ALL MEDICATION PRESCRIBED FOR HIM; SHALL SUBMIT TO ANY EXAMINATIONS OR THERAPY ORDERED BY BOARD; SHALL APPEAR BEFORE BOARD FOR INTERVIEWS UPON REQUEST; SHALL INFORM BOARD OF CHANGE OF ADDRESS OR IF AWAY FOR MORE THAN FIVE DAYS. ON 5/15/98 ORDER TERMINATED.

BRECHNER, ROSS J MD, WAS DISCIPLINED BY ARIZONA ON JULY 30, 1999
DISCIPLINARY ACTION: RESTRICTION PLACED ON LICENSE

NOTES: GRANTED LICENSE AND MAY NOT PRACTICE OPHTHALMOLOGIC SURGERY.

BRENNAN, MICHAEL JAMES MD, LICENSE NUMBER 0014591, WAS DISCIPLINED BY ARIZONA ON APRIL 10, 1992
DISCIPLINARY ACTION: REQUIRED TO TAKE ADDITIONAL MEDICAL EDUCATION; MONITORING OF PHYSICIAN PERFORMANCE
OFFENSE: SUBSTANDARD CARE, INCOMPETENCE OR NEGLIGENCE

NOTES: VOLUNTARILY SURRENDERED HIS CLINICAL PRIVILEGES AT SCOTTSDALE MEMORIAL HOSPITAL WHILE UNDER INVESTIGATION TO DETERMINE IF HIS PATIENT MANAGEMENT MET ACCEPTED STANDARDS OF CARE. SHALL OBTAIN A MANAGEMENT AND EDUCATIONAL CONSULTANT ACCEPTABLE TO THE BOARD TO REVIEW ALL DOCUMENTATION AND RECORDKEEPING POLICIES AND PROCEDURES AND RECOMMEND CONTINUING MEDICAL EDUCATION NECESSARY TO ASSIST HIS ASSIMILATION INTO THE PRACTICE OF MEDICINE IN THE UNITED STATES. THE CONTINUING MEDICAL EDUCATION SHALL INCLUDE, BUT NOT BE LIMITED TO, COURSES INVOLVING RECORDKEEPING, FLUID MANAGEMENT AND ANTIBIOTIC THERAPY. ORDER TERMINATED AS OF 1/26/94 AND IN SIX MONTHS A FOLLOW-UP PRACTICE

SURVEY SHALL BE CONDUCTED.

BRENNAN, MICHAEL JAMES MD, LICENSE NUMBER 14591 OF PHOENIX, AZ, WAS DISCIPLINED BY ARIZONA ON JULY 25, 1997
DISCIPLINARY ACTION: REPRIMAND
OFFENSE: PROFESSIONAL MISCONDUCT

NOTES: IN OCTOBER AND NOVEMBER 1996 HE ADVERTISED ON THE RADIO THAT HE WAS A BOARD CERTIFIED MEDICAL DOCTOR, BUT NEVER SUPPLIED THE FULL NAME OF THE SPECIFIC AGENCY, ORGANIZATION OR ENTITY GRANTING THIS STANDING OF BOARD CERTIFICATION, IN ADVERTISEMENTS FOR A WEIGHT MANAGEMENT CENTER.

BREWER, EDWARD A MD, LICENSE NUMBER C017672 OF PHOENIX, AZ, WAS DISCIPLINED BY CALIFORNIA ON JANUARY 18, 1990
DISCIPLINARY ACTION: LICENSE REVOCATION
OFFENSE: DISCIPLINARY ACTION BY ANOTHER STATE OR AGENCY

NOTES: DISCIPLINED BY ARIZONA FOR PRESCRIPTION VIOLATIONS; DEFAULT DECISION.

BREWER, EDWARD A MD, LICENSE NUMBER 0002822, WAS DISCIPLINED BY ARIZONA ON JULY 15, 1992
DISCIPLINARY ACTION: REQUIRED TO TAKE ADDITIONAL MEDICAL EDUCATION
OFFENSE: OVERPRESCRIBING OR MISPRESCRIBING DRUGS

NOTES: TREATED A PATIENT WITH CHRONIC PAIN FROM 11/26/69 THROUGH AT LEAST 6/19/91, PRESCRIBING CONTROLLED SUBSTANCES IN EXCESS OF A THERAPEUTIC AMOUNT EVEN AFTER PATIENT SHOWED SYMPTOMS THAT COULD HAVE BEEN DRUG-INDUCED. FAILED TO KEEP ADEQUATE MEDICAL RECORDS. HAD PREVIOUSLY BEEN DISCIPLINED ON 10/5/87 FOR PRESCRIBING PRELUDIN FOR MORE THAN 30 DAYS IN THE TREATMENT OF OBESITY WHEN HE AGREED TO CEASE PRESCRIBING, DISPENSING OR ADMINISTERING ANY SYMPATHOMIMETIC CONTROLLED SUBSTANCE DRUG SCHEDULE II THROUGH IV. CENSURED; SHALL SUCCESSFULLY COMPLETE (WITHIN SIX MONTHS) 40 HOURS OF CONTINUING MEDICAL EDUCATION IN THE SUBJECT OF PAIN CONTROL MANAGEMENT. ON 11/14/97 ORDER TERMINATED AS EDUCATION REQUIREMENTS MET.

BREWER, EDWARD A MD, LICENSE NUMBER 2822, WAS DISCIPLINED BY ARIZONA ON MAY 8, 1997
DISCIPLINARY ACTION: REPRIMAND
OFFENSE: FAILURE TO COMPLY WITH PREVIOUS BOARD ORDER

NOTES: IN EIGHT OF HIS PATIENTS, MOST OF WHOM HE HAD SEEN ON A LONG-TERM BASIS, DURING 1995 WHEN A PHARMACY SURVEY WAS DONE THE FOLLOWING DEFICIENCIES WERE FOUND: IN ONE CASE FAILED TO OBTAIN FURTHER NEUROLOGIC CONSULTATION AND FAILED TO OBTAIN A PSYCHIATRIC CONSULTATION OR PAIN CLINIC CONSULTATION FOR DETOXIFICATION OF A PATIENT; FOR ANOTHER PATIENT WHO INITIALLY PRESENTED A COMPLAINT OF MIGRAINE, HE FAILED TO MAKE ANY ASSESSMENT OF THE HEADACHE, FAILED TO NOTE ANY PREVIOUS WORK-UP AND FAILED TO USE STANDARD THERAPIES SUCH AS ERGOTS, BETA BLOCKERS, CALCIUM CHANNEL BLOCKERS OR IMITREX; WITH A CHILD ON RITALIN, HE FAILED TO MAKE ANY PROGRESS NOTES REFERABLE TO THE CHILD'S HYPERACTIVITY, FAILED TO RE-EVALUATE THE CHILD'S HYPERACTIVITY DURING THE COURSE OF TREATMENT AND FAILED TO INSTITUTE DRUG HOLIDAYS; IN ANOTHER PATIENT HE FAILED TO NOTE OBJECTIVE FINDINGS ON THE MAJORITY OF EXAMINATIONS CONDUCTED ON A PATIENT TREATED FOR INJURIES FROM AN AUTOMOBILE ACCIDENT; IN SEVERAL OF THESE CASES HE FAILED TO OBTAIN ADEQUATE HISTORIES OR PERFORM ADEQUATE EXAMINATIONS; IN 10/95 HE VIOLATED PREVIOUS BOARD ORDER BY PRESCRIBING DEXEDRINE.

BRIGGS, ROBERT C MD, LICENSE NUMBER 0004376 OF AZ, WAS DISCIPLINED BY ARIZONA ON JANUARY 19, 1995
DISCIPLINARY ACTION: RESTRICTION PLACED ON LICENSE; MONITORING OF PHYSICIAN PERFORMANCE

NOTES: SHALL PROMPTLY UNDERGO PSYCHOMETRIC AND PSYCHOLOGICAL EVALUATION BY BOARD-DESIGNATED EVALUATORS; SHALL SUBMIT TO PERIODIC RANDOM REVIEW OF HIS OFFICE RECORDS AND PRACTICES FOR ONE YEAR; SHALL UNDERGO ALCOHOL AND SUBSTANCE ABUSE EVALUATION FOR ONE YEAR, INCLUDING BUT NOT LIMITED TO, RANDOM BIOLOGICAL FLUID SPECIMENS; SHALL CEASE ADMITTING PATIENTS TO THE HOSPITAL AND SHALL SEE NO HOSPITAL PATIENTS UNTIL FURTHER ORDER OF THE BOARD; REQUIRED TO PASS THE SPECIAL PURPOSE EXAMINATION OR BE SUBJECT TO ADDITIONAL CONDITIONS. ON 1/22/97 BOARD RECOGNIZED HIS COMPLIANCE WITH ORDER.

BRIGGS, ROBERT C MD, LICENSE NUMBER 4525 OF 2146 E BELMONT, PHOENIX, AZ, WAS DISCIPLINED BY HAWAII ON MARCH 14, 1997
DISCIPLINARY ACTION: FINE; MONITORING OF PHYSICIAN PERFORMANCE
OFFENSE: NONCOMPLIANCE WITH A PROFESSIONAL RULE

NOTES: HE BELIEVED THAT THE ARIZONA MATTER WAS A COOPERATIVE AND REMEDIAL ACTION RATHER THAN A DISCIPLINARY ONE AND THEREFORE NOT REPORTABLE TO HAWAII. MUST COMPLY WITH ALL TERMS AND CONDITIONS OF ARIZONA ORDERS FROM 7/11/94 AND FROM 2/27/95 WHICH INCLUDE: SHALL TAKE AND PASS THE SPEX EXAM; SHALL SUBMIT TO PSYCHIATRIC AND PSYCHOLOGICAL EVALUATION BY A BOARD EVALUATOR; SHALL UNDERGO A RANDOM REVIEW OF HIS OFFICE RECORDS, OFFICE PRACTICES AND NURSING HOME CARE OF PATIENTS; SHALL UNDERGO ALCOHOL AND SUBSTANCE ABUSE EVALUATION, INCLUDING RANDOM BIOLOGICAL FLUID SPECIMENS; SHALL CEASE ADMITTING PATIENTS TO THE HOSPITAL AND SHALL SEE NO PATIENTS UNTIL FURTHER ORDER OF THE ARIZONA BOARD. IN HAWAII SHALL PAY A FINE OF $500.

BROADBENT, DAVID H MD OF PROVO, UT, WAS DISCIPLINED BY UTAH ON MARCH 22, 1990
DISCIPLINARY ACTION: 12-MONTH PROBATION
OFFENSE: SUBSTANDARD CARE, INCOMPETENCE OR NEGLIGENCE

NOTES: SECOND YEAR OF TWO YEAR PROBATION STAYED. LICENSE SHALL BE REINSTATED TO FULL PRIVILEGES AFTER ONE YEAR OF PROBATION UPON FULL COMPLIANCE WITH CONDITIONS. ON 10/9/91 PROBATION TERMINATED AND LICENSE REINSTATED WITH FULL PRIVILEGES.

BROADBENT, DAVID H MD, LICENSE NUMBER 0009129, WAS DISCIPLINED BY ARIZONA ON APRIL 10, 1992
DISCIPLINARY ACTION: RESTRICTION PLACED ON LICENSE
OFFENSE: DISCIPLINARY ACTION BY ANOTHER STATE OR AGENCY

NOTES: ON 3/22/90, DISCIPLINED BY UTAH BOARD FOR PERFORMING LIPOSUCTION PROCEDURES WHICH HE WAS NOT QUALIFIED TO DO. SHALL NOT PERFORM LIPOSUCTION PROCEDURES UNTIL FURTHER ORDER OF THE ARIZONA BOARD OF MEDICAL EXAMINERS,

AND SHALL CONFINE HIS MEDICAL PRACTICE TO OBSTETRICS AND GYNECOLOGY.

BROADBENT, DAVID H MD, LICENSE NUMBER 0G29387 OF PROVO, UT, WAS DISCIPLINED BY CALIFORNIA ON APRIL 13, 1994
DISCIPLINARY ACTION: 24-MONTH PROBATION
OFFENSE: DISCIPLINARY ACTION BY ANOTHER STATE OR AGENCY

NOTES: DISCIPLINED BY UTAH DIVISION OF OCCUPATIONAL AND PROFESSIONAL LICENSING FOR POOR MEDICAL JUDGMENT, INADEQUATE MEDICAL HISTORY OBTAINED OR DOCUMENTED, ON 2 LIPOSUCTION PATIENTS. IN CALIFORNIA, SUSPENSION STAYED.

BROCK, EDSON GEORGE II MD, LICENSE NUMBER 0054839 OF SCOTTSDALE, AZ, WAS DISCIPLINED BY FLORIDA ON DECEMBER 24, 1996
DISCIPLINARY ACTION: LICENSE SUSPENSION
OFFENSE: NONCOMPLIANCE WITH A PROFESSIONAL RULE

NOTES: VIOLATED A RULE OR A LAWFUL ORDER OF THE BOARD, OR FAILED TO COMPLY WITH A LAWFUL SUBPOENA OF THE BOARD. SUSPENSION UNTIL APPEARS BEFORE THE BOARD AND ANSWERS CHARGES IN THE ADMINISTRATIVE COMPLAINT.

BROCKWAY, STEPHEN S MD, LICENSE NUMBER 0017759, WAS DISCIPLINED BY ARIZONA ON MAY 10, 1994
DISCIPLINARY ACTION: RESTRICTION PLACED ON LICENSE; MONITORING OF PHYSICIAN PERFORMANCE

NOTES: RELATIVE TO RECENT TREATMENT FOR SEXUAL ADDICTION. SHALL HAVE A FEMALE CHAPERONE PRESENT AT ALL TIMES DURING WHICH HE SEES OR TREATS FEMALE PATIENTS; SHALL NOT PRESCRIBE MEDICATION FOR ANY PERSON WHO IS NOT UNDER HIS DIRECT CARE; SHALL NOT ENGAGE IN PRIVATE PRACTICE; INTERACTION WITH PATIENTS SHALL BE LIMITED TO THE THERAPEUTIC SETTING ONLY; SHALL OBTAIN A BOARD-APPROVED TREATING PHYSICIAN; SHALL SUBMIT TO ANY THERAPY ORDERED BY BOARD; SHALL HAVE HIS LITHIUM LEVEL DETERMINED AT LEAST ONCE EVERY TWO WEEKS; SHALL ABSTAIN COMPLETELY FROM THE CONSUMPTION OF ALCOHOLIC BEVERAGES AND DRUGS EXCEPT WHEN PRESCRIBED BY HIS TREATING PHYSICIAN; MUST SUBMIT TO WITNESSED RANDOM BIOLOGICAL FLUID COLLECTION; SHALL ATTEND A MINIMUM OF THREE WEEKLY MEETINGS IN A 12-STEP RECOVERY PROGRAM APPROPRIATE FOR SEXUAL ADDICTION; SHALL HAVE EMPLOYER SUBMIT QUARTERLY REPORTS TO THE BOARD.

BROCKWAY, STEPHEN S MD, LICENSE NUMBER 0017759, WAS DISCIPLINED BY ARIZONA ON JULY 15, 1994
DISCIPLINARY ACTION: MONITORING OF PHYSICIAN PERFORMANCE
OFFENSE: FAILURE TO COMPLY WITH PREVIOUS BOARD ORDER

NOTES: HE FAILED TO MEET TERM OF PREVIOUS STIPULATION AND ORDER OF OR ABOUT 05/10/94, BY SEEING APPROXIMATELY 25 FEMALE PATIENTS AS OF 07/15/94 WITHOUT HAVING A FEMALE CHAPERONE PRESENT DURING THOSE SESSIONS. ISSUED AN ORDER OF CENSURE. PREVIOUS ORDER MODIFIED SUCH THAT HIS LITHIUM LEVEL WILL BE CHECKED EVERY TWO MONTHS RATHER THAN EVERY TWO WEEKS. ON 4/7/95 ORDER MODIFIED AS FOLLOWS: SHALL OBTAIN A BOARD APPROVED TREATING PHYSICIAN; SHALL SUBMIT TO ANY THERAPY ORDERED BY THE BOARD; SHALL ABSTAIN COMPLETELY FROM THE CONSUMPTION OF ALCOHOLIC BEVERAGES AND DRUGS EXCEPT WHEN PRESCRIBED FOR HIM BY HIS APPROVED TREATING PHYSICIAN; SHALL SUBMIT TO WITNESSED RANDOM BIOLOGICAL FLUID COLLECTION; SHALL DIRECT HIS EMPLOYER TO PROVIDE QUARTERLY WRITTEN REPORTS TO THE BOARD REGARDING HIS JOB PERFORMANCE AND APPROPRIATENESS OF BEHAVIOR; SHALL ATTEND A MINIMUM OF THREE WEEKLY MEETINGS IN A 12-STEP RECOVERY PROGRAM APPROPRIATE FOR SEXUAL ADDICTION. ON 3/14/97 ORDER MODIFIED TO REMOVE THE FOLLOWING REQUIREMENTS: HAVING A BOARD APPROVED TREATING PHYSICIAN; ABSTAINING FROM THE CONSUMPTION OF ALCOHOL AND ANY DRUGS OR MEDICATIONS, EXCEPT FOR PLAIN ASPIRIN AND/OR PLAIN ACETAMINOPHEN AND THOSE PRESCRIBED BY HIS TREATING PHYSICIAN; SUBMITTING TO RANDOM BIOLOGICAL FLUID COLLECTION. ON 9/23/98 ORDER TERMINATED.

BROOKS, KENNETH L MD, DATE OF BIRTH OCTOBER 19, 1961, LICENSE NUMBER 1059207 OF 2858 EAST FOX STREET, MESA, AZ, WAS DISCIPLINED BY MICHIGAN ON DECEMBER 1, 1999
DISCIPLINARY ACTION: 24-MONTH PROBATION; FINE
OFFENSE: NONCOMPLIANCE WITH A PROFESSIONAL RULE

NOTES: FAILURE TO MEET CONTINUING EDUCATION REQUIREMENTS. $1,000 FINE; REPRIMAND.

BROWN, CHARLES MD, WAS DISCIPLINED BY ARIZONA ON JULY 17, 1996
OFFENSE: FAILURE TO COMPLY WITH PREVIOUS BOARD ORDER

NOTES: INTERVIEWED BY THE BOARD REGARDING HIS CARE AND TREATMENT OF A PATIENT AND THE MALPRACTICE CLAIM ALLEGING THAT HE FAILED TO DIAGNOSE TUBERCULOSIS; THE 11/16/95 ORDER THAT HE TAKE AND PASS THE SPECIAL PURPOSE EXAMINATION; AND HIS VIOLATION OF ORDER BY FAILING TO TAKE THE EXAM. WITHIN 10 WEEKS, SHALL TAKE AND PASS THE SPECIAL PURPOSE EXAMINATION WITH A SCORE OF 75 OR GREATER.

BROWN, CHARLES MD, WAS DISCIPLINED BY ARIZONA ON MAY 15, 1998

NOTES: HE FAILED THE SPEX. MAY NOT PRACTICE MEDICINE IN ARIZONA UNTIL HE HAS TAKEN AND PASSED THE SPEX EXAM.

BROWN, RICHARD C DO, LICENSE NUMBER 2760 OF 1521 E THUNDERHEAD, TUCZON, AZ, WAS DISCIPLINED BY ARIZONA ON OCTOBER 24, 1997
DISCIPLINARY ACTION: EMERGENCY SUSPENSION
OFFENSE: OVERPRESCRIBING OR MISPRESCRIBING DRUGS

NOTES: DR. BROWN ADMITTED TO TAKING 15 VICODIN OUT OF THE ORACLE FAMILY HEALTH CARE CENTER AFTER NORMAL WORK HOURS TO PRESCRIBE TO HIS WIFE USING ANOTHER PHYSICIAN'S NAME; ON NUMEROUS OCCASIONS HE PRESCRIBED VICODIN FOR HIS FATHER, BROTHER, HIS WIFE, THE PHYSICIAN WHOSE NAME HE USED, AND HIMSELF; HE ADMITTED TO SELF-PRESCRIBING VICODIN ES, ACTING AS BOTH PATIENT AND PHYSICIAN, ADMITTING TO TAKING 1-2 VICODIN TABLETS PER WORK DAY AND ALLOWING A NURSE PRACTITIONER TO USE HIS PRESCRIPTION PAD AND DRUG ENFORCEMENT AGENCY NUMBER PRIOR TO THE NURSE PRACTITIONER'S PRESCRIBING AUTHORIZATION. SHALL SUBMIT HIMSELF FOR SUCH MENTAL, PHYSICAL, ORAL OR WRITTEN MEDICAL COMPETENCY EXAMINATIONS AS DESIGNATED BY THE BOARD.

BROWN, RICHARD C DO, LICENSE NUMBER 2760, WAS

DISCIPLINED BY ARIZONA ON FEBRUARY 27, 1998
DISCIPLINARY ACTION: REQUIRED TO ENTER AN IMPAIRED PHYSICIAN PROGRAM OR SUBSTANCE ABUSE TREATMENT
OFFENSE: SUBSTANCE ABUSE

NOTES: SHALL REFRAIN FROM PRACTICE UNTIL HE HAS COMPLIED WITH THE FOLLOWING TERMS: WILL SUCCESSFULLY COMPLETE INPATIENT EVALUATION FOR CHEMICAL DEPENDENCY AND DEVELOP A PLAN FOR AFTERCARE TREATMENT AND MONITORING; SHALL SIGN A RELEASE ALLOWING TREATMENT PERSONNEL TO RELEASE HIS MEDICAL RECORDS; SHALL MEET WITH THE BOARD UPON COMPLIANCE WITH THESE CONDITIONS. LICENSE WILL THEN BE PLACED ON PROBATION WITH SPECIFIED CONDITIONS.

BROWN, RICHARD C DO, LICENSE NUMBER 2760 OF 1521 E THUNDERHEAD, TUCSON, AZ, WAS DISCIPLINED BY ARIZONA ON MAY 16, 1998
DISCIPLINARY ACTION: SURRENDER OF LICENSE
OFFENSE: PHYSICAL OR MENTAL ILLNESS INHIBITING THE ABILITY TO PRACTICE WITH SKILL AND SAFETY

NOTES: HE WAS EVALUATED IN 4/98 REGARDING HIS HISTORY OF HAND PROBLEMS AND NO LONGER WISHES TO COMPLETE REQUIREMENTS OF THE 1/31/98 STIPULATION HE IS UNDER. VOLUNTARY SURRENDER.

BROWNE, ALLEN MD, LICENSE NUMBER 14411, WAS DISCIPLINED BY ARIZONA ON MAY 21, 1999
DISCIPLINARY ACTION: PROBATION; FINE
OFFENSE: CRIMINAL CONVICTION OR PLEA OF GUILTY, NOLO CONTENDERE, OR NO CONTEST TO A CRIME

NOTES: CONVICTED OF A CLASS II FELONY; COMMITTED UNPROFESSIONAL CONDUCT. ISSUED A DECREE OF CENSURE; ADMINISTRATIVE PENALTY OF $5,000; LICENSE PLACED ON LIFETIME PROBATION AND SHALL HAVE A FEMALE CHAPERONE DURING ALL VISITS WITH FEMALE PATIENTS, WITH THE CHAPERONE NOTING HER PRESENCE ON THE PATIENT'S RECORD; MUST MAKE HIS RECORDS AVAILABLE TO THE BOARD FOR REVIEW TO ASCERTAIN COMPLIANCE; SHALL OBTAIN THE SERVICES OF A TREATING PSYCHIATRIST WITH THE BOARD'S APPROVAL, SUBMITTING QUARTERLY REPORTS FOR NOT LESS THAN TWO YEARS.

BRYANT, GEORGE DO, LICENSE NUMBER 0000974, WAS DISCIPLINED BY ARIZONA ON JANUARY 18, 1990
DISCIPLINARY ACTION: PROBATION; MONITORING OF PHYSICIAN PERFORMANCE
OFFENSE: SUBSTANCE ABUSE

NOTES: ADMITS TO A NARCOTIC ABUSE PROBLEM; COMPLETED AN INPATIENT CHEMICAL DEPENDENCY TREATMENT PROGRAM. MINIMUM THREE YEAR PROBATION UNDER TERMS AND CONDITIONS: SHALL REFRAIN FROM THE USE OF ALL ILLICIT DRUGS AND SHALL NOT TAKE PRESCRIPTION NARCOTIC DRUGS, EXCEPT UNDER EMERGENCY CIRCUMSTANCES AND ONLY UPON PRESCRIPTION OF A TREATING PHYSICIAN EXCEPT FOR ASPIRIN AND TYLENOL; SHALL NOT CONSUME ALCOHOL; SHALL ATTEND AT LEAST THREE AA/NARCOTICS ANONYMOUS MEETINGS PER WEEK AND KEEP A LOG OF ATTENDANCE TO BE SIGNED BY THE CHAIR OF EACH MEETING; SHALL APPEAR BEFORE THE BOARD UPON REQUEST; SHALL CONTINUE IN THE PHYSICIANS' MONITORED AFTERCARE PROGRAM; SHALL SUBMIT TO BIOLOGICAL FLUID TESTING UPON BOARD REQUEST; SHALL BE RESPONSIBLE FOR HAVING WRITTEN REPORTS SUBMITTED QUARTERLY TO THE BOARD BY HIS TREATING PSYCHIATRIST REGARDING HIS PROGRESS IN TREATMENT AND PROGNOSIS OR RECOMMENDATIONS. PROBATION SATISFIED IN FULL ON 1/18/93.

BUBIEN, JOHN F MD, WAS DISCIPLINED BY ARIZONA ON APRIL 11, 1992
DISCIPLINARY ACTION: REQUIRED TO ENTER AN IMPAIRED PHYSICIAN PROGRAM OR SUBSTANCE ABUSE TREATMENT; MONITORING OF PHYSICIAN PERFORMANCE
OFFENSE: SUBSTANCE ABUSE

NOTES: HE APPLIED FOR AN ARIZONA LICENSE AND HAS BEEN PREVIOUSLY TREATED FOR ALCOHOLISM. LICENSE WILL BE GRANTED FOLLOWING COMPLETION OF THE SPEX EXAMINATION ON THE FOLLOWING TERMS AND CONDITIONS: MUST IMMEDIATELY PARTICIPATE IN A BOARD-APPROVED MONITORED AFTERCARE TREATMENT PROGRAM WHOSE THERAPIST MUST SUBMIT QUARTERLY REPORTS; MUST PARTICIPATE IN 90 12-STEP MEETINGS FOR SUBSTANCE ABUSE WITHIN 90 DAYS; MUST THEN PARTICIPATE IN A 12-STEP RECOVERY PROGRAM AS DETERMINED BY HIS TREATING THERAPIST AND ATTEND AT LEAST 3 WEEKLY MEETINGS; SHALL OBTAIN A BOARD-APPROVED TREATING PHYSICIAN; SHALL ABSTAIN COMPLETELY FROM THE CONSUMPTION OF ALCOHOLIC BEVERAGES AND DRUGS EXCEPT WHEN PRESCRIBED BY HIS TREATING PHYSICIAN; MUST SUBMIT TO WITNESSED RANDOM BIOLOGICAL FLUID COLLECTION; KEEP A LOG OF ANY AND ALL MEDICATIONS PRESCRIBED FOR HIM; SHALL SUBMIT TO ANY EXAMINATIONS OR THERAPY ORDERED BY BOARD; SHALL APPEAR BEFORE BOARD FOR INTERVIEWS UPON REQUEST; SHALL INFORM BOARD OF CHANGE OF ADDRESS OR IF AWAY FOR MORE THAN 5 DAYS. AS OF 1/21/95 ORDER TO BE TERMINATED IN 90 DAYS.

BURKE, JAMES DO, LICENSE NUMBER 0001528, WAS DISCIPLINED BY ARIZONA ON JUNE 14, 1990
DISCIPLINARY ACTION: MONITORING OF PHYSICIAN PERFORMANCE

NOTES: SHALL UNDERGO NEUROPSYCHIATRIC AND SUBSTANCE ABUSE EXAMINATIONS AND/OR TESTING; SHALL SIGN A RELEASE ALLOWING THE RESULTS OF THE TESTING AND EXAMINATIONS TO BE FORWARDED TO THE BOARD; SHALL APPEAR BEFORE THE BOARD UPON REQUEST TO REVIEW THE RESULTS OF THE EXAMINATIONS.

BURKS, JAMES R MD, LICENSE NUMBER 0007877, WAS DISCIPLINED BY ARIZONA ON OCTOBER 12, 1990
DISCIPLINARY ACTION: REQUIRED TO ENTER AN IMPAIRED PHYSICIAN PROGRAM OR SUBSTANCE ABUSE TREATMENT; MONITORING OF PHYSICIAN PERFORMANCE
OFFENSE: SUBSTANCE ABUSE

NOTES: MUST IMMEDIATELY PARTICIPATE IN THE ARIZONA MEDICAL ASSOCIATION'S MONITORED AFTERCARE TREATMENT PROGRAM WITH QUARTERLY REPORTS TO THE BOARD; MUST HAVE A BOARD APPROVED TREATING PHYSICIAN; MUST ABSTAIN COMPLETELY FROM ALCOHOL AND ALL OTHER DRUGS; MUST SUBMIT TO RANDOM BIOLOGICAL FLUID TESTS; MUST SUBMIT TO ANY EXAMS OR THERAPY ORDERED BY THE BOARD; MUST PARTICIPATE IN A 12-STEP RECOVERY PROGRAM FOR SUBSTANCE ABUSE AS DETERMINED BY THERAPIST AND ATTEND AT LEAST 3 WEEKLY MEETINGS, INCLUDING AA OR NARCOTICS ANONYMOUS; MUST APPEAR BEFORE BOARD FOR INTERVIEWS UPON REQUEST; MUST MAINTAIN A LOG OF ALL MEDICATIONS; MUST ADVISE THE BOARD OF ANY CHANGE OF OFFICE OR HOME ADDRESS OR IF HE

PLANS TO BE AWAY FOR MORE THAN FIVE DAYS. ON 10/16/93 ORDER TERMINATED AFTER 90 DAYS.

BURNETT, DAVID W DO, LICENSE NUMBER 0001720 OF 304 11TH AVENUE, LUMBERTON, MS, WAS DISCIPLINED BY ARIZONA ON APRIL 20, 1991
DISCIPLINARY ACTION: REPRIMAND
OFFENSE: SUBSTANDARD CARE, INCOMPETENCE OR NEGLIGENCE

NOTES: FAILED TO EXAMINE THE RESULTS OF A MAMMOGRAM THAT HAD BEEN PERFORMED ON 3/16/89 PRIOR TO 1/19/90; MAMMOGRAM RECOMMENDED A BIOPSY WHICH WAS DONE ON 2/1/90 AND REVEALED BREAST CANCER.

BURNETT, DAVID W DO, DATE OF BIRTH JUNE 16, 1946, LICENSE NUMBER 0009227 OF 305 WEST MOODY STREET, POPLARVILLE, MS, WAS DISCIPLINED BY MISSISSIPPI ON JULY 21, 1994
DISCIPLINARY ACTION: PROBATION

NOTES: SUSPENSION STAYED.

BURNETT, DAVID W DO, DATE OF BIRTH JUNE 16, 1946, LICENSE NUMBER 0009227 OF 315 11TH STREET, LUMBERTON, MS, WAS DISCIPLINED BY MISSISSIPPI ON NOVEMBER 7, 1994

NOTES: ORDER ISSUED PROHIBITING HIM FROM PRACTICING MEDICINE UNTIL HE CONFORMS TO REQUIREMENTS OF CONSENT AGREEMENT.

BURNETT, DAVID W DO, LICENSE NUMBER 0001720 OF 304 11TH AVENUE, LUMBERTON, MS, WAS DISCIPLINED BY ARIZONA ON APRIL 22, 1996
DISCIPLINARY ACTION: LICENSE REVOCATION
OFFENSE: DISCIPLINARY ACTION BY ANOTHER STATE OR AGENCY

NOTES: FIVE YEAR SUSPENSION, STAYED TO PROBATION IN MISSISSIPPI ON 7/21/94; ADMITTED HE WAS CHEMICALLY DEPENDENT; UNLAWFUL USE OF CONTROLLED SUBSTANCES; ON 11/7/94 MISSISSIPPI PROHIBITS HIM FROM PRACTICING UNTIL HE COMPLETED TREATMENT FOR CHEMICAL DEPENDENCY; IN ARIZONA HIS LICENSE WAS PLACED ON SUSPENDED STATUS IN 1995 WHEN HE FAILED TO RENEW HIS LICENSE ON OR BEFORE 4/01/95 DUE TO THE FACT THERE WAS A PENDING BOARD INVESTIGATION OF UNPROFESSIONAL CONDUCT. MAY APPLY FOR A LICENSE TWO YEARS AFTER REVOCATION.

BURWELL, BEVERLY A MD, WAS DISCIPLINED BY ARIZONA ON MAY 15, 1998

NOTES: SHALL NOT PRACTICE MEDICINE IN ARIZONA UNTIL SHE MEETS WITH THE BOARD AND RECEIVES ITS AFFIRMATIVE APPROVAL TO DO SO; SHE WILL SEND A LETTER OF RESIGNATION TO HER RESIDENCY PROGRAM AND ADVISE STAFF WHEN THAT HAS BEEN ACCOMPLISHED; UPON HER RESIGNATION FROM HER RESIDENCY PROGRAM, HER PARTICIPATION IN THE MONITORED AFTERCARE PROGRAM WOULD TERMINATE.

CALKINS, GREGORY P MD, DATE OF BIRTH NOVEMBER 23, 1950, LICENSE NUMBER 0025811 OF JOLIET, IL, WAS DISCIPLINED BY KENTUCKY ON JANUARY 4, 1990
DISCIPLINARY ACTION: 24-MONTH PROBATION; FINE

NOTES: FINE $500.00. PROBATION TERMINATED ON 1/15/92.

CALKINS, GREGORY P MD OF CINCINNATI, OH, WAS DISCIPLINED BY OHIO ON MARCH 19, 1990
DISCIPLINARY ACTION: 1-MONTH LICENSE SUSPENSION; 60-MONTH PROBATION
OFFENSE: CRIMINAL CONVICTION OR PLEA OF GUILTY, NOLO CONTENDERE, OR NO CONTEST TO A CRIME

NOTES: FELONY CONVICTION (INCOME TAX EVASION). REVOCATION STAYED

CALKINS, GREGORY P MD, LICENSE NUMBER 0172708 OF HAMMOND, IN, WAS DISCIPLINED BY NEW YORK ON APRIL 17, 1990
DISCIPLINARY ACTION: 36-MONTH PROBATION

NOTES: THREE YEAR SUSPENSION STAYED.

CALKINS, GREGORY P MD, DATE OF BIRTH NOVEMBER 23, 1950, LICENSE NUMBER 0026343 OF 817 GLENWOOD AVENUE, JOLIET, IL, WAS DISCIPLINED BY IOWA ON DECEMBER 23, 1991
DISCIPLINARY ACTION: SURRENDER OF LICENSE
OFFENSE: DISCIPLINARY ACTION BY ANOTHER STATE OR AGENCY

CALKINS, GREGORY PAUL MD, LICENSE NUMBER 040120E, WAS DISCIPLINED BY PENNSYLVANIA ON JANUARY 26, 1990
DISCIPLINARY ACTION: REPRIMAND

CALKINS, GREGORY PAUL MD, LICENSE NUMBER 0017859, WAS DISCIPLINED BY ARIZONA ON JUNE 30, 1990
DISCIPLINARY ACTION: EMERGENCY SUSPENSION
OFFENSE: CRIMINAL CONVICTION OR PLEA OF GUILTY, NOLO CONTENDERE, OR NO CONTEST TO A CRIME

NOTES: PLED GUILTY TO INCOME TAX EVASION IN INDIANA 10/28/87 AND PLACED ON CRIMINAL PROBATION FOR FIVE YEARS WITH A $1000 FINE AND 500 HOURS OF COMMUNITY SERVICE. TEXAS BOARD ALSO REQUIRED HIM TO INFORM THEM OF ANY ACTION TAKEN BASED ON THIS CONVICTION.

CALKINS, GREGORY PAUL MD, WAS DISCIPLINED BY HAWAII ON JULY 18, 1990
DISCIPLINARY ACTION: LICENSE REVOCATION

CALKINS, GREGORY PAUL MD, WAS DISCIPLINED BY WASHINGTON ON OCTOBER 19, 1990
OFFENSE: DISCIPLINARY ACTION BY ANOTHER STATE OR AGENCY

NOTES: CONVICTED IN U.S. DISTRICT COURT FOR THE NORTHERN DISTRICT OF INDIANA OF INCOME TAX EVASION ON 12/18/87; TEXAS RESTRICTED HIS LICENSE ON 9/24/88. MUST COMPLY WITH TEXAS AND DISTRICT COURT ORDERS; MUST APPEAR BEFORE THE BOARD BEFORE PRACTICING IN WASHINGTON; MUST ADVISE BOARD OF ANY CHANGE OF ADDRESS.

CAPELLAN, TERESA MD, LICENSE NUMBER 0009127, WAS DISCIPLINED BY ARIZONA ON JUNE 2, 1995

NOTES: SHE MUST NOTIFY THE ARIZONA BOARD 90 DAYS PRIOR TO PRACTICING MEDICINE IN ARIZONA.

CAPPELLO, JOHN V DO, DATE OF BIRTH MARCH 11, 1941, LICENSE NUMBER 14523 OF 108 NORTH BLANDING STREET, LAKE CITY, SC, WAS DISCIPLINED BY MISSISSIPPI ON FEBRUARY 20, 1997

NOTES: AGREES NOT TO PRACTICE MEDICINE IN MISSISSIPPI AND UPON EXPIRATION OF HIS LICENSE ON 6/30/97 AGREES NEVER TO SEEK RENEWAL OF MISSISSIPPI MEDICAL LICENSE.

CAPPELLO, JOHN V DO, LICENSE NUMBER 3178 OF 108 N BLANDING STREET, LAKE CITY, SC, WAS DISCIPLINED BY ARIZONA

ON AUGUST 22, 1997
DISCIPLINARY ACTION: 60-MONTH PROBATION; MONITORING OF PHYSICIAN PERFORMANCE
OFFENSE: DISCIPLINARY ACTION BY ANOTHER STATE OR AGENCY

NOTES: ON 12/14/96 ACKNOWLEDGED THAT HE DID NOT PROVIDE COMPLETE AND ACCURATE INFORMATION ON HIS APPLICATION FORM REGARDING A PAST ARREST THAT HAD BEEN SUBSEQUENTLY EXPUNGED AND A DIAGNOSIS OF A MENTAL ILLNESS; HAS ENTERED INTO STIPULATED CONSENT ORDER IN PENNSYLVANIA AND SOUTH CAROLINA REGARDING THE MONITORING OF HIS MENTAL ILLNESS; HAS ENTERED INTO A STIPULATED CONSENT ORDER IN MISSISSIPPI THAT HE PROVIDED FALSE INFORMATION ON AN APPLICATION FORM AND WILL NOT PRACTICE MEDICINE IN MISSISSIPPI AND WILL NOT SEEK RENEWAL OF HIS MEDICAL LICENSE. TERMS OF PROBATION ARE AS FOLLOWS: SHALL REMAIN IN COMPLIANCE WITH ALL ORDERS ISSUED AND IMPOSED BY SOUTH CAROLINA WHILE RESIDING AND/OR PRACTICING IN THAT STATE AND REMAIN IN GOOD STANDING THERE; SHALL OBTAIN A TREATING THERAPIST APPROVED BY THE BOARD AND SHALL REMAIN IN TREATMENT UNTIL FURTHER ORDER OF THE BOARD WITH MONTHLY REPORTS FOR SIX MONTHS THEN QUARTERLY; SHALL PROVIDE A COPY OF THIS ORDER TO ANY HEALTH CARE ENTITY WHERE HE HAS PRIVILEGES; SHALL ABSTAIN COMPLETELY FROM THE CONSUMPTION OF ANY ILLICIT DRUGS OR CONTROLLED SUBSTANCES EXCEPT WHEN PRESCRIBED BY HIS TREATING PHYSICIAN; MUST KEEP A LOG OF ANY AND ALL MEDICATIONS PRESCRIBED FOR HIM; SHALL SUBMIT TO ANY EVALUATIONS ORDERED BY BOARD; SHALL APPEAR BEFORE BOARD FOR INTERVIEWS UPON REQUEST; SHALL INFORM BOARD OF CHANGE OF ADDRESS; MUST SUBMIT TO WITNESSED RANDOM BIOLOGICAL FLUID COLLECTION

CAPPELLO, JOHN V DO, LICENSE NUMBER 004190L OF PO BOX 70, LAHASKA, PA, WAS DISCIPLINED BY PENNSYLVANIA ON APRIL 8, 1998
DISCIPLINARY ACTION: 3-MONTH LICENSE SUSPENSION; 12-MONTH PROBATION
OFFENSE: DISCIPLINARY ACTION BY ANOTHER STATE OR AGENCY

NOTES: DISCIPLINED BY MISSISSIPPI ON 2/20/97 AND ARIZONA ON 8/22/97. REMAINDER OF 12 MONTH SUSPENSION, STAYED FOR PROBATION WITH THE FOLLOWING TERMS AND CONDITIONS: SHALL COOPERATE WITH THE BUREAU OF PROFESSIONAL AND OCCUPATIONAL AFFAIRS AND THE PROFESSIONAL HEALTH MONITORING PROGRAMS (PHMP); UPON RESUMING PRACTICE IN OKLAHOMA SHALL NOT BE ABSENT FOR MORE THAN 20 DAYS WITHOUT PERMISSION; SHALL INFORM BOARD OF CHANGE OF ADDRESS WITHIN 72 HOURS; WITHIN 30 DAYS PRIOR TO RESUMING PRACTICE IN OKLAHOMA WILL SUBMIT TO AN ASSESSMENT/TREATMENT EVALUATION; SHALL IDENTIFY A PRIMARY CARE PHYSICIAN WHO SHALL SEND WRITTEN REPORTS TO THE BOARD; SHALL ATTEND AND PARTICIPATE IN ANY SUPPORT GROUP PROGRAMS RECOMMENDED NO LESS THAN TWICE A WEEK; SHALL ABSTAIN FROM THE USE OF CONTROLLED SUBSTANCES, MOOD ALTERING DRUGS OR DRUGS OF ABUSE INCLUDING ALCOHOL UNLESS PRESCRIBED BY A TREATING PRACTITIONER; SHALL SUPPLY ANY CURRENT OR PROSPECTIVE EMPLOYER WITH A COPY OF THIS ORDER; SHALL EXECUTE THE RELEASE OF ANY MEDICAL RECORDS; SHALL SUBMIT TO EVALUATIONS, PHYSICAL EXAMINATION OR INTERVIEWS; SHALL PAY COSTS.

CARAWAY, LYNN DEAN MD, LICENSE NUMBER 0005572, WAS DISCIPLINED BY ARIZONA ON JANUARY 18, 1995

NOTES: INFORMATION RECEIVED THAT HE MAY BE SELF-MEDICATING WITH SCHEDULE IV CONTROLLED SUBSTANCES. SHALL NOT PRACTICE MEDICINE IN ARIZONA UNTIL HE MEETS WITH THE BOARD; SHALL NOT PRESCRIBE OR DISPENSE CONTROLLED SUBSTANCES TO MEMBERS OF HIS IMMEDIATE FAMILY; SHALL NOT USE CONTROLLED SUBSTANCES EXCEPT IF PRESCRIBED BY ANOTHER PHYSICIAN FOR USE DURING A PRESCRIBED COURSE OF TREATMENT.

CARIDEO, CAROL MD, LICENSE NUMBER 0016318, WAS DISCIPLINED BY ARIZONA ON OCTOBER 18, 1996
DISCIPLINARY ACTION: REPRIMAND
OFFENSE: OVERPRESCRIBING OR MISPRESCRIBING DRUGS

NOTES: PRESCRIBING, DISPENSING OR ADMINISTERING ANY CONTROLLED SUBSTANCES OR PRESCRIPTION-ONLY DRUG FOR OTHER THAN THERAPEUTIC PURPOSES IN THAT IN A PHARMACY SURVEY FOR PHYSICIAN'S PRESCRIPTIONS WRITTEN BETWEEN 2/94 AND 7/94, BOARD INVESTIGATOR FOUND AT LEAST 24 PRESCRIPTIONS FOR SCHEDULE II DRUGS AND 18 PRESCRIPTIONS FOR CONTROLLED SUBSTANCES OTHER THAN SCHEDULE II DRUGS WRITTEN FOR ONE PATIENT, A CO-WORKER OF THE PHYSICIAN'S AT A WOMEN'S SHELTER; REPORTED THAT SHE HAD TREATED PATIENT AND PRESCRIBED CONTROLLED SUBSTANCES TO HER IN 3/94, BUT THAT SHE HAD NO RECORD AND THAT MAJORITY OF PRESCRIPTIONS HAD BEEN FORGED BY PATIENT; FAILED TO RESPOND TO THREE LETTERS FROM THE BOARD BETWEEN 7/95 AND 3/96 REQUESTING HER TO RESPOND TO SPECIFIC FINDINGS REGARDING THE MATTER.

CARLSON, JOHN S MD, LICENSE NUMBER 0002455, WAS DISCIPLINED BY ARIZONA ON APRIL 4, 1995
DISCIPLINARY ACTION: RESTRICTION PLACED ON LICENSE; RESTRICTION PLACED ON CONTROLLED SUBSTANCE LICENSE
OFFENSE: PROFESSIONAL MISCONDUCT

NOTES: INTERVIEWED BY BOARD RELATIVE TO INFORMATION QUESTIONING HIS PRESCRIBING OF CONTROLLED SUBSTANCES. SHALL TAKE AND PASS THE SPECIAL PURPOSE EXAMINATION IN 6/95 WITH A SCORE OF 75 OR GREATER; SHALL NOT PRESCRIBE CONTROLLED SUBSTANCES; SHALL NOT PERFORM SURGERY OR ASSIST IN SURGERY. ON 10/19/95 THIS ORDER TERMINATED AND AN OFFICE PRACTICE SURVEY SHALL BE COMPLETED IN SIX MONTHS AND A PHARMACY SURVEY SHALL BE COMPLETED IN 18 MONTHS.

CARTER, H EUGENE MD, LICENSE NUMBER 0011460, WAS DISCIPLINED BY ARIZONA ON JULY 21, 1995
DISCIPLINARY ACTION: LICENSE REVOCATION
OFFENSE: SUBSTANDARD CARE, INCOMPETENCE OR NEGLIGENCE

NOTES: BETWEEN 10/89 AND 11/94, VIOLATIONS RELATING TO HIS PRACTICE OF PAIN MANAGEMENT AND OUTPATIENT ANESTHESIA IN SIX PATIENTS. ENGAGED IN MEDICAL RECORDS VIOLATIONS IN THAT HE CREATED AND MAINTAINED MEDICAL RECORDS WHICH HE DID NOT PREPARE CONTEMPORANEOUSLY; MECHANICALLY REPRODUCED SIGNATURES, CREATED RECORDS OF TREATMENT, WHICH WERE NOT ACCURATE AS TO THE INJECTION SITES FOR THE REGIONAL ANESTHETIC PROCEDURES AND THE DRUGS USED ARE NOT RECORDED, MAINTAINED INCOMPLETE OFFICE RECORDS WITH THE EXPECTATION THAT SUPPLEMENTARY TREATMENT INFORMATION COULD

BE OBTAINED; NO EVIDENCE THAT HE DID SO; MAINTAINED INCOMPLETE TREATMENT RECORDS, CONTAINING INSUFFICIENT INFORMATION FOR ANOTHER PRACTITIONER TO ASSUME CONTINUITY OF CARE; FAILURE TO RECORD A TREATMENT PLAN IN THE MEDICAL RECORDS WHEREBY THERE IS NO JUSTIFICATION FOR THE TREATMENTS PROVIDED; FAILURE TO UPDATE TREATMENT RECORDS; FAILURE TO DOCUMENT ADVICE AND CAUTIONARY WARNINGS TO PATIENTS; CHARGING VIOLATIONS FOR THESE SIX PATIENTS, FEES WERE UNREASONABLE OVER EXTENDED LENGTHS OF TIME AND NOT JUSTIFIED IN THE MEDICAL RECORDS. ENGAGED IN PRACTICE THAT IS OR MIGHT BE HARMFUL OR DANGEROUS TO THE HEALTH OF THE PATIENT IN THAT HE FAILED TO SEEK A PSYCHOLOGICAL EVALUATION OF THREE PATIENTS PRIOR TO IMPLANTING A DORSAL COLUMN STIMULATOR; FOR THREE PATIENTS, USED REGIONAL ANESTHETIC TECHNIQUES WHICH WERE NOT MEDICALLY NECESSARY AS SET FORTH IN MEDICARE GUIDELINES; AND PERFORMED A CAUDAL EPIDUREAL BLOCK ON A PATIENT WHICH LEFT PATIENT WEAK AND UNABLE TO WALK AND WHICH RESULTED IN HER HOSPITALIZATION. ENGAGED IN PRESCRIBING PRACTICES WHICH ARE OR MIGHT BE HARMFUL OR DANGEROUS TO THE HEALTH OF TWO PATIENTS IN THAT HE PRESCRIBED NUMEROUS NARCOTIC MEDICATIONS, INCLUDING ROXICET, HYDROCET, DEMEROL, LORCET AND DURAGESIC PATCHES FOR OTHER THAN ACCEPTED THERAPEUTIC PURPOSES. AS MEDICAL DIRECTOR OF PAIN GROUP, FAILED TO SUPERVISE THE MEDICAL TREATMENT PROVIDED TO TWO PATIENTS BY ANOTHER PHYSICIAN WHO WAS PERMITTED TO PERFORM A MYRIAD OF REGIONAL ANESTHETIC PROCEDURES WHICH WERE NOT MEDICALLY NECESSARY AND FAILED TO DIRECT PHYSICIAN'S CLINICAL ACTIONS. ON 9/23/98 ARIZONA SUPREME COURT DENIED HIS PETITION FOR REVIEW AND AFFIRMED BOARD'S REVOCATION ORDER.

CARTER, H EUGENE MD, WAS DISCIPLINED BY NEW MEXICO ON MAY 1, 1996
DISCIPLINARY ACTION: LICENSE REVOCATION
OFFENSE: NONCOMPLIANCE WITH A PROFESSIONAL RULE

NOTES: FAILED TO REPORT REVOCATION IN ANOTHER STATE.

CARTER, HERBERT EUGENE MD, DATE OF BIRTH JUNE 2, 1950 OF 2701 E CAMELBACK ROAD #510, PHOENIX, AZ, WAS DISCIPLINED BY MEDICARE ON DECEMBER 9, 1996
DISCIPLINARY ACTION: EXCLUSION FROM THE MEDICARE AND/OR MEDICAID PROGRAM
OFFENSE: DISCIPLINARY ACTION BY ANOTHER STATE OR AGENCY

NOTES: LICENSE REVOKED FOR REASONS BEARING ON PROFESSIONAL PERFORMANCE.

CARTER, HERBERT EUGENE MD, LICENSE NUMBER C43145 OF SAN DIEGO, CA, WAS DISCIPLINED BY CALIFORNIA ON NOVEMBER 13, 1997
DISCIPLINARY ACTION: LICENSE REVOCATION
OFFENSE: DISCIPLINARY ACTION BY ANOTHER STATE OR AGENCY

NOTES: DISCIPLINED BY ARIZONA FOR NEGLIGENT TREATMENT OF SIX PATIENTS UNDER HIS CARE FOR PAIN MANAGEMENT AND OUTPATIENT ANESTHESIA IN THAT HE FAILED TO MAINTAIN ADEQUATE MEDICAL RECORDS, PRESCRIBED AND ADMINISTERED CONTROLLED SUBSTANCES FOR OTHER THAN THERAPEUTIC PURPOSES, PROVIDED TREATMENT THAT WAS OR MIGHT BE HARMFUL OR DANGEROUS AND CHARGED FOR SERVICES NOT RENDERED.

CASTILLO, ROBERT DIAZ MD, LICENSE NUMBER 0011036, WAS DISCIPLINED BY ARIZONA ON MAY 15, 1990
DISCIPLINARY ACTION: MONITORING OF PHYSICIAN PERFORMANCE

NOTES: AMENDED ORDER. SHALL CONTINUE WITH THERAPIST WHO MUST SUBMIT QUARTERLY REPORTS TO THE BOARD; SHALL OBTAIN A BOARD APPROVED TREATING PHYSICIAN; SHALL NOT SELF-PRESCRIBE OR TAKE ANY DRUGS; SHALL APPEAR BEFORE THE BOARD UPON REQUEST; THIS ORDER WAS TERMINATED ON 10/12/90.

CASTILLO, ROBERT DIAZ MD, LICENSE NUMBER 11036, WAS DISCIPLINED BY ARIZONA ON MARCH 14, 1997
DISCIPLINARY ACTION: REPRIMAND; REQUIRED TO TAKE ADDITIONAL MEDICAL EDUCATION
OFFENSE: PROFESSIONAL MISCONDUCT

NOTES: IN 1995 AND 1996 BOARD RECEIVED COMPLAINTS FROM FOUR PATIENTS THAT HE FAILED TO PROVIDE MEDICAL RECORDS WHEN REQUESTED; WHEN PARTIAL MEDICAL RECORDS WERE PROVIDED IN ONE CASE, THEY WERE LARGELY ILLEGIBLE AND DID NOT APPEAR TO STATE A DIAGNOSIS, JUSTIFY TREATMENT, OR PROVIDE SUFFICIENT INFORMATION FOR ANOTHER PRACTITIONER TO ASSUME CONTINUITY OF THE PATIENTS' CARE; DID NOT RESPOND TO THE BOARD REQUESTS FOR INFORMATION ON THESE COMPLAINTS; REGARDING PRESCRIBING PRACTICE, HE GAVE ONE PATIENT A SIGNED, UNDATED PRESCRIPTION FORM THAT FAILED TO LIST THE PATIENT'S NAME OR THE MEDICATION PRESCRIBED; GAVE SAME PATIENT A SAMPLE PACKAGE OF EFFEXOR, AN ANTIDEPRESSANT, ON WHICH HE HAD WRITTEN THE NAME OF SOME OTHER PATIENT; SIGNED BLANK PRESCRIPTION FORMS IN ADVANCE AND INSTRUCTED ANOTHER DOCTOR TO USE THEM. WITHIN 60 DAYS SHALL SUBMIT TO PSYCHIATRIC AND PSYCHOMETRIC EVALUATIONS BY EVALUATORS DESIGNATED BY THE BOARD WHO SHALL PROVIDE WRITTEN EVALUATION REPORTS; SHALL ENGAGE, AT HIS OWN EXPENSE, THE SERVICES OF A PRACTICE MANAGEMENT CONSULTANT APPROVED BY THE BOARD REGARDING TIMELY AND APPROPRIATE RESPONSE TO REQUESTS FOR MEDICAL RECORDS AND CORRESPONDENCE; SHALL OBTAIN 30 HOURS OF CONTINUING MEDICAL EDUCATION IN PSYCHOPHARMACOLOGY WITHIN ONE YEAR.

CASTRO, RONALD J MD, LICENSE NUMBER 0012701, WAS DISCIPLINED BY ARIZONA ON OCTOBER 18, 1995
DISCIPLINARY ACTION: REQUIRED TO TAKE ADDITIONAL MEDICAL EDUCATION
OFFENSE: SUBSTANDARD CARE, INCOMPETENCE OR NEGLIGENCE

NOTES: INTERVIEWED BY THE BOARD REGARDING HIS CARE AND TREATMENT OF A PATIENT AND MALPRACTICE CLAIM ALLEGING PRE-ECLAMPSIA AND A BOARD-ORDERED PRACTICE REVIEW. WITHIN SIX MONTHS, SHALL SUCCESSFULLY COMPLETE A 100 HOUR MINI-RESIDENCY IN THE MANAGEMENT OF HIGH RISK PREGNANCIES, PARTICULARLY THOSE INVOLVING HYPERTENSION, AND SHALL CONSENT TO THE RELEASE OF ANY RECORDS FROM MINI-RESIDENCY TO THE BOARD.

CATENA, MICHAEL R MD, LICENSE NUMBER 0011218 OF 995 SUMMER PLACE, PITTSBURGH, PA, WAS DISCIPLINED BY WEST VIRGINIA ON JANUARY 23, 1990
DISCIPLINARY ACTION: FINE; REPRIMAND
OFFENSE: DISCIPLINARY ACTION BY ANOTHER STATE OR AGENCY

NOTES: ENTERED INTO STIPULATION AND CONSENT

AGREEMENT IN PENNSYLVANIA DATED 12/22/88. FINE OF $2500.

CATENA, MICHAEL R MD, LICENSE NUMBER 0013913, WAS DISCIPLINED BY ARIZONA ON JUNE 29, 1990
DISCIPLINARY ACTION: SURRENDER OF LICENSE
OFFENSE: DISCIPLINARY ACTION BY ANOTHER STATE OR AGENCY

NOTES: ON 12/22/88 HE ENTERED INTO A STIPULATION AGREEMENT WITH THE PENNSYLVANIA BOARD IN WHICH HE ADMITTED TO REUSING DISPOSABLE SYRINGES; PENNSYLVANIA REPRIMANDED HIM AND FINED HIM $1,000.

CATENA, MICHAEL ROBERT MD, DATE OF BIRTH JUNE 29, 1945, LICENSE NUMBER 0020347 OF 995 SUMMER PLACE, PITTSBURGH, PA, WAS DISCIPLINED BY IOWA ON JULY 2, 1991
DISCIPLINARY ACTION: SURRENDER OF LICENSE
OFFENSE: DISCIPLINARY ACTION BY ANOTHER STATE OR AGENCY

CATENA, WILLIAM P JR MD, LICENSE NUMBER 0010381, WAS DISCIPLINED BY ARIZONA ON JUNE 29, 1990
DISCIPLINARY ACTION: SURRENDER OF LICENSE
OFFENSE: DISCIPLINARY ACTION BY ANOTHER STATE OR AGENCY

NOTES: ON 12/22/88 HE ENTERED INTO A STIPULATION AGREEMENT WITH PENNSYLVANIA BOARD IN WHICH HE ADMITTED TO REUSING DISPOSABLE SYRINGES; PENNSYLVANIA REPRIMANDED HIM AND FINED HIM $1,000.

CAZARES, CARLOS DO, LICENSE NUMBER 0001700 OF 8607 N 59TH AVE SUITE A-3, GLENDALE, AZ, WAS DISCIPLINED BY ARIZONA ON AUGUST 2, 1993
DISCIPLINARY ACTION: 1-MONTH LICENSE SUSPENSION; 12-MONTH PROBATION
OFFENSE: SUBSTANDARD CARE, INCOMPETENCE OR NEGLIGENCE

NOTES: FROM 1987 TO 1989 DURING HIS SUPERVISION OF THE WEIGHT CONTROL TREATMENT PROGRAM OF VARIOUS PATIENTS FAILED TO TAKE OR MONITOR PATIENTS' BLOOD PRESSURE FOR EXTENDED PERIODS OF TIME; PRESCRIBED CONTROLLED SUBSTANCE ANOREXICS FOR NON-THERAPEUTIC PURPOSES IN THAT THEY LOST LITTLE OR NO WEIGHT; FAILED TO SUPERVISE OR DIRECT OFFICE PERSONNEL IN THE MEDICAL CARE OF HIS PROFESSIONAL WEIGHT PATIENTS, FOR EXAMPLE, ON NUMEROUS OCCASIONS HE NOTED THAT THE PATIENT WAS NOT TO RECEIVE CONTROLLED SUBSTANCE ANOREXICS HOWEVER, OFFICE STAFF WOULD THEREAFTER ORDER ANOREXICS FOR THE PATIENT IN VIOLATION OF HIS ORDERS. SUSPENSION EFFECTIVE 8/01/93. PROBATION UNDER TERMS AND CONDITIONS: SHALL NOT TREAT ANY PATIENT FOR OBESITY, METABOLIC DYSFUNCTION OR OTHER WEIGHT RELATED DISORDERS; SHALL NOT PRESCRIBE ANY ANOREXICS FOR WEIGHT CONTROL; SHALL NOT TESTIFY AS AN EXPERT WITNESS IN ANY PROCEEDING ON ANY ISSUE DIRECTLY OR INDIRECTLY RELATING TO METABOLIC DISORDERS, WEIGHT CONTROL, EXOGENOUS OBESITY OR THE USE OR EFFECT OF CONTROLLED SUBSTANCE ANOREXIC DRUGS. $1,500 ADMINISTRATIVE PENALTY; $3,358.30 INVESTIGATION COSTS.

CECIL, JOHN G MD, DATE OF BIRTH NOVEMBER 19, 1905 OF 625 DEER PASS DRIVE, SEDONA, AZ, WAS DISCIPLINED BY MEDICARE ON JULY 22, 1991
DISCIPLINARY ACTION: EXCLUSION FROM THE MEDICARE AND/OR MEDICAID PROGRAM
OFFENSE: DISCIPLINARY ACTION BY ANOTHER STATE OR AGENCY

NOTES: LICENSE REVOCATION OR SUSPENSION.

CHAVES, JESUS V JR MD, LICENSE NUMBER 0013281, WAS DISCIPLINED BY ARIZONA ON APRIL 6, 1992
DISCIPLINARY ACTION: REQUIRED TO TAKE ADDITIONAL MEDICAL EDUCATION; MONITORING OF PHYSICIAN PERFORMANCE
OFFENSE: OVERPRESCRIBING OR MISPRESCRIBING DRUGS

NOTES: OVERPRESCRIBING OF CONTROLLED SUBSTANCES. MUST COMPLETE BY 12/31/92 20 HOURS OF CATEGORY I CONTINUING MEDICAL EDUCATION IN THE AREA OF CONTROL OF ADDICTIVE DRUGS. BOARD WILL CONDUCT AN OFFICE REVIEW OF HIS RECORDKEEPING AND PREPARE A PHARMACY SURVEY WITHIN 9 MONTHS. EFFECTIVE 10/20/94 ORDER TERMINATED.

CHERISH, LAWRENCE DO, LICENSE NUMBER 2877 OF 4346 W VILA RITA DRIVE, GLENDALE, AZ, WAS DISCIPLINED BY ARIZONA ON MAY 4, 1999
DISCIPLINARY ACTION: LICENSE SUSPENSION; REQUIRED TO ENTER AN IMPAIRED PHYSICIAN PROGRAM OR SUBSTANCE ABUSE TREATMENT
OFFENSE: SUBSTANCE ABUSE

NOTES: ON 4/21/99 BOARD RECEIVED INFORMATION THAT HE HAD SHOWN UP AT THE EMERGENCY ROOM WITH ALCOHOL ON HIS BREATH, HAD BEEN UNCONSCIOUS IN HIS HOUSE THE NIGHT BEFORE AND HAD MISSED WORK TWICE DUE TO ALCOHOL; ON 4/26/99 VOLUNTARILY ENTERED INTO AN ASSESSMENT AND ACKNOWLEDGED AN ALCOHOL PROBLEM. SHALL NOT PRESCRIBE UNTIL HE HAS MET THE FOLLOWING CONDITIONS: MUST SUCCESSFULLY COMPLETE INPATIENT EVALUATION FOR POSSIBLE ALCOHOL OR CHEMICAL DEPENDENCY AND FOLLOW RECOMMENDATIONS FOR TREATMENT; WILL DEVELOP A PLAN FOR AFTERCARE TREATMENT AND MONITORING WHICH SHALL INCLUDE; WILL MEET WITH BOARD, UPON WRITTEN REQUEST AFTER HIS DISCHARGE FROM THE FACILITY TO DISCUSS WHETHER OR NOT HE SHOULD RESUME HIS PRACTICE.

CHERISH, LAWRENCE DO, LICENSE NUMBER 2877 OF 4346 2 VIA RITA DRIVE, GLENDALE, AZ, WAS DISCIPLINED BY ARIZONA ON OCTOBER 22, 1999
DISCIPLINARY ACTION: 60-MONTH PROBATION; MONITORING OF PHYSICIAN PERFORMANCE
OFFENSE: SUBSTANCE ABUSE

NOTES: ON OR ABOUT 4/21/99 SHOWED UP AT EMERGENCY ROOM WITH ALCOHOL ON HIS BREATH, HAD BEEN UNCONSCIOUS IN HIS HOUSE THE NIGHT BEFORE AND WAS UNABLE TO COME TO WORK, HE CALLED IN AT NOON AND SOUNDED INTOXICATED, HAS MISSED WORK TWICE DUE TO ALCOHOL, AND REFUSED TO TAKE A BLOOD ALCOHOL TEST AND WAS TERMINATED; ON 4/26/99 VOLUNTARILY ENTERED INTO A TREATMENT PROGRAM, ACKNOWLEDGING HIS ALCOHOL PROBLEM; ON 5/4/99 LICENSE WAS SUSPENDED; ON 8/20/99 SUCCESSFULLY COMPLETED TREATMENT AND SUBSEQUENTLY REQUESTED THAT HIS LICENSE BE PLACED ON PROBATION. LICENSE LIMITED AS FOLLOWS: SHALL IMMEDIATELY OBTAIN A TREATING THERAPIST APPROVED BY THE BOARD AND SHALL REMAIN IN TREATMENT UNTIL FURTHER ORDER OF THE BOARD; THERAPIST SHALL SEND MONTHLY REPORTS TO THE BOARD; SHALL PROVIDE A COPY OF THIS ORDER TO ANY HEALTH CARE ENTITY

WHERE HE HAS PRIVILEGES; SHALL ABSTAIN COMPLETELY FROM THE CONSUMPTION OF ALCOHOLIC BEVERAGES AND DRUGS EXCEPT WHEN PRESCRIBED BY HIS TREATING PHYSICIAN; MUST KEEP A LOG OF ANY AND ALL MEDICATIONS PRESCRIBED FOR HIM; SHALL SUBMIT TO ANY EVALUATIONS ORDERED BY BOARD; SHALL APPEAR BEFORE THE BOARD UPON REQUEST; SHALL SUBMIT TO RANDOM BIOLOGICAL FLUID TESTING; SHALL PARTICIPATE IN A MINIMUM OF TWO SELF-HELP MEETINGS PER WEEK THROUGH SUCH ORGANIZATIONS AS AA OR NARCOTICS ANONYMOUS; SHALL INFORM THE BOARD IF HE CEASES TO PRACTICE IN ARIZONA; SHALL PAY COSTS.

CHESHIRE, DAVID MD, LICENSE NUMBER 0008691, WAS DISCIPLINED BY ARIZONA ON SEPTEMBER 23, 1996
DISCIPLINARY ACTION: RESTRICTION PLACED ON LICENSE

NOTES: LICENSE REACTIVATED; SHALL NOT ENGAGE IN PRACTICE OF CLINICAL MEDICINE UNTIL FURTHER ORDER OF THE BOARD.

CHESTER, ALVIN A MD, WAS DISCIPLINED BY NEW MEXICO ON DECEMBER 2, 1992
DISCIPLINARY ACTION: LICENSE REVOCATION

CHESTER, ALVIN A MD, LICENSE NUMBER 0102512 OF 1305 TIJERAS AVENUE NW, ALBUQUERQUE, NM, WAS DISCIPLINED BY NEW YORK ON NOVEMBER 30, 1993
DISCIPLINARY ACTION: LICENSE REVOCATION
OFFENSE: DISCIPLINARY ACTION BY ANOTHER STATE OR AGENCY

NOTES: LICENSE REVOKED BY THE NEW MEXICO BOARD.

CHESTER, ALVIN A MD, DATE OF BIRTH JANUARY 16, 1937 OF 6611 W PEORIA AVENUE #5, GLENDALE, AZ, WAS DISCIPLINED BY MEDICARE ON APRIL 5, 1995
DISCIPLINARY ACTION: EXCLUSION FROM THE MEDICARE AND/OR MEDICAID PROGRAM
OFFENSE: DISCIPLINARY ACTION BY ANOTHER STATE OR AGENCY

NOTES: LICENSE REVOKED FOR REASONS BEARING ON PROFESSIONAL PERFORMANCE.

CHUBATY, ROMAN A MD, LICENSE NUMBER 0011316 OF PHOENIX, AZ, WAS DISCIPLINED BY ARIZONA ON OCTOBER 19, 1994
DISCIPLINARY ACTION: RESTRICTION PLACED ON LICENSE

NOTES: SHALL NOT PROVIDE MEDICAL CARE OR TREATMENT TO PATIENTS FIVE YEARS OF AGE OR UNDER, EXCEPT ON AN ACTUAL EMERGENCY BASIS. SHALL TAKE AND PASS THE SPECIAL PURPOSE EXAMINATION IN 12/94 WITH A SCORE OF 75 OR GREATER. ON 1/20/95 ORDER MODIFIED AS FOLLOWS: THE BOARD RESCINDED THE PART OF THIS ORDER DEALING WITH THE TREATMENT OF CHILDREN OF FIVE YEARS OF AGE AND YOUNGER; SHALL COMPLETE A PEDIATRIC MINI-RESIDENCY WITHIN 12 MONTHS; SHALL SUBMIT TO AN OFFICE PRACTICE SURVEY IN ONE YEAR. ON 4/17/96 TIME EXTENDED 12 MONTHS TO COMPLETE A MINI-RESIDENCY IN PEDIATRICS. HIS REQUEST TO PARTICIPATE IN THE COLORADO PERSONALIZED EDUCATION FOR PHYSICIANS IN LIEU OF A MINI-RESIDENCY AND AN EXTENSION TO FULFILL THE REQUIREMENTS OF THE ORDER DENIED ON 10/16/96.

CLARK, RANDALL L MD, WAS DISCIPLINED BY ARIZONA ON MAY 21, 1996
DISCIPLINARY ACTION: RESTRICTION PLACED ON LICENSE; REQUIRED TO TAKE ADDITIONAL MEDICAL EDUCATION

NOTES: FOLLOWING REVIEW OF HIS REQUEST FOR REACTIVATION OF LICENSE, BOARD ORDERED HIM TO TAKE AND PASS AN ORAL COMPETENCY EXAMINATION IN OPHTHALMOLOGY THE RESULTS OF WHICH WERE PRESENTED AT BOARD MEETING. SHALL NOT PERFORM SURGERY; PRIOR TO THE REACTIVATION OF HIS LICENSE, HE SHALL COMPLETE A TWO-WEEK MINI-RESIDENCY IN OPHTHALMOLOGY APPROVED BY THE BOARD; REACTIVATION SHALL NOT BE EFFECTIVE UNTIL ORDERED BY THE BOARD. ON 4/16/96 OFFERED STIPULATION FOR RESTRICTION AND EDUCATION. ACCEPTED AND MADE EFFECTIVE 5/21/96.

CLARK, ROBERT W SR MD, LICENSE NUMBER 0002030 OF TEMPE, AZ, WAS DISCIPLINED BY ARIZONA ON JULY 14, 1994
OFFENSE: OVERPRESCRIBING OR MISPRESCRIBING DRUGS

NOTES: ON 11/15/92 PHARMACY SURVEY INDICATED HE IS PRESCRIBING LARGE AMOUNTS OF SCHEDULED DRUGS TO PATIENTS. SHALL PROMPTLY UNDERGO PSYCHOMETRIC AND PSYCHOLOGICAL EVALUATION BY EVALUATORS DESIGNATED BY BOARD STAFF; SHALL NOT PRACTICE MEDICINE IN ARIZONA UNTIL THE BOARD REVIEWS THE EVALUATION AND UNTIL FURTHER ORDER OF THE BOARD.

CLARK, ROBERT W MD OF 2055 E SOUTHERN AVE, TEMPE, AZ, WAS DISCIPLINED BY DEA ON NOVEMBER 28, 1994
DISCIPLINARY ACTION: SURRENDER OF CONTROLLED SUBSTANCE LICENSE
OFFENSE: DISCIPLINARY ACTION BY ANOTHER STATE OR AGENCY

NOTES: STATE BOARD.

CLARKE, GEORGE MD, LICENSE NUMBER 0004071, WAS DISCIPLINED BY ARIZONA ON JANUARY 21, 1995
DISCIPLINARY ACTION: 60-MONTH PROBATION; REQUIRED TO ENTER AN IMPAIRED PHYSICIAN PROGRAM OR SUBSTANCE ABUSE TREATMENT
OFFENSE: SUBSTANCE ABUSE

NOTES: FROM 8/88 UNTIL 7/92, HE WAS UNDER A STIPULATION AND ORDER WITH THE BOARD FOR CHEMICAL DEPENDENCY; IN 8/94, HAD RELAPSED IN THE USE OF DRUGS AND ALCOHOL AT WHICH HIS MEDICAL LICENSE WAS INACTIVATED; PARTICIPATED IN OUTPATIENT, INPATIENT AND CHEMICAL TREATMENT PROGRAMS BETWEEN 8/94 AND 12/94 AND REQUESTED REACTIVATION OF LICENSE IN 12/94. REACTIVATION TO PROBATION WITH CONDITIONS: MUST IMMEDIATELY PARTICIPATE IN A BOARD-APPROVED MONITORED AFTERCARE TREATMENT PROGRAM WHOSE THERAPIST MUST SUBMIT QUARTERLY REPORTS; MUST PARTICIPATE IN A 12-STEP RECOVERY PROGRAM AS DETERMINED BY HIS TREATING THERAPIST AND ATTEND AT LEAST THREE WEEKLY MEETINGS; SHALL OBTAIN A BOARD-APPROVED TREATING PHYSICIAN; SHALL ABSTAIN COMPLETELY FROM THE CONSUMPTION OF ALCOHOLIC BEVERAGES AND DRUGS EXCEPT WHEN PRESCRIBED BY HIS TREATING PHYSICIAN; MUST SUBMIT TO WITNESSED RANDOM BIOLOGICAL FLUID COLLECTION; SHALL KEEP A LOG OF ANY AND ALL MEDICATIONS PRESCRIBED FOR HIM; SHALL SUBMIT TO ANY EXAMINATIONS OR THERAPY ORDERED BY BOARD; SHALL APPEAR BEFORE BOARD FOR INTERVIEWS UPON REQUEST; SHALL INFORM BOARD OF CHANGE OF ADDRESS OR IF AWAY FOR MORE THAN FIVE DAYS.

CLARKE, GEORGE M MD, LICENSE NUMBER A020090 OF KINGMAN, AZ, WAS DISCIPLINED BY CALIFORNIA ON NOVEMBER 1, 1990

DISCIPLINARY ACTION: LICENSE REVOCATION
OFFENSE: DISCIPLINARY ACTION BY ANOTHER STATE OR AGENCY

NOTES: ARIZONA BOARD IMPOSED RESTRICTIONS AND CONDITIONS ON PRACTICE. DEFAULT DECISION.

CLAYTON, DEANNA MD, WAS DISCIPLINED BY ARIZONA ON JANUARY 29, 1999
DISCIPLINARY ACTION: PROBATION; RESTRICTION PLACED ON LICENSE

NOTES: LICENSE REACTIVATED UNDER FOLLOWING PROBATIONARY CONDITIONS: MUST COMPLY WITH THE TERMS OF THE MONITORED AFTERCARE PROGRAM AGREEMENT; TAKE AND PASS THE SPEX EXAM AND WORK UNDER SUPERVISION. THE BOARD DID NOT DISCUSS SPECIFICS OF THIS MOTION. ON 3/24/99 ORDER WAS CLARIFIED, SHE WAS PLACED ON A FIVE YEAR PROBATION WITH THE FOLLOWING TERMS: SHE IS ALLOWED TO REVIEW RECORDS, DO HEALTH HISTORY AND PHYSICALS AT SPECIFIED FACILITY; SHE PRACTICE A LIMITED SCOPE OF MEDICINE, WHILE SUPERVISED AT SPECIFIED FACILITY; IF SHE WANTS TO EXPAND HER SCOPE OF PRACTICE, SHE MUST TAKE AND PASS THE SPEX AND APPEAR BEFORE THE BOARD.

CLAYTON, DEANNA D MD, LICENSE NUMBER 23639, WAS DISCIPLINED BY ARIZONA ON JANUARY 25, 1997
DISCIPLINARY ACTION: LICENSE SUSPENSION; REQUIRED TO ENTER AN IMPAIRED PHYSICIAN PROGRAM OR SUBSTANCE ABUSE TREATMENT
OFFENSE: FAILURE TO COMPLY WITH PREVIOUS BOARD ORDER

NOTES: DRANK ALCOHOL AND INGESTED COCAINE IN VIOLATION OF THE TERMS OF THE 1/19/96 REHABILITATION ORDER. CONDITIONS OF INACTIVE LICENSE: SHE AGREES TO ENTER LONG TERM INPATIENT TREATMENT FOR CHEMICAL DEPENDENCY AND ALCOHOLISM AND TO SUCCESSFULLY COMPLETE ALL TREATMENT RECOMMENDED BY THE TREATMENT FACILITY; SHE AGREES NOT TO PRACTICE IN ARIZONA OR ANY OTHER STATE WHILE HER ARIZONA LICENSE IS IN INACTIVE STATUS; SHE MAY NOT HOLD OR MAINTAIN A CONTROLLED SUBSTANCE CERTIFICATE WITH THE DRUG ENFORCEMENT ADMINISTRATION OR WRITE OR REFILL PRESCRIPTIONS AS LONG AS HER LICENSE IS CLASSIFIED AS INACTIVE; PRIOR TO HER LICENSE BEING PLACED ON INACTIVE STATUS, SHE WILL PAY ALL FEES REQUIRED BY THE MEDICAL PRACTICE ACT; SHE MAY NOT REQUEST REACTIVATION OF HER LICENSE UNTIL SHE MEETS WITH THE BOARD AT A REGULARLY SCHEDULED MEETING AND COMPLIES WITH ALL REQUESTS OF THE BOARD WHICH MAY INCLUDE, BUT ARE NOT LIMITED TO, EXTENDED INPATIENT TREATMENT, PSYCHIATRIC AND PSYCHOMETRIC EVALUATION, PHYSICAL EXAMINATION AND TESTING, AND WRITTEN AND/OR ORAL COMPETENCY EXAMINATIONS. LICENSE PLACED ON INACTIVE STATUS.

CLEMANS, WILLIAM MD, LICENSE NUMBER 3395, WAS DISCIPLINED BY ARIZONA ON SEPTEMBER 23, 1999
DISCIPLINARY ACTION: PROBATION
OFFENSE: NONCOMPLIANCE WITH A PROFESSIONAL RULE

NOTES: FAILURE TO MAINTAIN ADEQUATE PATIENT RECORDS. DECREE OF CENSURE ISSUED.

CLEMENTS, MARK DO, LICENSE NUMBER 0002355, WAS DISCIPLINED BY ARIZONA ON NOVEMBER 21, 1990
DISCIPLINARY ACTION: 36-MONTH PROBATION; REQUIRED TO ENTER AN IMPAIRED PHYSICIAN PROGRAM OR SUBSTANCE ABUSE TREATMENT
OFFENSE: SUBSTANCE ABUSE

NOTES: PRIOR TO 10/23/90 SELF-ADMINISTERED LORTABS AND XANAX FOR THE RELIEF OF PAIN DUE TO BACK INJURY WHILE NOT UNDER A PHYSICIAN'S CARE AND HAD NOT BEEN PRESCRIBED LORTABS AND XANAX; ON VARIOUS OCCASIONS PRIOR TO 10/23/90 REMOVED VARIOUS AMOUNTS OF LORTABS AND DARVOCET FROM BOTTLES OF MEDICATIONS AT HIS PLACE OF EMPLOYMENT; HIS URINE SAMPLE TAKEN ON 10/23/90 TESTED POSITIVE FOR XANAX, DARVOCET, AND CANNABINOID; ADMITTED TO PROBLEM WITH ABUSE OF CONTROLLED SUBSTANCES. PROBATION UNDER TERMS AND CONDITIONS: SHALL SUBMIT TO BIOLOGICAL FLUID TESTING UPON BOARD REQUEST; SHALL COMPLETE A CHEMICAL ABUSE TREATMENT PROGRAM CONSISTING OF AT LEAST TWO INDIVIDUAL AND TWO GROUP COUNSELING SESSIONS PER MONTH AND UNDER THE SUPERVISION OF A BOARD APPROVED PSYCHIATRIST OR PSYCHOLOGIST WHO SHALL SUBMIT TO THE BOARD AN INITIAL EVALUATION AND DIAGNOSIS AND HIS OR HER TREATMENT PLAN WITH QUARTERLY REPORTS THEREAFTER; SHALL USE NO CONTROLLED SUBSTANCE OR PRESCRIPTION ONLY MEDICATION UNLESS PRESCRIBED BY HIS ATTENDING PHYSICIAN; SHALL NOT CONSUME ALCOHOL; SHALL MEET REGULARLY WITH THE BOARD TO REVIEW HIS COMPLIANCE; SHALL AUTHORIZE ANY ATTENDING PHYSICIAN, PSYCHIATRIST, OR PSYCHOLOGIST TO RELEASE TO THE BOARD ALL RECORDS PERTAINING TO HIS CARE AND TREATMENT. PROBATION SATISFIED IN FULL ON 11/21/93.

CLOUSE, RICHARD G MD, LICENSE NUMBER 0014929, WAS DISCIPLINED BY ARIZONA ON OCTOBER 30, 1990
DISCIPLINARY ACTION: LICENSE REVOCATION
OFFENSE: SEXUAL ABUSE OF OR SEXUAL MISCONDUCT WITH A PATIENT

NOTES: INAPPROPRIATE CONTACT WITH PATIENT DURING GYNECOLOGICAL EXAMINATION. SHALL NOT REAPPLY FOR 3 YEARS.

CLOUSE, RICHARD G MD, DATE OF BIRTH JUNE 27, 1956 OF 3700 WEST KENT DR, CHANDLER, AZ, WAS DISCIPLINED BY MEDICARE ON NOVEMBER 4, 1991
DISCIPLINARY ACTION: EXCLUSION FROM THE MEDICARE AND/OR MEDICAID PROGRAM
OFFENSE: DISCIPLINARY ACTION BY ANOTHER STATE OR AGENCY

NOTES: LICENSE REVOCATION OR SUSPENSION.

COBB, CHARLES R MD, LICENSE NUMBER 0010147, WAS DISCIPLINED BY ARIZONA ON JULY 15, 1993
DISCIPLINARY ACTION: LICENSE REVOCATION
OFFENSE: NONCOMPLIANCE WITH A PROFESSIONAL RULE

NOTES: FAILED TO KEEP BOARD INFORMED OF HIS CURRENT ADDRESS; FAILED TO PRODUCE RECORDS IN RESPONSE TO SUBPOENAS ISSUED BY THE BOARD REGARDING TWO PENDING MALPRACTICE CLAIMS, WHERE SUBPOENAS WERE LEGALLY ISSUED AND SENT TO HIM ON 3/31/92; INFORMED ON 5/6/92 THAT LICENSE HAD BEEN SUSPENDED BECAUSE HE HAD NOT RENEWED IT; FAILED TO APPEAR AT THIS HEARING.

COBB, CHARLES R MD, LICENSE NUMBER 0A22892 OF SAIPAN, GUAM, WAS DISCIPLINED BY CALIFORNIA ON APRIL 27, 1995
DISCIPLINARY ACTION: LICENSE REVOCATION

OFFENSE: DISCIPLINARY ACTION BY ANOTHER STATE OR AGENCY

NOTES: DEFAULT REVOCATION BY ARIZONA BOARD FOR FAILING TO RESPOND TO BOARD SUBPOENAS FOR RECORDS RELATED TO TWO MALPRACTICE CLAIMS. FAILING TO ANSWER ARIZONA BOARD CORRESPONDENCE OR PROVIDE HIS NEW ADDRESS. DEFAULT DECISION.

COBB, CHARLES R MD, DATE OF BIRTH AUGUST 22, 1939 OF COMMON WEALTH HEALTH CENTER, GUAM, SAIPAN MP, WAS DISCIPLINED BY MEDICARE ON FEBRUARY 14, 1996
DISCIPLINARY ACTION: EXCLUSION FROM THE MEDICARE AND/OR MEDICAID PROGRAM
OFFENSE: DISCIPLINARY ACTION BY ANOTHER STATE OR AGENCY

NOTES: LICENSE REVOKED FOR REASONS BEARING ON PROFESSIONAL PERFORMANCE.

COCHRAN, WILLIAM M MD, LICENSE NUMBER 0015469, WAS DISCIPLINED BY ARIZONA ON OCTOBER 20, 1994
DISCIPLINARY ACTION: LICENSE SUSPENSION; REQUIRED TO ENTER AN IMPAIRED PHYSICIAN PROGRAM OR SUBSTANCE ABUSE TREATMENT
OFFENSE: FAILURE TO COMPLY WITH PREVIOUS BOARD ORDER

NOTES: USED FENTANYL AND VERSED IN 9/94 IN VIOLATION OF THE TERMS OF THE BOARD'S ORDER DATED 12/21/93. CONDITIONS AND TERMS INCLUDE: HE AGREES NOT TO PRACTICE MEDICINE IN ARIZONA OR ANY OTHER STATE IN U.S. OR FOREIGN COUNTRY WHILE ARIZONA LICENSE IS ON INACTIVE STATUS; MAY NOT HOLD REGISTRATION WITH THE DRUG ENFORCEMENT ADMINISTRATION OR WRITE PRESCRIPTIONS AS LONG AS HIS LICENSE IS CLASSIFIED AS INACTIVE; HE AGREES NOT TO REQUEST REACTIVATION OF HIS LICENSE UNTIL HE ENTERS A LONG-TERM RESIDENTIAL/IN-PATIENT TREATMENT FOR CHEMICAL DEPENDENCY AND UNTIL HE SUCCESSFULLY COMPLETES ALL TREATMENT RECOMMENDED BY THE FACILITY; AGREES THAT HE SHALL NOT REQUEST REACTIVATION UNTIL HE MEETS WITH THE BOARD AT A REGULARLY SCHEDULED MEETING OF THE BOARD AND COMPLIES WITH ANY REQUESTS OF THE BOARD.

COCHRAN, WILLIAM M MD, LICENSE NUMBER 0015469, WAS DISCIPLINED BY ARIZONA ON APRIL 8, 1995
DISCIPLINARY ACTION: 60-MONTH PROBATION; RESTRICTION PLACED ON LICENSE
OFFENSE: FAILURE TO COMPLY WITH PREVIOUS BOARD ORDER

NOTES: IN 10/94, HOSPITAL MEMBERSHIP AND CLINICAL PRIVILEGES WERE SUMMARILY SUSPENDED BASED ON SUSPENSION BY ANOTHER HOSPITAL FOR SELF-ADMINISTRATION OF MEDICINE WHILE PERFORMING A CASE FOR WHICH THERE WAS A SIGNIFICANT RISK; DRUG USE VIOLATED PREVIOUS BOARD ORDER; ON 2/95, HOSPITAL PRIVILEGES REVOKED. HAS NOT PRACTICED CLINICAL PEDIATRICS SINCE 1982. COMPLETED INPATIENT CHEMICAL DEPENDENCY TREATMENT IN 1/95. REINSTATEMENT TO PROBATION WITH CONDITIONS: MUST IMMEDIATELY PARTICIPATE IN A BOARD-APPROVED MONITORED AFTERCARE TREATMENT PROGRAM WHOSE THERAPIST MUST SUBMIT QUARTERLY REPORTS; HAS PREVIOUSLY PARTICIPATED IN 90 12-STEP MEETINGS IN 90 DAYS AND SHALL PARTICIPATE IN A 12-STEP RECOVERY PROGRAM AS DETERMINED BY HIS TREATING THERAPIST AND ATTEND AT LEAST THREE WEEKLY MEETINGS; SHALL OBTAIN A BOARD-APPROVED TREATING PHYSICIAN; SHALL ABSTAIN COMPLETELY FROM THE CONSUMPTION OF ALCOHOLIC BEVERAGES AND DRUGS EXCEPT WHEN PRESCRIBED BY HIS TREATING PHYSICIAN; MUST SUBMIT TO WITNESSED RANDOM BIOLOGICAL FLUID COLLECTION; MUST KEEP A LOG OF ANY AND ALL MEDICATIONS PRESCRIBED FOR HIM; SHALL SUBMIT TO ANY EXAMINATIONS OR THERAPY ORDERED BY BOARD; SHALL APPEAR BEFORE BOARD FOR INTERVIEWS UPON REQUEST; SHALL INFORM BOARD OF CHANGE OF ADDRESS OR IF AWAY FOR MORE THAN FIVE DAYS; SHALL ENROLL IN AND SUCCESSFULLY COMPLETE FORMAL TRAINING OF NOT LESS THAN THREE MONTHS AT A BOARD-APPROVED INSTITUTE IN AN AREA OF MEDICINE OTHER THAN ANESTHESIOLOGY AND SHALL PRACTICE MEDICINE ONLY IN THE APPROVED TRAINING PROGRAM UNTIL FURTHER ORDER OF THE BOARD; SHALL NOT PRACTICE ANESTHESIOLOGY. ON 10/21/95 HIS REQUEST THAT THIS ORDER BE MODIFIED WAS DENIED. ON 4/20/96 ORDER AMENDED ALLOWING HIM TO PERFORM INTAKE HISTORIES AND PHYSICALS, WRITE ORDERS FOR DISPENSING MEDICATION FROM THE FACILITY PHARMACY AND SIGN ORDERS FOR ALCOHOL DETOXIFICATION; HIS PERFORMANCE AND ORDERS SHALL BE REVIEWED AND HE SHALL PROVIDE QUARTERLY WRITTEN REPORTS TO THE BOARD. ON 1/24/97 ORDER AMENDED ALLOWING HIM TO PRACTICE ADDICTION MEDICINE. ON 3/15/97 SECOND AMENDMENT TO ORDER OF PROBATION: MAY PERFORM INTAKE HISTORIES AND PHYSICALS, WRITE OR TELEPHONE PRESCRIPTION ORDERS AND REFILLS, AND ISSUE ORDERS FOR CHEMICAL DETOXIFICATION FOR VARIOUS SPECIFIED FACILITIES.

COCHRAN, WILLIAM MICHAEL MD OF 3390 N. CAMPBELL AVE. STE. 110, TUCSON, AZ, WAS DISCIPLINED BY DEA ON DECEMBER 28, 1994
DISCIPLINARY ACTION: SURRENDER OF CONTROLLED SUBSTANCE LICENSE
OFFENSE: DISCIPLINARY ACTION BY ANOTHER STATE OR AGENCY

COELHO, ALDEMIR T MD, DATE OF BIRTH JULY 14, 1942 OF 1444 E COLT ROAD, TEMPE, AZ, WAS DISCIPLINED BY MEDICARE ON NOVEMBER 21, 1993
DISCIPLINARY ACTION: 12-MONTH EXCLUSION FROM THE MEDICARE AND/OR MEDICAID PROGRAM

NOTES: EXCLUDED BASED ON A RECOMMENDATION FROM A PEER REVIEW ORGANIZATION THAT HE VIOLATED STATUTORY OBLIGATIONS.

COHEN, EDWIN CHARLES MD, DATE OF BIRTH MARCH 13, 1930 OF 6855 E PARADISE LANE, PHOENIX, AZ, WAS DISCIPLINED BY MEDICARE ON OCTOBER 20, 1999
DISCIPLINARY ACTION: EXCLUSION FROM THE MEDICARE AND/OR MEDICAID PROGRAM
OFFENSE: CRIMINAL CONVICTION OR PLEA OF GUILTY, NOLO CONTENDERE, OR NO CONTEST TO A CRIME

NOTES: CONVICTED OF A CRIME INVOLVING THE MEDICARE, MEDICAID, MATERNAL AND CHILD HEALTH SERVICES BLOCK GRANT OR BLOCK GRANTS TO STATES FOR SOCIAL SERVICES PROGRAMS.

COHEN, NATHANIEL M MD, DATE OF BIRTH AUGUST 24, 1922, LICENSE NUMBER 0028463 OF SALT LAKE CITY, UT, WAS DISCIPLINED BY KENTUCKY ON DECEMBER 1, 1992
DISCIPLINARY ACTION: FINE
OFFENSE: NONCOMPLIANCE WITH A PROFESSIONAL RULE

NOTES: FAILED TO COMPLETE REQUIRED CONTINUING MEDICAL EDUCATION IN THE AREA OF HIV/AIDS.

COHEN, NATHANIEL M MD, DATE OF BIRTH AUGUST 24, 1922, LICENSE NUMBER 0021299 OF 258 HARVARD ST #323, BROOKLINE, MA, WAS DISCIPLINED BY MASSACHUSETTS ON JULY 26, 1995
DISCIPLINARY ACTION: RESTRICTION PLACED ON LICENSE
OFFENSE: LOSS OR RESTRICTION OF HOSPITAL PRIVILEGES

NOTES: LOSS OF HOSPITAL PRIVILEGES.

COHEN, NATHANIEL M MD, DATE OF BIRTH AUGUST 24, 1922, LICENSE NUMBER 1062523 OF 5655 EAST RIVER RD, STE 101-207, TUCSON, AZ, WAS DISCIPLINED BY MICHIGAN ON APRIL 17, 1996
DISCIPLINARY ACTION: RESTRICTION PLACED ON LICENSE
OFFENSE: DISCIPLINARY ACTION BY ANOTHER STATE OR AGENCY

NOTES: FAILURE TO REPORT/COMPLY.

COHEN, NATHANIEL M MD, DATE OF BIRTH AUGUST 24, 1922, LICENSE NUMBER 0028463 OF TUCSON, AZ, WAS DISCIPLINED BY KENTUCKY ON MAY 20, 1996
DISCIPLINARY ACTION: RESTRICTION PLACED ON LICENSE
OFFENSE: DISCIPLINARY ACTION BY ANOTHER STATE OR AGENCY

NOTES: DISCIPLINARY ACTION TAKEN BY THE MASSACHUSETTS BOARD. MAY NOT ATTEND DELIVERIES, PRACTICE IN AN EMERGENCY ROOM, NEONATAL OR PEDIATRIC INTENSIVE CARE UNIT OR ANY CRITICAL CARE SETTING; PROHIBITED FROM PRACTICING MEDICINE EXCEPT IN A GROUP PRACTICE OR INSTITUTIONAL SETTING WHERE SUPERVISION AND BACKUP ARE READILY AVAILABLE.

COHEN, NATHANIEL M MD, LICENSE NUMBER 0425680 OF 5655 EAST RIVER RD SUITE 101-207, TUCSON, AZ, WAS DISCIPLINED BY KANSAS ON JULY 23, 1996
DISCIPLINARY ACTION: RESTRICTION PLACED ON LICENSE
OFFENSE: DISCIPLINARY ACTION BY ANOTHER STATE OR AGENCY

NOTES: ACTION IN MASSACHUSETTS ON 7/26/95 LIMITING HIS KANSAS LICENSE FOR AN INDEFINITE PERIOD, BUT AT LEAST AS LONG AS THE MASSACHUSETTS BOARD MAINTAINS ITS LIMITATIONS. KANSAS PROHIBITS HIM FROM: ATTENDING DELIVERIES; PRACTICING IN AN EMERGENCY ROOM, NEONATAL OR PEDIATRIC INTENSIVE CARE UNIT, OR ANY CRITICAL CARE SETTING; AND PRACTICING MEDICINE EXCEPT IN A GROUP PRACTICE OR INSTITUTIONAL SETTING WHERE SUPERVISION AND BACK-UP ARE READILY AVAILABLE.

COHEN, NATHANIEL M MD, DATE OF BIRTH AUGUST 24, 1922, LICENSE NUMBER 0032717 OF 5655 EAST RIVER ROAD #107-207, TUCSON, AZ, WAS DISCIPLINED BY WISCONSIN ON AUGUST 22, 1996
DISCIPLINARY ACTION: RESTRICTION PLACED ON LICENSE; MONITORING OF PHYSICIAN PERFORMANCE
OFFENSE: DISCIPLINARY ACTION BY ANOTHER STATE OR AGENCY

NOTES: ON 7/25/95 THE MASSACHUSETTS BOARD IMPOSED DISCIPLINE UPON HIS LICENSE TO PRACTICE MEDICINE. HIS WISCONSIN LICENSE IS LIMITED AS FOLLOWS: SHALL REFRAIN FROM PRACTICING OBSTETRICS, EMERGENCY MEDICINE, NEONATAL MEDICINE, SURGERY, PEDIATRIC INTENSIVE CARE OR IN ANY OTHER CRITICAL CARE SETTING; SHALL REFRAIN FROM THE PRACTICE OF MEDICINE IN WISCONSIN OR THE PRACTICE OF MEDICINE ELSEWHERE UNDER THE USE OF HIS WISCONSIN LICENSE EXCEPT IN A GROUP PRACTICE OR INSTITUTIONAL SETTING AND UNDER SUPERVISION BY OTHER LICENSED PHYSICIANS; PRIOR TO ENGAGING IN THE PRACTICE OF MEDICINE IN WISCONSIN, SHALL SUBMIT AND OBTAIN APPROVAL BY THE BOARD OF A PLAN OF SUPERVISION FOR HIS PRACTICE; SHALL IMMEDIATELY SURRENDER ALL INDICIA OF WISCONSIN REGISTRATION TO THE DEPARTMENT MONITOR WHO SHALL REISSUE CREDENTIALS MARKED "LIMITED."

COHEN, NATHANIEL M MD, LICENSE NUMBER 00G1904 OF TUCSON, AZ, WAS DISCIPLINED BY CALIFORNIA ON AUGUST 30, 1996
DISCIPLINARY ACTION: SURRENDER OF LICENSE

NOTES: WHILE CHARGES PENDING.

COHEN, NATHANIEL M MD, DATE OF BIRTH AUGUST 24, 1922, LICENSE NUMBER J5730, WAS DISCIPLINED BY TEXAS ON MAY 10, 1997
OFFENSE: DISCIPLINARY ACTION BY ANOTHER STATE OR AGENCY

NOTES: ON 7/26/95 ENTERED INTO AN AGREED ORDER WITH THE MASSACHUSETTS BOARD RESTRICTING HIS LICENSE BASED ON SOME HOSPITAL PRIVILEGES BEING WITHDRAWN FOLLOWING TWO INCIDENTS IN WHICH HIS RESPONSE TO TWO CESAREAN SECTIONS WAS DEEMED TO BE INSUFFICIENTLY AGGRESSIVE; FAILED TO REPORT RESTRICTION TO THE BOARD WITHIN 30 DAYS SHALL NOT PRACTICE MEDICINE IN TEXAS UNTIL HE REQUESTS PERMISSION IN WRITING TO RESUME THE PRACTICE OF MEDICINE THERE, AND PERSONALLY APPEARS BEFORE THE BOARD TO PROVIDE SUFFICIENT EVIDENCE THAT HE IS OTHERWISE COMPETENT TO PRACTICE MEDICINE SAFELY INCLUDING AT A MINIMUM: EVIDENCE THAT THE 7/26/95 ORDER'S TERMS AND CONDITIONS HAVE BEEN TERMINATED/LIFTED OR MODIFIED; AND EVIDENCE THAT HE IS NOT THE SUBJECT OF ANY OTHER STATE DISCIPLINARY ACTION, INVESTIGATION, OR PROCEEDINGS; SHALL COOPERATE WITH THE BOARD IN VERIFYING COMPLIANCE INCLUDING PROVIDING COPIES OF ANY DOCUMENTS SUBMITTED TO MASSACHUSETTS UPON REQUEST; SHALL GIVE A COPY OF THIS ORDER TO ANY HEALTH CARE ENTITY WHERE HE HAS PRIVILEGES; SHALL INFORM THE BOARD OF CHANGE OF ADDRESS WITHIN 10 DAYS; SHALL NOT SEEK MODIFICATION FOR ONE YEAR.

COHEN, NATHANIEL MAURICE MD, DATE OF BIRTH AUGUST 24, 1922, LICENSE NUMBER 0003379 OF 5655 EAST RIVER ROAD NO. 101-207, TUCSON, AZ, WAS DISCIPLINED BY HAWAII ON OCTOBER 30, 1996
DISCIPLINARY ACTION: RESTRICTION PLACED ON LICENSE; MONITORING OF PHYSICIAN PERFORMANCE
OFFENSE: DISCIPLINARY ACTION BY ANOTHER STATE OR AGENCY

NOTES: RESTRICTIONS ON LICENSES IN MICHIGAN (4/17/96), KANSAS (7/23/96), AND KENTUCKY (5/17/96). HAWAII ORDER FOR INDEFINITE LIMITED LICENSE. TERMS AND CONDITIONS: SHALL COMPLY WITH MICHIGAN, KANSAS, AND KENTUCKY TERMS AND CONDITIONS: PROHIBITED FROM ATTENDING DELIVERIES OR PRACTICING IN AN EMERGENCY ROOM, NEONATAL, OR PEDIATRIC INTENSIVE CARE UNIT, OR ANY CRITICAL CARE SETTING; SHALL ONLY PRACTICE MEDICINE IN A GROUP PRACTICE OR INSTITUTIONAL SETTING WHERE SUPERVISION AND BACK-UP ARE READILY AVAILABLE; RESTRICTIONS IN HAWAII FOR AT LEAST AS LONG AS MASSACHUSETTS MAINTAINS LIMITATIONS.

COHN, FREDERICK MD, LICENSE NUMBER 0003778, WAS DISCIPLINED BY ARIZONA ON OCTOBER 14, 1993
DISCIPLINARY ACTION: RESTRICTION PLACED ON LICENSE

NOTES: LICENSE REACTIVATED UNDER THE FOLLOWING TERMS: SHALL NOT PRACTICE OBSTETRICS OR GYNECOLOGY AND SHALL NOT PERFORM ELECTIVE TERMINATION OF PREGNANCIES EXCEPT ON AN EMERGENCY BASIS ONLY; SHALL PROMPTLY SUPPLY

THE BOARD WITH EVIDENCE THAT HE HAS SATISFIED THIS BOARD'S CONTINUING MEDICAL EDUCATION REQUIREMENTS TO DATE.

COLLETTE, DAVID J MD OF FLAGSTAFF, AZ, WAS DISCIPLINED BY UTAH ON DECEMBER 4, 1990
DISCIPLINARY ACTION: CONTROLLED SUBSTANCE LICENSE PLACED ON PROBATION

NOTES: LICENSE TO PRESCRIBE SCHEDULES II THROUGH V PLACED ON FIVE YEAR PROBATION WITH THE CONDITION THAT HE MAY ONLY PRESCRIBE CONTROLLED SUBSTANCES IN THE WORK CARE INDUSTRIAL CLINIC AND EMERGICARE CLINIC. ON 8/28/95 PROBATION TERMINATED IN FAVOR OF HIM AGREEING TO CERTAIN TERMS AND CONDITIONS REGARDING HIS RETURN TO MEDICINE IN UTAH.

COMAS, THOMAS E MD, LICENSE NUMBER A022420 OF PHOENIX, AZ, WAS DISCIPLINED BY CALIFORNIA ON AUGUST 8, 1991
DISCIPLINARY ACTION: SURRENDER OF LICENSE

NOTES: VOLUNTARY SURRENDER WHILE CHARGES PENDING.

COMPTON, SAMUEL P JR MD, LICENSE NUMBER 0004318 OF PHOENIX, AZ, WAS DISCIPLINED BY ARIZONA ON APRIL 14, 1993
DISCIPLINARY ACTION: 60-MONTH PROBATION; RESTRICTION PLACED ON CONTROLLED SUBSTANCE LICENSE
OFFENSE: OVERPRESCRIBING OR MISPRESCRIBING DRUGS

NOTES: PRACTICE OF PRESCRIBING PAIN MEDICATION AND OTHER CONTROLLED SUBSTANCES FOR OTHER THAN THERAPEUTIC USES IN SEVERAL PATIENTS WHOM HE HAD BEEN SEEING FOR PERIODS OF 12 TO 20 YEARS SOME OF WHOM HE KNEW TO BE ABUSERS; ALSO POOR RECORD KEEPING WITH REGARD TO WHY THE DRUGS WERE PRESCRIBED. PROBATION WITH FOLLOWING TERMS AND CONDITIONS: WITHIN 21 DAYS SHALL SURRENDER TO THE DRUG ENFORCEMENT ADMINISTRATION HIS CONTROLLED SUBSTANCES REGISTRATION CERTIFICATE FOR SCHEDULE II AND SCHEDULE III CONTROLLED SUBSTANCES AND SHALL PROVIDE WRITTEN EVIDENCE TO THE BOARD OF SUCH SURRENDER. WITHIN 12 MONTHS SHALL OBTAIN 40 HOURS CONTINUING MEDICAL EDUCATION ACCEPTABLE TO THE BOARD IN PAIN MANAGEMENT OR A MINI-RESIDENCY IN PAIN MANAGEMENT. THESE HOURS SHALL BE IN ADDITION TO THE 20 HOURS CONTINUING MEDICAL EDUCATION REQUIRED BY LAW FOR ANNUAL RENEWAL OF AN ARIZONA MEDICAL LICENSE. WITHIN NINE MONTHS HE SHALL TAKE AND PASS WITH A GRADE OF 75 OR MORE THE SPECIAL PURPOSE LICENSING EXAMINATION.

CONE, JOHN A MD, LICENSE NUMBER 0021884, WAS DISCIPLINED BY ARIZONA ON JANUARY 18, 1995

NOTES: SHALL CEASE FROM THE SELF-ADMINISTRATION OF VALIUM OR ANY OTHER CONTROLLED SUBSTANCE OR PRESCRIPTION-ONLY DRUG. SHALL OBTAIN A REGULAR TREATING PHYSICIAN FOR PURPOSES OF OBTAINING PRESCRIPTIONS FOR VALIUM AND ANY OTHER CONTROLLED SUBSTANCE OR PRESCRIPTION-ONLY DRUG.

CONN, VICTORIA ANN MD, WAS DISCIPLINED BY ARIZONA ON APRIL 14, 1993
DISCIPLINARY ACTION: RESTRICTION PLACED ON LICENSE

NOTES: SHALL BE OFFERED A LICENSE WITH THE FOLLOWING STIPULATIONS: SHALL CONTINUE IN PSYCHIATRIC THERAPY WITH HER CURRENT THERAPIST OR OTHER THERAPIST APPROVED BY THE BOARD ON A FREQUENCY DETERMINED BY THE THERAPIST; SHALL NOT PRACTICE MEDICINE (INCLUDING PSYCHIATRY) IN A SOLO PRACTICE SETTING; SHALL PRACTICE MEDICINE (INCLUDING PSYCHIATRY) ONLY IN ASSOCIATION WITH ANOTHER PHYSICIAN OR PHYSICIANS; PRIOR TO PRACTICING MEDICINE IN ARIZONA SHE SHALL NOTIFY THE BOARD OF HER INTENTION TO PRACTICE IN ARIZONA AND SHALL MEET WITH THE BOARD; SHALL GIVE WRITTEN AUTHORIZATION TO HER THERAPIST AND EMPLOYERS TO PROVIDE MEDICAL RECORDS AND INFORMATION TO THE BOARD. ON 4/12/94 ORDER MODIFIED TO ONLY REQUIRE THAT PRIOR TO PRACTICING (INCLUDING PSYCHIATRY) IN ARIZONA SHE SHALL NOTIFY THE BOARD AND MEET WITH THEM.

COOPER, LAVONT L MD, LICENSE NUMBER 0017051, WAS DISCIPLINED BY ARIZONA ON JULY 31, 1990
DISCIPLINARY ACTION: RESTRICTION PLACED ON LICENSE

NOTES: MUST PERFORM NO EXAM OF ANY KIND, INCLUDING BUT NOT LIMITED TO PELVIC OR BREAST EXAM, OF ANY FEMALE PATIENT WITHOUT PRESENCE OF A FEMALE ATTENDANT. MUST CAUSE ATTENDANT TO INITIAL EACH PATIENT'S CHART INDICATING HER ATTENDANCE.

COOPER, LAVONT L MD, LICENSE NUMBER 0017051, WAS DISCIPLINED BY ARIZONA ON APRIL 4, 1995
DISCIPLINARY ACTION: MONITORING OF PHYSICIAN PERFORMANCE
OFFENSE: FAILURE TO COMPLY WITH PREVIOUS BOARD ORDER

NOTES: INTERVIEWED REGARDING FAILURE TO ADHERE TO THE BOARD'S 7/31/90 ORDER; AFTER BEING TOLD OF AN OMINOUS TRACING AND NEGATIVE CONTRACTION STRESS TEST, SHOULD HAVE EVALUATED A PATIENT EARLIER; MISMANAGED SEVERAL CASES, ONE WITH INTRAUTERINE FETAL DEMISE AND OTHERS WITH VAGINAL LACERATIONS FOLLOWING DELIVERY. SHALL TAKE AND PASS THE AMERICAN COLLEGE OF OBSTETRICS AND GYNECOLOGY WRITTEN CERTIFICATION EXAMINATION IN 6/95 AND FORWARD HIS SCORE TO THE BOARD. SHALL MEET WITH THE BOARD AT A FUTURE MEETING. STAFF WILL CONDUCT A RANDOM HOSPITAL CHART SURVEY OF HIS OBSTETRICAL CASES.

COOPER, LAVONT L MD, LICENSE NUMBER 0017051, WAS DISCIPLINED BY ARIZONA ON MAY 1, 1996
DISCIPLINARY ACTION: LICENSE SUSPENSION; REQUIRED TO TAKE ADDITIONAL MEDICAL EDUCATION
OFFENSE: FAILURE TO COMPLY WITH PREVIOUS BOARD ORDER

NOTES: HAS NOT ADHERED TO THE REQUIREMENT OF THE 7/90 ORDER TO HAVE A FEMALE ATTENDANT INITIAL PATIENT'S CHART INDICATING THE PRESENCE OF AN ATTENDANT DURING EACH FEMALE PATIENT EXAMINATION; IN 4/93, BOARD RECEIVED INFORMATION THAT A HOSPITAL HAD SUMMARILY SUSPENDED HIS CLINICAL PRIVILEGES FOR A PERIOD NOT TO EXCEED 30 DAYS AND BASED ON HIS CARE AND TREATMENT OF THE FOLLOWING PATIENTS: HE DID NOT ORDER ANY LABORATORY TESTS THROUGHOUT LABOR AND DID NOT CONSIDER PLACENTAL ABRUPTION AS THE SOURCE OF FETAL DEMISE IN A PATIENT ADMITTED TO LABOR AND DELIVERY IN 4/92 WITH SHARP PAIN, WHO HAD SIGNIFICANT HEMORRHAGE FOLLOWING DELIVERY AND WAS TAKEN TO THE INTENSIVE CARE UNIT FOR MONITORING AND THERAPY AND SUSTAINED A CARDIOPULMONARY ARREST; IN A PATIENT FAILED TO NOTE VAGINAL, CERVICAL OR RECTAL LACERATIONS,

WHEN AN HOUR LATER SHE WAS FOUND BY ANOTHER PHYSICIAN TO HAVE A SECOND DEGREE DEEP VAGINAL LACERATION AND BILATERAL PERIUTERAL LACERATION WITH BLEEDING; FAILED TO NOTE VAGINAL LACERATIONS IN A PATIENT FOLLOWING A FORCEPS DELIVERY; IN ANOTHER PATIENT WHO WAS ADMITTED AT 39 WEEKS GESTATION, HE FAILED TO EVALUATE THE PATIENT AFTER BEING PAGED BY NURSES AT 9:50 AM REGARDING OMINOUS FETAL MONITOR SIGNS; ONE HOUR AND FORTY MINUTES AFTER INITIAL PAGE, HE ARRIVED AND PERFORMED A CESAREAN SECTION; INFANT WAS BRAIN DAMAGED AND DIED AT APPROXIMATELY 18 MONTHS OF AGE; IN 4/95 BOARD ORDERED TO PASS EXAM; IN 6/95, HE FAILED THE AMERICAN BOARD OF OBSTETRICS AND GYNECOLOGY CERTIFICATION EXAMINATION WITH A SCORE OF 66; AT THE TIME, HE WAS SEVERELY CLINICALLY DEPRESSED AND UNDER THE CARE OF A PSYCHIATRIST AND TAKING XANAX, PROZAC, VERAPAMIL, CORDORA, TRAZODONE AND RESTORIL; HOSPITALIZED FROM 7/95 FOR CLINICAL DEPRESSION BUT HAS SINCE BEEN DISCHARGED. SUSPENSION UNTIL HE PASSES THE SPECIAL PURPOSE EXAMINATION WITH A SCORE OF 75 OR GREATER; SHALL OBTAIN A TREATING PSYCHIATRIST APPROVED BY THE BOARD, WHO SHALL SUBMIT QUARTERLY REPORTS; SHALL SUCCESSFULLY COMPLETE 100 HOURS OF CONTINUING MEDICAL EDUCATION IN GENERAL OBSTETRICS.

COPPELLI, LUIS A MD, LICENSE NUMBER 9535, WAS DISCIPLINED BY ARIZONA ON SEPTEMBER 26, 1997
DISCIPLINARY ACTION: REPRIMAND
OFFENSE: SEXUAL ABUSE OF OR SEXUAL MISCONDUCT WITH A PATIENT

NOTES: HE NEVER FORMALLY TERMINATED THE DOCTOR-PATIENT RELATIONSHIP WITH A PATIENT HE SAW TWICE BETWEEN 10/4/93 AND 12/23/93 AND BECAME SEXUALLY INTIMATE WITH HER BEGINNING IN 4/94.

CORDES, DORIAN H MD, LICENSE NUMBER 0012403, WAS DISCIPLINED BY ARIZONA ON APRIL 11, 1992
DISCIPLINARY ACTION: REQUIRED TO ENTER AN IMPAIRED PHYSICIAN PROGRAM OR SUBSTANCE ABUSE TREATMENT; MONITORING OF PHYSICIAN PERFORMANCE

NOTES: MUST IMMEDIATELY PARTICIPATE IN A BOARD-APPROVED MONITORED AFTERCARE TREATMENT PROGRAM WHOSE THERAPIST MUST SUBMIT QUARTERLY REPORTS; MUST PARTICIPATE IN 90 12-STEP MEETINGS APPROPRIATE FOR SUBSTANCE ABUSE WITHIN 90 DAYS; MUST THEN PARTICIPATE IN A 12-STEP RECOVERY PROGRAM AS DETERMINED BY HIS TREATING THERAPIST AND ATTEND AT LEAST 3 WEEKLY MEETINGS; SHALL OBTAIN A BOARD-APPROVED TREATING PHYSICIAN; SHALL ABSTAIN COMPLETELY FROM THE CONSUMPTION OF ALCOHOLIC BEVERAGES AND DRUGS EXCEPT WHEN PRESCRIBED BY HIS TREATING PHYSICIAN; MUST SUBMIT TO WITNESSED RANDOM BIOLOGICAL FLUID COLLECTION; KEEP A LOG OF ANY AND ALL MEDICATIONS PRESCRIBED FOR HIM; SHALL SUBMIT TO ANY EXAMINATIONS OR THERAPY ORDERED BY THE BOARD; SHALL APPEAR BEFORE BOARD FOR INTERVIEWS UPON REQUEST; SHALL INFORM BOARD OF CHANGE OF ADDRESS OR IF AWAY FOR MORE THAN 5 DAYS. AS OF 1/21/95, ORDER TO BE TERMINATED IN 90 DAYS.

CORDES, DORIAN H MD, DATE OF BIRTH SEPTEMBER 27, 1938, LICENSE NUMBER 0019089 OF 1609 EAST LESTER, TUCSON, AZ, WAS DISCIPLINED BY WISCONSIN ON APRIL 26, 1995
DISCIPLINARY ACTION: SURRENDER OF LICENSE
OFFENSE: DISCIPLINARY ACTION BY ANOTHER STATE OR AGENCY

NOTES: ACTION IN ARIZONA EFFECTIVE 4/03/92 FORMALIZING HIS PARTICIPATION IN AN ALCOHOL REHABILITATION TREATMENT PROGRAM. THE ORDER WAS COMPLETED AND TERMINATED ON 4/21/95. HE HAS NOT PRACTICED IN WISCONSIN SINCE 1976 AND HAS NO INTENTION OF RENEWING HIS REGISTRATION OR RETURNING TO THE STATE. VOLUNTARY SURRENDER

CORDON, RICARDO M MD, LICENSE NUMBER 0015499, WAS DISCIPLINED BY ARIZONA ON JULY 15, 1993
OFFENSE: DISCIPLINARY ACTION BY ANOTHER STATE OR AGENCY

NOTES: FAILURE TO REPORT RESTRICTION IN PRIVILEGES BY THE MILITARY IN 1989 ON HIS LICENSE RENEWAL FORM; FAILED THE SPEX EXAMINATION IN ARIZONA. SHALL NOT ENGAGE IN THE PRACTICE OF MEDICINE IN ARIZONA UNTIL HE HAS FIRST ADVISED THE BOARD OF HIS INTENTION TO DO SO. THE BOARD MAY REQUIRE ADDITIONAL EXAMS OR INVESTIGATION IN ORDER TO SATISFY ITSELF THAT HE IS MEDICALLY COMPETENT TO PRACTICE.

CORDON, RICARDO M MD OF 1211 E AZTEC, GALLUP, NM, WAS DISCIPLINED BY DEA ON MAY 17, 1995
DISCIPLINARY ACTION: SURRENDER OF CONTROLLED SUBSTANCE LICENSE
OFFENSE: DISCIPLINARY ACTION BY ANOTHER STATE OR AGENCY

NOTES: STATE BOARD.

CORRAL, MARTHA ELENA RAMIREZ MD, WAS DISCIPLINED BY ARIZONA ON NOVEMBER 14, 1997
DISCIPLINARY ACTION: RESTRICTION PLACED ON LICENSE; MONITORING OF PHYSICIAN PERFORMANCE

NOTES: SHALL PRACTICE MEDICINE ONLY IN A GROUP SETTING; SHALL UNDERGO THERAPY BY A BOARD-APPROVED THERAPIST AND SHALL REMAIN IN THERAPY UNTIL FURTHER ORDER OF THE BOARD; SHALL INSTRUCT THE THERAPIST TO RELEASE TO THE BOARD, ALL RECORDS RELATING TO HER TREATMENT, AND TO SUBMIT QUARTERLY WRITTEN REPORTS.

CORRIGAN, JAMES P DO, LICENSE NUMBER 0002664 OF P.O. BOX 89, CHESTER SPRINGS, PA, WAS DISCIPLINED BY ARIZONA ON JULY 25, 1996
DISCIPLINARY ACTION: 6-MONTH PROBATION

NOTES: SHALL PREPARE AN INVENTORY LIST OF ALL PATIENT FILES BELONGING TO TWO SPECIFIED HEALTH PLANS WITHIN 10 DAYS; SHALL SUBMIT A COPY TO SPECIFIC HEALTH CARE PLAN ADMINISTRATORS WHO SHALL BE ASKED TO VERIFY THEM.

CORRIGAN, JAMES PATRICK DO, DATE OF BIRTH OCTOBER 25, 1951 OF 1 MATTHEW RUN, CHESTER SPRINGS, PA, WAS DISCIPLINED BY MEDICARE ON SEPTEMBER 3, 1997
DISCIPLINARY ACTION: EXCLUSION FROM THE MEDICARE AND/OR MEDICAID PROGRAM
OFFENSE: NONCOMPLIANCE WITH A PROFESSIONAL RULE

NOTES: DEFAULTED ON PUBLIC HEALTH SERVICE EDUCATION LOAN.

COSBY, ROBERT L MD, DATE OF BIRTH SEPTEMBER 10, 1954, LICENSE NUMBER 0027190 OF PHOENIX, AZ, WAS DISCIPLINED BY COLORADO ON JUNE 19, 1992
DISCIPLINARY ACTION: SURRENDER OF LICENSE

OFFENSE: PROFESSIONAL MISCONDUCT

NOTES: PATIENT ABANDONMENT.

COY, JOHN R MD, LICENSE NUMBER 5932, WAS DISCIPLINED BY ARIZONA ON JANUARY 24, 1997
DISCIPLINARY ACTION: 60-MONTH PROBATION; FINE
OFFENSE: CRIMINAL CONVICTION OR PLEA OF GUILTY, NOLO CONTENDERE, OR NO CONTEST TO A CRIME

NOTES: ON RENEWAL APPLICATIONS FOR STAFF RADIOLOGY PRIVILEGES AT A HOSPITAL BETWEEN 1980 & 1992 AND ON LICENSE RENEWAL APPLICATIONS IN 1990 & 1991 HE MISREPRESENTED THAT HE WAS CERTIFIED BY THE AMERICAN BOARD OF RADIOLOGY; ALSO MISREPRESENTED THIS FACT TO OBTAIN PERMISSION FOR HIS PRACTICE TO DO MAMMOGRAPHY SCREENING FOR THE MEDICARE PROGRAM; BECAUSE OF THIS HE WAS CONVICTED OF MAKING FALSE STATEMENTS OR ENTRIES AND PLACED ON THREE YEARS PROBATION AND FINED $1,500. CONDITIONS OF HIS PROBATION ARE AS FOLLOWS: SHALL PAY A CIVIL PENALTY OF $5,000; SHALL PERFORM 100 HOURS OF BOARD APPROVED COMMUNITY SERVICE PER YEAR FOR THE TERM OF HIS PROBATION; ISSUED A DECREE OF CENSURE.

COY, JOHN ROSS MD, DATE OF BIRTH MAY 23, 1941 OF 423 MAIN STREET, SAFFORD, AZ, WAS DISCIPLINED BY MEDICARE ON JULY 18, 1996
DISCIPLINARY ACTION: 60-MONTH EXCLUSION FROM THE MEDICARE AND/OR MEDICAID PROGRAM
OFFENSE: CRIMINAL CONVICTION OR PLEA OF GUILTY, NOLO CONTENDERE, OR NO CONTEST TO A CRIME

NOTES: CONVICTED OF A CRIME INVOLVING THE MEDICARE, MEDICAID, MATERNAL AND CHILD HEALTH SERVICES BLOCK GRANT OR BLOCK GRANTS TO STATES FOR SOCIAL SERVICES PROGRAMS.

COYLE, RADCLIFFE J MD, LICENSE NUMBER 0010924, WAS DISCIPLINED BY ARIZONA ON JULY 15, 1994
OFFENSE: PROFESSIONAL MISCONDUCT

NOTES: WROTE FIVE TO SEVEN PRESCRIPTIONS FOR ARIZONA RESIDENTS BUT SAW ONLY THREE OF THESE PATIENTS, EXAMINED NONE OF THEM AND IN THE CASE OF AT LEAST TWO PATIENTS, SIMPLY MAILED A PRESCRIPTION TO HIS SISTER. IN 1990-1992 SISTER OPERATED A CLINIC IN MEXICO WHICH LISTED HIS YUMA PHONE NUMBER WHILE HE WAS IN PENSACOLA FLORIDA. DID NOT MAINTAIN ANY RECORDS ON ANY OF THE PATIENTS FOR WHOM HE WROTE PRESCRIPTIONS, BUT STATED THAT HE REQUESTED HIS SISTER TO MAKE A RECORD IN HER FILES OF THE PRESCRIPTIONS WRITTEN BY HIM. A PHARMACY SURVEY FOUND 24 PRESCRIPTIONS WRITTEN FROM THE CLINIC, AT LEAST 4 OF WHICH WERE FILLED WITH HIS DEA NUMBER. 1,552 LAB STUDIES WERE ORDERED IN HIS NAME OF WHICH 200 WERE RECEIVED BY HIM. ORDER OF CENSURE ISSUED.

COYLE, RADCLIFFE JOHN MD, LICENSE NUMBER 0006346 OF LILLIAN, AL, WAS DISCIPLINED BY ALABAMA ON JULY 10, 1995
DISCIPLINARY ACTION: REPRIMAND
OFFENSE: DISCIPLINARY ACTION BY ANOTHER STATE OR AGENCY

NOTES: ACTION IN ARIZONA.

CUDAK, SOPHIA MD OF 9239 S OAK STREET, TEMPE, AZ, WAS DISCIPLINED BY DEA ON OCTOBER 7, 1997
DISCIPLINARY ACTION: SURRENDER OF CONTROLLED SUBSTANCE LICENSE

CUDAK, SOPHIA MD, WAS DISCIPLINED BY ARIZONA ON SEPTEMBER 25, 1998
DISCIPLINARY ACTION: PROBATION; RESTRICTION PLACED ON LICENSE
OFFENSE: NONCOMPLIANCE WITH A PROFESSIONAL RULE

NOTES: DISPENSED LARGE AMOUNTS OF CONTROLLED SUBSTANCES WITHOUT MAINTAINING THE APPROPRIATE DOCUMENTATION AND COMPLYING WITH THE FEDERAL STATUTES AND DRUG ENFORCEMENT ADMINISTRATION REGULATIONS. PRACTICE LIMITED TO SOLELY REVIEWING, EVALUATING AND REPORTING ON PATIENTS CHARTS AND MEDICAL CARE AND TREATMENTS; REPRIMAND.

CUNNIEN, ALAN J MD, LICENSE NUMBER 0016180, WAS DISCIPLINED BY ARIZONA ON JANUARY 25, 1991
DISCIPLINARY ACTION: REQUIRED TO ENTER AN IMPAIRED PHYSICIAN PROGRAM OR SUBSTANCE ABUSE TREATMENT; MONITORING OF PHYSICIAN PERFORMANCE
OFFENSE: SUBSTANCE ABUSE

NOTES: MISUSING CHEMICAL SUBSTANCES. MUST IMMEDIATELY PARTICIPATE IN THE ARIZONA MEDICAL ASSOCIATION'S MONITORED AFTERCARE TREATMENT PROGRAM WHOSE THERAPIST MUST SUBMIT QUARTERLY REPORTS; SHALL PARTICIPATE IN 90 12-STEP MEETINGS APPROPRIATE FOR SUBSTANCE ABUSE AND ACCEPTABLE TO THE BOARD WITHIN 90 DAYS; MUST THEN PARTICIPATE IN A 12-STEP RECOVERY PROGRAM AND ATTEND A MINIMUM OF THREE WEEKLY MEETINGS; MUST OBTAIN A BOARD-APPROVED SOLE TREATING PHYSICIAN; SHALL ABSTAIN COMPLETELY FROM THE CONSUMPTION OF ALCOHOLIC BEVERAGES; SHALL TAKE NO DRUGS OR MEDICATIONS WHATEVER; SHALL SUBMIT TO RANDOM BIOLOGICAL FLUID TESTS; SHALL MAINTAIN A LOG OF ANY AND ALL MEDICATIONS PRESCRIBED FOR HIM; SHALL SUBMIT TO MENTAL, PHYSICAL OR MEDICAL COMPETENCY EXAMINATIONS OR ANY COMBINATION THEREOF; SHALL SUBMIT TO ANY BOARD-ORDERED THERAPY; SHALL APPEAR BEFORE BOARD FOR INTERVIEWS UPON REQUEST; MUST ADVISE BOARD OF CHANGE OF ADDRESS OR IF HE IS AWAY FOR MORE THAN FIVE DAYS. ON 10/16/93 ORDER TERMINATED AFTER 90 DAYS.

CUNNIEN, ALAN J MD, DATE OF BIRTH OCTOBER 6, 1953, LICENSE NUMBER 0025622 OF MAYO CLINIC 13400 E SHEA BLVD, SCOTTSDALE, AZ, WAS DISCIPLINED BY MINNESOTA ON SEPTEMBER 12, 1992
OFFENSE: DISCIPLINARY ACTION BY ANOTHER STATE OR AGENCY

NOTES: SUSPENSION STAYED UPON COMPLIANCE WITH THE FOLLOWING: SHALL COMPLY WITH ALL TERMS AND CONDITIONS IMPOSED ON ARIZONA LICENSE. IF HE MOVES TO MINNESOTA TO PRACTICE, SHALL MEET WITH COMPLAINT REVIEW COMMITTEE WHICH MAY THEN CONDITION OR RESTRICT HIS LICENSE. UNCONDITIONAL LICENSE AS OF 3/12/94.

CURTIS, BRUCE NELSON MD, LICENSE NUMBER 0003160 OF SAFFORD, AZ, WAS DISCIPLINED BY ARIZONA ON JANUARY 22, 1993
DISCIPLINARY ACTION: RESTRICTION PLACED ON LICENSE; REQUIRED TO TAKE ADDITIONAL MEDICAL EDUCATION
OFFENSE: SUBSTANDARD CARE, INCOMPETENCE OR NEGLIGENCE

NOTES: ALLEGATIONS OF DELAY IN C-SECTION WHICH RESULTED IN DELIVERY OF A BRAIN DAMAGED FEMALE INFANT 17 YEARS AGO. SHALL COMPLETE WITHIN SIX MONTHS A MINI-RESIDENCY IN THE

NORMAL OBSTETRIC AND PRENATAL CLINIC WHICH WILL INCLUDE SCREENING FOR HIGH RISK DELIVERY, INDICATIONS FOR CESAREAN SECTIONS, FETAL MONITORING AND THE MANAGEMENT OF LABOR AND DELIVERY; PENDING SUCCESSFUL COMPLETION OF THIS RESIDENCY SHALL NOT PRACTICE OBSTETRICAL MEDICINE. ON 10/15/93 THIS ORDER WAS TERMINATED AS HE HAD COMPLETED THE REQUIREMENTS.

DAS, AJAY K MD, LICENSE NUMBER 0156589 OF 8211 NORTH KEATING AVENUE, SKOKIE, IL, WAS DISCIPLINED BY NEW YORK ON AUGUST 25, 1994
DISCIPLINARY ACTION: SURRENDER OF LICENSE
OFFENSE: DISCIPLINARY ACTION BY ANOTHER STATE OR AGENCY

NOTES: CONVICTED OF VENDOR FRAUD (MEDICAID) AND DISCIPLINED BY ILLINOIS BOARD.

DAS, AJAY K MD, LICENSE NUMBER 0036114 OF SKOKIE, IL, WAS DISCIPLINED BY VIRGINIA ON AUGUST 11, 1995
DISCIPLINARY ACTION: LICENSE REVOCATION
OFFENSE: CRIMINAL CONVICTION OR PLEA OF GUILTY, NOLO CONTENDERE, OR NO CONTEST TO A CRIME

NOTES: FELONY CONVICTION FOR VENDOR FRAUD.

DAS, AJAY K MD, LICENSE NUMBER 0036114 OF SKOKIE, IL, WAS DISCIPLINED BY VIRGINIA ON NOVEMBER 6, 1995
DISCIPLINARY ACTION: LICENSE REINSTATEMENT; PROBATION

NOTES: LICENSE REINSTATED ON INDEFINITE PROBATION UNDER TERMS AND CONDITIONS. ON 8/22/97 PROBATION TERMINATED; FULL AND UNRESTRICTED LICENSE GRANTED.

DAS, AJAY KUMAR MD OF GLENVIEW, IL, WAS DISCIPLINED BY ILLINOIS ON JULY 1, 1991
DISCIPLINARY ACTION: 6-MONTH LICENSE SUSPENSION; 6-MONTH SUSPENSION OF CONTROLLED SUBSTANCE LICENSE
OFFENSE: CRIMINAL CONVICTION OR PLEA OF GUILTY, NOLO CONTENDERE, OR NO CONTEST TO A CRIME

NOTES: FINED $25,000 AFTER HE WAS CONVICTED OF VENDOR FRAUD. MEDICAL AND CONTROLLED SUBSTANCES LICENSES PLACED ON FIVE YEARS PROBATION UPON TERMINATION OF SUSPENSION.

DAS, AJAY KUMAR MD, LICENSE NUMBER 0014432, WAS DISCIPLINED BY ARIZONA ON JULY 15, 1993
DISCIPLINARY ACTION: 6-MONTH LICENSE SUSPENSION; PROBATION
OFFENSE: DISCIPLINARY ACTION BY ANOTHER STATE OR AGENCY

NOTES: ON 6/4/91 SIGNED STIPULATION WITH ILLINOIS BOARD ADMITTING THAT HE HAD BEEN CONVICTED OF VENDOR FRAUD IN THAT HE BILLED INVOICES TO THE ILLINOIS DEPARTMENT OF PUBLIC AID WHICH FALSELY STATED THAT HE HAD PROVIDED MEDICAL CARE TO PEOPLE HE HAD NOT AND FOR WHOM HE RECEIVED PAYMENT; ILLINOIS LICENSE SUSPENDED FOR SIX MONTHS FOLLOWED BY PROBATION FOR FIVE YEARS. UNDER ARIZONA ORDER DR. DAS SHALL COMPLY IN ALL RESPECTS WITH THE ORDER OF PROBATION OF ILLINOIS AND SHALL PROVIDE ARIZONA WITH ALL REPORTS PROVIDED TO ILLINOIS; SHALL MEET WITH THE BOARD PRIOR TO PRACTICING IN ARIZONA OR TERMINATION OF THE ILLINOIS PROBATION, WHICHEVER OCCURS FIRST. ON 7/26/97 PROBATION TERMINATED.

DAS, AJAY KUMAR MD, LICENSE NUMBER 1033077 OF 3356 THORNWOOD DRIVE, GLENVIEW, IL, WAS DISCIPLINED BY INDIANA ON JULY 29, 1993
DISCIPLINARY ACTION: PROBATION; REQUIRED TO TAKE ADDITIONAL MEDICAL EDUCATION
OFFENSE: DISCIPLINARY ACTION BY ANOTHER STATE OR AGENCY

NOTES: ON 5/28/93 RENEWAL APPLICATION, DAS RESPONDED POSITIVELY TO QUESTIONS REGARDING CONVICTION FOR A CRIME AND DISCIPLINARY ACTION IN ANOTHER STATE. HE WAS DISCIPLINED IN ILLINOIS BASED ON A CONVICTION OF VENDOR FRAUD AGAINST ILLINOIS DEPARTMENT OF PUBLIC AID FOR EMPLOYING A PHYSICIAN ASSISTANT WHO WAS NOT LICENSED IN ILLINOIS FOR WHICH HE HAD TO REIMBURSE THE ILLINOIS DEPARTMENT OF PUBLIC AID $150,000; ON JUNE 4, 1991, ILLINOIS MEDICAL BOARD SUSPENDED DAS'S LICENSE FOR 6 MONTH AND PLACED IT ON PROBATION FOR 5 YEARS WITH CONDITIONS. INDIANA LICENSE ON INDEFINITE PROBATION; SHALL COMPLY WITH THE TERMS IMPOSED BY ILLINOIS INCLUDING SUBMITTING QUARTERLY REPORTS TO THE BOARD REGARDING HIS EMPLOYMENT STATUS; KEEPING THE BOARD INFORMED OF HIS HOME AND BUSINESS ADDRESSES; SHALL COMPLETE 50 HOURS CONTINUING MEDICAL EDUCATION PER YEAR OR A TOTAL OF 250 HOURS. IF ILLINOIS MODIFIES THEIR ORDER INDIANA WILL DO THE SAME; SHALL NOT APPLY FOR WITHDRAWAL OF PROBATION UNTIL ALL RESTRICTIONS ARE REMOVED FROM ILLINOIS LICENSE. ON 4/24/97 ORDER TERMINATED. ON 5/14/97 PROBATION WITHDRAWN.

DAS, AJAY KUMAR MD OF GLENVIEW, IL, WAS DISCIPLINED BY ILLINOIS ON SEPTEMBER 1, 1993
DISCIPLINARY ACTION: REPRIMAND
OFFENSE: FAILURE TO COMPLY WITH PREVIOUS BOARD ORDER

NOTES: VIOLATED A PREVIOUS DEPARTMENT ORDERED PROBATION. IN 07/15/93 MINUTES OF BOARD IT WAS DETERMINED THAT DR. DAS BE OFFERED THE OPPORTUNITY TO ENTER INTO A STIPULATION CONSENTING TO ORDER OF PROBATION IN ARIZONA UNDER SAME TERMS OF ILLINOIS AGREEMENT. IT WAS DECIDED THAT THE PROBATION IN ARIZONA WOULD GO THROUGH.

DAS, AJAY KUMAR MD, DATE OF BIRTH MAY 14, 1946, LICENSE NUMBER 0025571 OF 8211 NORTH KEATING AVENUE, SKOKIE, IL, WAS DISCIPLINED BY WISCONSIN ON MAY 25, 1995
DISCIPLINARY ACTION: 6-MONTH LICENSE SUSPENSION; REQUIRED TO TAKE ADDITIONAL MEDICAL EDUCATION
OFFENSE: DISCIPLINARY ACTION BY ANOTHER STATE OR AGENCY

NOTES: ON 4/20/90 CONVICTED BY COOK COUNTY CIRCUIT COURT IN ILLINOIS OF VENDOR FRAUD FOR CAUSING TO BE MADE BILLING INVOICES THAT FALSELY CLAIMED HE HAD PROVIDED MEDICAL CARE WHEN IN FACT HIS EMPLOYEE WHO WAS NOT LICENSED DID; PLACED ON PROBATION FOR A PERIOD OF TWO YEARS AND ORDERED TO PAY RESTITUTION OF $150,000. ON 7/29/91 THE ILLINOIS BOARD SUSPENDED HIS LICENSE FOR SIX MONTHS, IMPOSED CERTAIN LIMITATIONS ON HIS LICENSE, AND ORDERED HIM TO PAY FINE OF $25,000 BASED ON THIS CONVICTION. ON 9/30/93 THE ILLINOIS BOARD REPRIMANDED HIM FOR FAILING TO PAY ONE INSTALLMENT OF THE FINE IMPOSED. HE HAS SINCE PAID THE FINE; IN 5/93 INDIANA RENEWED HIS LICENSE WITH RESTRICTIONS. WISCONSIN RESTRICTIONS OF THE ORDER ARE AS FOLLOWS: SHALL SUBMIT QUARTERLY REPORTS TO THE BOARD INDICATING WHERE HE IS EMPLOYED, THE NATURE OF THE WORK HE IS DOING, THE NUMBER OF HOURS THAT HE IS WORKING, WHO HE EMPLOYS AND IN WHAT CAPACITY; SHALL INFORM BOARD OF ADDRESSES

AND PHONE NUMBER AND OF ANY CHANGES; SHALL IMMEDIATELY INFORM BOARD IF HE IS NAMED AS A DEFENDANT IN A MEDICAL MALPRACTICE LAWSUIT, IF HIS PRIVILEGES ARE REVOKED, SUSPENDED OF LIMITED AT ANY HOSPITAL OR MANAGED CARE ORGANIZATION OR IF HE IS SUBJECT TO AN INVESTIGATION CONCERNING HIS PRACTICE; SHALL SUBMIT PROOF OF ATTENDANCE AND COMPLETION OF A MINIMUM OF 12 HOURS OF CONTINUING MEDICAL EDUCATION IN MEDICAL OR BI0-ETHICS; SHALL COMPLY WITH ALL TERMS OF THE ILLINOIS ORDER; SHALL PAY COSTS OF $500. LIMITATIONS SHALL REMAIN IN EFFECT UNTIL 1/31/97. ON 3/12/97 ORDER TERMINATED AND HE IS RETURNED TO FULL LICENSURE.

DAS, AJAY KUMAR MD, DATE OF BIRTH MAY 14, 1946, LICENSE NUMBER 1046766 OF 8211 N KEATING AVE, SKOKIE, IL, WAS DISCIPLINED BY MICHIGAN ON AUGUST 23, 1995
DISCIPLINARY ACTION: RESTRICTION PLACED ON LICENSE
OFFENSE: PROFESSIONAL MISCONDUCT

NOTES: UNETHICAL BUSINESS PRACTICE.

DAVE, CHAITANYA V MD, WAS DISCIPLINED BY ARIZONA ON MAY 19, 1999
DISCIPLINARY ACTION: DENIAL OF NEW LICENSE
OFFENSE: PROVIDING FALSE INFORMATION TO THE BOARD OR OTHER HEALTH AGENCY

NOTES: FALSIFICATION OF HIS LICENSE APPLICATION.

DAVIS, NANCY L MD, LICENSE NUMBER 0005881, WAS DISCIPLINED BY RHODE ISLAND ON JUNE 14, 1995
DISCIPLINARY ACTION: SURRENDER OF LICENSE
OFFENSE: SUBSTANCE ABUSE

NOTES: DEPENDENCY ON CONTROLLED SUBSTANCES; HABITUAL DRUNKENNESS. VOLUNTARY SURRENDER WHILE UNDER INVESTIGATION. ADMINISTRATIVE FEE LEVIED.

DAVIS, NANCY L MD, LICENSE NUMBER 085187 OF 9642 EAST PINE VALLEY ROAD, SCOTTSDALE, AZ, WAS DISCIPLINED BY NEW YORK ON MARCH 13, 1997
DISCIPLINARY ACTION: SURRENDER OF LICENSE
OFFENSE: DISCIPLINARY ACTION BY ANOTHER STATE OR AGENCY

NOTES: DISCIPLINED BY THE RHODE ISLAND BOARD FOR BEING NONCOMPLIANT WITH THE RECOMMENDATIONS OF THE RHODE ISLAND PHYSICIAN'S HEALTH COMMITTEE REGARDING HER USE OF ALCOHOL.

DAVIS, ROBERT C MD OF 1519 WEST 90TH SOUTH, WEST JORDAN, UT, WAS DISCIPLINED BY NEW MEXICO ON DECEMBER 15, 1993
DISCIPLINARY ACTION: LICENSE REVOCATION
OFFENSE: CRIMINAL CONVICTION OR PLEA OF GUILTY, NOLO CONTENDERE, OR NO CONTEST TO A CRIME

NOTES: CRIMINAL CONVICTION IN ANOTHER STATE.

DAVIS, ROBERT CHARLES MD, DATE OF BIRTH OCTOBER 25, 1953, LICENSE NUMBER 0005035 OF 1781 WEST 90TH S, WEST JORDAN, UT, WAS DISCIPLINED BY MONTANA ON JANUARY 24, 1991
DISCIPLINARY ACTION: SURRENDER OF LICENSE
OFFENSE: NONCOMPLIANCE WITH A PROFESSIONAL RULE

NOTES: FAILURE TO DISCLOSE UTAH DISCIPLINARY ACTION IN A TIMELY MANNER.

DAVIS, ROBERT CHARLES MD OF SANDY, UT, WAS DISCIPLINED BY UTAH ON JULY 19, 1993
DISCIPLINARY ACTION: LICENSE REVOCATION; REVOCATION OF CONTROLLED SUBSTANCE LICENSE
OFFENSE: CRIMINAL CONVICTION OR PLEA OF GUILTY, NOLO CONTENDERE, OR NO CONTEST TO A CRIME

NOTES: CONVICTION OF CRIMES OF MORAL TURPITUDE WHICH RELATE TO HIS PRACTICE OF MEDICINE AND DEMONSTRATE A THREAT TO THE PUBLIC HEALTH, SAFETY AND WELFARE. HE FILED A REQUEST FOR AGENCY REVIEW ON 07/08/93 AND THE REVOCATION WAS STAYED PENDING THE ISSUANCE OF AN ORDER ON THE REQUEST. ORDER WAS UPHELD IN ITS ENTIRETY.

DAVIS, ROBERT CHARLES MD, DATE OF BIRTH OCTOBER 25, 1953, LICENSE NUMBER 0023956 OF 1519 WEST 90TH STREET, WEST JORDAN, UT, WAS DISCIPLINED BY IOWA ON JUNE 6, 1994
DISCIPLINARY ACTION: LICENSE REVOCATION
OFFENSE: DISCIPLINARY ACTION BY ANOTHER STATE OR AGENCY

NOTES: CHARGES THAT UTAH TOOK ACTION FOR FRAUD.

DAVIS, ROBERT CHARLES MD, DATE OF BIRTH OCTOBER 25, 1953 OF RR 2 BOX 9000, SAFFORD, AZ, WAS DISCIPLINED BY MEDICARE ON OCTOBER 10, 1994
DISCIPLINARY ACTION: 300-MONTH EXCLUSION FROM THE MEDICARE AND/OR MEDICAID PROGRAM
OFFENSE: CRIMINAL CONVICTION OR PLEA OF GUILTY, NOLO CONTENDERE, OR NO CONTEST TO A CRIME

NOTES: CONVICTED OF A CRIME INVOLVING THE MEDICARE, MEDICAID, MATERNAL AND CHILD HEALTH SERVICES BLOCK GRANT OR BLOCK GRANTS TO STATES FOR SOCIAL SERVICES PROGRAMS.

DAVIS, ROGER MD, LICENSE NUMBER 5798, WAS DISCIPLINED BY ARIZONA ON NOVEMBER 17, 1999
DISCIPLINARY ACTION: REPRIMAND
OFFENSE: SUBSTANDARD CARE, INCOMPETENCE OR NEGLIGENCE

NOTES: FAILURE TO DIAGNOSE COLON CANCER, AND FAILURE TO PERFORM AN ADEQUATE EXAMINATION.

DE ALVA, WILLIAM E MD, DATE OF BIRTH APRIL 2, 1925, LICENSE NUMBER 0015060 OF TUCSON, AZ, WAS DISCIPLINED BY COLORADO ON FEBRUARY 19, 1993
DISCIPLINARY ACTION: REPRIMAND
OFFENSE: SUBSTANDARD CARE, INCOMPETENCE OR NEGLIGENCE

NOTES: SUBSTANDARD CARE.

DE LA PAVA, DANIEL MD, LICENSE NUMBER 0011945, WAS DISCIPLINED BY ARIZONA ON DECEMBER 23, 1996
DISCIPLINARY ACTION: MONITORING OF PHYSICIAN PERFORMANCE

NOTES: WITHIN 90 DAYS SHALL ENGAGE THE SERVICES OF A PRACTICE MANAGEMENT CONSULTANT REGARDING MEDICAL RECORDS; SHALL CAUSE THE CONSULTANT TO PROVIDE A WRITTEN REPORT TO THE BOARD; WITHIN NINE MONTHS THE BOARD SHALL CONDUCT A SURVEY OF HIS MEDICAL RECORDS. ON 9/26/97 ORDER TERMINATED BASED ON RESULTS OF SURVEY AND CONSULTANT'S REPORT.

DEAN, ROBERT T MD, LICENSE NUMBER 0002812, WAS DISCIPLINED BY ARIZONA ON MAY 17, 1996
DISCIPLINARY ACTION: RESTRICTION PLACED ON LICENSE
OFFENSE: FAILURE TO COMPLY WITH PREVIOUS BOARD ORDER

NOTES: ALLEGATIONS THAT HE IS DISPENSING MEDICATIONS TO PATIENTS AND NOT WRITING PRESCRIPTIONS AND THAT HE IS NOT REGISTERED AS A DISPENSING

PHYSICIAN; A PATIENT MAY HAVE BECOME ADDICTED TO DRUGS HE PRESCRIBED; DELIVERED AND CHARGED LARGE AMOUNTS OF MONEY FOR MEDICATIONS BROUGHT TO THIS PATIENT; DID NOT PASS SPEX EXAM AS REQUIRED BY 10/16/95 ORDER. SHALL NOT PRACTICE CLINICAL MEDICINE.

DECADY, LEE MD, LICENSE NUMBER 081863 OF 2737 E. ARIZONA BILTMORE CIRCLE, PHOENIX, AZ, WAS DISCIPLINED BY NEW YORK ON JUNE 27, 1997
DISCIPLINARY ACTION: SURRENDER OF LICENSE
OFFENSE: DISCIPLINARY ACTION BY ANOTHER STATE OR AGENCY

NOTES: DISCIPLINED BY THE CALIFORNIA BOARD FOR MAKING MISLEADING ADVERTISEMENTS, EXCESSIVELY USING DIAGNOSTIC PROCEDURES, SUBMITTING FRAUDULENT INSURANCE CLAIMS, CREATING FALSE MEDICAL RECORDS, AIDING AND ABETTING THE UNLICENSED PRACTICE OF MEDICINE AND FAILING TO PROPERLY SUPERVISE A PHYSICIAN ASSISTANT.

DEMARSE, CORWIN F MD, LICENSE NUMBER 0009287, WAS DISCIPLINED BY ARIZONA ON JUNE 30, 1990
DISCIPLINARY ACTION: REQUIRED TO ENTER AN IMPAIRED PHYSICIAN PROGRAM OR SUBSTANCE ABUSE TREATMENT; MONITORING OF PHYSICIAN PERFORMANCE
OFFENSE: SUBSTANCE ABUSE

NOTES: MUST IMMEDIATELY PARTICIPATE IN THE ARIZONA MEDICAL ASSOCIATION PHYSICIAN'S HEALTH COMMITTEE PROGRAM WITH QUARTERLY REPORTS TO THE BOARD; MUST OBTAIN BOARD APPROVED TREATING PHYSICIAN; MUST ABSTAIN COMPLETELY FROM ALCOHOL AND ALL OTHER DRUGS; MUST COMPLY WITH REQUESTS FOR RANDOM BIOLOGICAL FLUID TESTS; MUST SUBMIT TO ANY EXAMS OR THERAPY ORDERED BY THE BOARD; MUST PARTICIPATE IN 12-STEP RECOVERY PROGRAM FOR SUBSTANCE ABUSE AS DETERMINED BY THERAPIST AND ATTEND AT LEAST 3 WEEKLY MEETINGS; MUST APPEAR BEFORE BOARD FOR INTERVIEWS ON REQUEST; MUST ADVISE BOARD OF CHANGE OF OFFICE OR HOME ADDRESS AND IF AWAY FOR MORE THAN FIVE DAYS; MUST MAINTAIN A LOG OF ALL MEDICATIONS TAKEN. ON 4/11/92, FOLLOWING DISCUSSION OF HIS ONGOING REHABILITATION EFFORTS, BOARD MODIFIED PREVIOUS ORDER AUTHORIZING HIM TO DISCONTINUE HIS WEEKLY THERAPY SESSIONS BUT ENCOURAGING HIM TO VOLUNTARILY ATTEND SUCH GROUP THERAPY. THE BOARD TERMINATED THIS ORDER ON 10/15/93.

DENICOLE, MICHAEL A DO, LICENSE NUMBER 0002103 OF 7111 NORTH 59TH PLACE, PARADISE VALLEY, AZ, WAS DISCIPLINED BY ARIZONA ON FEBRUARY 22, 1996
DISCIPLINARY ACTION: 60-MONTH PROBATION; RESTRICTION PLACED ON CONTROLLED SUBSTANCE LICENSE
OFFENSE: SUBSTANCE ABUSE

NOTES: RECEIVED TREATMENT FOR SUBSTANCE ABUSE. ON 11/29/95 ACKNOWLEDGED THAT HE HAD IMPROPERLY DIVERTED QUANTITIES OF CONTROLLED SUBSTANCE FOR HIS PERSONAL USE FOR APPROXIMATELY ONE YEAR AND HAD BECOME DEPENDENT UPON THE USE OF SAID CONTROLLED SUBSTANCES. PROBATION UNDER TERMS AND CONDITIONS: SHALL OBTAIN PSYCHIATRIC OR PSYCHOLOGICAL TREATMENT BY A BOARD APPROVED THERAPIST WHO SHALL SUBMIT TO THE BOARD A WRITTEN PROGRESS REPORT EVERY MONTH FOR THE FIRST SIX MONTHS, THEN EVERY THREE MONTHS FOR THE REMAINDER OF THE PROBATION; SHALL PROVIDE A COPY OF THIS ORDER TO ALL FACILITIES WHERE HE IS CURRENTLY EMPLOYED AS A PHYSICIAN AND/OR HAS PRIVILEGES TO ENGAGE IN THE PRACTICE OF MEDICINE; SHALL ABSTAIN FROM THE CONSUMPTION OF ALCOHOL AND SHALL NOT CONSUME ILLICIT DRUGS OR TAKE ANY CONTROLLED SUBSTANCES UNLESS PRESCRIBED BY HIS TREATING PHYSICIAN; SHALL MAINTAIN A LOG OF SUCH PRESCRIPTIONS AND PROVIDE A COPY TO THE BOARD MONTHLY; SHALL SUBMIT TO AND COOPERATE IN ANY INDEPENDENT MEDICAL OR PSYCHOLOGICAL EVALUATION THAT IS ORDERED BY THE BOARD; SHALL APPEAR BEFORE THE BOARD UPON REQUEST; SHALL SUBMIT TO RANDOM BIOLOGICAL FLUID TESTING; SHALL PARTICIPATE IN A MINIMUM OF TWO SELF-HELP MEETINGS PER WEEK THROUGH SUCH ORGANIZATIONS SUCH AS AA, NARCOTICS ANONYMOUS, AND DOCTOR'S CADUCEUS GROUP WITH MONTHLY REPORTS; SHALL NOTIFY THE BOARD WITHIN 20 DAYS IF HE CEASES TO RESIDE IN ARIZONA; SHALL NOT PRESCRIBE ANY CONTROLLED SUBSTANCES EXCEPT FOR SCHEDULE IV AND V SUBSTANCES; HIS PRESCRIPTIONS FOR THESE DRUGS, PER PATIENT, SHALL NOT EXCEED A DOSAGE AMOUNT FOR MORE THAN SEVEN DAYS AND THE PRESCRIPTION MAY NOT BE RENEWED BY HIM; SHALL COMPLY WITH CONDITIONS IMPOSED BY DEA AND SHALL DISCLOSE TO THE BOARD A COMPLETE COPY OF ALL DEA ORDERS; UPON APPROVAL OF PRESCRIPTION PRIVILEGES, MUST USE TRIPLICATE COPIES OF PRESCRIPTION PADS AND SUBMIT COPIES TO THE BOARD MONTHLY; SHALL COMPLY WITH ANY CONDITIONS PLACED ON HOSPITAL PRIVILEGES.

DENICOLE, MICHAEL A DO, LICENSE NUMBER 628, WAS DISCIPLINED BY HAWAII ON AUGUST 22, 1997
DISCIPLINARY ACTION: SURRENDER OF LICENSE
OFFENSE: DISCIPLINARY ACTION BY ANOTHER STATE OR AGENCY

NOTES: ALLEGATIONS THAT ARIZONA TOOK DISCIPLINARY ACTION AGAINST HIS LICENSE AND HE FAILED TO REPORT THIS ACTION TO HAWAII. VOLUNTARY SURRENDER; MAY NOT APPLY FOR A NEW LICENSE FOR FIVE YEARS.

DENOVELLIS, ANNA MD, LICENSE NUMBER 0012578, WAS DISCIPLINED BY ARIZONA ON JULY 20, 1995
OFFENSE: SUBSTANCE ABUSE

NOTES: INTERVIEWED BY BOARD RELATIVE TO INFORMATION RECEIVED BY THE BOARD ALLEGING THAT SHE IS INCOMPETENT AND MAY BE SUFFERING FROM POSSIBLE MENTAL PROBLEMS OR IMPAIRMENT; INFORMATION ALLEGING THAT SHE WAS INAPPROPRIATELY PRESCRIBING CONTROLLED SUBSTANCES FOR A PERSON LIVING IN HER HOME; HER ADMITTED DRUG PROBLEM. SHE SHALL NOT PRACTICE MEDICINE IN ARIZONA UNTIL FURTHER ORDER OF THE BOARD.

DENSON, MARK L MD, LICENSE NUMBER 0015740, WAS DISCIPLINED BY ARIZONA ON JULY 21, 1995
OFFENSE: SUBSTANCE ABUSE

NOTES: DID NOT INFORM THE BOARD ON HIS RENEWAL FORMS THAT HE WAS TREATED FOR CHEMICAL DEPENDENCY. SHALL SUBMIT TO EVALUATION FOR CHEMICAL DEPENDENCY WITHIN TWO WEEKS.

DENSON, MARK L MD, LICENSE NUMBER 15740, WAS DISCIPLINED BY ARIZONA ON MARCH 15, 1997
DISCIPLINARY ACTION: REQUIRED TO ENTER AN IMPAIRED PHYSICIAN PROGRAM OR SUBSTANCE ABUSE TREATMENT; MONITORING OF PHYSICIAN PERFORMANCE
OFFENSE: SUBSTANCE ABUSE

NOTES: ON 12/5/96 CITED FOR DRIVING UNDER THE INFLUENCE OF INTOXICATING BEVERAGE. CONDITIONS OF PROBATION: MUST IMMEDIATELY PARTICIPATE IN A BOARD-APPROVED MONITORED AFTERCARE TREATMENT PROGRAM WHOSE THERAPIST MUST SUBMIT QUARTERLY REPORTS; MUST PARTICIPATE IN A 12-STEP RECOVERY PROGRAM AS DETERMINED BY HIS TREATING THERAPIST AND ATTEND AT LEAST THREE WEEKLY MEETINGS; SHALL OBTAIN A BOARD-APPROVED TREATING PHYSICIAN; SHALL ABSTAIN COMPLETELY FROM THE CONSUMPTION OF ALCOHOLIC BEVERAGES AND DRUGS EXCEPT WHEN PRESCRIBED BY HIS TREATING PHYSICIAN; MUST SUBMIT TO WITNESSED RANDOM BIOLOGICAL FLUID COLLECTION; MUST KEEP A LOG OF ANY AND ALL MEDICATIONS PRESCRIBED FOR HIM; SHALL SUBMIT TO ANY EXAMINATIONS OR THERAPY ORDERED BY BOARD; SHALL APPEAR BEFORE BOARD FOR INTERVIEWS UPON REQUEST; SHALL INFORM BOARD OF CHANGE OF ADDRESS OR IF AWAY FOR MORE THAN FIVE DAYS.

DENSON, MARK L MD, LICENSE NUMBER 15740, WAS DISCIPLINED BY ARIZONA ON MAY 21, 1999
DISCIPLINARY ACTION: PROBATION
OFFENSE: NONCOMPLIANCE WITH A PROFESSIONAL RULE

NOTES: ALLEGATIONS THAT HE VIOLATED TERMS OF HIS MONITORED AFTERCARE PROGRAM. INTERIM ORDER.

DENSON, MARK L MD, LICENSE NUMBER 15740, WAS DISCIPLINED BY ARIZONA ON JULY 30, 1999
DISCIPLINARY ACTION: 60-MONTH PROBATION; MONITORING OF PHYSICIAN PERFORMANCE

NOTES: PROBATION WITH THE FOLLOWING TERMS: THE STANDARD REHABILITATION TERMS INCLUDE PSYCHIATRIC MONITORING; SHALL PARTICIPATE IN THE SUBSTANCE ABUSE MONITORING PROGRAM.

DESAI, JASUBHAI K MD, DATE OF BIRTH SEPTEMBER 29, 1941, LICENSE NUMBER 1031425 OF 1675 KINGSWAY COURT, TRENTON, MI, WAS DISCIPLINED BY MICHIGAN ON APRIL 5, 1995
DISCIPLINARY ACTION: EMERGENCY SUSPENSION
OFFENSE: CRIMINAL CONVICTION OR PLEA OF GUILTY, NOLO CONTENDERE, OR NO CONTEST TO A CRIME

NOTES: CRIMINAL CONVICTION.

DESAI, JASUBHAI K MD, DATE OF BIRTH SEPTEMBER 29, 1941, LICENSE NUMBER 1031425 OF 1675 KINGSWAY COURT, TRENTON, MI, WAS DISCIPLINED BY MICHIGAN ON APRIL 5, 1995
DISCIPLINARY ACTION: LICENSE REVOCATION
OFFENSE: CRIMINAL CONVICTION OR PLEA OF GUILTY, NOLO CONTENDERE, OR NO CONTEST TO A CRIME

NOTES: CRIMINAL CONVICTION. REVOCATION EFFECTIVE AS OF DATE OF EMERGENCY SUSPENSION.

DESAI, JASUBHAI K MD, DATE OF BIRTH SEPTEMBER 29, 1941 OF 2975 STEWART ROAD, MONROE, MI, WAS DISCIPLINED BY MEDICARE ON FEBRUARY 27, 1997
DISCIPLINARY ACTION: EXCLUSION FROM THE MEDICARE AND/OR MEDICAID PROGRAM
OFFENSE: DISCIPLINARY ACTION BY ANOTHER STATE OR AGENCY

NOTES: LICENSE SUSPENDED FOR REASONS BEARING ON PROFESSIONAL PERFORMANCE.

DESAI, JASUBHAI K MD, LICENSE NUMBER 13529, WAS DISCIPLINED BY ARIZONA ON JULY 30, 1999
DISCIPLINARY ACTION: LICENSE REVOCATION
OFFENSE: DISCIPLINARY ACTION BY ANOTHER STATE OR AGENCY

NOTES: LICENSE REVOKED IN MICHIGAN FOR UNPROFESSIONAL CONDUCT.

DESMARAIS, GILLES M K MD, LICENSE NUMBER 0030536 OF 2975 S RAINBOW, LAS VEGAS, NV, WAS DISCIPLINED BY MASSACHUSETTS ON DECEMBER 28, 1994
DISCIPLINARY ACTION: NONRENEWAL OF LICENSE
OFFENSE: PROFESSIONAL MISCONDUCT

NOTES: SEXUAL RELATIONS. REVOCATION OF INCHOATE RIGHT TO RENEW LICENSE.

DESMARAIS, GILLES MARK KILDA MD, LICENSE NUMBER 0017915, WAS DISCIPLINED BY ARIZONA ON APRIL 16, 1996
OFFENSE: DISCIPLINARY ACTION BY ANOTHER STATE OR AGENCY

NOTES: DISCIPLINARY ACTION BY MASSACHUSETTS. SHALL NOT PRACTICE MEDICINE IN ARIZONA.

DEWILDE, STEVEN B DO, LICENSE NUMBER 0002611 OF 5696 WINDJAMMER, ALGONAC, MI, WAS DISCIPLINED BY ARIZONA ON JANUARY 25, 1994
DISCIPLINARY ACTION: SURRENDER OF LICENSE; REPRIMAND
OFFENSE: PROFESSIONAL MISCONDUCT

NOTES: IN 1992 THE BOARD RECEIVED INFORMATION SUGGESTING THAT HE MIGHT HAVE ABANDONED PATIENTS AND FAILED TO MAKE PATIENT RECORDS AVAILABLE IN A TIMELY MANNER; DURING THE INVESTIGATION HE FAILED TO TIMELY PAY FOR RENEWAL OF HIS BOARD LICENSE ON OR BEFORE 4/01/93; HIS LICENSE WAS SUSPENDED ON THE DATE IT WOULD HAVE EXPIRED. SHALL VOLUNTARILY TERMINATE THE PRACTICE OF OSTEOPATHIC MEDICINE WITHIN 10 DAYS; SHALL DELIVER TO THE BOARD ALL DOCUMENTS IN HIS POSSESSION INDICATING HE IS A LICENSEE OF THE BOARD.

DEWILDE, STEVEN B DO, DATE OF BIRTH JULY 13, 1957 OF 5696 WINDJAMMER STREET, ALGONAC, MI, WAS DISCIPLINED BY MEDICARE ON MAY 24, 1994
DISCIPLINARY ACTION: EXCLUSION FROM THE MEDICARE AND/OR MEDICAID PROGRAM
OFFENSE: NONCOMPLIANCE WITH A PROFESSIONAL RULE

NOTES: DEFAULTED ON PUBLIC HEALTH SERVICE EDUCATION LOAN. REINSTATED ON 4/19/95.

DEWILDE, STEVEN B DO, DATE OF BIRTH JULY 13, 1957, LICENSE NUMBER 1009688 OF 1209 10TH ST, PORT HURON, MI, WAS DISCIPLINED BY MICHIGAN ON JANUARY 8, 1996
DISCIPLINARY ACTION: 12-MONTH PROBATION
OFFENSE: SUBSTANDARD CARE, INCOMPETENCE OR NEGLIGENCE

NOTES: NEGLIGENCE; INCOMPETENCE.

DHILLON, CHARANJIT MD, LICENSE NUMBER 0011273, WAS DISCIPLINED BY ARIZONA ON JULY 19, 1995
DISCIPLINARY ACTION: MONITORING OF PHYSICIAN PERFORMANCE
OFFENSE: PROFESSIONAL MISCONDUCT

NOTES: INTERVIEWED BY BOARD RELATIVE TO THE CARE AND TREATMENT OF A PATIENT, COMPLAINT REGARDING PHYSICIAN'S FEES, AND ALLEGATIONS THAT PHYSICIAN MADE RUDE REMARKS TO THE PATIENT. WITHIN 45 DAYS, SHALL BEGIN COUNSELING WITH A BOARD-APPROVED COUNSELOR REGARDING THE ISSUE OF INTERPERSONAL RELATIONSHIPS. COUNSELOR SHALL SUBMIT QUARTERLY REPORTS TO THE BOARD. ON 9/24/97 ORDER TERMINATED BASED

ON THE THERAPIST'S REPORT.

DIDES, JURJI W MD OF MINNEAPOLIS, MN, WAS DISCIPLINED BY NORTH DAKOTA ON NOVEMBER 22, 1991
DISCIPLINARY ACTION: LICENSE REVOCATION
OFFENSE: CRIMINAL CONVICTION OR PLEA OF GUILTY, NOLO CONTENDERE, OR NO CONTEST TO A CRIME

NOTES: CONVICTED OF "SEXUAL EXPLOITATION BY A THERAPIST".

DIDES, JURJI W MD, WAS DISCIPLINED BY ARIZONA ON SEPTEMBER 10, 1992
DISCIPLINARY ACTION: LICENSE REVOCATION
OFFENSE: DISCIPLINARY ACTION BY ANOTHER STATE OR AGENCY

NOTES: ACTION TAKEN AGAINST HIS LICENSE IN NORTH DAKOTA. BOARD ACCEPTED HIS REQUEST FOR CANCELLATION OF HIS ARIZONA LICENSE WITH CAUSE.

DIDES, JURJI W MD, DATE OF BIRTH JANUARY 30, 1944 OF 515 E GRANT ST #801, MINNEAPOLIS, MN, WAS DISCIPLINED BY MEDICARE ON NOVEMBER 20, 1992
DISCIPLINARY ACTION: EXCLUSION FROM THE MEDICARE AND/OR MEDICAID PROGRAM
OFFENSE: CRIMINAL CONVICTION OR PLEA OF GUILTY, NOLO CONTENDERE, OR NO CONTEST TO A CRIME

NOTES: CONVICTION FOR PATIENT ABUSE OR NEGLECT.

DIDES, JURJI W MD, LICENSE NUMBER 0164006 OF 515 EAST GRANT STREET #801, MINNEAPOLIS, MN, WAS DISCIPLINED BY NEW YORK ON JANUARY 5, 1993
DISCIPLINARY ACTION: LICENSE REVOCATION
OFFENSE: SEXUAL ABUSE OF OR SEXUAL MISCONDUCT WITH A PATIENT

NOTES: CONDUCT EVIDENCING MORAL UNFITNESS TO PRACTICE HAVING ENGAGED IN PHYSICAL CONDUCT OF A SEXUAL NATURE WITH A PATIENT AND WILLFULLY PHYSICALLY ABUSING A PATIENT.

DIDES, JURJI W MD, LICENSE NUMBER 0031500, WAS DISCIPLINED BY MINNESOTA ON MAY 8, 1993
DISCIPLINARY ACTION: LICENSE REVOCATION

DIEHL, CRAIG MD, WAS DISCIPLINED BY ARIZONA ON APRIL 16, 1993
DISCIPLINARY ACTION: REQUIRED TO ENTER AN IMPAIRED PHYSICIAN PROGRAM OR SUBSTANCE ABUSE TREATMENT; MONITORING OF PHYSICIAN PERFORMANCE
OFFENSE: SUBSTANCE ABUSE

NOTES: ALLEGATIONS THAT HE MAY HAVE A SUBSTANCE ABUSE PROBLEM WITH ALCOHOL. WITHIN 30 DAYS MUST ENTER INTO A 30 DAY IN-PATIENT TREATMENT PROGRAM FOR ALCOHOL DEPENDENCY AT A BOARD APPROVED FACILITY AND SUCCESSFULLY COMPLETE THE PROGRAM. AFTER SATISFACTORY COMPLETION OF THE 30 DAY TREATMENT PROGRAM, HE MUST ENTER INTO A STANDARD STIPULATION AND ORDER WITHOUT A REQUIREMENT THAT HE GO TO 90 AA MEETINGS IN 90 DAYS SINCE HE HAS ALREADY COMPLETED THIS REQUIREMENT.

DIEHL, CRAIG D MD, DATE OF BIRTH JULY 30, 1947, LICENSE NUMBER 0024696 OF 1951 MESQUITE AVE, SUITE 1, LAKE HAVASU CITY, AZ, WAS DISCIPLINED BY IOWA ON SEPTEMBER 8, 1994
DISCIPLINARY ACTION: PROBATION
OFFENSE: DISCIPLINARY ACTION BY ANOTHER STATE OR AGENCY

NOTES: SETTLEMENT TO CHARGES THAT LICENSE IN ARIZONA RESTRICTED. INDEFINITE PROBATION.

DIFATTA, ANTHONY S DO OF AZ, WAS DISCIPLINED BY LOUISIANA ON FEBRUARY 17, 1998
DISCIPLINARY ACTION: 24-MONTH LICENSE SUSPENSION; 60-MONTH PROBATION
OFFENSE: CRIMINAL CONVICTION OR PLEA OF GUILTY, NOLO CONTENDERE, OR NO CONTEST TO A CRIME

NOTES: DECEIT OR PERJURY IN OBTAINING ANY LICENSE ISSUED BY THE BOARD; HABITUAL OR RECURRING ABUSE OF DRUGS; PRESCRIBING, DISPENSING OR ADMINISTERING CONTROLLED OR DEPENDENCY-INDUCING SUBSTANCES WITHOUT LEGITIMATE MEDICAL JUSTIFICATION; EFFORTS TO DECEIVE OR DEFRAUD THE PUBLIC; UNPROFESSIONAL CONDUCT; VIOLATION OF THE RULES OR PRIOR ORDERS OF THE BOARD. CONDITIONS OF PROBATION: COMPLETION OF SPECIFIED CONTINUING MEDICAL EDUCATION; SUCCESSFUL PASSAGE OF THE SPEX EXAMINATION; LIFETIME MAINTENANCE OF ABSTINENCE FROM THE USE OF ALCOHOL, CONTROLLED AND MOOD-ALTERING SUBSTANCES AS WELL AS THE DRUGS STADOL, NUBAIN AND DALGAN; CONTINUING PSYCHIATRIC EVALUATION AND/OR TREATMENT BY A PHYSICIAN APPROVED BY THE BOARD; THE RECEIPT OF FAVORABLE MEDICAL REPORTS FROM TWO PSYCHIATRISTS ACCEPTABLE TO THE BOARD; PARTICIPATION IN PHYSICIANS HEALTH PROGRAM; UNANNOUNCED DRUG SCREENS; MUST SUBMIT TO INPATIENT EVALUATION OF EMOTIONAL AND/OR POTENTIALLY ADDICTIVE DISORDERS IF DEEMED APPROPRIATE.

DIFATTA, ANTHONY S DO, DATE OF BIRTH APRIL 3, 1961 OF 4412 E UNION HILLS DRIVE, PHOENIX, AZ, WAS DISCIPLINED BY MEDICARE ON DECEMBER 20, 1998
DISCIPLINARY ACTION: EXCLUSION FROM THE MEDICARE AND/OR MEDICAID PROGRAM
OFFENSE: DISCIPLINARY ACTION BY ANOTHER STATE OR AGENCY

NOTES: LICENSE REVOKED, SUSPENDED, SURRENDERED OR OTHERWISE LOST FOR REASONS BEARING ON PROFESSIONAL PERFORMANCE, PROFESSIONAL COMPETENCE OR FINANCIAL INTEGRITY.

DIMITROPLOS, GEORGE C MD, LICENSE NUMBER 0005449, WAS DISCIPLINED BY ARIZONA ON NOVEMBER 26, 1990
DISCIPLINARY ACTION: 60-MONTH PROBATION; RESTRICTION PLACED ON LICENSE
OFFENSE: PROFESSIONAL MISCONDUCT

NOTES: IN FIVE CASES BETWEEN APRIL 1989 AND SEPTEMBER 1989 WHILE EMPLOYED BY THE CENTER FOR ADVANCED MEDICAL SPECIALTIES HE TREATED PATIENTS WHO WERE SENT FOR TESTS THAT WERE UNNECESSARY GIVEN THEIR STATED SYMPTOMS; HE CLAIMED THAT HE WAS EMPLOYED BY CENTER TO PERFORM PHYSICAL EXAMS AND TREAT ANY UNDERLYING DISEASE AND THAT HE HAD NO CONTROL OVER CHARGES MADE OR OF THE INITIAL LAB TESTING, ALTHOUGH HE ADMITTED HE ROUTINELY ALLOWED THE CENTER TO USE HIS NAME ON THEIR INSURANCE CLAIM FORMS. CONDITIONS OF PROBATION ARE THAT HE WILL TAKE THE SPEX EXAM AT THE FIRST AVAILABLE OPPORTUNITY; WILL NOT PARTICIPATE IN ANY WEIGHT REDUCTION PROGRAM OR SMOKING CESSATION PROGRAMS; WILL LIMIT PRACTICE TO OBSTETRICS AND GYNECOLOGY. HE REQUESTED A REHEARING IN 1991 AND THE BOARD DETERMINED TO RESCIND THIS ORDER AND DIRECTED THE CASE TO A FORMAL HEARING TO DETERMINE IF HIS LICENSE SHOULD BE SUSPENDED

OR REVOKED.

DIMITROPLOS, GEORGE C MD, WAS DISCIPLINED BY ARIZONA ON DECEMBER 31, 1991
DISCIPLINARY ACTION: LICENSE SUSPENSION

NOTES: REQUEST FOR INACTIVE STATUS OF LICENSE WITH CAUSE ACCEPTED.

DINE, MAX E MD, LICENSE NUMBER 0019587, WAS DISCIPLINED BY ARIZONA ON OCTOBER 9, 1991
DISCIPLINARY ACTION: MONITORING OF PHYSICIAN PERFORMANCE
OFFENSE: PHYSICAL OR MENTAL ILLNESS INHIBITING THE ABILITY TO PRACTICE WITH SKILL AND SAFETY

NOTES: INTERVIEWED BY THE BOARD RELATIVE TO AN INQUIRY CONCERNING HIS CURRENT TREATMENT FOR BIPOLAR AFFECTIVE DISORDER AND THE RESULTS OF BOARD-ORDERED EVALUATIONS. SHALL IMMEDIATELY OBTAIN A BOARD-APPROVED TREATING PHYSICIAN; SHALL VISIT HIS TREATING PHYSICIAN AS OFTEN AS DIRECTED AND COMPLY WITH THE RECOMMENDATIONS AND TREATMENT PLANS COMMUNICATED TO HIM BY THE PHYSICIAN; THE TREATING PHYSICIAN SHALL PROVIDE QUARTERLY REPORTS TO THE BOARD, WHICH SHALL INCLUDE LABORATORY STUDIES DONE, HIS CURRENT LEVEL OF FUNCTIONING, ANY EVIDENCE OF RECURRENT SYMPTOMS AND THE CURRENT TREATMENT PROTOCOL AND RECOMMENDATIONS; ANY AND ALL INFORMATION REGARDING HIS TREATMENT SHALL BE RELEASED TO THE BOARD; SHALL APPEAR BEFORE BOARD FOR INTERVIEWS UPON REQUEST; SHALL INFORM BOARD OF CHANGE OF ADDRESS OR IF AWAY FOR MORE THAN 10 DAYS. ON 7/18/92 BOARD DENIED REQUEST TO TERMINATE THIS ORDER.

DINGLE, STEVEN MD, LICENSE NUMBER 17697 OF 4127 E HOLMES AVENUE, MESA, AZ, WAS DISCIPLINED BY ARIZONA ON APRIL 16, 1997
DISCIPLINARY ACTION: REPRIMAND
OFFENSE: PROFESSIONAL MISCONDUCT

NOTES: IN 1994 AND 1995 MADE INAPPROPRIATE REMARKS TO AND TOUCHED INAPPROPRIATELY THREE RESIDENTS UNDER HIS PSYCHIATRY RESIDENCY TRAINING PROGRAM INCLUDING: TOUCHING A RESIDENT'S BREAST AS HE PASSED HER IN THE HALLWAY; INAPPROPRIATELY RUBBING A RESIDENT'S SHOULDERS.

DIOGUARDI, JEREMIA MD, LICENSE NUMBER 0004001 OF PHOENIX, AZ, WAS DISCIPLINED BY ARIZONA ON JULY 13, 1993
DISCIPLINARY ACTION: PROBATION
OFFENSE: PROFESSIONAL MISCONDUCT

NOTES: ALLOWING UNLICENSED PERSONS TO EVALUATE AND PRESCRIBE TREATMENT FOR HIS PATIENTS; MANY PATIENTS WERE SEEN FOR ILLNESSES, WHERE TREATMENT WAS OUTLINED OR PRESCRIBED BY THE OFFICE PERSONNEL (MANY OF THESE INCLUDED RECOMMENDATIONS FOR ANTIBIOTICS, TOPICAL STEROID CREAMS, ORAL STEROIDS, AND ORAL ANTIHISTAMINES; ALSO ON CHARTS APPEARED TO BE A LACK OF APPROPRIATE EXAMS FOR LONG PERIODS OF TIME, POOR DEVELOPMENTAL HISTORIES AND INAPPROPRIATE PRESCRIBING OF STEROIDS. CENSURED AND PLACED ON PROBATION, WHICH TERMS ARE THAT HE SHALL TAKE AND PASS THE SPECIAL PURPOSE EXAMINATION WITHIN SIX MONTHS.

DIOGUARDI, JEREMIA MD, LICENSE NUMBER 0004001, WAS DISCIPLINED BY ARIZONA ON NOVEMBER 7, 1994
DISCIPLINARY ACTION: LICENSE REVOCATION
OFFENSE: FAILURE TO COMPLY WITH PREVIOUS BOARD ORDER

NOTES: DID NOT PASS THE SPEX EXAM AS 07/13/93 ORDER REQUIRED HIM TO STATING THAT NOT PRACTICING INPATIENT MEDICINE FOR MANY YEARS HAS PUT HIM AT A DISADVANTAGE IN ANSWERING CERTAIN QUESTIONS ON THE SPEX. ON 1/20/95 REQUEST FOR RECONSIDERATION OF ORDER DENIED. ON 4/3/95 COURT OF APPEALS MANDATED RECONSIDERATION OF THE ORDER BY THE BOARD. COMPLAINT AND MOTION FOR STAY FILED IN COURT ON 5/6/95; BOARD FILED APPLICATION FOR INJUNCTION ON 5/31/95; APPLICATION FOR STAY TAKEN UNDER ADVISEMENT 6/29/95. ON 7/18/95 THE BOARD DENIED HIS MOTION FOR RECONSIDERATION.

DIOGUARDI, JERRY MD OF 3530 WEST MCDOWELL ROAD, PHOENIX, AZ, WAS DISCIPLINED BY DEA ON SEPTEMBER 8, 1995
DISCIPLINARY ACTION: SURRENDER OF CONTROLLED SUBSTANCE LICENSE

NOTES: IN LIEU OF ORDER TO SHOW CAUSE.

DISNEY, THOMAS F MD, LICENSE NUMBER 0014341, WAS DISCIPLINED BY ARIZONA ON OCTOBER 22, 1994
DISCIPLINARY ACTION: REQUIRED TO ENTER AN IMPAIRED PHYSICIAN PROGRAM OR SUBSTANCE ABUSE TREATMENT; MONITORING OF PHYSICIAN PERFORMANCE
OFFENSE: SUBSTANCE ABUSE

NOTES: RECENTLY TREATED FOR AMPHETAMINE DEPENDENCE AND CURRENTLY AT TALBOTT-MARSH RECOVERY SYSTEMS. MUST IMMEDIATELY ENGAGE IN TREATMENT WITH A BOARD-APPROVED PSYCHIATRIST WITH QUARTERLY REPORTS; SHALL NOT PRACTICE UNTIL HE MEETS WITH THE BOARD AND RECEIVES PERMISSION TO; MUST IMMEDIATELY PARTICIPATE IN A BOARD-APPROVED MONITORED AFTERCARE TREATMENT PROGRAM WHOSE THERAPIST MUST SUBMIT QUARTERLY REPORTS; MUST PARTICIPATE IN A 12-STEP RECOVERY PROGRAM AS DETERMINED BY HIS TREATING THERAPIST AND ATTEND AT LEAST THREE WEEKLY MEETINGS; SHALL OBTAIN A BOARD-APPROVED TREATING PHYSICIAN; SHALL ABSTAIN COMPLETELY FROM THE CONSUMPTION OF ALCOHOLIC BEVERAGES AND DRUGS EXCEPT WHEN PRESCRIBED BY HIS TREATING PHYSICIAN; MUST SUBMIT TO WITNESSED RANDOM BIOLOGICAL FLUID COLLECTION; KEEP A LOG OF ANY AND ALL MEDICATIONS PRESCRIBED FOR HIM; SHALL SUBMIT TO ANY EXAMINATIONS OR THERAPY ORDERED BY BOARD; SHALL APPEAR BEFORE BOARD FOR INTERVIEWS UPON REQUEST; SHALL INFORM BOARD OF CHANGE OF ADDRESS OR IF AWAY FOR MORE THAN FIVE DAYS. ON 7/30/99 ORDER TERMINATED.

DISNEY, THOMAS FREDERICK MD, LICENSE NUMBER 0G18361 OF PHOENIX, AZ, WAS DISCIPLINED BY CALIFORNIA ON NOVEMBER 22, 1996
DISCIPLINARY ACTION: 60-MONTH PROBATION
OFFENSE: DISCIPLINARY ACTION BY ANOTHER STATE OR AGENCY

NOTES: DISCIPLINED BY ARIZONA FOR SELF-USE OF RITALIN. REVOCATION STAYED, PRIOR CONDITION UNDER TERMS AND CONDITIONS.

DITTEMORE, DENISE MD, LICENSE NUMBER 0022383, WAS DISCIPLINED BY ARIZONA ON JULY 19, 1996
DISCIPLINARY ACTION: RESTRICTION PLACED ON LICENSE; MONITORING OF PHYSICIAN PERFORMANCE

NOTES: INTERVIEWED BY THE BOARD REGARDING HER RETURN TO HER RESIDENCY PROGRAM. SHALL CONTINUE PSYCHIATRIC TREATMENT WITH A BOARD-APPROVED TREATING PSYCHIATRIST AND SHALL REMAIN IN TREATMENT UNTIL FURTHER ORDER OF THE BOARD; TREATING PSYCHIATRIST SHALL SUBMIT QUARTERLY REPORTS TO THE BOARD; SHALL PRACTICE ONLY IN A BOARD-APPROVED RESIDENCY PROGRAM; QUARTERLY REPORTS RELATING TO HER PARTICIPATION AND PERFORMANCE IN RESIDENCY PROGRAM SHALL BE SUBMITTED TO THE BOARD. ON 7/25/97 ORDER TERMINATED.

DOBBS, ROBERT MAYS JR MD, LICENSE NUMBER 0008422 OF 6015 E EXETER BLVD, SCOTTSDALE, AZ, WAS DISCIPLINED BY GEORGIA ON MAY 3, 1990
DISCIPLINARY ACTION: PROBATION; MONITORING OF PHYSICIAN PERFORMANCE
OFFENSE: DISCIPLINARY ACTION BY ANOTHER STATE OR AGENCY

NOTES: HE IS REQUIRED TO ABIDE BY RESTRICTIONS OF ARIZONA BOARD. 0N 6/24/88 HIS LICENSE WAS RESTRICTED BY ARIZONA BOARD WITH FOLLOWING PROVISIONS: WILL PARTICIPATE IN PHYSICIANS HEALTH COMMITTEE PROGRAM WITH QUARTERLY REPORTS TO THE BOARD; SHALL OBTAIN A BOARD APPROVED TREATING PHYSICIAN; SHALL ABSTAIN FROM ALCOHOL; SHALL TAKE NO DRUGS FOR PAIN EXCEPT FOR PLAIN ASPIRIN OR ACETAMINOPHEN, OR WHEN PRESCRIBED BY HIS TREATING PHYSICIAN; SHALL SUBMIT TO RANDOM BIOLOGICAL FLUID TESTS; SHALL SUBMIT TO MEDICAL, MENTAL OR PHYSICAL COMPETENCY TESTS; SHALL PARTICIPATE IN AN AFTERCARE GROUP AT LEAST 3 TIMES A WEEK; SHALL MAINTAIN A LOG OF DRUGS PRESCRIBED FOR HIM. HE HAS NOT PRACTICED IN GEORGIA AND IF HE DESIRES TO HE WILL GIVE NOTICE IN WRITING 90 DAYS PRIOR TO ANTICIPATED DATE OF INITIAL PRACTICE AND SHALL PROVIDE BOARD WITH COMPLETE REPORT ON STATUS OF AND COMPLIANCE WITH ARIZONA'S ORDER.

DOKE, ANTHONY P MD, WAS DISCIPLINED BY ARIZONA ON APRIL 14, 1994
DISCIPLINARY ACTION: RESTRICTION PLACED ON LICENSE; MONITORING OF PHYSICIAN PERFORMANCE

NOTES: SHALL PRACTICE MEDICINE ONLY IN A CLINICAL SETTING IN WHICH HIS CARE AND TREATMENT OF PATIENTS IS CONCURRENTLY SUPERVISED BY A LICENSED ARIZONA MEDICAL DOCTOR WITH QUARTERLY REPORTS REGARDING THE ADEQUACY OF HIS CARE AND TREATMENT OF PATIENTS; SHALL CONTINUE RECEIVING PSYCHOLOGICAL OR PSYCHIATRIC CARE AND TREATMENT AT A FREQUENCY TO BE DETERMINED BY HIS TREATING THERAPIST WITH QUARTERLY REPORTS; SHALL SUBMIT TO FOLLOW-UP PSYCHOLOGICAL OR PSYCHIATRIC EVALUATION AS DIRECTED BY BOARD STAFF; SHALL OBTAIN A SOLE TREATING PHYSICIAN WHO SHALL BE APPROVED BY THE BOARD; SHALL ADVISE HIS APPROVED TREATING PHYSICIAN OF HIS REHABILITATION EFFORTS AND PROVIDE A COPY OF THE BOARD'S ORDER TO HIM.

DOKE, ANTHONY P MD, WAS DISCIPLINED BY ARIZONA ON AUGUST 8, 1998
DISCIPLINARY ACTION: LICENSE SUSPENSION

NOTES: PLACED ON INACTIVE STATUS WITH CAUSE.

DOLORES, MICHAEL A MD, LICENSE NUMBER 0018942, WAS DISCIPLINED BY ARIZONA ON JULY 16, 1992
DISCIPLINARY ACTION: LICENSE REVOCATION
OFFENSE: SUBSTANCE ABUSE

NOTES: ON 2/28/91, VOLUNTARILY ADMITTED HIMSELF TO A DRUG TREATMENT FACILITY IN MINNESOTA WHERE HE UNDERWENT TREATMENT UNTIL 3/30/91. ON 5/3/91, INDICATED THAT HE WAS USING MARIJUANA DAILY, AS WELL AS FIORINOL, A SCHEDULE III CONTROLLED SUBSTANCE, AND USING ALCOHOL TWO OR THREE TIMES A WEEK. ALSO ON 5/3/91, EXECUTED A TREATMENT AGREEMENT WITH MONITORED AFTERCARE TREATMENT PROGRAM, PART OF WHICH WAS TO ACKNOWLEDGE HIS ALCOHOLISM AND/OR DRUG DEPENDENCY. ON 5/28/91, GAVE A URINE SAMPLE WHICH TESTED POSITIVE FOR A GENERIC EQUIVALENT OF FIORINOL, WHICH HAD NOT BEEN PRESCRIBED FOR HIM. ON 6/13/91, INFORMED BOARD INVESTIGATOR HE WOULD NOT SUBMIT TO PROVIDING ADDITIONAL URINE SAMPLES ON THE ADVICE OF HIS ATTORNEY.

DOLORES, MICHAEL A MD, LICENSE NUMBER 0058620 OF 6650 WEST SUNSET ROAD, TUCSON, AZ, WAS DISCIPLINED BY MASSACHUSETTS ON JULY 14, 1993
DISCIPLINARY ACTION: EMERGENCY SUSPENSION

DOLORES, MICHAEL A MD, LICENSE NUMBER 0058620 OF 6650 WEST SUNSET ROAD, TUCSON, AZ, WAS DISCIPLINED BY MASSACHUSETTS ON DECEMBER 29, 1993
DISCIPLINARY ACTION: LICENSE REVOCATION
OFFENSE: SUBSTANCE ABUSE

NOTES: IMPAIRMENT BY CONTROLLED SUBSTANCES; LICENSE FRAUD: FALSE STATEMENT.

DOLORES, MICHAEL A MD, DATE OF BIRTH APRIL 30, 1951 OF 35 SUSSEX STREET, SAN FRANCISCO, CA, WAS DISCIPLINED BY MEDICARE ON SEPTEMBER 11, 1995
DISCIPLINARY ACTION: EXCLUSION FROM THE MEDICARE AND/OR MEDICAID PROGRAM
OFFENSE: DISCIPLINARY ACTION BY ANOTHER STATE OR AGENCY

NOTES: LICENSE REVOKED FOR REASONS BEARING ON PROFESSIONAL PERFORMANCE.

DONOVAN, HAROLD E D0 OF 7055 EAST MCDONALD DRIVE, SCOTTSDALE, AZ, WAS DISCIPLINED BY DEA ON JANUARY 13, 1994
DISCIPLINARY ACTION: SURRENDER OF CONTROLLED SUBSTANCE LICENSE
OFFENSE: PROFESSIONAL MISCONDUCT

NOTES: ALLEGED VIOLATION OF CONTROLLED SUBSTANCE ACT. SURRENDERED REGISTRATION DUE TO RETIREMENT AND DEMENTIA.

DORN, JANICE B MD, LICENSE NUMBER 0015548, WAS DISCIPLINED BY ARIZONA ON JANUARY 19, 1990
DISCIPLINARY ACTION: REQUIRED TO ENTER AN IMPAIRED PHYSICIAN PROGRAM OR SUBSTANCE ABUSE TREATMENT; MONITORING OF PHYSICIAN PERFORMANCE
OFFENSE: SUBSTANCE ABUSE

NOTES: MUST IMMEDIATELY PARTICIPATE IN THE ARIZONA MEDICAL ASSOCIATION PHYSICIAN'S HEALTH COMMITTEE PROGRAM WITH QUARTERLY REPORTS TO THE BOARD; MUST OBTAIN A BOARD-APPROVED TREATING PHYSICIAN; MUST ABSTAIN COMPLETELY FROM ALCOHOL AND ALL OTHER DRUGS; MUST COMPLY WITH REQUESTS FOR RANDOM BIOLOGICAL FLUIDS TESTS; MUST SUBMIT TO ANY EXAMS OR THERAPY ORDERED BY THE BOARD; MUST PARTICIPATE IN A 12-STEP RECOVERY PROGRAM FOR SUBSTANCE ABUSE AS DETERMINED BY THERAPIST

AND ATTEND AT LEAST 3 WEEKLY MEETINGS; MUST APPEAR BEFORE THE BOARD FOR INTERVIEWS UPON REQUEST; MUST ADVISE THE BOARD OF ANY CHANGE OF OFFICE OR HOME ADDRESS OR IF PLANS TO BE AWAY FOR MORE THAN FIVE DAYS; MUST MAINTAIN A LOG OF ALL MEDICATIONS TAKEN. ON 10/24/92, FOLLOWING DISCUSSION OF SUCCESSFUL COMPLETION OF THE STIPULATION AND ORDER, THE BOARD TERMINATED THE STIPULATION AND ORDER TO BECOME EFFECTIVE IN 90 DAYS.

DORN, JANICE B MD, LICENSE NUMBER 0015548, WAS DISCIPLINED BY ARIZONA ON APRIL 14, 1994
DISCIPLINARY ACTION: LICENSE SUSPENSION
OFFENSE: SUBSTANCE ABUSE

NOTES: RELAPSED SINCE THE TERMINATION OF HER REHABILITATION ORDER IN 10/92.

DORN, JANICE B MD OF 4647 NORTH 32ND ST. SUITE 250, PHOENIX, AZ, WAS DISCIPLINED BY DEA ON NOVEMBER 28, 1994
DISCIPLINARY ACTION: SURRENDER OF CONTROLLED SUBSTANCE LICENSE

NOTES: IN LIEU OF PUBLIC INTEREST REVOCATION.

DORN, JANICE B MD, LICENSE NUMBER 0015548, WAS DISCIPLINED BY ARIZONA ON JANUARY 21, 1995
DISCIPLINARY ACTION: RESTRICTION PLACED ON CONTROLLED SUBSTANCE LICENSE; 60-MONTH PROBATION
OFFENSE: SUBSTANCE ABUSE

NOTES: ON 3/6/94 SHE ENTERED LONG-TERM RESIDENTIAL TREATMENT FOR SUBSTANCE ABUSE AND WAS DISCHARGED IN 8/94 AFTER SUCCESSFUL COMPLETION. LICENSE REACTIVATED ON PROBATION WITH FOLLOWING CONDITIONS: MUST IMMEDIATELY PARTICIPATE IN A BOARD-APPROVED MONITORED AFTERCARE TREATMENT PROGRAM WHOSE THERAPIST MUST SUBMIT QUARTERLY REPORTS; SHALL PARTICIPATE IN A 12-STEP RECOVERY PROGRAM AS DETERMINED BY HER TREATING THERAPIST AND ATTEND AT LEAST THREE WEEKLY MEETINGS; SHALL OBTAIN A BOARD-APPROVED TREATING PHYSICIAN; SHALL ABSTAIN COMPLETELY FROM THE CONSUMPTION OF ALCOHOLIC BEVERAGES AND DRUGS EXCEPT WHEN PRESCRIBED BY HER TREATING PHYSICIAN; MUST SUBMIT TO WITNESSED RANDOM BIOLOGICAL FLUID COLLECTION; MUST KEEP A LOG OF ANY AND ALL MEDICATIONS PRESCRIBED FOR HER; SHALL SUBMIT TO ANY EXAMINATIONS OR THERAPY ORDERED BY BOARD; SHALL APPEAR BEFORE THE BOARD FOR INTERVIEWS UPON REQUEST; SHALL INFORM BOARD OF CHANGE OF ADDRESS OR IF AWAY FOR MORE THAN FIVE DAYS; SHALL NOT PRACTICE ADDICTION MEDICINE OR CHRONIC PAIN MEDICINE FOR A MINIMUM OF TWO YEARS; SHALL LIMIT HER PRACTICE OF PSYCHIATRY TO A PART-TIME 20 HOUR WORK WEEK WITH A MAXIMUM OF FOUR HOURS PER DAY; SHALL PRACTICE MEDICINE ONLY IN A GROUP SETTING; WITHIN FIVE DAYS SHALL SURRENDER HER FEDERAL CONTROLLED SUBSTANCE REGISTRATION CERTIFICATES TO THE DEA AND SHALL NOT REAPPLY FOR ANY REGISTRATION CERTIFICATE FOR A MINIMUM OF TWO YEARS.

DOTSON, RODNEY N MD, WAS DISCIPLINED BY ARIZONA ON APRIL 10, 1991
DISCIPLINARY ACTION: DENIAL OF NEW LICENSE
OFFENSE: DISCIPLINARY ACTION BY ANOTHER STATE OR AGENCY

NOTES: ACTION BASED ON LICENSE RESTRICTION IN TEXAS.

DOTSON, RODNEY N MD, WAS DISCIPLINED BY ARIZONA ON JUNE 21, 1991
DISCIPLINARY ACTION: DENIAL OF NEW LICENSE

NOTES: FAILURE TO MEET STATUTORY REQUIREMENTS FOR LICENSURE.

DOTSON, RODNEY NORMAN MD, LICENSE NUMBER 00D9988 OF TEXARKANA, TX, WAS DISCIPLINED BY TEXAS ON JANUARY 12, 1991
DISCIPLINARY ACTION: 60-MONTH PROBATION; RESTRICTION PLACED ON LICENSE

NOTES: IMMEDIATE CESSATION OF CERVICAL CAUTERY EXCEPT UNDER DIRECT SUPERVISION OF A PHYSICIAN AS PART OF AN APPROVED FAMILY PRACTICE RESIDENCY OR PRECEPTORSHIP, PRESCRIBING OR ADMINISTERING CERTAIN DRUGS, OR PROVIDING ONGOING PRENATAL CARE, EXCEPT WITH PRIOR ARRANGEMENTS FOR DELIVERY AND FOLLOW-UP; LIMITATION OF MANAGEMENT OF YEAST INFECTION PATIENTS; NO TREATMENT OF ATTENTION DEFICIT DISORDER OR HYPERACTIVE PATIENTS WITHOUT ONGOING CONSULTATION WITH A PEDIATRICIAN; PERFORMANCE OF CIRCUMCISIONS LIMITED TO NEONATAL PATIENTS UNLESS UNDER DIRECT SUPERVISION OF A PHYSICIAN AS PART OF A FAMILY PRACTICE RESIDENCY OR PRECEPTORSHIP; OBTAINING AN ARIZONA LICENSE TO PRACTICE MEDICINE IMMEDIATELY, OR SURRENDER OF TEXAS MEDICAL LICENSE EFFECTIVE 7/1/91 UNLESS ENTERED INTO A ONE-YEAR PRECEPTORSHIP OR FAMILY PRACTICE RESIDENCY WITH TIMELY AND SUCCESSFUL COMPLETION.

DOTSON, RODNEY NORMAN MD, LICENSE NUMBER D9988 OF HEREFORD, TX, WAS DISCIPLINED BY TEXAS ON AUGUST 22, 1998
DISCIPLINARY ACTION: 60-MONTH PROBATION; REQUIRED TO TAKE ADDITIONAL MEDICAL EDUCATION
OFFENSE: OVERPRESCRIBING OR MISPRESCRIBING DRUGS

NOTES: IN 1983 HE SIGNED AN AFFIDAVIT WITH THE BOARD WHICH INVOLVED ALLEGATIONS OF NON-THERAPEUTIC PRESCRIBING AND FAILURE TO PRACTICE MEDICINE IN AN ACCEPTABLE MANNER; IN 1/91 THE BOARD AND HE ENTERED INTO AN AGREED ORDER OF PROVISIONS WHICH HE SUCCESSFULLY COMPLETED; A BOARD CONSULTANT DETERMINED THAT HIS ADMINISTRATION/PRESCRIPTION OF DONNAGEL PG WAS CONTRAINDICATED AND DANGEROUS; HE MAINTAINS THAT HE WITHDREW THE PRESCRIPTIONS AFTER HE WAS INFORMED BY A PHARMACIST THAT THE MEDICATION WAS NO LONGER AVAILABLE IN THE FORM HE WISHED TO USE IT AND, THEREFORE, USE AS PRESCRIBED WAS CONTRAINDICATED; HIS MEDICAL RECORDS FOR TREATMENT OF SEVERAL PATIENTS DID NOT CLEARLY INDICATE HIS ASSESSMENTS AND TREATMENT PLANS; DID NOT KEEP ADEQUATE RECORDS OF DRUGS; PHARMACY RECORDS INDICATE THAT HE ORDERED PRESCRIPTIONS FOR MEMBERS OF HIS FAMILY WITHOUT DOCUMENTING THESE PRESCRIPTIONS; HE HAS NO RECORDS FOR HIS TREATMENT OF FAMILY MEMBERS; UNTIL AT LEAST 4/97 HE HAD NOT CONTRACTED WITH A HAZARDOUS WASTE DISPOSAL COMPANY TO REMOVE HAZARDOUS WASTE FROM HIS OFFICE; CITY HEALTH INSPECTORS DETERMINED THAT HE WAS DISPOSING OF NEEDLES, USED SPECULUMS, BODY WASTE, AND SYRINGES, IN THE TRASH AND ALLEY BEHIND HIS OFFICE; HE HELD HIMSELF OUT TO BE A " BOARD TRAINED" PEDIATRICIAN; THIS VAGUE DISTINCTION IS INACCURATE AND HE MAINTAINS THAT HE NO LONGER HOLDS HIMSELF OUT TO BE "BOARD

TRAINED"; HE MAINTAINS THAT HE HAS ENROLLED IN A COURSE OF STUDY OFFERED BY THE AMERICAN COLLEGE OF GENERAL MEDICINE, THROUGH THE COLLEGE OF WILLIAM AND MARY, WHICH WILL SUPPORT HIS CONTINUED RETRAINING; HE FURTHER MAINTAINS THAT THIS COURSE OF STUDY EVIDENCES HIS COMMITMENT TO EXCELLENCE IN HIS PRACTICE. SUSPENSION STAYED FOR PROBATION WITH FOLLOWING TERMS AND CONDITIONS: WITHIN 1 YEAR SHALL TAKE AND PASS THE SPEX WITHIN 3 ATTEMPTS; HIS MEDICAL PRACTICE SHALL BE MONITORED BY A BOARD APPROVED TEXAS PHYSICIAN WHO SHALL PROVIDE QUARTERLY REPORTS TO THE BOARD; SHALL OBTAIN 50 HOURS PER YEAR OF CONTINUING MEDICAL EDUCATION IN FAMILY PRACTICE AND/OR PEDIATRICS; SHALL BECOME FAMILIAR WITH AND COMPLY WITH THE LAWS OF THE TEXAS DEPARTMENT OF HEALTH AND OSHA PERTAINING TO BIO-HAZARDOUS WASTE DISPOSAL; SHALL MAINTAIN ADEQUATE MEDICAL RECORDS WHICH SHALL BE AVAILABLE FOR REVIEW; SHALL APPEAR BEFORE THE BOARD AT LEAST ONCE A YEAR; SHALL COOPERATE WITH THE BOARD IN VERIFYING COMPLIANCE; TIME SPENT OUT OF TEXAS DOES NOT COUNT TOWARD PROBATION; SHALL INFORM THE BOARD OF CHANGE OF ADDRESS WITHIN 10 DAYS OR IF HE LEAVES THE STATE; SHALL NOT SEEK MODIFICATION FOR ONE YEAR.

DRYE, ROBERT MD, WAS DISCIPLINED BY ARIZONA ON DECEMBER 9, 1999
DISCIPLINARY ACTION: DENIAL OF NEW LICENSE

NOTES: BY HIS OWN ADMISSION, HE COMMITTED CONDUCT THAT IS GROUNDS TO DENY LICENSURE.

DRYE, ROBERT C MD, LICENSE NUMBER G003618 OF OIL CITY, PA, WAS DISCIPLINED BY CALIFORNIA ON OCTOBER 25, 1991
DISCIPLINARY ACTION: SURRENDER OF LICENSE

NOTES: VOLUNTARY SURRENDER WHILE CHARGES PENDING.

DRYE, ROBERT C MD, DATE OF BIRTH OCTOBER 1, 1927, LICENSE NUMBER 0040091 OF TEMPE, AZ, WAS DISCIPLINED BY PENNSYLVANIA ON AUGUST 24, 1993
DISCIPLINARY ACTION: SURRENDER OF LICENSE
OFFENSE: DISCIPLINARY ACTION BY ANOTHER STATE OR AGENCY

NOTES: GUILTY PLEA TO A MISDEMEANOR CHARGE UNDER THE PENNSYLVANIA CONTROLLED SUBSTANCES ACT; VOLUNTARY SURRENDER OF HIS CALIFORNIA MEDICAL LICENSE. VOLUNTARY SURRENDER.

DVORAK, B ANTHONY MD, WAS DISCIPLINED BY ARIZONA ON AUGUST 9, 1991
OFFENSE: PHYSICAL OR MENTAL ILLNESS INHIBITING THE ABILITY TO PRACTICE WITH SKILL AND SAFETY

NOTES: INFORMATION RECEIVED QUESTIONING HIS ABILITY TO SAFELY ENGAGE IN THE PRACTICE OF MEDICINE AS A RESULT OF A RECURRENCE OF BIPOLAR DISORDER. WITHIN 10 DAYS, SHALL MAKE AN APPOINTMENT FOR A PSYCHIATRIC EVALUATION, A PSYCHOMETRIC EVALUATION AND A PHYSICAL EXAMINATION, ALL TO BE CONDUCTED WITHIN 30 DAYS.

DVORAK, BENJAMIN ANTHONY MD, LICENSE NUMBER 0004757, WAS DISCIPLINED BY ARIZONA ON FEBRUARY 28, 1992
DISCIPLINARY ACTION: LICENSE SUSPENSION
OFFENSE: FAILURE TO COMPLY WITH PREVIOUS BOARD ORDER

NOTES: FAILED TO COMPLY WITH 8/9/91 BOARD ORDER STATING THAT HE BE EXAMINED AND EVALUATED PSYCHIATRICALLY; HAS CHANGED TREATING PHYSICIAN WITHOUT PRIOR BOARD APPROVAL AND HAS FAILED TO PROMPTLY NOTIFY THE BOARD OF HIS ABSENCE FROM THE STATE AND IS MENTALLY AND/OR PHYSICALLY UNABLE TO PRACTICE MEDICINE DUE TO A RECURRENCE OF HIS BIPOLAR DISORDER IN 5/91. HE HAD PREVIOUSLY, IN 1985 AND 1987 ENTERED INTO AGREEMENTS WITH THE BOARD DETAILING TREATMENT AND MONITORING FOR THIS CONDITION. LICENSE SHALL BE PLACED ON INACTIVE STATUS; SHALL NOT PRACTICE IN ARIZONA OR ANY OTHER STATE, TERRITORY OR DISTRICT OF THE U.S. WHILE LICENSE IS INACTIVE; SHALL NOT REQUEST REACTIVATION UNTIL HE MEETS WITH THE BOARD AND COMPLIES WITH ANY AND ALL REQUESTS THEY MAY HAVE; SHALL NOT HOLD REGISTRATION WITH THE DEA OR WRITE PRESCRIPTIONS AS LONG AS LICENSE IS INACTIVE.

DYE, ROBERT A MD, LICENSE NUMBER 0016904 OF MESA, AZ, WAS DISCIPLINED BY ARIZONA ON JANUARY 20, 1993

NOTES: FAILED THE OREGON SPEX EXAM. SHALL NOT PRACTICE MEDICINE IN ARIZONA UNTIL HE HAS TAKEN AND PASSED THE SPEX EXAM AND MET WITH THE BOARD.

DYE, ROBERT ARTHUR MD, LICENSE NUMBER MD16553 OF PARADISE VALLEY, OR, WAS DISCIPLINED BY OREGON ON MAY 16, 1990
DISCIPLINARY ACTION: RESTRICTION PLACED ON LICENSE

NOTES: VOLUNTARY LIMITATION. AS OF 3/10/94 NO LONGER LISTED AS RESTRICTED.

EASLEY, S FOSTER DO, LICENSE NUMBER 3212 OF 7810 N. 14TH PLACE #3010, PHOENIX, AZ, WAS DISCIPLINED BY ARIZONA ON OCTOBER 18, 1999
DISCIPLINARY ACTION: 60-MONTH PROBATION; MONITORING OF PHYSICIAN PERFORMANCE
OFFENSE: PROVIDING FALSE INFORMATION TO THE BOARD OR OTHER HEALTH AGENCY

NOTES: ON OR ABOUT 1/28/99 PROVIDED A FALSE ANSWER ON RENEWAL APPLICATION IN REGARDS TO A QUESTION ASKING WHETHER HE HAD BEEN ARRESTED, PLED GUILTY TO OR NO CONTEST TO OR BEEN CONVICTED OF A FELONY OR A MISDEMEANOR INVOLVING MORAL TURPITUDE WHEN IN FACT HE WAS ARRESTED FOR POSSESSION OF NARCOTICS ON OR ABOUT 9/15/97; ON 4/21/98 HE WAS CHARGED FOR KNOWINGLY POSSESSING OR USING COCAINE, AND LESS THAN TWO POUNDS OF MARIJUANA, AND RECKLESSLY DEFACING OR DAMAGING PROPERTY, A CAMERA, CAUSING DAMAGE IN THE AMOUNT OF $250 OR LESS; ADMITTED IN THE SAME RENEWAL APPLICATION THAT HE HAD ENROLLED IN A DIVERSION PROGRAM AS ORDERED BY THE COUNTY ATTORNEY; TREATMENT. LICENSE LIMITED AS FOLLOWS: SHALL IMMEDIATELY OBTAIN A TREATING THERAPIST APPROVED BY THE BOARD AND SHALL REMAIN IN TREATMENT UNTIL FURTHER ORDER OF THE BOARD; THERAPIST SHALL SEND MONTHLY REPORTS TO BOARD; SHALL PROVIDE A COPY OF THIS ORDER TO ANY HEALTH CARE FACILITY WHERE HE HAS PRIVILEGES; SHALL ABSTAIN COMPLETELY FROM THE CONSUMPTION OF ALCOHOLIC BEVERAGES AND DRUGS EXCEPT WHEN PRESCRIBED BY HIS TREATING PHYSICIAN; MUST SUBMIT TO RANDOM BIOLOGICAL FLUID COLLECTION; MUST KEEP A LOG OF ANY AND ALL MEDICATIONS PRESCRIBED FOR HIM; SHALL SUBMIT TO ANY EXAMINATIONS ORDERED BY BOARD; SHALL APPEAR

BEFORE BOARD UPON REQUEST; SHALL PARTICIPATE IN A MINIMUM OF TWO SELF-HELP MEETINGS PER WEEK THROUGH SUCH ORGANIZATIONS AS AA OR NARCOTICS ANONYMOUS; SHALL INFORM THE BOARD IF HE CEASES TO PRACTICE IN ARIZONA; SHALL PAY COSTS.

EDELSTEIN, MITCHELL E DO, LICENSE NUMBER 003308L OF 2101 NORTH COUNTRY CLUB ROAD, TUCSON, AZ, WAS DISCIPLINED BY PENNSYLVANIA ON FEBRUARY 26, 1991
DISCIPLINARY ACTION: FINE; REPRIMAND
OFFENSE: DISCIPLINARY ACTION BY ANOTHER STATE OR AGENCY

NOTES: IN 4/88 THE ARIZONA BOARD ISSUED A DECREE OF CENSURE FOR PRESCRIBING A CLASS II CONTROLLED SUBSTANCE FOR TWO PATIENTS IN EXCESS OF 30 DAYS IN ONE CALENDAR YEAR. PENNSYLVANIA BOARD ISSUED $1,000 FINE.

EDWARDS, DONALD C MD, WAS DISCIPLINED BY ARIZONA ON JANUARY 20, 1995
DISCIPLINARY ACTION: MONITORING OF PHYSICIAN PERFORMANCE

NOTES: INTERVIEWED BY BOARD MEMBERS RELATIVE TO HIS PARTICIPATION IN THE FLORIDA PHYSICIANS HEALTH PROGRAM AND HIS APPLICATION FOR AN ARIZONA LICENSE. SHALL OBTAIN A BOARD-APPROVED TREATING PSYCHIATRIST WHO SHALL PROVIDE QUARTERLY REPORTS TO THE BOARD REGARDING HIS DIAGNOSIS, PROGNOSIS AND COMPLIANCE WITH THE TREATMENT OF DEPRESSION PROGRAM; SHALL ABSTAIN COMPLETELY FROM THE CONSUMPTION OF ALCOHOL; SHALL COMPLY IMMEDIATELY WITH REQUESTS TO SUBMIT TO WITNESSED RANDOM BIOLOGICAL FLUID COLLECTION.

EICHER, WALTER R MD, WAS DISCIPLINED BY ARIZONA ON FEBRUARY 1, 1992
DISCIPLINARY ACTION: LICENSE SUSPENSION

NOTES: REQUESTED INACTIVE STATUS OF HIS LICENSE WITH CAUSE.

EL-TOUKHY, MOHAMMED S MD, WAS DISCIPLINED BY ARIZONA ON AUGUST 6, 1998
DISCIPLINARY ACTION: REPRIMAND; REQUIRED TO TAKE ADDITIONAL MEDICAL EDUCATION
OFFENSE: PROFESSIONAL MISCONDUCT

NOTES: EXCESSIVE BILLING AND INADEQUATE RECORD KEEPING. SHALL COMPLETE 10 HOURS OF CONTINUING MEDICAL EDUCATION IN RECORD KEEPING, BILLING, PROCEDURE CODES AND NERVE BLOCKS TO BE COMPLETED WITHIN 12 MONTHS.

ELTOUKHY, MOHAMED SAMY MD, LICENSE NUMBER 0015892 OF LAKE HAVASU/NEEDLES, CA, WAS DISCIPLINED BY ARIZONA ON OCTOBER 18, 1994
DISCIPLINARY ACTION: REQUIRED TO TAKE ADDITIONAL MEDICAL EDUCATION
OFFENSE: SUBSTANDARD CARE, INCOMPETENCE OR NEGLIGENCE

NOTES: ALLEGATIONS THAT HE DID NOT APPROPRIATELY MONITOR A PATIENT'S THEOPHYLLINE DOSAGE AND DID NOT ADEQUATELY TREAT THIS PATIENT'S ASTHMATIC CONDITION. SHALL COMPLETE 20 CREDIT HOURS OF CONTINUING MEDICAL EDUCATION IN PHARMACOLOGICAL TREATMENT OF ACUTE INFECTIOUS AND RESPIRATORY DISEASES WITHIN 9 MONTHS OF THE DATE OF THIS ORDER; SUCH HOURS SHALL BE IN ADDITION TO THE 20 CREDIT HOURS REQUIRED FOR THE ANNUAL RENEWAL OF MEDICAL LICENSE. ON 4/05/95 THE BOARD MODIFIED ORDER SUCH THAT AFTER 10/95 THEY SHALL CONDUCT A FOLLOW-UP OFFICE SURVEY OF FIVE TO TEN CHARTS OF PATIENTS, SELECTED AT RANDOM, WHO WERE INITIALLY SEEN AFTER 1/27/95. AS A RESULT OF PRACTICE SURVEY ORDER TERMINATED ON 7/18/96.

EMBRY, THOMAS L MD, LICENSE NUMBER 0013084, WAS DISCIPLINED BY ARIZONA ON OCTOBER 19, 1992
DISCIPLINARY ACTION: RESTRICTION PLACED ON LICENSE
OFFENSE: SUBSTANDARD CARE, INCOMPETENCE OR NEGLIGENCE

NOTES: COMPLAINT ALLEGING NEGLIGENT TREATMENT OF ELDERLY PATIENTS. SHALL NOT ADMIT OR TRANSFER ANY OF HIS PATIENTS TO A NURSING HOME, UNLESS HE CANNOT FIND ANOTHER PHYSICIAN TO TAKE OVER CARE, IN WHICH CASE HE SHALL PROVIDE CARE AND TREATMENT UNTIL THE PATIENT CAN BE TRANSFERRED TO ANOTHER PHYSICIAN. UNTIL CARE IS TRANSFERRED, SHALL SEE PATIENT AT LEAST ONCE WEEKLY AND, IF NECESSARY, SHALL GO TO NURSING HOME TO PERSONALLY SEE PATIENT.

ENCISO, VINCENTE O JR MD, LICENSE NUMBER 6706, WAS DISCIPLINED BY ARIZONA ON JULY 25, 1997
DISCIPLINARY ACTION: REPRIMAND
OFFENSE: NONCOMPLIANCE WITH A PROFESSIONAL RULE

NOTES: A PATIENT IN WHOM HE HAD INSERTED A NORPLANT DEVICE IN 4/93 RETURNED ABOUT NINE MONTHS LATER, COMPLAINING OF WEIGHT GAIN, IRREGULAR HEAVY BLEEDING AND CRAMPING AND NO PHYSICAL EXAMINATION WAS NOTED IN THE CHART. THE PATIENT LATER REQUESTED HER MEDICAL RECORDS AND DR. ENCISCO TOLD HER HE WOULD NOT RELEASE A COPY OF THE RECORDS TO HER BECAUSE IT WOULD BE HARMFUL TO HER HEALTH; HE TOLD THE BOARD HE DID NOT GIVE HER THE RECORDS BECAUSE OF HER ATTITUDE AND IRREGULAR FOLLOW-UP.

ERDOES, LUKE S MD, DATE OF BIRTH FEBRUARY 5, 1958, LICENSE NUMBER 0027079 OF TUCSON, AZ, WAS DISCIPLINED BY COLORADO ON NOVEMBER 19, 1993
DISCIPLINARY ACTION: REPRIMAND

FANCHER, JOHN H MD, WAS DISCIPLINED BY WYOMING ON APRIL 2, 1995
DISCIPLINARY ACTION: DENIAL OF NEW LICENSE

FANCHER, JOHN H MD, LICENSE NUMBER 198654 OF 11045 NORTH 19TH AVENUE, PHOENIX, AZ, WAS DISCIPLINED BY NEW YORK ON MARCH 26, 1999
DISCIPLINARY ACTION: LICENSE REVOCATION
OFFENSE: SUBSTANDARD CARE, INCOMPETENCE OR NEGLIGENCE

NOTES: ORDERED EXCESSIVE TESTS; CONDUCT WHICH EVIDENCES MORAL UNFITNESS; PRACTICED WITH NEGLIGENCE AND INCOMPETENCE ON MORE THAN ONE OCCASION; FAILED TO MAINTAIN ACCURATE PATIENT RECORDS.

FANDINO, ROMEO BANZUELA MD, LICENSE NUMBER 0027981 OF CASA GRANDE, AZ, WAS DISCIPLINED BY FLORIDA ON MAY 7, 1991
DISCIPLINARY ACTION: LICENSE SUSPENSION; PROBATION
OFFENSE: DISCIPLINARY ACTION BY ANOTHER STATE OR AGENCY

NOTES: $1,000 FINE; LICENSE SUSPENDED UNTIL HE APPEARS BEFORE BOARD AND ESTABLISHES ABILITY TO PRACTICE WITH SKILL AND SAFETY, WHICH SHALL INCLUDE DOCUMENTATION THAT ARIZONA LICENSE IS UNENCUMBERED. UPON REINSTATEMENT,

PROBATION WITH TERMS, CONDITIONS AND PERIOD OF TIME TO BE ESTABLISHED.

FELLENS, THOMAS E MD, WAS DISCIPLINED BY ARIZONA ON JUNE 19, 1991
DISCIPLINARY ACTION: DENIAL OF NEW LICENSE
OFFENSE: SUBSTANCE ABUSE

NOTES: WAS REQUIRED TO REPEAT HIS SECOND YEAR OF RESIDENCY TRAINING DUE TO A LEAVE OF ABSENCE WHEN HE ENTERED INPATIENT THEN OUTPATIENT TREATMENT FOR CHEMICAL DEPENDENCY. HE DECLINED TO ENTER INTO STANDARD REHABILITATION AGREEMENT.

FERNANDO, RAWINSON C D MD OF LORAIN, OH, WAS DISCIPLINED BY OHIO ON JANUARY 12, 1990
DISCIPLINARY ACTION: 72-MONTH PROBATION; REPRIMAND
OFFENSE: NONCOMPLIANCE WITH A PROFESSIONAL RULE

NOTES: FAILURE TO COMPLY WITH CONTINUING MEDICAL EDUCATION REQUIREMENTS. SIX YEARS PROBATION.

FERNANDO, RAWINSON C D MD, LICENSE NUMBER 17475, WAS DISCIPLINED BY ARIZONA ON MAY 8, 1997
DISCIPLINARY ACTION: REPRIMAND
OFFENSE: DISCIPLINARY ACTION BY ANOTHER STATE OR AGENCY

NOTES: ON 10/11/89 HE WAS CITED BY THE OHIO BOARD FOR FRAUDULENT MISREPRESENTATIONS IN HIS RENEWAL APPLICATION; LIED ABOUT THIS ON HIS 11/89 RENEWAL APPLICATION IN ARIZONA; ON 1/12/90 HE WAS REPRIMANDED AND PLACED ON PROBATION FOR SIX YEARS BY OHIO BOARD FOR FAILURE TO COMPLY WITH CONTINUING MEDICAL EDUCATION REQUIREMENTS; LIED ABOUT THIS ON 4/90 RENEWAL APPLICATION IN ARIZONA.

FERRIS, JOHN DELOS MD, LICENSE NUMBER 0015102, WAS DISCIPLINED BY ARIZONA ON JUNE 29, 1990
DISCIPLINARY ACTION: RESTRICTION PLACED ON LICENSE

NOTES: MUST CEASE PERFORMING ELECTRICAL HEMORRHOIDOLYSIS ON PATIENTS IN ARIZONA INVOLVING THE USE OF LOW LEVEL DIRECT CURRENT FOR THE DESTRUCTION OF INTERNAL HEMORRHOIDS. ACCEPTANCE OF ORDER DOES NOT CONSTITUTE ADMISSION OF WRONGDOING.

FINE, JOEL F MD, LICENSE NUMBER 0015746, WAS DISCIPLINED BY ARIZONA ON APRIL 20, 1996
OFFENSE: DISCIPLINARY ACTION BY ANOTHER STATE OR AGENCY

NOTES: INTERVIEWED BY THE BOARD REGARDING ACTION TAKEN AGAINST HIS CALIFORNIA LICENSE. SHALL NOT PRACTICE MEDICINE IN ARIZONA PRIOR TO MEETING WITH THE BOARD AND RECEIVING ITS APPROVAL TO PRACTICE.

FINE, JOEL F MD, LICENSE NUMBER 0005376 OF P.O. BOX 2328, KEALAKEKUA, HI, WAS DISCIPLINED BY HAWAII ON AUGUST 21, 1996
DISCIPLINARY ACTION: MONITORING OF PHYSICIAN PERFORMANCE
OFFENSE: SUBSTANCE ABUSE

NOTES: ENGAGED IN THE PRACTICE OF MEDICINE WHILE HIS ABILITY TO PRACTICE WAS IMPAIRED BY DRUGS. VOLUNTARILY ENTERED INTO MONITORING AGREEMENTS AND CONTRACTS WITH THE TALBOTT-MARSH RECOVERY CENTER, COMPLETED ON 3/13/96, AND THE HAWAII MEDICAL ASSOCIATION (HMA); HIS CONTRACT WITH HMA SHALL CONTINUE FOR THE NEXT FIVE YEARS; WITHIN TEN DAYS OF BOARD APPROVAL OF THIS ORDER SHALL NOTIFY AND DIRECT THE HMA TO IMMEDIATELY REPORT TO THE BOARD ANY FAILURE TO ABIDE BY THE TERMS OF THE MEMORANDUM OF UNDERSTANDING WITH THE PHYSICIANS HEALTH COMMITTEE. MEMORANDUM OF UNDERSTANDING DATED 11/29/95: SHALL NOT TAKE MIND-ALTERING DRUGS ON ANY OCCASION UNLESS HOSPITALIZED AS A PATIENT OR UNDER TREATMENT BY A PHYSICIAN; SHALL NOT DRINK ANY ALCOHOL; SHALL ATTEND 90 NARCOTICS ANONYMOUS/AA MEETINGS IN 90 DAYS, AFTER WHICH FIVE MEETINGS A WEEK, ONE OF WHICH WITH THE MD/AA GROUP; SHALL PARTICIPATE IN PSYCHOTHERAPY SESSIONS AT LEAST QUARTERLY; SHALL MAINTAIN CONTACT WITH AN AA SPONSOR WHO WILL REPORT VERBALLY AT LEAST MONTHLY; SHALL SUBMIT WEEKLY RANDOM URINE SCREENINGS AS DETERMINED BY THE HMA; SHALL MEET MONTHLY WITH THE HMA FOR THE FIRST THREE MONTHS AND THEN ON A QUARTERLY BASIS UNTIL TERMINATION OF THIS AGREEMENT; WRITTEN COMPLIANCE REPORTS SHALL BE MADE QUARTERLY BY HIS PHYSICIAN TO THE HMA UNTIL TERMINATION OF THIS AGREEMENT.

FINLEY, LIEUTENANT WAYNE MD, LICENSE NUMBER 0014434, WAS DISCIPLINED BY ARIZONA ON JULY 1, 1993
DISCIPLINARY ACTION: 60-MONTH PROBATION; FINE
OFFENSE: CRIMINAL CONVICTION OR PLEA OF GUILTY, NOLO CONTENDERE, OR NO CONTEST TO A CRIME

NOTES: ON 8/24/90 ENTERED A PLEA OF GUILTY TO A FELONY CHILD ABUSE CHARGE REGARDING AN INCIDENT INVOLVING HIS SON; CHARGE WILL BE DISMISSED UPON COMPLETION OF PROBATION. KEPT INADEQUATE MEDICAL RECORDS IN THAT THEY RARELY CONTAINED A HISTORY OR PHYSICAL FINDINGS; IN ONE CASE, ALTERED PATIENT RECORDS PROVIDING FALSE OR MISLEADING INFORMATION TO THE BOARD REGARDING THE QUALITY OF HIS MEDICAL RECORDS. CENSURED; CONDITIONS OF PROBATION INCLUDE: SHALL SUCCESSFULLY COMPLETE 20 HOURS OF CONTINUING MEDICAL EDUCATION IN THE TOPIC OF MEDICAL RECORDS MANAGEMENT ON OR BEFORE 12/31/93; ASSESSED AN ADMINISTRATIVE PENALTY IN THE AMOUNT OF $5,000. MAY ALTERNATIVELY ELECT TO PROVIDE 50 HOURS OF COMMUNITY SERVICE PER YEAR FOR FIVE YEARS FOR A BOARD APPROVED ORGANIZATION IN PLACE OF PAYING THE FINE. ON 11/1/98 PROBATION TERMINATED.

FISHER, KENNETH M MD, LICENSE NUMBER 0012762, WAS DISCIPLINED BY ARIZONA ON APRIL 18, 1996
DISCIPLINARY ACTION: RESTRICTION PLACED ON LICENSE; MONITORING OF PHYSICIAN PERFORMANCE

NOTES: SHALL OBTAIN A CHAPERONE FOR ALL PATIENT PHYSICAL EXAMINATIONS; SHALL OBTAIN A BOARD-APPROVED TREATING THERAPIST TO ADDRESS BOUNDARY ISSUES AND OTHER ISSUES IDENTIFIED BY THERAPIST, WHO WILL SUBMIT QUARTERLY REPORTS; SHALL SUBMIT TO ANY EXAMINATIONS OR THERAPY ORDERED BY THE BOARD; SHALL APPEAR BEFORE THE BOARD FOR INTERVIEWS UPON REQUEST; SHALL IMMEDIATELY ADVISE BOARD OF ANY CHANGE IN OFFICE OR HOME ADDRESSES.

FISHER, KENNETH M MD, LICENSE NUMBER 12762, WAS DISCIPLINED BY ARIZONA ON SEPTEMBER 24, 1999
DISCIPLINARY ACTION: PROBATION; RESTRICTION PLACED ON LICENSE
OFFENSE: FAILURE TO COMPLY WITH PREVIOUS BOARD ORDER

NOTES: VIOLATED A BOARD ORDER; SEXUAL INTIMACIES WITH A PATIENT. REVOCATION STAYED; BOARD RESTITUTION; CHAPERONE FOR ALL PATIENT PHYSICALS; THERAPY WITH QUARTERLY REPORTS.

FITZGERALD, JANIS K MD, LICENSE NUMBER 0017132 OF TUCSON, AZ, WAS DISCIPLINED BY ARIZONA ON OCTOBER 23, 1993
DISCIPLINARY ACTION: SURRENDER OF CONTROLLED SUBSTANCE LICENSE; RESTRICTION PLACED ON LICENSE

NOTES: SHE SHALL IMMEDIATELY SURRENDER HER DRUG ENFORCEMENT ADMINISTRATION CONTROLLED SUBSTANCE REGISTRATION CERTIFICATE TO THE DEA; SHALL NOT PRACTICE CLINICAL MEDICINE; SHALL OBTAIN A SOLE TREATING PHYSICIAN WHO SHALL BE APPROVED BY THE BOARD; SHALL TAKE NO CONTROLLED SUBSTANCES OR PRESCRIPTION-ONLY MEDICATION UNLESS THEY WERE PRESCRIBED FOR HER BY HER APPROVED TREATING PHYSICIAN; SHALL SUBMIT TO WITNESSED RANDOM BIOLOGICAL FLUID COLLECTION.

FLEISCHER, ALAN S MD, LICENSE NUMBER 0013932, WAS DISCIPLINED BY ARIZONA ON JANUARY 17, 1990
DISCIPLINARY ACTION: RESTRICTION PLACED ON LICENSE; MONITORING OF PHYSICIAN PERFORMANCE
OFFENSE: SUBSTANDARD CARE, INCOMPETENCE OR NEGLIGENCE

NOTES: HE ADMITTED THAT CERTAIN SURGICAL CASES IN LATE 1986 AND EARLY 1987 WERE NOT ADEQUATELY HANDLED. ON 3/20/87 HE SUFFERED A SEVERE HAND INJURY FOR WHICH HE HAS UNDERGONE 3 SURGERIES; ADVISED HE WILL NOT BE ABLE TO PRACTICE NEUROSURGERY AGAIN. SHALL NOT PERFORM ANY TYPE OF CLINICAL MEDICAL PRACTICE, INCLUDING SURGERY, WITHOUT WRITTEN PERMISSION OF THE BOARD; MUST SUBMIT TO ANY AND ALL PHYSICAL, MENTAL, PSYCHOLOGICAL, AND/OR COMPETENCY EXAMS DIRECTED BY THE BOARD; CONSENTS TO RELEASE OF ALL MEDICAL RECORDS TO THE BOARD.

FLEISCHER, ALAN SELIG MD, LICENSE NUMBER 0016598 OF ARIZONA HLTH SCIENCES, TUCSON, AZ, WAS DISCIPLINED BY GEORGIA ON OCTOBER 10, 1990
DISCIPLINARY ACTION: LICENSE REVOCATION
OFFENSE: NONCOMPLIANCE WITH A PROFESSIONAL RULE

NOTES: HIS DAUGHTER TOLD HER PSYCHIATRIST SHE WAS SEXUALLY MOLESTED BY HER FATHER. THE PHYSICAL EXAM YIELDED NO EVIDENCE OF VAGINAL PENETRATION. HE WAS INDICTED BY SUPERIOR COURT OF DEKALB COUNTY FOR CHILD MOLESTATION BUT THIS WAS NOT CONSIDERED AS EVIDENCE HAVING PROBATIVE VALUE. HE DENIES ALL ALLEGATIONS. HIS LICENSE IS CURRENTLY DELINQUENT FOR FAILURE TO RENEW AND IS THEREFORE REVOKED. IF HE WISHES TO APPLY FOR REINSTATEMENT, HE MUST MAKE A PERSONAL APPEARANCE BEFORE THE BOARD AND ANSWER QUESTIONS REGARDING THESE ALLEGATIONS. ON 4/3/97 THE BOARD REPORTED THAT NO FURTHER DISCIPLINARY ORDERS HAD BEEN TAKEN AGAINST DR. FLEISCHER IN GEORGIA. HE THUS HAS ONLY BEEN DISCIPLINED FOR NON-RENEWAL OF HIS MEDICAL LICENSE. AS OF 4/3/97, HIS GEORGIA LICENSE IS NOT CURRENT.

FLOREZ, JUAN B G MD, WAS DISCIPLINED BY ARIZONA ON OCTOBER 8, 1991
DISCIPLINARY ACTION: REQUIRED TO TAKE ADDITIONAL MEDICAL EDUCATION
OFFENSE: FAILURE TO COMPLY WITH PREVIOUS BOARD ORDER

NOTES: FAILED THE BOARD-ORDERED SPEX EXAMINATION FOR THE SECOND TIME. BOARD SHALL CONTINUE ITS INVESTIGATION IN THIS MATTER AND HE SHALL COMPLETE A MINI-RESIDENCY COURSE IN PHARMACOLOGY, WITH EMPHASIS ON PSYCHOTROPIC DRUGS WITHIN SIX MONTHS; SHALL TAKE AND PASS THE SPEX EXAM ON 12/5/91. HE SHALL APPEAR FOR FURTHER INTERVIEW BEFORE THE BOARD AT A FUTURE MEETING WHEN THE ABOVE HAS BEEN COMPLETED. HE VOLUNTARILY AGREED NOT TO PRACTICE IN THE STATE UNTIL HE COMPLETED THE ABOVE.

FLOREZ, JUAN BAUTISTA MD, LICENSE NUMBER 0015040, WAS DISCIPLINED BY ARIZONA ON JULY 19, 1993
DISCIPLINARY ACTION: LICENSE SUSPENSION; RESTRICTION PLACED ON LICENSE
OFFENSE: PROFESSIONAL MISCONDUCT

NOTES: INADEQUATE DOCUMENTATION AND INAPPROPRIATE PSYCHO-PHARMACOLOGICAL PRACTICES IN TREATING TWO PSYCHIATRIC PATIENTS; PRESCRIBED AND/OR DISPENSED XANAX TO HIS WIFE; BOARD ORDERED HIM TO TAKE THE SPEX EXAM WHICH HE FAILED 4 TIMES. TEMPORARILY SUSPENDED EXCEPT, HE MAY BE RETAINED OR EMPLOYED TO ENGAGE IN ADMINISTRATIVE MEDICINE WHICH DOES NOT INVOLVE DIRECT PATIENT CARE. SHALL TAKE AND PASS THE SPEX WITH A SCORE OF 75 OR MORE IN ONE ATTEMPT WITHIN ONE YEAR AFTER THE EFFECTIVE DATE OF THIS ORDER. IF HE FAILS TO COMPLY WITH THIS, BOARD MAY REVOKE HIS LICENSE TO PRACTICE MEDICINE IN ARIZONA.

FLOREZ, JUAN BAUTISTA MD, LICENSE NUMBER 0014204 OF 333 EAST MEDLOCK DRIVE, PHOENIX, AZ, WAS DISCIPLINED BY OKLAHOMA ON JULY 31, 1995
DISCIPLINARY ACTION: LICENSE REVOCATION
OFFENSE: DISCIPLINARY ACTION BY ANOTHER STATE OR AGENCY

NOTES: ON 7/20/93 ARIZONA SUSPENDED HIS LICENSE UNTIL HE PASSED THE SPEX EXAMINATION WITH A SCORE OF 75 BASED ON HIS ALLEGEDLY PRESCRIBING AND/OR DISPENSING XANAX TO HIS WIFE, INAPPROPRIATE TREATMENT OF TWO PSYCHIATRIC PATIENTS, FOCUSING ON INADEQUATE DOCUMENTATION AND INAPPROPRIATE PSYCO-PHARMACOLOGICAL PRACTICES.

FLOREZ, JUAN BAUTISTA MD, LICENSE NUMBER 0015040, WAS DISCIPLINED BY ARIZONA ON APRIL 19, 1996
DISCIPLINARY ACTION: LICENSE REVOCATION
OFFENSE: FAILURE TO COMPLY WITH PREVIOUS BOARD ORDER

NOTES: VIOLATION OF 7/93 BOARD ORDER IN THAT HE FAILED THE SPECIAL PURPOSE EXAMINATION WITH A SCORE OF 72. ON 4/19/96 MOTION FOR REHEARING/REVIEW DENIED.

FLYNN, PATRICK WILLIAM MD, LICENSE NUMBER 0004384, WAS DISCIPLINED BY ARIZONA ON JANUARY 19, 1990
DISCIPLINARY ACTION: 60-MONTH PROBATION; REQUIRED TO ENTER AN IMPAIRED PHYSICIAN PROGRAM OR SUBSTANCE ABUSE TREATMENT
OFFENSE: FAILURE TO COMPLY WITH PREVIOUS BOARD ORDER

NOTES: ON 4/10/87 ENTERED INTO BOARD ORDER WITH TERMS INCLUDING ABSTAINING FROM ALCOHOL AND ALL OTHER DRUGS AND CONTINUING CARE AND TREATMENT FOR SUBSTANCE ABUSE. CEASED PRACTICING MEDICINE IN ARIZONA ON OR BEFORE 12/87. ON OR ABOUT 12/11/87 ENTERED INTO STIPULATION WITH NEVADA BOARD, WHICH WAS

AMENDED ON OR ABOUT 11/21/88. ON 10/24/88 SUBMITTED URINE SAMPLE WHICH TESTED POSITIVE FOR ALCOHOL AND ON 6/19/89 SUBMITTED URINE SAMPLE WHICH TESTED POSITIVE FOR BARBITURATES. ENTERED SUBSTANCE ABUSE PROGRAM IN ATLANTA IN 10/89. CONDITIONS OF PROBATION: MUST HAVE NEVADA BOARD SUBMIT EVALUATIONS OF HIS PROGRESS EVERY SIX MONTHS AND IMMEDIATELY INFORM THE ARIZONA BOARD IN THE EVENT HE VIOLATES THE NEVADA STIPULATION; MUST NOT PRACTICE IN ARIZONA WITHOUT BOARD APPROVAL; MUST OBTAIN CARE FROM BOARD APPROVED PRIMARY CARE PHYSICIAN WHO IS A CERTIFIED ADDICTIONOLOGIST AND WHO MUST SUBMIT QUARTERLY REPORTS TO THE BOARD; MUST ABSTAIN FROM USE OF ALCOHOL AND ANY OTHER DRUGS; MUST COMPLY WITH REQUESTS FOR RANDOM BIOLOGICAL FLUID TESTS; MUST SUBMIT TO ANY EXAMS AND THERAPY ORDERED BY BOARD; MUST PARTICIPATE IN 12-STEP RECOVERY PROGRAM FOR SUBSTANCE ABUSE AS DETERMINED BY THERAPIST AND ATTEND AT LEAST THREE WEEKLY MEETINGS; MUST IMMEDIATELY PARTICIPATE IN ARIZONA MEDICAL ASSOCIATION PHYSICIAN'S HEALTH COMMITTEE PROGRAM WITH QUARTERLY REPORTS TO BOARD; MUST APPEAR BEFORE BOARD FOR INTERVIEWS UPON REQUEST; MUST MAINTAIN A LOG OF ALL MEDICATIONS TAKEN; MUST ADVISE BOARD OF CHANGE IN OFFICE OR HOME ADDRESSES OR IF PLANS TO BE AWAY FOR MORE THAN FIVE DAYS. ON 4/17/93 ORDER TERMINATED.

FLYNN, STEPHEN E JR MD, LICENSE NUMBER 0003351, WAS DISCIPLINED BY ARIZONA ON NOVEMBER 19, 1990
DISCIPLINARY ACTION: REQUIRED TO ENTER AN IMPAIRED PHYSICIAN PROGRAM OR SUBSTANCE ABUSE TREATMENT; MONITORING OF PHYSICIAN PERFORMANCE
OFFENSE: SUBSTANCE ABUSE

NOTES: MUST IMMEDIATELY PARTICIPATE IN ARIZONA MEDICAL ASSOCIATION'S MONITORED AFTERCARE TREATMENT PROGRAM WITH QUARTERLY REPORTS TO THE BOARD; MUST PARTICIPATE IN 90 12-STEP MEETINGS APPROPRIATE FOR SUBSTANCE ABUSE WITHIN 90 DAYS; MUST THEN PARTICIPATE IN RECOVERY PROGRAM AS DETERMINED BY THERAPIST AND ATTEND AT LEAST FIVE WEEKLY MEETINGS; MUST OBTAIN A BOARD APPROVED TREATING PHYSICIAN; MUST ABSTAIN COMPLETELY FROM ALCOHOL AND ANY OTHER DRUGS; MUST COMPLY WITH REQUESTS FOR RANDOM BIOLOGICAL FLUID TESTS; MUST MAINTAIN A LOG OF ALL MEDICATIONS TAKEN; MUST SUBMIT TO ANY EXAMS OR THERAPY ORDERED BY THE BOARD; MUST APPEAR BEFORE BOARD FOR INTERVIEWS UPON REQUEST; MUST ADVISE BOARD OF CHANGE IN OFFICE OR HOME ADDRESS OR PLANS TO BE AWAY FOR MORE THAN FIVE DAYS. ON 4/17/93 BOARD CONTINUED ORDER AND DROPPED THE REQUIREMENT FOR GROUP THERAPY. ON 1/29/94 ORDER TERMINATED AFTER 90 DAYS.

FLYNN, STEPHEN E JR MD, LICENSE NUMBER 0003351, WAS DISCIPLINED BY ARIZONA ON OCTOBER 17, 1995
OFFENSE: PROVIDING FALSE INFORMATION TO THE BOARD OR OTHER HEALTH AGENCY

NOTES: IN 12/93, SUBMITTED FALSE INFORMATION TO A HOSPITAL IN THAT IN APPLICATION FOR REAPPOINTMENT TO THE MEDICAL STAFF, HE FALSELY STATED THAT HE HAD A PROFESSIONAL LIABILITY INSURANCE POLICY; HE SUBMITTED TWO FRAUDULENT CERTIFICATES OF INSURANCE WHICH HE HAD PREPARED FROM AN OLD CERTIFICATE; IN 11/94, BOARD INFORMED HIM THAT HIS REAPPLICATION FOR HOSPITAL PRIVILEGES HAD BEEN DENIED AND REQUESTED THAT HE PROVIDE WRITTEN COMMENTS WITHIN 15 DAYS, IN WHICH HE ADMITTED THAT HE HAD SENT FALSE DOCUMENTS WITH HIS APPLICATION, BUT THAT HE HAD BEEN ISSUED A POLICY IN 5/94 WHICH HE HAD APPLIED FOR IN 3/94. CENSURED.

FLYNN, STEPHEN EUGENE MD, LICENSE NUMBER 00C6937 OF PHOENIX, AZ, WAS DISCIPLINED BY TEXAS ON MARCH 6, 1992
DISCIPLINARY ACTION: 60-MONTH PROBATION
OFFENSE: DISCIPLINARY ACTION BY ANOTHER STATE OR AGENCY

NOTES: DISCIPLINARY ACTION TAKEN BY ANOTHER STATE BOARD AND INTEMPERATE USE OF ALCOHOL OR DRUGS. LICENSE SUSPENDED, SUSPENSION STAYED; PROBATION UNDER TERMS AND CONDITIONS.

FLYNN, STEPHEN EUGENE MD, LICENSE NUMBER 00C6937 OF PHOENIX, AZ, WAS DISCIPLINED BY TEXAS ON OCTOBER 9, 1992
DISCIPLINARY ACTION: SURRENDER OF LICENSE

NOTES: PERMANENTLY SURRENDERED.

FORD, ARTHUR MD, LICENSE NUMBER 0011461, WAS DISCIPLINED BY ARIZONA ON OCTOBER 19, 1992
OFFENSE: SUBSTANDARD CARE, INCOMPETENCE OR NEGLIGENCE

NOTES: ON 8/3/87 USED A CONTRAINDICATED CONCENTRATION OF MARCAINE, AN ANESTHESIA, IN AN OBSTETRICAL PATIENT IN AN ATTEMPT TO ANESTHETIZE HER DURING CHILDBIRTH WHICH LED TO A SEIZURE. CENSURED.

FORD, ARTHUR MD, LICENSE NUMBER 0011461 OF PHOENIX, AZ, WAS DISCIPLINED BY ARIZONA ON JANUARY 19, 1995
OFFENSE: SUBSTANDARD CARE, INCOMPETENCE OR NEGLIGENCE

NOTES: WITH REGARDS TO SURGERY PERFORMED ON 2/4/93 AT NO TIME PRIOR OR DURING ABDOMINAL SURGERY DID HE PLACE A NASO-GASTRIC TUBE DESPITE PATIENT'S ACUTE ABDOMEN AND MULTIPLE EPISODES OF VOMITING, INCLUDING AN EMESIS OF FOUL-SMELLING GASTRIC CONTENTS MOMENTS BEFORE INDUCTION OF ANESTHESIA; FAILED TO EXTUBATE THE PATIENT POST-SURGERY IN A LATERAL POSITION TO MINIMIZE THE EFFECTS OF POSSIBLE VOMITING AND ASPIRATION; FAILED TO AGGRESSIVELY TREAT PATIENT ONCE THE SIGNIFICANT ASPIRATION HAD OCCURRED AND INSTEAD HAD BLOOD GASES DRAWN AND CHEST X-RAYS TAKEN, DURING WHICH TIME PATIENT WORSENED TO THE POINT WHERE RECOVERY WAS IMPOSSIBLE AND DIED OF PULMONARY FAILURE DUE TO ASPIRATION OF GASTRIC CONTENTS. CENSURED.

FORD, LAVELL MD, LICENSE NUMBER 0010360, WAS DISCIPLINED BY ARIZONA ON JANUARY 19, 1995
DISCIPLINARY ACTION: MONITORING OF PHYSICIAN PERFORMANCE

NOTES: SHALL TAKE AND PASS THE SPEX IN MARCH 1995 WITH A SCORE OF 75 OR GREATER; SHALL SUBMIT TO A RANDOM RECORD REVIEW OF HIS OFFICE RECORDS BY THE BOARD STAFF.

FORD, LAVELL MD, LICENSE NUMBER 0010360, WAS DISCIPLINED BY ARIZONA ON APRIL 6, 1995
DISCIPLINARY ACTION: LICENSE REVOCATION
OFFENSE: SUBSTANDARD CARE, INCOMPETENCE OR NEGLIGENCE

NOTES: UNDER INVESTIGATION BY THE BOARD FOR

INAPPROPRIATELY GIVING INTRA-ARTICULAR INJECTIONS OF KENALOG AND XYLOCAINE.

FORSBERG, GARY ROY DO, LICENSE NUMBER 0003983 OF LONGWOOD, FL, WAS DISCIPLINED BY FLORIDA ON APRIL 5, 1995
DISCIPLINARY ACTION: FINE; REQUIRED TO TAKE ADDITIONAL MEDICAL EDUCATION
OFFENSE: SUBSTANDARD CARE, INCOMPETENCE OR NEGLIGENCE

NOTES: CHARGED WITH FAILING TO PRACTICE MEDICINE WITH AN ACCEPTABLE LEVEL OF CARE AND SKILL. $1,000 FINE; SHALL COMPLETE 30 HOURS OF CONTINUING MEDICAL EDUCATION.

FORSBERG, GARY ROY DO, DATE OF BIRTH OCTOBER 28, 1946, LICENSE NUMBER 002970L OF 2948 CARDINAL DRIVE, SIERRA VISTA, AZ, WAS DISCIPLINED BY PENNSYLVANIA ON JULY 17, 1996
DISCIPLINARY ACTION: FINE
OFFENSE: DISCIPLINARY ACTION BY ANOTHER STATE OR AGENCY

NOTES: ON 9/14/94 FLORIDA BOARD ASSESSED A CIVIL PENALTY OF $1,000 AND REQUIRED HIM TO COMPLETE 30 HOURS OF CONTINUING MEDICAL EDUCATION. PENNSYLVANIA ASSESSED A $1,000 CIVIL PENALTY.

FOSDICK, CLAUDE C III MD, LICENSE NUMBER 0044681 OF CASA GRANDE, AZ, WAS DISCIPLINED BY FLORIDA ON MARCH 3, 1992
DISCIPLINARY ACTION: LICENSE SUSPENSION; PROBATION
OFFENSE: SUBSTANDARD CARE, INCOMPETENCE OR NEGLIGENCE

NOTES: CHARGED WITH FAILING TO PRACTICE MEDICINE WITH AN ACCEPTABLE LEVEL OF CARE AND SKILL; ADMINISTERING A LEGEND DRUG IN INAPPROPRIATE OR EXCESSIVE QUANTITIES; FAILING TO KEEP MEDICAL RECORDS JUSTIFYING THE COURSE OF TREATMENT OF A PATIENT. $5,000 FINE; REPRIMAND; WITHIN ONE YEAR SHALL ATTEND 30 HOURS CONTINUING MEDICAL EDUCATION IN DELIVERY OF ANESTHESIA; LICENSE SUSPENDED UNTIL SUCH TIME AS HE WANTS TO RETURN TO HIS PRACTICE OF MEDICINE IN FLORIDA AND APPEARS BEFORE THE BOARD AND DEMONSTRATES HIS ABILITY TO PRACTICE WITH SKILL AND SAFETY. TERMS AND CONDITIONS OF PROBATION TO BE SET AT THAT TIME.

FOSDICK, CLAUDE C III MD, LICENSE NUMBER 0013210 OF CASA GRANDE, AZ, WAS DISCIPLINED BY ARIZONA ON JANUARY 27, 1994
DISCIPLINARY ACTION: RESTRICTION PLACED ON LICENSE; REQUIRED TO TAKE ADDITIONAL MEDICAL EDUCATION
OFFENSE: DISCIPLINARY ACTION BY ANOTHER STATE OR AGENCY

NOTES: FLORIDA TOOK ACTION AGAINST HIS MEDICAL LICENSE.
SHALL BE PERMANENTLY RESTRICTED FROM PERFORMING MAJOR SURGERY AND COSMETIC SURGERY; SHALL COMPLETE 60 HOURS OF CONTINUING MEDICAL EDUCATION PER YEAR IN GENERAL MEDICINE FOR THE NEXT FIVE YEARS, 30 HOURS PER YEAR OF WHICH SHALL BE IN THE FIELD OF PEDIATRICS. HIS MOTION TO MODIFY AGREEMENT DENIED ON 4/11/94. AS OF 4/06/95 HE MET CONTINUING EDUCATION REQUIREMENTS.

FOSDICK, WILLIAM M MD, LICENSE NUMBER 0003985 OF TUCSON, AZ, WAS DISCIPLINED BY ARIZONA ON JANUARY 17, 1995
OFFENSE: SUBSTANDARD CARE, INCOMPETENCE OR NEGLIGENCE

NOTES: ENGAGED IN CONDUCT WHICH WAS HARMFUL OR DANGEROUS TO THE HEALTH OF A PATIENT THAT HE SAW FOR AT LEAST THREE YEARS DURING 1986 THROUGH 1988 IN THAT HE DID NOT PERFORM ANY BASELINE STUDIES REGARDING THE PATIENT'S EYES BEFORE PRESCRIBING CHLOROQUINE, A DRUG KNOWN TO POSE A RISK FOR VISION LOSS AND RETINAL LESIONS, AND PERIODIC OPTHALMOLOGICAL EXAMINATIONS WHILE PRESCRIBING HIGHER THAN NORMAL DOSES OF CHLOROQUINE; PATIENT WAS FOUND TO HAVE CORNEAL ABNORMALITIES AS EARLY AS SEVEN MONTHS BEFORE CHLOROQUINE WAS DISCONTINUED AND ULTIMATELY EXPERIENCED PERMANENTLY DIMINISHED VISION IN BOTH EYES. FAILED TO MAINTAIN ADEQUATE RECORDS ON THIS PATIENT BY FAILING TO INDICATE IN RECORDS AN INCREASE IN DOSE OF CHLOROQUINE AND HAVING NO WRITTEN ENTRY IN THE RECORDS INDICATING THAT THE PATIENT WAS TOLD THAT SHE WAS ON A HIGHER DOSE THAN RECOMMENDED. CENSURED.

FRASER, KENNETH R MD, LICENSE NUMBER 0007913 OF SCOTTSDALE, AZ, WAS DISCIPLINED BY ARIZONA ON JULY 16, 1993
DISCIPLINARY ACTION: FINE
OFFENSE: SUBSTANDARD CARE, INCOMPETENCE OR NEGLIGENCE

NOTES: MANAGEMENT OF SEVERAL GYNECOLOGICAL PATIENTS DURING 1991 WAS INAPPROPRIATE -- TREATMENTS DONE AT WRONG TIME AND INAPPROPRIATELY; HOSPITALIZATIONS WERE OF EXCESSIVE DURATION; PROCEDURES DONE SEPARATELY THAT SHOULD HAVE BEEN DONE TOGETHER; SURGERY PERFORMED PRIOR TO ADEQUATE OBSERVATION; OVERCHARGED FOR VARIOUS SURGICAL PROCEDURES IN 2 CASES. CENSURED AND SHALL PAY A $7,500 ADMINISTRATIVE PENALTY WITHIN 6 MONTHS. REQUEST FOR RECONSIDERATION DENIED ON 4/15/94.

FREMER, EDWARD DO, LICENSE NUMBER 2925 OF 2000 HIGHWAY 95, #216, BULLHEAD CITY, AZ, WAS DISCIPLINED BY ARIZONA ON MARCH 25, 1998
DISCIPLINARY ACTION: 60-MONTH PROBATION
OFFENSE: PROFESSIONAL MISCONDUCT

NOTES: ON 4/27/95 HE CONSPIRED WITH ANOTHER INDIVIDUAL TO INFLICT PHYSICAL HARM TO ANOTHER DOCTOR; THE OTHER PERSON TAPE RECORDED THEIR CONVERSATION AND DR. FREMER WITHDREW FROM THE CONSPIRACY THE SAME EVENING; HE IS CENSURED FOR UNPROFESSIONAL CONDUCT. TERMS AND CONDITIONS OF PROBATION ARE AS FOLLOWS: WITHIN 45 DAYS MUST OBTAIN A NEUROPSYCHOLOGICAL EXAMINATION BY EITHER A LICENSED PSYCHIATRIST OR PSYCHOLOGIST WHO IS APPROVED BY THE BOARD AND COMPLY WITH ANY RECOMMENDATION MADE FOR TREATMENT OR COUNSELING; SHALL WAIVE ANY CONFIDENTIALITY WITH REGARD TO EVALUATION OR TREATMENT; SHALL PROVIDE A COPY OF THIS ORDER TO ALL HEALTH CARE FACILITIES WHERE HE IS EMPLOYED AS A PHYSICIAN; SHALL SUBMIT TO ANY EVALUATIONS ORDERED BY THE BOARD; SHALL APPEAR BEFORE THE BOARD UPON REQUEST; SHALL NOTIFY THE BOARD IF HE CEASES TO RESIDE IN ARIZONA; SHALL PAY COSTS.

FREMER, EDWARD DO, LICENSE NUMBER 2925 OF 1895 CORWIN ROAD, BULLHEAD CITY, AZ, WAS DISCIPLINED BY ARIZONA ON APRIL 10, 1999
DISCIPLINARY ACTION: LICENSE SUSPENSION; MONITORING OF PHYSICIAN PERFORMANCE
OFFENSE: PHYSICAL OR MENTAL ILLNESS INHIBITING THE ABILITY TO PRACTICE WITH SKILL AND SAFETY

NOTES: NOT CURRENTLY COMPETENT TO PRACTICE DUE TO HIS EXISTING MEDICAL CONDITION BASED ON PSYCHIATRIC AND PSYCHOLOGICAL EVALUATIONS. SHALL OBTAIN AN IME PERFORMED BY AN IME

PHYSICIAN TO DETERMINE HIS MENTAL STATUS AND COMPETENCE WHO SHALL SEND A COPY OF THE EVALUATION TO THE BOARD; SHALL SUBMIT TO ANY EXAMINATIONS ORDERED BY BOARD; SHALL APPEAR BEFORE BOARD FOR INTERVIEWS UPON REQUEST; MUST SUBMIT TO RANDOM BIOLOGICAL FLUID COLLECTION; SHALL INFORM THE BOARD IF HE CEASES TO PRACTICE IN ARIZONA; SHALL PAY COSTS; SHALL CONTINUE TO MEET CONDITIONS OF THE 3/25/98 ORDER.

FREMER, EDWARD DO, LICENSE NUMBER 2925 OF 1895 CORWIN ROAD, BULLHEAD CITY, AZ, WAS DISCIPLINED BY ARIZONA ON MAY 16, 1999
DISCIPLINARY ACTION: LICENSE SUSPENSION; SUSPENSION OF CONTROLLED SUBSTANCE LICENSE
OFFENSE: PHYSICAL OR MENTAL ILLNESS INHIBITING THE ABILITY TO PRACTICE WITH SKILL AND SAFETY

NOTES: AGREED TO VOLUNTARILY WITHDRAW FROM THE PRACTICE OF MEDICINE BECAUSE HE WAS NOT CURRENTLY COMPETENT TO PRACTICE DUE TO HIS EXISTING MEDICAL CONDITIONS BASED ON PSYCHIATRIC AND PSYCHOLOGICAL EVALUATIONS; ALLEGATIONS OF UNPROFESSIONAL CONDUCT. DURING THE PERIOD OF SUSPENSION: SHALL OBTAIN AN IME PERFORMED BY A PHYSICIAN THE RESULTS OF WHICH SHALL BE SENT TO THE BOARD; SHALL SUBMIT TO ANY EVALUATIONS ORDERED BY THE BOARD; SHALL APPEAR BEFORE THE BOARD UPON REQUEST; SHALL CONTINUE TO MEET REQUIREMENTS OF 3/25/98 ORDER; HIS PRESCRIPTION WRITING AUTHORITY IS SUSPENDED FOR THE DURATION OF THIS ORDER; SHALL SUBMIT TO RANDOM BIOLOGICAL FLUID TESTING; SHALL NOTIFY THE BOARD IF HE CEASES TO RESIDE IN ARIZONA; SHALL PAY COSTS.

FREMER, EDWARD M DO, LICENSE NUMBER 20A6944 OF BULLHEAD CITY, AZ, WAS DISCIPLINED BY CALIFORNIA ON NOVEMBER 24, 1998
DISCIPLINARY ACTION: 48-MONTH PROBATION
OFFENSE: DISCIPLINARY ACTION BY ANOTHER STATE OR AGENCY

NOTES: ACTION TAKEN BY ANOTHER STATE; COMMISSION OF DISHONEST ACTS; CONDUCT WARRANTING DENIAL OF CERTIFICATE; ATTEMPTING TO VIOLATE STATUTE. SUSPENSION STAYED.

FREMER, EDWARD M DO, LICENSE NUMBER 189379 OF PO BOX 376, STEGER, IL, WAS DISCIPLINED BY NEW YORK ON JULY 13, 1999
DISCIPLINARY ACTION: LICENSE SUSPENSION; PROBATION
OFFENSE: DISCIPLINARY ACTION BY ANOTHER STATE OR AGENCY

NOTES: DISCIPLINED BY THE ARIZONA BOARD FOR ENGAGING IN CONDUCT WHICH IS CONTRARY TO THE RECOGNIZED STANDARDS OF MEDICAL ETHICS. SUSPENSION UNTIL PROVEN FIT TO PRACTICE; PROBATION FOR NO LESS THAN FIVE YEARS.

FROST, ALAN P MD, LICENSE NUMBER 0041480 OF MT DORA, FL, WAS DISCIPLINED BY FLORIDA ON JULY 17, 1991
DISCIPLINARY ACTION: FINE; REQUIRED TO TAKE ADDITIONAL MEDICAL EDUCATION
OFFENSE: SUBSTANDARD CARE, INCOMPETENCE OR NEGLIGENCE

NOTES: CHARGED WITH FAILING TO PRACTICE MEDICINE WITH AN ACCEPTABLE LEVEL OF CARE AND SKILL. IN LIEU OF FURTHER PROSECUTION, STIPULATED TO $1000 FINE; COMPLETION OF 20 HOURS CONTINUING MEDICAL EDUCATION WITHIN ONE YEAR IN DIAGNOSTIC MEASURES AND/OR RISK MANAGEMENT; MUST WRITE AN ARTICLE SUITABLE FOR PUBLICATION WITHIN 180 DAYS ON THE PITFALLS IN INTERPRETING MAMMOGRAPHIES AND BREAST ULTRASOUNDS.

FROST, ALAN P MD, LICENSE NUMBER 0018967, WAS DISCIPLINED BY ARIZONA ON JULY 15, 1994
OFFENSE: DISCIPLINARY ACTION BY ANOTHER STATE OR AGENCY

NOTES: FLORIDA MEDICAL BOARD TOOK ACTION AGAINST HIS LICENSE, REQUIRING THAT HE PAY AN ADMINISTRATION FINE, WRITE AN ARTICLE ON "PITFALLS OF MAMMOGRAPHY AND BREAST ULTRASOUNDS" AND COMPLETE ADDITIONAL CONTINUING MEDICAL EDUCATION REQUIREMENTS. SHALL NOT ENGAGE IN THE PRACTICE OF MEDICINE IN ARIZONA UNTIL HE HAS FIRST INFORMED THE ARIZONA BOARD OF HIS INTENTION TO DO SO, APPEARED AT AN INFORMAL INTERVIEW AT THE INVITATION OF THE BOARD, AND RECEIVED AUTHORIZATION BY THE BOARD TO PRACTICE MEDICINE IN ARIZONA.

FRY, PHILLIP E MD, LICENSE NUMBER 5325, WAS DISCIPLINED BY ARIZONA ON JULY 29, 1999
DISCIPLINARY ACTION: 6-MONTH PROBATION; REPRIMAND

NOTES: SHALL OBTAIN 20 HOURS OF BOARD APPROVED CONTINUING MEDICAL EDUCATION IN ANESTHETIC MANAGEMENT FOR HIGH RISK PATIENTS.

FUSCO, MICHAEL CARL DR, LICENSE NUMBER 0017666, WAS DISCIPLINED BY ARIZONA ON JULY 15, 1994
DISCIPLINARY ACTION: LICENSE SUSPENSION
OFFENSE: NONCOMPLIANCE WITH A PROFESSIONAL RULE

NOTES: FAILURE TO PAY RENEWAL FEE DURING PENDING INVESTIGATION.

GABRIELLE, DENIS MICHAEL STEPHEN MD, LICENSE NUMBER 0010295, WAS DISCIPLINED BY ARIZONA ON JULY 19, 1996
DISCIPLINARY ACTION: LICENSE REVOCATION
OFFENSE: DISCIPLINARY ACTION BY ANOTHER STATE OR AGENCY

NOTES: DISCIPLINARY ACTION TAKEN BY THE COLLEGE OF PHYSICIANS AND SURGEONS OF ONTARIO, CANADA: ON 11/29/95, LICENSE SUSPENDED FOR 18 MONTHS RETROACTIVE TO 6/1/94 AND HIS PRACTICE RESTRICTED INDEFINITELY TO ASSIST AT SURGERY AT ONE HOSPITAL; BASED ON FINDINGS THAT HE DISPLAYED A DISREGARD FOR THE WELFARE OF HIS PATIENTS; FOUND GUILTY OF SEXUAL IMPROPRIETY IN HIS BEHAVIOR TOWARD FOUR PATIENTS; FOUND GUILTY OF SEXUAL ABUSE IN HIS BEHAVIOR TOWARD TWO PATIENTS; IN 2/95, REQUESTED TO ENTER INTO A STIPULATION AND ORDER WITH THE ARIZONA BOARD, WHICH WOULD RESTRICT HIS LICENSE UNTIL MEETING WITH THE BOARD; IN 5/95, ASKED BY THE BOARD TO SUBMIT STATEMENTS REGARDING THE ONTARIO ACTION; FAILED TO FURNISH INFORMATION IN A TIMELY MANNER TO THE BOARD IN THAT HE FEIGNED CONFUSION OVER WHAT THE BOARD WAS REQUESTING AND DECLINED TO STIPULATE; ORDERED BY THE BOARD TO APPEAR FOR AN INFORMAL INTERVIEW ON 1/18/96; VIOLATED A BOARD ORDER IN THAT HE FAILED TO APPEAR BEFORE THE BOARD FOR AN INFORMAL INTERVIEW. REVOCATION IS PERMANENT.

GABROY, JAMES B MD, LICENSE NUMBER 0012491 OF CASA GRANDE, AZ, WAS DISCIPLINED BY ARIZONA ON JULY 14, 1993
DISCIPLINARY ACTION: REQUIRED TO TAKE ADDITIONAL MEDICAL EDUCATION
OFFENSE: OVERPRESCRIBING OR MISPRESCRIBING DRUGS

NOTES: ALLEGATIONS OF OVERPRESCRIBING OF MULTIPLE

DRUGS. SHALL WITHIN ONE YEAR, SUCCESSFULLY COMPLETE 20 HOURS OF CONTINUING MEDICAL EDUCATION ACCEPTABLE TO THE BOARD IN THE SUBJECT OF PRESCRIBING PSYCHOACTIVE MEDICATIONS. ON 1/20/95 ORDER TERMINATED.

GALLAGHER, WILLIAM B MD, LICENSE NUMBER 0010814, WAS DISCIPLINED BY ARIZONA ON APRIL 18, 1996
DISCIPLINARY ACTION: 24-MONTH PROBATION; REQUIRED TO TAKE ADDITIONAL MEDICAL EDUCATION
OFFENSE: SUBSTANDARD CARE, INCOMPETENCE OR NEGLIGENCE

NOTES: GROSS NEGLIGENCE, REPEATED NEGLIGENCE OR NEGLIGENCE RESULTING IN HARM TO OR THE DEATH OF A PATIENT IN THAT THREE TIMES BETWEEN 5/5/92 AND 5/13/92, HE TREATED A PATIENT WHO HAD A HISTORY OF CARDIAC DISEASE FOR MUSCULO-SKELETAL PAIN WITHOUT CONDUCTING A FULL EXAMINATION WHICH COULD HAVE REVEALED CARDIAC CAUSES OF THE PAIN; ON TWO OF THESE OCCASIONS, PATIENT WAS PLACED ON PAIN MEDICATIONS FOR HIS BACK PAIN AND ON THE THIRD VISIT WAS PLACED ON ERYTHROMYCIN AND TUSSI-ORGANIDIN FOR AN IMPRESSION OF PNEUMONITIS; ON 5/14/92, PARAMEDICS WERE CALLED TO PATIENT'S HOUSE WHERE HE WAS EXPERIENCING RESPIRATORY DISTRESS AND WAS ADMITTED TO THE EMERGENCY ROOM WHERE HE DEVELOPED RESPIRATORY ARREST AND COMPLETE HEART BLOCK AND ULTIMATELY DIED FROM ACUTE MYOCARDIAL INFARCTION. PROBATION WITH TERMS: WITHIN ONE YEAR, SHALL COMPLETE A 60-DAY BOARD-APPROVED MINI-RESIDENCY IN EMERGENCY MEDICINE; WITHIN ONE YEAR, SHALL OBTAIN 20 HOURS OF BOARD-APPROVED CONTINUING MEDICAL EDUCATION IN RECORD KEEPING; WITHIN 60 DAYS, SHALL SUBMIT TO PSYCHIATRIC, PSYCHOLOGICAL AND PHYSICAL EXAMINATIONS BY BOARD-DESIGNATED EVALUATORS. ON 4/18/96 PROBATION TERMINATED. ON 1/22/97 REQUEST THAT HE BE ALLOWED TO PARTICIPATE IN A ONE MONTH MINI-RESIDENCY IN CARDIOLOGY IN LIEU OF THE BOARD-ORDERED 60 DAY MINI-RESIDENCY IN EMERGENCY MEDICINE GRANTED. ON 5/14/98 ORDER TERMINATED.

GALLAGHER, WILLIAM B MD, LICENSE NUMBER 10814, WAS DISCIPLINED BY ARIZONA ON NOVEMBER 14, 1997
DISCIPLINARY ACTION: LICENSE SUSPENSION

NOTES: UNDER INVESTIGATION BY THE BOARD. REQUESTED LICENSE BE PLACED ON INACTIVE STATUS WITH CAUSE. MAY NOT REQUEST REACTIVATION OF HIS LICENSE UNTIL HE MEETS WITH THE BOARD AND COMPLIES WITH ALL BOARD REQUESTS WHICH MAY INCLUDE PSYCHIATRIC AND PSYCHOMETRIC EVALUATION, INPATIENT EVALUATION, PHYSICAL EXAMINATION AND TESTING AND WRITTEN AND/OR ORAL COMPETENCY EXAMINATIONS. HE IS CURRENTLY ON PROBATION AND UNDERGOING VOLUNTARY RANDOM WITNESSED BIOLOGICAL TESTING. LICENSE PLACED ON INACTIVE STATUS.

GANNON, GEORGE W MD, LICENSE NUMBER 0003909, WAS DISCIPLINED BY ARIZONA ON APRIL 10, 1991
OFFENSE: NONCOMPLIANCE WITH A PROFESSIONAL RULE

NOTES: CENSURED FOR UNPROFESSIONAL CONDUCT IN FAILING OR REFUSING TO MAINTAIN ADEQUATE RECORDS ON A PATIENT, OR FAILING OR REFUSING TO MAKE SUCH RECORDS PROMPTLY AVAILABLE TO ANOTHER PHYSICIAN UPON REQUEST AND RECEIPT OF PROPER AUTHORIZATION; ANY CONDUCT OR PRACTICE WHICH IS OR MIGHT BE HARMFUL OR DANGEROUS TO THE HEALTH OF THE PATIENT OR THE PUBLIC.

GANNON, GEORGE W MD, LICENSE NUMBER 0003909 OF PHOENIX, AZ, WAS DISCIPLINED BY ARIZONA ON APRIL 13, 1993
OFFENSE: NONCOMPLIANCE WITH A PROFESSIONAL RULE

NOTES: REPEATED FAILURE TO SEND MEDICAL RECORDS OF TWO PATIENTS TO ANOTHER PHYSICIAN UPON REQUEST AND RECEIPT OF PROPER AUTHORIZATION; HAD PREVIOUSLY FAILED TO SEND RECORDS WITHOUT PRIOR PAYMENT OF A FEE. CENSURED.

GARCIA, FRANCISCO A MD, LICENSE NUMBER 0015551, WAS DISCIPLINED BY ARIZONA ON NOVEMBER 20, 1996
DISCIPLINARY ACTION: MONITORING OF PHYSICIAN PERFORMANCE

NOTES: MUST IMMEDIATELY OBTAIN COUNSELING FROM A BOARD- APPROVED THERAPIST REGARDING INTERPERSONAL ISSUES; SHALL REMAIN IN THERAPY UNTIL THERAPEUTICALLY DISCHARGED BY THAT THERAPIST AND SHALL AUTHORIZE RELEASE OF QUARTERLY REPORTS TO THE BOARD. ON 11/14/97 ORDER TERMINATED.

GARLAND, DONALD J MD, LICENSE NUMBER 11505, WAS DISCIPLINED BY ARIZONA ON MARCH 27, 1998
DISCIPLINARY ACTION: REPRIMAND
OFFENSE: SUBSTANDARD CARE, INCOMPETENCE OR NEGLIGENCE

NOTES: IN 5/96 FAMILY MEMBERS OF ONE OF HIS PATIENTS ALLEGED THAT HE HAD INAPPROPRIATELY TREATED AND DIAGNOSED THEIR SISTER WITH MULTIPLE PERSONALITY DISORDER BASED ON FALSE MEMORIES OF CHILDHOOD PHYSICAL, SEXUAL AND RITUAL OR SATANIC ABUSE BY HER FAMILY MEMBERS; PATIENT WAS EXCLUSIVELY UNDER HIS CARE FROM LATE 1991 AND WAS HOSPITALIZED SEVERAL TIMES DUE TO DEPRESSIVE SYMPTOMS WITH SUICIDAL PLANS; WITH REGARD TO HIS DIAGNOSTIC CRITERIA, HIS RECORDS VAGUELY REFERENCE THE PRESENCE OF THE PATIENT'S MULTIPLE PERSONALITIES AND DO NOT MENTION ANY SPECIFICITY OF THE SYMPTOMATOLOGY OR DURATION OF THESE PERSONALITY STATES; HIS RECORDS DO NOT DEFINE THE TREATMENT PROTOCOL HE WAS FOLLOWING OR THE BENEFITS, RISKS AND ALTERNATIVES OF HIS TREATMENT PLAN; BASED ON THE PATIENT'S MULTIPLE HOSPITALIZATIONS, HER POSSIBLE COMPLICATIONS OF MULTIPLE PERSONALITY DISORDER AND THE FACT SHE HAD CUT OFF TIES WITH HER FAMILY AND WAS ALONE CARING FOR HER CHILDREN, HE SHOULD HAVE MORE ACTIVELY PURSUED PROVISIONS FOR HER CHILDREN'S CARE; ANOTHER PHYSICIAN SAW THIS PATIENT AND COULD FIND NO VISIBLE PHYSICAL EVIDENCE OF PREVIOUS SEXUAL MOLESTATION TRAUMA, BUT DR. GARLAND DID NOT INITIALLY INCLUDE THESE RECORDS IN RESPONSE TO THE BOARD'S SUBPOENA FOR ALL RECORDS IN HIS POSSESSION; IN AT LEAST 21 INSTANCES HE ADMITTED THAT HE HAD NOT DOCUMENTED INFORMATION THAT WAS PERTINENT TO THE PATIENT'S DIAGNOSIS, MEDICATION AND TREATMENT.

GARRETT, ROBERT LYNDEL MD, LICENSE NUMBER 0010927, WAS DISCIPLINED BY ARIZONA ON JANUARY 1, 1995
DISCIPLINARY ACTION: LICENSE SUSPENSION; REQUIRED TO ENTER AN IMPAIRED PHYSICIAN PROGRAM OR SUBSTANCE ABUSE TREATMENT
OFFENSE: FAILURE TO COMPLY WITH PREVIOUS BOARD ORDER

NOTES: IN 11/94, CONSUMED ALCOHOL IN VIOLATION OF

11/15/93 STIPULATION. SHALL NOT PRACTICE MEDICINE ANYWHERE WHILE LICENSE IS INACTIVE; MAY NOT HOLD DEA REGISTRATION OR WRITE PRESCRIPTIONS WHILE LICENSE IS INACTIVE; AGREES TO ENTER LONG-TERM/INPATIENT TREATMENT FOR CHEMICAL DEPENDENCY AND ALCOHOLISM AND TO SUCCESSFULLY COMPLETE ALL TREATMENT RECOMMENDED. AGREES TO NOT REQUEST REACTIVATION UNTIL HAS MET WITH THE BOARD AND HAS SIX MONTHS DOCUMENTED SOBRIETY FOLLOWING SUCCESSFUL COMPLETION OF ALL RECOMMENDED TREATMENT.

GARRETT, ROBERT LYNDEL MD, LICENSE NUMBER 0010927, WAS DISCIPLINED BY ARIZONA ON APRIL 8, 1995
DISCIPLINARY ACTION: 60-MONTH PROBATION; REQUIRED TO ENTER AN IMPAIRED PHYSICIAN PROGRAM OR SUBSTANCE ABUSE TREATMENT
OFFENSE: FAILURE TO COMPLY WITH PREVIOUS BOARD ORDER

NOTES: TREATMENT FOR ALCOHOL DEPENDENCY BETWEEN 11/25/94 AND 3/13/95 WHICH HE COMPLETED. REINSTATEMENT TO PROBATION WITH CONDITIONS: MUST IMMEDIATELY PARTICIPATE IN A BOARD-APPROVED MONITORED AFTERCARE TREATMENT PROGRAM WHOSE THERAPIST MUST SUBMIT QUARTERLY REPORTS; HAS PREVIOUSLY PARTICIPATED IN 90 12-STEP MEETINGS IN 90 DAYS AND SHALL PARTICIPATE IN A 12-STEP RECOVERY PROGRAM AS DETERMINED BY HIS TREATING THERAPIST AND ATTEND AT LEAST THREE WEEKLY MEETINGS; SHALL OBTAIN A BOARD-APPROVED TREATING PHYSICIAN; SHALL ABSTAIN COMPLETELY FROM THE CONSUMPTION OF ALCOHOLIC BEVERAGES AND DRUGS EXCEPT WHEN PRESCRIBED BY HIS TREATING PHYSICIAN; MUST SUBMIT TO WITNESSED RANDOM BIOLOGICAL FLUID COLLECTION; MUST KEEP A LOG OF ANY AND ALL MEDICATIONS PRESCRIBED FOR HIM; SHALL SUBMIT TO ANY EXAMINATIONS OR THERAPY ORDERED BY BOARD; SHALL APPEAR BEFORE BOARD FOR INTERVIEWS UPON REQUEST; SHALL INFORM BOARD OF CHANGE OF ADDRESS OR IF AWAY FOR MORE THAN FIVE DAYS.

GARRETT, ROBERT LYNDEL MD, LICENSE NUMBER 10927, WAS DISCIPLINED BY ARIZONA ON JANUARY 25, 1997
DISCIPLINARY ACTION: 84-MONTH PROBATION; RESTRICTION PLACED ON LICENSE

NOTES: ORDER AMENDS 4/8/95 ORDER AS FOLLOWS: TIME OF PROBATION EXTENDED; SHALL IMMEDIATELY OBTAIN A BOARD-APPROVED TREATING PSYCHIATRIST AND REMAIN IN TREATMENT UNTIL FURTHER ORDER OF THE BOARD; THE PSYCHIATRIST SHALL SUBMIT QUARTERLY WRITTEN REPORTS; SHALL LIMIT HIS PRACTICE OF MEDICINE TO NOT MORE THAN AN AVERAGE OF 40 HOURS PER WEEK; HE SHALL NOT TAKE CALL ON DAYS THAT HE HAS SCHEDULED PROCEDURES.

GARTNER, CHARLES H MD, DATE OF BIRTH JUNE 12, 1942, LICENSE NUMBER 0016580 OF DENVER, CO, WAS DISCIPLINED BY COLORADO ON APRIL 14, 1995
DISCIPLINARY ACTION: 60-MONTH PROBATION; RESTRICTION PLACED ON LICENSE
OFFENSE: SUBSTANDARD CARE, INCOMPETENCE OR NEGLIGENCE

NOTES: SUBSTANDARD CARE. PROBATION INCLUDES RESTRICTIONS, PRACTICE MONITORING AND REEDUCATION ACTIVITIES.

GARTNER, CHARLES H MD, LICENSE NUMBER 0017295, WAS DISCIPLINED BY ARIZONA ON SEPTEMBER 19, 1996

NOTES: SHALL NOT PRACTICE MEDICINE IN ARIZONA UNTIL FIRST MEETING WITH THE BOARD AND UNTIL ORDER OF THE BOARD.

GEAR, PHILLIP E MD, LICENSE NUMBER 0015896, WAS DISCIPLINED BY ARIZONA ON APRIL 12, 1991
DISCIPLINARY ACTION: REQUIRED TO ENTER AN IMPAIRED PHYSICIAN PROGRAM OR SUBSTANCE ABUSE TREATMENT; MONITORING OF PHYSICIAN PERFORMANCE
OFFENSE: SUBSTANCE ABUSE

NOTES: ACTION BASED ON INFORMATION RECEIVED ALLEGING THAT HE WAS SELF-PRESCRIBING CONTROLLED SUBSTANCES. SHALL IMMEDIATELY PARTICIPATE IN THE ARIZONA MEDICAL ASSOCIATION'S MONITORED AFTERCARE TREATMENT PROGRAM WHOSE THERAPIST MUST SUBMIT QUARTERLY REPORTS; SHALL PARTICIPATE IN 90 12-STEP MEETINGS APPROPRIATE FOR SUBSTANCE ABUSE WITHIN 90 DAYS; MUST THEN PARTICIPATE IN A 12-STEP RECOVERY PROGRAM APPROPRIATE FOR SUBSTANCE ABUSE AS DETERMINED BY HIS TREATING THERAPIST AND ATTEND A MINIMUM OF THREE WEEKLY MEETINGS; SHALL OBTAIN A BOARD APPROVED SOLE TREATING PHYSICIAN; SHALL COMPLETELY ABSTAIN FROM ALCOHOL CONSUMPTION; SHALL TAKE NO DRUGS OR MEDICATIONS WHATEVER UNLESS PRESCRIBED FOR HIM BY HIS TREATING PHYSICIAN; SHALL SUBMIT TO WITNESSED RANDOM BIOLOGICAL FLUID COLLECTIONS; SHALL MAINTAIN A LOG OF ANY AND ALL MEDICATIONS PRESCRIBED TO HIM; SHALL SUBMIT TO ANY EXAMS OR THERAPY ORDERED BY THE BOARD; SHALL APPEAR BEFORE THE BOARD FOR INTERVIEWS UPON REQUEST AND INFORM THE BOARD IF HE'S AWAY FOR MORE THAN FIVE DAYS. ON 1/24/94 ORDER TERMINATED AFTER 90 DAYS.

GERMAN, CHARLES MD, WAS DISCIPLINED BY ARIZONA ON APRIL 10, 1991
DISCIPLINARY ACTION: RESTRICTION PLACED ON LICENSE
OFFENSE: DISCIPLINARY ACTION BY ANOTHER STATE OR AGENCY

NOTES: ACTION BASED ON INFORMATION RECEIVED FROM THE COLORADO BOARD INVOLVING ANESTHESIA COMPLICATIONS DURING A PATIENT'S SURGERY; COLORADO PLACED HIM ON THREE YEARS PROBATION AND LICENSE RESTRICTED. STIPULATION AGREEMENT ISSUED UNDER THE FOLLOWING TERMS: SHALL PERFORM NO SURGERY PROCEDURES WITHOUT A BOARD-APPROVED MD/D.O. ANESTHESIOLOGIST IN ATTENDANCE (THIS REQUIREMENT SHALL NOT APPLY TO MINOR SURGICAL PROCEDURES); SHALL PERFORM NO SURGERY WITHOUT THE PROPER MONITORING AND RESUSCITATIVE EQUIPMENT PRESENT AND PROPERLY FUNCTIONING; SHALL NOT CONDUCT EXAMINATIONS OF, NOR TAKE PHOTOGRAPHS OF, AND SHALL NOT TREAT FEMALE PATIENTS EXCEPT IN THE PRESENCE OF A FEMALE OBSERVER.

GERMAN, CHARLES MD, WAS DISCIPLINED BY ARIZONA ON OCTOBER 19, 1995
DISCIPLINARY ACTION: LICENSE SUSPENSION

NOTES: SIGNED A CONSENT AGREEMENT ADMITTING ALLEGATIONS AND ACCEPTS INACTIVE STATUS WITH CAUSE AND ORDER IN LIEU OF A FORMAL HEARING.

GERSTENBERGER, DEAN L MD, LICENSE NUMBER 0010490, WAS

DISCIPLINED BY ARIZONA ON OCTOBER 30, 1990
DISCIPLINARY ACTION: LICENSE REVOCATION
OFFENSE: SEXUAL ABUSE OF OR SEXUAL MISCONDUCT WITH A PATIENT

NOTES: ASPEN HILL HOSPITAL IN FLAGSTAFF REVOKED HIS HOSPITAL PRIVILEGES ON 7/17/90; ALSO HAD SEXUAL RELATIONS WITH 2 PATIENTS.

GERSTENBERGER, DEAN L MD, DATE OF BIRTH OCTOBER 17, 1948 OF 1355 NO BEAVER, FLAGSTAFF, AZ, WAS DISCIPLINED BY MEDICARE ON NOVEMBER 4, 1991
DISCIPLINARY ACTION: EXCLUSION FROM THE MEDICARE AND/OR MEDICAID PROGRAM
OFFENSE: DISCIPLINARY ACTION BY ANOTHER STATE OR AGENCY

NOTES: LICENSE REVOCATION OR SUSPENSION.

GERTZ, EDWARD W MD, LICENSE NUMBER 0019590 OF 222 W THOMAS RD, PHOENIX, AZ, WAS DISCIPLINED BY ARIZONA ON OCTOBER 1, 1991
DISCIPLINARY ACTION: EMERGENCY SUSPENSION
OFFENSE: SEXUAL ABUSE OF OR SEXUAL MISCONDUCT WITH A PATIENT

NOTES: ENGAGED IN CONDUCT WHICH DEMONSTRATES THAT THE PUBLIC HEALTH, SAFETY AND WELFARE IMPERATIVELY REQUIRE EMERGENCY ACTION AND CONSTITUTES UNPROFESSIONAL CONDUCT WHICH IS OR MIGHT BE HARMFUL OR DANGEROUS TO THE HEALTH OF PATIENTS IN THAT ON 11/26/90, MASTURBATED A COMATOSE OR SEMI-COMATOSE PATIENT; IN ANOTHER CASE ON 8/20/91, HE CONDUCTED A CARDIAC CONSULTATION OF A 16-YEAR-OLD PATIENT WITHOUT AUTHORIZATION AND ON THE NIGHT OF 8/21/91, TOLD PATIENT AND NURSE THAT HE WAS GOING TO TAKE THIS PATIENT FOR AN ECHOCARDIOGRAM, DESPITE THE FACT THAT EARLIER THAT DAY A PREVIOUS ECHOCARDIOGRAM WAS FOUND TO BE WITHIN NORMAL LIMITS AND THE LAB WAS CLOSED; HE THEN ORDERED PAIN MEDICATION FOR THE SAME PATIENT EVEN THOUGH THE PATIENT DID NOT WANT OR NEED THE MEDICATION; THE PATIENT REPORTED TO THE NURSE THAT DR. GERTZ HAD KISSED HIM AND TOUCHED HIM INAPPROPRIATELY WHILE THEY WERE OUT OF THE ROOM. SUMMARILY SUSPENDED PENDING FURTHER DISCIPLINARY PROCEEDINGS OR UNTIL FURTHER ORDER OF THE BOARD. SHALL SUBMIT HIMSELF FOR SUCH MENTAL OR PHYSICAL EXAMINATIONS DESIGNATED BY THE BOARD STAFF AND CONDUCTED BY PERSONS SPECIFIED BY THE BOARD STAFF.

GERTZ, EDWARD W MD, LICENSE NUMBER 0019590 OF 222 W THOMAS RD, PHOENIX, AZ, WAS DISCIPLINED BY ARIZONA ON JUNE 20, 1992
DISCIPLINARY ACTION: LICENSE REVOCATION
OFFENSE: SEXUAL ABUSE OF OR SEXUAL MISCONDUCT WITH A PATIENT

NOTES: SEXUALLY ABUSED TWO MALE PATIENTS, ONE IN 1990 WHILE HE WAS IN A COMA, THE OTHER IN 1991 WHILE HE WAS SEDATED DUE TO AN INJECTION OF DEMEROL. ON 4/16/93 IT WAS REPORTED TO THE BOARD THAT SUPERIOR COURT AFFIRMED BOARD'S FINDINGS AND ORDER.

GERTZ, EDWARD W MD, LICENSE NUMBER 0G26476 OF PARADISE VALLEY, AZ, WAS DISCIPLINED BY CALIFORNIA ON NOVEMBER 26, 1993
DISCIPLINARY ACTION: LICENSE REVOCATION
OFFENSE: DISCIPLINARY ACTION BY ANOTHER STATE OR AGENCY

NOTES: DISCIPLINED BY ARIZONA BOARD. DEFAULT DECISION.

GERTZ, EDWARD W MD, LICENSE NUMBER 0031552 OF 3411 EAST RANCHO DRIVE, PARADISE VALLEY, AZ, WAS DISCIPLINED BY MASSACHUSETTS ON MAY 4, 1994
DISCIPLINARY ACTION: NONRENEWAL OF LICENSE
OFFENSE: DISCIPLINARY ACTION BY ANOTHER STATE OR AGENCY

NOTES: DISCIPLINE BY ARIZONA; SEXUAL MISCONDUCT. REVOCATION OF INCHOATE RIGHT TO RENEW LICENSE.

GHARAGOZLOO, FARID MD, LICENSE NUMBER 20565, WAS DISCIPLINED BY ARIZONA ON MAY 21, 1999
DISCIPLINARY ACTION: REPRIMAND

GHARAVI, NAJM M MD OF 1700 SOUTH EASTERN, LAS VEGAS, NV, WAS DISCIPLINED BY MEDICARE ON AUGUST 10, 1994
DISCIPLINARY ACTION: 60-MONTH EXCLUSION FROM THE MEDICARE AND/OR MEDICAID PROGRAM
OFFENSE: CRIMINAL CONVICTION OR PLEA OF GUILTY, NOLO CONTENDERE, OR NO CONTEST TO A CRIME

NOTES: CONVICTED OF A CRIME INVOLVING THE MEDICARE, MEDICAID, MATERNAL AND CHILD HEALTH SERVICES BLOCK GRANT OR BLOCK GRANTS TO STATES FOR SOCIAL SERVICES PROGRAMS.

GHARAVI, NAJM M MD, WAS DISCIPLINED BY NEVADA ON DECEMBER 7, 1994
DISCIPLINARY ACTION: REPRIMAND; COMMUNITY SERVICE
OFFENSE: CRIMINAL CONVICTION OR PLEA OF GUILTY, NOLO CONTENDERE, OR NO CONTEST TO A CRIME

NOTES: CONVICTED IN THE JUSTICE COURT OF LAS VEGAS FOR MEDICAID FRAUD. MUST COMPLETE 20 HOURS OF UNCOMPENSATED PUBLIC SERVICE WITHIN 6 MONTHS.

GHARAVI, NAJM M MD, LICENSE NUMBER 0008065, WAS DISCIPLINED BY ARIZONA ON JANUARY 18, 1996
DISCIPLINARY ACTION: LICENSE REVOCATION
OFFENSE: DISCIPLINARY ACTION BY ANOTHER STATE OR AGENCY

NOTES: IN 6/94, EXCLUDED BY THE NEVADA DEPARTMENT OF HUMAN RESOURCES, WELFARE DIVISION-NEVADA MEDICAID FROM THE MEDICAID PROGRAM FOR THREE YEARS DUE TO A GUILTY PLEA TO MEDICAID FRAUD; IN 8/94, EXCLUDED FOR FIVE YEARS FROM PARTICIPATION IN THE MEDICARE, MEDICAID, MATERNAL AND CHILD HEALTH SERVICES BLOCK GRANT AND BLOCK GRANTS TO STATES FOR SOCIAL SERVICES PROGRAMS; EXCLUSION BASED ON CONVICTION IN NEVADA OF A CRIMINAL OFFENSE RELATED TO THE DELIVERY OF AN ITEM OR SERVICE UNDER THE MEDICAID PROGRAM; IN 5/95, RECEIVED NOTIFICATION THAT A COMPLAINT AGAINST HIM HAD BEEN FILED WITH THE BOARD; WITH NOTIFICATION RECEIVED A COPY OF THE DHHS CORRESPONDENCE; ON FOUR OCCASIONS BETWEEN 5/95 AND 10/95, HE WAS REQUESTED TO FILE A NARRATIVE STATEMENT CONCERNING THE MATTER WITH SUPPORTING DOCUMENTATION REGARDING THE COMPLAINT, BUT FAILED TO PROVIDE THIS INFORMATION AS HE WAS LEGALLY REQUESTED; IN 9/95, INTERVIEWED BY THE BOARD, BUT FAILED TO PROVIDE MEANINGFUL INFORMATION OR DOCUMENTATION; ATTEMPTS BY THE BOARD TO COMMUNICATE WITH HIM HAVE BEEN UNSUCCESSFUL, WITH ALL CORRESPONDENCE TO HIS HOME OR OFFICE RETURNED UNCLAIMED; HAS FAILED TO KEEP THE BOARD INFORMED OF HIS CURRENT OFFICE AND/OR RESIDENCE ADDRESS AS REQUIRED; IN 1/96, BOARD RECEIVED INFORMATION THAT IN 12/94, HE WAS REPRIMANDED BY THE

NEVADA BOARD AND REQUIRED TO COMPLETE 20 HOURS OF PUBLIC SERVICE.

GHARAVI, NAJM MOOSAVI MD, LICENSE NUMBER C41322 OF LAS VEGAS, NV, WAS DISCIPLINED BY CALIFORNIA ON JANUARY 6, 1997
DISCIPLINARY ACTION: LICENSE REVOCATION
OFFENSE: DISCIPLINARY ACTION BY ANOTHER STATE OR AGENCY

NOTES: DISCIPLINED BY NEVADA FOR MEDICAID FRAUD.

GHAZI-ASKAR, MEHDI MD, LICENSE NUMBER 0019065, WAS DISCIPLINED BY ARIZONA ON APRIL 18, 1996
DISCIPLINARY ACTION: MONITORING OF PHYSICIAN PERFORMANCE
OFFENSE: SUBSTANDARD CARE, INCOMPETENCE OR NEGLIGENCE

NOTES: INTERVIEWED BY THE BOARD REGARDING ALLEGED NEGLIGENCE IN PATIENT TREATMENT, AND RUDE AND OFFENSIVE BEHAVIOR. SHALL PROMPTLY OBTAIN COUNSELING FOR SENSITIVITY TRAINING AND INTERPERSONAL RELATIONSHIPS BY A BOARD-APPROVED COUNSELOR, WHO SHALL DETERMINE FREQUENCY AND DURATION OF COUNSELING; SHALL REMAIN IN COUNSELING UNTIL HE HAS MET THE THERAPEUTIC GOALS SET BY THE COUNSELOR AND IS THERAPEUTICALLY DISCHARGED; SHALL RELEASE QUARTERLY REPORTS TO THE BOARD REGARDING HIS PARTICIPATION AND PROGRESS IN COUNSELING. ON 3/14/97 THIS ORDER WAS TERMINATED BASED ON A RECOMMENDATION FROM THE THERAPIST.

GHEBLEH, FARID MD, LICENSE NUMBER 0015863, WAS DISCIPLINED BY ARIZONA ON APRIL 14, 1993
DISCIPLINARY ACTION: MONITORING OF PHYSICIAN PERFORMANCE

NOTES: SHALL WITHIN 15 DAYS ENTER INTO THERAPY WITH A THERAPIST APPROVED BY THE BOARD REGARDING ISSUES OF SEXUAL HARASSMENT, APPROPRIATE INTERACTION WITH WOMEN IN A PROFESSIONAL SETTING, STRESS, AND SUCH OTHER ISSUES AS THE THERAPIST DEEMS APPROPRIATE AT LEAST TWICE A WEEK AND SHALL PROVIDE THE THERAPIST WITH A COPY OF ORDER. SHALL INSTRUCT THE THERAPIST TO PROVIDE QUARTERLY WRITTEN REPORTS TO THE BOARD; SHALL NOT SELF-PRESCRIBE, SELF-ADMINISTER OR SELF-DISPENSE CONTROLLED SUBSTANCES. ORDER TERMINATED ON 10/16/96.

GIERKE, KLAUS DETLEV MD, LICENSE NUMBER 3850 OF 9485 EAST PLACITA OAXACA, TUCSON, AZ, WAS DISCIPLINED BY HAWAII ON SEPTEMBER 12, 1997
DISCIPLINARY ACTION: REQUIRED TO ENTER AN IMPAIRED PHYSICIAN PROGRAM OR SUBSTANCE ABUSE TREATMENT; MONITORING OF PHYSICIAN PERFORMANCE
OFFENSE: SUBSTANCE ABUSE

NOTES: ON 12/20/95 SIGNED A NONDISCIPLINARY REHABILITATION STIPULATION AND ORDER WITH ARIZONA BOARD; SHALL ABIDE BY THE PROVISIONS OF THIS ORDER WHICH INCLUDE BUT ARE NOT LIMITED TO: A MONITORED AFTERCARE TREATMENT PROGRAM, A 12-STEP RECOVERY PROGRAM, ABSTENTION FROM ALCOHOL AND DRUGS, MAINTENANCE OF A LOG OF ANY MEDICATIONS PRESCRIBED FOR HIM AND MENTAL, PHYSICAL OR MEDICAL COMPETENCY EXAMINATIONS. SHALL SUPPLY HAWAII WITH ANY REQUESTED REPORTS, AND NOTIFICATION OF ANY DISCIPLINARY DECISION WITHIN 30 DAYS.

GILBARD, STEVEN M MD, LICENSE NUMBER 0015552, WAS DISCIPLINED BY ARIZONA ON APRIL 19, 1996
DISCIPLINARY ACTION: RESTRICTION PLACED ON LICENSE; MONITORING OF PHYSICIAN PERFORMANCE
OFFENSE: PROFESSIONAL MISCONDUCT

NOTES: INTERVIEWED BY BOARD REGARDING MALPRACTICE CASE ALLEGING HIS INAPPROPRIATE BEHAVIOR IN THE OPERATING ROOM. SHALL CONTINUE IN THERAPY WITH A BOARD-APPROVED PSYCHIATRIST WHO SHALL SUBMIT QUARTERLY REPORTS TO THE BOARD; SHALL PRACTICE ONLY OPHTHALMOLOGY AND OCULOPLASTIC RECONSTRUCTIVE AND ORBITAL SURGERY, INCLUDING BROW SURGERY AND LIFTS AND ALL ORBITAL FRACTURES INCLUDING TRIMALAR FRACTURES AND INCLUDING THE ABILITY TO HARVEST NECESSARY TISSUE FROM OUTSIDE THE ORBITAL AREA IN OCULOPLASTIC PROCEDURES. ON 5/21/96 ORDER TERMINATED. ON 1/22/98 STIPULATION AND ORDER FOR INVESTIGATION TERMINATED.

GILLETTE, WARREN JR MD, LICENSE NUMBER 0020124, WAS DISCIPLINED BY ARIZONA ON JULY 5, 1991
DISCIPLINARY ACTION: REQUIRED TO ENTER AN IMPAIRED PHYSICIAN PROGRAM OR SUBSTANCE ABUSE TREATMENT; MONITORING OF PHYSICIAN PERFORMANCE
OFFENSE: SUBSTANCE ABUSE

NOTES: INFORMATION RECEIVED THAT HE HAD BEEN TREATED FOR SUBSTANCE ABUSE. MUST IMMEDIATELY PARTICIPATE IN A BOARD-APPROVED MONITORED AFTERCARE TREATMENT PROGRAM WHOSE THERAPIST MUST SUBMIT QUARTERLY REPORTS; MUST PARTICIPATE IN 90 12-STEP MEETINGS FOR SUBSTANCE ABUSE WITHIN 90 DAYS; MUST THEN PARTICIPATE IN A 12-STEP RECOVERY PROGRAM AS DETERMINED BY HIS TREATING THERAPIST AND ATTEND AT LEAST THREE WEEKLY MEETINGS; SHALL OBTAIN A BOARD-APPROVED TREATING PHYSICIAN; SHALL ABSTAIN COMPLETELY FROM THE CONSUMPTION OF ALCOHOLIC BEVERAGES AND DRUGS EXCEPT WHEN PRESCRIBED BY HIS TREATING PHYSICIAN; MUST SUBMIT TO WITNESSED RANDOM BIOLOGICAL FLUID COLLECTION; MUST KEEP A LOG OF ANY AND ALL MEDICATIONS PRESCRIBED FOR HIM; SHALL SUBMIT TO ANY EXAMINATIONS OR THERAPY ORDERED BY THE BOARD; SHALL APPEAR BEFORE THE BOARD FOR INTERVIEWS UPON REQUEST; SHALL INFORM BOARD OF CHANGE OF ADDRESS OR IF AWAY FOR MORE THAN FIVE DAYS.

GLADHART, RODNEY MD, LICENSE NUMBER 4503, WAS DISCIPLINED BY ARIZONA ON DECEMBER 9, 1999
DISCIPLINARY ACTION: REPRIMAND
OFFENSE: SUBSTANDARD CARE, INCOMPETENCE OR NEGLIGENCE

NOTES: FAILURE TO DIAGNOSE COLON CANCER.

GLEASON, VINSON W DO OF SCOTTSDALE, AZ, HAD ACTION TAKEN BY MISSOURI ON AUGUST 21, 1990
OFFENSE: DISCIPLINARY ACTION BY ANOTHER STATE OR AGENCY

NOTES: ACTION TAKEN BY THE KANSAS BOARD. RETIREMENT AGREEMENT SIGNED IN LIEU OF DISCIPLINARY ACTION BY MISSOURI.

GLENN, THOMAS W MD, LICENSE NUMBER 0005328, WAS DISCIPLINED BY ARIZONA ON JUNE 20, 1991
DISCIPLINARY ACTION: DENIAL OF LICENSE REINSTATEMENT; MONITORING OF PHYSICIAN PERFORMANCE
OFFENSE: FAILURE TO COMPLY WITH PREVIOUS BOARD ORDER

NOTES: IN NOVEMBER 1981 HE NOTIFIED THE BOARD THAT HE HAD BEEN SELF-ADMINISTERING MEPERIDINE (DEMEROL), A SCHEDULE II CONTROLLED SUBSTANCE. A 3/17/82 ORDER REQUIRED HIM TO

ABSTAIN COMPLETELY FROM THE PERSONAL USE OR POSSESSION OF CONTROLLED SUBSTANCES. THE BOARD ENTERED SIMILAR ORDERS ON 11/1/82 AND 12/29/82. ON 12/24/82 THE BOARD TERMINATED THE STIPULATION DATED 12/29/82. FROM 6/6/85 THROUGH 9/3/85 HE ORDERED AND RECEIVED 210 CC. OF MEPERIDINE FOR OFFICE USE. A VOLUNTARILY PROVIDED SAMPLE OF HIS URINE TAKEN ON 9/6/85 TESTED POSITIVE FOR MEPERIDINE. ON 9/13/85 HE ENTERED A TREATMENT PROGRAM FOR NARCOTIC DEPENDENCY AND SUCCESSFULLY COMPLETED THE PROGRAM ON 10/4/85. ON 12/6/85 HE WAS PLACED ON PROBATION FOR FIVE YEARS FOR USING MEPERIDINE. VIOLATED THE TERMS OF THIS AGREEMENT ON 4/29/86 AND 6/5/86 BY USING COCAINE. VOLUNTARILY SURRENDERED HIS LICENSE ON 6/20/86 AND THEN USED LICENSE AFTER THAT DATE BY ORDERING A PRESCRIPTION FOR MEPERIDINE. FAILED TO SUCCESSFULLY COMPLETE TREATMENT PROGRAM MANDATED BY ORDER OF 6/20/86. LICENSE WAS REVOKED ON 5/11/87 AND HE WAS PROHIBITED FROM REAPPLYING FOR 2 YEARS. BEFORE APPLYING FOR A NEW LICENSE HE WOULD HAVE TO SUBMIT TO RANDOM BIOLOGICAL FLUID TESTING; SUCCESSFULLY PASS AN ORAL COMPETENCY EXAM; STIPULATE TO PROBATION; SUBMIT TO EVALUATION; COMPLETE A CHEMICAL DEPENDENCY PROGRAM. WHEN APPLYING FOR RELICENSURE HE SUBMITTED A URINE SAMPLE ON 11/28/90 THAT TESTED POSITIVE FOR COCAINE.

GOLDBERG, MARK D MD, LICENSE NUMBER 0018592, WAS DISCIPLINED BY ARIZONA ON JANUARY 17, 1996
OFFENSE: INSURANCE, MEDICARE OR MEDICAID FRAUD

NOTES: IN 1/94, UNDERCOVER AGENT PRESENTED HERSELF TO HIM AS A DANCER WHO HAD SUSTAINED KNEE INJURY ON THE JOB AND PLANNED TO PURSUE A LAWSUIT AGAINST HER EMPLOYER OR A WORKER'S COMPENSATION CLAIM THROUGH THE INDUSTRIAL COMMISSION OF ARIZONA (ICA); ON FIVE OCCASIONS BETWEEN 3/94 AND 4/94, HE CHARGED OR ATTEMPTED TO CHARGE THE ICA FOR DETAILED EXAMINATIONS WHICH HE DID NOT PERFORM AND, ON TWO OCCASIONS, FOR ULTRASOUNDS WHICH HE DID NOT PERFORM; ON THE SECOND VISIT HE ENCOURAGED THE AGENT TO COME IN A FEW MORE TIMES TO CREATE A PICTURE FOR THE LAWSUIT AND OVER THE TELEPHONE A MONTH LATER HE ADVISED HER TO WAIT A FEW WEEKS BEFORE SUBMITTING A CLAIM IN ORDER TO "JUST LET THE CASE BUILD." CENSURED; WITH REGARD TO CHARGES STEMMING FROM AN INVESTIGATION INTO PRESCRIBING PRACTICES, CARE AND TREATMENT OF TWO PATIENTS AND AN OFFICE RECORD REVIEW, SHALL TAKE AND PASS THE SPECIAL PURPOSE EXAMINATION WITHIN 60 DAYS WITH A SCORE OF 75 OR GREATER.

GOLDBERG, MARK D MD, LICENSE NUMBER 0018592, WAS DISCIPLINED BY ARIZONA ON JULY 18, 1996
DISCIPLINARY ACTION: 60-MONTH PROBATION; REQUIRED TO TAKE ADDITIONAL MEDICAL EDUCATION
OFFENSE: FAILURE TO COMPLY WITH PREVIOUS BOARD ORDER

NOTES: FAILED TO RECORD THE RESULTS OF ANY X-RAYS TAKEN FOR A PATIENT BETWEEN 10/89 AND 1/94; FAILED TO READ THE RESULTS OF PATIENT'S X-RAY TAKEN IN 1/94, WHICH WOULD HAVE REVEALED A DEFINITE LESION IN THE LUNG; WHEN PATIENT RETURNED IN 3/94 WITH SYMPTOMS, HE CHECKED HIS LUNGS, BUT HAD STILL NOT CHECKED HIS PREVIOUS 1/94 X-RAY; X-RAYS TAKEN IN MARCH REVEALED A LARGER TUMOR AND THE PATIENT DIED OF LUNG CANCER IN 5/94; IN RESPONSE TO THE BOARD, PHYSICIAN INDICATED THAT HE CUSTOMARILY PUTS ROUTINE SCREENING X-RAYS ASIDE AND DOES NOT READ THEM FOR 4-6 WEEKS; IN 7/95, BOARD ORDERED A SURVEY OF HIS PRACTICE WHICH NOTED THE FOLLOWING DEFICIENCIES: FOR A PATIENT TREATED FROM 7/95 THROUGH 10/95, HE PLACED HER ON AMOXIL WITHOUT DOCUMENTING ANY APPROPRIATE EXAMINATIONS OR DIAGNOSTIC PROCEDURES; IN 3/95, HE DIAGNOSED A PATIENT WITH PERNICIOUS ANEMIA WITHOUT PERFORMING ANY EVALUATION FOR THIS DIAGNOSIS AND WITHOUT EVIDENCE OF THE CONDITION; A PHARMACY SURVEY CONDUCTED FOR THE PERIOD OF 12/1/95 THROUGH 5/31/95, IT WAS REVEALED THAT FOR ONE PATIENT, HE WROTE 116 PRESCRIPTIONS FOR CONTROLLED SUBSTANCES AND PRESCRIPTION-ONLY DRUGS FOR A TOTAL OF 1,995 DOSAGE UNITS; FOLLOWING THE ABOVE SURVEY, CHARTS WERE OBTAINED ON SEVERAL PATIENTS TO EVALUATE HIS MANAGEMENT AND EVALUATION REGARDING THE NEED FOR SCHEDULE DRUGS AND THE FOLLOWING DEFICIENCIES WERE NOTED IN THE CHARTS OF EIGHT PATIENTS SEEN BETWEEN 8/90 AND 7/95: FOR THREE PATIENTS, THERE WAS NO DOCUMENTATION OF APPROPRIATE EXAMINATIONS; FOR THREE PATIENTS, THERE WERE NO APPROPRIATE REFERRALS; FOR ONE PATIENT HE HAD NEVER SEEN, PRESCRIBED RITALIN MULTIPLE TIMES; FOR ONE PATIENT, INDICATED NO ATTEMPT TO WEAN FROM MEDICATIONS DESPITE OBVIOUS DRUG-SEEKING BEHAVIOR; AND FOR TWO PATIENTS, CONDUCTED NO APPROPRIATE DIAGNOSTIC PROCEDURES; VIOLATED A PREVIOUS BOARD ORDER IN THAT HE DID NOT TAKE THE SPECIAL PURPOSE EXAMINATION UNTIL 4/25/96, WHEN HE WAS ORDERED TO TAKE IT WITHIN 60 DAYS OF A 1/29/96 ORDER. PROBATION WITH TERMS: SHALL OBTAIN 30 HOURS OF CONTINUING MEDICAL EDUCATION ANNUALLY IN PAIN MANAGEMENT AND PRESCRIBING OF CONTROLLED SUBSTANCES AND AN ADDITIONAL 30 HOURS OF GENERAL CONTINUING MEDICAL EDUCATION ANNUALLY OVER AND ABOVE THE ANNUAL REQUIREMENTS; WITHIN 90 DAYS, SHALL OBTAIN A BOARD-APPROVED PRACTICE MANAGEMENT CONSULTANT TO REVIEW HIS PRACTICE AND MAKE RECOMMENDATIONS; SHALL COMPLY WITH RECOMMENDATIONS AND PROVIDE A COPY OF REPORT TO THE BOARD; SHALL SUBMIT TO AN ANNUAL OFFICE SURVEY BY BOARD. ON 3/26/98 BOARD RECOGNIZED HIS COMPLIANCE WITH PROBATION AND THAT THE REMAINDER OF THE TERMS OF THE ORDER REMAIN IN FULL FORCE AND EFFECT.

GOLDBERG, MARK DANIEL MD, DATE OF BIRTH JUNE 30, 1958, LICENSE NUMBER 48277 OF 5616 EAST MAIN STREET, MESA, AZ, WAS DISCIPLINED BY NEW JERSEY ON APRIL 22, 1999
DISCIPLINARY ACTION: REPRIMAND
OFFENSE: DISCIPLINARY ACTION BY ANOTHER STATE OR AGENCY

NOTES: DISCIPLINARY ACTION IN ARIZONA WHERE HE WAS PLACED ON PROBATION FOR FIVE YEARS AND ORDERED TO TAKE ADDITIONAL CONTINUING MEDICAL EDUCATION IN THE MANAGEMENT OF PAIN AND PRESCRIBING OF CONTROLLED SUBSTANCES, AMONG OTHER THINGS. PRIOR TO BEGINNING PRACTICE IN NEW JERSEY, HE SHALL BE REQUIRED TO APPEAR BEFORE BOARD TO DEMONSTRATE SUCCESSFUL COMPLIANCE WITH AND COMPLETION OF THE REQUIREMENTS OF THE ARIZONA BOARD AND HIS POSSESSION OF AN UNRESTRICTED LICENSE TO PRACTICE IN ALL OTHER JURISDICTIONS. A PROVISIONAL ORDER OF DISCIPLINE WAS FILED 11/13/98.

GOLDSTEIN, MARK J DO, LICENSE NUMBER 0001572 OF 7701 EAST INDIAN SCHOOL #E, SCOTTSDALE, AZ, WAS DISCIPLINED BY ARIZONA ON FEBRUARY 26, 1992
DISCIPLINARY ACTION: 3-MONTH LICENSE SUSPENSION; 36-MONTH PROBATION
OFFENSE: FAILURE TO COMPLY WITH PREVIOUS BOARD ORDER

NOTES: NONCOMPLIANCE TO A PREVIOUS PROBATION ORDER IN THAT ON 12/14/92 ARRESTED FOR DRIVING WHILE UNDER THE INFLUENCE OF INTOXICATING LIQUOR AND EXCESSIVE SPEED; ADMITTED TO DRINKING THREE OR FOUR GLASSES OF WINE. SUSPENSION COMMENCING 1/18/92. PROBATION EXTENDED FROM ITS PREVIOUS TERMINATION DATE OF 12/03/92 UNDER TERMS AND CONDITIONS: SHALL ENROLL AND PARTICIPATE IN THE MONITORED PHYSICIANS AFTERCARE PROGRAM AND PROVIDE THE BOARD A COPY OF HIS CONTRACT; SHALL SUBMIT TO BIOLOGICAL FLUID TESTING UPON BOARD REQUEST; SHALL USE NO CONTROLLED SUBSTANCE OR PRESCRIPTION-ONLY MEDICATION UNLESS PRESCRIBED BY HIS ATTENDING PHYSICIAN; SHALL NOT CONSUME ALCOHOL; SHALL ATTEND 90 AA OR NARCOTICS ANONYMOUS MEETINGS IN THE FIRST 90 DAYS OF HIS AFTERCARE PROGRAM; SHALL ATTEND NO LESS THAN ONE PSYCHIATRIC TREATMENT PER WEEK UNTIL FURTHER NOTICE FROM THE BOARD; SHALL COMPLETE 40 HOURS OF COMMUNITY SERVICE PER MONTH AT A BOARD APPROVED SITE; SHALL APPEAR BEFORE THE BOARD UPON REQUEST TO REVIEW HIS COMPLIANCE WITH THIS ORDER; SHALL AUTHORIZE ANY ATTENDING PHYSICIAN, PSYCHIATRIST OR PSYCHOLOGIST TO RELEASE TO THE BOARD ALL RECORDS PERTAINING TO HIS CARE AND TREATMENT.

GOLDSTEIN, MARK J DO, LICENSE NUMBER 0124251 OF 4020 N SCOTTSDALE ROAD, SCOTTSDALE, AZ, WAS DISCIPLINED BY NEW YORK ON OCTOBER 22, 1996
DISCIPLINARY ACTION: SURRENDER OF LICENSE
OFFENSE: DISCIPLINARY ACTION BY ANOTHER STATE OR AGENCY

NOTES: DISCIPLINED BY ARIZONA FOR PRACTICING WHILE IMPAIRED AND FOR HAVING VIOLATED THE TERMS OF HIS ARIZONA PROBATION.

GOODMAN, HERBERT MD, LICENSE NUMBER 0015871 OF SCOTTSDALE, AZ, WAS DISCIPLINED BY CONNECTICUT ON AUGUST 24, 1993
DISCIPLINARY ACTION: REPRIMAND
OFFENSE: SUBSTANDARD CARE, INCOMPETENCE OR NEGLIGENCE

NOTES: INCOMPETENCE/NEGLIGENCE.

GOODMAN, HERBERT D MD, LICENSE NUMBER 0007607, WAS DISCIPLINED BY ARIZONA ON JANUARY 21, 1992
OFFENSE: SUBSTANDARD CARE, INCOMPETENCE OR NEGLIGENCE

NOTES: INADEQUATE AND INCOMPLETE MANAGEMENT OF A PATIENT, SPECIFICALLY, FAILURE TO EVALUATE PERSISTENT ANEMIA AND PAINFUL PROTRUDING HEMORRHOIDS, LEADING TO AN ADVANCED CARCINOMA OF THE RECTUM WHICH HAD TO BE TREATED BY AN ABDOMINAL PERINEAL RESECTION. AFTER A MEDICAL MALPRACTICE ACTION WAS INITIATED AGAINST HIM CONCERNING HIS TREATMENT IN THIS CASE, HE SENT COPIES OF THIS PATIENT'S MEDICAL RECORDS TO HIS INSURANCE CARRIER THAT HE HAD ALTERED TO INCLUDE A TEST WHICH HE HAD NOT IN FACT ORDERED. DECREE OF CENSURE.

GOODMAN, HERBERT D MD, WAS DISCIPLINED BY NEVADA ON JANUARY 16, 1993
DISCIPLINARY ACTION: FINE; REPRIMAND
OFFENSE: NONCOMPLIANCE WITH A PROFESSIONAL RULE

NOTES: ON 12/16/92 COMPLAINT FILED WHERE HE WAS CHARGED WITH FAILURE TO REPORT TO THE BOARD A CLAIM OF NEGLIGENCE AGAINST HIM BY THE ARIZONA MEDICAL BOARD, AND THE SUBSEQUENT DISPOSITION THEREOF WITHIN 90 DAYS AFTER THE CLAIM WAS FILED OR THE DISPOSITION OF THE CLAIM. MUST PAY A $1,000 FINE.

GOODMAN, HERBERT D MD, DATE OF BIRTH FEBRUARY 2, 1940, LICENSE NUMBER 0028104 OF 6726 E. MONTECITO AVENUE, SCOTTSDALE, AZ, WAS DISCIPLINED BY NEW JERSEY ON FEBRUARY 1, 1994
DISCIPLINARY ACTION: REPRIMAND
OFFENSE: DISCIPLINARY ACTION BY ANOTHER STATE OR AGENCY

NOTES: DISCIPLINARY ACTION TAKEN IN THE STATE OF ARIZONA. PRIOR TO RESUMING PRACTICE, MUST APPEAR FOR A STATUS CONFERENCE BEFORE A COMMITTEE OF THE NEW JERSEY BOARD.

GOTTESMAN, JOSEPH R MD, LICENSE NUMBER 0008308 OF SCOTTSDALE, AZ, WAS DISCIPLINED BY ARIZONA ON OCTOBER 18, 1994
DISCIPLINARY ACTION: REQUIRED TO TAKE ADDITIONAL MEDICAL EDUCATION
OFFENSE: OVERPRESCRIBING OR MISPRESCRIBING DRUGS

NOTES: RELATIVE TO PRESCRIBING OF SCHEDULE II MEDICATIONS. SHALL, WITHIN ONE YEAR COMPLETE 12 WEEKS OF MINI-RESIDENCY TRAINING SPONSORED BY THE UNIVERSITY OF ARIZONA COLLEGE OF MEDICINE IN CHRONIC PAIN MANAGEMENT; SHALL PROMPTLY SIGN A WRITTEN AUTHORIZATION DIRECTING RELEASE TO THE BOARD OF ALL RECORDS REQUESTED REGARDING HIS MINI-RESIDENCY TRAINING. ON 9/26/97 ORDER TERMINATED AS EDUCATION WAS COMPLETED.

GOTTESMAN, JOSEPH R MD, LICENSE NUMBER 8308, WAS DISCIPLINED BY ARIZONA ON NOVEMBER 19, 1999
DISCIPLINARY ACTION: 12-MONTH LICENSE SUSPENSION; REQUIRED TO TAKE ADDITIONAL MEDICAL EDUCATION

NOTES: LICENSE SUSPENDED BEGINNING ON THE DATE OF HIS INCARCERATION AT A FEDERAL INSTITUTION; DECREE OF CENSURE; WITHIN SIX MONTHS OF RETURNING TO PRACTICE, SHALL TAKE A BOARD-APPROVED ETHICS CLASS.

GRADE, THOMAS J MD, LICENSE NUMBER 0010424, WAS DISCIPLINED BY ARIZONA ON JUNE 22, 1991
DISCIPLINARY ACTION: REQUIRED TO ENTER AN IMPAIRED PHYSICIAN PROGRAM OR SUBSTANCE ABUSE TREATMENT; MONITORING OF PHYSICIAN PERFORMANCE
OFFENSE: SUBSTANCE ABUSE

NOTES: MUST IMMEDIATELY PARTICIPATE IN THE ARIZONA MEDICAL ASSOCIATION'S MONITORED AFTERCARE TREATMENT PROGRAM WHOSE THERAPIST MUST SUBMIT QUARTERLY REPORTS; MUST PARTICIPATE IN 90 12-STEP MEETINGS FOR SUBSTANCE ABUSE WITHIN 90 DAYS; MUST THEN PARTICIPATE IN A 12-STEP RECOVERY PROGRAM AS DETERMINED BY HIS TREATING THERAPIST AND ATTEND AT LEAST 3 WEEKLY MEETINGS; SHALL OBTAIN A BOARD APPROVED TREATING PHYSICIAN; SHALL ABSTAIN COMPLETELY FROM THE CONSUMPTION OF ALCOHOLIC BEVERAGES AND DRUGS EXCEPT WHEN PRESCRIBED BY HIS TREATING PHYSICIAN; MUST

SUBMIT TO RANDOMIZED BIOLOGICAL FLUID COLLECTION; KEEP A LOG OF ANY AND ALL MEDICATIONS PRESCRIBED; SHALL SUBMIT TO ANY EXAMINATIONS OR THERAPY ORDERED BY BOARD; SHALL APPEAR BEFORE BOARD FOR INTERVIEWS UPON REQUEST. SHALL INFORM BOARD OF CHANGE OF ADDRESS OR IF AWAY FOR MORE THAN 5 DAYS. ON 10/16/93 STIPULATION TERMINATED AFTER 90 DAYS.

GRAHAM, CURTIS G MD, LICENSE NUMBER 007157E OF CONCORD, CA, WAS DISCIPLINED BY PENNSYLVANIA ON APRIL 27, 1993
DISCIPLINARY ACTION: FINE
OFFENSE: CRIMINAL CONVICTION OR PLEA OF GUILTY, NOLO CONTENDERE, OR NO CONTEST TO A CRIME

NOTES: PLED GUILTY TO ONE FELONY COUNT OF MAKING A FALSE STATEMENT FOR THE PURPOSE OF INFLUENCING THE ACTION OF THE U.S. DEPARTMENT OF HOUSING AND URBAN DEVELOPMENT. $500 FINE.

GRAHAM, CURTIS G MD, LICENSE NUMBER 00G9793 OF KALAMAZOO, MI, WAS DISCIPLINED BY CALIFORNIA ON AUGUST 10, 1994
DISCIPLINARY ACTION: 60-MONTH PROBATION
OFFENSE: DISCIPLINARY ACTION BY ANOTHER STATE OR AGENCY

NOTES: FEDERAL CONVICTION FOR MAIL FRAUD IN FALSIFYING AT LEAST 10 MORTGAGE APPLICATIONS MAILED TO THE DEPARTMENT OF HOUSING AND URBAN DEVELOPMENT. RESTRICTIONS PLACED ON HIS ARIZONA LICENSE BY THE ARIZONA BOARD. REVOCATION STAYED.

GRAHAM, CURTIS G MD, DATE OF BIRTH MAY 31, 1937, LICENSE NUMBER 1062866 OF 252 E LOVELL ST, KALAMAZOO, MI, WAS DISCIPLINED BY MICHIGAN ON SEPTEMBER 15, 1995
DISCIPLINARY ACTION: 24-MONTH PROBATION
OFFENSE: DISCIPLINARY ACTION BY ANOTHER STATE OR AGENCY

NOTES: FAILURE TO REPORT/COMPLY.

GRAHAM, CURTIS G MD, DATE OF BIRTH MAY 31, 1937, LICENSE NUMBER 0020875 OF 9039 WEST END DRIVE, KALAMAZOO, MI, WAS DISCIPLINED BY NEW JERSEY ON JUNE 3, 1996
DISCIPLINARY ACTION: SURRENDER OF LICENSE
OFFENSE: DISCIPLINARY ACTION BY ANOTHER STATE OR AGENCY

NOTES: ACTION IN CALIFORNIA. PERMANENTLY SURRENDERED WITH PREJUDICE TO ANY APPLICATION FOR REINSTATEMENT IN THE FUTURE.

GRAHAM, CURTIS G MD, LICENSE NUMBER 8809, WAS DISCIPLINED BY HAWAII ON DECEMBER 12, 1997
DISCIPLINARY ACTION: SURRENDER OF LICENSE

NOTES: VOLUNTARY SURRENDER; MAY NOT APPLY FOR A NEW LICENSE FOR 10 YEARS.

GRAHAM, CURTIS GALE MD, WAS DISCIPLINED BY ARIZONA ON OCTOBER 22, 1992
DISCIPLINARY ACTION: RESTRICTION PLACED ON LICENSE; MONITORING OF PHYSICIAN PERFORMANCE

NOTES: GRANTED LICENSE WITH STIPULATION: SHALL OBTAIN TREATING THERAPIST, WHO WILL SUBMIT QUARTERLY REPORTS TO BOARD; SHALL NOT PRACTICE OBSTETRICS, EXCEPT TO PROVIDE ROUTINE GYNECOLOGICAL CARE AND TREATMENT TO PREGNANT WOMEN DURING THE FIRST 12 WEEKS OF PREGNANCY.

GRAHAM, WILLIAM C MD, LICENSE NUMBER 0015753, WAS DISCIPLINED BY ARIZONA ON OCTOBER 16, 1993
DISCIPLINARY ACTION: EMERGENCY SUSPENSION
OFFENSE: FAILURE TO COMPLY WITH PREVIOUS BOARD ORDER

NOTES: USED ALCOHOL IN 9/92 IN VIOLATION OF A STIPULATION ORDER OF 06/23/89 WHICH INCLUDED A PROVISION THAT HE WAS TO ABSTAIN FROM ALCOHOL. IN 9/93, HE RELAPSED AND RE-ENTERED TREATMENT.

GRAHAM, WILLIAM C MD, WAS DISCIPLINED BY ARIZONA ON APRIL 14, 1994
DISCIPLINARY ACTION: LICENSE SUSPENSION
OFFENSE: FAILURE TO COMPLY WITH PREVIOUS BOARD ORDER

NOTES: ENTERED INTO A REHABILITATION STIPULATION AND ORDER WITH THE BOARD ON 06/23/89 AND EXPERIENCED A RELAPSE.

GRAHAM, WILLIAM C MD OF 926 E. MCDOWELL ST. SUITE 205, PHOENIX, AZ, WAS DISCIPLINED BY DEA ON OCTOBER 4, 1994
DISCIPLINARY ACTION: SURRENDER OF CONTROLLED SUBSTANCE LICENSE

NOTES: IN LIEU OF ORDER TO SHOW CAUSE.

GRAY, LEO D MD, LICENSE NUMBER 0019592 OF NJ, WAS DISCIPLINED BY ARIZONA ON OCTOBER 15, 1993

NOTES: BOARD HAS INVESTIGATED ALLEGATIONS CONCERNING HIS HEALTH AND HE NOW RESIDES IN NEW JERSEY. SHALL NOT PRACTICE IN ARIZONA UNTIL HE ADVISES THE BOARD IN WRITING OF HIS INTENTION TO DO SO, APPEARS BEFORE THE BOARD AND RECEIVES AUTHORIZATION.

GRAY, MICHAEL R MD, LICENSE NUMBER 11623, WAS DISCIPLINED BY ARIZONA ON JANUARY 23, 1997
DISCIPLINARY ACTION: REPRIMAND
OFFENSE: LOSS OR RESTRICTION OF HOSPITAL PRIVILEGES

NOTES: IN 5/94 HOSPITAL SUSPENDED HIS ADMITTING PRIVILEGES DUE TO FAILING TO COMPLETE MEDICAL RECORDS ON A TIMELY BASIS; PRIVILEGES REINSTATED ON 7/29/94; FAILED TO PROVIDE A WRITTEN STATEMENT REGARDING HOSPITAL'S ACTION IN SUSPENDING HIS PRIVILEGES IN A TIMELY MANNER AS REQUESTED BY BOARD ON 8/8/94; HE DID RESPOND TO A FURTHER REQUEST ON 10/12/94; IN ANOTHER CASE OF A PATIENT WHO HE FIRST SAW ON 11/13/95, HANDWRITTEN PROGRESS NOTES ARE LARGELY ILLEGIBLE; REPORTS FOR VARIOUS LABORATORY STUDIES ORDERED ARE NOT FOUND IN THE PATIENT CHART; ASIDE FROM PATIENT'S INITIAL VISIT, THERE IS NO EVIDENCE IN THE PATIENT MEDICAL RECORD THAT HE HAD ANY INVOLVEMENT IN THE CARE AND TREATMENT OF THIS PATIENT OR THAT HE PROVIDED ANY MEANINGFUL SUPERVISION OF THE NURSE PRACTITIONER HANDLING THAT PATIENT'S CARE AND TREATMENT; THE PATIENT EVENTUALLY WAS BROUGHT TO A HOSPITAL WHERE THE DOCTOR'S IMPRESSION WAS DEHYDRATION, HYPOTHERMIA, BRADYCARDIA, ATRIAL FIBRILLATION, RENAL FAILURE AND CORONARY ARTERY DISEASE. ON 11/21/98 REQUEST FOR RECONSIDERATION DENIED.

GRAYSON, JOHN G DO, LICENSE NUMBER 0001989 OF 7550 N 19TH AVENUE #104, PHOENIX, AZ, WAS DISCIPLINED BY ARIZONA ON

JANUARY 11, 1991
DISCIPLINARY ACTION: 12-MONTH PROBATION; MONITORING OF PHYSICIAN PERFORMANCE
OFFENSE: PROFESSIONAL MISCONDUCT

NOTES: FROM 9/88 TO 8/02/90 ADMINISTERED TO HIMSELF THE CONTROLLED SUBSTANCES TYLENOL III AT A FREQUENCY OF TWO TO FOUR TIME PER WEEK AND VALIUM ON ONE OCCASION; ADMITTED THAT HE HAD SELF-ADMINISTERED CONTROLLED SUBSTANCES ON VARIOUS OCCASIONS PRIOR TO 10/90; STATED THAT SUCH SELF-MEDICATION WAS FOR THE PURPOSE OF THE RELIEF OF NECK PAIN RESULTING FROM A PRIOR AUTOMOBILE ACCIDENT. PROBATION UNDER TERMS AND CONDITIONS: SHALL SUBMIT TO BIOLOGICAL FLUID TESTING UPON BOARD REQUEST; SHALL USE NO CONTROLLED SUBSTANCE OR PRESCRIPTION-ONLY MEDICATION UNLESS PRESCRIBED BY HIS ATTENDING PHYSICIAN; SHALL MEET REGULARLY WITH THE BOARD TO REVIEW HIS COMPLIANCE; SHALL AUTHORIZE ANY ATTENDING PHYSICIAN, PSYCHIATRIST, OR PSYCHOLOGIST TO RELEASE TO THE BOARD ALL RECORDS PERTAINING TO HIS CARE AND TREATMENT. AMENDED ON 1/11/91 TO SPECIFY A ONE YEAR TERM FOR ALL CONDITIONS THEREIN IMPOSED. AMENDED AT THE 7/12-13/91 BOARD MEETING TO ELIMINATE THE REQUIREMENT OF PSYCHIATRIC COUNSELING. PROBATION SATISFIED IN FULL ON 1/11/92.

GREEN, JAMES C DO, LICENSE NUMBER 0001623, WAS DISCIPLINED BY ARIZONA ON JANUARY 11, 1991
DISCIPLINARY ACTION: 12-MONTH LICENSE SUSPENSION; 60-MONTH PROBATION
OFFENSE: OVERPRESCRIBING OR MISPRESCRIBING DRUGS

NOTES: FROM 8/18/85 TO 12/05/89 PRESCRIBED CONTROLLED SUBSTANCES AND/OR PRESCRIPTION-ONLY DRUGS TO THREE PATIENTS OF WHICH THE AMOUNTS AND FREQUENCY IN WHICH SUCH SUBSTANCES AND/OR DRUGS WERE PRESCRIBED CANNOT BE JUSTIFIED BASED ON HIS DIAGNOSIS AS SET FORTH IN THE RECORDS. SUSPENSION RETROACTIVE TO 11/01/90. PROBATION UNDER TERMS AND CONDITIONS: SHALL ATTEND A BOARD-APPROVED CONTINUING MEDICAL EDUCATION COURSE CONCERNING ADEQUATE RECORDKEEPING AND EXAMINATIONS OF PATIENTS RELATING TO THE DISPENSING AND WRITING OF PRESCRIPTIONS FOR CONTROLLED SUBSTANCES AND PRESCRIPTION-ONLY DRUGS AND SUBMIT PROOF TO THE BOARD; $1,000 CIVIL PENALTY; $2,500 INVESTIGATION COSTS. PROBATION SATISFIED IN FULL ON 7/16/94.

GREEN, JAMES C DO, DATE OF BIRTH DECEMBER 4, 1933, LICENSE NUMBER 0005291 OF 2655 W GUADALUPE ROAD, MESA, AZ, WAS DISCIPLINED BY MICHIGAN ON AUGUST 4, 1994
DISCIPLINARY ACTION: 6-MONTH LICENSE SUSPENSION
OFFENSE: PROFESSIONAL MISCONDUCT

NOTES: DIVERSION OR MISPRESCRIBING OF DRUGS.

GREENBERG, RICHARD PAUL MD, LICENSE NUMBER 0013656, WAS DISCIPLINED BY ARIZONA ON NOVEMBER 1, 1991
DISCIPLINARY ACTION: RESTRICTION PLACED ON LICENSE; MONITORING OF PHYSICIAN PERFORMANCE
OFFENSE: PROFESSIONAL MISCONDUCT

NOTES: INADEQUATE DOCUMENTATION SHOWING THE NEED FOR SURGERY AND INFORMED CONSENT AND INADEQUATE POST-OPERATIVE DOCUMENTATION FOR ONE PATIENT; INADEQUATE OBJECTIVE INFORMATION INDICATING THE NEED FOR AN ELECTIVE ANTERIOR CERVICAL DECOMPRESSION AND FUSION FOR ANOTHER PATIENT. FOR THREE YEARS, SHALL OBTAIN AN INDEPENDENT SECOND MEDICAL OPINION PRIOR TO PERFORMING ANY ELECTIVE ANTERIOR CERVICAL FUSION SURGERY FOR DEGENERATIVE DISC DISEASE; PRIOR TO THIS SURGERY, SHALL OBTAIN AND REVIEW ALL PAST MEDICAL RECORDS OF THE PATIENT WHICH RELATE TO THOSE CONDITIONS WHICH REQUIRE SURGICAL INTERVENTION; SHALL NOT USE THE REFERRING PHYSICIAN AS AN ASSISTING PHYSICIAN DURING THIS KIND OF SURGERY; SHALL MAINTAIN LEGIBLE MEDICAL RECORDS CONTAINING SUFFICIENT INFORMATION TO IDENTIFY THE PATIENT, SUPPORT THE DIAGNOSIS, JUSTIFY THE TREATMENT, DOCUMENT THE RESULTS, INDICATE ADVICE AND WARNINGS PROVIDED TO THE PATIENT SUFFICIENT TO ESTABLISH INFORMED CONSENT AND PROVIDE SUFFICIENT INFORMATION FOR ANOTHER PRACTITIONER TO ASSUME CONTINUITY OF THE PATIENT'S CARE; SHALL SUBMIT TO A RANDOM EXAMINATION AND REVIEW OF HIS MEDICAL TREATMENT RECORDS IN TWO YEARS AT WHICH TIME THE BOARD WILL DETERMINE COMPLIANCE WITH THE CONDITIONS; IF HE HAS COMPLIED WITH CONDITIONS, EFFECTIVE LENGTH OF THIS ORDER SHALL BE REDUCED FROM THREE YEARS TO THE DATE OF BOARD'S DETERMINATION OF COMPLIANCE.

GRIFFITH, LARRY L MD, LICENSE NUMBER 0005334, WAS DISCIPLINED BY ARIZONA ON OCTOBER 16, 1996
DISCIPLINARY ACTION: MONITORING OF PHYSICIAN PERFORMANCE

NOTES: INTERVIEWED BY THE BOARD REGARDING HIS CARE AND TREATMENT OF THREE PATIENTS AND THE RESULTS OF BOARD-ORDERED EVALUATIONS. SHALL PROMPTLY ENGAGE IN PSYCHOTHERAPY REGARDING APPROPRIATE INTERPERSONAL RELATIONSHIPS WITH A BOARD APPROVED THERAPIST; THERAPIST WILL SUBMIT QUARTERLY REPORTS TO THE BOARD; SHALL REMAIN IN PSYCHOTHERAPY ON A REGULAR BASIS UNTIL ORDER IS TERMINATED BY THE BOARD. ON 3/26/99 STIPULATION TO REMAIN IN THERAPY TERMINATED.

GRIGGS, JAMES A DO, LICENSE NUMBER 0002604 OF 200 EL CAMINO REAL, SIERRA VISTA, AZ, WAS DISCIPLINED BY ARIZONA ON FEBRUARY 7, 1996
DISCIPLINARY ACTION: 60-MONTH PROBATION; RESTRICTION PLACED ON CONTROLLED SUBSTANCE LICENSE
OFFENSE: SUBSTANCE ABUSE

NOTES: RECEIVED TREATMENT FOR SUBSTANCE ABUSE FROM 9/06/95 TO 10/03/95. PROBATION UNDER TERMS AND CONDITIONS: SHALL OBTAIN PSYCHIATRIC OR PSYCHOLOGICAL TREATMENT BY A BOARD APPROVED THERAPIST WHO SHALL SUBMIT TO THE BOARD A WRITTEN PROGRESS REPORT EVERY MONTH FOR THE FIRST SIX MONTHS AND THEN EVERY THREE MONTHS FOR THE REMAINDER OF THE PROBATION; SHALL PROVIDE A COPY OF THIS ORDER TO ALL FACILITIES WHERE HE IS CURRENTLY EMPLOYED AS A PHYSICIAN AND/OR HAS PRIVILEGES TO ENGAGE IN THE PRACTICE OF MEDICINE; SHALL ABSTAIN FROM THE CONSUMPTION OF ALCOHOL AND SHALL NOT CONSUME ILLICIT DRUGS OR TAKE ANY CONTROLLED SUBSTANCES UNLESS SUCH MEDICATION IS PRESCRIBED FOR HIM BY HIS TREATING PHYSICIAN; SHALL MAINTAIN A LOG OF THESE PRESCRIPTIONS AND PROVIDE A COPY TO THE BOARD MONTHLY; SHALL SUBMIT TO AND COOPERATE IN ANY INDEPENDENT MEDICAL OR PSYCHOLOGICAL EVALUATION ORDERED BY THE BOARD; SHALL APPEAR BEFORE THE BOARD UPON

REQUEST; SHALL SUBMIT TO RANDOM BIOLOGICAL FLUID TESTING; SHALL PARTICIPATE IN A MINIMUM OF TWO SELF-HELP MEETINGS PER WEEK THROUGH SUCH ORGANIZATIONS AS AA, NARCOTICS ANONYMOUS, AND DOCTOR'S CADUCEUS GROUP; SHALL NOTIFY THE BOARD WITHIN 20 DAYS IF HE CEASES TO RESIDE IN ARIZONA; MAY ONLY PRESCRIBE CONTROLLED SUBSTANCES PURSUANT TO THOSE TERMS AND CONDITIONS IMPOSED BY THE DEA; SHALL PROVIDE THE BOARD WITH A COPY OF ALL DEA ORDERS AND AGREEMENTS APPLICABLE TO HIS PRESCRIBING PRIVILEGES OR DEA REGISTRATION; UPON APPROVAL OF PRESCRIPTION PRIVILEGES MUST USE TRIPLICATE COPIES OF PRESCRIPTION PADS AND SUPPLY COPIES TO THE BOARD.

GRIGGS, JAMES ALLAN DO OF 155 CALLS PORTAL #300, SIERRA VISTA, AZ, WAS DISCIPLINED BY DEA ON NOVEMBER 15, 1996
DISCIPLINARY ACTION: SURRENDER OF CONTROLLED SUBSTANCE LICENSE

GROH, JACK MD, WAS DISCIPLINED BY ARIZONA ON OCTOBER 21, 1992
DISCIPLINARY ACTION: LICENSE REVOCATION
OFFENSE: NONCOMPLIANCE WITH A PROFESSIONAL RULE

NOTES: FAILED TO PASS THE SPEX EXAM. BOARD ACCEPTED HIS REQUEST FOR CANCELLATION OF LICENSE WITH CAUSE.

GROH, JACK E MD, WAS DISCIPLINED BY ARIZONA ON JULY 14, 1994
DISCIPLINARY ACTION: LICENSE SUSPENSION
OFFENSE: NONCOMPLIANCE WITH A PROFESSIONAL RULE

NOTES: NONPAYMENT OF HIS LICENSE RENEWAL FEES DURING A PENDING INVESTIGATION.

GROVES, THOMAS J MD, LICENSE NUMBER 0005104, WAS DISCIPLINED BY ARIZONA ON OCTOBER 20, 1992
OFFENSE: SUBSTANDARD CARE, INCOMPETENCE OR NEGLIGENCE

NOTES: ON 7/20/88, HIS ANESTHESIA PATIENT SUFFERED INTRAOPERATIVE HYPOTENSION DURING SURGERY AND SUBSEQUENT POSTOPERATIVE ENCEPHALOPATHY. ALSO FAILED TO MAINTAIN ADEQUATE MEDICAL RECORD. CENSURED.

GUIDA, JOSEPH MD, WAS DISCIPLINED BY ARIZONA ON JULY 15, 1993
DISCIPLINARY ACTION: RESTRICTION PLACED ON LICENSE
OFFENSE: PHYSICAL OR MENTAL ILLNESS INHIBITING THE ABILITY TO PRACTICE WITH SKILL AND SAFETY

NOTES: HAS MENIERE'S DISEASE WHICH CAUSES HIM TO HAVE PERIODIC VERTIGO AND NAUSEA. BECAUSE OF THE VERTIGINOUS EPISODES, HE SHALL NOT PRACTICE CLINICAL ANESTHESIA.

GUIDA, JOSEPH MD, DATE OF BIRTH MAY 31, 1955, LICENSE NUMBER 0045247 OF 8311 EAST VIA DEDORADO, SCOTTSDALE, AZ, WAS DISCIPLINED BY NEW JERSEY ON DECEMBER 12, 1994
OFFENSE: DISCIPLINARY ACTION BY ANOTHER STATE OR AGENCY

NOTES: MUST COMPLY WITH ALL REQUIREMENTS OF AN ORDER DATED 08/06/93 ISSUED BY THE BOARD OF MEDICAL EXAMINERS OF ARIZONA. SHALL PROVIDE NOTICE TO THE NEW JERSEY STATE BOARD OF ANY CHANGE IN THE TERMS OF THE ARIZONA AGREEMENT OR HIS MEDICAL CONDITION. PRIOR TO ENGAGING IN ACTIVE PRACTICE IN NEW JERSEY, HE SHALL APPEAR BEFORE A COMMITTEE OF THE BOARD FOR A STATUS CONFERENCE TO DISCUSS HIS HEALTH AND PLANS TO PRACTICE MEDICINE.

GUMEINER, STEVEN C MD, LICENSE NUMBER 0D29288, WAS DISCIPLINED BY MARYLAND ON APRIL 24, 1990
DISCIPLINARY ACTION: REPRIMAND
OFFENSE: SUBSTANDARD CARE, INCOMPETENCE OR NEGLIGENCE

NOTES: HE ADMINISTERED SUCCINYLCHOLINE INAPPROPRIATELY TO A PATIENT WHO HAD EXHIBITED SIGNS OF PARAPLEGIA FOR APPROXIMATELY 3 WEEKS PRIOR TO ADMINISTRATION AFTER WHICH PATIENT DEVELOPED TACHYCARDIA FOLLOWED BY CARDIAC ARREST AND DEATH; USE OF DRUG IS CONTRAINDICATED EXCEPT WITHIN 48 HOURS AFTER MAJOR SPINAL CORD INJURY.

GUMEINER, STEVEN C MD, LICENSE NUMBER 0015898 OF OH, WAS DISCIPLINED BY ARIZONA ON JANUARY 20, 1993
OFFENSE: DISCIPLINARY ACTION BY ANOTHER STATE OR AGENCY

NOTES: ON 04/24/90, MARYLAND BOARD OF PHYSICIAN QUALITY ASSURANCE CONCLUDED THAT DR. GUMEINER'S ADMINISTRATION OF SUCCINYLCHOLINE TO A PATIENT MAY HAVE CAUSED CARDIAC ARREST AND DEATH AND REPRIMANDED HIM. DR. GUMEINER DID NOT ADMIT THIS. ARIZONA CENSURED HIM AND ORDERED THAT HE SHALL NOT PRACTICE MEDICINE IN ARIZONA.

GUMEINER, STEVEN C MD, LICENSE NUMBER 043129E OF MD, WAS DISCIPLINED BY PENNSYLVANIA ON JANUARY 26, 1993
DISCIPLINARY ACTION: REPRIMAND
OFFENSE: DISCIPLINARY ACTION BY ANOTHER STATE OR AGENCY

NOTES: MARYLAND LICENSE REPRIMANDED FOR FAILING TO MEET APPROPRIATE STANDARDS FOR THE DELIVERY OF QUALITY ANESTHESIA CARE.

GURLAND, DAVID B MD, DATE OF BIRTH SEPTEMBER 2, 1939 OF 4703 NORTH FIRST AVE, TUCSON, AZ, WAS DISCIPLINED BY MEDICARE ON MARCH 26, 1990
DISCIPLINARY ACTION: EXCLUSION FROM THE MEDICARE AND/OR MEDICAID PROGRAM
OFFENSE: DISCIPLINARY ACTION BY ANOTHER STATE OR AGENCY

NOTES: LICENSE REVOCATION OR SUSPENSION.

GURLAND, DAVID B MD OF 4703 NORTH FIRST AVE, TUCSON, AZ, WAS DISCIPLINED BY DEA ON MAY 29, 1990
DISCIPLINARY ACTION: SURRENDER OF CONTROLLED SUBSTANCE LICENSE
OFFENSE: OVERPRESCRIBING OR MISPRESCRIBING DRUGS

NOTES: PRESCRIBED EXCESSIVE QUANTITIES OF CONTROLLED AND NON-CONTROLLED SUBSTANCES FOUND TO BE HARMFUL AND CONTRIBUTED TO DEATH OF A PATIENT.

GUSTAVSON, ANDREW MD, WAS DISCIPLINED BY ARIZONA ON AUGUST 8, 1998
DISCIPLINARY ACTION: REPRIMAND
OFFENSE: PROFESSIONAL MISCONDUCT

NOTES: EXCEEDED APPROPRIATE DOCTOR/PATIENT BOUNDARIES DURING HIS PSYCHIATRIC RESIDENCY.

HADE, RALPH D MD, LICENSE NUMBER 22264 OF LAKE HAVASU, AZ, WAS DISCIPLINED BY WASHINGTON ON MARCH 18, 1998
OFFENSE: DISCIPLINARY ACTION BY ANOTHER STATE OR AGENCY

NOTES: COMMITTED UNPROFESSIONAL CONDUCT.

SUSPENSION STAYED ON CONDITION THAT HE COMPLY WITH AN ORDER ISSUED BY THE ARIZONA MEDICAL BOARD, AND THAT HE APPEAR BEFORE THE COMMISSION PRIOR TO PRACTICING MEDICINE IN WASHINGTON.

HADE, RALPH DOUGLAS MD, LICENSE NUMBER 0018114, WAS DISCIPLINED BY ARIZONA ON JANUARY 1, 1995
DISCIPLINARY ACTION: LICENSE SUSPENSION; REQUIRED TO ENTER AN IMPAIRED PHYSICIAN PROGRAM OR SUBSTANCE ABUSE TREATMENT
OFFENSE: FAILURE TO COMPLY WITH PREVIOUS BOARD ORDER

NOTES: VIOLATED PREVIOUS BOARD ORDER IN THAT IN 11/94, CONSUMED DRUGS AND EXPERIENCED A RELAPSE. BOARD ACCEPTED HIS REQUEST FOR INACTIVE STATUS. AGREES NOT TO PRACTICE IN ANY STATE WHILE ARIZONA LICENSE IS INACTIVE. MAY NOT HOLD DEA REGISTRATION OR WRITE PRESCRIPTIONS WHILE LICENSE IS CLASSIFIED AS INACTIVE. AGREES TO ENTER LONG-TERM RESIDENTIAL/INPATIENT TREATMENT FOR CHEMICAL DEPENDENCY AND ALCOHOLISM AND TO SUCCESSFULLY COMPLETE ALL TREATMENT RECOMMENDED.

HADE, RALPH DOUGLAS MD, LICENSE NUMBER 0018114, WAS DISCIPLINED BY ARIZONA ON APRIL 8, 1995
DISCIPLINARY ACTION: 60-MONTH PROBATION; REQUIRED TO ENTER AN IMPAIRED PHYSICIAN PROGRAM OR SUBSTANCE ABUSE TREATMENT
OFFENSE: FAILURE TO COMPLY WITH PREVIOUS BOARD ORDER

NOTES: ACKNOWLEDGED THAT HE HAD CONSUMED DRUGS IN VIOLATION OF 10/94 ORDER. ON 3/18/95 DISCHARGED FROM RECOVERY PROGRAM AFTER SUCCESSFULLY COMPLETING TREATMENT FOR CHEMICAL DEPENDENCY. REINSTATED TO PROBATION WITH CONDITIONS: MUST IMMEDIATELY PARTICIPATE IN A BOARD-APPROVED MONITORED AFTERCARE TREATMENT PROGRAM WHOSE THERAPIST MUST SUBMIT QUARTERLY REPORTS; HAS PREVIOUSLY PARTICIPATED IN 90 12-STEP MEETINGS FOR SUBSTANCE ABUSE; MUST PARTICIPATE IN A 12-STEP RECOVERY PROGRAM AS DETERMINED BY HIS TREATING THERAPIST AND ATTEND AT LEAST THREE WEEKLY MEETINGS; SHALL OBTAIN A BOARD-APPROVED TREATING PHYSICIAN; SHALL ABSTAIN COMPLETELY FROM THE CONSUMPTION OF ALCOHOLIC BEVERAGES AND DRUGS EXCEPT WHEN PRESCRIBED BY HIS TREATING PHYSICIAN; MUST SUBMIT TO WITNESSED RANDOM BIOLOGICAL FLUID COLLECTION; MUST KEEP A LOG OF ANY AND ALL MEDICATIONS PRESCRIBED FOR HIM; SHALL SUBMIT TO ANY EXAMINATIONS OR THERAPY ORDERED BY THE BOARD; SHALL APPEAR BEFORE BOARD FOR INTERVIEWS UPON REQUEST; SHALL INFORM BOARD OF CHANGE OF ADDRESS OR IF AWAY FOR MORE THAN FIVE DAYS.

HADE, RALPH DOUGLAS MD, LICENSE NUMBER 0054413 OF LAKE HAVERSU CITY, AZ, WAS DISCIPLINED BY FLORIDA ON NOVEMBER 2, 1995
DISCIPLINARY ACTION: LICENSE SUSPENSION
OFFENSE: DISCIPLINARY ACTION BY ANOTHER STATE OR AGENCY

NOTES: CHARGED WITH HAVING LICENSE ACTED AGAINST BY THE LICENSING AUTHORITY OF ANOTHER JURISDICTION; FAILING TO REPORT THIS TO THE BOARD WITHIN 30 DAYS. SUSPENSION UNLESS AND UNTIL HE APPEARS BEFORE THE BOARD AND DEMONSTRATES THAT HE IS ABLE TO PRACTICE WITH SKILL AND SAFETY.

HALCOMB, WILLIAM W DO, LICENSE NUMBER 00E5774 OF MESA, AZ, WAS DISCIPLINED BY TEXAS ON SEPTEMBER 28, 1990
DISCIPLINARY ACTION: SURRENDER OF LICENSE

HALCOMB, WILLIAM W MD, LICENSE NUMBER 0A27934 OF MESA, AZ, WAS DISCIPLINED BY CALIFORNIA ON JANUARY 17, 1995
DISCIPLINARY ACTION: 60-MONTH PROBATION
OFFENSE: DISCIPLINARY ACTION BY ANOTHER STATE OR AGENCY

NOTES: SURRENDER OF LICENSE TO TEXAS BOARD WHILE UNDER INVESTIGATION. REVOCATION STAYED.

HALL, GARY WAYNE MD, LICENSE NUMBER 0012977, WAS DISCIPLINED BY ARIZONA ON JANUARY 19, 1996
DISCIPLINARY ACTION: 36-MONTH PROBATION; MONITORING OF PHYSICIAN PERFORMANCE
OFFENSE: NONCOMPLIANCE WITH A PROFESSIONAL RULE

NOTES: IN SIX CASES FAILED TO DOCUMENT THAT HE HAD ADVISED PATIENTS ABOUT REQUIRED RISKS OF THEIR CARE AND PROCEDURES, INCLUDING GETTING PROPER INFORMED CONSENT; FAILED TO DOCUMENT THAT HE HAD INFORMED THESE PATIENTS WHO WOULD PERFORM POSTOPERATIVE CARE; AND FAILED TO DOCUMENT PROCEDURE IN THEIR MEDICAL CHARTS IN ONE OF THESE PATIENTS. PROBATION WITH THE FOLLOWING TERMS: SHALL PRACTICE RADIAL KERATOTOMY (RK) WITHIN PRACTICE GUIDELINES; FOR EACH RK PERFORMED HE SHALL REVIEW THE RESULTS OF THE PREOPERATIVE EXAMINATIONS WITH THE PATIENT AND DOCUMENT THAT REVIEW APPROPRIATELY; EACH PATIENT TO RECEIVE RK MUST VIEW AN INSTRUCTIONAL VIDEOTAPE REGARDING THE SURGERY AND GIVE PROPER INFORMED CONSENT BEFORE THE SURGERY; IN CASES WHERE PERFORMING RK WOULD FALL OUTSIDE THE GUIDELINES, HE SHALL PERSONALLY CONDUCT A PREOPERATIVE EXAMINATION AND INFORMED CONSENT DISCUSSION WITH THE PATIENT ON A DAY OTHER THAN THE DAY OF SURGERY AND HE, OR ANOTHER OPHTHALMOLOGIST SHALL CONDUCT A POSTOPERATIVE EXAMINATION OF THE PATIENT. IF THE PATIENT IS COMING FROM OUT OF TOWN, THE PREOPERATIVE EXAM/INFORMED CONSENT DISCUSSION SHALL OCCUR AT LEAST SIX HOURS IN ADVANCE OF SURGERY; IF HE IS NOT PERFORMING THE POST OPERATIVE CARE, SHALL INFORM THE PATIENT WHO WILL BE PERFORMING IT AND DOCUMENT THAT IN THE PATIENT'S CHART; SHALL PERFORM 80 HOURS OF COMMUNITY SERVICE DURING THE FIRST YEAR OF PROBATION AND PROVIDE DOCUMENTATION OF THIS SERVICE; SHALL PRACTICE WITHIN THE MEDICARE GUIDELINES IN THE PRACTICE OF CATARACT SURGERY AND YAG LASER CAPSULOTOMIES; THE BOARD SHALL HAVE THE RIGHT TO CONDUCT A RANDOM OFFICE PRACTICE SURVEY OF CHARTS INVOLVING RK AND CATARACT SURGERY ON A QUARTERLY BASIS; WITHIN 90 DAYS HE SHALL PAY $10,000 COSTS OF PROCEEDINGS. ON 1/24/97 REQUEST FOR THREE MONTH EXTENSION TO THE TIME IN WHICH HE IS TO PERFORM COMMUNITY SERVICES GRANTED; NO FURTHER EXTENSIONS TO BE GRANTED. ON 11/14/97 BOARD RECOGNIZED HIS COMPLIANCE WITH THE 80 HOUR COMMUNITY SERVICE REQUIREMENT.

HALL, GARY WAYNE MD, LICENSE NUMBER 12977, WAS DISCIPLINED BY ARIZONA ON JANUARY 23, 1997
DISCIPLINARY ACTION: REPRIMAND
OFFENSE: PROFESSIONAL MISCONDUCT

NOTES: ON 5/95 IN A PRINT AD HE IS DEFINED AS "THE RK

EXPERT," AND ENCOURAGED SENIOR CITIZENS THE OPPORTUNITY TO "SEE THE BEST EYE DOCTORS FOR FREE" WITH NO OBJECTIVE CRITERIA TO SUPPORT THESE CONTENTIONS; AN ADVERTISEMENT FOR HIS PRACTICE THAT RAN ON THE RADIO ON 1/22/96 IMPLIED THAT EVERY PERSON WITH NEARSIGHTEDNESS, FARSIGHTEDNESS OR ASTIGMATISM IS A CANDIDATE FOR EITHER "BIOSENSORY RK OR THE NEWEST LASER PROCEDURE" WHEN SUCH IS NOT THE CASE; ADVERTISEMENTS OF 1/28/96 IN PRINT INDICATES THAT HE IS A BOARD CERTIFIED OPHTHALMOLOGIST BUT DOES NOT SUPPLY THE FULL NAME OF THE SPECIFIC AGENCY, ORGANIZATION OR ENTITY GRANTING THIS STANDING; THE 11/95 ADVERTISEMENT DID NOT MENTION THE REFUNDABILITY OR NON-REFUNDABILITY OF A GIFT CERTIFICATE PURCHASED PRIOR TO THE EXPIRATION DATE FOR RK SURGERY; AN INDIVIDUAL WHO PURCHASED A GIFT CERTIFICATE OVER THE PHONE DECIDED AGAINST THE SURGERY, ASKING FOR A REFUND AND WAS NOT GRANTED THE REFUND UNTIL AFTER A COMPLAINT WAS MADE WITH THE ARIZONA BOARD OF MEDICAL EXAMINERS.

HALL, GARY WAYNE MD, LICENSE NUMBER 12977, WAS DISCIPLINED BY ARIZONA ON SEPTEMBER 24, 1999
DISCIPLINARY ACTION: 36-MONTH PROBATION; FINE

NOTES: SHALL NO LONGER BE ABLE TO PERFORM RADIAL KERATOTOMY, BOTH PRIMARY PROCEDURE OR ENHANCEMENT; SHALL TAKE A COMPREHENSIVE BOARD-APPROVED CRS COURSE IN LASIK, AND SHALL REFRAIN FROM LASIK SURGERY UNTIL COURSE COMPLETED; SHALL PAY A $15,000 FINE; SHALL COMPLY WITH ALL INVESTIGATIONS OF NON-RADIAL KERATOTOMY CHARTS.

HALL, SHANNA D MD, LICENSE NUMBER 0018449, WAS DISCIPLINED BY ARIZONA ON MARCH 24, 1990
DISCIPLINARY ACTION: RESTRICTION PLACED ON LICENSE; REQUIRED TO TAKE ADDITIONAL MEDICAL EDUCATION

NOTES: SUMMARY SUSPENSION ORDER OF 8/3/89 RESCINDED AND LICENSE TO PRACTICE IS REINSTATED SUBJECT TO FOLLOWING TERMS AND CONDITIONS: MUST OBTAIN CARE AND TREATMENT FOR AFFECTIVE DISORDERS FROM A BOARD-APPROVED THERAPIST WHO MUST SUBMIT QUARTERLY REPORTS TO THE BOARD; MUST SUBMIT TO ANY EXAMS ORDERED BY THE BOARD; MUST TAKE NO DRUGS; MUST APPEAR BEFORE BOARD FOR INTERVIEWS UPON REQUEST; MUST AUTHORIZE RELEASE OF ALL DOCUMENTS CONCERNING PROFESSIONAL CONDUCT; MUST PRACTICE ONLY WITHIN A MEDICAL CARE GROUP, HOSPITAL OR MEDICAL FACILITY WITH FOLLOWING CONDITIONS: MUST HAVE IMMEDIATE ACCESS TO A LICENSED PEDIATRICIAN FOR CONSULTATION; A FORMAL PEER REVIEW MECHANISM IN PLACE; MUST HAVE QUARTERLY REPORTS SUBMITTED TO THE BOARD. MUST ALSO TAKE 35 HOURS OF CONTINUING MEDICAL EDUCATION IN PEDIATRICS WITHIN 18 MONTHS FROM AT LEAST 3 DIFFERENT PROVIDERS; SHALL PROVIDE COPY OF ORDER TO THERAPIST AND EMPLOYER. ON 7/17/92 BOARD ACCEPTED THE CONTINUING MEDICAL EDUCATION SUBMITTED BY HER AS FULFILLMENT OF THE REQUIREMENTS OF THIS STIPULATION ORDER.

HALL, SHANNA D MD, DATE OF BIRTH JUNE 24, 1951, LICENSE NUMBER 0033893 OF DENVER, CO, WAS DISCIPLINED BY COLORADO ON OCTOBER 9, 1992
DISCIPLINARY ACTION: DENIAL OF NEW LICENSE
OFFENSE: SUBSTANCE ABUSE

NOTES: MENTAL DISABILITY, EXCESSIVE USE OF A CONTROLLED SUBSTANCE. APPLICATION FOR AN UNRESTRICTED LICENSE DENIED. BOARD WILLING TO OFFER LICENSURE UNDER PROBATIONARY TERMS. THE DENIAL OF THE APPLICATION HAS BEEN APPEALED TO THE COLORADO COURT OF APPEALS.

HALL, SHANNA D MD OF COLUMBIA, MO, WAS DISCIPLINED BY MISSOURI ON JUNE 28, 1993
DISCIPLINARY ACTION: DENIAL OF NEW LICENSE
OFFENSE: DISCIPLINARY ACTION BY ANOTHER STATE OR AGENCY

NOTES: DENIAL BASED ON A DENIAL OF LICENSURE BY ANOTHER STATE.

HALL, SHANNA D MD, DATE OF BIRTH JUNE 24, 1951, LICENSE NUMBER 0033893 OF DENVER, CO, WAS DISCIPLINED BY COLORADO ON JULY 14, 1994
DISCIPLINARY ACTION: 36-MONTH PROBATION; RESTRICTION PLACED ON LICENSE
OFFENSE: SUBSTANCE ABUSE

NOTES: SUBSTANCE ABUSE ISSUES AND MENTAL/PHYSICAL DISABILITY. PROBATION PERIOD INCLUDES TREATMENT AND PRACTICE MONITORING. MAY PRACTICE ONLY WITHIN A HOSPITAL OR MEDICAL CARE GROUP SETTING OF THREE OR MORE PHYSICIANS.

HAMMER, RAYMOND EUGENE MD, LICENSE NUMBER G29528 OF KINGMAN, AZ, WAS DISCIPLINED BY CALIFORNIA ON AUGUST 29, 1997
DISCIPLINARY ACTION: REPRIMAND
OFFENSE: DISCIPLINARY ACTION BY ANOTHER STATE OR AGENCY

NOTES: DISCIPLINED BY ARIZONA FOR INAPPROPRIATE PRESCRIBING OF ATIVAN AND DALMANE TO ONE PATIENT.

HARGIS, THOMAS C MD, LICENSE NUMBER 0008441, WAS DISCIPLINED BY ARIZONA ON JUNE 20, 1991
DISCIPLINARY ACTION: REQUIRED TO ENTER AN IMPAIRED PHYSICIAN PROGRAM OR SUBSTANCE ABUSE TREATMENT; MONITORING OF PHYSICIAN PERFORMANCE
OFFENSE: SUBSTANCE ABUSE

NOTES: MUST IMMEDIATELY PARTICIPATE IN THE ARIZONA MEDICAL ASSOCIATION'S MONITORED AFTERCARE TREATMENT PROGRAM WHOSE THERAPIST MUST SUBMIT QUARTERLY REPORTS; SHALL PARTICIPATE IN 90 12-STEP MEETINGS APPROPRIATE FOR SUBSTANCE ABUSE AND ACCEPTABLE TO THE BOARD WITHIN 90 DAYS OF THIS ORDER; AFTER COMPLETION OF THIS REQUIREMENT, MUST PARTICIPATE IN A 12-STEP RECOVERY PROGRAM FOR SUBSTANCE ABUSE AND ATTEND AT LEAST 3 WEEKLY MEETINGS; SHALL OBTAIN A SOLE BOARD-APPROVED TREATING PHYSICIAN; SHALL ABSTAIN COMPLETELY FROM THE CONSUMPTION OF ALCOHOLIC BEVERAGES AND SHALL TAKE NO DRUGS OR MEDICATIONS UNLESS PRESCRIBED BY HIS TREATING PHYSICIAN; SHALL COMPLY WITH REQUESTS FOR RANDOM BODILY FLUID TESTS; SHALL MAINTAIN A LOG OF ANY AND ALL MEDICATIONS TAKEN; SHALL SUBMIT TO MENTAL, PHYSICAL OR MEDICAL COMPETENCY EXAMINATIONS, OR ANY THERAPY ORDERED BY THE BOARD; SHALL COMPLY WITH REQUESTS FOR RANDOM BIOLOGICAL FLUID TESTS; SHALL APPEAR BEFORE THE BOARD FOR INTERVIEWS UPON REQUEST AND MUST INFORM BOARD OF ADDRESS CHANGE OR IF AWAY FOR MORE THAN FIVE DAYS.

HARGIS, THOMAS C MD, LICENSE NUMBER 0008441, WAS DISCIPLINED BY ARIZONA ON JULY 15, 1994
DISCIPLINARY ACTION: 60-MONTH PROBATION; REQUIRED TO ENTER AN IMPAIRED PHYSICIAN PROGRAM OR SUBSTANCE ABUSE TREATMENT
OFFENSE: FAILURE TO COMPLY WITH PREVIOUS BOARD ORDER

NOTES: ON 6/20/91, ENTERED INTO A REHABILITATION STIPULATION INCLUDING A REQUIREMENT THAT HE TAKE NO DRUGS; SEVEN TIMES BETWEEN 8/91 AND 11/93 HE TESTED POSITIVE FOR DRUGS NOT PRESCRIBED BY TREATING PHYSICIAN; AS A RESULT, BOARD ORDERED EVALUATION FOR SUBSTANCE ABUSE; ENTERED LONG TERM RESIDENTIAL TREATMENT ON 3/2/94. MUST IMMEDIATELY PARTICIPATE IN A BOARD-APPROVED MONITORED AFTERCARE TREATMENT PROGRAM WHOSE THERAPIST MUST SUBMIT QUARTERLY REPORTS; MUST PARTICIPATE IN A 12-STEP RECOVERY PROGRAM AS DETERMINED BY HIS TREATING THERAPIST AND ATTEND AT LEAST THREE WEEKLY MEETINGS; SHALL OBTAIN A BOARD-APPROVED TREATING PHYSICIAN; SHALL ABSTAIN COMPLETELY FROM THE CONSUMPTION OF ALCOHOLIC BEVERAGES AND DRUGS EXCEPT WHEN PRESCRIBED BY HIS TREATING PHYSICIAN; MUST SUBMIT TO WITNESSED RANDOM BIOLOGICAL FLUID COLLECTION; KEEP A LOG OF ANY AND ALL MEDICATIONS PRESCRIBED FOR HIM; SHALL SUBMIT TO ANY EXAMINATIONS OR THERAPY ORDERED BY BOARD; SHALL APPEAR BEFORE BOARD FOR INTERVIEWS UPON REQUEST; SHALL INFORM BOARD OF CHANGE OF ADDRESS OR IF AWAY FOR MORE THAN FIVE DAYS. ON 1/25/97 SECOND AMENDMENT TO PROBATION ORDER: SHALL TAKE NO DRUGS, MEDICATIONS, OR HERBAL SUBSTANCE WHATEVER (EXCEPT FOR PLAIN ASPIRIN AND/OR PLAIN ACETAMINOPHEN), WHETHER CONTROLLED SUBSTANCES, PRESCRIPTION-ONLY DRUGS OR OVER-THE-COUNTER PREPARATIONS, UNLESS SUCH DRUG, MEDICATION, OR HERBAL SUBSTANCE WAS PRESCRIBED FOR HIM BY HIS SOLE TREATING PHYSICIAN. ON 11/19/99 ORDER TERMINATED.

HARPSTER, GENE O MD, LICENSE NUMBER 0007897, WAS DISCIPLINED BY ARIZONA ON JULY 15, 1993
DISCIPLINARY ACTION: 600-MONTH PROBATION
OFFENSE: DISCIPLINARY ACTION BY ANOTHER STATE OR AGENCY

NOTES: THE KANSAS BOARD FOUND EVIDENCE THAT HE WAS GUILTY OF 65 VIOLATIONS OF THE KANSAS HEALING ARTS ACT. EXCLUDED FROM THE MEDICARE AND SOCIAL SECURITY PROGRAMS BY THE DEPT. OF HEALTH AND HUMAN SERVICES, FOR A PERIOD OF SEVEN YEARS. SHALL NOT PRACTICE MEDICINE IN ARIZONA UNTIL HE HAS ACHIEVED REINSTATEMENT OF HIS LICENSE TO PRACTICE MEDICINE IN KANSAS AND MET WITH THE ARIZONA BOARD OF MEDICAL EXAMINERS AT AN INFORMAL INTERVIEW.

HARRIS, DENNIS HOWARD MD OF 1402 N MILLER ROAD SUITE F-4, SCOTTSDALE, AZ, WAS DISCIPLINED BY DEA ON OCTOBER 5, 1990
DISCIPLINARY ACTION: RESTRICTION PLACED ON CONTROLLED SUBSTANCE LICENSE
OFFENSE: CRIMINAL CONVICTION OR PLEA OF GUILTY, NOLO CONTENDERE, OR NO CONTEST TO A CRIME

NOTES: PLED GUILTY 09/16/83 TO CONSPIRACY AND ATTEMPT TO MANUFACTURE MDA. SENTENCED TO FIVE YEARS PROBATION, ORDERED TO RENDER FOUR HOURS WEEKLY COMMUNITY SERVICE AND $8,000 FINE.

HAUK, MARTHA L MD, LICENSE NUMBER 0005915 OF 1516 E. COLTER STREET #222, PHOENIX, AZ, WAS DISCIPLINED BY HAWAII ON OCTOBER 19, 1994
DISCIPLINARY ACTION: FINE
OFFENSE: NONCOMPLIANCE WITH A PROFESSIONAL RULE

NOTES: FAILED TO APPRISE THE BOARD OF CHANGES TO ADDRESS AND HAS NOT ADVISED BOARD OF CURRENT ADDRESS. SETTLEMENT AGREEMENT: $500 FINE; COMPLIANCE WITH ALL CONDITIONS, RESTRICTIONS AND REQUIREMENTS OF THE FEDERAL GOVERNMENT AND OTHER STATE MEDICAL BOARDS.

HAYASHI, JOE T MD, LICENSE NUMBER 0012865, WAS DISCIPLINED BY ARIZONA ON APRIL 13, 1993
OFFENSE: SUBSTANDARD CARE, INCOMPETENCE OR NEGLIGENCE

NOTES: FAILED TO TIMELY NOTIFY PATIENT OF HER MAY 1989 MAMMOGRAM REPORT SHOWING AN IRREGULAR MASS AND FAILED TO PURSUE THE RECOMMENDATION THAT EARLIER MAMMOGRAMS BE OBTAINED FOR COMPARISON. THE MASS LATER PROVED MALIGNANT RESULTING IN A MODIFIED RADICAL MASTECTOMY. CONSTITUTES ACTIVITY WHICH WAS HARMFUL TO THE HEALTH OF THE PATIENT. CENSURED.

HEARTER, WILLIAM R JR MD, LICENSE NUMBER 0016116, WAS DISCIPLINED BY ARIZONA ON OCTOBER 17, 1995
DISCIPLINARY ACTION: 60-MONTH PROBATION; MONITORING OF PHYSICIAN PERFORMANCE
OFFENSE: OVERPRESCRIBING OR MISPRESCRIBING DRUGS

NOTES: OVER THE COURSE OF MORE THAN ONE YEAR, HE PRESCRIBED MEDICATIONS INAPPROPRIATELY TO HIS CHILD WHO WAS UNDER THE AGE OF 12, WITHOUT CONSULTING HER ALLERGIST OR PEDIATRICIAN. IN 7/93, COMMENCED STEROID TREATMENT RECOMMENDED FOR SEVERE ALLERGIES WITH ANAPHYLACTOID REACTIONS, WHICH, ACCORDING TO HER PEDIATRICIAN, WAS NOT JUSTIFIED FOR HIS CHILD WHO DID NOT OFTEN HAVE ALLERGIC SYMPTOMS AND NEVER HAD SEVERE REACTIONS; IN 4/94, PRESCRIBED CLARITIN WITHOUT STATING THE FREQUENCY OF ADMINISTRATION; SAFETY AND EFFECTIVENESS OF THIS DRUG WAS NOT ESTABLISHED IN CHILDREN UNDER 12; DID NOT MAINTAIN ADEQUATE RECORDS ON MEDICATIONS PRESCRIBED TO HIS CHILD; IN 4/94, REQUESTED TO READ HIS ESTRANGED WIFE'S MEDICAL CHARTS WITHOUT HER CONSENT AND WITHOUT HOSPITAL PRIVILEGES; USED ANOTHER PHYSICIAN'S NAME TO PRESCRIBE MEDICATIONS TO HIMSELF AND TO HIS CHILD; IN 1/95, ORDERED BY THE BOARD IN AN INFORMAL INTERVIEW TO BE EVALUATED WITHIN 60 DAYS BY A PSYCHIATRIST AND PSYCHOLOGIST, WHICH HE FAILED TO DO; IN 4/95, ORDERED BY BOARD TO BE EVALUATED WITHIN SIX WEEKS BY A BOARD-APPROVED PSYCHIATRIST AND PSYCHOLOGIST; COMPLIED WITH 4/95 ORDER. PROBATION WITH CONDITIONS: SHALL NOT PRESCRIBE, ADMINISTER OR DISPENSE ANY PRESCRIPTION-ONLY MEDICATION OR CONTROLLED SUBSTANCE TO HIS CHILDREN OR ANY OTHER MEMBER OF HIS IMMEDIATE FAMILY, EXCEPT IN A LIFE-THREATENING EMERGENCY; SHALL IMMEDIATELY ENTER INTO PSYCHOTHERAPY WITH A BOARD-APPROVED THERAPIST WHO SHALL SUBMIT QUARTERLY REPORTS TO THE BOARD. ON 7/18/96 ORDER AMENDED TO DELETE THE REQUIREMENT THAT HE ENTER INTO PSYCHOTHERAPY BASED ON REPORTS SUBMITTED BY HIS THERAPIST.

HEARTER, WILLIAM R JR MD, LICENSE NUMBER 0138028 OF STE C-

128 10575 N. TATUM BLVD, PARADISE VALLEY, AZ, WAS DISCIPLINED BY NEW YORK ON NOVEMBER 7, 1996
DISCIPLINARY ACTION: SURRENDER OF LICENSE
OFFENSE: DISCIPLINARY ACTION BY ANOTHER STATE OR AGENCY

NOTES: ACTION IN ARIZONA FOR DISCLOSING CONFIDENTIAL PATIENT INFORMATION WITHOUT AUTHORIZATION; FAILED TO MAINTAIN ADEQUATE PATIENT RECORDS; AND PRESCRIBED A CONTROLLED DRUG FOR OTHER THAN THERAPEUTIC PURPOSES.

HEFFRON, PATRICK THOMAS MD, LICENSE NUMBER 0002442, WAS DISCIPLINED BY ARIZONA ON JULY 18, 1992
DISCIPLINARY ACTION: REQUIRED TO ENTER AN IMPAIRED PHYSICIAN PROGRAM OR SUBSTANCE ABUSE TREATMENT; MONITORING OF PHYSICIAN PERFORMANCE

NOTES: ISSUED PERMANENT LICENSE WITH THE FOLLOWING ORDER: MUST IMMEDIATELY PARTICIPATE IN A BOARD-APPROVED MONITORED AFTERCARE TREATMENT PROGRAM WHOSE THERAPIST MUST SUBMIT QUARTERLY REPORTS; MUST PARTICIPATE IN 90 12-STEP MEETINGS FOR SUBSTANCE ABUSE WITHIN 90 DAYS; MUST THEN PARTICIPATE IN A 12-STEP RECOVERY PROGRAM AS DETERMINED BY HIS TREATING THERAPIST AND ATTEND AT LEAST THREE WEEKLY MEETINGS; SHALL OBTAIN A BOARD-APPROVED TREATING PHYSICIAN; SHALL ABSTAIN COMPLETELY FROM THE CONSUMPTION OF ALCOHOLIC BEVERAGES AND DRUGS EXCEPT WHEN PRESCRIBED BY HIS TREATING PHYSICIAN; MUST SUBMIT TO WITNESSED RANDOM BIOLOGICAL FLUID COLLECTION; KEEP A LOG OF ANY AND ALL MEDICATIONS PRESCRIBED FOR HIM; SHALL SUBMIT TO ANY EXAMINATIONS OR THERAPY ORDERED BY BOARD; SHALL APPEAR BEFORE BOARD FOR INTERVIEWS UPON REQUEST; SHALL INFORM BOARD OF CHANGE OF ADDRESS OR IF AWAY FOR MORE THAN 5 DAYS. ON 10/16/93 ORDER TERMINATED AFTER 90 DAYS.

HEISELT, LAWRENCE R MD, LICENSE NUMBER 0C23995 OF TUCSON, AZ, WAS DISCIPLINED BY CALIFORNIA ON OCTOBER 23, 1995
DISCIPLINARY ACTION: SURRENDER OF LICENSE

NOTES: WHILE CHARGES PENDING.

HERMAN, RICHARD M MD, LICENSE NUMBER 0017228 OF PHOENIX, AZ, WAS DISCIPLINED BY ARIZONA ON OCTOBER 18, 1994
DISCIPLINARY ACTION: REQUIRED TO TAKE ADDITIONAL MEDICAL EDUCATION; MONITORING OF PHYSICIAN PERFORMANCE
OFFENSE: SEXUAL ABUSE OF OR SEXUAL MISCONDUCT WITH A PATIENT

NOTES: ALLEGATIONS OF SEXUAL ADVANCES TOWARD A PATIENT. SHALL OBTAIN EDUCATION BY A THERAPIST DESIGNATED BY THE BOARD IN AREAS OF BOUNDARY ISSUES, UNDUE FAMILIARITY WITH PATIENTS AND THE GENERAL ISSUES OF TRANSFERENCE AND COUNTER-TRANSFERENCE IN PHYSICIAN/PATIENT RELATIONSHIPS; SHALL MAINTAIN ADEQUATE RECORDS OF ALL PATIENT CONTACTS INCLUDING PHONE CALLS ON ALL PATIENTS FOR WHOM HE PROVIDES MEDICAL CONSULTATION OR ADVICE; SHALL FORMALLY DISCHARGE ANY PATIENT WITH WHOM HE HAS OR ANTICIPATES HAVING A RELATIONSHIP OTHER THAN A PHYSICIAN-PATIENT RELATIONSHIP. ORDER TERMINATED ON 4/16/96.

HEYWOOD, JAMES R MD, LICENSE NUMBER 0A24877 OF TEMPE, AZ, WAS DISCIPLINED BY CALIFORNIA ON DECEMBER 7, 1995
DISCIPLINARY ACTION: SURRENDER OF LICENSE

NOTES: WHILE CHARGES PENDING.

HEYWOOD, JAMES ROBERT MD, DATE OF BIRTH JANUARY 1, 1943, LICENSE NUMBER 0930040 OF WILSON, NC, WAS DISCIPLINED BY NORTH CAROLINA ON OCTOBER 26, 1993

NOTES: MUST COMPLY WITH CONDITIONS OF CONSENT ORDER (TEMPORARY LICENSE ISSUED ON 09/18/93). ON 2/14/94 LICENSE EXTENDED UNTIL 7/31/94 AND ON 8/22/94 LICENSE EXTENDED UNTIL 8/31/95.

HICKS, WILLIAM, WAS DISCIPLINED BY ARIZONA ON OCTOBER 18, 1996
DISCIPLINARY ACTION: LICENSE SUSPENSION

NOTES: INACTIVE STATUS WITH CAUSE.

HICKS, WILLIAM R MD, LICENSE NUMBER 0014516, WAS DISCIPLINED BY ARIZONA ON OCTOBER 20, 1994
DISCIPLINARY ACTION: LICENSE SUSPENSION; REQUIRED TO ENTER AN IMPAIRED PHYSICIAN PROGRAM OR SUBSTANCE ABUSE TREATMENT
OFFENSE: FAILURE TO COMPLY WITH PREVIOUS BOARD ORDER

NOTES: DRANK ALCOHOL IN VIOLATION OF THE TERMS OF THE BOARD'S REHABILITATION STIPULATION AND ORDER OF 1/27/94. LICENSE PLACED ON INACTIVE STATUS WITH FOLLOWING TERMS AND CONDITIONS: HE AGREES NOT TO PRACTICE MEDICINE IN ARIZONA OR ANY OTHER STATE OR FOREIGN COUNTRY WHILE ARIZONA LICENSE IS IN AN INACTIVE STATUS CATEGORY; MAY NOT HOLD REGISTRATION WITH THE DRUG ENFORCEMENT ADMINISTRATION OR WRITE PRESCRIPTIONS AS LONG AS LICENSE IS INACTIVE; HE AGREES TO ENTER LONG-TERM RESIDENTIAL/IN-PATIENT TREATMENT FOR CHEMICAL DEPENDENCY AND ALCOHOLISM, AND SUCCESSFULLY COMPLETE ALL TREATMENT RECOMMENDED BY THE FACILITY; SHALL NOT REQUEST REACTIVATION OF LICENSE TO PRACTICE MEDICINE UNTIL HE MEETS WITH THE BOARD AT A REGULARLY SCHEDULED MEETING.

HICKS, WILLIAM R MD, LICENSE NUMBER 0014516, WAS DISCIPLINED BY ARIZONA ON JULY 22, 1995
DISCIPLINARY ACTION: 60-MONTH PROBATION; RESTRICTION PLACED ON LICENSE
OFFENSE: SUBSTANCE ABUSE

NOTES: TREATMENT FOR CHEMICAL DEPENDENCY FROM 1/9/95 UNTIL 5/13/95. LICENSE REACTIVATED TO PROBATION WITH CONDITIONS: MUST IMMEDIATELY PARTICIPATE IN A BOARD-APPROVED MONITORED AFTERCARE TREATMENT PROGRAM WHOSE THERAPIST MUST SUBMIT QUARTERLY REPORTS; MUST PARTICIPATE IN 90 12-STEP MEETINGS FOR SUBSTANCE ABUSE WITHIN 90 DAYS; MUST THEN PARTICIPATE IN A 12-STEP RECOVERY PROGRAM AS DETERMINED BY HIS TREATING THERAPIST AND ATTEND AT LEAST THREE WEEKLY MEETINGS; SHALL OBTAIN A BOARD-APPROVED TREATING PHYSICIAN; SHALL ABSTAIN COMPLETELY FROM THE CONSUMPTION OF ALCOHOLIC BEVERAGES AND DRUGS EXCEPT WHEN PRESCRIBED BY HIS TREATING PHYSICIAN; MUST SUBMIT TO WITNESSED RANDOM BIOLOGICAL FLUID COLLECTION; MUST KEEP A LOG OF ANY AND ALL MEDICATIONS PRESCRIBED FOR HIM; SHALL SUBMIT TO ANY EXAMINATIONS OR THERAPY ORDERED BY THE BOARD; SHALL APPEAR BEFORE BOARD FOR INTERVIEWS UPON REQUEST; SHALL INFORM BOARD OF CHANGE OF ADDRESS OR IF AWAY FOR MORE THAN FIVE DAYS; SHALL NOT PRACTICE MEDICINE AS A SOLE PRACTITIONER; WITHIN 45 DAYS, SHALL OBTAIN TREATMENT FOR DEPRESSION FROM A

BOARD-APPROVED PSYCHOLOGIST OR PSYCHIATRIST AND SHALL CONTINUE TREATMENT FOR A DURATION AND AT A FREQUENCY TO BE DETERMINED BY THE THERAPIST, WHO SHALL SUBMIT QUARTERLY REPORTS TO THE BOARD. ON 2/15/96, ORDER AMENDED AS FOLLOWS: HE WILL NOT PRACTICE MEDICINE AS A SOLE PRACTITIONER FOR MORE THAN EIGHT HOURS A WEEK; HE WILL MEET WITH HE MONITORED AFTERCARE PROGRAM COMMITTEE IN THREE MONTHS; HE WILL SUBMIT QUARTERLY REPORTS FROM HIS PRIMARY TREATING PSYCHIATRIST.

HIDALGO, MERLIN Z MD, LICENSE NUMBER 0146234 OF WESLEY HILLS, NY, WAS DISCIPLINED BY NEW YORK ON DECEMBER 12, 199(
DISCIPLINARY ACTION: LICENSE REVOCATION

HIDALGO, MERLIN Z MD, DATE OF BIRTH FEBRUARY 9, 1941 OF 12 ASTOR PLACE, WESLEY HILLS, NY, WAS DISCIPLINED BY MEDICARE ON FEBRUARY 25, 1991
DISCIPLINARY ACTION: 120-MONTH EXCLUSION FROM THE MEDICARE AND/OR MEDICAID PROGRAM
OFFENSE: CRIMINAL CONVICTION OR PLEA OF GUILTY, NOLO CONTENDERE, OR NO CONTEST TO A CRIME

NOTES: PROGRAM-RELATED CONVICTION.

HIDALGO, MERLIN Z MD, LICENSE NUMBER 0013512, WAS DISCIPLINED BY ARIZONA ON JANUARY 23, 1992
DISCIPLINARY ACTION: LICENSE REVOCATION
OFFENSE: DISCIPLINARY ACTION BY ANOTHER STATE OR AGENCY

NOTES: ON 10/13/89 PLED GUILTY IN NEW YORK TO 63 COUNTS OF OFFERING A FALSE INSTRUMENT FOR FILING, THE UNAUTHORIZED PRACTICE OF MEDICINE AND SECOND DEGREE GRAND LARCENY DUE TO FILING OF MEDICAID CLAIMS DR. HIDALGO KNEW CONTAINED FALSE INFORMATION. WAS PLACED ON PROBATION FOR FIVE YEARS AND ORDERED TO PAY RESTITUTION IN THE SUM OF $500,000. HIS ACTIONS, IN VIOLATION OF THE LAW, WHICH FORMED THE BASIS FOR REVOCATION OF HIS LICENSE BY NEW YORK ON 11/16/90 CONSTITUTES UNPROFESSIONAL CONDUCT IN ARIZONA.

HIDALGO, MERLIN Z MD, DATE OF BIRTH FEBRUARY 9, 1941, LICENSE NUMBER 0039993 OF 12 ASTOR PL, WESLEY HILLS, NY, WAS DISCIPLINED BY NEW JERSEY ON MAY 12, 1992
DISCIPLINARY ACTION: RESTRICTION PLACED ON LICENSE; MONITORING OF PHYSICIAN PERFORMANCE
OFFENSE: DISCIPLINARY ACTION BY ANOTHER STATE OR AGENCY

NOTES: CONVICTED OF MEDICAID FRAUD AND NEW YORK LICENSE SANCTION. FIVE-YEAR SUSPENSION, STAYED, PROVIDED FULL COMPLIANCE WITH CONDITIONS AND LIMITATIONS. RESTRICTED TO SUPERVISED SETTING, CURRENTLY ST. CLAIRE'S RIVERSIDE MEDICAL CENTER. SHALL NOT DIRECTLY BILL PATIENTS. SUPERVISOR MUST SUBMIT QUARTERLY REPORTS TO BOARD REGARDING PERFORMANCE/FITNESS BEGINNING 7/1/92.

HIDALGO, MERLIN Z MD, DATE OF BIRTH FEBRUARY 9, 1941, LICENSE NUMBER 0039993 OF 12 ASTOR PLACE, WESTLEY HILLS, NY, WAS DISCIPLINED BY NEW JERSEY ON JULY 10, 1992
DISCIPLINARY ACTION: LICENSE REVOCATION
OFFENSE: CRIMINAL CONVICTION OR PLEA OF GUILTY, NOLO CONTENDERE, OR NO CONTEST TO A CRIME

NOTES: CONVICTED IN NEW YORK OF MEDICAID FRAUD.

HIDALGO, MERLIN Z MD, LICENSE NUMBER 0A38777 OF WESLEY HILLS, NY, WAS DISCIPLINED BY CALIFORNIA ON MARCH 5, 1993
DISCIPLINARY ACTION: LICENSE REVOCATION

HIDALGO, MERLIN Z MD, WAS DISCIPLINED BY MAINE ON DECEMBER 11, 1996
DISCIPLINARY ACTION: FINE; REPRIMAND
OFFENSE: DISCIPLINARY ACTION BY ANOTHER STATE OR AGENCY

NOTES: ACTION IN NEW YORK. RECIPROCAL ACTION.

HIDALGO, MERLIN Z MD, LICENSE NUMBER 010556, WAS DISCIPLINED BY MAINE ON JULY 1, 1999
OFFENSE: PROVIDING FALSE INFORMATION TO THE BOARD OR OTHER HEALTH AGENCY

NOTES: GAVE FALSE ANSWERS IN HIS MEDICAL STAFF APPLICATION; FAILED TO DISCLOSE PRIOR DISCIPLINARY ACTIONS. SHALL RECEIVE A CENSURE.

HIGUERA, JOSE A MD, LICENSE NUMBER 0012358, WAS DISCIPLINED BY ARIZONA ON OCTOBER 20, 1994
OFFENSE: SUBSTANDARD CARE, INCOMPETENCE OR NEGLIGENCE

NOTES: COMPLAINT ALLEGING DELAY IN SCHEDULING SURGERY FOR PATIENT WITH A HEMATURIA. SHALL OBTAIN THE SERVICES OF AN OFFICE MANAGEMENT CONSULTANT.

HIGUERA, JOSE A MD, LICENSE NUMBER 12358, WAS DISCIPLINED BY ARIZONA ON JANUARY 23, 1998
DISCIPLINARY ACTION: 60-MONTH PROBATION; RESTRICTION PLACED ON LICENSE
OFFENSE: LOSS OR RESTRICTION OF HOSPITAL PRIVILEGES

NOTES: IN 4/95 BOARD WAS NOTIFIED BY A HEALTH PLAN THAT ONE OF ITS MEMBERS HAD MADE A COMPLAINT AGAINST DR. HIGUERA WHICH INVOLVED INAPPROPRIATE TOUCHING OF A SEXUAL NATURE; WHEN THE BOARD CONTACTED THIS PERSON SHE WOULD NOT MAKE A COMPLAINT WITH BOARD UNLESS IT WAS ANONYMOUS; ON 7/17/95 HIS PROVIDER CONTRACT WAS TERMINATED AFTER "COMPLAINTS OF MISCONDUCT WITH FEMALE PATIENTS"; HE UNDERWENT BOARD REQUESTED PHYSICAL AND PSYCHOMETRIC TESTING. THE TERMS OF THE PROBATION ARE AS FOLLOWS: HE CANNOT SEE OR TREAT ANY FEMALE PATIENT WITHOUT A FEMALE CHAPERONE PRESENT AND WILL LEGIBLY ENTER THE NAME IN THE PATIENT CHART AT THE TIME OF PATIENT CONTACT AND HAVE A CHAPERONE INITIAL THIS ENTRY; SHALL SUBMIT TO THERAPY WITH A PSYCHIATRIST OR PSYCHOLOGIST APPROVED BY THE BOARD AND PAY THE COST OF THERAPY WITH QUARTERLY WRITTEN REPORTS.

HILDING, RONALD MD, WAS DISCIPLINED BY ARIZONA ON JANUARY 21, 1993

NOTES: REQUESTED REACTIVATION OF HIS LICENSE; HAD PREVIOUSLY REQUESTED TAKING ORAL COMPETENCY EXAMINATION IN PSYCHIATRY RATHER THAN A WRITTEN GENERAL MEDICAL EXAM PRIOR TO A REQUEST FOR REACTIVATION OF HIS LICENSE. BOARD APPROVED ORAL EXAM REQUEST BUT HE FAILED THE EXAM GIVEN.

HILDING, RONALD F MD, LICENSE NUMBER 0G12500 OF PARADISE VALLEY, AZ, WAS DISCIPLINED BY CALIFORNIA ON DECEMBER 4, 1995
DISCIPLINARY ACTION: LICENSE REVOCATION
OFFENSE: DISCIPLINARY ACTION BY ANOTHER STATE OR AGENCY

NOTES: ACTION IN ARIZONA. PLACED ON INACTIVE STATUS WITH CAUSE. DEFAULT ACTION.

HILL, RICHARD J MD, LICENSE NUMBER 0002802, WAS DISCIPLINED BY ARIZONA ON APRIL 18, 1996
OFFENSE: SUBSTANDARD CARE, INCOMPETENCE OR NEGLIGENCE

NOTES: INTERVIEWED BY THE BOARD REGARDING ALLEGATIONS OF NEGLIGENT PATIENT CARE, POOR RECORD KEEPING, THE BOARD'S ORDER THAT HE TAKE AND PASS THE SPECIAL PURPOSE EXAMINATION AND HIS FAILURE OF EXAMINATION. SHALL NOT PRACTICE CLINICAL MEDICINE UNTIL HE TAKES AND PASSES THE SPECIAL PURPOSE EXAMINATION WITH A SCORE OF 75 AND MEETS WITH THE BOARD.

HILLER, CRAIG DO, LICENSE NUMBER 3127 OF 12425 N 84TH STREET, SCOTTSDALE, AZ, WAS DISCIPLINED BY ARIZONA ON MARCH 26, 1998
DISCIPLINARY ACTION: 60-MONTH PROBATION; MONITORING OF PHYSICIAN PERFORMANCE
OFFENSE: LOSS OR RESTRICTION OF HOSPITAL PRIVILEGES

NOTES: ON 12/13/96 A COMPLAINT WAS RECEIVED THAT HE HAD PERFORMED AN IMPROPER PHYSICAL EXAMINATION WHICH MAY HAVE BEEN SEXUALLY INAPPROPRIATE AND CONSUMED ALCOHOL WHILE ENGAGING IN PRACTICE; ON 8/16/96 HE WAS INVOLUNTARILY TERMINATED FROM A MEDICAL CENTER DUE TO INAPPROPRIATE AND UNPROFESSIONAL BEHAVIOR; ON 1/29/98 HE WAS TERMINATED FROM A MEDICAL RECRUITMENT GROUP DUE TO BEHAVIORAL PROBLEMS AND ABANDONMENT OF PATIENTS. HE IS CENSURED FOR UNPROFESSIONAL CONDUCT. CONDITIONS OF PROBATION AS FOLLOWS: WITHIN 30 DAYS WILL OBTAIN AN EXAMINATION BY A LICENSED PSYCHIATRIST AND/OR PSYCHOLOGIST WHO IS APPROVED BY THE BOARD; SHALL WAIVE ANY CONFIDENTIALITY WITH REGARD TO EVALUATION OR TREATMENT; WILL COMPLY WITH ANY RECOMMENDATION FOR TREATMENT AND/OR COUNSELING; PROVIDE A COPY OF THIS ORDER TO ALL HEALTH CARE FACILITIES WHERE HE HAS PRIVILEGES; SHALL BE SUBJECT TO RANDOM BIOLOGICAL FLUID TESTING; SHALL SUBMIT TO ANY EVALUATIONS ORDERED BY THE BOARD; SHALL APPEAR BEFORE THE BOARD UPON REQUEST; SHALL NOTIFY THE BOARD IF HE CEASES TO RESIDE IN ARIZONA; SHALL PAY COSTS.

HILLER, CRAIG DO, LICENSE NUMBER 3127 OF 12425 N 84TH STREET, SCOTTSDALE, AZ, WAS DISCIPLINED BY ARIZONA ON MARCH 4, 1999
DISCIPLINARY ACTION: LICENSE REVOCATION
OFFENSE: FAILURE TO COMPLY WITH PREVIOUS BOARD ORDER

NOTES: HE VIOLATED THE TERMS AND CONDITIONS OF THE 3/28/98 ORDER AS FOLLOWS: ON 9/21/98 HE PROVIDED WRITTEN AND VERBAL NOTICE THAT HE WAS RELOCATING TO ARKANSAS IN FIVE DAYS BUT WAS STILL IN ARIZONA ON 10/15/98; HE WAS REQUESTED TO PROVIDE A URINE DRUG SCREEN AND TOLD BOARD THAT HE WAS NO LONGER HAVING HIS REQUIRED THERAPY NOR WAS HE PRACTICING MEDICINE BUT THE BOARD INFORMED HIM HE WAS STILL BOUND BY THE TERMS AND CONDITIONS OF HIS PRIOR ORDER; HE DID NOT SIGN OR RETURN THE STIPULATED CONSENT ORDER FOR SURRENDER OF HIS LICENSE; IN ADDITION ONE OF HIS PATIENTS TOLD ANOTHER PHYSICIAN THAT HE HAD PROVIDED A PRESCRIPTION TO HER FOR PERCODAN FOR A CASH PAYMENT "ON THE SIDE" FOR MANY MONTHS; THIS PATIENT STATED THAT HE MADE SEXUAL ADVANCES TOWARD HER. ON 4/28/99, 6/15/99 AND 7/6/99 MOTIONS FOR REHEARING DENIED.

HINSON, CHRISTOPHER MD OF SCOTTSDALE, AZ, WAS DISCIPLINED BY ILLINOIS ON OCTOBER 1, 1990
DISCIPLINARY ACTION: 3-MONTH LICENSE SUSPENSION
OFFENSE: PROFESSIONAL MISCONDUCT

NOTES: HE AIDED, ABETTED, ENCOURAGED AND ASSISTED AN UNLICENSED INDIVIDUAL TO PRACTICE MEDICINE.

HOFFERT, KEVIN G MD, LICENSE NUMBER 0013766, WAS DISCIPLINED BY ARIZONA ON JUNE 21, 1991
DISCIPLINARY ACTION: REQUIRED TO ENTER AN IMPAIRED PHYSICIAN PROGRAM OR SUBSTANCE ABUSE TREATMENT; MONITORING OF PHYSICIAN PERFORMANCE
OFFENSE: SUBSTANCE ABUSE

NOTES: MUST IMMEDIATELY PARTICIPATE IN THE ARIZONA MEDICAL ASSOCIATION'S MONITORED AFTERCARE TREATMENT PROGRAM WHOSE THERAPIST MUST SUBMIT QUARTERLY REPORTS; SHALL PARTICIPATE IN 90 12-STEP MEETINGS APPROPRIATE FOR SUBSTANCE ABUSE AND ACCEPTABLE TO THE BOARD IN 90 DAYS FROM THE EFFECTIVE DATE OF THIS ORDER; MUST THEN PARTICIPATE IN A 12-STEP RECOVERY PROGRAM AS DETERMINED BY HIS TREATING THERAPIST AND ATTEND AT LEAST 3 WEEKLY MEETINGS; SHALL OBTAIN A SOLE TREATING PHYSICIAN APPROVED BY THE BOARD; SHALL ABSTAIN COMPLETELY FROM THE CONSUMPTION OF ALCOHOLIC BEVERAGES AND TAKE NO DRUGS UNLESS PRESCRIBED BY HIS TREATING PHYSICIAN; SHALL COMPLY WITH REQUESTS TO SUBMIT TO RANDOM BIOLOGICAL FLUID TESTS; SHALL MAINTAIN A LOG OF ANY AND ALL MEDICATIONS; SHALL SUBMIT TO ANY EXAMINATIONS OR THERAPY ORDERED BY BOARD; SHALL APPEAR BEFORE BOARD FOR INTERVIEWS UPON REQUEST. SHALL ADVISE THE BOARD IF HE CHANGES ADDRESS OR IS AWAY FOR MORE THAN FIVE DAYS. ON 4/11/94 ORDER TERMINATED AFTER 180 DAYS.

HOLMES, HENRY H MD, LICENSE NUMBER 0002262 OF ELOY, AZ, WAS DISCIPLINED BY ARIZONA ON APRIL 15, 1993

NOTES: ON OR BEFORE 12/31/93 HE SHALL TAKE AND PASS THE SPECIAL PURPOSE LICENSING EXAMINATION WITH A GRADE OF 75 OR HIGHER. IF HE FAILS TO TAKE AND PASS THIS EXAM, IT SHALL BE TAKEN AS A REQUEST TO INACTIVATE HIS LICENSE AND ON 01/01/94 HIS MEDICAL LICENSE SHALL BE PLACED ON INACTIVE STATUS WITH CAUSE. ON 1/26/94 THIS WAS DONE AS HE DID NOT PASS SPEX.

HOOPER, GERRY R MD OF 2155 E DECATUR, MESA, AZ, WAS DISCIPLINED BY DEA ON OCTOBER 29, 1990
DISCIPLINARY ACTION: RESTRICTION PLACED ON CONTROLLED SUBSTANCE LICENSE

NOTES: SURRENDER OF CLASS A REGISTRATION. PROBATION AMENDED AND CONTINUED. APPROVAL OF CLASS A APPLICATION; SURRENDERED SCHEDULES II THROUGH IV; ISSUED AMENDED REGISTRATION FOR SCHEDULE V.

HOPKIN, JEFFREY MD, LICENSE NUMBER 0016117, WAS DISCIPLINED BY ARIZONA ON JULY 19, 1995
DISCIPLINARY ACTION: MONITORING OF PHYSICIAN PERFORMANCE
OFFENSE: PROFESSIONAL MISCONDUCT

NOTES: ALLEGATIONS THAT HE EXHIBITED DISRUPTIVE BEHAVIOR AT HOSPITAL. WITHIN 45 DAYS, SHALL BEGIN COUNSELING WITH A BOARD-APPROVED COUNSELOR REGARDING THE ISSUE OF INTERPERSONAL RELATIONSHIPS. COUNSELOR SHALL SUBMIT QUARTERLY REPORTS TO THE BOARD. 1/1/96 ORDER TERMINATED.

HOPWOOD, DON M MD, LICENSE NUMBER 0019013, WAS DISCIPLINED BY ARIZONA ON APRIL 19, 1996
DISCIPLINARY ACTION: FINE
OFFENSE: INSURANCE, MEDICARE OR MEDICAID FRAUD

NOTES: BETWEEN 2/95 AND 2/96, HE ALLOWED AN UNLICENSED INDIVIDUAL TO TREAT PATIENTS AT THE OFFICE AND IN THE HOSPITAL, MAKE ENTRIES IN THEIR MEDICAL RECORDS AND PRESCRIBE AND REFILL MEDICATIONS; SIGNED HIS INITIALS TO RECORDS OF PATIENTS WHO WERE TREATED BY THIS PERSON; LEFT HIM IN CHARGE OF HIS PATIENTS WHILE HE WAS AWAY FROM THE OFFICE, INCLUDING DURING A WEEK VACATION AND PRESENTED TO PATIENTS AS A PHYSICIAN; IN A SEARCH OF HIS HOME, POLICE FOUND A PLASTIC BAG CONTAINING DISCARDED PAGES FROM HIS OFFICE MEDICAL RECORDS FOR 17 PATIENTS; ALL PAGES WERE INITIALED BY THE UNLICENSED INDIVIDUAL; UPON SEARCH OF HIS OFFICE, POLICE SEIZED RECORDS IN WHICH THE DISCARDED PAGES FOUND IN HIS HOME HAD BEEN REWRITTEN IN PHYSICIAN'S HANDWRITING AND INITIALED BY HIM, DESPITE THE FACT THAT HE HAD NOT SEEN OR TREATED ALL OF THE PATIENTS; HE SUBMITTED BILLS TO HEALTH INSURANCE COMPANIES AND MEDICARE FOR SERVICES PERFORMED BY UNLICENSED INDIVIDUAL AND FALSELY INDICATED THAT HE HAD PERFORMED SERVICES FOR PATIENTS. CENSURED; SHALL PAY FINE OF $10,000. ON 7/25/97 BOARD ACKNOWLEDGED THAT HE HAD PAID THE CIVIL PENALTY.

HOPWOOD, DON M MD, LICENSE NUMBER 19013, WAS DISCIPLINED BY ARIZONA ON NOVEMBER 18, 1999
OFFENSE: SUBSTANDARD CARE, INCOMPETENCE OR NEGLIGENCE

NOTES: FAILURE TO PROPERLY MANAGE A HIGH-RISK CARDIAC PATIENT, WHICH LED TO THE PATIENT'S DEATH. DECREE OF CENSURE ISSUED.

HORSLEY, WILLIAM W MD, LICENSE NUMBER 0010876, WAS DISCIPLINED BY ARIZONA ON APRIL 13, 1991
DISCIPLINARY ACTION: REQUIRED TO ENTER AN IMPAIRED PHYSICIAN PROGRAM OR SUBSTANCE ABUSE TREATMENT; MONITORING OF PHYSICIAN PERFORMANCE
OFFENSE: SUBSTANCE ABUSE

NOTES: BOARD RECEIVED INFORMATION FROM DR. HORSLEY THAT HE HAD BEEN ADMITTED FOR INPATIENT TREATMENT OF SUBSTANCE ABUSE. MUST IMMEDIATELY PARTICIPATE IN THE ARIZONA MEDICAL ASSOCIATION'S MONITORED AFTERCARE TREATMENT PROGRAM WITH QUARTERLY REPORTS TO THE BOARD. SHALL PARTICIPATE IN 90 12-STEP MEETINGS APPROPRIATE FOR SUBSTANCE ABUSE AND ACCEPTABLE TO THE BOARD IN 90 DAYS; MUST THEN PARTICIPATE IN A 12-STEP RECOVERY PROGRAM APPROPRIATE FOR SUBSTANCE ABUSE AS DETERMINED BY HIS TREATING THERAPIST, AND ATTEND A MINIMUM OF THREE WEEKLY MEETINGS; SHALL OBTAIN A SOLE TREATING PHYSICIAN APPROVED BY THE BOARD; SHALL ABSTAIN COMPLETELY FROM THE CONSUMPTION OF ALCOHOLIC BEVERAGES AND SHALL TAKE NO DRUGS OR MEDICATIONS WHATEVER UNLESS PRESCRIBED FOR HIM BY HIS TREATING PHYSICIAN; SHALL COMPLY IMMEDIATELY WITH REQUESTS TO SUBMIT TO WITNESSED RANDOM BIOLOGICAL FLUID COLLECTION; SHALL MAINTAIN A LOG OF ALL MEDICATIONS WHATEVER PRESCRIBED FOR HIM BY HIS TREATING PHYSICIAN AND SHALL MAKE SUCH LOG AVAILABLE TO THE BOARD; SHALL SUBMIT TO MENTAL, PHYSICAL, OR MEDICAL COMPETENCY EXAMS, OR ANY COMBINATION THEREOF, OR ANY THERAPY, AS ORDERED OR RECOMMENDED; SHALL APPEAR IN PERSON BEFORE BOARD FOR INTERVIEWS UPON REQUEST. SHALL ADVISE BOARD OF CHANGE OF ADDRESS OR IF AWAY FOR MORE THAN FIVE DAYS. ON 4/16/94 ORDER TERMINATED AFTER 90 DAYS

HOWARD, MILES WAYNE MD, WAS DISCIPLINED BY ARIZONA ON APRIL 6, 1990
DISCIPLINARY ACTION: REQUIRED TO ENTER AN IMPAIRED PHYSICIAN PROGRAM OR SUBSTANCE ABUSE TREATMENT; MONITORING OF PHYSICIAN PERFORMANCE
OFFENSE: SUBSTANCE ABUSE

NOTES: MUST IMMEDIATELY PARTICIPATE IN THE ARIZONA MEDICAL ASSOCIATION PHYSICIAN'S HEALTH COMMITTEE PROGRAM WITH QUARTERLY REPORTS TO THE BOARD; MUST OBTAIN A BOARD-APPROVED TREATING PHYSICIAN; MUST ABSTAIN FROM ALCOHOL AND ALL OTHER DRUGS; MUST COMPLY WITH REQUESTS FOR RANDOM BIOLOGICAL FLUID TESTS; MUST SUBMIT TO ANY EXAMS OR THERAPY ORDERED BY THE BOARD; MUST PARTICIPATE IN A 12-STEP RECOVERY PROGRAM FOR SUBSTANCE ABUSE AS DETERMINED BY THERAPIST AND ATTEND AT LEAST 3 WEEKLY MEETINGS; MUST APPEAR BEFORE THE BOARD FOR INTERVIEWS UPON REQUEST; MUST ADVISE THE BOARD OF ANY CHANGE IN OFFICE OR HOME ADDRESSES AND IF AWAY FOR MORE THAN FIVE DAYS; MUST MAINTAIN A LOG OF ALL MEDICATIONS TAKEN. ON 10/15/93 BOARD RECOMMENDED THAT HE COMPLY WITH THE SUGGESTIONS OF TALBOT RECOVERY PROGRAM AND ENROLL IN COUPLES THERAPY WITH HIS WIFE AND PURSUE OBTAINING WORK WHICH IS LIMITED TO 40 HOURS PER WEEK.

HOWARD, MILES WAYNE MD, LICENSE NUMBER 0021113, WAS DISCIPLINED BY ARIZONA ON JULY 17, 1993
DISCIPLINARY ACTION: PROBATION; RESTRICTION PLACED ON LICENSE
OFFENSE: FAILURE TO COMPLY WITH PREVIOUS BOARD ORDER

NOTES: IN VIOLATION OF 4/6/90 BOARD ORDER HAD A URINE SPECIMEN TEST POSITIVE FOR COCAINE ON 9/16/91 AND OBTAINED A PRESCRIPTION FOR PERCOCET FROM SOMEONE OTHER THAN HIS DESIGNATED TREATING PHYSICIAN. THEN WROTE 16 PRESCRIPTIONS FOR HIMSELF; ENTERED TREATMENT FOR CHEMICAL DEPENDENCY IN 3/93 WAS TERMINATED FROM HIS RESIDENCY PROGRAM. MUST IMMEDIATELY PARTICIPATE IN A BOARD-APPROVED MONITORED AFTERCARE TREATMENT PROGRAM WHOSE THERAPIST MUST SUBMIT QUARTERLY REPORTS; MUST PARTICIPATE IN A 12-STEP RECOVERY PROGRAM AS DETERMINED BY HIS TREATING THERAPIST AND ATTEND AT LEAST THREE WEEKLY MEETINGS; SHALL OBTAIN A BOARD-APPROVED TREATING PHYSICIAN; SHALL ABSTAIN COMPLETELY FROM THE CONSUMPTION OF ALCOHOLIC BEVERAGES AND DRUGS EXCEPT WHEN PRESCRIBED BY HIS TREATING PHYSICIAN; MUST SUBMIT TO WITNESSED RANDOM BIOLOGICAL FLUID COLLECTION; KEEP A LOG OF ANY AND ALL MEDICATIONS PRESCRIBED FOR HIM; SHALL SUBMIT

TO ANY EXAMINATIONS OR THERAPY ORDERED BY BOARD; SHALL APPEAR BEFORE BOARD FOR INTERVIEWS UPON REQUEST; SHALL INFORM BOARD OF CHANGE OF ADDRESS OR IF AWAY FOR MORE THAN FIVE DAYS; SHALL PRACTICE ONLY IN A SUPERVISED PRACTICE SETTING WITH NO NIGHT CALL. ON 1/20/95 ORDER AMENDED AS FOLLOWS: SHALL PRACTICE MEDICINE ONLY IN A GROUP PRACTICE SETTING INSTEAD OF ONLY IN A SUPERVISED SETTING; REFERS TO ABILITY TO PRACTICE IN AN OUTPATIENT SETTING AS WELL. PROBATION AND RESTRICTIONS TERMINATED ON 4/20/96; REMAINDER OF MONITORING CONDITIONS REMAIN. ON 3/28/98 ORDER TERMINATED EFFECTIVE IN 90 DAYS.

HOWARD, MILES WAYNE MD, LICENSE NUMBER 0008560 OF 5203 NORTH 24TH STREET #102, PHOENIX, AZ, WAS DISCIPLINED BY HAWAII ON JULY 19, 1996
DISCIPLINARY ACTION: FINE; RESTRICTION PLACED ON LICENSE
OFFENSE: DISCIPLINARY ACTION BY ANOTHER STATE OR AGENCY

NOTES: ACTION IN ARIZONA. FAILED TO INFORM HAWAII OF THE DISCIPLINARY ACTION IN ARIZONA. HIS HAWAII LICENSE EXPIRED ON 1/31/96. SHALL COMPLY WITH ALL TERMS, CONDITIONS, RESTRICTIONS, AND REQUIREMENTS IMPOSED BY ARIZONA IN 4/90 AND 7/93 ORDERS TO CONTINUE TO BE LICENSED IN HAWAII INCLUDING SHALL ONLY PRACTICE IN A GROUP SETTING IN HAWAII. $500 FINE.

HUANG, DONALD J MD, LICENSE NUMBER 425219 OF 620 NORTH PINECLIFF DRIVE, FLAGSTAFF, AZ, WAS DISCIPLINED BY KANSAS ON OCTOBER 19, 1998
DISCIPLINARY ACTION: REPRIMAND
OFFENSE: SUBSTANDARD CARE, INCOMPETENCE OR NEGLIGENCE

NOTES: FAILURE TO ADHERE TO THE APPLICABLE STANDARD OF CARE TO A DEGREE WHICH CONSTITUTES ORDINARY NEGLIGENCE IN THREE CASES: ON APPROXIMATELY 1/30 AND 1/31/98 FAILED TO DIAGNOSE THE CONDITION OF A PATIENT PREOPERATIVELY, WHICH ALSO RESULTED IN UNNECESSARY SURGERY; ON 2/2/98 FAILED TO ENSURE AN ADEQUATE BLOOD SUPPLY FOR THE SURGERY AND/OR FAILED TO TRANSFER ANOTHER PATIENT AS APPROPRIATE; ON 1/8/98, WHEN HE FAILED TO OBTAIN THE INFORMED CONSENT OF ANOTHER PATIENT BEFORE THE EXCISION OF A FACIAL LESION.

HUBBARD, JOHN R MD, LICENSE NUMBER 0016346, WAS DISCIPLINED BY ARIZONA ON JULY 30, 1992
DISCIPLINARY ACTION: 24-MONTH PROBATION; RESTRICTION PLACED ON CONTROLLED SUBSTANCE LICENSE
OFFENSE: OVERPRESCRIBING OR MISPRESCRIBING DRUGS

NOTES: MAINTAINING INADEQUATE MEDICAL RECORDS FOR FOUR PATIENTS REGARDING PRESCRIPTIONS WRITTEN DURING 1990 AND 1991. SHALL NOT DISPENSE OR PRESCRIBE, BUT MAY ADMINISTER, SCHEDULE II, III, AND IV CONTROLLED SUBSTANCES; SHALL ATTEND WITHIN ONE YEAR A MINI-RESIDENCY IN THE PHARMACOLOGICAL MANAGEMENT OF CHRONIC PAIN; SHALL PERFORM OR OBTAIN APPROPRIATE DIAGNOSTIC WORKUPS OF ALL PAIN PATIENTS PRIOR TO TREATING SUCH PATIENTS.

HUBBARD, JOHN R MD, LICENSE NUMBER 0016346, WAS DISCIPLINED BY ARIZONA ON JULY 14, 1994
DISCIPLINARY ACTION: LICENSE REVOCATION
OFFENSE: FAILURE TO COMPLY WITH PREVIOUS BOARD ORDER

NOTES: IN ONE CASE DURING 1991 A PATIENT'S MEDICAL RECORDS WERE OFTEN CONFUSING AND OF AN UNACCEPTABLE QUALITY; IN ONE CASE DURING 1992 OVERPRESCRIBED DRUGS TO A PATIENT HE SHOULD HAVE KNOWN HAD A PROBLEM WITH DRUG SEEKING BEHAVIOR; HE HAD BEEN PLACED ON PROBATION 7/16/92 WITH THE REQUIREMENT THAT HE OBTAIN A MINI-RESIDENCY IN THE PHARMACOLOGICAL MANAGEMENT OF CHRONIC PAIN AND PROVIDE VERIFICATION OF THIS; HAS NOT DONE SO.

HUBBARD, JOHN R MD, LICENSE NUMBER 0097831 OF 205-B KINO SPRINGS DRIVE, NOGALES, AZ, WAS DISCIPLINED BY NEW YORK ON JUNE 30, 1995
DISCIPLINARY ACTION: SURRENDER OF LICENSE
OFFENSE: DISCIPLINARY ACTION BY ANOTHER STATE OR AGENCY

NOTES: DISCIPLINED IN ARIZONA FOR INAPPROPRIATE PRESCRIBING OF CONTROLLED SUBSTANCES; FAILING TO MAINTAIN ADEQUATE PATIENT RECORDS; AND VIOLATED THE TERMS OF PROBATION IMPOSED BY THE ARIZONA BOARD; VIOLATED THE TERMS OF PROBATION IMPOSED BY THE NEW YORK BOARD; FAILED TO RESPOND TO WRITTEN COMMUNICATION FROM THEM.

HUBBARD, JOHN R MD, WAS DISCIPLINED BY ARIZONA ON JULY 30, 1999
DISCIPLINARY ACTION: 60-MONTH PROBATION; REQUIRED TO TAKE ADDITIONAL MEDICAL EDUCATION
OFFENSE: DISCIPLINARY ACTION BY ANOTHER STATE OR AGENCY

NOTES: DISCIPLINED BY REVOCATION BY PENNSYLVANIA. PROBATION WITH THE FOLLOWING TERMS: THAT HE COMPLETE A ONE YEAR RESIDENCY IN A BOARD APPROVED PRIMARY CARE AREA, THAT HE MEET WITH THE BOARD UPON SUCCESSFUL COMPLETION OF THE RESIDENCY AND RECEIVE AFFIRMATIVE APPROVAL TO PRACTICE UNSUPERVISED MEDICINE, THAT HE MEET WITH THE MAP DIRECTORS AND ARRANGE FOR SATISFACTORY ACCORDS WITH THE MAP PROGRAM, AND THAT HE PAY FOR ANY RECOMMENDED TREATMENTS OR EVALUATIONS BY THE MAP PROGRAM. ON 11/19/99 HE WAS GRANTED A MOTION FOR REVIEW AND AGREED TO THESE TERMS.

HUBBARD, JOHN ROLAND MD, DATE OF BIRTH SEPTEMBER 14, 1933, LICENSE NUMBER 016397E OF 205B KINO SPRINGS DRIVE, NOGALES, AZ, WAS DISCIPLINED BY PENNSYLVANIA ON MAY 20, 1999
DISCIPLINARY ACTION: LICENSE SUSPENSION
OFFENSE: DISCIPLINARY ACTION BY ANOTHER STATE OR AGENCY

NOTES: DISCIPLINARY ACTION TAKEN BY NEW YORK.

HUDAK, DEBORAH DO, LICENSE NUMBER 3363 OF PO BOX 24557, TEMPE, AZ, WAS DISCIPLINED BY ARIZONA ON OCTOBER 3, 1998
DISCIPLINARY ACTION: 12-MONTH PROBATION; MONITORING OF PHYSICIAN PERFORMANCE

NOTES: LICENSE GRANTED UNDER THE FOLLOWING TERMS AND CONDITIONS: SHALL OBTAIN A CONSULTATION WITH AN ADDICTION SPECIALIST AS APPROVED BY THE BOARD; SHALL COMPLY WITH ANY RECOMMENDATION FOR FURTHER THERAPY; SHALL PROVIDE A COPY OF THIS ORDER TO ALL HEALTH CARE FACILITIES WHERE SHE PRACTICES; SHALL ABSTAIN COMPLETELY FROM THE CONSUMPTION OF ALCOHOLIC BEVERAGES AND SHALL NOT CONSUME ILLICIT DRUGS OR TAKE ANY MEDICATION UNLESS PRESCRIBED FOR HER BY HER TREATING PHYSICIAN; SHALL MAINTAIN A MONTHLY LOG OF ALL MEDICATIONS TAKEN BY HER AND PROVIDE A COPY

TO THE BOARD; SHALL SUBMIT TO ANY EVALUATIONS ORDERED BY BOARD; SHALL APPEAR BEFORE THE BOARD UPON REQUEST; SHALL SUBMIT TO RANDOM BIOLOGICAL FLUID TESTING; SHALL INFORM THE BOARD IF SHE CEASES TO PRACTICE MEDICINE IN ARIZONA; SHALL PAY COSTS. ON 10/16/99 PROBATION TERMINATED; FULL AND UNRESTRICTED LICENSE.

HUGHES, THOMAS J JR MD, LICENSE NUMBER 0001749, WAS DISCIPLINED BY ARIZONA ON OCTOBER 10, 1991
DISCIPLINARY ACTION: FINE
OFFENSE: PROFESSIONAL MISCONDUCT

NOTES: ENGAGED IN ANY CONDUCT OR PRACTICE WHICH IS OR MIGHT BE HARMFUL OR DANGEROUS TO THE HEALTH OF THE PATIENT OR THE PUBLIC IN THAT HE FAILED TO NOTIFY HIS ON-CALL PHYSICIAN OF A SERIOUSLY ILL 27-YEAR OLD PATIENT ADMITTED TO THE HOSPITAL AFTER BEING BROUGHT TO THE EMERGENCY ROOM ON THE MORNING OF 11/16/89; HE FAILED TO RESPOND TO FIVE ATTEMPTS TO REACH HIM BETWEEN 12.30PM AND 3.30PM; ARRIVED AT 6.00 PM AND ORDERED A SURGICAL CONSULTATION, WHICH COULD NOT BE OBTAINED UNTIL THE NEXT MORNING; AFTER TRANSFERRING TO ANOTHER HOSPITAL FOR SURGICAL PROCEDURES PATIENT FOUND TO HAVE A PERFORATED VISCUS AND AN ABDOMINAL LYMPHOMA, HAD POST-SURGICAL COMPLICATIONS AND EXPIRED IN 1/90. CENSURED. $1,000 FINE.

HUGHES, THOMAS J JR MD, LICENSE NUMBER 0001749, WAS DISCIPLINED BY ARIZONA ON OCTOBER 21, 1992
DISCIPLINARY ACTION: REQUIRED TO TAKE ADDITIONAL MEDICAL EDUCATION
OFFENSE: OVERPRESCRIBING OR MISPRESCRIBING DRUGS

NOTES: ALLEGATIONS THAT HE WAS PRESCRIBING LARGE QUANTITIES OF PERCOCET OVER A LONG PERIOD OF TIME TO A PATIENT. SHALL OBTAIN 20 HOURS CONTINUING MEDICAL EDUCATION IN THE SUBJECT OF CHRONIC PAIN MANAGEMENT PRIOR TO 4/30/93. ON 7/15/93 BOARD TERMINATED THIS ORDER SINCE HE HAD FULFILLED THE CONTINUING MEDICAL EDUCATION REQUIREMENT.

HUNTER, RUSSELL L MD, LICENSE NUMBER 6167, WAS DISCIPLINED BY ARIZONA ON NOVEMBER 14, 1997
DISCIPLINARY ACTION: REPRIMAND
OFFENSE: PROFESSIONAL MISCONDUCT

NOTES: AFTER RECEIVING A COMPLAINT FROM AN ARIZONA PHARMACIST, BOARD INVESTIGATORS CONDUCTED A PHARMACY SURVEY ON 10 1-2/96 FOR THE TIME PERIOD 4/96 THROUGH 9/96; AND WITH THREE EXCEPTIONS, ALL 98 PRESCRIPTIONS RECEIVED BY THE BOARD BEAR THE SIGNATURE OF SOMEONE OTHER THAN DR. HUNTER; HE ADMITTED THAT HE HAD HIS RN SIGN THE PRESCRIPTIONS UNDER HIS SUPERVISION.

HUNTER, WILLARD S MD, LICENSE NUMBER 0002933 OF PHOENIX, AZ, WAS DISCIPLINED BY ARIZONA ON FEBRUARY 23, 1992
DISCIPLINARY ACTION: 36-MONTH PROBATION; RESTRICTION PLACED ON CONTROLLED SUBSTANCE LICENSE
OFFENSE: OVERPRESCRIBING OR MISPRESCRIBING DRUGS

NOTES: FAILING OR REFUSING TO MAINTAIN ADEQUATE RECORDS; PRESCRIBING, DISPENSING OR ADMINISTERING CONTROLLED SUBSTANCES FOR OTHER THAN ACCEPTED THERAPEUTIC PURPOSES AND IN EXCESSIVE AMOUNTS TO NUMEROUS PATIENTS; SUCH SUBSTANCES INCLUDED VALIUM, TYLENOL #4, SOMA, DEMEROL AND PERCOCET. DURING TERM OF PROBATION: SHALL NOT PRESCRIBE, ADMINISTER OR DISPENSE SCHEDULE II OR III CONTROLLED SUBSTANCES EXCEPT FOR HOSPITALIZED OR POSTOPERATIVE PATIENTS FOR UP TO TWO MONTHS AFTER SURGERY; SHALL OBTAIN 80 HOURS CONTINUING MEDICAL EDUCATION IN THE PRESCRIBING OF CONTROLLED SUBSTANCES. EFFECTIVE 1/26/94 BOARD ORDER TERMINATED AND IN SIX AND EIGHTEEN MONTHS AFTER TERMINATION, STAFF SHALL CONDUCT AN OFFICE AND PHARMACY SURVEY TO REVIEW HIS PRESCRIBING OF CONTROLLED SUBSTANCES.

HUNTER, WILLARD S MD OF PHOENIX, AZ, WAS DISCIPLINED BY UTAH ON DECEMBER 7, 1992
DISCIPLINARY ACTION: PROBATION; RESTRICTION PLACED ON CONTROLLED SUBSTANCE LICENSE
OFFENSE: DISCIPLINARY ACTION BY ANOTHER STATE OR AGENCY

NOTES: ARIZONA MEDICAL BOARD TOOK ACTION UPON FINDING THAT HE PRESCRIBED, DISPENSED OR ADMINISTERED CONTROLLED SUBSTANCES IN AMOUNTS AND IN A MANNER INCONSISTENT WITH THERAPEUTIC PURPOSES. SCHEDULE II AND III CONTROLLED SUBSTANCE LICENSE IS RESTRICTED. ON 9/2/94 PROBATION ON LICENSE TO PRACTICE MEDICINE AND PRESCRIBE AND ADMINISTER CONTROLLED SUBSTANCES WAS TERMINATED AND LICENSE WAS REINSTATED WITH FULL PRIVILEGES.

HUNTER, WILLARD S MD, LICENSE NUMBER 0C23614 OF PHOENIX, AZ, WAS DISCIPLINED BY CALIFORNIA ON FEBRUARY 20, 1995
DISCIPLINARY ACTION: REPRIMAND
OFFENSE: DISCIPLINARY ACTION BY ANOTHER STATE OR AGENCY

NOTES: DISCIPLINE BY ARIZONA BOARD FOR FAILING TO MAINTAIN ADEQUATE RECORDS REGARDING DRUGS TO PATIENTS, AND FOR DISPENSING DRUGS FOR OTHER THAN THERAPEUTIC PURPOSES. ALSO, DISCIPLINED BY UTAH BOARD BASED ON ARIZONA ACTION. BOTH BOARDS REINSTATED FULL PRIVILEGES.

HUNTER, WILLARD SMITH MD OF TEMPE, AZ, WAS DISCIPLINED BY UTAH ON JULY 11, 1996
OFFENSE: DISCIPLINARY ACTION BY ANOTHER STATE OR AGENCY

NOTES: ACTION IN ARIZONA. SUSPENSION WITH A STAY OF ENFORCEMENT ON THE SUSPENSION DURING THE ARIZONA PERIOD OF PROBATION SO LONG AS HE REMAINS IN FULL COMPLIANCE WITH THE TERMS AND CONDITIONS OF HIS ARIZONA PROBATION. HE HAS CONDITIONS TO BE MET DURING THIS PERIOD OF TIME.

HURLEY, JAMES M E MD, LICENSE NUMBER 0003191, WAS DISCIPLINED BY ARIZONA ON APRIL 8, 1992
DISCIPLINARY ACTION: REQUIRED TO TAKE ADDITIONAL MEDICAL EDUCATION; MONITORING OF PHYSICIAN PERFORMANCE
OFFENSE: OVERPRESCRIBING OR MISPRESCRIBING DRUGS

NOTES: CONCERNING PRESCRIBING PRACTICES. SHALL SUCCESSFULLY COMPLETE 40 HOURS OF CONTINUING MEDICAL EDUCATION IN THE FIELD OF PAIN CONTROL MANAGEMENT BEFORE 2/1/93. A FOLLOW-UP PHARMACY SURVEY WILL BE PERFORMED ONE YEAR FOLLOWING COMPLETION OF CONTINUING MEDICAL EDUCATION. BOARD TERMINATED THIS ORDER ON 10/15/93 SINCE HE SUCCESSFULLY COMPLETED HIS 40 HOURS OF CONTINUING MEDICAL EDUCATION IN PAIN MANAGEMENT.

HURM, RAYMOND A MD, LICENSE NUMBER 0007498, WAS DISCIPLINED BY ARIZONA ON APRIL 20, 1996
OFFENSE: SUBSTANDARD CARE, INCOMPETENCE OR NEGLIGENCE

NOTES: IN 1989, TREATED A PATIENT SURGICALLY FOR ERECTILE DYSFUNCTION AND ERRONEOUSLY REMOVED A PORTION OF THE URETHRA, WHICH RESULTED IN ACUTE URINARY RETENTION AND NECESSITATED THE USE OF REPEATED SUPRA-PUBIC CATHERIZATIONS; PRIOR TO THE SURGERY, DID NOT INFORM THE PATIENT THAT HE HAD NEVER PERFORMED OR ASSISTED WITH DEEP DORSAL VEIN LIGATION; DID NOT INFORM PATIENT THAT A PART OF HIS URETHRA HAD BEEN REMOVED, BUT INSTEAD TOLD HIM THAT THE URETHRA HAD BEEN COMPROMISED; IN DISCHARGE SUMMARY DICTATED 30 DAYS FOLLOWING DISCHARGE, DID NOT ACKNOWLEDGE THAT HE HAD INADVERTENTLY REMOVED A PORTION OF URETHRA, BUT STATED CONSIDERING URETHRAL IMPINGEMENT SYNDROME AS BEING THE CAUSE OF THE PATIENT'S URINARY RETENTION; PRIOR TO SURGERY, FAILED TO RULE OUT THE PRESENCE OF ARTERIAL DISEASE IN ORDER TO DETERMINE THAT PATIENT WAS GOOD CANDIDATE IN THAT HIS PATIENT'S FAMILY HISTORY SHOWED DIABETES, HEART DISEASE, AND HIGH BLOOD PRESSURE AND HIS PERSONAL HISTORY SHOWED HIGH BLOOD PRESSURE AND HIGH TRIGLYCERIDES; FAILED TO NOTE PATIENT'S ALLERGY TO CATGUT SUTURES MENTIONED TO HIM BY THE PATIENT AND PROMINENTLY DISPLAYED IN THREE PLACES IN HIS MEDICAL RECORDS; USED CATGUT SUTURES WHICH RESULTED IN PATIENT'S STITCHES TO SEPARATE; 18 MONTHS AFTER THE SURGERY, PATIENT SEEN FOR SYMPTOMS HE HAD NOT HAD BEFORE SURGERY BY EXPERT IN VEIN LIGATION, WHO REPORTED THAT THE PATIENT'S HISTORY AND VESSEL INJURIES WERE CONSISTENT WITH DAMAGE THAT COULD HAVE OCCURRED AT THE TIME OF THE SURGERY; FALSELY REPRESENTED HIMSELF TO THE PATIENT AND ON HIS CURRICULUM VITAE AS THE CHIEF OF THE UROLOGY SECTION OF THE HOSPITAL, WHICH DID NOT ACTUALLY HAVE A UROLOGY SECTION. CENSURED.

HYDE, ROBERT L MD, LICENSE NUMBER 0004247, WAS DISCIPLINED BY ARIZONA ON JULY 19, 1996
DISCIPLINARY ACTION: PROBATION
OFFENSE: SUBSTANDARD CARE, INCOMPETENCE OR NEGLIGENCE

NOTES: FOR A PATIENT HE SAW CONSISTENTLY BETWEEN 6/84 AND 9/90 FOR A VARIETY OF AILMENTS, HIS MEDICAL RECORDS ARE GENERALLY SUBSTANDARD IN THAT HE FAILED TO CONDUCT BREAST EXAMINATIONS WHEN INDICATED, FAILED TO CONDUCT A PAP SMEAR EVEN THOUGH HE REALIZED THAT SHE HAD NOT HAD ONE IN FOUR YEARS AND AT NO TIME RECORDED A PHYSICAL EXAMINATION; ADMINISTERED B-12 INJECTIONS ON SEVERAL OCCASIONS WITHOUT ANY DIAGNOSTIC DOCUMENTATION AND TREATED HER SINUSITIS WITH ROCEPHIN, KEFLEX AND PREDNISONE WITHOUT BENEFIT OF A DOCUMENTED EXAMINATION OR NOTING VITAL SIGNS; ON 8/27/90, ADMINISTERED TRIGGER POINT INJECTIONS TO HER TRAPEZIUS AND SACROILIAC JOINTS WITHOUT EVIDENCE OF APPROPRIATE EXAMINATION; ON 8/29/90, PATIENT COMPLAINED OF DIFFICULTY BREATHING AND HE MERELY CHECKED HER VITAL SIGNS, NOTED A PNEUMOTHORAX AND ADMINISTERED AN INJECTION OF ROCEPHIN; RECORDS LACK X-RAYS TO SUBSTANTIATE HIS DIAGNOSIS AND INCLUDE NO EXAMINATION OF THE LUNGS OR HEART; AROUND 9/2/90, PATIENT ADMITTED TO THE HOSPITAL IN SEVERE CARDIO-RESPIRATORY DISTRESS; HIS PRESCRIBING OF PSYCHOACTIVE DRUGS TO THIS PATIENT WAS INAPPROPRIATE. CENSURED; SHALL NOTIFY AND MEET WITH THE BOARD PRIOR TO RESUMING PRACTICE IN ARIZONA.

HYDE, ROBERT L MD, LICENSE NUMBER G8979 OF LOWER LAKE, CA, WAS DISCIPLINED BY CALIFORNIA ON APRIL 10, 1998
DISCIPLINARY ACTION: 60-MONTH PROBATION
OFFENSE: DISCIPLINARY ACTION BY ANOTHER STATE OR AGENCY

NOTES: DISCIPLINED BY ARIZONA FOR UNPROFESSIONAL CONDUCT, GROSS NEGLIGENCE, AND REPEATED ACTS OF NEGLIGENCE IN THE TREATMENT OF ONE PATIENT; FAILING OR REFUSING TO MAINTAIN ADEQUATE MEDICAL RECORDS ON A PATIENT. REVOCATION STAYED.

HYDE, ROBERT L MD, LICENSE NUMBER 0009150 OF KELSEYVILLE, CA, WAS DISCIPLINED BY WASHINGTON ON DECEMBER 28, 1999
DISCIPLINARY ACTION: LICENSE SUSPENSION
OFFENSE: DISCIPLINARY ACTION BY ANOTHER STATE OR AGENCY

NOTES: LICENSE DISCIPLINED IN TWO OTHER STATES.

HYDE, ROBERT LOGAN MD, LICENSE NUMBER 06637 OF LOWER LAKE, OR, WAS DISCIPLINED BY OREGON ON JULY 27, 1998
DISCIPLINARY ACTION: PROBATION; FINE

NOTES: MUST PAY $2,000 CIVIL PENALTY AND COST OF HEARING. PROBATION UPON COMMENCING PRACTICE IN OREGON.

INFORZATO, NANCY M MD, LICENSE NUMBER 0020893 OF PHOENIX, AZ, WAS DISCIPLINED BY ARIZONA ON JULY 14, 1993
DISCIPLINARY ACTION: RESTRICTION PLACED ON LICENSE; MONITORING OF PHYSICIAN PERFORMANCE
OFFENSE: SUBSTANCE ABUSE

NOTES: TESTED POSITIVELY FOR AMPHETAMINES. MUST WITHIN 15 DAYS OBTAIN A BOARD-APPROVED THERAPIST AND HAVE THERAPY AT LEAST ONCE A WEEK WITH MONTHLY REPORTS; SHALL OBTAIN A BOARD-APPROVED TREATING PHYSICIAN; SHALL ABSTAIN COMPLETELY FROM THE CONSUMPTION OF ALCOHOLIC BEVERAGES AND DRUGS EXCEPT WHEN PRESCRIBED BY HER TREATING PHYSICIAN; MUST SUBMIT TO WITNESSED RANDOM BIOLOGICAL FLUID COLLECTION; KEEP A LOG OF ANY AND ALL MEDICATIONS PRESCRIBED FOR HER; SHALL PROVIDE A COPY OF THE ORDER TO ANY TRAINING PROGRAM OR EMPLOYER; IF INVOLVED IN DIRECT PATIENT CARE SHALL BE SUPERVISED; SHALL COMPLY WITH THE TERMS AND CONDITIONS OF THE STIPULATION AND ORDER WHETHER SHE RESIDES AND/OR PRACTICES MEDICINE IN ARIZONA OR ELSEWHERE. ORDER MODIFIED ON 7/15/94 SUCH THAT SHE SHALL ENGAGE IN THERAPY AT LEAST TWICE WEEKLY FOR A PERIOD OF ONE YEAR; SHALL REPEAT THE MMPI-2 AND THE MCMI PREVIOUSLY ADMINISTERED AT ANCHOR HOSPITAL.

INFORZATO, NANCY M MD, LICENSE NUMBER 0020893, WAS DISCIPLINED BY ARIZONA ON APRIL 16, 1994
DISCIPLINARY ACTION: REQUIRED TO ENTER AN IMPAIRED PHYSICIAN PROGRAM OR SUBSTANCE ABUSE TREATMENT
OFFENSE: OVERPRESCRIBING OR MISPRESCRIBING DRUGS

NOTES: WRITING PRESCRIPTIONS FOR AMPHETAMINES FOR ANOTHER PHYSICIAN FOR REASONS THAT WERE NOT THERAPEUTIC AND INAPPROPRIATELY TAKING AMPHETAMINES HERSELF. SHALL, WITHIN 30 DAYS ENTER INTO A LONG-TERM RESIDENTIAL OR IN-

PATIENT TREATMENT FOR CHEMICAL DEPENDENCY AT A TREATMENT FACILITY ACCEPTABLE TO THE BOARD AND SHALL REMAIN IN TREATMENT UNTIL THERAPEUTICALLY DISCHARGED BY THE TREATMENT CENTER. THIS ORDER RESCINDED ON 7/15/94.

INJEIAN, ABRAHAM V MD, LICENSE NUMBER 0007736, WAS DISCIPLINED BY ARIZONA ON OCTOBER 23, 1992
DISCIPLINARY ACTION: EMERGENCY SUSPENSION

NOTES: SHALL NOT PRACTICE MEDICINE UNTIL BOARD RESOLVES CURRENTLY PENDING FORMAL HEARING REGARDING A PATIENT, WHICH SHALL NOT OCCUR EARLIER THAN JANUARY 1993. SHALL BE ADMITTED FOR IN-PATIENT NEURO-PSYCHOLOGICAL EVALUATION, AND TREATMENT IF NEEDED, AT FACILITY OF BOARD'S CHOICE.

INJEIAN, ABRAHAM V MD, LICENSE NUMBER 0007736, WAS DISCIPLINED BY ARIZONA ON JANUARY 22, 1993
DISCIPLINARY ACTION: LICENSE REVOCATION

NOTES: AGREES NOT TO RE-APPLY FOR LICENSURE TO PRACTICE IN ARIZONA FOR A PERIOD OF AT LEAST FIVE YEARS.

INJEIAN, ABRAHAM V MD, LICENSE NUMBER 0104931 OF 475 NORTH 16TH STREET, YUMA, AZ, WAS DISCIPLINED BY NEW YORK ON DECEMBER 8, 1993
DISCIPLINARY ACTION: LICENSE REVOCATION
OFFENSE: DISCIPLINARY ACTION BY ANOTHER STATE OR AGENCY

NOTES: DISCIPLINED BY THE ARIZONA BOARD.

INJEIAN, ABRAHAM V MD, DATE OF BIRTH JUNE 6, 1931 OF 1656 ATHENS AVENUE, YUMA, AZ, WAS DISCIPLINED BY MEDICARE ON MARCH 14, 1996
DISCIPLINARY ACTION: EXCLUSION FROM THE MEDICARE AND/OR MEDICAID PROGRAM
OFFENSE: DISCIPLINARY ACTION BY ANOTHER STATE OR AGENCY

NOTES: LICENSE SURRENDERED FOR REASONS BEARING ON PROFESSIONAL COMPETENCE.

JABCZENSKI, FELIX MD, WAS DISCIPLINED BY ARIZONA ON MARCH 24, 1999

NOTES: ISSUES A DECREE OF CENSURE. HIS APPEAL FOR A REHEARING WAS DENIED ON 5/21/99.

JABCZENSKI, MARION MD, WAS DISCIPLINED BY ARIZONA ON JANUARY 23, 1998
DISCIPLINARY ACTION: FINE

NOTES: INTERIM ORDER. MUST UNDERGO PSYCHIATRIC, PSYCHOLOGICAL/PSYCHOMETRIC, AND PHYSICAL EVALUATIONS AT THE BOARD'S EXPENSE WITHIN 90 DAYS; MUST MAKE AN INITIAL DOWN PAYMENT OF $500 TOWARDS HIS ADMINISTRATIVE PENALTY AND THEN SET UP A BOARD APPROVED PAYMENT SCHEDULE.

JABCZENSKI, MARION A MD, LICENSE NUMBER 0003812 OF PHOENIX, AZ, WAS DISCIPLINED BY ARIZONA ON JANUARY 19, 1993
DISCIPLINARY ACTION: FINE
OFFENSE: OVERCHARGING

NOTES: FAILED TO SUPPLY REQUESTED INFORMATION IN A TIMELY MANNER TO THE BOARD REGARDING ORIGINAL MAMMOGRAMS WHICH THE BOARD SUBPOENAED SEVERAL TIMES BETWEEN 6/26/91 AND 1/14/92. ALSO CHARGED ADDITIONAL EXAMINATION FEE IN CONNECTION WITH MAMMOGRAMS IN SEVERAL CASES. MUST PAY AN ADMINISTRATIVE FINE OF $5,000 WITHIN SIX MONTHS. CENSURED. FOLLOWING THE BOARD'S REVIEW AND DISCUSSION OF THIS MATTER AT A HEARING REQUESTED BY DR. JABCZENSKI TO RECONSIDER THIS ACTION, HIS REQUEST FOR RECONSIDERATION WAS DENIED ON 4/14/93. ON 4/15/94 IT WAS REPORTED TO THE BOARD THAT THE JUDICIAL REVIEW HE FILED WAS DISMISSED BY THE COURT.

JABCZENSKI, MARION A MD, LICENSE NUMBER 3812, WAS DISCIPLINED BY ARIZONA ON NOVEMBER 18, 1999
DISCIPLINARY ACTION: MONITORING OF PHYSICIAN PERFORMANCE

NOTES: INTERIM CONSENT ORDER WITH FOLLOWING TERMS: THE OFFICE PROCEDURES IN HIS PRACTICE SHALL BE REVIEWED; HE SHALL PRODUCE THE REQUESTED MAMMOGRAMS WITHIN 30 DAYS; HE SHALL RETURN TO THE BOARD, AT ITS FEBRUARY MEETING, FOR A CONTINUATION OF THE FORMAL INTERVIEW; ALL FINES MUST BE PAID IN FULL, PRIOR TO THE FEBRUARY MEETING.

JACOBS, WALTER L JR MD, LICENSE NUMBER 0003829, WAS DISCIPLINED BY ARIZONA ON JANUARY 22, 1992
OFFENSE: PROFESSIONAL MISCONDUCT

NOTES: UNPROFESSIONAL CONDUCT FOR CHARGING A FEE FOR SERVICES NOT RENDERED TO A PATIENT HE VISITED SOCIALLY AT A HOSPITAL WHERE HE HAD NO ADMITTING PRIVILEGES; HE HAD PREVIOUSLY TREATED HER ON AN OUT-PATIENT BASIS. ISSUED A DECREE OF CENSURE.

JADAV, BIPINCHANDRA K MD, LICENSE NUMBER 0011907, WAS DISCIPLINED BY ARIZONA ON OCTOBER 16, 1996
DISCIPLINARY ACTION: 60-MONTH PROBATION; RESTRICTION PLACED ON LICENSE
OFFENSE: PROVIDING FALSE INFORMATION TO THE BOARD OR OTHER HEALTH AGENCY

NOTES: CHARGING A FEE FOR SERVICES NOT RENDERED IN THAT A PATIENT WAS BILLED FOR TWO VISITS ON 1/29/93 AND 2/2/93 FOR WHICH THERE IS NO NOTE IN PATIENT'S CHART THAT HE SAW THE PATIENT HIMSELF; FOR A PATIENT SEEN BETWEEN 3/93 AND 2/94, HE BILLED PATIENT FOR NUMEROUS OFFICE VISITS EVEN THOUGH HIS OFFICE RECORDS DO NOT SUBSTANTIATE THAT HE SAW THE PATIENT; ENGAGING IN PRACTICE WHICH IS OR MIGHT BE HARMFUL TO THE HEALTH OF PATIENTS IN THAT FOR A CHILD HE SAW FROM 11/92 UNTIL 7/94 HE FAILED TO REFER HER TO AN OTOLARYNGOLOGIST FOR EVALUATION OF RECURRENT EAR INFECTIONS; HE FAILED TO OBTAIN A URINE CULTURE OR SENSITIVITY OR OTHER TESTS REGARDING HER URINARY TRACT INFECTION AND HIS RECORDS DID NOT INDICATE ANY PLAN FOR FOLLOW-UP OF THE INFECTION; RECORDS FAILED TO SHOW SHE HAD RECEIVED THE REQUIRED CHILDHOOD IMMUNIZATIONS; FAILING TO MAINTAIN ADEQUATE RECORDS ON PATIENTS IN THAT FOR A PATIENT HE SAW TWICE IN 1993, THERE WAS NO NOTE IN THE CHART THAT HE HAD SEEN HER; FOR A PATIENT FOR WHOM HE HAD PRESCRIBED MULTIPLE INJECTIONS OF MEDICATIONS OVER LONG PERIODS OF TIME, THERE WAS NO INDICATION IN THE PATIENT'S CHART THAT HE HAD SEEN OR EXAMINED THE PATIENT; PRESCRIBING, DISPENSING OR ADMINISTERING ANY CONTROLLED SUBSTANCES OR PRESCRIPTION-ONLY DRUGS FOR OTHER THAN THERAPEUTIC PURPOSES IN THAT FOR ONE PATIENT BETWEEN 1987 AND 1993, HE ADMINISTERED MULTIPLE INJECTIONS INCLUDING NUBAIN, STADOL,

THORAZINE, DEMEROL, VISTARIL AND VERSED AND PRESCRIBED PERCOCET, FLORINEF, XANAX, SOMA, PREDNISONE, FIORINAL, BUMEX AND CIPRO; KNOWINGLY MAKING ANY FALSE STATEMENT IN CONNECTION WITH THE PRACTICE OF MEDICINE IN THAT IN 4/92, HE SUBMITTED A PROVIDER CREDENTIALING APPLICATION TO A HEALTH PLAN IN WHICH HE CLAIMED TO HAVE PRIVILEGES AT TWO HOSPITALS, WHERE HE DID NOT ACTUALLY HAVE PRIVILEGES. PROBATION WITH TERMS: SHALL NOT PRACTICE ANESTHESIA; ON OR BEFORE 7/1/97, MAY ENTER INTO AN APPROVED FAMILY PRACTICE RESIDENCY PROGRAM AND SHALL SUCCESSFULLY COMPLETE THREE YEARS OF RESIDENCY. AT ANY TIME DURING PROBATION THAT HE IS NOT IN RESIDENCY PROGRAM, SHALL COMPLY WITH THE FOLLOWING: WITHIN SEVEN DAYS, SHALL SURRENDER HIS CONTROLLED SUBSTANCE REGISTRATION CERTIFICATE FOR SCHEDULES II, III AND IV CONTROLLED SUBSTANCES TO THE DRUG ENFORCEMENT ADMINISTRATION; SHALL NOT PRESCRIBE, ADMINISTER OR DISPENSE ANY SCHEDULE II, III OR IV CONTROLLED SUBSTANCES AND SHALL NOT REAPPLY FOR REGISTRATION WITHOUT PRIOR CONSENT OF THE BOARD; SHALL NOT PRESCRIBE, ADMINISTER OR DISPENSE ANY ANTIPSYCHOTIC OR SYNTHETIC OPIOID MEDICATION; EACH YEAR FOR THE TERM OF PROBATION, SHALL OBTAIN 20 HOURS CONTINUING MEDICAL EDUCATION IN MEDICAL RECORD KEEPING AND 40 HOURS IN PHARMACOLOGY AND PROPER PRESCRIBING; IF HE ENGAGES IN THE PRIVATE PRACTICE OF MEDICINE IN WHICH HE IS THE OWNER OR PRINCIPAL PHYSICIAN IN THE PRACTICE, HE SHALL ENGAGE THE SERVICES OF A BOARD-APPROVED MEDICAL PRACTICE MANAGEMENT CONSULTANT; WITHIN NINE MONTHS, SHALL SUCCESSFULLY COMPLETE ADVANCED CARDIAC LIFE SUPPORT TRAINING AND PROVIDE BOARD WITH EVIDENCE OF COMPLETION.

JAFFE, MARC DO, LICENSE NUMBER 0002406 OF 1442 SOUTHWIND WAY, DRESHER, PA, WAS DISCIPLINED BY ARIZONA ON JUNE 14, 1990
DISCIPLINARY ACTION: LICENSE REVOCATION; FINE
OFFENSE: PROFESSIONAL MISCONDUCT

NOTES: FROM 1979 TO 1983 WHILE IN PENNSYLVANIA ENTERED INTO RELATIONSHIPS WITH LAWYERS, DURING WHICH TIME HE PROVIDED FRAUDULENT MEDICAL BILLS TO THESE LAWYERS WHICH THEY IN TURN USED TO PREPARE FRAUDULENT PERSONAL INJURY CLAIMS; ALSO SUPPLIED THESE LAWYERS WITH FRAUDULENTLY INFLATED MEDICAL BILLS IN ORDER TO MEET MINIMUM FILING AND CUT OFF LIMITS; SUBSEQUENTLY COOPERATED WITH INVESTIGATION OF THESE MATTERS IN EXCHANGE FOR AN IMMUNITY AGREEMENT; FALSELY CLAIMED HE WAS NOT AWARE THAT HIS BILLING PRACTICE WAS FRAUDULENT IN A LETTER DATED 8/18/88. $1,000 ADMINISTRATIVE PENALTY. ISSUED LICENSE NUMBER 3078 ON 1/25/96.

JAFFE, ROBERT T MD, LICENSE NUMBER 0016832, WAS DISCIPLINED BY ARIZONA ON NOVEMBER 19, 1990
DISCIPLINARY ACTION: REQUIRED TO TAKE ADDITIONAL MEDICAL EDUCATION

NOTES: SHALL OBTAIN, PRIOR TO 6/12/91, 100 HOURS OF BOARD-APPROVED CONTINUING MEDICAL EDUCATION IN GENERAL ALLOPATHIC MEDICINE.

JAIN, SATYENDRA K MD, LICENSE NUMBER 0016809, WAS DISCIPLINED BY ARIZONA ON AUGUST 23, 1990
DISCIPLINARY ACTION: REQUIRED TO TAKE ADDITIONAL MEDICAL EDUCATION

NOTES: SHALL COMPLETE 30 CREDIT HOURS OF CONTINUING MEDICAL EDUCATION ON THE SUBJECT OF PHARMACOLOGY, WITH EMPHASIS ON THE USE OF CONTROLLED SUBSTANCES BEFORE 6/26/91.

JAIN, SATYENDRA K MD, LICENSE NUMBER 0016809, WAS DISCIPLINED BY ARIZONA ON JULY 19, 1995
DISCIPLINARY ACTION: RESTRICTION PLACED ON CONTROLLED SUBSTANCE LICENSE; MONITORING OF PHYSICIAN PERFORMANCE
OFFENSE: PROFESSIONAL MISCONDUCT

NOTES: COMPLAINT REGARDING HIS CARE AND TREATMENT OF A PATIENT AND COMPLAINT ALLEGING THAT HE DISPENSED PERCOCET AND VALIUM FROM HIS OFFICE. INTERIM ORDER: SHALL MEET WITH THE BOARD AS REQUESTED REGARDING HIS SCORE ON THE 6/95 SPECIAL PURPOSE EXAMINATION. MUST NOT REGISTER WITH THE BOARD AS A DISPENSING PHYSICIAN, NOR DISPENSE DRUGS OR DEVICES FROM HIS OFFICE UNTIL THE BOARD GRANTS HIM PERMISSION TO DO SO; SHALL ABSTAIN COMPLETELY FROM THE CONSUMPTION OF DRUGS EXCEPT WHEN PRESCRIBED BY HIS TREATING PHYSICIAN; SHALL SUBMIT TO WITNESSED RANDOM BIOLOGICAL FLUID COLLECTION; ACKNOWLEDGES THAT HE HAS ENGAGED THE SERVICES OF A PRACTICE MANAGEMENT CONSULTANT AND AGREES TO RELEASE THE RESULTS OF THAT CONSULTATION TO THE BOARD AS PART OF ITS ONGOING INVESTIGATION

JAIN, SATYENDRA K MD, WAS DISCIPLINED BY ARIZONA ON OCTOBER 20, 1995
DISCIPLINARY ACTION: RESTRICTION PLACED ON CONTROLLED SUBSTANCE LICENSE; REPRIMAND
OFFENSE: PROFESSIONAL MISCONDUCT

NOTES: INTERVIEWED BY THE BOARD REGARDING HIS CARE AND TREATMENT OF A PATIENT AND THE COMPLAINT ALLEGING THAT HE DISPENSED PERCOCET AND VALIUM FROM HIS OFFICE, HIS INTERIM STIPULATION AND ORDER OF 8/95, AND HIS PASSING THE SPEX WITH A SCORE OF 80. SHALL NOT REGISTER WITH THE BOARD AS A DISPENSING PHYSICIAN; WITHIN 30 DAYS, SHALL SURRENDER TO THE DEA HIS CONTROLLED SUBSTANCE REGISTRATION CERTIFICATE FOR SCHEDULES II, III, AND IV; FOR TWO YEARS, SHALL OBTAIN 20 HOURS PER YEAR OF CONTINUING MEDICAL EDUCATION IN PHARMACOLOGY OF PAIN CONTROL; WITHIN NINE MONTHS, SHALL COMPLETE A BOARD-APPROVED ONE MONTH MINI-RESIDENCY IN FAMILY PRACTICE; BOARD SHALL CONDUCT A FOLLOW-UP SURVEY OF HIS PRACTICE ON OR ABOUT ONE YEAR FROM THIS ORDER. ON 1/24/97 ORDER WAS TERMINATED BASED ON THE RESULTS OF THE CHART SURVEY.

JAIN, SATYENDRA K MD OF 1195 NORTH ARIZONA BLVD, COLLIDGE, AZ, WAS DISCIPLINED BY DEA ON NOVEMBER 27, 1995
DISCIPLINARY ACTION: RESTRICTION PLACED ON CONTROLLED SUBSTANCE LICENSE
OFFENSE: DISCIPLINARY ACTION BY ANOTHER STATE OR AGENCY

NOTES: STATE BOARD.

JANIKOWSKI, MARY DARIN DO, LICENSE NUMBER 2596 OF 1402 BAILEY AVENUE, NEEDLES, CA, WAS DISCIPLINED BY ARIZONA ON SEPTEMBER 11, 1997
DISCIPLINARY ACTION: 60-MONTH PROBATION; RESTRICTION PLACED ON LICENSE
OFFENSE: SUBSTANCE ABUSE

NOTES: ON 2/27/97 SHE INFORMED BOARD SHE HAD VOLUNTARILY ENTERED INTO A DIVERSION PROGRAM FOR SUBSTANCE ABUSE AND ON 3/13/97 VOLUNTARILY ENTERED INTO A DIVERSION AGREEMENT WITH CALIFORNIA BOARD. CONDITIONS OF THE ARIZONA PROBATION ARE AS FOLLOWS: SHALL IMMEDIATELY OBTAIN A TREATING PSYCHIATRIST APPROVED BY THE BOARD AND SHALL REMAIN IN TREATMENT WITH THE PSYCHIATRIST UNTIL FURTHER ORDER OF THE BOARD WITH MONTHLY REPORTS; SHALL PROVIDE A COPY OF THIS ORDER TO ANY HEALTH CARE ENTITY SHE HAS PRIVILEGES; SHALL ABSTAIN COMPLETELY FROM THE CONSUMPTION OF ALCOHOLIC BEVERAGES AND DRUGS EXCEPT WHEN PRESCRIBED BY HER TREATING PHYSICIAN; MUST SUBMIT TO WITNESSED RANDOM BIOLOGICAL FLUID COLLECTION; MUST KEEP A LOG OF ANY AND ALL MEDICATIONS PRESCRIBED FOR HER; SHALL SUBMIT TO ANY MEDICAL OR PSYCHOLOGICAL EVALUATIONS ORDERED BY BOARD; SHALL APPEAR BEFORE BOARD FOR INTERVIEWS UPON REQUEST; SHALL INFORM THE BOARD OF ANY CHANGE OF ADDRESS; SHALL PARTICIPATE IN A MINIMUM OF TWO SELF-HELP MEETINGS PER WEEK THROUGH SUCH ORGANIZATIONS AS AA, NARCOTICS ANONYMOUS, AND DOCTOR'S CADUCEUS GROUP; SHALL LIMIT HER WORK HOURS TO AN AVERAGE OF 24 PER WEEK AND MAY REQUEST IN WRITING THAT THIS TERM BE MODIFIED; SHALL REIMBURSE THE BOARD FOR ALL EXPENSES ASSOCIATED WITH THIS MATTER.

JAREM, BOHDAN J MD, WAS DISCIPLINED BY ARIZONA ON DECEMBER 2, 1993
OFFENSE: DISCIPLINARY ACTION BY ANOTHER STATE OR AGENCY

NOTES: TEXAS ISSUED AN ORDER IN 01/93 SUSPENDING HIS LICENSE FOR FIVE YEARS. HE SIGNED AND ENTERED INTO A STIPULATION AND ORDER NOT TO PRACTICE MEDICINE IN ARIZONA.

JAREM, BOHDAN JOHN MD, DATE OF BIRTH JULY 22, 1941, LICENSE NUMBER 00D9829 OF 5400 PRESTON OAKS #2003, DALLAS, TX, WAS DISCIPLINED BY TEXAS ON JANUARY 30, 1993
DISCIPLINARY ACTION: EMERGENCY SUSPENSION
OFFENSE: PHYSICAL OR MENTAL ILLNESS INHIBITING THE ABILITY TO PRACTICE WITH SKILL AND SAFETY

NOTES: SUFFERS FROM A BIPOLAR DISORDER IN THE MANIC PHASE AND IS IN NEED OF PSYCHIATRIC COUNSELING.

JAREM, BOHDAN JOHN MD, DATE OF BIRTH JULY 22, 1941, LICENSE NUMBER 00D9829 OF 4118 KEYSTONE, GARLAND, TX, WAS DISCIPLINED BY TEXAS ON JUNE 15, 1993
DISCIPLINARY ACTION: 60-MONTH PROBATION; MONITORING OF PHYSICIAN PERFORMANCE
OFFENSE: PHYSICAL OR MENTAL ILLNESS INHIBITING THE ABILITY TO PRACTICE WITH SKILL AND SAFETY

NOTES: FROM 1/7/93-2/22/93 HE RECEIVED INPATIENT PSYCHIATRIC TREATMENT FOR A BIPOLAR DISORDER IN THE MANIC PHASE; DISORDER IS CURRENTLY IN REMISSION AND HE IS RECEIVING PSYCHIATRIC COUNSELING. FIVE YEAR SUSPENSION STAYED. CONDITIONS OF PROBATION: SHALL CONTINUE TO RECEIVE PSYCHIATRIC TREATMENT WITH QUARTERLY REPORTS TO THE BOARD; SHALL OBTAIN A BOARD-APPROVED PSYCHIATRIST AND CONTINUE TREATMENT IF HE RELOCATES; SHALL SUBMIT HIMSELF FOR RANDOM LAB TESTING OF HIS LITHIUM LEVEL; SHALL APPEAR BEFORE THE BOARD TWICE A YEAR; SHALL GIVE A COPY OF THIS ORDER TO ANY HEALTH CARE ENTITY WHERE HE HAS PRIVILEGES; SHALL COOPERATE WITH THE BOARD IN VERIFYING COMPLIANCE; SHALL INFORM BOARD OF CHANGE OF ADDRESS WITHIN 10 DAYS OR IF HE LEAVES TEXAS; TIME SPENT OUT OF TEXAS DOES NOT COUNT TOWARD PROBATION. SHALL NOT SEEK MODIFICATION FOR ONE YEAR. ON 6/28/95 HIS PETITION FOR TERMINATION OF THIS ORDER DENIED.

JAREM, BOHDAN JOHN MD, LICENSE NUMBER 0029241 OF GARLAND, TX, WAS DISCIPLINED BY OHIO ON MARCH 16, 1994
DISCIPLINARY ACTION: LICENSE SUSPENSION; PROBATION
OFFENSE: DISCIPLINARY ACTION BY ANOTHER STATE OR AGENCY

NOTES: PRIOR ACTION BY TEXAS BOARD DUE TO HIS BIPOLAR DISORDER. INDEFINITE SUSPENSION. CONDITIONS FOR REINSTATEMENT ESTABLISHED; PROBATION FOR AT LEAST TWO YEARS.

JOHNSON, BRENT E MD OF PRESCOTT, AZ, WAS DISCIPLINED BY IOWA ON FEBRUARY 12, 1997
DISCIPLINARY ACTION: PROBATION
OFFENSE: DISCIPLINARY ACTION BY ANOTHER STATE OR AGENCY

NOTES: CHARGED IN CONNECTION WITH A VOLUNTARY AGREEMENT HE HAD ENTERED INTO WITH THE ARIZONA BOARD OF MEDICAL EXAMINERS WHICH PLACED RESTRICTIONS ON HIS ARIZONA LICENSE. PROBATION FOR NOT MORE THAN 17 MONTHS.

JOHNSON, PATRICIA MD, WAS DISCIPLINED BY ARIZONA ON APRIL 16, 1994
DISCIPLINARY ACTION: REQUIRED TO ENTER AN IMPAIRED PHYSICIAN PROGRAM OR SUBSTANCE ABUSE TREATMENT
OFFENSE: SUBSTANCE ABUSE

NOTES: SHALL WITHIN 14 DAYS ENTER INTO LONG-TERM RESIDENTIAL TREATMENT FOR SUBSTANCE ABUSE AT A TREATMENT FACILITY APPROVED BY THE BOARD AND SHALL REMAIN IN TREATMENT UNTIL THERAPEUTICALLY DISCHARGED BY THE TREATMENT CENTER.

JOHNSON, PATRICIA MD, WAS DISCIPLINED BY ARIZONA ON OCTOBER 22, 1994
DISCIPLINARY ACTION: 120-MONTH PROBATION; RESTRICTION PLACED ON CONTROLLED SUBSTANCE LICENSE

NOTES: INTERVIEWED REGARDING TREATMENT AT CHANDLER VALLEY HOSPITAL AND SPRINGBROOK NORTHWEST. CONDITIONS AND TERMS OF PROBATION ARE AS FOLLOWS: ALL PRESCRIPTIONS FOR PRESCRIPTION-ONLY MEDICATIONS AND CONTROLLED SUBSTANCES SHALL BE IN WRITING AND SHALL BE COUNTERSIGNED BY HER SUPERVISING PHYSICIAN; SHALL NOT APPLY FOR A CONTROLLED SUBSTANCE REGISTRATION CERTIFICATE FROM THE DRUG ENFORCEMENT ADMINISTRATION; MUST IMMEDIATELY PARTICIPATE IN A BOARD-APPROVED MONITORED AFTERCARE TREATMENT PROGRAM WHOSE THERAPIST MUST SUBMIT QUARTERLY REPORTS; MUST PARTICIPATE IN 90 12-STEP MEETINGS FOR SUBSTANCE ABUSE WITHIN 90 DAYS; MUST THEN PARTICIPATE IN A 12-STEP RECOVERY PROGRAM AS DETERMINED BY HER TREATING THERAPIST AND ATTEND AT LEAST THREE WEEKLY MEETINGS; SHALL OBTAIN A BOARD-APPROVED TREATING PHYSICIAN; SHALL ABSTAIN COMPLETELY FROM THE CONSUMPTION OF ALCOHOLIC BEVERAGES AND DRUGS EXCEPT WHEN PRESCRIBED BY HER TREATING PHYSICIAN; MUST SUBMIT TO WITNESSED RANDOM BIOLOGICAL FLUID COLLECTION; KEEP A LOG OF ANY AND ALL MEDICATIONS PRESCRIBED FOR HER; SHALL SUBMIT

TO ANY EXAMINATIONS OR THERAPY ORDERED BY BOARD; SHALL APPEAR BEFORE BOARD FOR INTERVIEWS UPON REQUEST; SHALL INFORM BOARD OF CHANGE OF ADDRESS OR IF AWAY FOR MORE THAN FIVE DAYS.

JOHNSON, WILLIAM MD OF 1501 N. CAMPBELL AVENUE, TUCSON, AZ, WAS DISCIPLINED BY DEA ON DECEMBER 16, 1999
DISCIPLINARY ACTION: SURRENDER OF CONTROLLED SUBSTANCE LICENSE
OFFENSE: OVERPRESCRIBING OR MISPRESCRIBING DRUGS

NOTES: INAPPROPRIATE PRESCRIBING.

JOHNSTON, JAMES C MD, LICENSE NUMBER 0022573, WAS DISCIPLINED BY ARIZONA ON OCTOBER 18, 1995

NOTES: SHALL NOT PRACTICE MEDICINE IN ARIZONA PRIOR TO MEETING WITH THE BOARD.

JOHNSTON, JAMES C MD, LICENSE NUMBER 25337 OF SAN ANTONIO, TX, WAS DISCIPLINED BY WASHINGTON ON JANUARY 24, 1997

NOTES: AGREED ORDER TO APPEAR BEFORE THE COMMISSION PRIOR TO PRACTICING MEDICINE IN WASHINGTON. ON 1/21/99 REQUEST TO TERMINATE THE CONDITIONS OF THIS ORDER GRANTED AND LICENSE IS NOW UNRESTRICTED.

JOHNSTON, JAMES C MD, DATE OF BIRTH NOVEMBER 20, 1954, LICENSE NUMBER 33573, WAS DISCIPLINED BY COLORADO ON APRIL 17, 1997
DISCIPLINARY ACTION: SURRENDER OF LICENSE

NOTES: NO UNPROFESSIONAL CONDUCT IDENTIFIED.

JOHNSTON, JAMES CHRISTOPHER MD, DATE OF BIRTH NOVEMBER 20, 1959, LICENSE NUMBER 00G8880 OF NACOGDOCHES, TX, WAS DISCIPLINED BY TEXAS ON JUNE 22, 1994
DISCIPLINARY ACTION: RESTRICTION PLACED ON LICENSE
OFFENSE: SEXUAL ABUSE OF OR SEXUAL MISCONDUCT WITH A PATIENT

NOTES: AS RECENTLY AS 6/8/94 CRIMINAL COMPLAINTS WERE FILED AGAINST HIM ALLEGING HE ENGAGED IN BEHAVIOR CONSTITUTING ATTEMPTED SEXUAL ASSAULT AGAINST INDIVIDUALS WHO WERE PATIENTS; DENIES ALLEGATIONS; BECAUSE HE DESIRES TO FOCUS RESOURCES AND TIME ON DEFENSE OF THE CRIMINAL CASE. AGREES TO THIS ORDER WITH THE BOARD. LICENSE IS RESTRICTED AS FOLLOWS: SHALL NOT EXAMINE OR TREAT PATIENTS AFTER THE ORDER DATE; WITHIN 30 DAYS SHALL SUBMIT HIMSELF FOR ASSESSMENT THROUGH THE BEHAVIOR CARE NETWORK PROGRAM OR OTHER BOARD-APPROVED PROGRAM WHICH WILL FOCUS ON THE DISPARITY BETWEEN THE COMPLAINTS AGAINST HIM AND HIS OWN VERSION OF EVENTS AND ATTEMPT TO DETERMINE THE DEGREE OF RISK TO THE PUBLIC INVOLVED IN HIS CONTINUED PRACTICE; SHOULD THIS EVALUATION INDICATE HIS PRACTICE CONSTITUTES NO THREAT TO THE PUBLIC HEALTH HE SHALL BE PERMITTED TO RESUME PRACTICE PENDING FURTHER ORDER OF THE BOARD PROVIDED HE SEES PATIENTS ONLY WHEN ACCOMPANIED BY A CHAPERONE APPROVED IN ADVANCE WHO WILL SIGN ALL CHARTS TO INDICATE PRESENCE; SHALL COOPERATE WITH THE BOARD IN VERIFYING COMPLIANCE; SHALL INFORM BOARD OF CHANGE OF ADDRESS WITHIN 10 DAYS.

JOHNSTON, JAMES CHRISTOPHER MD, DATE OF BIRTH NOVEMBER 20, 1959, LICENSE NUMBER 00G8880 OF 5601 BANDERA ROAD SUITE 416, SAN ANTONIO, TX, WAS DISCIPLINED BY TEXAS ON SEPTEMBER 30, 1994
DISCIPLINARY ACTION: RESTRICTION PLACED ON LICENSE
OFFENSE: SEXUAL ABUSE OF OR SEXUAL MISCONDUCT WITH A PATIENT

NOTES: CRIMINAL COMPLAINTS HAVE BEEN FILED AGAINST HIM ALLEGING THAT HE HAS ENGAGED IN BEHAVIOR CONSTITUTING ATTEMPTED SEXUAL ASSAULT AGAINST INDIVIDUALS WHO WERE PATIENTS; HE DENIES ALL OF THESE ALLEGATIONS; AS A CONDITION OF 6/22/94 AGREEMENT HAS UNDERGONE AN EXTENSIVE EVALUATION WHICH CONCLUDED THAT THERE WAS NOTHING TO SUGGEST THAT HE WOULD BE UNABLE TO PROVIDE CLINICAL SERVICES UNDER CERTAIN RESTRICTIONS AND SUPERVISION. CONDITIONS OF RESTRICTION WHICH SUPERSEDE PREVIOUS ORDER: SHALL NOT EXAMINE OR TREAT ANY PATIENT WITHOUT BEING ACCOMPANIED BY A BOARD APPROVED CHAPERONE WHO SHALL VERIFY PRESENCE BY SIGNING ALL CHARTS; SHALL OBTAIN AN EXAM TABLE WITH SPECIFICATIONS; SHALL REPOSITION THIS TABLE SO HE MAY WALK BEHIND PATIENTS TO EXAMINE THE SHOULDER AND PROXIMAL AREAS; SHALL NOT PLACE A PAGER OR INSTRUMENTS IN HIS POCKETS DURING EXAMS; PATIENTS SHALL ONLY BE REPOSITIONED BY A NURSE OR TECHNICIAN; SHALL EXPLAIN TO ALL PATIENTS PROCEDURES WHICH INVOLVE CONTACT AND ASK THEM IN DETAIL REGARDING ANY PROBLEMS OR CONCERNS REGARDING HIS EXAM; WITHIN 60 DAYS SHALL UNDERGO ADDITIONAL PHALLOMETRIC TESTING; SHALL COOPERATE WITH THE BOARD IN VERIFYING COMPLIANCE; SHALL INFORM THE BOARD OF CHANGE OF ADDRESS WITHIN 10 DAYS; SHALL HAVE THE RIGHT TO PETITION FOR AMENDMENT OR TERMINATION UPON DISMISSAL OR ACQUITTAL ON THE CRIMINAL CHARGES; OTHERWISE MAY SEEK MODIFICATIONS ONCE A YEAR. ON 1/29/99 ORDER TERMINATED.

JOHNSTON, JAMES CHRISTOPHER MD, LICENSE NUMBER 00M5411, WAS DISCIPLINED BY IDAHO ON DECEMBER 14, 1994
DISCIPLINARY ACTION: RESTRICTION PLACED ON LICENSE; MONITORING OF PHYSICIAN PERFORMANCE
OFFENSE: DISCIPLINARY ACTION BY ANOTHER STATE OR AGENCY

NOTES: ON 9/30/94 TEXAS RESTRICTED HIS LICENSE BASED ON CRIMINAL ALLEGATIONS THAT HE HAD ENGAGED IN BEHAVIOR CONSTITUTING ATTEMPTED SEXUAL ASSAULT AGAINST PATIENTS. IDAHO BOARD ADOPTS AND INCORPORATES ALL TERMS AND CONDITIONS OF THE TEXAS ORDER WHICH INCLUDE: SHALL NOT EXAMINE OR TREAT ANY PATIENTS WITHOUT BEING ACCOMPANIED AT ALL TIMES BY A PROCTOR OR CHAPERONE APPROVED BY THE BOARD; SHALL OBTAIN AN EXAM TABLE THAT IS SPECIFICALLY DESIGNED FOR THE PERFORMANCE OF ELECTROMYOGRAPHY WITH A STANDARD ARM BOARD AND THE ABILITY TO ELEVATE THE HEAD OF THE PATIENT; SHALL REPOSITION HIS EXAMINATION TABLE SO THAT HE MAY WALK BEHIND PATIENTS TO EXAMINE THE SHOULDER AND PROXIMAL AREAS; SHALL NOT PLACE A PAGER OR INSTRUMENTS IN HIS POCKETS DURING EXAMINATION OF PATIENTS; PATIENTS SHALL BE REPOSITIONED DURING EVALUATIONS ONLY BY A NURSE OR TECHNICIAN; SHALL EXPLAIN TO ALL PATIENTS THOSE PROCEDURES WHICH INVOLVE CONTACT WITH HIM PRIOR TO SUCH CONTACT; SHALL ASK PATIENTS IN DETAIL REGARDING ANY PROBLEMS OR CONCERNS WHICH THEY MIGHT HAVE CONCERNING HIS

EXAMINATIONS OR ANY PROCEDURES PERFORMED; SHALL UNDERGO ADDITIONAL PHALLOMETRIC TESTING WITHIN 60 DAYS. ON 1/13/99 ORDER TERMINATED.

JOHNSTON, JAMES CHRISTOPHER MD, LICENSE NUMBER 0A44527 OF NACOGDOCHES, TX, WAS DISCIPLINED BY CALIFORNIA ON DECEMBER 30, 1995
DISCIPLINARY ACTION: SURRENDER OF LICENSE
NOTES: WHILE CHARGES PENDING.

JOHNSTON, JAMES CHRISTOPHER MD, LICENSE NUMBER 0018716 OF SAN ANTONIO, TX, WAS DISCIPLINED BY OREGON ON NOVEMBER 4, 1996
DISCIPLINARY ACTION: SURRENDER OF LICENSE
NOTES: VOLUNTARY SURRENDER.

JOLLY, MICHAEL J MD, DATE OF BIRTH MAY 16, 1954 OF 810 CAMINO SANTIAGO AVE, TUCSON, AZ, WAS DISCIPLINED BY MEDICARE ON MAY 10, 1991
DISCIPLINARY ACTION: EXCLUSION FROM THE MEDICARE AND/OR MEDICAID PROGRAM
OFFENSE: DISCIPLINARY ACTION BY ANOTHER STATE OR AGENCY
NOTES: LICENSE REVOCATION OR SUSPENSION.

JOLLY, MICHAEL JAMES MD, WAS DISCIPLINED BY ARIZONA ON JUNE 27, 1990
DISCIPLINARY ACTION: DENIAL OF NEW LICENSE
OFFENSE: DISCIPLINARY ACTION BY ANOTHER STATE OR AGENCY
NOTES: CALIFORNIA REVOKED HIS LICENSE 12/27/89 BECAUSE OF THE FINDING THAT HIS ABILITY TO PRACTICE SAFELY WAS IMPAIRED BECAUSE HE WAS MENTALLY ILL. TWO PHYSICIANS SELECTED BY ARIZONA BOARD DETERMINED HE WAS NOT FIT TO PRACTICE. PLED NO CONTEST TO CHARGES IN ARIZONA OF USE AND POSSESSION OF NARCOTIC PARAPHERNALIA AND RESISTING ARREST. ADMITTED TO SELF-MEDICATING WITH METHAMPHETAMINE. ALSO PROVIDED AMPHETAMINES TO DRUG ADDICTS AND DRUG DEALERS AND FAILED TO KEEP RECORDS OF HIS DISTRIBUTION OF CONTROLLED SUBSTANCES.

JOSEPH, RONALD B MD, LICENSE NUMBER 8699, WAS DISCIPLINED BY ARIZONA ON NOVEMBER 12, 1997
DISCIPLINARY ACTION: 24-MONTH PROBATION; REQUIRED TO TAKE ADDITIONAL MEDICAL EDUCATION
OFFENSE: PROFESSIONAL MISCONDUCT
NOTES: ON ONE OR MORE OCCASIONS DURING THE BOARD'S INVESTIGATION, HE FAILED TO RESPOND TO SUBPOENAS TO PRODUCE DOCUMENTS OR TO TIMELY OBJECT TO THE SUBPOENAS. THE FOLLOWING CASES WERE INVOLVED IN THE INVESTIGATION: ON 6/22/92, HE PERFORMED SURGERY ON A FEMALE PATIENT; ALTHOUGH THE PATIENT HAD SIGNED A CONSENT FORM, THERE WAS NO DOCUMENTATION INDICATING THAT THE PATIENT HAD REQUESTED THE PROCEDURE, THAT HE HAD EXPLAINED THE RISKS ASSOCIATED WITH THE PROCEDURE OR THAT HE HAD REVIEWED X-RAYS; HE ALSO FAILED TO TIMELY DICTATE A MEDICAL RECORD THAT ANOTHER SURGERY, SCHEDULED FOR THE PATIENT ON 7/2/92, HAD BEEN CANCELED. IN A SECOND CASE ON 8/11/93, A HOSPITAL EMERGENCY DEPARTMENT PHYSICIAN ATTEMPTED TO CONTACT DR. JOSEPH REGARDING A MALE PATIENT THAT HE HAD TREATED ON SEVERAL OCCASIONS BETWEEN JULY AND AUGUST 1993 AND PERFORMED AN ARTHROSCOPY; ON 8/6/93; THE EMERGENCY PHYSICIAN WAS ABLE TO REACH THE DOCTOR'S NURSE; ACCORDING TO THE NURSE, DR. JOSEPH WAS OUT OF TOWN, WAS NOT AVAILABLE, AND THAT TO HER KNOWLEDGE, HE HAD NO ONE COVERING FOR HIM. IN A DEPOSITION HE GAVE ON 6/26/95, IN A THIRD CASE DR. JOSEPH PROVIDED TESTIMONY CONTRARY TO HIS OFFICE NOTES REGARDING A PATIENT HE TREATED BETWEEN 6/11/93 AND 2/15/95. CONDITIONS OF PROBATION: WITHIN 30 DAYS, HE SHALL ENGAGE A BOARD APPROVED OFFICE MANAGEMENT AND BILLING CONSULTANT WHO WITHIN 150 DAYS SHALL MAKE A WRITTEN REPORT, INCLUDING RECOMMENDATIONS, OF HIS EVALUATION OF DR. JOSEPH'S OFFICE AND BILLING PRACTICES; SHALL PERFORM 20 MAJOR SURGERIES WHICH SHALL BE CONCURRENTLY SUPERVISED BY AT LEAST FOUR DIFFERENT BOARD APPROVED SUPERVISORS WHO SHALL SUBMIT A WRITTEN REPORT TO THE BOARD WITHIN 60 DAYS AFTER EACH SURGICAL CASE; THE BOARD SHALL CONDUCT A REVIEW OF HIS PATIENT CARE AND BILLING PRACTICES AT THE END OF ONE YEAR; WITHIN ONE YEAR, SHALL TAKE EIGHT HOURS OF CONTINUING MEDICAL EDUCATION IN FORENSIC ETHICS. WITHIN 90 DAYS, HE SHALL PAY RESTITUTION TO A SPECIFIED PATIENT OF ALL FEES PAID TO THE DOCTOR AND HIS MEDICAL PRACTICE, SHALL REIMBURSE THE PATIENT'S INSURANCE CARRIER(S), AND SHALL PROVIDE SATISFACTORY EVIDENCE TO THE BOARD OF PAYMENT IN FULL.

JOSEPH, RONALD B MD, DATE OF BIRTH OCTOBER 9, 1944, LICENSE NUMBER 19422, WAS DISCIPLINED BY COLORADO ON AUGUST 18, 1999
DISCIPLINARY ACTION: REPRIMAND

JOSEPHS, GORDON HARVEY DO, LICENSE NUMBER 0001272 OF 7315 E EVANS, SCOTTSDALE, AZ, WAS DISCIPLINED BY ARIZONA ON JULY 5, 1992
DISCIPLINARY ACTION: LICENSE REVOCATION
OFFENSE: FAILURE TO COMPLY WITH PREVIOUS BOARD ORDER
NOTES: REFUSED TO TAKE THE SPECIAL PURPOSE EXAMINATION ON 6/18/92 AS ORDERED BY THE BOARD.

JOZSEF, STEPHEN M MD, WAS DISCIPLINED BY ARIZONA ON OCTOBER 11, 1991
DISCIPLINARY ACTION: MONITORING OF PHYSICIAN PERFORMANCE; REQUIRED TO ENTER AN IMPAIRED PHYSICIAN PROGRAM OR SUBSTANCE ABUSE TREATMENT
OFFENSE: DISCIPLINARY ACTION BY ANOTHER STATE OR AGENCY
NOTES: INFORMATION RECEIVED THAT HE WAS DENIED LICENSURE BY THE COLORADO BOARD AND THAT HE MIGHT BE INAPPROPRIATELY USING CONTROLLED SUBSTANCES IN TREATMENT FOR HIS HEADACHES AND THAT HE HAD VOLUNTARILY ENTERED AN INPATIENT TREATMENT PROGRAM AT AN ADDICTION RECOVERY UNIT IN COLORADO. SHALL NOT PRACTICE MEDICINE IN ARIZONA BEFORE MEETING WITH THE BOARD; SHALL AUTHORIZE THE COLORADO IMPAIRED PHYSICIANS' PROGRAM TO FORWARD TO THE BOARD QUARTERLY AFTERCARE REPORTS ON HIS PROGRESS; SHALL PARTICIPATE IN THE SPEX EXAMINATION ON 3/19/92; SHALL UNDERGO PSYCHIATRIC, PSYCHOMETRIC, PSYCHOLOGICAL AND PHYSICAL EVALUATIONS; SHALL RETURN FOR FURTHER REVIEW AT THE 4/92 BOARD MEETING.

KAHLE, JOHN F MD, LICENSE NUMBER 0002789, WAS DISCIPLINED BY ARIZONA ON APRIL 6, 1992
DISCIPLINARY ACTION: REQUIRED TO TAKE ADDITIONAL MEDICAL EDUCATION

OFFENSE: OVERPRESCRIBING OR MISPRESCRIBING DRUGS

NOTES: TWO INSTANCES OF OVERPRESCRIBING OF CONTROLLED SUBSTANCES AND PRESCRIBING PRELUDIN IN EXCESS OF STATUTORY LIMITS. SHALL SUCCESSFULLY COMPLETE BEFORE 12/31/92 A COURSE INVOLVING CONTINUING MEDICAL EDUCATION IN THE TOPIC OF DOCUMENTATION AND RECORDKEEPING. EFFECTIVE 4/14/94 ORDER TERMINATED.

KANAS, RONNIE J MD, LICENSE NUMBER 22902, WAS DISCIPLINED BY ARIZONA ON MAY 15, 1998
DISCIPLINARY ACTION: LICENSE SUSPENSION
OFFENSE: DISCIPLINARY ACTION BY ANOTHER STATE OR AGENCY

NOTES: ON 10/16/97, VOLUNTARILY PLACED NEW YORK LICENSE ON INACTIVE STATUS; TERMS OF NEW YORK ORDER REQUIRE THAT HE NOT PRACTICE MEDICINE IN NEW YORK OR ANY OTHER STATE. ARIZONA LICENSE PLACED ON INACTIVE STATUS WITH CAUSE. SHALL NOT REQUEST REACTIVATION OF LICENSE UNTIL HE MEETS WITH THE BOARD AT A REGULARLY SCHEDULED MEETING AND COMPLIES WITH ALL BOARD REQUESTS.

KANAS, RONNIE J MD, LICENSE NUMBER 63122 OF VESTAL, NY, WAS DISCIPLINED BY FLORIDA ON JUNE 28, 1999
OFFENSE: DISCIPLINARY ACTION BY ANOTHER STATE OR AGENCY

NOTES: CHARGED WITH HAVING A DISCIPLINARY ACTION IN ANOTHER STATE AND FAILING TO REPORT THIS. SHALL REMAIN IN CONTINUAL COMPLIANCE WITH ALL PROVISIONS OF THE NEW YORK RESTORATION ORDER; PRIOR TO COMMENCING ANY PRACTICE IN FLORIDA, HE SHALL APPEAR BEFORE THE BOARD AND DEMONSTRATE CAPABILITY TO PRACTICE MEDICINE WITH SKILL AND SAFETY.

KANAS, RONNIE JAMES MD, DATE OF BIRTH JULY 10, 1956, LICENSE NUMBER 9500109 OF VESTAL, NY, WAS DISCIPLINED BY NORTH CAROLINA ON JANUARY 24, 1998
DISCIPLINARY ACTION: SURRENDER OF LICENSE

NOTES: VOLUNTARY SURRENDER OF LICENSE.

KANGSUMRITH, SURIYUN MD, LICENSE NUMBER 0015115, WAS DISCIPLINED BY ARIZONA ON OCTOBER 17, 1995
DISCIPLINARY ACTION: 60-MONTH PROBATION; FINE
OFFENSE: DISCIPLINARY ACTION BY ANOTHER STATE OR AGENCY

NOTES: IN 12/92 RENEWAL APPLICATION FOR ARIZONA LICENSE, HE DENIED ANY RESTRICTIONS BY LICENSING BOARDS WHEN IN FACT IN 5/92, HE SURRENDERED HIS DEA CERTIFICATION AND HIS ALABAMA STATE CONTROLLED SUBSTANCES REGISTRATION CERTIFICATE BECAUSE HE AND ONE OF HIS EMPLOYEES DISPENSED CONTROLLED AND NON-CONTROLLED SUBSTANCES IN THE FORM OF TYLENOL #3, DARVOCET, HYDROCODONE AND LORTABS TO KNOWN DRUG ADDICTS AND WITHOUT PROPER MEDICAL EXAMINATIONS; AFTER INVESTIGATION BY THE ALABAMA BOARD AND THE DEA, HE SURRENDERED ALL CONTROLLED SUBSTANCES IN HIS POSSESSION AND SURRENDERED HIS DEA CERTIFICATION; IN 12/93, IN ANTICIPATION OF OBTAINING A JOB WITH THE PUBLIC HEALTH SERVICE, HE COMPLETED AN APPLICATION FOR DEA CERTIFICATION USING HIS HOME ADDRESS IN MESA AND DECLARING TO THE BOARD THAT HE WAS RETIRED FROM PRACTICE IN ALL STATES IN WHICH HE IS LICENSED. CENSURED; $1,000 FINE; PROBATION WITH TERMS: SHALL NOT POSSESS OR APPLY FOR A DEA REGISTRATION; SHALL PARTICIPATE IN A 30 HOUR MINI-RESIDENCY IN APPROPRIATE PRESCRIBING OF NARCOTICS TO KNOWN DRUG ADDICTS; SHALL PARTICIPATE IN A FIVE-HOUR MINI-RESIDENCY REGARDING THE LEGAL AND ETHICAL ASPECTS OF COMPLETING APPLICATIONS FOR LICENSURE AND STAFF PRIVILEGES. ON 3/26/99 REQUEST TO TERMINATE ORDER DENIED.

KANGSUMRITH, SURIYUN MD, LICENSE NUMBER 115178 OF 943 SOUTH POWER ROAD, MESA, AZ, WAS DISCIPLINED BY NEW YORK ON JANUARY 15, 1997
DISCIPLINARY ACTION: LICENSE REVOCATION
OFFENSE: DISCIPLINARY ACTION BY ANOTHER STATE OR AGENCY

NOTES: DISCIPLINED BY THE ARIZONA BOARD FOR MAKING FALSE STATEMENTS ON HIS MEDICAL LICENSE RENEWAL APPLICATION.

KANSHEPOLSKY, JOSE MD, WAS DISCIPLINED BY ARIZONA ON JANUARY 23, 1992
OFFENSE: DISCIPLINARY ACTION BY ANOTHER STATE OR AGENCY

NOTES: BOARD OFFERED A STIPULATED AGREEMENT THAT DR. KANSHEPOLSKY WOULD NOT PRACTICE MEDICINE IN ARIZONA UNTIL SUCH TIME AS DISCIPLINARY ACTION PENDING IN WISCONSIN WAS RESOLVED. THE COURT HAS ORDERED THAT HIS WISCONSIN MEDICAL LICENSE BE REVOKED AS ORIGINALLY DETERMINED BY THE WISCONSIN MEDICAL BOARD. HOWEVER, HE IS APPEALING THIS DECISION. MUST MEET BEFORE THE BOARD PRIOR TO PRACTICING MEDICINE IN ARIZONA.

KANSHEPOLSKY, JOSE MD OF 10120 E. CINNABAR AVENUE, SCOTTSDALE, AZ, WAS DISCIPLINED BY DEA ON JULY 30, 1999
DISCIPLINARY ACTION: SURRENDER OF CONTROLLED SUBSTANCE LICENSE
OFFENSE: DISCIPLINARY ACTION BY ANOTHER STATE OR AGENCY

NOTES: STATE BOARD.

KASA, ROBERT MD, WAS DISCIPLINED BY ARIZONA ON MAY 19, 1999
DISCIPLINARY ACTION: PROBATION; MONITORING OF PHYSICIAN PERFORMANCE

NOTES: MUST ENTER A MONITORED AFTERCARE PROGRAM FOR SUBSTANCE ABUSE.

KAZAN, ALAN P MD OF CHANDLER, AZ, WAS DISCIPLINED BY ILLINOIS ON SEPTEMBER 1, 1990
DISCIPLINARY ACTION: 60-MONTH PROBATION
OFFENSE: DISCIPLINARY ACTION BY ANOTHER STATE OR AGENCY

NOTES: DISCIPLINED IN ARIZONA.

KAZAN, ALAN PETER MD, LICENSE NUMBER 0010092, WAS DISCIPLINED BY ARIZONA ON JANUARY 19, 1990
DISCIPLINARY ACTION: 60-MONTH PROBATION; REQUIRED TO ENTER AN IMPAIRED PHYSICIAN PROGRAM OR SUBSTANCE ABUSE TREATMENT
OFFENSE: FAILURE TO COMPLY WITH PREVIOUS BOARD ORDER

NOTES: ENTERED INTO ORDER WITH BOARD ON 4/14/89 REQUIRING THAT HE TAKE NO DRUGS OR MEDICATION NOT PRESCRIBED BY TREATING PHYSICIAN. BODILY FLUID SPECIMENS TAKEN IN 7/89 TESTED POSITIVE FOR BENZODIAZEPINES. AT MEETING IN SEPTEMBER 1989 ARIZONA BOARD DIRECTED HIM TO OBTAIN TREATMENT AT A GEORGIA TREATMENT CENTER, WHERE HE PARTICIPATED IN TREATMENT FROM 10/6/89 THROUGH 10/27/89 AND SUCCESSFULLY COMPLETED PROGRAM. CONDITIONS

OF PROBATION: MUST IMMEDIATELY PARTICIPATE IN ARIZONA MEDICAL ASSOCIATION PHYSICIAN'S HEALTH COMMITTEE PROGRAM WITH QUARTERLY REPORTS SUBMITTED TO THE BOARD; MUST OBTAIN A BOARD APPROVED TREATING PHYSICIAN; MUST ABSTAIN FROM ALCOHOL AND ANY OTHER DRUGS; MUST COMPLY WITH REQUESTS FOR RANDOM BIOLOGICAL FLUID TESTS; MUST SUBMIT TO ANY EXAMS OR THERAPY ORDERED BY BOARD; MUST PARTICIPATE IN 12-STEP AA RECOVERY PROGRAM AND ATTEND AT LEAST 4 WEEKLY MEETINGS; MUST APPEAR BEFORE BOARD FOR INTERVIEW UPON REQUEST; MUST MAINTAIN A LOG OF ALL MEDICATIONS TAKEN; MUST ADVISE BOARD OF CHANGE IN OFFICE OR HOME ADDRESSES OR IF HE PLANS TO BE AWAY FOR MORE THAN FIVE DAYS. EFFECTIVE 7/17/93 PROBATION TERMINATED DUE TO SUCCESSFUL ONGOING REHABILITATION EFFORTS.

KAZMI, MOHAMMAD A MD, LICENSE NUMBER 0018563, WAS DISCIPLINED BY ARIZONA ON JULY 20, 1995
DISCIPLINARY ACTION: MONITORING OF PHYSICIAN PERFORMANCE

NOTES: WITHIN 75 DAYS, SHALL OBTAIN THE SERVICES OF A PRACTICE MANAGEMENT CONSULTANT APPROVED BY THE BOARD REGARDING BILLING AND CODING, MEDICAL RECORD KEEPING AND SUPERVISION OF NON-LICENSED PERSONNEL.

KAZMI, MOHAMMAD A MD, LICENSE NUMBER 18563, WAS DISCIPLINED BY ARIZONA ON MAY 8, 1997
DISCIPLINARY ACTION: PROBATION
OFFENSE: FAILURE TO COMPLY WITH PREVIOUS BOARD ORDER

NOTES: AS A CONDITION OF A 7/20/95 ORDER, HE WAS TO OBTAIN THE SERVICES OF A BOARD-APPROVED PRACTICE MANAGEMENT CONSULTANT BUT INSTEAD, ENGAGED THE SERVICES OF A BILLING AND COLLECTION AGENCY TO CONDUCT A PRACTICE EVALUATION THAT WAS NOT APPROVED BY BOARD STAFF AND CONFINED ITS CONSULTATION LARGELY TO INTERNAL BILLING PRACTICES AND DID NOT ADDRESS CODING, RECORD KEEPING OR THE SUPERVISION OF NON-LICENSED PERSONNEL. WITHIN 45 DAYS, MUST UNDERGO A PRACTICE MANAGEMENT CONSULTATION BY A PRACTICE MANAGEMENT CONSULTANT APPOINTED BY THE BOARD REGARDING BILLING AND CODING, MEDICAL RECORD-KEEPING, AND SUPERVISION OF NON-LICENSED PERSONNEL; HE SHALL PAY THE COST OF THE CONSULTANT, OR CAUSE TO BE PROVIDED, A COPY OF THE CONSULTANT'S REPORT TO THE BOARD. ON 8/8/98 PROBATION TERMINATED.

KAZMI, MOHAMMAD A MD, LICENSE NUMBER A41156 OF LAKE HAVASU CITY, AZ, WAS DISCIPLINED BY CALIFORNIA ON APRIL 17, 1998
DISCIPLINARY ACTION: REPRIMAND
OFFENSE: DISCIPLINARY ACTION BY ANOTHER STATE OR AGENCY

NOTES: DISCIPLINED BY ARIZONA FOR UNPROFESSIONAL CONDUCT FOR VIOLATING A PRIOR ORDER ENTERED INTO WITH ARIZONA.

KEHLE, A PAUL MD, LICENSE NUMBER 0004239 OF PHOENIX, AZ, WAS DISCIPLINED BY ARIZONA ON JULY 13, 1994
DISCIPLINARY ACTION: RESTRICTION PLACED ON LICENSE
OFFENSE: LOSS OR RESTRICTION OF HOSPITAL PRIVILEGES

NOTES: PRIVILEGES TO SEE FHP PATIENTS AND AT CHANDLER REGIONAL HOSPITAL SUSPENDED. SHALL NOT PERFORM TERM OBSTETRICAL PROCEDURES, INCLUDING, BUT NOT LIMITED TO, VAGINAL OR CESAREAN SECTION DELIVERIES; SHALL NOT PERFORM MAJOR SURGERY, INCLUDING BUT NOT LIMITED TO, GYNECOLOGICAL SURGERY.

KELLY, JOHN D DR OF ST CHARLES, IL, WAS DISCIPLINED BY ILLINOIS ON FEBRUARY 1, 1995
DISCIPLINARY ACTION: FINE; REPRIMAND
OFFENSE: PRACTICING WITHOUT A VALID LICENSE

NOTES: PRACTICING ON A NON-RENEWED LICENSE. $1,400 FINE.

KELLY, JOHN D MD, LICENSE NUMBER 17496, WAS DISCIPLINED BY ARIZONA ON MAY 8, 1997
DISCIPLINARY ACTION: FINE; REPRIMAND
OFFENSE: DISCIPLINARY ACTION BY ANOTHER STATE OR AGENCY

NOTES: DISCIPLINED BY ILLINOIS ON 2/24/95 BECAUSE HE FAILED TO TIMELY RENEW HIS LICENSE AND PRACTICED WITHOUT A LICENSE FROM 7/31/93 TO 1/27/94; IN 11/95 LIED ON HIS RENEWAL FOR ARIZONA LICENSURE. ASSESSED A CIVIL PENALTY OF $1,000.

KENOYER, MARSHALL R MD, WAS DISCIPLINED BY ARIZONA ON SEPTEMBER 12, 1991

NOTES: BOARD DIRECTED STAFF TO TERMINATE DR. KENOYER'S STIPULATION AND ORDER; STAFF FURTHER DIRECTED TO ADVISE THE DOCTOR THAT IF HE RETURNS TO PRACTICE MEDICINE IN ARIZONA, THE BOARD WOULD LIKE TO MEET WITH HIM FIRST.

KERR, EUBULUS W MD, LICENSE NUMBER 0013357, WAS DISCIPLINED BY ARIZONA ON APRIL 6, 1995
DISCIPLINARY ACTION: LICENSE SUSPENSION
OFFENSE: LOSS OR RESTRICTION OF HOSPITAL PRIVILEGES

NOTES: HOSPITAL PRIVILEGES SUMMARILY SUSPENDED AT AN INSTITUTION, WHERE HE RESIGNED HIS PRIVILEGES BECAUSE OF HIS HEALTH. WHILE ARIZONA LICENSE IS INACTIVE: SHALL NOT PRACTICE MEDICINE ANYWHERE; MAY NOT HOLD DEA REGISTRATION OR WRITE PRESCRIPTIONS.

KHAN, MUHAMMED AZAM MD, LICENSE NUMBER 0009994 OF KINGMAN, AZ, WAS DISCIPLINED BY ARIZONA ON JANUARY 19, 1995
DISCIPLINARY ACTION: 60-MONTH PROBATION; FINE
OFFENSE: SUBSTANDARD CARE, INCOMPETENCE OR NEGLIGENCE

NOTES: GROSS OR REPEATED NEGLIGENCE IN SPECIFIED CASES INCLUDING A CASE IN 2/93 WHERE HE FAILED TO PLACE A NASO-GASTRIC TUBE PRIOR TO OR DURING SURGERY IN A PATIENT, DESPITE THE PATIENT'S ACUTE ABDOMEN AND MULTIPLE EPISODES OF VOMITING, INCLUDING MOMENTS BEFORE INDUCTION OF ANESTHESIA; PATIENT LATER DIED OF CARDIAC ARREST; IN 9/92 ORDERED AN EXCESSIVE AMOUNT OF POTASSIUM CHLORIDE AND OTHERWISE MAY HAVE INAPPROPRIATELY HANDLED A CASE REQUIRING MONITORING OF SERUM POTASSIUM LEVELS IN A PATIENT WHO LATER WAS FOUND WITH NO RESPIRATIONS, PULSE OR HEART SOUNDS; ALSO IN 9/92 PERFORMED A PROXIMAL GASTRECTOMY WITH DESPHGOGASTROSTOMY, VAGOTOMY AND PYLOROPLASTY, LEFT HEPATIC LOBECTOMY, SPLENECTOMY AND FEEDING JEJUNOSTOMY ON A PATIENT WITHOUT A PRE-OPERATIVE CT SCAN WHICH MAY HAVE AVOIDED A MAJOR SURGICAL PROCEDURE, AND POST-OPERATIVELY, HE DID NOT EVALUATE SYMPTOMS BY EITHER ULTRASOUND OR CT SCAN TO LOOK FOR CAUSE; IN 2/91 DIAGNOSED A PATIENT WITH SUSPECTED PULMONARY EMBOLISM, YET DID NOT

ADMIT TO A TELEMETRY BED; IN 5/91 FAILED TO OBTAIN LAB STUDIES AT ADMISSION FOR A PATIENT, FAILED TO OBTAIN SPUTUM FOR CULTURE AND SENSITIVITY PRIOR TO ORDERING AN ANTIBIOTIC, FAILED TO ORDER TWO MEDICATIONS PATIENT WAS ON AS AN OUTPATIENT, FAILED TO GIVE A COMPLETE DICTATED HISTORY AND PHYSICAL AND FAILED TO COMPLETE A DISCHARGE SUMMARY UNTIL A MONTH AFTER DISCHARGE; IN 3/92 OVERCHARGED A PATIENT FOR SERVICES RENDERED; IN 5/94 CHOSE AN ILL-ADVISED METHOD OF SURGERY FOR A KNEE FRACTURE THAT WAS DETRIMENTAL TO THE PATIENT AND WITHOUT BEING AN ORTHOPEDIST; PATIENT REQUIRED A SECOND SURGERY. PROBATION WITH CONDITIONS: FOR THE FIRST NINE MONTHS OF PROBATION, SHALL SUBMIT A MONTHLY REPORT OF ALL OF HIS SURGICAL CASES; BOARD SHALL SUBMIT TO THE HEALTH SERVICES ADVISORY GROUP A MINIMUM OF FIVE CASES EACH MONTH FOR COMPREHENSIVE REVIEW; SHALL EMPLOY WITHIN 30 DAYS, A BOARD-APPROVED PRACTICE MANAGEMENT CONSULTANT, WHO SHALL EVALUATE HIS CURRENT LEVEL OF PRACTICE MANAGEMENT AND SUBMIT A REPORT TO THE BOARD WITH RECOMMENDATIONS FOR IMPROVEMENT; $3,000 FINE WITHIN 90 DAYS.

KHAN, MUHAMMED AZAM MD, LICENSE NUMBER 0009994, WAS DISCIPLINED BY ARIZONA ON APRIL 4, 1995
DISCIPLINARY ACTION: FINE
OFFENSE: SUBSTANDARD CARE, INCOMPETENCE OR NEGLIGENCE

NOTES: ON 8/6/90 DURING A LAPAROSCOPIC CHOLECYSTECTOMY, THE GRASPING FORCEPS FELL OFF THE PATIENT'S GALLBLADDER AND INTO THE MORISON'S POUCH, INJURING THE PATIENT'S COLON. SEVERAL AREAS WHERE THIS PROCEDURE FELL BELOW ACCEPTED STANDARDS OF CARE: ALTHOUGH THE PROCEDURE PERFORMED ON THIS PATIENT WAS HIS THIRD DR. KHAN FAILED TO HAVE THE PROCEDURE SUPERVISED, ASSISTED OR OBSERVED BY A SURGEON EXPERIENCED IN THE PROCEDURE AND DID NOT EVALUATE THE POSSIBILITY THAT THE COLON HAD BEEN INJURED UNTIL THE FOURTH POSTOPERATIVE DAY ALTHOUGH DIFFICULTIES WERE LISTED IN HIS POSTOPERATIVE REPORT. $1000 FINE.

KHAN, MUHAMMED AZAM MD, LICENSE NUMBER 9994, WAS DISCIPLINED BY ARIZONA ON MARCH 14, 1997
DISCIPLINARY ACTION: 60-MONTH PROBATION; RESTRICTION PLACED ON LICENSE
OFFENSE: SUBSTANDARD CARE, INCOMPETENCE OR NEGLIGENCE

NOTES: RESULTS OF BOARD ORDERED REVIEW OF FILES REVEALED FOLLOWING DEFICIENCIES IN PATIENTS HE SAW BETWEEN 1/95 AND 9/95; PROVIDED SUBSTANDARD CARE TO SEVERAL PATIENTS WHICH INCLUDED: NOT GETTING RESULTS OF A TEST PRIOR TO SURGICAL INTERVENTION ON A PATIENT; CHARGING A PATIENT FOR THREE PRE-OPERATIVE HOSPITAL VISITS YET THERE IS NO DOCUMENTATION THAT THESE VISITS TOOK PLACE; PATIENT RECORDS ARE INCOMPLETE AND DISCHARGE SUMMARIES WERE NOT WRITTEN IN A TIMELY MANNER. IN SEVERAL OF THESE CASES CHARGES WERE NOT APPROPRIATE INCLUDING BILLING FOR SERVICES WHICH HE DID NOT PERFORM AS PER REQUIREMENTS AND BILLING SEPARATELY FOR PROCEDURES THAT SHOULD HAVE BEEN BILLED TOGETHER. DURING A LAPAROSCOPIC CHOLECYSTECTOMY, HE FAILED TO PERFORM AN INTRAOPERATIVE CHOLANGIOGRAM AND FILED TO BIOPSY THE PATIENT'S LIVER EVEN THOUGH IT WAS ENLARGED, FIBROTIC AND NODULAR; IN SEVERAL CASES HIS RECORDS DID NOT CONTAIN SUFFICIENT INFORMATION TO JUSTIFY PERFORMING SURGERY ON A PATIENT. CONDITIONS OF PROBATION ARE AS FOLLOWS: SHALL ENROLL IN AND SUCCESSFULLY COMPLETE A THREE MONTH MINI-RESIDENCY IN GENERAL SURGERY WITHIN SIX MONTHS; WHILE ENROLLED, SHALL PRACTICE MEDICINE ONLY IN CONNECTION WITH THE MINI-RESIDENCY; FOLLOWING SUCCESSFUL COMPLETION OF THE PROGRAM, SHALL COMPLETE ADDITIONAL DIDACTIC TRAINING ON A ONE DAY PER WEEK BASIS OVER A PERIOD OF NINE MONTHS; SHALL TAKE AND PASS THE BOARD RECERTIFICATION EXAMINATION IN GENERAL SURGERY IN ONE SITTING; AFTER THE FIRST YEAR OF PROBATION, SHALL SUBMIT TO PERIODIC OFFICE AND PRACTICE SURVEYS AT A FREQUENCY TO BE DETERMINED BY THE BOARD; MUST PAY $7,500 AS REIMBURSEMENT TOWARD EXPENSES INCURRED BY THE BOARD WITHIN 90 DAYS; THE 1/30/95 ORDER IS TERMINATED. ON 5/8/97 THIS ORDER MODIFIED.

KIM, CHRISTOPHER Y MD, WAS DISCIPLINED BY ARIZONA ON OCTOBER 14, 1993
DISCIPLINARY ACTION: RESTRICTION PLACED ON LICENSE; REQUIRED TO TAKE ADDITIONAL MEDICAL EDUCATION

NOTES: SHALL COMPLETE 160 CREDIT HOURS OF CONTINUING MEDICAL EDUCATION IN GYNECOLOGY AND/OR INFERTILITY WITHIN TWO YEARS AND SHALL PROVIDE THE BOARD WITH SATISFACTORY EVIDENCE OF COMPLETION; SHALL NOTIFY THE BOARD IN WRITING IF HE INTENDS TO PRACTICE OBSTETRICS IN ARIZONA; SHALL AT ALL TIMES HAVE A FEMALE ATTENDANT PRESENT WHEN HE EXAMINES FEMALE PATIENTS.

KINCAID, JOSEPH P MD, WAS DISCIPLINED BY ARIZONA ON DECEMBER 10, 1991
DISCIPLINARY ACTION: REQUIRED TO ENTER AN IMPAIRED PHYSICIAN PROGRAM OR SUBSTANCE ABUSE TREATMENT; MONITORING OF PHYSICIAN PERFORMANCE
OFFENSE: SUBSTANCE ABUSE

NOTES: VOLUNTARILY ENTERED A TREATMENT PROGRAM FOR ALCOHOL ABUSE. MUST IMMEDIATELY PARTICIPATE IN A BOARD-APPROVED MONITORED AFTERCARE TREATMENT PROGRAM WHOSE THERAPIST MUST SUBMIT QUARTERLY REPORTS; MUST PARTICIPATE IN 90 12-STEP MEETINGS FOR SUBSTANCE ABUSE WITHIN 90 DAYS; MUST THEN PARTICIPATE IN A 12-STEP RECOVERY PROGRAM AS DETERMINED BY HIS TREATING THERAPIST AND ATTEND AT LEAST THREE WEEKLY MEETINGS; SHALL OBTAIN A BOARD-APPROVED TREATING PHYSICIAN; SHALL ABSTAIN COMPLETELY FROM THE CONSUMPTION OF ALCOHOLIC BEVERAGES AND DRUGS EXCEPT WHEN PRESCRIBED BY HIS TREATING PHYSICIAN; MUST SUBMIT TO WITNESSED RANDOM BIOLOGICAL FLUID COLLECTION; KEEP A LOG OF ANY AND ALL MEDICATIONS PRESCRIBED FOR HIM; SHALL SUBMIT TO ANY EXAMINATIONS OR THERAPY ORDERED BY BOARD; SHALL APPEAR BEFORE BOARD FOR INTERVIEWS UPON REQUEST; SHALL INFORM BOARD OF CHANGE OF ADDRESS OR IF AWAY FOR MORE THAN 5 DAYS. ORDER TERMINATED ON 4/16/96.

KINCAID, JOSEPH P MD, WAS DISCIPLINED BY WASHINGTON ON JULY 13, 1992
DISCIPLINARY ACTION: RESTRICTION PLACED ON LICENSE

NOTES: CONDITIONAL LICENSE ISSUED WITH SPECIFIC CONDITIONS.

KING, KEITH M MD, DATE OF BIRTH JANUARY 29, 1945, LICENSE NUMBER 0021831, WAS DISCIPLINED BY KENTUCKY ON JANUARY 25, 1990
DISCIPLINARY ACTION: LICENSE REVOCATION
OFFENSE: DISCIPLINARY ACTION BY ANOTHER STATE OR AGENCY

NOTES: BASED ON DISCIPLINARY ACTION TAKEN BY HIGHLANDS REGIONAL HOSPITAL, PRESTONSBURG KENTUCKY AND THE ARIZONA BOARD OF MEDICAL EXAMINERS; CASE BEING APPEALED IN JEFFERSON CIRCUIT COURT AS OF MARCH 1, 1990 .

KING, KEITH M MD, DATE OF BIRTH JANUARY 29, 1945 OF 6530 WEST GLENROSA, PHOENIX, AZ, WAS DISCIPLINED BY MEDICARE ON AUGUST 1, 1990
DISCIPLINARY ACTION: EXCLUSION FROM THE MEDICARE AND/OR MEDICAID PROGRAM
OFFENSE: DISCIPLINARY ACTION BY ANOTHER STATE OR AGENCY

NOTES: LICENSE REVOCATION OR SUSPENSION. NO LONGER LISTED AS EXCLUDED AS OF 9/30/92.

KING, KEITH M MD, DATE OF BIRTH JANUARY 29, 1945, LICENSE NUMBER 0012299, WAS DISCIPLINED BY ARIZONA ON APRIL 12, 1991
DISCIPLINARY ACTION: 12-MONTH MONITORING OF PHYSICIAN PERFORMANCE
OFFENSE: DISCIPLINARY ACTION BY ANOTHER STATE OR AGENCY

NOTES: LICENSE IN ILLINOIS WAS INDEFINITELY SUSPENDED BASED ON ARIZONA'S 1986 DECREE OF CENSURE; KENTUCKY ORDERED HIM TO UNDERGO PSYCHIATRIC AND PSYCHOMETRIC EXAMS AS A RESULT OF SUSPENSION OF HOSPITAL PRIVILEGES FOR REPEATED VIOLATIONS OF HOSPITAL RULES AND REGULATIONS; INFORMATION RECEIVED THAT HE MAY BE ABUSING DRUGS AND/OR ALCOHOL. THIS ORDER DOES NOT CONSTITUTE THE FINAL DISPOSITION OF THE BOARD'S INQUIRY INTO THE KENTUCKY ORDER OF 1/25/90 REVOKING HIS LICENSE, PENDING APPEAL. MUST OBTAIN A SOLE TREATING PHYSICIAN ACCEPTABLE TO THE BOARD; SHALL ABSTAIN FROM THE CONSUMPTION OF ALCOHOL AND ALL OTHER DRUGS; SHALL COMPLY WITH REQUESTS FOR RANDOM BIOLOGICAL FLUID TESTING; SHALL PROVIDE A MONTHLY SCHEDULE OF HIS MEDICAL PRACTICE; SHALL SUBMIT TO MENTAL, PHYSICAL OR MEDICAL COMPETENCY EXAMS REQUESTED BY BOARD; MUST APPEAR IN PERSON BEFORE BOARD UPON REQUEST; MUST ADVISE THE BOARD OF ANY CHANGE OF ADDRESS OR IF HE PLANS TO BE AWAY FOR MORE THAN FIVE DAYS.

KING, KEITH M MD, DATE OF BIRTH JANUARY 29, 1945, LICENSE NUMBER 0021831 OF PHOENIX, AZ, WAS DISCIPLINED BY KENTUCKY ON AUGUST 1, 1991
DISCIPLINARY ACTION: 60-MONTH PROBATION

NOTES: IF HE REACTIVATES HIS KENTUCKY MEDICAL LICENSE, AGREED ORDER WILL PLACE LICENSE ON PROBATION FOR A PERIOD OF FIVE YEARS.

KING, KEITH M MD, DATE OF BIRTH JANUARY 29, 1945, LICENSE NUMBER 0012299, WAS DISCIPLINED BY ARIZONA ON APRIL 9, 1992
DISCIPLINARY ACTION: MONITORING OF PHYSICIAN PERFORMANCE

NOTES: SHALL RETAIN AND MAINTAIN A PSYCHIATRIST ACCEPTABLE TO THE BOARD AND SHALL DIRECT HIS PSYCHIATRIST TO PROVIDE REPORTS TO THE BOARD; SHALL COMPLY WITH REQUESTS FROM THE BOARD TO SUBMIT TO WITNESSED RANDOM BIOLOGICAL FLUID TESTS; SHALL SUBMIT TO MENTAL OR PHYSICAL EXAMINATIONS AT SUCH TIMES AND UNDER SUCH CONDITIONS AS DIRECTED BY THE BOARD TO ASSIST THE BOARD IN MONITORING HIS ABILITY TO SAFELY ENGAGE IN THE PRACTICE OF MEDICINE; SHALL IMMEDIATELY ADVISE THE BOARD OF ANY CHANGE IN ADDRESS OR IF AWAY FOR MORE THAN FIVE DAYS. THIS ORDER WILL REMAIN IN FORCE FOR A TWO YEAR PERIOD UNLESS EARLIER TERMINATED BY THE BOARD. EFFECTIVE 10/16/93, ORDER TERMINATED DUE TO SUCCESSFUL REHABILITATION EFFORTS.

KING, KEITH M MD, DATE OF BIRTH JANUARY 29, 1945, LICENSE NUMBER 0012299 OF PHOENIX, AZ, WAS DISCIPLINED BY ARIZONA ON JANUARY 17, 1995
DISCIPLINARY ACTION: RESTRICTION PLACED ON LICENSE

NOTES: SHALL LIMIT HIS PRACTICE TO ADMINISTRATIVE DUTIES AND BLOOD BANKING DUTIES UNTIL HE MEETS WITH BOARD TO RESOLVE INVESTIGATION. BOARD HAD INFORMATION THAT THE GOVERNING BODY OF INDIAN HEALTH SERVICES WAS REQUESTED TO REVOKE THE DOCTOR'S PRIVILEGES.

KING, KELLY S MD, WAS DISCIPLINED BY ARIZONA ON NOVEMBER 21, 1998

NOTES: UNSPECIFIED INTERIM STIPULATION. SHALL NOT PRACTICE UNTIL MEETING WITH THE BOARD AND RECEIVING AUTHORIZATION TO DO SO.

KLIEWER, PAUL MD, LICENSE NUMBER 2914, WAS DISCIPLINED BY ARIZONA ON NOVEMBER 17, 1999
DISCIPLINARY ACTION: REPRIMAND
OFFENSE: SUBSTANDARD CARE, INCOMPETENCE OR NEGLIGENCE

NOTES: FAILURE TO DIAGNOSE AND TREAT A MYOCARDIAL INFARCTION.

KNIGHT, PATRICK L MD, LICENSE NUMBER 00E7638 OF PHOENIX, AZ, WAS DISCIPLINED BY TEXAS ON AUGUST 18, 1990
OFFENSE: DISCIPLINARY ACTION BY ANOTHER STATE OR AGENCY

NOTES: STIPULATED ORDER. MUST COMPLY WITH ARIZONA BOARD ORDER, OBTAIN PERMISSION OF BOARD BEFORE PRACTICING IN TEXAS, AND FOLLOW SUCH TERM AS MAY BE IMPOSED.

KOERPEL, BARRY J MD, LICENSE NUMBER 0008981, WAS DISCIPLINED BY ARIZONA ON OCTOBER 17, 1995
DISCIPLINARY ACTION: RESTRICTION PLACED ON LICENSE; REQUIRED TO TAKE ADDITIONAL MEDICAL EDUCATION
OFFENSE: DISCIPLINARY ACTION BY ANOTHER STATE OR AGENCY

NOTES: KNOWINGLY MADE FALSE OR FRAUDULENT STATEMENTS IN CONNECTION WITH APPLICATION FOR HOSPITAL PRIVILEGES IN THAT WHEN APPLYING FOR PRIVILEGES AT AN ARIZONA HOSPITAL IN 10/93. HE FAILED TO REPORT ACTION BY THE BOARD OF A UTAH HOSPITAL INITIATED IN 10/83 THAT INCLUDED A LETTER SENT IN 12/84 FOR INADEQUATE RESPONSE TIME, PROVIDING INADEQUATE CALL COVERAGE, POOR COMMUNICATION WITH COLLEAGUES AND FAILURE TO MAKE ROUNDS ON SIGNIFICANTLY ILL PATIENTS; ANOTHER SUSPENSION IN 4/86 FOR POOR RECORDKEEPING; AND ANOTHER LETTER IN 11/86 REGARDING INADEQUATE RESPONSE TIMES TO CRITICALLY ILL PATIENTS; DENIED THAT HIS LICENSE HAD EVER BEEN SUSPENDED, MODIFIED OR TERMINATED DESPITE 6/84 PROBATION BY UTAH BOARD FOR UNPROFESSIONAL CONDUCT INCLUDING THAT IN 1981 AND 1982, CONTINUED TO TREAT FOUR PATIENTS ON CHRONIC DIALYSIS TREATMENT WHEN SUCH TREATMENT WAS CONTRARY TO MEDICAL STANDARDS; PERMITTED SEVEN PATIENTS TO CONTINUE DIALYSIS TREATMENTS AFTER THEY WERE

NOTES: NO LONGER MEDICALLY NECESSARY; INITIATED UNNECESSARY DIALYSIS TREATMENT ON ONE PATIENT; AND ALLOWED 10 PATIENTS TO RECEIVE INADEQUATE AND SUBSTANDARD DIALYSIS TREATMENTS; UTAH PROBATION TERMINATED ON 5/26/87. IN 4/85, HE WAS EXCLUDED FROM THE MEDICARE PROGRAM FOR 10 YEARS BY THE DEPARTMENT OF HEALTH AND HUMAN SERVICES FOR FURNISHING SERVICES FOUND TO BE IN EXCESS OF THE NEEDS OF HIS PATIENTS AND FURNISHING CARE WHICH DOES NOT MEET PROFESSIONALLY RECOGNIZED STANDARDS OF HEALTH CARE; TWO YEARS AFTER AN UNSUCCESSFUL APPEAL, REQUESTED REINSTATEMENT AS A MEDICARE PROVIDER WHICH WAS APPROVED ON 4/25/89; HAS NOT PRACTICED CLINICAL MEDICINE SINCE 1989. SHALL NOT PRACTICE CLINICAL MEDICINE IN ARIZONA UNTIL HE SUCCESSFULLY COMPLETES A BOARD-APPROVED ONE YEAR TRAINING EXPERIENCE; CENSURED.

KOERPEL, BARRY JON MD OF HAYWARD, WI, WAS DISCIPLINED BY UTAH ON JUNE 18, 1996
DISCIPLINARY ACTION: LICENSE SUSPENSION
OFFENSE: DISCIPLINARY ACTION BY ANOTHER STATE OR AGENCY

NOTES: DISCIPLINARY ACTION TAKEN AGAINST HIS LICENSE TO PRACTICE MEDICINE IN ARIZONA. UTAH MEDICAL LICENSE SUSPENDED DURING ARIZONA RESTRICTION PERIOD. HE HAS CONDITIONS TO BE MET DURING THE PERIOD OF SUSPENSION.

KOGIANES, MICHAEL G MD, LICENSE NUMBER 0014597, WAS DISCIPLINED BY ARIZONA ON AUGUST 17, 1990
DISCIPLINARY ACTION: REQUIRED TO TAKE ADDITIONAL MEDICAL EDUCATION

NOTES: SHALL COMPLETE 40 HOURS OF CONTINUING MEDICAL EDUCATION IN OBSTETRICS AND GYNECOLOGY BY THE END OF 1990 AND AGAIN IN 1991

KOGIANES, MICHAEL G MD, LICENSE NUMBER 0014597, WAS DISCIPLINED BY ARIZONA ON JANUARY 26, 1991
DISCIPLINARY ACTION: PROBATION; RESTRICTION PLACED ON LICENSE
OFFENSE: PROFESSIONAL MISCONDUCT

NOTES: ACTION BASED ON UNPROFESSIONAL CONDUCT. PLACED ON PERMANENT PROBATION AND IS PERMANENTLY RESTRICTED FROM AND SHALL NOT ENGAGE IN ANY OBSTETRICAL PRACTICE OF MEDICINE INCLUDING ALL ASPECTS OF DIAGNOSIS, TREATMENT OR SURGERY ASSOCIATED THEREWITH. FURTHER RESTRICTIONS ARE AS FOLLOWS: SHALL NOTIFY ALL CURRENT OBSTETRICAL PATIENTS THAT ARE NOT MORE THAN TWENTY-EIGHT WEEKS OF GESTATION IN THEIR PREGNANCY OF THE TERMINATION OF HIS OBSTETRICAL MEDICAL SERVICES TO BE EFFECTIVE 30 DAYS FROM THE DATE OF THIS ORDER; MAY ONLY CONTINUE TO PROVIDE OBSTETRICAL SERVICES TO HIS CURRENT PATIENTS THAT ARE BEYOND 28 WEEKS AND WHO GIVE THEIR EXPRESS WRITTEN CONSENT; MAY PROVIDE EMERGENCY OBSTETRICAL CARE IF THE PATIENT IS HOSPITALIZED OR BEING TREATED AT A HOSPITAL EMERGENCY ROOM; MAY ENGAGE IN THE GYNECOLOGICAL PRACTICE OF MEDICINE SUBJECT TO RESTRICTIONS FOR A MINIMUM OF TWO YEARS. MUST SUBMIT TO SUPERVISED REVIEW OF PRACTICE; SHALL TAKE IN ARIZONA PRIOR TO 6/30/91, AND PASS, THE SPECIAL PURPOSE LICENSING EXAMINATION (SPEX); FAILURE TO PASS THIS EXAM SHALL CONSTITUTE GROUNDS FOR SUMMARY SUSPENSION WITHOUT NOTICE AND HEARING.

KOGIANES, MICHAEL G MD, LICENSE NUMBER 0014597, WAS DISCIPLINED BY ARIZONA ON AUGUST 24, 1991
DISCIPLINARY ACTION: LICENSE SUSPENSION
OFFENSE: FAILURE TO COMPLY WITH PREVIOUS BOARD ORDER

NOTES: FAILURE TO MEET THE CONDITIONS OF THE BOARD ORDER OF 1/26/91 IN THAT HE DID NOT PASS THE SPEX EXAM. LICENSE SHALL REMAIN SUSPENDED UNTIL THE BOARD ORDERS IT TERMINATED PURSUANT TO THE 1/26/91 ORDER. ON 7/15/92 THE BOARD ACCEPTED A MINI-RESIDENCY PROGRAM AT THE UNIVERSITY OF ARIZONA IN FAMILY PRACTICE, PEDIATRICS, INTERNAL MEDICINE, AND GYNECOLOGY/UROLOGY (ORIGINALLY REJECTED THIS PROPOSAL ON 6/20/92) IN LIEU OF THE CURRENT STIPULATED ORDER REQUIRING HIM TO PARTICIPATE IN A ONE YEAR RESIDENCY PROGRAM FOLLOWING HIS FAILURE OF THE SPEX EXAM.

KOGIANES, MICHAEL G MD, LICENSE NUMBER 0014597, WAS DISCIPLINED BY ARIZONA ON APRIL 4, 1995
DISCIPLINARY ACTION: LICENSE REVOCATION
OFFENSE: CRIMINAL CONVICTION OR PLEA OF GUILTY, NOLO CONTENDERE, OR NO CONTEST TO A CRIME

NOTES: ON 2/9/94, FOUND GUILTY OF TWO COUNTS OF FIRST DEGREE MURDER IN THE DEATHS OF HIS ESTRANGED WIFE AND HER BOYFRIEND AND ON 3/9/94, SENTENCED TO TWO CONCURRENT LIFE SENTENCES.

KOPPULA, SAMPURNARAO MD, LICENSE NUMBER 0013707, WAS DISCIPLINED BY ARIZONA ON JANUARY 22, 1992
DISCIPLINARY ACTION: REQUIRED TO ENTER AN IMPAIRED PHYSICIAN PROGRAM OR SUBSTANCE ABUSE TREATMENT; MONITORING OF PHYSICIAN PERFORMANCE
OFFENSE: SUBSTANCE ABUSE

NOTES: ALLEGATIONS OF ALCOHOL MISUSE. MUST IMMEDIATELY PARTICIPATE IN A BOARD-APPROVED MONITORED AFTERCARE TREATMENT PROGRAM WHOSE THERAPIST MUST SUBMIT QUARTERLY REPORTS; MUST PARTICIPATE IN 90 12-STEP MEETINGS FOR SUBSTANCE ABUSE WITHIN 90 DAYS; MUST THEN PARTICIPATE IN A 12-STEP RECOVERY PROGRAM AS DETERMINED BY HIS TREATING THERAPIST AND ATTEND AT LEAST 3 WEEKLY MEETINGS; SHALL OBTAIN A BOARD-APPROVED TREATING PHYSICIAN; SHALL ABSTAIN COMPLETELY FROM THE CONSUMPTION OF ALCOHOLIC BEVERAGES AND DRUGS EXCEPT WHEN PRESCRIBED BY TREATING PHYSICIAN; MUST SUBMIT TO WITNESSED RANDOM BIOLOGICAL FLUID COLLECTION; KEEP A LOG OF ANY AND ALL MEDICATIONS PRESCRIBED TO DR. KOPPULA; SHALL SUBMIT TO ANY EXAMINATIONS OR THERAPY ORDERED BY BOARD; SHALL APPEAR BEFORE BOARD FOR INTERVIEWS UPON REQUEST; SHALL INFORM BOARD OF CHANGE OF ADDRESS OR IF AWAY FOR MORE THAN 5 DAYS. ON 1/29/94 ORDER TERMINATED AFTER 90 DAYS.

KOSIOREK, J ROBERT MD, LICENSE NUMBER 7500 OF 4145 E. GRANDVIEW CIRCLE, MESA, AZ, WAS DISCIPLINED BY HAWAII ON FEBRUARY 13, 1998
DISCIPLINARY ACTION: FINE

NOTES: $500 FINE.

KOSIOREK, JOHN R MD OF 30 W CARTER DR #15206, TEMPE, AZ, WAS DISCIPLINED BY VERMONT ON JULY 24, 1991

DISCIPLINARY ACTION: DENIAL OF NEW LICENSE
OFFENSE: NONCOMPLIANCE WITH A PROFESSIONAL RULE

NOTES: HAS NOT PASSED BOTH PARTS OF FLEX EXAM AS REQUIRED.

KOSIOREK, JOHN R MD, LICENSE NUMBER 0020136, WAS DISCIPLINED BY ARIZONA ON APRIL 17, 1996
DISCIPLINARY ACTION: FINE
OFFENSE: PROVIDING FALSE INFORMATION TO THE BOARD OR OTHER HEALTH AGENCY

NOTES: KNOWINGLY MADE FALSE STATEMENT ON RENEWAL APPLICATION IN THAT IN RENEWAL APPLICATION FOR LICENSE IN 11/91, ANSWERED "NO" TO A QUESTION REGARDING PREVIOUS DISCIPLINARY ACTION AGAINST HIS LICENSE, DESPITE HAVING HIS APPLICATION FOR LICENSURE DENIED BY THE VERMONT BOARD IN 6/91; ENGAGED IN CONDUCT WHICH IS OR MIGHT BE HARMFUL TO THE HEALTH OF A PATIENT IN THAT IN 10/94, IN TREATING AN EIGHT YEAR OLD BOY FOR A WART ON HIS HAND, FAILED TO EXPLAIN PROCEDURE TO THE BOY OR HIS MOTHER AND SPRAYED WART WITH LIQUID NITROGEN; MOTHER REFUSED FURTHER NITROGEN TREATMENT FOR BOY; THE NEXT DAY, BOY WAS UNABLE TO MOVE HIS HAND AND WAS EXAMINED IN THE EMERGENCY ROOM THREE DAYS AFTER THE PROCEDURE FOR A 2-3 CM BLISTER IN THE PREVIOUS LOCATION OF THE WART; IN 11/94 AND 6/95, INFORMED BOARD THAT HE HAD APPLIED NITROGEN WITH A COTTON SWAB AND DENIED HAVING USED A SPRAY; IN 2/95, BOARD INVESTIGATOR VISITED HIS OFFICE AND INSPECTED THE SPRAY CANISTER USED AT THE TIME OF THE BOY'S TREATMENT WHICH COULD ONLY HAVE BEEN USED AS A SPRAY; MEDICAL RECORD REQUESTED BY BOY'S MOTHER WAS BRIEF, MAKING NO MENTION OF TREATMENT OF THE WART; WHEN REQUESTED RECORDS WERE SUBMITTED TO THE BOARD IN 11/94 IT WAS A DIFFERENT MEDICAL RECORD THAN HE HAD GIVEN MOTHER WHICH WAS LONGER, DESCRIBED THE WART PROCEDURE IN DETAIL AND WAS WRITTEN IN A DIFFERENT HANDWRITING; VIOLATED RULES AND REGULATIONS APPLICABLE TO THE PRACTICE OF MEDICINE IN THAT THE RECORDS WERE EXAMINED AND IT WAS DETERMINED THAT HE HAD GIVEN THE BOY'S MOTHER THE ORIGINAL RECORDS AND HAD MANUFACTURED THE REPORT FOR THE BOARD. CENSURED; $5,000 FINE.

KOTLER, EVERETT G MD, DATE OF BIRTH APRIL 1, 1932, LICENSE NUMBER 0018793 OF 616 DAWES HIGHWAY, POMPTON LAKES, NJ, WAS DISCIPLINED BY NEW JERSEY ON FEBRUARY 18, 1994
DISCIPLINARY ACTION: REPRIMAND
OFFENSE: OVERPRESCRIBING OR MISPRESCRIBING DRUGS

NOTES: PRESCRIBED SYMPATHOMIMETIC AMINES TO A PATIENT, FAILING TO MAINTAIN THOROUGH AND ADEQUATE PATIENT RECORDS AND FAILING TO MONITOR PATIENTS BY MEANS OF LABORATORY TESTING. MAY CONTINUE TO PRESCRIBE OR DISPENSE SYMPATHOMIMETIC AMINES FOR HIS PATIENTS FOR WEIGHT LOSS OR WEIGHT CONTROL, PROVIDED THAT HE COMPLIES WITH THE RESTRICTIONS AND LIMITATIONS SPECIFIED IN THIS ORDER.

KOTLER, EVERETT G MD, DATE OF BIRTH APRIL 1, 1932, LICENSE NUMBER 0D06560 OF 616 DAWES HIGHWAY, POMPTON LAKES, NJ, WAS DISCIPLINED BY MARYLAND ON DECEMBER 20, 1994
DISCIPLINARY ACTION: REPRIMAND
OFFENSE: DISCIPLINARY ACTION BY ANOTHER STATE OR AGENCY

NOTES: RECIPROCAL ACTION BASED ON A NEW JERSEY ORDER ISSUED DUE TO HIS PRESCRIBING PRACTICES. MUST COMPLY WITH ALL TERMS AND CONDITIONS OF NEW JERSEY ORDER OF 2/9/94; MUST OBTAIN APPROVAL OF THE MARYLAND BOARD BEFORE PRACTICING IN MARYLAND.

KOTLER, EVERETT G MD, DATE OF BIRTH APRIL 1, 1932, LICENSE NUMBER 0D06560 OF 616 DAWES HIGHWAY, POMPTON LAKES, NJ, WAS DISCIPLINED BY MARYLAND ON FEBRUARY 21, 1995
OFFENSE: DISCIPLINARY ACTION BY ANOTHER STATE OR AGENCY

NOTES: PRACTICES AND RESIDES IN NEW JERSEY; THE NEW JERSEY BOARD CONTINUES TO MONITOR HIS PRESCRIBING FOR WEIGHT LOSS OR WEIGHT CONTROL. GRANTED AN INACTIVE LICENSE. HE SHALL NOT PRACTICE MEDICINE IN MARYLAND UNTIL HE APPEARS BEFORE THE BOARD. PROBATION IMPOSED ON 12/20/94 IS TOLLED UNTIL LICENSE IS REINSTATED. (HELD IN ABEYANCE).

KOTLER, EVERETT G MD, DATE OF BIRTH APRIL 1, 1932, LICENSE NUMBER 0005670, WAS DISCIPLINED BY ARIZONA ON JULY 22, 1995
DISCIPLINARY ACTION: PROBATION; RESTRICTION PLACED ON CONTROLLED SUBSTANCE LICENSE
OFFENSE: DISCIPLINARY ACTION BY ANOTHER STATE OR AGENCY

NOTES: DISCIPLINED BY NEW JERSEY IN 2/94; PRESCRIBED, DISPENSED OR ADMINISTERED ANY CONTROLLED SUBSTANCE OR PRESCRIPTION-ONLY DRUG FOR OTHER THAN ACCEPTED THERAPEUTIC PURPOSES IN THAT HE HAS BEEN ENGAGED IN A PRACTICE OF PRESCRIBING AND DISPENSING LARGE QUANTITIES OF SCHEDULE III AND SCHEDULE IV CONTROLLED DANGEROUS SUBSTANCES OVER EXTENDED PERIODS OF TIME TO PATIENTS OF HIS WEIGHT CONTROL PRACTICE; NEW JERSEY BOARD HAS HAD ONGOING CONCERNS ABOUT HIS POOR RECORD KEEPING, THE ABSENCE OF ADEQUATE LABORATORY TESTING AND THE LARGE QUANTITY OF DRUGS DISPENSED TO PATIENTS, MANY OF WHOM HAD NO APPRECIABLE WEIGHT LOSS AFTER SEVERAL YEARS; MANY CHARTS REVIEWED BY THE NEW JERSEY BOARD LACKED LABORATORY TESTS, HISTORIES AND PHYSICALS, AND VITAL SIGNS, PARTICULARLY HEART RATE; IN 1987, NEW JERSEY BOARD EVALUATED HIS DISPENSING OF PHENTERMINE TO A PATIENT WITH HYPERTENSION BETWEEN 1979 AND 1987 AND CONCLUDED THAT HE FAILED TO MAINTAIN A THOROUGH PATIENT RECORD, FAILED TO PERFORM NECESSARY AND APPROPRIATE TESTS AND INAPPROPRIATELY DISPENSED PHENTERMINE IN LIGHT OF THE PATIENT'S HYPERTENSION. CENSURED BY ARIZONA. INDEFINITE PROBATION WITH CONDITIONS: MAY NOT PRESCRIBE OR DISTRIBUTE MORE THAN A ONE-WEEK SUPPLY OF CONTROLLED DANGEROUS SUBSTANCES IN CONNECTION WITH A WEIGHT LOSS OR WEIGHT CONTROL PROGRAM TO ANY PATIENT WITHOUT HAVING REVIEWED THE RESULTS OF CURRENT BLOOD TESTING; IF HE CONTINUES TO PRESCRIBE DRUGS TO THAT PATIENT, BLOOD TESTING MUST BE REPEATED AT LEAST ONCE EVERY NINE MONTHS; COPIES OF ALL LABORATORY REPORTS MUST BE MAINTAINED IN PATIENT'S CHART; MAY NOT PRESCRIBE OR DISTRIBUTE CONTROLLED SUBSTANCES TO ANY PATIENT UNLESS PATIENT IS AT LEAST 20 PERCENT OVERWEIGHT, OR PROVES THAT HE OR SHE IS CURRENTLY TAKING APPETITE SUPPRESSANT MEDICATIONS PRESCRIBED OR DISPENSED BY ANOTHER PHYSICIAN AND IS NOT UNDERWEIGHT; LABELS ON ANY MEDICATIONS DISPENSED MUST CLEARLY CONTAIN ALL INFORMATION REQUIRED; PATIENT RECORDS MUST LEGIBLY INDICATE FOR EACH VISIT THAT A PHYSICAL

EXAMINATION WAS CONDUCTED; MAY NOT DISPENSE OR PRESCRIBE MORE THAN A 30 DAY SUPPLY OF ANY CONTROLLED DANGEROUS SUBSTANCE. SHALL NOT PRESCRIBE OR DISPENSE SYMPATHOMIMETIC AMINES TO ANY HYPERTENSIVE PATIENT; SHALL NOT PRACTICE MEDICINE IN ARIZONA UNTIL HE HAS INFORMED THE BOARD OF HIS INTENTION TO DO SO, APPEARED AT AN INTERVIEW WITH THE BOARD AND RECEIVED AUTHORIZATION BY THE BOARD TO PRACTICE.

KRAMOLC, NICHOLAS I MD, LICENSE NUMBER 0009553, WAS DISCIPLINED BY ARIZONA ON APRIL 18, 1996
DISCIPLINARY ACTION: RESTRICTION PLACED ON LICENSE
OFFENSE: SEXUAL ABUSE OF OR SEXUAL MISCONDUCT WITH A PATIENT

NOTES: INTERVIEWED BY THE BOARD REGARDING ALLEGED INAPPROPRIATE SEXUAL REMARKS HE MADE TO A PATIENT. SHALL PERFORM NO PELVIC EXAMS WITHOUT THE PRESENCE OF A FEMALE CHAPERONE, WHO SHALL DOCUMENT HER PRESENCE DURING THE EXAMINATION IN THE PATIENT'S CHART.

KRASNER, BERNARD MD, LICENSE NUMBER 0023691 OF SCOTTSDALE, AZ, WAS DISCIPLINED BY FLORIDA ON FEBRUARY 6, 1990
DISCIPLINARY ACTION: SURRENDER OF LICENSE
OFFENSE: SUBSTANDARD CARE, INCOMPETENCE OR NEGLIGENCE

NOTES: CHARGED WITH FAILURE TO PRACTICE WITH AN ACCEPTABLE LEVEL OF CARE AND SKILL; FAILING TO KEEP WRITTEN MEDICAL RECORDS JUSTIFYING THE COURSE OF TREATMENT OF A PATIENT. AGREES TO NEVER AGAIN APPLY FOR LICENSURE IN FLORIDA TO AVOID THE NECESSITY OF FURTHER ADMINISTRATIVE ACTION.

KRASNER, BERNARD MD, LICENSE NUMBER 00G2470 OF SCOTTSDALE, AZ, WAS DISCIPLINED BY CALIFORNIA ON JUNE 18, 1993
DISCIPLINARY ACTION: SURRENDER OF LICENSE

NOTES: VOLUNTARY SURRENDER WHILE CHARGES PENDING.

KREMPEN, JOHN MD OF 1712 W. ANKLAM RD. #101, TUCSON, AZ, WAS DISCIPLINED BY DEA ON OCTOBER 5, 1999
DISCIPLINARY ACTION: SURRENDER OF CONTROLLED SUBSTANCE LICENSE
OFFENSE: DISCIPLINARY ACTION BY ANOTHER STATE OR AGENCY

NOTES: STATE BOARD.

KREUZER, FREDERICK A MD, LICENSE NUMBER 0008375 OF TUCSON, AZ, WAS DISCIPLINED BY ARIZONA ON APRIL 6, 1990
DISCIPLINARY ACTION: REQUIRED TO ENTER AN IMPAIRED PHYSICIAN PROGRAM OR SUBSTANCE ABUSE TREATMENT; MONITORING OF PHYSICIAN PERFORMANCE
OFFENSE: SUBSTANCE ABUSE

NOTES: MUST IMMEDIATELY PARTICIPATE IN THE ARIZONA MEDICAL ASSOCIATION PHYSICIAN'S HEALTH COMMITTEE PROGRAM WITH QUARTERLY REPORTS TO THE BOARD; MUST OBTAIN A BOARD APPROVED TREATING PHYSICIAN; MUST ABSTAIN FROM ALCOHOL AND ALL OTHER DRUGS; MUST COMPLY WITH REQUESTS FOR RANDOM BIOLOGICAL FLUID TESTS; MUST SUBMIT TO ANY EXAMS OR THERAPY ORDERED BY BOARD; MUST PARTICIPATE IN 12-STEP RECOVERY PROGRAM FOR SUBSTANCE ABUSE AS DETERMINED BY THERAPIST AND ATTEND AT LEAST 3 WEEKLY MEETINGS; MUST APPEAR BEFORE BOARD FOR INTERVIEWS UPON REQUEST; MUST NOTIFY THE BOARD OF CHANGE IN OFFICE OR HOME ADDRESSES AND IF PLANS TO BE AWAY FOR MORE THAN FIVE DAYS; MUST MAINTAIN A LOG OF ALL MEDICATIONS TAKEN. ON 1/20/93 BOARD ORDERED THAT THIS ORDER BE TERMINATED IN 90 DAYS BECAUSE HE HAS SATISFACTORILY DEMONSTRATED HIS COMMITMENT TO RECOVERY SO FORMAL MONITORING IS NO LONGER NEEDED.

KROFT, VADEE MD, LICENSE NUMBER 0008662, WAS DISCIPLINED BY ARIZONA ON JANUARY 26, 1994
DISCIPLINARY ACTION: LICENSE REVOCATION
OFFENSE: CRIMINAL CONVICTION OR PLEA OF GUILTY, NOLO CONTENDERE, OR NO CONTEST TO A CRIME

NOTES: CONVICTED OF CONSPIRACY TO POSSESS WITH INTENT TO DISTRIBUTE MARIJUANA. SENTENCED TO 30 MONTHS IMPRISONMENT, FINED $20,000 AND ORDERED UPON RELEASE TO SERVE A 48 MONTH TERM OF SUPERVISED RELEASE, PARTICIPATE IN MENTAL HEALTH COUNSELING AS DESIGNATED AND CONTRIBUTE 300 HOURS OF COMMUNITY WORK.

KRONEN, FREDERICK LLOYD MD, LICENSE NUMBER G51034 OF FLAGSTAFF, AZ, WAS DISCIPLINED BY CALIFORNIA ON NOVEMBER 23, 1999
DISCIPLINARY ACTION: REPRIMAND

KUMAR, RAJIV MD, LICENSE NUMBER 15116, WAS DISCIPLINED BY ARIZONA ON MARCH 15, 1997
DISCIPLINARY ACTION: FINE; REPRIMAND
OFFENSE: PROFESSIONAL MISCONDUCT

NOTES: FOR A PATIENT HE TREATED FOR DEPRESSION IN 2/91, HE BILLED TWICE FOR PROVIDING FAMILY MEDICAL PSYCHOTHERAPY WHEN HE DID NOT PROVIDE IT, AND FIVE TIMES WHEN HIS MEDICAL RECORDS ON A PATIENT DO NOT SATISFY PROPER CRITERIA FOR CHARGES; HE PAID ANOTHER PERSON $40 TO PROVIDE FAMILY MEDICAL PSYCHOTHERAPY WHEN THAT PERSON WAS NOT HIS EMPLOYEE. $2,500 FINE. ON 9/26/97 BOARD ACKNOWLEDGED COMPLIANCE WITH ORDER AS HE HAD PAID THE PENALTY.

KUNZ, ARTHUR MD, LICENSE NUMBER 0C42551 OF TUCSON, AZ, WAS DISCIPLINED BY CALIFORNIA ON NOVEMBER 30, 1994
DISCIPLINARY ACTION: 60-MONTH PROBATION
OFFENSE: DISCIPLINARY ACTION BY ANOTHER STATE OR AGENCY

NOTES: DISCIPLINED BY THE U.S. NAVY FOR FALSIFYING A DOCUMENT ALLOWING HIM, AS A NAVY PHYSICIAN, TO MOONLIGHT IN A CIVILIAN HOSPITAL EMERGENCY ROOM. ALCOHOL ABUSE PROBLEM IN THE RECENT PAST. REVOCATION STAYED.

KWEE, JAMES-YEN T MD, LICENSE NUMBER C37261 OF FLAGSTAFF, AZ, WAS DISCIPLINED BY CALIFORNIA ON JULY 10, 1997
DISCIPLINARY ACTION: 60-MONTH PROBATION
OFFENSE: SUBSTANDARD CARE, INCOMPETENCE OR NEGLIGENCE

NOTES: CHARGED WITH INCOMPETENCE AND NEGLIGENCE IN THE CARE AND TREATMENT OF THREE PATIENTS. AGREES HIS LICENSE IS SUBJECT TO DISCIPLINE FOR GROSS NEGLIGENCE. REVOCATION STAYED.

LABARRE, LISE A MD, LICENSE NUMBER 0011152 OF PHOENIX, AZ, WAS DISCIPLINED BY ARIZONA ON JANUARY 23, 1992
OFFENSE: NONCOMPLIANCE WITH A PROFESSIONAL RULE

NOTES: ALLEGED UNSANITARY CONDITIONS IN HER OFFICE

AND DELAY IN RESPONDING TO THE BOARD'S REQUEST FOR INFORMATION. SHALL HAVE HER OFFICE MANAGEMENT PROCEDURES EVALUATED BY AN OUTSIDE MANAGEMENT CONSULTANT AND REPORT TO THE BOARD ON THE CONSULTANT'S RECOMMENDATIONS, AND ANY CHANGES IN HER OFFICE PRACTICES INITIATED BY HER AS A RESULT, WITHIN SIX MONTHS OF THIS ORDER.

LAFLEUR, MELANIE KOHOUT MD, LICENSE NUMBER 00H3482 OF MESA, AZ, WAS DISCIPLINED BY TEXAS ON JANUARY 6, 1995
DISCIPLINARY ACTION: MONITORING OF PHYSICIAN PERFORMANCE
OFFENSE: DISCIPLINARY ACTION BY ANOTHER STATE OR AGENCY

NOTES: ENTERED INTO A REHABILITATION STIPULATION AND ORDER WITH THE ARIZONA BOARD ON 5/25/93 WHICH PLACED HER UNDER TERMS AND CONDITIONS BUT DOES NOT CONSTITUTE A DISCIPLINARY ORDER. SHALL NOT PRACTICE IN TEXAS UNTIL SHE PERSONALLY APPEARS BEFORE THE BOARD AND PROVIDES SUFFICIENT EVIDENCE THAT SHE IS PHYSICALLY, MENTALLY AND OTHERWISE COMPETENT TO SAFELY PRACTICE INCLUDING AT A MINIMUM REPORTS FROM TREATING PHYSICIAN, COMPETENCY EXAMS OR ANY THERAPIST; SHALL COMPLY WITH TERMS OF ARIZONA ORDER; SHALL PROVIDE COPIES OF REPORTS SENT TO OR RECEIVED FROM ARIZONA BOARD UPON REQUEST; SHALL SURRENDER TEXAS CONTROLLED SUBSTANCES CERTIFICATES AND UNUSED TRIPLICATE PRESCRIPTION FORMS; SHALL NOT SEEK REREGISTRATION WITHOUT PERMISSION.

LAIRD, C ANDREW MD, LICENSE NUMBER 0007044, WAS DISCIPLINED BY ARIZONA ON OCTOBER 20, 1995
DISCIPLINARY ACTION: MONITORING OF PHYSICIAN PERFORMANCE

NOTES: INTERIM INVESTIGATIVE ORDER; WITHIN 21 DAYS, SHALL PRESENT HIMSELF FOR EVALUATION AND SHALL COMPLETE THE EVALUATION; SHALL COMPLY WITH REQUESTS FROM THE BOARD TO SUBMIT TO WITNESSED RANDOM BIOLOGICAL FLUID COLLECTION WITHIN TWO HOURS OF REQUEST; SHALL AUTHORIZE ANY PERSON OR ORGANIZATION CONDUCTING THE TESTS ON COLLECTED SAMPLES TO PROVIDE THE RESULTS TO THE BOARD.

LANSING, CORNELIUS MD, LICENSE NUMBER 0008604, WAS DISCIPLINED BY ARIZONA ON JUNE 28, 1990
DISCIPLINARY ACTION: 120-MONTH PROBATION; RESTRICTION PLACED ON CONTROLLED SUBSTANCE LICENSE
OFFENSE: OVERPRESCRIBING OR MISPRESCRIBING DRUGS

NOTES: BETWEEN 1/88 AND 7/88 PRESCRIBED DRUGS FOR A PATIENT WITHOUT EXAMINATION, KNOWING PATIENT WAS A RECOVERING ALCOHOLIC. IN 1/88 PRESCRIBED A COMBINATION OF DRUGS FOR A PATIENT WITH NO REQUEST FOR EKG, DESPITE THE FACT THAT SEVERAL OF THESE MEDICATIONS HAD A DIRECT EFFECT ON THE CARDIAC SYSTEM. IN 6/87 ADMITTED PATIENT TO HOSPITAL PSYCHIATRIC UNIT BECAUSE OF COMBATIVE AND PSYCHOTIC BEHAVIOR. LEFT PATIENT IN THE CARE OF A DOCTOR WITH NO PRIVILEGES AT HOSPITAL; PATIENT EVENTUALLY DIED. PRESCRIBED DRUGS FOR PATIENT WHO HE WAS AWARE HAD A 25 YEAR HISTORY OF SEVERE ALCOHOLISM WITHOUT MONITORING VITAL SIGNS OR MAINTAINING ADEQUATE TREATMENT RECORDS. MUST IMMEDIATELY SURRENDER CONTROLLED SUBSTANCES LICENSE FOR CLASS II, III, AND IV SUBSTANCES; MUST COMPLETE 50 HOURS OF CONTINUING MEDICAL EDUCATION PER YEAR FOR TWO YEARS IN CLINICAL PSYCHIATRY AND ADDICTION MEDICINE. MAY ONLY PRACTICE PSYCHIATRY.

LANSING, CORNELIUS MD OF 525 E BROADWAY, APACHE JUNCTION, AZ, WAS DISCIPLINED BY DEA ON AUGUST 20, 1990
DISCIPLINARY ACTION: SURRENDER OF CONTROLLED SUBSTANCE LICENSE
OFFENSE: OVERPRESCRIBING OR MISPRESCRIBING DRUGS

NOTES: DEA REGISTRATION SURRENDERED IN SCHEDULES II, III AND IV BASED IN PART ON CHARGE OF PRESCRIBING CONTROLLED SUBSTANCES FOR OTHER THAN LEGITIMATE THERAPEUTIC PURPOSES.

LANSING, CORNELIUS MD OF APACHE JUNCTION, AZ, WAS DISCIPLINED BY NORTH CAROLINA ON DECEMBER 27, 1991
DISCIPLINARY ACTION: SURRENDER OF LICENSE

LANSING, CORNELIUS MD, LICENSE NUMBER 0008604, WAS DISCIPLINED BY ARIZONA ON JANUARY 21, 1993
DISCIPLINARY ACTION: 6-MONTH LICENSE SUSPENSION; RESTRICTION PLACED ON LICENSE
OFFENSE: FAILURE TO COMPLY WITH PREVIOUS BOARD ORDER

NOTES: ALLEGED VIOLATIONS OF 6/28/90 PROBATION; HIS CONDUCT CONSTITUTES UNPROFESSIONAL CONDUCT. SHALL NOT SEE, TREAT, EVALUATE, PROVIDE CARE FOR, OR PRESCRIBE FOR PATIENTS WHO ARE 18 YEARS OF AGE OR YOUNGER; SHALL BE MONITORED BY A BOARD-APPROVED PSYCHIATRIST WHO WILL REVIEW HIS CARE AND TREATMENT OF PATIENTS FROM THE DATE OF THIS CONSENT ORDER AND SUBMIT QUARTERLY REPORTS TO THE BOARD REGARDING ALL SUCH CARE AND TREATMENT; ADDITIONAL CONDITIONS OF 6/28/9O PROBATION SHALL REMAIN IN EFFECT.

LAORR, ANAN K MD, LICENSE NUMBER 0012510 OF GLENDALE, AZ, WAS DISCIPLINED BY ARIZONA ON OCTOBER 19, 1994
OFFENSE: SUBSTANDARD CARE, INCOMPETENCE OR NEGLIGENCE

NOTES: CARE AND TREATMENT OF ONE PATIENT REGARDING A MALPRACTICE CLAIM ALLEGING THAT HE FAILED TO PROPERLY INVESTIGATE THE POSSIBILITY OF COMMON DUCT STONES DURING THE CHOLECYSTECTOMY AND CARE AND TREATMENT OF ANOTHER PATIENT REGARDING THE MALPRACTICE CLAIM ALLEGING INAPPROPRIATE CARE IN PERFORMING A VEIN LIGATION AND STRIPPING IN JUNE AND JULY 1990. ALSO DID NOT DICTATE OPERATIVE REPORTS AND DISCHARGE SUMMARIES IN A TIMELY MANNER. DOCTOR IS CENSURED.

LAORR, ANAN KAO MD, LICENSE NUMBER 0099984 OF 7115 WEST BEHREND DRIVE, GLENDALE, AZ, WAS DISCIPLINED BY NEW YORK ON FEBRUARY 20, 1996
DISCIPLINARY ACTION: REPRIMAND
OFFENSE: DISCIPLINARY ACTION BY ANOTHER STATE OR AGENCY

NOTES: ACTION IN ARIZONA FOR NOT COMPLETING A PATIENT'S MEDICAL RECORDS IN A TIMELY MANNER.

LAPRADE, PAUL W JR MD, LICENSE NUMBER 0013306, WAS DISCIPLINED BY ARIZONA ON JULY 15, 1993
DISCIPLINARY ACTION: MONITORING OF PHYSICIAN PERFORMANCE

NOTES: WITH REGARDS TO THE PSYCHOLOGICAL, PSYCHIATRIC AND PSYCHOMETRIC EVALUATIONS, SHALL ENTER INTO PSYCHOTHERAPY WITH A PSYCHOTHERAPIST APPROVED BY BOARD AND SHALL CONTINUE AT A FREQUENCY DETERMINED BY THE PSYCHOTHERAPIST WHO SHALL PROVIDE WRITTEN QUARTERLY REPORTS TO THE BOARD. ON 1/22/97

ORDER TERMINATED.

LAPRADE, PAUL W JR MD, LICENSE NUMBER 0013306, WAS DISCIPLINED BY ARIZONA ON JULY 20, 1995
OFFENSE: SUBSTANDARD CARE, INCOMPETENCE OR NEGLIGENCE

NOTES: IN A LETTER RECEIVED BY BOARD 8/19/94 HE ADMITTED TECHNICAL ERROR IN PERFORMING AN ANTERIOR CERVICAL FUSION AT THE WRONG LEVEL OF A PATIENT'S BACK IN AN OPERATION IN 6/91. CENSURED.

LARSON, DEBORAH J DO, LICENSE NUMBER 0002714 OF 10390 EAST LAKEVIEW DRIVE #203, SCOTTSDALE, AZ, WAS DISCIPLINED BY ARIZONA ON JUNE 26, 1996
DISCIPLINARY ACTION: 60-MONTH PROBATION; MONITORING OF PHYSICIAN PERFORMANCE
OFFENSE: SUBSTANCE ABUSE

NOTES: ON 5/14/96 AGREED TO ENTER A TREATMENT PROGRAM OR ALCOHOL DEPENDENCY. PROBATION UNDER TERMS AND CONDITIONS: SHALL OBTAIN PSYCHIATRIC OR PSYCHOLOGICAL TREATMENT BY A BOARD APPROVED THERAPIST WHO SHALL SUBMIT TO THE BOARD A WRITTEN PROGRESS REPORT EVERY MONTH FOR THE FIRST SIX MONTHS AND THEN EVERY THREE MONTHS FOR THE REMAINDER OF THE PROBATION; SHALL PARTICIPATE IN A MINIMUM OF THREE SELF-HELP MEETINGS PER WEEK THROUGH SUCH ORGANIZATIONS AS AA, AND DOCTOR'S CADUCEUS GROUP WITH MONTHLY REPORTS; SHALL PROVIDE A COPY OF THIS ORDER TO ALL FACILITIES WHERE SHE IS EMPLOYED AS A PHYSICIAN AND/OR HAS PRIVILEGES TO ENGAGE IN THE PRACTICE OF MEDICINE; SHALL ABSTAIN FROM THE CONSUMPTION OF ALCOHOL AND SHALL NOT CONSUME ILLICIT DRUGS OR TAKE ANY CONTROLLED SUBSTANCES UNLESS SUCH MEDICATION IS PRESCRIBED FOR HER BY HER TREATING PHYSICIAN; SHALL MAINTAIN A LOG OF SUCH PRESCRIPTIONS AND PROVIDE A COPY TO THE BOARD MONTHLY; SHALL SUBMIT TO AND COOPERATE IN ANY INDEPENDENT MEDICAL OR PSYCHOLOGICAL EVALUATION THAT IS ORDERED BY THE BOARD; SHALL APPEAR BEFORE THE BOARD UPON REQUEST; SHALL SUBMIT TO RANDOM BIOLOGICAL FLUID TESTING; SHALL NOTIFY THE BOARD WITHIN 20 DAYS IF SHE CEASES TO RESIDE IN ARIZONA; SHALL COMPLY WITH CONDITIONS IMPOSED BY DEA; SHALL COMPLY WITH ANY CONDITIONS IMPOSED ON HOSPITAL PRIVILEGES.

LARSON, DEBORAH J DO OF SCOTTSDALE, AZ, WAS DISCIPLINED BY IOWA ON MARCH 12, 1998
DISCIPLINARY ACTION: 42-MONTH PROBATION
OFFENSE: DISCIPLINARY ACTION BY ANOTHER STATE OR AGENCY

NOTES: CHARGED WITH BEING DISCIPLINED BY THE ARIZONA BOARD DUE TO SUBSTANCE ABUSE PROBLEMS.

LAWSON, DONALD A MD, LICENSE NUMBER 0007367, WAS DISCIPLINED BY ARIZONA ON OCTOBER 22, 1994
DISCIPLINARY ACTION: MONITORING OF PHYSICIAN PERFORMANCE
OFFENSE: PROFESSIONAL MISCONDUCT

NOTES: ALLEGATIONS THAT HE ORDERED LARGE AMOUNTS OF CONTROLLED SUBSTANCES. SHALL OBTAIN A BOARD-APPROVED TREATING PHYSICIAN; SHALL ABSTAIN COMPLETELY FROM THE CONSUMPTION OF ALCOHOLIC BEVERAGES AND DRUGS EXCEPT WHEN PRESCRIBED BY HIS TREATING PHYSICIAN; MUST SUBMIT TO WITNESSED RANDOM BIOLOGICAL FLUID COLLECTION; SHALL TAKE NO OVER-THE-COUNTER MEDICATIONS WHICH ARE TAKEN INTERNALLY UNLESS APPROVED IN ADVANCE BY HIS TREATING PHYSICIAN. KEEP A LOG OF ANY AND ALL MEDICATIONS PRESCRIBED FOR HIM; SHALL SUBMIT TO ANY EXAMINATIONS ORDERED BY BOARD; SHALL APPEAR BEFORE BOARD FOR INTERVIEWS UPON REQUEST; SHALL INFORM BOARD OF CHANGE OF ADDRESS OR IF AWAY FOR MORE THAN FIVE DAYS. ORDER MODIFIED ON 7/18/96 SUCH THAT METHOD OF COLLECTING FLUID SAMPLES WAS MODIFIED. RETROACTIVE TO 12/28/94. ON 10/18/96 ORDER TERMINATED.

LAWSON, DONALD A MD, LICENSE NUMBER 0A21755 OF PHOENIX, AZ, WAS DISCIPLINED BY CALIFORNIA ON MAY 20, 1996
DISCIPLINARY ACTION: SURRENDER OF LICENSE

NOTES: WHILE CHARGES PENDING.

LEAVITT, J ALLEN DO, LICENSE NUMBER 0000356, WAS DISCIPLINED BY ARIZONA ON MARCH 22, 1993
DISCIPLINARY ACTION: PROBATION; REQUIRED TO TAKE ADDITIONAL MEDICAL EDUCATION
OFFENSE: SUBSTANDARD CARE, INCOMPETENCE OR NEGLIGENCE

NOTES: ON 5/13/91 STARTED TO PROVIDE PRENATAL MEDICAL SERVICES TO A PATIENT AND CONTINUED UNTIL 9/30/91; ON 5/23/91 PRESCRIBED DEPO PROVERA TO THE PATIENT FOR TREATMENT OF A THREATENED MISCARRIAGE WHICH IS NOT IN ACCORDANCE WITH COMMUNITY STANDARDS; ALSO DETERMINED PATIENT WAS BLOOD TYPE RH NEGATIVE BUT DID NOT PERFORM ANY ANTIBODY TESTING ON THE FETUS OR THE PATIENT. MINIMUM TWO YEAR PROBATION UNDER TERMS AND CONDITIONS: SHALL COMPLETE A MINIMUM OF 40 HOURS OF CONTINUING MEDICAL EDUCATION IN THE TREATMENT AND MANAGEMENT OF HIGH-RISK OBSTETRICAL PATIENTS; SHALL MEET WITH THE BOARD UPON REQUEST TO REVIEW HIS COMPLIANCE WITH THIS ORDER; SHALL MAKE AVAILABLE UPON BOARD REQUEST PATIENT MEDICAL RECORDS FOR REVIEW. PROBATION SATISFIED IN FULL ON 3/22/95.

LEAVITT, JOSEPH A DO, LICENSE NUMBER 20A1954 OF MESA, AZ, WAS DISCIPLINED BY CALIFORNIA ON NOVEMBER 8, 1993
DISCIPLINARY ACTION: LICENSE REVOCATION
OFFENSE: DISCIPLINARY ACTION BY ANOTHER STATE OR AGENCY

NOTES: ACTION TAKEN BY ANOTHER STATE.

LEBEIS, KERWIN J MD, LICENSE NUMBER 16331, WAS DISCIPLINED BY ARIZONA ON JANUARY 22, 1997
DISCIPLINARY ACTION: 24-MONTH PROBATION; REQUIRED TO TAKE ADDITIONAL MEDICAL EDUCATION
OFFENSE: OVERPRESCRIBING OR MISPRESCRIBING DRUGS

NOTES: FROM 1/95-8/95 HE PRESCRIBED LARGE QUANTITIES OF POTENTIALLY TOXIC DOSES OF ACETAMINOPHEN WITH CODEINE TO ONE PATIENT. HIS MEDICAL RECORDS DO NOT DOCUMENT DIAGNOSIS AND GENERAL TREATMENT PLANS FOR THIS PATIENT WHEN FIRST SEEN ON 9/10/92; HE HAS NO RECORDS TO INDICATE THE CAUSE OF THIS PATIENT'S CHRONIC PAIN, PRIOR EVALUATIONS OR TREATMENT, OR INFORMATION REGARDING OTHER DOCTORS WHO MIGHT BE PRESCRIBING FOR THIS PATIENT; HE REPEATEDLY PRESCRIBED LITHIUM AND TEGRETOL YET THERE WAS NOT ONE LITHIUM LEVEL OR TEGRETOL LEVEL IN THE RECORDS; HE REPORTS THAT HIS PATIENT'S LIVER AND KIDNEY FUNCTIONS ARE NORMAL YET THERE IS NO LABORATORY DATA WITHIN THE ENTIRE RECORD TO DEMONSTRATE THIS. CONDITIONS OF PROBATION ARE AS FOLLOWS:

WITHIN NINE MONTHS SHALL SUCCESSFULLY COMPLETE 30 HOURS OF CONTINUING MEDICAL EDUCATION IN ADDICTION MEDICINE AND PSYCHOPHARMACOLOGY AND 10 HOURS IN RECORD KEEPING AND DOCUMENTATION; SHALL SUBMIT 15 CASES FOR REVIEW BY A BOARD CONSULTANT WITHIN ONE YEAR.

LEE, JOHN JOON MD, LICENSE NUMBER 12631, WAS DISCIPLINED BY ARIZONA ON NOVEMBER 19, 1999
DISCIPLINARY ACTION: LICENSE REVOCATION

LEE, KEVIN H DO, LICENSE NUMBER 0002275, WAS DISCIPLINED BY ARIZONA ON MAY 19, 1992
DISCIPLINARY ACTION: 60-MONTH PROBATION; REQUIRED TO ENTER AN IMPAIRED PHYSICIAN PROGRAM OR SUBSTANCE ABUSE TREATMENT
OFFENSE: PROVIDING FALSE INFORMATION TO THE BOARD OR OTHER HEALTH AGENCY

NOTES: ON 10/07/90 REQUESTED A CO-WORKER TO OBTAIN PRESCRIPTION-ONLY MEDICATION ON HIS BEHALF; WROTE TWO PRESCRIPTIONS FOR THIS CO-WORKER AND HER MOTHER WITHOUT ANY MEDICAL EXAMINATION FOR PERCOCET AND SOMA; THE CO-WORKER KEPT ONE PRESCRIPTION OF PERCOCET FOR HERSELF AND DELIVERED ONE TO HIM; HAS REQUESTED OTHER PERSONNEL TO OBTAIN PRESCRIPTION-ONLY MEDICATION ON HIS BEHALF; ON 6/12/91 ACKNOWLEDGED THAT HE SELF-ADMINISTERED MEDICATIONS, INCLUDING CONTROLLED SUBSTANCES AND THAT HE HAS WRITTEN PRESCRIPTIONS FOR PRESCRIPTION-ONLY MEDICATION FOR HIS BROTHER; ON 3/17/91 AND 5/06/91 WROTE PRESCRIPTIONS FOR 40 TABLETS AND 60 TABLETS OF PERCOCET FOR A PERSON HE WAS NOT THE PHYSICIAN FOR; DURING THE AUTUMN OF 1990 HE WAS ENROLLED IN A SUBSTANCE ABUSE TREATMENT PROGRAM, BUT ON 12/06/90 IN THE COURSE OF SEEKING RENEWAL OF HIS LICENSE HE STATED THAT HE HAD RECEIVED NO TREATMENT FOR SUBSTANCE ABUSE DURING THE PRECEDING 12 MONTHS. PROBATION UNDER TERMS AND CONDITIONS: SHALL COMPLETE A PROGRAM OF TREATMENT FOR SUBSTANCE ABUSE AND CHEMICAL DEPENDENCY FOR NO FEWER THAN TWO MONTHS AND NO MORE THAN FOUR MONTHS; MAY RESUME PRACTICE AFTER SUCCESSFUL COMPLETION OF THIS PROGRAM; SHALL ENROLL IN THE MICHIGAN PHYSICIAN'S RECOVERY NETWORK AFTERCARE PROGRAM AND SHALL PROVIDE THE BOARD WITH A COPY OF THE CONTRACT; THEY SHALL PROVIDE QUARTERLY REPORTS TO THE BOARD; SHALL SUBMIT TO BIOLOGICAL FLUID TESTING; SHALL USE NO CONTROLLED SUBSTANCE OR PRESCRIPTION-ONLY MEDICATION UNLESS PRESCRIBED BY HIS ATTENDING PHYSICIAN; SHALL NOT CONSUME ALCOHOL; SHALL ATTEND 90 AA OR NARCOTICS ANONYMOUS MEETINGS IN 90 DAYS; SHALL ATTEND FIVE AA OR NARCOTICS ANONYMOUS MEETINGS PER WEEK FOLLOWING THE INITIAL 90 DAY PERIOD; SHALL MAINTAIN AN AA OR NARCOTICS ANONYMOUS SPONSOR; SHALL ATTEND NO LESS THAN TWO CADUCEUS CLUB MEETINGS MONTHLY; SHALL NOTIFY THE APPROPRIATE SUPERVISORY PERSONNEL AT HIS EMPLOYMENT OF THIS ORDER; SHALL ATTEND NO LESS THAN ONE AFTERCARE GROUP MEETING PER WEEK FOR THREE MONTHS; SHALL APPEAR BEFORE THE BOARD UPON REQUEST TO REVIEW HIS COMPLIANCE WITH THIS ORDER; AS LONG AS HE RESIDES IN ARIZONA SHALL MEET IN PERSON ON A MONTHLY BASIS WITH THE BOARD; SHALL AUTHORIZE ANY ATTENDING PHYSICIAN, PSYCHIATRIST, OR PSYCHOLOGIST TO RELEASE TO THE BOARD ALL RECORDS PERTAINING TO HIS CARE AND TREATMENT.

LEE, KEVIN HARRY DO, DATE OF BIRTH JUNE 6, 1952, LICENSE NUMBER 0008929 OF 3814 JEFFERSON, MIDLAND, MI, WAS DISCIPLINED BY MICHIGAN ON FEBRUARY 28, 1994
DISCIPLINARY ACTION: 48-MONTH PROBATION; RESTRICTION PLACED ON LICENSE
OFFENSE: SUBSTANCE ABUSE

LEE, KEVIN HARRY DO, DATE OF BIRTH JUNE 6, 1952, LICENSE NUMBER 1008929 OF 3814 JEFFERSON, MIDLAND, MI, WAS DISCIPLINED BY MICHIGAN ON JULY 8, 1996
DISCIPLINARY ACTION: 6-MONTH LICENSE SUSPENSION; FINE
OFFENSE: SUBSTANDARD CARE, INCOMPETENCE OR NEGLIGENCE

NOTES: NEGLIGENCE/INCOMPETENCE; LACK OF GOOD MORAL CHARACTER. $1,000 FINE.

LEE, KEVIN HARRY DO, DATE OF BIRTH JUNE 6, 1952, LICENSE NUMBER 1008929 OF 3814 JEFFERSON, MIDLAND, MI, WAS DISCIPLINED BY MICHIGAN ON MAY 5, 1998
DISCIPLINARY ACTION: 60-MONTH PROBATION; 60-MONTH RESTRICTION PLACED ON LICENSE

LEFF, ALAN M MD, DATE OF BIRTH APRIL 3, 1940, LICENSE NUMBER 0024607 OF 8 PARK HILL DRIVE, MENANDS, NY, WAS DISCIPLINED BY NEW JERSEY ON JUNE 23, 1993
OFFENSE: DISCIPLINARY ACTION BY ANOTHER STATE OR AGENCY

NOTES: SANCTIONED IN ARIZONA. SHALL REFRAIN FROM PRACTICE OF MEDICINE AND SURGERY IN NEW JERSEY UNTIL HE INFORMS THE BOARD OF HIS INTENT TO SO PRACTICE, APPEARS BEFORE THE BOARD AND RECEIVES APPROVAL TO COMMENCE PRACTICE IN NEW JERSEY.

LEFF, ALAN MICHAEL MD, LICENSE NUMBER 0014051, WAS DISCIPLINED BY ARIZONA ON OCTOBER 10, 1991
DISCIPLINARY ACTION: FINE
OFFENSE: NONCOMPLIANCE WITH A PROFESSIONAL RULE

NOTES: FAILED TO FURNISH INFORMATION TO THE BOARD IN A TIMELY MANNER IN THAT HE TOOK MORE THAN THREE MONTHS (FROM 5/90 TO 8/90) TO RESPOND TO A REQUEST BY THE BOARD TO SUBMIT COMMENTS AND RECORDS CONCERNING THE COMPLAINT OF A PATIENT OVER BILLING. PREVIOUSLY BOARD HAD EXPRESSED CONCERN REGARDING HIS FAILURE TO COMMUNICATE WITH BOARD CORRESPONDENCE AND REQUEST FOR INFORMATION. SHALL UNDERGO PSYCHOLOGICAL, PSYCHIATRIC AND PHYSICAL EXAMINATIONS AND SHALL APPEAR FOR FURTHER INTERVIEW AT THE BOARD'S 1/92 MEETING. CENSURED. $1,000 FINE.

LEIBSOHN, STEVEN MD, LICENSE NUMBER 0017701, WAS DISCIPLINED BY ARIZONA ON OCTOBER 16, 1996
OFFENSE: SUBSTANDARD CARE, INCOMPETENCE OR NEGLIGENCE

NOTES: IN 10/93, HE PERFORMED A MAJOR ELECTIVE SURGERY ON A PATIENT WITH A MARKEDLY ABNORMAL WHITE COUNT; FAILED TO INVESTIGATE THE WHITE COUNT TO REVEAL A POSSIBLE UNTREATED URINARY TRACT INFECTION; AFTER SURGERY, PATIENT BECAME COMATOSE AND HAD A CONSUMPTIVE COAGULOPHATHY, SEPTIC SHOCK AND THEN MULTI-SYSTEM FAILURE; IN 10/92, HE PERFORMED A TOTAL ABDOMINAL HYSTERECTOMY AND BILATERAL SALPINGO-OOPHORECTOMY ON A PATIENT WHO HAD UNDERGONE A D&C AND

HYSTEROSCOPY ONLY 36 HOURS EARLIER, NOT ALLOWING HER TIME TO RECOVER BETWEEN THE TWO PROCEDURES AND NOT GIVING HER SUFFICIENT ANTIBIOTICS FOR THE SECOND PROCEDURE; PATIENT BECAME FEBRILE TWO DAYS AFTER SURGERY AND DIED FROM ACUTE RESPIRATORY DISTRESS SYNDROME; IN 11/90, FAILED TO EVALUATE A PATIENT IN ACUTE RESPIRATORY DISTRESS WITH MARKEDLY ABNORMAL ARTERIAL BLOOD GASES AND CYANOSIS FOR AT LEAST FIVE HOURS; PATIENT WAS TRANSFERRED TO THE ICU IN APPARENT RESPIRATORY FAILURE WITH CENTRAL AND PERIPHERAL CYANOSIS AND SPENT 28 DAYS IN THE HOSPITAL; FAILED TO MAINTAIN ADEQUATE RECORDS ON THE FIRST TWO PATIENTS, THERE IS NO RECORD OF LAB VALUES WHICH COULD HAVE CHANGED THE OUTCOME OF THEIR SITUATIONS. CENSURED.

LEKANDER, GARY M MD, LICENSE NUMBER 0024094, WAS DISCIPLINED BY ARIZONA ON APRIL 20, 1996
DISCIPLINARY ACTION: MONITORING OF PHYSICIAN PERFORMANCE

NOTES: MUST OBTAIN COUNSELING WITHIN 60 DAYS IN THE AREAS OF INTERPERSONAL RELATIONSHIPS AND THE USE OF ALCOHOL; HIS THERAPIST SHALL SUBMIT REPORTS REGARDING HIS PROGRESS IN THERAPY STARTING 7/1/96 AND QUARTERLY THEREAFTER. ON 3/14/97 BOARD DID NOT APPROVE HIS CURRENT THERAPIST AND ORDERED HIM TO OBTAIN A DIFFERENT THERAPIST WHO CAN BETTER ADDRESS THE PROBLEMS IDENTIFIED BY THE BOARD; THERAPIST SHALL BE APPROVED BY BOARD. ON 9/24/97 ORDER TERMINATED.

LEMCKE, RALPH A MD, LICENSE NUMBER 0007116 OF 6542 E CARONDELET DRIVE, TUCSON, AZ, WAS DISCIPLINED BY ARIZONA ON SEPTEMBER 19, 1996
DISCIPLINARY ACTION: MONITORING OF PHYSICIAN PERFORMANCE

NOTES: WITHIN THREE MONTHS SHALL OBTAIN THE SERVICES OF A BOARD-APPROVED OFFICE MANAGEMENT CONSULTANT AND AUTHORIZE THAT CONSULTANT TO RELEASE ANY AND ALL REPORTS TO THE BOARD FOR ITS CONSIDERATION. ON 3/14/97 ORDER WAS TERMINATED.

LEPPERD, FLOYD CHARLES MD, LICENSE NUMBER 0006931, WAS DISCIPLINED BY ARIZONA ON APRIL 6, 1995
DISCIPLINARY ACTION: LICENSE SUSPENSION
OFFENSE: SUBSTANCE ABUSE

NOTES: UNDERGOING LONG-TERM TREATMENT FOR ALCOHOL ABUSE OR DEPENDENCY PROBLEM. BOARD ACCEPTED REQUEST FOR LICENSE TO BE IN INACTIVE STATUS. EFFECTIVE 11/1/95 WHILE ARIZONA LICENSE IS IN AN INACTIVE STATUS CATEGORY: AGREES NOT TO PRACTICE MEDICINE ANYWHERE; MAY NOT HOLD DEA REGISTRATION OR WRITE PRESCRIPTIONS.

LEVITT, MICHAEL K MD, LICENSE NUMBER 0017231, WAS DISCIPLINED BY ARIZONA ON OCTOBER 19, 1992

NOTES: AGREES NOT TO SEE, TREAT, CLINICALLY EVALUATE OR PROVIDE DIRECT CARE TO ANY PATIENT PENDING A FINAL DECISION BY THE ARIZONA BOARD.

LEVITT, MICHAEL K MD, LICENSE NUMBER 0017231 OF FLAGSTAFF, AZ, WAS DISCIPLINED BY ARIZONA ON JULY 12, 1993
DISCIPLINARY ACTION: LICENSE SUSPENSION
OFFENSE: FAILURE TO COMPLY WITH PREVIOUS BOARD ORDER

NOTES: IN 3/92 HE AND A PATIENT ENGAGED IN SEXUAL INTIMACIES; UNABLE TO WORK IN 4/92 AND 5/92 BECAUSE HE WAS IMPAIRED BY ALCOHOL, STRESS, DEPRESSION AND/OR OTHER CAUSES; ON 10/19/92 HE ENTERED INTO A STIPULATION WITH THE BOARD THAT HE WOULD NOT TREAT PATIENTS PENDING FINAL ACTION; SAW 3 PATIENTS ON 10/22/92; WAS TREATED FOR CHEMICAL DEPENDENCY AND DEPRESSION IN 11/92 AND 12/92. SUSPENSION RETROACTIVE UNTIL 10/22/92. SHALL SUBMIT TO MENTAL AND PHYSICAL EVALUATIONS.

LEVITT, MICHAEL K MD, LICENSE NUMBER 0017231, WAS DISCIPLINED BY ARIZONA ON JULY 12, 1994
DISCIPLINARY ACTION: LICENSE SUSPENSION
OFFENSE: FAILURE TO COMPLY WITH PREVIOUS BOARD ORDER

NOTES: FAILED TO SEND A CERTIFIED LETTER TO THE BOARD WITHIN SEVEN DAYS OF HIS CHANGE OF ADDRESS AS REQUIRED BY THE 07/13/93 ORDER; BOARD DID NOT RECEIVE TIMELY REPORTS FROM HIS THERAPIST, TREATING PHYSICIAN, OR THE MARYLAND REHABILITATION PROGRAM. UPON APPROVAL OF THIS STIPULATION AND ORDER HIS PROBATION AND SUSPENSION SHALL TERMINATE AND LICENSE IS INACTIVATED. LICENSE SURRENDERED ON 7/94. HIS REQUEST FOR REACTIVATION OF HIS LICENSE DENIED ON 7/17/96.

LEVITT, MICHAEL KENT MD, DATE OF BIRTH MAY 6, 1941, LICENSE NUMBER 0023947 OF GAMBRILLS, MD, WAS DISCIPLINED BY NORTH CAROLINA ON JANUARY 5, 1996
DISCIPLINARY ACTION: LICENSE REVOCATION
OFFENSE: DISCIPLINARY ACTION BY ANOTHER STATE OR AGENCY

NOTES: LICENSE SUSPENDED BY THE ARIZONA BOARD.

LEWIS, CAROL E MD, DATE OF BIRTH DECEMBER 27, 1958 OF 6661 N 78TH PLACE, SCOTTSDALE, AZ, WAS DISCIPLINED BY MEDICARE ON OCTOBER 9, 1993
DISCIPLINARY ACTION: EXCLUSION FROM THE MEDICARE AND/OR MEDICAID PROGRAM
OFFENSE: NONCOMPLIANCE WITH A PROFESSIONAL RULE

NOTES: DEFAULTED ON PUBLIC HEALTH SERVICE EDUCATION LOAN. REINSTATED ON 11/10/94.

LEWIS, CAROL E MD, DATE OF BIRTH DECEMBER 27, 1958 OF 6661 NORTH 78TH PLACE, SCOTTSDALE, AZ, WAS DISCIPLINED BY MEDICARE ON DECEMBER 22, 1997
DISCIPLINARY ACTION: EXCLUSION FROM THE MEDICARE AND/OR MEDICAID PROGRAM
OFFENSE: NONCOMPLIANCE WITH A PROFESSIONAL RULE

NOTES: DEFAULTED ON PUBLIC HEALTH SERVICE EDUCATION LOAN.

LEWIS, LEO MD, WAS DISCIPLINED BY ARIZONA ON APRIL 9, 1992
DISCIPLINARY ACTION: LICENSE SUSPENSION
OFFENSE: SUBSTANCE ABUSE

NOTES: FOLLOWING HIS RETIREMENT BOARD RECEIVED CONCERNS REGARDING HIS MISUSE OF ALCOHOL AND LATER THAT HE WAS MISUSING CONTROLLED SUBSTANCES. ENTERED INTO TREATMENT AND THEN SIGNED HIMSELF OUT BUT RE-ENTERED THE TREATMENT PROGRAM. BOARD ACCEPTED DOCTOR'S REQUEST FOR INACTIVE STATUS OF MEDICAL LICENSE WITH CAUSE.

LI, WILLIAM K P MD, WAS DISCIPLINED BY ARIZONA ON JULY 25, 1997
DISCIPLINARY ACTION: REQUIRED TO TAKE ADDITIONAL MEDICAL EDUCATION; MONITORING OF PHYSICIAN PERFORMANCE

NOTES: MUST OBTAIN 20 HOURS OF CONTINUING MEDICAL EDUCATION IN THE AREA OF RECORD KEEPING AND CODING WITHIN SIX MONTHS; BOARD WILL CONDUCT A FOLLOW-UP SURVEY IN NINE MONTHS.

LINDEN, HEINZ RALPH MD, LICENSE NUMBER 0026866 OF SOMERTON, AZ, WAS DISCIPLINED BY OHIO ON AUGUST 8, 1990
DISCIPLINARY ACTION: PROBATION
OFFENSE: DISCIPLINARY ACTION BY ANOTHER STATE OR AGENCY

NOTES: PROBATIONARY TERMS, CONDITIONS, AND LIMITATIONS IMPOSED BASED ON PRIOR LIMITATIONS OF MEDICAL LICENSE BY ARIZONA ORDERING DOCTOR NOT TO PRACTICE ANESTHESIOLOGY.

LINDEN, HEINZ RALPH MD, LICENSE NUMBER 0026866 OF SOMERTON, AZ, WAS DISCIPLINED BY OHIO ON JULY 10, 1991
DISCIPLINARY ACTION: LICENSE REVOCATION
OFFENSE: DISCIPLINARY ACTION BY ANOTHER STATE OR AGENCY

NOTES: PRIOR DISCIPLINARY ACTION BY ARIZONA BOARD OF MEDICAL EXAMINERS RELATING TO DOCTOR'S FATAL ADMINISTRATION OF ANESTHESIA TO A PATIENT; FAILURE TO COMPLY WITH TERMS OF 8/8/90 CONSENT AGREEMENT ENTERED INTO WITH OHIO BOARD ON THE BASIS OF ARIZONA ACTION. PERMANENT REVOCATION. HIS APPEAL OF REVOCATION WAS DISMISSED BY A COMMON PLEAS COURT DECISION OF 4/10/92 DUE TO HIS FAILURE TO EXHAUST ADMINISTRATIVE REMEDIES.

LINDEN, HEINZ RALPH MD, LICENSE NUMBER 0006340, WAS DISCIPLINED BY ARIZONA ON APRIL 16, 1993
DISCIPLINARY ACTION: LICENSE REVOCATION
OFFENSE: PROFESSIONAL MISCONDUCT

NOTES: IN 1/88 CENSURED FOR UNPROFESSIONAL CONDUCT RELATED TO HIS PRACTICE OF ANESTHESIOLOGY RESULTING IN THE DEATH OF A PATIENT; IN 3/89 BOARD PROHIBITED HIM FROM PRACTICING ANESTHESIOLOGY. BECAUSE OF THIS, OHIO BOARD REQUIRED HIM TO SUBMIT QUARTERLY REPORTS; OHIO LICENSE REVOKED IN 5/91 BASED ON HIS FAILURE TO SUBMIT THESE REPORTS. ON 6/25/92 BOARD ISSUED A COMPLAINT BASED ON THE FACT THAT DURING 1989 AND 1990 HE HAD SIX PATIENTS IN A WEIGHT LOSS PROGRAM IN WHICH THEY WERE INJECTED WITH HUMAN CHORIONIC GONADOTROPIN (HCG). TOGETHER WITH ORAL DOSES OF THYROID AND PHENTERMINE; BEFORE STARTING THESE PATIENTS IN THE PROGRAM DR. LINDEN DID NOT PERFORM A COMPLETE PHYSICAL EXAM NOR DID HE TAKE A FULL HISTORY; WAS INFORMED ON 7/2/90 THAT HE WAS IN VIOLATION OF THE LAW WHEN INJECTING HCG AS IT WAS NOT KNOWN TO BE EFFECTIVE; TOOK SPEX EXAM AS DIRECTED BY BOARD IN 1991 AND 1992 AND FAILED.

LINGENFELTER, JOHN MD, LICENSE NUMBER 0003604, WAS DISCIPLINED BY ARIZONA ON JANUARY 17, 1996
DISCIPLINARY ACTION: REQUIRED TO TAKE ADDITIONAL MEDICAL EDUCATION
OFFENSE: OVERPRESCRIBING OR MISPRESCRIBING DRUGS

NOTES: INTERVIEWED BY THE BOARD REGARDING HIS TREATMENT OF A PATIENT AND THE BOARD'S 7/20/95 VOTE THAT HE TAKE AND PASS THE SPECIAL PURPOSE EXAMINATION; HIS CARE AND TREATMENT OF A SECOND PATIENT AND THE MALPRACTICE CLAIM ALLEGING INAPPROPRIATE PRESCRIBING OF SCHEDULE DRUGS; AND THE RESULTS OF A PHARMACY AND OFFICE PRACTICE SURVEY. WITHIN SIX MONTHS SHALL SUCCESSFULLY COMPLETE 60 HOURS OF CONTINUING MEDICAL EDUCATION IN LONG TERM CARE WITH A FOCUS ON GERIATRICS WITH 50% DIDACTIC AND 50% CLINICAL COMPONENTS; SHALL SUBMIT PROOF OF SUCCESSFUL COMPLETION TO THE BOARD. ON 7/18/96 BOARD APPROVED HIS REQUEST FOR AN EXTENSION UNTIL 10/31/96 TO FULFILL THE TERMS OF HIS STIPULATION. ON 10/18/96 BOARD APPROVED HIS REQUEST FOR ANOTHER EXTENSION UNTIL 2/1/97 TO FULFILL THE TERMS OF HIS STIPULATION. ON 1/22/97 BOARD TERMINATED ORDER AS HE HAD COMPLETED THE EDUCATION REQUIREMENTS AND RESCINDED THE ORDER REQUIRING HIM TO TAKE THE SPEX EXAM.

LINGENFELTER, JOHN G MD, LICENSE NUMBER 16297 OF KINGMAN, AZ, WAS DISCIPLINED BY IOWA ON MARCH 28, 1997
DISCIPLINARY ACTION: REPRIMAND
OFFENSE: DISCIPLINARY ACTION BY ANOTHER STATE OR AGENCY

NOTES: DISCIPLINED BY THE MEDICAL LICENSING AUTHORITIES OF ARIZONA. MUST COMPLY WITH THE CONDITIONS OF A VOLUNTARY AGREEMENT HE HAD ENTERED INTO WITH THE ARIZONA BOARD OF MEDICAL EXAMINERS.

LOCNIKAR, STEVEN DO, LICENSE NUMBER 0002669 OF 3201 W. PEORIA, #D805, PHOENIX, AZ, WAS DISCIPLINED BY ARIZONA ON MAY 20, 1996
DISCIPLINARY ACTION: 60-MONTH PROBATION; MONITORING OF PHYSICIAN PERFORMANCE
OFFENSE: SUBSTANCE ABUSE

NOTES: POSSESSION AND USE OF AN ILLICIT SUBSTANCE AND SUBSTANCE ADDICTION; ON 4/26/96 VOLUNTARILY CEASED THE PRACTICE OF OSTEOPATHIC MEDICINE UNTIL AFTER THE 5/15/96 BOARD MEETING. PROBATION UNDER TERMS AND CONDITIONS: SHALL OBTAIN PSYCHIATRIC OR PSYCHOLOGICAL TREATMENT BY A BOARD APPROVED PSYCHIATRIST AND OR PSYCHOLOGIST WHO SHALL PROVIDE THE BOARD WITH A WRITTEN PROGRESS REPORT EVERY MONTH FOR THE FIRST SIX MONTHS AND THEN EVERY THREE MONTHS FOR THE REMAINDER OF THE PROBATION; SHALL PARTICIPATE IN A MINIMUM OF TWO SELF-HELP MEETINGS PER WEEK THROUGH SUCH ORGANIZATIONS AS AA, NARCOTICS ANONYMOUS AND DOCTOR'S CADUCEUS GROUP WITH MONTHLY REPORTS; SHALL PROVIDE A COPY OF THIS ORDER TO ALL FACILITIES WHERE HE IS EMPLOYED AS A PHYSICIAN AND/OR HAS PRIVILEGES TO ENGAGE IN THE PRACTICE OF MEDICINE; SHALL ABSTAIN FROM THE CONSUMPTION OF ALCOHOL AND SHALL NOT CONSUME ILLICIT DRUGS OR TAKE ANY CONTROLLED SUBSTANCES UNLESS SUCH MEDICATION IS PRESCRIBED FOR HIM BY HIS TREATING PHYSICIAN; SHALL MAINTAIN A LOG OF SUCH PRESCRIPTIONS AND PROVIDE A COPY TO THE BOARD MONTHLY; SHALL SUBMIT TO AND COOPERATE IN ANY INDEPENDENT MEDICAL OR PSYCHOLOGICAL EVALUATION THAT IS ORDERED BY THE BOARD; SHALL APPEAR BEFORE THE BOARD UPON REQUEST; SHALL SUBMIT TO RANDOM BIOLOGICAL FLUID TESTING; SHALL NOTIFY THE BOARD WITHIN 20 DAYS IF HE CEASES TO RESIDE IN ARIZONA; SHALL COMPLY WITH CONDITIONS IMPOSED BY DEA; SHALL COMPLY WITH ANY CONDITIONS PLACED ON HOSPITAL PRIVILEGES.

LOCNIKAR, STEVEN DO, LICENSE NUMBER 0002669 OF 3201 WEST PEORIA, #D805, PHOENIX, AZ, WAS DISCIPLINED BY ARIZONA ON OCTOBER 1, 1996
DISCIPLINARY ACTION: MONITORING OF PHYSICIAN PERFORMANCE
OFFENSE: FAILURE TO COMPLY WITH PREVIOUS BOARD ORDER

NOTES: USED CONTROLLED DANGEROUS SUBSTANCES OR PRESCRIPTION ONLY DRUGS NOT PROVIDED BY A MEDICAL PRACTITIONER WHICH VIOLATED 5/20/96 ORDER. SHALL ATTEND 90 ONE HOUR SELF-HELP MEETINGS FOR 90 DAYS BEGINNING ON 8/09/96 THROUGH SUCH ORGANIZATIONS AS AA, NARCOTICS ANONYMOUS, AND DOCTOR'S CADUCEUS GROUP WITH MONTHLY REPORTS; SHALL PROVIDE A COPY OF THIS ORDER TO ALL FACILITIES WHERE HE IS EMPLOYED AS A PHYSICIAN AND/OR HAS PRIVILEGES TO ENGAGE IN THE PRACTICE OF MEDICINE.

LOCNIKAR, STEVEN DO, LICENSE NUMBER 2669 OF 3201 W PEORIA AVENUE, SUITE D-85, GLENDALE, AZ, WAS DISCIPLINED BY ARIZONA ON JANUARY 13, 1997
DISCIPLINARY ACTION: LICENSE SUSPENSION; 60-MONTH PROBATION
OFFENSE: FAILURE TO COMPLY WITH PREVIOUS BOARD ORDER

NOTES: VIOLATED A 5/20/96 PROBATIONARY ORDER BY CONSUMING ALCOHOL AND FAILING TO TIMELY COMPLY WITH INSTRUCTIONS TO SUBMIT TO BIOLOGICAL FLUID TESTING; A HOSPITAL INFORMED HIM HE HAD FORFEITED HIS "ON CALL" SCHEDULE PRIVILEGES BECAUSE HE FAILED TO TIMELY AND APPROPRIATELY RESPOND TO CALLS FROM A HOSPITAL EMERGENCY DEPARTMENT; HE ARRIVED LATE FOR A SURGICAL PROCEDURE. SUSPENSION SUBJECT TO SUCCESSFUL COMPLETION OF A BOARD-APPROVED MONITORED AFTERCARE TREATMENT PROGRAM; UPON REINSTATEMENT TO PROBATION: SHALL OBTAIN A BOARD-APPROVED TREATING THERAPIST WHO SHALL SEND THE BOARD A WRITTEN PROGRESS REPORT EVERY THREE MONTHS; SHALL ABSTAIN COMPLETELY FROM THE CONSUMPTION OF ALCOHOLIC BEVERAGES AND DRUGS EXCEPT WHEN PRESCRIBED BY HIS TREATING PHYSICIAN; MUST SUBMIT TO WITNESSED RANDOM BIOLOGICAL FLUID COLLECTION; MUST KEEP A LOG OF ANY AND ALL MEDICATIONS PRESCRIBED FOR HIM; SHALL SUBMIT TO ANY EVALUATIONS ORDERED BY BOARD; SHALL APPEAR BEFORE BOARD FOR INTERVIEWS UPON REQUEST; SHALL INFORM BOARD OF CHANGE OF ADDRESS IF HE LEAVES ARIZONA; LICENSE REINSTATED TO PROBATION ON 4/3/97 AND HE IS ABLE TO ENGAGE IN THE PRACTICE OF MEDICINE, ADHERING TO ALL PROBATIONARY REQUIREMENTS PREVIOUSLY ENTERED.

LOCNIKAR, STEVEN DO, LICENSE NUMBER 2669 OF 3201 W PEORIA AVENUE, SUITE D-85, GLENDALE, AZ, WAS DISCIPLINED BY ARIZONA ON JANUARY 17, 1997
DISCIPLINARY ACTION: EMERGENCY SUSPENSION
OFFENSE: FAILURE TO COMPLY WITH PREVIOUS BOARD ORDER

NOTES: HE VIOLATED 5/20/96 PROBATIONARY ORDER BY CONSUMING ALCOHOL, MARIJUANA AND COCAINE ON 1/2/97 AS EVIDENCED BY BIOLOGICAL FLUID TESTING CONDUCTED 7/15/96, 10/7/96 AND 1/2/97; HE PRACTICED MEDICINE WHILE UNDER THE INFLUENCE OF ALCOHOL TO APPROXIMATELY 17 PATIENTS; HE FAILED TO TIMELY COMPLY WITH INSTRUCTIONS TO SUBMIT TO RANDOM BIOLOGICAL FLUID TESTING. ORDER TERMINATED EFFECTIVE 1/13/97.

LOCNIKAR, STEVEN DO OF PHOENIX, AZ, WAS DISCIPLINED BY MISSOURI ON AUGUST 17, 1998
DISCIPLINARY ACTION: LICENSE REVOCATION
OFFENSE: DISCIPLINARY ACTION BY ANOTHER STATE OR AGENCY

NOTES: CALIFORNIA LICENSE REVOKED. MAY NOT APPLY FOR REINSTATEMENT OF LICENSE FOR TWO YEARS AND ONE DAY.

LOCNIKAR, STEVEN JOSEPH DO, LICENSE NUMBER 20A6192 OF PHOENIX, AZ, WAS DISCIPLINED BY CALIFORNIA ON DECEMBER 2, 1996
DISCIPLINARY ACTION: LICENSE REVOCATION
OFFENSE: DISCIPLINARY ACTION BY ANOTHER STATE OR AGENCY

NOTES: ACTION TAKEN BY ANOTHER STATE.

LOGAN, MARK MD OF 12722 NORTH 100TH STREET, SCOTTSDALE, AZ, WAS DISCIPLINED BY DEA ON SEPTEMBER 21, 1999
DISCIPLINARY ACTION: SURRENDER OF CONTROLLED SUBSTANCE LICENSE
OFFENSE: DISCIPLINARY ACTION BY ANOTHER STATE OR AGENCY

NOTES: STATE BOARD.

LOGAN, MARK E MD, LICENSE NUMBER 22621, WAS DISCIPLINED BY ARIZONA ON JANUARY 23, 1998
DISCIPLINARY ACTION: PROBATION; REPRIMAND
OFFENSE: FAILURE TO COMPLY WITH PREVIOUS BOARD ORDER

NOTES: IN 1/95 & 2/95 HE PRESCRIBED CONTROLLED SUBSTANCES TO A MEMBER OF HIS IMMEDIATE FAMILY BUT CLAIMED THAT HE DID NOT KNOW IT WAS AGAINST THE LAW; IN 2/96 HE DID SO AGAIN AND HE INDICATED THAT THE PRESCRIPTION WAS FOR HIS OWN USE; HE SURRENDERED DEA PRIVILEGES AND ARIZONA LICENSE WAS INACTIVATED IN 2/96, AFTER WHICH HE UNDERWENT TREATMENT; LICENSE REINSTATED WITH CONDITIONS IN 11/96; ON 11/17/97 BOARD WAS INFORMED HE HAD BEEN RELAPSING FOR TWO MONTHS, WRITING AND FILLING CONTROLLED SUBSTANCE PRESCRIPTIONS IN THE NAME OF FAMILY MEMBERS; SAID HE DID NOT TAKE THE DRUGS; MUST IMMEDIATELY PARTICIPATE IN A BOARD-APPROVED MONITORED AFTERCARE TREATMENT PROGRAM WHOSE THERAPIST MUST SUBMIT MONTHLY REPORTS; MUST THEN PARTICIPATE IN A 12-STEP RECOVERY PROGRAM AS DETERMINED BY HIS TREATING THERAPIST AND ATTEND AT LEAST THREE WEEKLY MEETINGS; SHALL OBTAIN A BOARD-APPROVED TREATING PHYSICIAN; SHALL ABSTAIN COMPLETELY FROM THE CONSUMPTION OF ALCOHOLIC BEVERAGES AND DRUGS EXCEPT WHEN PRESCRIBED BY HIS TREATING PHYSICIAN; SHALL NOT CONSUME FOOD OR SUBSTANCES CONTAINING POPPYSEEDS; MUST SUBMIT TO WITNESSED RANDOM BIOLOGICAL FLUID COLLECTION; MUST KEEP A LOG OF ANY AND ALL MEDICATIONS PRESCRIBED FOR HIM; SHALL SUBMIT TO ANY EXAMINATIONS OR THERAPY ORDERED BY BOARD; SHALL APPEAR BEFORE BOARD FOR INTERVIEWS UPON REQUEST; SHALL INFORM BOARD OF CHANGE OF ADDRESS OR IF AWAY FOR MORE THAN FIVE DAYS. SHALL CONTINUE IN THERAPY WITH A TREATING PSYCHIATRIST APPROVED BY THE BOARD AND SHALL REMAIN IN TREATMENT WITH THE PSYCHIATRIST UNTIL FURTHER ORDER OF THE BOARD WITH QUARTERLY REPORTS. THIS ORDER SUPERSEDES REHABILITATION ORDER OF 11/96. ON 3/24/99, LICENSE WAS INACTIVATED.

LONG, AARON E MD, LICENSE NUMBER 0040931 OF TAMPA, FL, WAS DISCIPLINED BY FLORIDA ON APRIL 11, 1990
DISCIPLINARY ACTION: 12-MONTH LICENSE SUSPENSION; 60-MONTH PROBATION
OFFENSE: CRIMINAL CONVICTION OR PLEA OF GUILTY, NOLO CONTENDERE, OR NO CONTEST TO A CRIME

NOTES: FOUND GUILTY OF BEING CONVICTED OR FOUND GUILTY OF A CRIME IN ANY JURISDICTION WHICH DIRECTLY RELATES TO THE PRACTICE OF MEDICINE OR TO THE ABILITY TO PRACTICE MEDICINE. MUST

PAY $400 FINE; UPON REINSTATEMENT, FIVE YEARS PROBATION, SUBJECT TO TERMS AND CONDITIONS TO BE SET AT THAT TIME. STAY GRANTED ON 05/16/90.

LONG, AARON E MD OF CALUMET CITY, IL, WAS DISCIPLINED BY ILLINOIS ON DECEMBER 1, 1990
DISCIPLINARY ACTION: 3-MONTH LICENSE SUSPENSION; 60-MONTH PROBATION
OFFENSE: CRIMINAL CONVICTION OR PLEA OF GUILTY, NOLO CONTENDERE, OR NO CONTEST TO A CRIME

NOTES: PLEADED GUILTY TO THREE FELONY COUNTS CONCERNING THE SUBMISSION OF FRAUDULENT CLAIMS TO INSURANCE COMPANIES,

LONG, AARON E MD, LICENSE NUMBER 1032632 OF 16202 FANTASIA DRIVE, TAMPA, FL, WAS DISCIPLINED BY INDIANA ON MAY 23, 1991
DISCIPLINARY ACTION: LICENSE REVOCATION
OFFENSE: DISCIPLINARY ACTION BY ANOTHER STATE OR AGENCY

NOTES: ENTERED INTO A VOLUNTARY GUILTY PLEA IN U.S. DISTRICT COURT, NORTHERN DISTRICT OF ILLINOIS FOR KNOWINGLY DIAGNOSING AND PROVIDING "TREATMENT" FOR NONEXISTENT INJURIES TO "VICTIMS" OF STAGED FAKE AUTO ACCIDENTS AND SUBMITTING FALSE MEDICAL BILLS TO INSURANCE COMPANIES; CONVICTED OF KNOWINGLY, WILLFULLY AND UNLAWFULLY USING THE MAILS FOR THE PURPOSE OF EXECUTING A SCHEME TO DEFRAUD AND/OR CONSPIRACY TO COMMIT THE OFFENSE ON 08/26/88. ON 4/11/90 FLORIDA SUSPENDED HIS LICENSE FOR ONE YEAR. DEFAULTED. ORDERED TO PAY $370 FOR COSTS OF PROCEEDINGS.

LONG, AARON E MD, LICENSE NUMBER 0017372, WAS DISCIPLINED BY ARIZONA ON APRIL 7, 1992
DISCIPLINARY ACTION: LICENSE REVOCATION
OFFENSE: DISCIPLINARY ACTION BY ANOTHER STATE OR AGENCY

NOTES: ON 10/23/87 ENTERED A GUILTY PLEA IN ILLINOIS TO THREE COUNTS OF CONDUCTING A SCHEME TO DEFRAUD INSURANCE COMPANIES; HIS PARTICIPATION INVOLVED "TREATING" "VICTIMS" INVOLVED IN STAGED ACCIDENTS AND THEREAFTER PREPARED INFLATED AND FRAUDULENT MEDICAL BILLS; SENTENCED TO PRISON FOR FOUR YEARS WITH SUBSEQUENT FIVE YEAR PROBATION ON CONDITION OF PERFORMING 1500 HOURS OF COMMUNITY SERVICE AND AT LEAST $11,650 RESTITUTION. ILLINOIS BOARD SUSPENDED HIS LICENSE FOR THREE MONTHS FOLLOWED BY A FIVE YEAR PROBATION ON 12/11/90.

LONG, AARON E MD, LICENSE NUMBER 0040931 OF VALRICO, FL, WAS DISCIPLINED BY FLORIDA ON FEBRUARY 16, 1995
DISCIPLINARY ACTION: FINE
OFFENSE: DISCIPLINARY ACTION BY ANOTHER STATE OR AGENCY

NOTES: CHARGED WITH HAVING A LICENSE ACTED AGAINST BY ANOTHER JURISDICTION AND FAILING TO REPORT THIS TO THE BOARD WITHIN 30 DAYS. $500 FINE.

LOPEZLIRA, JESUS MD, LICENSE NUMBER 1026809 OF 3301 WEST GLENN DRIVE, PHOENIX, AZ, WAS DISCIPLINED BY INDIANA ON FEBRUARY 9, 1990
DISCIPLINARY ACTION: LICENSE REVOCATION

LOPEZLIRA, JESUS MD, LICENSE NUMBER 0013124, WAS DISCIPLINED BY ARIZONA ON FEBRUARY 3, 1992
DISCIPLINARY ACTION: RESTRICTION PLACED ON LICENSE; REQUIRED TO TAKE ADDITIONAL MEDICAL EDUCATION

NOTES: SHALL NOT ENGAGE IN THE PRACTICE OF BARIATRIC MEDICINE (OBESITY TREATMENT) UNTIL HE COMPLIES WITH THE FOLLOWING: COMPLETE A MINIMUM ONE WEEK LONG MINI-RESIDENCY IN PHARMACOLOGY; COMPLETE A MINIMUM ONE WEEK LONG INTENSIVE COURSE IN BARIATRIC MEDICINE. WITHIN SIX MONTHS OF HIS RETURN TO BARIATRICS, BOARD SHALL CONDUCT A PRACTICE SURVEY TO DETERMINE THE QUALITY OF HIS PRACTICE.

LOPEZLIRA, JESUS MD, LICENSE NUMBER 0013124, WAS DISCIPLINED BY ARIZONA ON APRIL 19, 1996
DISCIPLINARY ACTION: 36-MONTH PROBATION; REPRIMAND
OFFENSE: FAILURE TO COMPLY WITH PREVIOUS BOARD ORDER

NOTES: IN 4/95, ORDERED TO TAKE AND PASS THE SPECIAL PURPOSE EXAMINATION (SPEX) IN 6/95 WITH A SCORE OF 75 OR GREATER; HAS NOT TAKEN OR PASSED THE SPEX. PROBATION WITH TERMS: SHALL NOT PRACTICE MEDICINE UNLESS AND UNTIL HE SUCCESSFULLY PASSES THE SPEX AND COMPLETES 10 HOURS OF CONTINUING MEDICAL EDUCATION IN RECORD-KEEPING; TWO PREVIOUS STIPULATIONS REGARDING PRACTICE OF BARIATRICS OR OBSTETRICS STILL IN EFFECT.

LOVE, BRUCE MD OF 4432 E MOCKINGBIRD LANE, PARADISE VALLEY, AZ, WAS DISCIPLINED BY DEA ON DECEMBER 9, 1999
DISCIPLINARY ACTION: SURRENDER OF CONTROLLED SUBSTANCE LICENSE
OFFENSE: DISCIPLINARY ACTION BY ANOTHER STATE OR AGENCY

NOTES: STATE BOARD.

LOVE, BRUCE D MD, WAS DISCIPLINED BY ARIZONA ON MARCH 25, 1999
DISCIPLINARY ACTION: RESTRICTION PLACED ON LICENSE
OFFENSE: PHYSICAL OR MENTAL ILLNESS INHIBITING THE ABILITY TO PRACTICE WITH SKILL AND SAFETY

NOTES: ON THE BASIS OF MENTAL IMPAIRMENT, HE CONSENTS THAT HE WILL NOT PRACTICE CLINICAL MEDICINE WITH PATIENT CONTACT UNTIL DEMONSTRATING HIS MENTAL AND PHYSICAL COMPETENCE. THE BOARD MAY REQUIRE ANY NUMBER OF EXAMINATIONS TO DETERMINE COMPETENCY AND HIS CONTINUING MEDICAL EDUCATION MUST BE UP-TO-DATE PRIOR TO HIS RESUMING PRACTICE.

LOVE, BRUCE DENNIS MD OF PHOENIX, AZ, WAS DISCIPLINED BY OHIO ON OCTOBER 11, 1995
OFFENSE: PROVIDING FALSE INFORMATION TO THE BOARD OR OTHER HEALTH AGENCY

NOTES: ADMITTED PROVIDING INCORRECT INFORMATION ON APPLICATIONS, CONSTITUTING MISREPRESENTATION. AUTHORIZED TO WITHDRAW APPLICATION FOR OHIO MEDICAL LICENSURE; PERMANENTLY INELIGIBLE TO APPLY IN THE FUTURE.

LUKE, WILLIAM J DO, LICENSE NUMBER 0001202 OF 4660 W THOMAS RD SUITE A, PHOENIX, AZ, WAS DISCIPLINED BY ARIZONA ON NOVEMBER 15, 1993
DISCIPLINARY ACTION: PROBATION; FINE
OFFENSE: OVERPRESCRIBING OR MISPRESCRIBING DRUGS

NOTES: BETWEEN 4/76 AND 11/91 PRESCRIBED, DISPENSED, OR ADMINISTERED CONTROLLED SUBSTANCES OR PRESCRIPTION-ONLY DRUGS TO 14 PATIENTS IN AMOUNTS AND FREQUENCY THAT CANNOT BE JUSTIFIED BASED ON THE DIAGNOSIS SET FORTH IN THE RECORDS. PROBATION BEGINNING 12/15/93

UNDER TERMS AND CONDITIONS: FOR THE FIRST 30 DAYS MAY NOT PROVIDE DIAGNOSIS AND TREATMENT OF ANY KIND AND PRESCRIBING OR ADMINISTERING MEDICATIONS; MAY NOT PRESCRIBE ANY SCHEDULE II AND II MEDICATIONS; SHALL COMPLETE 20 HOURS OF CONTINUING MEDICAL EDUCATION PER YEAR FOR TWO YEARS IN THE AREA OF APPROPRIATE PRESCRIBING OF NARCOTIC AND CONTROLLED SUBSTANCES AND SUBSTANCE ADDICTION; DURING THE FIRST THREE YEARS OF PROBATION SHALL BE SUBJECT TO REVIEW OF ALL ASPECTS OF HIS MEDICAL PRACTICE, BUT PRIMARILY IN THE AREA OF DIAGNOSIS AND TREATMENT OF PATIENTS AND MAINTENANCE OF PATIENT RECORDS; A RANDOM REVIEW OF AT LEAST 10 PATIENT RECORDS SHALL BE CONDUCTED EVERY 120 DAYS; THE SUPERVISING PHYSICIAN SHALL PROVIDE THE BOARD WITH A REPORT REFLECTING ANY RELEVANT FINDINGS OR OPINIONS CONCERNING HIS MEDICAL PRACTICE ACTIVITY AND COMPLIANCE WITH THIS ORDER; SHALL APPEAR BEFORE THE BOARD UPON REQUEST BUT NOT MORE THAN THREE TIMES A YEAR; AFTER THREE YEARS OF PROBATION AND COMPLETION OF CONTINUING EDUCATION REQUIREMENTS MAY PETITION THE BOARD TO TERMINATE PROBATION AND REINSTATE HIS PRESCRIBING PRIVILEGES. $15,000 CIVIL PENALTY; REPRIMAND. ON 4/10/99 CONDITIONS SATISFIED; FULL AND UNRESTRICTED LICENSE.

LUKE, WILLIAM J DO OF 4660 WEST THOMAS ROAD SUITE A, PHOENIX, AZ, WAS DISCIPLINED BY DEA ON MAY 2, 1995
DISCIPLINARY ACTION: RESTRICTION PLACED ON CONTROLLED SUBSTANCE LICENSE
OFFENSE: DISCIPLINARY ACTION BY ANOTHER STATE OR AGENCY

NOTES: STATE BOARD.

LUTHRA, ADARSH MD, LICENSE NUMBER 0010415, WAS DISCIPLINED BY ARIZONA ON OCTOBER 23, 1992
DISCIPLINARY ACTION: REQUIRED TO TAKE ADDITIONAL MEDICAL EDUCATION
OFFENSE: SUBSTANDARD CARE, INCOMPETENCE OR NEGLIGENCE

NOTES: MALPRACTICE CLAIM ALLEGING FAILURE TO PROPERLY INSERT A SUBCLAVIAN CATHETER FOR RENAL DIALYSIS RESULTING IN SEVERE INJURIES TO THE PATIENT. SHALL SUCCESSFULLY COMPLETE WITHIN SIX MONTHS A TWO-WEEK MINI-RESIDENCY IN INFECTIOUS DISEASES.

LYNN, HARVEY D MD, DATE OF BIRTH SEPTEMBER 8, 1912, LICENSE NUMBER 1013903 OF 7525 E GAINEY RANCH RD #147, SCOTTSDALE, AZ, WAS DISCIPLINED BY MICHIGAN ON NOVEMBER 27, 1997
DISCIPLINARY ACTION: SURRENDER OF LICENSE
OFFENSE: NONCOMPLIANCE WITH A PROFESSIONAL RULE

NOTES: FAILURE TO MEET CONTINUING EDUCATION REQUIREMENTS. VOLUNTARY SURRENDER.

LYNN, HARVEY D MD OF 27451 LAKEHILLS DRIVE, FRANKLIN, MI, WAS DISCIPLINED BY DEA ON FEBRUARY 18, 1998
DISCIPLINARY ACTION: SURRENDER OF CONTROLLED SUBSTANCE LICENSE

NOTES: IN LIEU OF PUBLIC INTEREST REVOCATION.

MAC, DALJIT SINGH MD, LICENSE NUMBER 0015117 OF PHOENIX, AZ, WAS DISCIPLINED BY ARIZONA ON OCTOBER 12, 1993
DISCIPLINARY ACTION: REQUIRED TO TAKE ADDITIONAL MEDICAL EDUCATION

NOTES: RELATIVE TO HIS CARE AND TREATMENT OF A PATIENT AND PRESCRIBING PRACTICES. SHALL COMPLETE 20 CREDIT HOURS OF CONTINUING MEDICAL EDUCATION IN PSYCHOPHARMACOLOGY. THESE HOURS SHALL BE IN ADDITION TO THE 20 HOURS OF CONTINUING MEDICAL EDUCATION REQUIRED ANNUALLY. COMPLETED THESE REQUIREMENTS AND STIPULATION TERMINATED ON 7/16/94.

MAC, DALJIT SINGH MD, LICENSE NUMBER 0015117 OF CHANDLER, AZ, WAS DISCIPLINED BY ARIZONA ON APRIL 13, 1994

NOTES: WITHIN 120 DAYS HE SHALL TAKE AND PASS AN ORAL COMPETENCY EXAMINATION IN PSYCHIATRY ADMINISTERED BY EXAMINERS APPOINTED BY THE BOARD; AND SHALL ENGAGE THE SERVICES OF A PRACTICE MANAGEMENT CONSULTANT WHO SHALL ADVISE HIM REGARDING NECESSARY AND APPROPRIATE OFFICE MANAGEMENT PROCEDURES. ON 1/20/95 ORDER TERMINATED.

MACCABE, FREDERICK MD, LICENSE NUMBER 0004715, WAS DISCIPLINED BY ARIZONA ON JANUARY 17, 1996
DISCIPLINARY ACTION: LICENSE SUSPENSION
OFFENSE: PROFESSIONAL MISCONDUCT

NOTES: TREATED A PATIENT FOR 18 MONTHS WITH PERPHENAZINE AND OTHER MEDICATIONS IN THE ABSENCE OF A NEUROLOGICAL ASSESSMENT REGARDING THE POSSIBILITY OF TARDIVE DYSKINESIA. LICENSE PLACED ON INACTIVE STATUS WITH CAUSE. SHALL NOT HOLD OR MAINTAIN A DEA CONTROLLED SUBSTANCE CERTIFICATE; SHALL NOT REQUEST REACTIVATION UNTIL MEETS WITH BOARD AND COMPLIES WITH ALL BOARD REQUESTS.

MACGILLIVRAY, IAN DO OF PHOENIX, AZ, WAS DISCIPLINED BY MISSOURI ON SEPTEMBER 17, 1990
DISCIPLINARY ACTION: LICENSE REVOCATION
OFFENSE: DISCIPLINARY ACTION BY ANOTHER STATE OR AGENCY

NOTES: REVOCATION OF LICENSE IN ARIZONA BASED ON CONVICTION OF FRAUDULENT INSURANCE CLAIMS AND THEFT OF PROPERTY VALUED AT $1,000 OR MORE.

MACLACHLAN, ROBERT T MD, LICENSE NUMBER 0012776, WAS DISCIPLINED BY ARIZONA ON JANUARY 31, 1995
DISCIPLINARY ACTION: LICENSE SUSPENSION; REQUIRED TO ENTER AN IMPAIRED PHYSICIAN PROGRAM OR SUBSTANCE ABUSE TREATMENT
OFFENSE: SUBSTANCE ABUSE

NOTES: RELEASED FROM TREATMENT CENTER IN EARLY 1/95 AFTER HE WAS TREATED FOR ALCOHOLISM; RELAPSED AND A BIOLOGICAL FLUID SPECIMEN OBTAINED BY THE BOARD ON 1/11/95 TESTED POSITIVE FOR ALCOHOL; DID NOT YET HAVE A PERMANENT SPONSOR AND MISSED AFTERCARE MEETINGS. BOARD ACCEPTED HIS REQUEST FOR INACTIVE STATUS. MAY NOT HOLD DEA REGISTRATION OR WRITE PRESCRIPTIONS WHILE LICENSE IS CLASSIFIED AS INACTIVE. PRIOR TO REACTIVATING LICENSE, AGREES TO ENTER LONG-TERM RESIDENTIAL/INPATIENT TREATMENT FOR CHEMICAL DEPENDENCY AND ALCOHOLISM AT A BOARD-APPROVED FACILITY, AND TO SUCCESSFULLY COMPLETE ALL TREATMENT RECOMMENDED. DID NOT COMPLETE LONG TERM TREATMENT. ON 1/18/96 REQUEST GRANTED ALLOWING HIM TO PARTICIPATE IN THE BOARD'S MONITORED AFTERCARE PROGRAM AS LONG AS HE PAYS THE PARTICIPATION FEES.

MACLACHLAN, ROBERT T MD OF 7119 E 1ST AVE, SCOTTSDALE, AZ, WAS DISCIPLINED BY DEA ON APRIL 25, 1995
DISCIPLINARY ACTION: SURRENDER OF CONTROLLED SUBSTANCE LICENSE
OFFENSE: SUBSTANCE ABUSE

NOTES: ALCOHOL ABUSE.

MADRID, EDWARD J MD, LICENSE NUMBER 0016602, WAS DISCIPLINED BY ARIZONA ON OCTOBER 12, 1991
DISCIPLINARY ACTION: REQUIRED TO ENTER AN IMPAIRED PHYSICIAN PROGRAM OR SUBSTANCE ABUSE TREATMENT; MONITORING OF PHYSICIAN PERFORMANCE
OFFENSE: SUBSTANCE ABUSE

NOTES: INFORMATION RECEIVED THAT HE WAS ABUSING CHEMICAL SUBSTANCES. MUST IMMEDIATELY PARTICIPATE IN A BOARD-APPROVED MONITORED AFTERCARE TREATMENT PROGRAM WHOSE THERAPIST MUST SUBMIT QUARTERLY REPORTS; MUST PARTICIPATE IN 90 12-STEP MEETINGS FOR SUBSTANCE ABUSE WITHIN 90 DAYS; MUST THEN PARTICIPATE IN A 12-STEP RECOVERY PROGRAM AS DETERMINED BY HIS TREATING THERAPIST AND ATTEND AT LEAST THREE WEEKLY MEETINGS; SHALL OBTAIN A BOARD-APPROVED TREATING PHYSICIAN; SHALL ABSTAIN COMPLETELY FROM THE CONSUMPTION OF ALCOHOLIC BEVERAGES AND DRUGS EXCEPT WHEN PRESCRIBED BY HIS TREATING PHYSICIAN; MUST SUBMIT TO WITNESSED RANDOM BIOLOGICAL FLUID COLLECTION; SHALL KEEP A LOG OF ANY AND ALL MEDICATIONS PRESCRIBED FOR HIM; SHALL SUBMIT TO ANY EXAMINATIONS OR THERAPY ORDERED BY BOARD; SHALL APPEAR BEFORE BOARD FOR FURTHER INTERVIEW UPON REQUEST; SHALL INFORM BOARD OF CHANGE OF ADDRESS OR IF AWAY FOR MORE THAN FIVE DAYS.

MADRID, EDWARD J MD, LICENSE NUMBER 0G70631 OF TEMPE, AZ, WAS DISCIPLINED BY CALIFORNIA ON OCTOBER 9, 1995
DISCIPLINARY ACTION: 60-MONTH PROBATION
OFFENSE: DISCIPLINARY ACTION BY ANOTHER STATE OR AGENCY

NOTES: ACTION IN ARIZONA FOR SUBSTANCE ABUSE. REVOCATION, STAYED.

MAESTAS, ANDREW L MD, LICENSE NUMBER 0046499 OF HOLBROOK, AZ, WAS DISCIPLINED BY FLORIDA ON APRIL 15, 1994
DISCIPLINARY ACTION: FINE
OFFENSE: NONCOMPLIANCE WITH A PROFESSIONAL RULE

NOTES: CHARGED WITH FAILING TO PROVIDE REQUESTED MEDICAL RECORDS AND INSURANCE INFORMATION IN A TIMELY MANNER; FAILING TO NOTIFY THE DEPARTMENT OF HIS NEW ADDRESS PRIOR TO CHANGING HIS PRIMARY PLACE OF PRACTICE. $500 FINE; SHALL DEMONSTRATE THAT THE MEDICAL RECORDS IN QUESTION HAVE BEEN PROVIDED TO A PATIENT, THAT HE HAS COMPLIED WITH THE RULES OF THE BOARD REGARDING NOTIFICATION OF PATIENTS WHEN A PRACTICE IS MOVED OR TERMINATED AND THAT A METHOD HAS BEEN SET UP FOR PATIENTS TO RECEIVE REQUESTED MEDICAL RECORDS IN A TIMELY MANNER.

MAHL, MICHAEL MD, WAS DISCIPLINED BY ARIZONA ON MAY 15, 1998
DISCIPLINARY ACTION: REQUIRED TO ENTER AN IMPAIRED PHYSICIAN PROGRAM OR TREATMENT

NOTES: MUST SUCCESSFULLY COMPLETE INPATIENT TREATMENT AT A FACILITY FOR SEXUAL COMPULSIVITY AND CHEMICAL DEPENDENCY AND THAT THE FACILITY BE APPROVED BY THE BOARD STAFF PRIOR TO HIS ADMISSION; HE MUST SIGN A RELEASE OF RECORDS TO THE ARIZONA BOARD FROM ALL TREATMENT FACILITIES; HE MAY NOT PRACTICE MEDICINE UNTIL HE MEETS WITH THE BOARD AND RECEIVES AFFIRMATIVE APPROVAL TO DO SO.

MALONE, WILLIAM WARREN MD, DATE OF BIRTH APRIL 13, 1930, LICENSE NUMBER 0006241, WAS DISCIPLINED BY ARIZONA ON JANUARY 24, 1992
DISCIPLINARY ACTION: PROBATION; FINE
OFFENSE: FAILURE TO COMPLY WITH PREVIOUS BOARD ORDER

NOTES: FAILED TO INFORM EMPLOYERS OF HIS SUSPENSION FOR SEVEN YEARS (STARTING 8/31/87) FROM THE MEDICARE PROGRAM, AND PROVIDED SERVICES TO SENIOR PLAN MEMBERS WHOSE TREATMENT WAS TIED TO MEDICARE BENEFITS. CENSURED; $392 ADMINISTRATIVE PENALTY; ON PROBATION UNTIL EXPIRATION OF HIS EXCLUSION FROM THE MEDICARE PROGRAM, AND DURING THIS TIME HE SHALL NOT TREAT ANY PATIENTS AGE 65 OR OLDER.

MALONE, WILLIAM WARREN MD, DATE OF BIRTH APRIL 13, 1930, LICENSE NUMBER 0006241, WAS DISCIPLINED BY ARIZONA ON JANUARY 31, 1994
DISCIPLINARY ACTION: LICENSE REVOCATION

NOTES: AGREES NOT TO RE-APPLY FOR LICENSURE TO PRACTICE MEDICINE IN ARIZONA FOR A FIVE YEAR PERIOD.

MALONE, WILLIAM WARREN MD, DATE OF BIRTH APRIL 13, 1930 OF PHOENIX, AZ, WAS DISCIPLINED BY DEA ON APRIL 6, 1995
DISCIPLINARY ACTION: REVOCATION OF CONTROLLED SUBSTANCE LICENSE
OFFENSE: DISCIPLINARY ACTION BY ANOTHER STATE OR AGENCY

NOTES: LICENSE SUSPENDED BY THE ARIZONA BOARD ON 1/31/94.

MANSON, JONATHAN DAVID MD OF 5755 EAST RIVER ROAD APT 3105, TUCSON, AZ, WAS DISCIPLINED BY MARYLAND ON DECEMBER 9, 1998
DISCIPLINARY ACTION: DENIAL OF NEW LICENSE
OFFENSE: PROVIDING FALSE INFORMATION TO THE BOARD OR OTHER HEALTH AGENCY

NOTES: LACKS THE REQUISITE MORAL CHARACTER; HE FRAUDULENTLY AND DECEPTIVELY ATTEMPTED TO OBTAIN A LICENSE AND HAS WILLFULLY MADE FALSE REPRESENTATIONS WHEN SEEKING LICENSURE.

MARAS, ANCA M MD, LICENSE NUMBER 0013103, WAS DISCIPLINED BY ARIZONA ON JULY 17, 1996
DISCIPLINARY ACTION: REPRIMAND
OFFENSE: LOSS OR RESTRICTION OF HOSPITAL PRIVILEGES

NOTES: INTERVIEWED BY THE BOARD REGARDING THE TERMINATION OF HER PRIVILEGES AT A HOSPITAL, HER ANESTHESIA CARE PROVIDED TO PATIENTS AND THE ADEQUACY OF HER PATIENT RECORDS; IN 1/91, HOSPITAL PRIVILEGES TERMINATED BASED ON HER FAILED SUPERVISORY REPORTS SUBMITTED FOR FOUR MEDICAL RECORDS, WHICH INDICATED INACCURATE OR FALSE RECORDING IN PATIENTS' CHARTS IN THREE CASES, A FAILURE TO RESPOND APPROPRIATELY TO A PATIENT'S OXYGEN DESATURATION IN ONE CASE AND INAPPROPRIATE ADMINISTRATION OF ANESTHESIA IN TWO CASES; IN 7/94, BOARD ORDERED HER TO BE EXAMINED BY THE COLORADO PERSONALIZED EDUCATION PROGRAM FOR PHYSICIANS; UNDERWENT ASSESSMENT IN 9/94

WITH TWO INTERVIEWERS, THE FIRST OF WHICH FOUND HER KNOWLEDGE OF ANESTHESIA SATISFACTORY AND HER RECORD-KEEPING TO BE ABOVE AVERAGE AND THE SECOND OF WHICH EXPRESSED CONCERN ABOUT HER RECORD-KEEPING AND LACK OF FUNDAMENTAL KNOWLEDGE OF ANESTHESIA; RECEIVED A SCORE OF 45% ON A MULTIPLE CHOICE EXAMINATION ABOUT ANESTHESIOLOGY ADMINISTERED BY THE COLORADO PERSONALIZED EDUCATION AS AN INDICATOR, RATHER THAN AS A BENCHMARK TEST OF KNOWLEDGE OR COMPETENCE; SHE BECAME A DIPLOMATE OF THE AMERICAN BOARD OF ANESTHESIOLOGY IN 1990 AFTER PREVIOUSLY FAILING THE WRITTEN PART OF THE EXAMINATION TWICE.

MARAS, ANCA M MD, LICENSE NUMBER 147761 OF 7840 E. CAMELBACK ROAD APT 440, SCOTTSDALE, AZ, WAS DISCIPLINED BY NEW YORK ON MAY 21, 1998
DISCIPLINARY ACTION: LICENSE SUSPENSION
OFFENSE: DISCIPLINARY ACTION BY ANOTHER STATE OR AGENCY

NOTES: DISCIPLINED BY THE ARIZONA BOARD FOR UNPROFESSIONAL CONDUCT AND FAILING TO MAINTAIN ADEQUATE PATIENT RECORDS. SUSPENSION UNTIL THE SUCCESSFUL COMPLETION OF A TRAINING PROGRAM DETERMINED BY THE NEW YORK STATE ANESTHESIOLOGISTS' SOCIETY.

MARCHESKY, WILLIAM D MD, LICENSE NUMBER 0015907, WAS DISCIPLINED BY ARIZONA ON APRIL 16, 1996
DISCIPLINARY ACTION: REQUIRED TO TAKE ADDITIONAL MEDICAL EDUCATION

NOTES: SHALL COMPLETE 50 HOURS OF CONTINUING MEDICAL EDUCATION, 30 ON MANAGEMENT OF DIABETES AND 20 OF PRACTICAL EXPERIENCE IN A DIABETIC CLINIC. ON 1/22/97 ORDER WAS TERMINATED.

MARLON, ANTHONY MD, LICENSE NUMBER 0008072, WAS DISCIPLINED BY ARIZONA ON OCTOBER 20, 1994
DISCIPLINARY ACTION: FINE
OFFENSE: DISCIPLINARY ACTION BY ANOTHER STATE OR AGENCY

NOTES: ON 09/20/91, THE NEVADA BOARD ISSUED AN ORDER FINDING THAT HIS MISDEMEANOR CONVICTIONS WERE A VIOLATION OF THE NEVADA MEDICAL PRACTICE ACT. CENSURED AND SHALL PAY A CIVIL PENALTY OF $2,500 TO THE ARIZONA BOARD ON OR BEFORE 03/01/95.

MARON, BARRY R MD, DATE OF BIRTH NOVEMBER 30, 1938, LICENSE NUMBER 0020300 OF IA, WAS DISCIPLINED BY ARIZONA ON APRIL 15, 1993

NOTES: BOARD HAS INVESTIGATED INFORMATION THAT HE HAS BIPOLAR DISORDER AND SELF MEDICATES HIMSELF. CURRENTLY PRACTICING IN IOWA. SHALL NOT PRACTICE MEDICINE IN ARIZONA UNTIL HE HAS FIRST ADVISED THE BOARD OF HIS INTENTION TO DO SO AND RECEIVED AUTHORIZATION.

MARON, BARRY R MD, DATE OF BIRTH NOVEMBER 30, 1938, LICENSE NUMBER 0021140 OF BOX 1707, BORGER, TX, WAS DISCIPLINED BY NEW JERSEY ON NOVEMBER 2, 1994

NOTES: AGREES TO COMPLY WITH ALL REQUIREMENTS OF AN ORDER DATED 06/16/93 ISSUED BY THE BOARD OF MEDICAL EXAMINERS OF ARIZONA. SHALL PROVIDE NOTICE TO NEW JERSEY OF ANY CHANGE IN ANY OF THE TERMS OF THE ARIZONA AGREEMENT OR HIS MEDICAL CONDITION. PRIOR TO ENGAGING IN ACTIVE PRACTICE IN NEW JERSEY, SHALL APPEAR BEFORE THE BOARD OR A COMMITTEE OF THE BOARD TO RESPOND TO QUESTIONS CONCERNING HIS STATUS, HEALTH AND PLANS.

MARON, BARRY R MD, LICENSE NUMBER 0G16120 OF ALBUQUERQUE, NM, WAS DISCIPLINED BY CALIFORNIA ON MAY 19, 1995
DISCIPLINARY ACTION: 60-MONTH PROBATION
OFFENSE: DISCIPLINARY ACTION BY ANOTHER STATE OR AGENCY

NOTES: ARIZONA ORDER RESTRICTING RESUMPTION OF PRACTICE WITH PRECONDITIONS, SUCH AS PSYCHIATRIC EVALUATION FOR SAFE PRACTICE. REVOCATION STAYED.

MARON, BARRY R MD, DATE OF BIRTH NOVEMBER 30, 1938, LICENSE NUMBER 0028935 OF 408 NORTH MAIN STREET, WARSAW, NY, WAS DISCIPLINED BY IOWA ON AUGUST 8, 1996

NOTES: AGREED THAT HE WILL NOT RETURN TO PRACTICE IN IOWA UNLESS HE GIVES THE BOARD 30 DAYS NOTICE IN WRITING AND IF HE DOES RETURN SHALL ENTER INTO A CONSENT AGREEMENT PLACING ANY RESTRICTIONS ON HIS LICENSE THAT THE BOARD DEEMS NECESSARY.

MARQUEZ, ALBERTO B MD, LICENSE NUMBER 0004243 OF TUCSON, AZ, WAS DISCIPLINED BY ARIZONA ON JULY 16, 1992
DISCIPLINARY ACTION: 60-MONTH PROBATION; RESTRICTION PLACED ON LICENSE
OFFENSE: SUBSTANDARD CARE, INCOMPETENCE OR NEGLIGENCE

NOTES: ON 3/1/90, IMPROPERLY HANDLED AN EXAMINATION OF A SIX YEAR OLD GIRL WHO HAD BEEN SEXUALLY ASSAULTED; STATED TO THE PATIENT'S PARENTS AND THE POLICE THAT HE THOUGHT THERE HAD BEEN PENILE PENETRATION AND THAT SHE HAD GONORRHEA WHEN IN FACT THERE WAS INSUFFICIENT EVIDENCE FOR EITHER OF THESE STATEMENTS. ALSO FAILED TO PERFORM AN ADEQUATE PHYSICAL EXAMINATION, OBTAIN A HISTORY, OR ORDER PROPER DIAGNOSTIC TESTING. FROM 2/87 THROUGH AT LEAST 10/90, PRESCRIBED EXCESSIVE AMOUNTS OF CONTROLLED SUBSTANCES TO A PATIENT, AND KEPT INADEQUATE MEDICAL RECORDS. BOARD HAD PREVIOUSLY CENSURED HIM ON 4/11/85 FOR FAILING TO CONDUCT PHYSICAL EXAMS AND RELYING SOLELY ON LAB TEST RESULTS. HAS RECENTLY RECEIVED TREATMENT FOR ALCOHOLIC CIRRHOSIS; BOARD DETERMINED THAT HIS HEALTH IS SEVERELY IMPAIRED. SHALL PERFORM NO PEDIATRIC TREATMENT ON PATIENTS LESS THAN 12 YEARS OLD; SHALL NOT CONDUCT AN EXAM, OR OTHERWISE MANAGE THE CARE AND TREATMENT OF ANY PATIENT IN A CASE INVOLVING SEXUAL ABUSE; SHALL SURRENDER DEA REGISTRATION FOR ALL SCHEDULE II CONTROLLED SUBSTANCES WITHIN 30 DAYS; SHALL PASS THE SPEX WITHIN SIX MONTHS; SHALL UNDERGO PHYSICAL, PSYCHIATRIC AND PSYCHOMETRIC EVALUATION, AND EVALUATION FOR ALCOHOLISM WITHIN 45 DAYS; SHALL SUBMIT TO REQUESTS FOR RANDOM BIOLOGICAL FLUID COLLECTION; SHALL APPEAR BEFORE THE BOARD FOR INTERVIEWS UPON REQUEST.

MARQUEZ, ALBERTO B MD, LICENSE NUMBER 0004243 OF TUCSON, AZ, WAS DISCIPLINED BY ARIZONA ON JANUARY 20, 1993
DISCIPLINARY ACTION: PROBATION; REQUIRED TO ENTER AN IMPAIRED PHYSICIAN PROGRAM OR SUBSTANCE ABUSE TREATMENT
OFFENSE: SUBSTANCE ABUSE

NOTES: FAILED TO COMPLY WITH 7/16/92 ORDER IN THAT HE DID NOT TAKE AND PASS SPEX EXAM; SEVERAL EVALUATIONS DIAGNOSED ALCOHOL RELATED DIFFICULTIES AND RECOMMENDED INPATIENT TREATMENT; NO BIOLOGICAL FLUID MONITORING WAS POSITIVE FOR ALCOHOL FOR FIVE MONTHS; HAS BEEN VOLUNTARILY ATTENDING TREATMENT. CONDITIONS OF PROBATION: SHALL SUCCESSFULLY COMPLETE PRESENT OUTPATIENT TREATMENT WITH REPORT TO THE BOARD; SHALL PASS THE SPEX BEFORE 4/1/93; MUST IMMEDIATELY PARTICIPATE IN A BOARD-APPROVED MONITORED AFTERCARE TREATMENT PROGRAM WHOSE THERAPIST MUST SUBMIT QUARTERLY REPORTS; MUST PARTICIPATE IN 90 12-STEP MEETINGS FOR SUBSTANCE ABUSE WITHIN 90 DAYS; MUST THEN PARTICIPATE IN A 12-STEP RECOVERY PROGRAM AS DETERMINED BY HIS TREATING THERAPIST AND ATTEND AT LEAST THREE WEEKLY MEETINGS; SHALL OBTAIN A BOARD-APPROVED TREATING PHYSICIAN; SHALL ABSTAIN COMPLETELY FROM THE CONSUMPTION OF ALCOHOLIC BEVERAGES AND DRUGS EXCEPT WHEN PRESCRIBED BY HIS TREATING PHYSICIAN; MUST SUBMIT TO WITNESSED RANDOM BIOLOGICAL FLUID COLLECTION; KEEP A LOG OF ANY AND ALL MEDICATIONS PRESCRIBED FOR HIM; SHALL SUBMIT TO ANY EXAMINATIONS OR THERAPY ORDERED BY BOARD; SHALL APPEAR BEFORE BOARD FOR INTERVIEWS UPON REQUEST; SHALL INFORM BOARD OF CHANGE OF ADDRESS OR IF AWAY FOR MORE THAN 5 DAYS.

MARQUEZ, ALBERTO B MD, LICENSE NUMBER 0004243, WAS DISCIPLINED BY ARIZONA ON JULY 17, 1993
OFFENSE: FAILURE TO COMPLY WITH PREVIOUS BOARD ORDER

NOTES: FAILED SPEX IN VIOLATION OF 1/20/93 ORDER. SHALL TAKE AND PASS IT PRIOR TO 12/31/93. THIS ORDER SHALL HAVE NO EFFECT ON THE PREVIOUS ORDER OF PROBATION.

MARQUEZ, ALBERTO B MD, LICENSE NUMBER 0004243, WAS DISCIPLINED BY ARIZONA ON FEBRUARY 5, 1994
DISCIPLINARY ACTION: LICENSE SUSPENSION
OFFENSE: FAILURE TO COMPLY WITH PREVIOUS BOARD ORDER

NOTES: TOOK SPECIAL PURPOSE EXAMINATION (SPEX) AGAIN IN DECEMBER 1993 AND RECEIVED A FAILING SCORE OF 57 -- PASSING SCORE IS 75; THIS WAS A REQUIREMENT OF PREVIOUS BOARD ORDER OF 8/9/93. MOTION FOR RECONSIDERATION WAS DENIED ON 4/13/94.

MARQUEZ, ALBERTO B MD OF 4107 SOUTH 6TH AVENUE, TUCSON, AZ, WAS DISCIPLINED BY MEDICARE ON SEPTEMBER 1, 1994
DISCIPLINARY ACTION: EXCLUSION FROM THE MEDICARE AND/OR MEDICAID PROGRAM
OFFENSE: DISCIPLINARY ACTION BY ANOTHER STATE OR AGENCY

NOTES: LICENSE SUSPENDED FOR REASONS BEARING ON PROFESSIONAL COMPETENCE.

MARQUEZ, ALBERTO RAMON BADILLA MD OF 4107 SOUTH 6TH AVENUE, TUCSON, AZ, WAS DISCIPLINED BY DEA ON AUGUST 25, 1994
DISCIPLINARY ACTION: SURRENDER OF CONTROLLED SUBSTANCE LICENSE
OFFENSE: DISCIPLINARY ACTION BY ANOTHER STATE OR AGENCY

NOTES: STATE BOARD.

MARSH, PATRICK DO OF 801 SOUTH POWER ROAD, MESA, AZ, WAS DISCIPLINED BY DEA ON JULY 13, 1999
DISCIPLINARY ACTION: SURRENDER OF CONTROLLED SUBSTANCE LICENSE

MARSH, PATRICK J DO, LICENSE NUMBER 0002502 OF 801 SOUTH POWER, MESA, AZ, WAS DISCIPLINED BY ARIZONA ON FEBRUARY 14, 1992
DISCIPLINARY ACTION: REQUIRED TO ENTER AN IMPAIRED PHYSICIAN PROGRAM OR SUBSTANCE ABUSE TREATMENT
OFFENSE: SUBSTANCE ABUSE

NOTES: ON 1/28/92 TESTED POSITIVE FOR HYDROCODONE (CODEINE), ALPRAZOLAM METABOLITE (XANAX) AND PHENTERMINE; AND ON 2/04/92 ADMITTED THAT HE HAD SELF-MEDICATED WITH CONTROLLED AND/OR PRESCRIPTION ONLY MEDICATIONS ON ONE OR MORE OCCASIONS; WAS NOT UNDER THE CARE AND TREATMENT OF A DOCTOR AT THAT TIME; SHALL REFRAIN FROM THE PRACTICE OF OSTEOPATHIC MEDICINE AND SURGERY UNTIL THE BOARD HAS DETERMINED THAT HE HAS SUCCESSFULLY COMPLETED A TREATMENT PROGRAM FOR SUBSTANCE ABUSE AND CHEMICAL DEPENDENCE FOR NO LESS THAN ONE MONTH AND NO MORE THAN TWO MONTHS; SHALL MEET WITH THE BOARD AFTER SUCCESSFUL COMPLETION OF THE TREATMENT PROGRAM; SHALL USE NO CONTROLLED SUBSTANCES OR PRESCRIPTION-ONLY MEDICATION UNLESS PRESCRIBED BY HIS ATTENDING PHYSICIAN; SHALL REFRAIN COMPLETELY FROM THE USE OF ALCOHOL.

MARSH, PATRICK J DO, LICENSE NUMBER 0002502 OF 801 SOUTH POWER, MESA, AZ, WAS DISCIPLINED BY ARIZONA ON MARCH 30, 1992
DISCIPLINARY ACTION: 36-MONTH PROBATION; REQUIRED TO ENTER AN IMPAIRED PHYSICIAN PROGRAM OR SUBSTANCE ABUSE TREATMENT
OFFENSE: SUBSTANCE ABUSE

NOTES: HAS COMPLIED WITH THE TERMS OF 2/14/92 ORDER; AUTHORIZED TO RESUME THE PRACTICE OF OSTEOPATHIC MEDICINE AND SURGERY UNDER TERMS AND CONDITIONS: SHALL SUBMIT TO RANDOM URINALYSIS TESTING BY THE BOARD; SHALL USE NO CONTROLLED SUBSTANCE OR PRESCRIPTION-ONLY MEDICATION UNLESS PRESCRIBED BY HIS ATTENDING PHYSICIAN; SHALL REFRAIN COMPLETELY FROM THE USE OF ALCOHOL; SHALL MEET REGULARLY WITH THE BOARD; SHALL AUTHORIZE ANY ATTENDING PHYSICIAN, PSYCHIATRIST, OR PSYCHOLOGIST TO RELEASE TO THE BOARD ALL RECORDS PERTAINING TO HIS CARE AND TREATMENT; SHALL REGULARLY ATTEND AA OR NARCOTICS ANONYMOUS OR A SIMILAR BOARD APPROVED 12 STEP PROGRAM ON A WEEKLY BASIS AND SHALL ATTEND NO FEWER THAN 90 MEETINGS THE FIRST 90 DAYS; SHALL OBTAIN AND MAINTAIN A SPONSOR FOR HIS PARTICIPATION IN A 12 STEP RECOVERY PROGRAM; SHALL ATTEND A GROUP THERAPY MEETING WITH A BOARD APPROVED COUNSELOR NO LESS THAN ONCE PER WEEK WHO SHALL PROVIDE REGULAR REPORTS TO THE BOARD; SHALL ATTEND A BOARD APPROVED IMPAIRED PROFESSIONALS GROUP THERAPY PROGRAM SESSION NO LESS THAN ONCE PER MONTH AND AUTHORIZE THE GROUP LEADER TO PROVIDE REGULAR REPORTS TO THE BOARD; SHALL ATTEND A PRIVATE COUNSELING SESSION NO LESS THAN ONCE PER WEEK WITH A BOARD APPROVED COUNSELOR WHO SHALL PROVIDE REGULAR REPORTS TO THE BOARD.

MARSH, PATRICK J DO, LICENSE NUMBER 0002502 OF 801 SOUTH POWER, MESA, AZ, WAS DISCIPLINED BY ARIZONA ON SEPTEMBER 2, 1994
OFFENSE: PROFESSIONAL MISCONDUCT

NOTES: INFORMATION RECEIVED BY THE BOARD THAT HE MAY BE PHYSICALLY AND/OR PSYCHOLOGICALLY UNABLE TO SAFELY AND SKILLFULLY ENGAGE IN THE PRACTICE OF MEDICINE AND MAY HAVE COMMITTED ONE OR MORE ACTS OF UNPROFESSIONAL CONDUCT. SHALL REFRAIN COMPLETELY FROM THE PRACTICE OF MEDICINE UNTIL HE HAS MET THE FOLLOWING CONDITIONS: SHALL PROVIDE AUTHORIZATIONS FOR ALL PHYSICIANS, PSYCHOLOGISTS, AND OTHER HEALTH CARE PROVIDERS INVOLVED IN HIS CARE AND TREATMENT TO RELEASE ANY INFORMATION ON HIS DIAGNOSIS, CARE, AND TREATMENT UPON BOARD REQUEST; BEEN EVALUATED AND RECEIVED CLEARANCE FROM ANY AND ALL PHYSICIANS INVOLVED IN/OR CHARGED WITH HIS CARE AND TREATMENT, TO RETURN TO THE PRACTICE OF MEDICINE; PROVIDED THE BOARD WITH COPIES OF RELEASE FORMS AND/OR DISCHARGE DIAGNOSIS AND TREATMENT PLANS DOCUMENTING THAT HE HAS RECEIVED CLEARANCE TO RETURN TO THE PRACTICE OF MEDICINE; MET WITH THE BOARD AFTER SUBMITTING WRITTEN REQUEST FOR APPROVAL TO RESUME PRACTICE.

MARSH, PATRICK J DO, LICENSE NUMBER 0002502 OF 801 SOUTH POWER, MESA, AZ, WAS DISCIPLINED BY ARIZONA ON JULY 14, 1995
DISCIPLINARY ACTION: PROBATION; RESTRICTION PLACED ON LICENSE
OFFENSE: FAILURE TO COMPLY WITH PREVIOUS BOARD ORDER

NOTES: RECEIVED TREATMENT FROM 9/6/94 TO 12/8/94; ADMITTED ON 3/10/95 TO USING VICODIN, A SCHEDULE III CONTROLLED SUBSTANCES, WITHOUT RECEIVING IT IN THE COURSE OF REGULAR MEDICAL TREATMENT. ALLOWED TO RETURN TO THE PRACTICE OF MEDICINE UNDER REVISED PROBATIONARY TERMS AND CONDITIONS: SHALL ATTEND AT LEAST ONE INDIVIDUAL COUNSELING SESSION PER WEEK WITH A PSYCHIATRIST OR PSYCHOLOGIST WHO SHALL SEND PROGRESS REPORTS TO THE BOARD ON A MONTHLY BASIS; SHALL OBTAIN AND MAINTAIN AN ACTIVE SPONSOR FOR HIS AA OR NARCOTICS ANONYMOUS PARTICIPATION; SHALL BE SUBJECT TO RANDOM BODILY FLUID TESTING FOR DRUGS; SHALL ENGAGE IN THE PRACTICE OF MEDICINE FOR NO MORE THAN 40 HOURS A WEEK; SHALL REFRAIN COMPLETELY FROM THE CONSUMPTION OF ALCOHOL; SHALL USE NO CONTROLLED SUBSTANCE OR PRESCRIPTION ONLY MEDICATIONS UNLESS PRESCRIBED BY A LICENSED PHYSICIAN; ALL PRESCRIPTIONS FOR CONTROLLED DRUGS IN DEA SCHEDULES II THROUGH V SHALL BE IN WRITTEN FORM ONLY AND SHALL BE ISSUED ONLY ON MULTIPLE COPY, AND SEQUENTIALLY NUMBERED BOARD APPROVED PRESCRIPTION PADS AND SHALL PROVIDE COPIES TO THE BOARD ON A WEEKLY BASIS; SHALL NOT ISSUE ORIGINAL PRESCRIPTIONS OR AUTHORIZE REFILLS OF CONTROLLED DRUG PRESCRIPTIONS VIA TELEPHONE CONTACT WITH ANY PHARMACY; SHALL KEEP A LOG OF ALL PRESCRIPTIONS WRITTEN AND SUBMIT THIS TO THE BOARD ON A MONTHLY BASIS; AND SHALL MEET REGULARLY WITH THE BOARD. SHALL INFORM THE BOARD IF HE LEAVES THE STATE. ALL OTHER TERMS OF 9/2/94 ORDER REMAIN IN EFFECT.

MARSH, PATRICK J DO, LICENSE NUMBER 2502 OF 6745 E SUPERSTITION SPRINGS BLVD, MESA, AZ, WAS DISCIPLINED BY ARIZONA ON MAY 4, 1999
DISCIPLINARY ACTION: LICENSE SUSPENSION; REQUIRED TO ENTER AN IMPAIRED PHYSICIAN PROGRAM OR SUBSTANCE ABUSE TREATMENT
OFFENSE: SUBSTANCE ABUSE

NOTES: SINCE 2/99 WAS ACQUIRING PRESCRIPTION MEDICINE FROM PHARMACIES UNDER A FALSE NAME FOR PERSONAL USE; ON 4/29/99 VOLUNTARILY ENTERED AN ASSESSMENT AT AN ALCOHOL AND DRUG TREATMENT CENTER. SHALL REFRAIN FROM THE PRACTICE OF OSTEOPATHIC MEDICINE UNTIL HE HAS COMPLIED WITH THE FOLLOWING: WILL SUCCESSFULLY COMPLETE THE IN-PATIENT EVALUATION FOR POSSIBLE ALCOHOL OR CHEMICAL DEPENDENCY AND FOLLOW RECOMMENDATIONS FOR TREATMENT; WILL DEVELOP A PLAN FOR AFTERCARE TREATMENT AND MONITORING; SHALL DEVELOP A PLAN FOR AFTERCARE; SHALL MEET WITH THE BOARD UPON WRITTEN REQUEST AFTER HIS DISCHARGE FROM THE FACILITY TO DISCUSS WHETHER OR NOT HE WILL RESUME PRACTICE.

MARSH, PATRICK J DO, LICENSE NUMBER 2502 OF 6745 SUPERSTITION SPRINGS BLVD., MESA, AZ, WAS DISCIPLINED BY ARIZONA ON OCTOBER 22, 1999
DISCIPLINARY ACTION: 60-MONTH PROBATION
OFFENSE: PROFESSIONAL MISCONDUCT

NOTES: HAS MET REQUIREMENTS OF 5/4/99 ORDER FOR REINSTATEMENT, INCLUDING INPATIENT TREATMENT. TERMS AND CONDITIONS OF LICENSE: SHALL IMMEDIATELY OBTAIN A TREATING THERAPIST APPROVED BY THE BOARD AND SHALL REMAIN IN TREATMENT UNTIL FURTHER ORDER OF THE BOARD; THERAPIST SHALL SUBMIT MONTHLY REPORTS TO THE BOARD; SHALL PROVIDE A COPY OF THIS ORDER TO ANY HEALTH CARE ENTITY WHERE HE HAS PRIVILEGES; SHALL ABSTAIN COMPLETELY FROM THE CONSUMPTION OF ALCOHOLIC BEVERAGES AND DRUGS EXCEPT WHEN PRESCRIBED BY HIS TREATING PHYSICIAN; SHALL SUBMIT TO ANY EXAMINATIONS ORDERED BY BOARD; SHALL APPEAR BEFORE BOARD UPON REQUEST; SHALL SUBMIT TO RANDOM BIOLOGICAL FLUID COLLECTION; SHALL PARTICIPATE IN A MINIMUM OF TWO SELF-HELP MEETINGS PER WEEK THROUGH SUCH ORGANIZATIONS AS AA OR NARCOTICS ANONYMOUS; SHALL INFORM THE BOARD IF HE CEASES TO PRACTICE IN ARIZONA; SHALL PAY COSTS.

MARTIN, ANTHONY MD, LICENSE NUMBER 22394, WAS DISCIPLINED BY ARIZONA ON MARCH 14, 1997
DISCIPLINARY ACTION: RESTRICTION PLACED ON LICENSE; MONITORING OF PHYSICIAN PERFORMANCE

NOTES: PRIOR TO TREATING ANY PATIENT WHO IS 13 YEARS OF AGE OR OLDER FOR ATTENTION DEFICIT DISORDER SHALL OBTAIN A SECOND OPINION REGARDING THE PATIENT FROM A PSYCHIATRIST WHO SHALL BE BOARD CERTIFIED BY THE AMERICAN BOARD OF PSYCHIATRY AND NEUROLOGY; THE PSYCHIATRIST SHALL PROVIDE WRITTEN EVIDENCE OF THE CONSULTATION TO DR. MARTIN WHO SHALL THEN PROVIDE IT TO THE BOARD; HE SHALL PAY ALL COSTS OF THE SECOND OPINION.

MARTIN, RICHARD J MD, LICENSE NUMBER 0003788, WAS DISCIPLINED BY ARIZONA ON JULY 17, 1992
DISCIPLINARY ACTION: MONITORING OF PHYSICIAN PERFORMANCE

NOTES: HAS IN THE PAST SUCCESSFULLY COMPLETED A CHEMICAL SUBSTANCE REHABILITATION PROGRAM

WITH THE BOARD. WAS RECEIVING A VARIETY OF CONTROLLED SUBSTANCES FROM NUMEROUS PHYSICIANS RELATING TO VARIOUS ILLNESSES FOR A TWO YEAR PERIOD. DENIED ANY RELAPSE OF DRUG DEPENDENCE. TO SATISFY BOARD THAT NO RELAPSE HAS OCCURRED, ENTERED INTO VOLUNTARY AGREEMENT: SHALL OBTAIN BOARD-APPROVED TREATING PHYSICIAN WHO WILL ACT AS GATEKEEPER FOR ALL TREATMENT WITH REPORTS EVERY SIX MONTHS FOR A YEAR; SHALL SUBMIT TO WITNESSED RANDOM BIOLOGICAL FLUID COLLECTION; SHALL TAKE NO DRUGS EXCEPT THOSE PRESCRIBED BY HIS TREATING PHYSICIAN; SHALL KEEP A LOG OF ANY AND ALL MEDICATIONS PRESCRIBED FOR HIM; SHALL MEET WITH BOARD IN ONE YEAR.

MARTIN, RICHARD J MD, LICENSE NUMBER 0003788 OF TUCSON, AZ, WAS DISCIPLINED BY ARIZONA ON JULY 16, 1993
DISCIPLINARY ACTION: MONITORING OF PHYSICIAN PERFORMANCE

NOTES: THIS ORDER REPLACES ORDER OF 8/14/92. SHALL OBTAIN A BOARD-APPROVED TREATING PHYSICIAN; SHALL ALSO OBTAIN A BOARD CERTIFIED PULMONOLOGIST TO TREAT HIS PULMONARY MEDICAL PROBLEMS (WHO MAY BE THE SAME PERSON); SHALL ADVISE HIS TREATING PULMONOLOGIST AND TREATING PHYSICIAN OF HIS CHEMICAL DEPENDENCY AND SUPPLY THEM WITH A COPY OF THIS DOCUMENT; MUST SUBMIT TO WITNESSED RANDOM BIOLOGICAL FLUID COLLECTION; SHALL ABSTAIN COMPLETELY FROM THE CONSUMPTION OF DRUGS EXCEPT WHEN PRESCRIBED BY HIS TREATING PHYSICIAN; SHALL MAINTAIN NO SAMPLES OF CONTROLLED SUBSTANCES; KEEP A LOG OF ANY AND ALL MEDICATIONS PRESCRIBED FOR HIM.

MARTIN, RICHARD J MD, LICENSE NUMBER 0003788 OF 4540 E GRANT ROAD, TUCSON, AZ, WAS DISCIPLINED BY ARIZONA ON OCTOBER 17, 1995

NOTES: SHALL MEET WITH A PERSON APPROVED BY BOARD STAFF FOR SENSITIVITY TRAINING, INCLUDING BOUNDARY ISSUES AT A FREQUENCY AND FOR A DURATION DETERMINED BY THE TRAINER. ON 4/17/96 ORDER WAS TERMINATED.

MATHIS, EDDIE GENE DR, LICENSE NUMBER 0016394, WAS DISCIPLINED BY ARIZONA ON JULY 15, 1994
DISCIPLINARY ACTION: LICENSE SUSPENSION
OFFENSE: NONCOMPLIANCE WITH A PROFESSIONAL RULE

NOTES: FAILURE TO PAY RENEWAL FEE DURING PENDING INVESTIGATION.

MATSON, GUSTAVE MD, WAS DISCIPLINED BY ARIZONA ON JANUARY 22, 1998
DISCIPLINARY ACTION: RESTRICTION PLACED ON LICENSE

NOTES: TERMS OF THE ORDER ARE AS FOLLOWS: MUST HAVE A FEMALE CHAPERONE PRESENT DURING ALL PHYSICAL EXAMINATIONS OF FEMALE PATIENTS, WHETHER IN HIS OFFICE OR AT ANY OTHER LOCATION, THE CHAPERONE WILL CONFIRM HER PRESENCE BY INITIALING AND SIGNING EACH PATIENT'S CHART AT THE TIME OF THE EXAMINATION.

MATTHEW, BURLEIGH J MD, LICENSE NUMBER 0008489, WAS DISCIPLINED BY ARIZONA ON APRIL 19, 1996
DISCIPLINARY ACTION: 24-MONTH PROBATION; FINE
OFFENSE: PROFESSIONAL MISCONDUCT

NOTES: FAILING TO MAINTAIN ADEQUATE RECORDS ON PATIENTS IN THAT FOLLOWING INVESTIGATION OF HIS TREATMENT OF A PATIENT, BOARD ORDERED A CHART REVIEW IN 10/93 OF 10 RANDOM CHARTS FROM 4/88 TO 9/93, ALL OF WHICH LACKED RECORDS OF GENERAL PHYSICAL EXAMINATIONS AND CONTAINED UNDATED OR INCOMPLETE REPORTS AND NOTES; A FOLLOW-UP CHART REVIEW OF 11 RANDOM CHARTS WAS ORDERED IN 10/94 REVEALING DEFICIENCIES: NO OPERATIVE REPORTS CONTAINED A DATE OF DICTATION, NINE QUESTIONNAIRES WERE UNDATED, THREE CHARTS LACKED A DESCRIPTION OF LESIONS OR OTHER PHYSICAL FINDINGS, THREE CHARTS HAD IDENTICAL CONSULTATION NOTES AND FIVE CHARTS DESCRIBED PRESCRIPTIONS WITHOUT DESCRIPTIONS ON HOW THEY WERE TO BE USED; IN HIS TREATMENT OF A PATIENT, CHARGED FOR 12 VISITS BETWEEN 5/26/94 AND 9/27/94, WHEN THERE WAS NO RECORD THAT HE HAD SEEN PATIENT, BUT HAD PERMITTED SURGICAL ASSISTANT TO SEE PATIENT WHO LISTED HIMSELF AS A PHYSICIAN'S ASSISTANT WHEN HE WAS NOT; PRESCRIBING OR DISPENSING CONTROLLED SUBSTANCES TO MEMBERS OF HIS IMMEDIATE FAMILY IN THAT HE ADMINISTERED DEMEROL TO HIS WIFE DURING AN OPERATIVE PROCEDURE AND ADMINISTERED VALIUM TO HER AS WELL. PROBATION WITH TERMS: WITHIN TWO MONTHS SHALL OBTAIN AN OFFICE PRACTICE CONSULTANT TO REVIEW AND ADVISE ON HIS BILLING, PERSONNEL AND RECORD KEEPING PRACTICES; REVIEW SHALL BE COMPLETED WITHIN ONE YEAR; WITHIN 30 DAYS, SHALL OBTAIN A TREATING PHYSICIAN TO TREAT HIS ENDOCRINE DISORDER; TREATING PHYSICIAN WILL SUBMIT QUARTERLY REPORTS; SHALL MAINTAIN A LOG OF ALL NARCOTICS RECEIVED AND WASTED IN HIS PRACTICE; WITHIN TWO MONTHS, SHALL PAY FINE OF $1,000.

MAUK, JOHN D JR MD, LICENSE NUMBER 0011213, WAS DISCIPLINED BY ARIZONA ON OCTOBER 12, 1990
DISCIPLINARY ACTION: REQUIRED TO ENTER AN IMPAIRED PHYSICIAN PROGRAM OR SUBSTANCE ABUSE TREATMENT; MONITORING OF PHYSICIAN PERFORMANCE
OFFENSE: SUBSTANCE ABUSE

NOTES: MUST IMMEDIATELY PARTICIPATE IN THE ARIZONA MEDICAL ASSOCIATION'S MONITORED AFTERCARE TREATMENT PROGRAM WITH QUARTERLY REPORTS TO THE BOARD; MUST OBTAIN A BOARD APPROVED TREATING PHYSICIAN; MUST ABSTAIN COMPLETELY FROM ALCOHOL AND ALL OTHER DRUGS; MUST COMPLY WITH REQUESTS FOR RANDOM BIOLOGICAL FLUID TESTS; MUST SUBMIT TO ANY EXAMS OR THERAPY ORDERED BY BOARD; MUST PARTICIPATE IN A 12-STEP RECOVERY PROGRAM FOR SUBSTANCE ABUSE AS DETERMINED BY THERAPIST AND ATTEND AT LEAST 3 WEEKLY MEETINGS; MUST APPEAR BEFORE THE BOARD FOR INTERVIEWS UPON REQUEST; MUST ADVISE BOARD OF CHANGE IN OFFICE OR HOME ADDRESSES OR OF PLANS TO BE AWAY FOR MORE THAN FIVE DAYS; MUST MAINTAIN A LOG OF ALL MEDICATIONS TAKEN. ON 7/16/94 THIS ORDER WAS TERMINATED EFFECTIVE IN 90 DAYS.

MAXWELL, ROBERT RICHARD MD, LICENSE NUMBER 7468, WAS DISCIPLINED BY ARIZONA ON MAY 7, 1997
DISCIPLINARY ACTION: FINE
OFFENSE: PROFESSIONAL MISCONDUCT

NOTES: IN 11/95 THE STATE COMPENSATION FUND RAISED CONCERNS REGARDING HIS BILLINGS STATING THAT NOTES PROVIDED TO THEM WITH HIS BILLINGS WERE

NOT SIGNED WHICH LEFT NO MEANS OF VERIFYING WHO PERFORMED THE TREATMENT; THE NOTES FAILED TO CONTAIN EVEN THE NAME OR LOCATION OF THE FACILITY WHERE TREATMENT WAS PERFORMED; THE RECORDS WERE NOT LEGIBLE AND THE NOTES FAILED TO SUPPORT HIS BILLED CHARGES. IN ONE CASE, IN 1995, HE DID NOT BILL MULTIPLE MODALITIES AND PROCEDURES IN ACCORDANCE WITH LISTED PERCENTAGES AND IN FIVE CASES DURING 1994 AND 1995, HIS RECORDS DID NOT SUPPORT HIS BILLINGS; IN SOME OF THESE CASES HIS OFFICE RECORDS WERE INADEQUATE OR ILLEGIBLE; HE DID NOT RESPOND TO THE BOARD IN A TIMELY MANNER WHEN ASKED FOR INFORMATION ON THESE MATTERS. HE IS ISSUED A DECREE OF CENSURE AND MUST PAY A CIVIL PENALTY OF $10,000 WITHIN SIX MONTHS. ON 6/1/99 BOARD VOTED TO REVIEW THE MERITS OF THE CASE AFTER DR. MAXWELL APPEALED THE DECISION TO THE COURTS.

MAYER, JOEL H MD, DATE OF BIRTH AUGUST 11, 1947, LICENSE NUMBER 0050843 OF 214 E COLLEGE STREET, KEWANEE, IL, WAS DISCIPLINED BY MICHIGAN ON JANUARY 2, 1995
DISCIPLINARY ACTION: 12-MONTH PROBATION; RESTRICTION PLACED ON LICENSE
OFFENSE: PHYSICAL OR MENTAL ILLNESS INHIBITING THE ABILITY TO PRACTICE WITH SKILL AND SAFETY

MAYER, JOEL H MD, DATE OF BIRTH AUGUST 11, 1947, LICENSE NUMBER 1050843 OF 714 WHITE SPAR RD, LOT 9, PRESCOTT, AZ, WAS DISCIPLINED BY MICHIGAN ON JANUARY 12, 1996
DISCIPLINARY ACTION: LICENSE REVOCATION; FINE
OFFENSE: FAILURE TO COMPLY WITH PREVIOUS BOARD ORDER

NOTES: PROBATION VIOLATION. $1,000 FINE.

MAYER, JOEL HENRY MD, LICENSE NUMBER 0157177 OF 6714 GATESHEAD LANE, INDIANAPOLIS, IN, WAS DISCIPLINED BY NEW YORK ON NOVEMBER 7, 1995
DISCIPLINARY ACTION: LICENSE REVOCATION
OFFENSE: DISCIPLINARY ACTION BY ANOTHER STATE OR AGENCY

NOTES: ACTION IN MICHIGAN. ACTION IN KENTUCKY WHICH DENIED HIM A MEDICAL LICENSE DUE TO A PSYCHIATRIC CONDITION WHICH IMPAIRS HIS ABILITY TO PRACTICE MEDICINE; PRACTICING WHILE IMPAIRED, AND FILING FALSE REGISTRATION APPLICATIONS.

MCBRIDE, CRIS D MD, LICENSE NUMBER 8522, WAS DISCIPLINED BY ARIZONA ON MAY 7, 1997
DISCIPLINARY ACTION: 12-MONTH LICENSE SUSPENSION; 60-MONTH PROBATION
OFFENSE: OVERPRESCRIBING OR MISPRESCRIBING DRUGS

NOTES: FROM 1990 THROUGH 1995 HE COMMITTED VIOLATIONS OF PRESCRIBING REGULATIONS: HE ADMINISTERED MULTIPLE INJECTIONS OF STADOL, DEMEROL AND MORPHINE SULFATE TO A PATIENT WITH LITTLE OR NO HISTORY OR PHYSICAL EXAMINATION NOTED IN THE MEDICAL RECORDS TO SUBSTANTIATE THE NEED OR REASON FOR THE INJECTIONS; PRESCRIBED MULTIPLE DRUGS TO A MEMBER OF HIS FAMILY FOR WHOM HE HAD ANOTHER PHYSICIAN INITIAL MEDICAL RECORDS; AFTER BOARD STAFF CONDUCTED A PHARMACY SURVEY, IT WAS FOUND THAT MANY OF HIS PRESCRIPTIONS WERE NOT DOCUMENTED AT ALL IN HIS MEDICAL RECORDS; PRESCRIBED RITALIN TO FOUR PATIENTS FOR AN EXTENDED PERIOD OF TIME WITHOUT TAKING A HISTORY OR CONDUCTING AN EXAMINATION TO DETERMINE WHETHER ATTENTION DEFICIT DISORDER WAS A VERIFIABLE DIAGNOSIS AND WITHOUT OBTAINING A CONSULTATION OR THE PATIENTS' PREVIOUS MEDICAL RECORDS. HIS INACTIVE LICENSE IS SUSPENDED AND PLACED ON PROBATION WITH THE FOLLOWING CONDITIONS: SHALL NOT PRESCRIBE, ADMINISTER, OR DISPENSE ANY CONTROLLED SUBSTANCE TO ANY MEMBER OF HIS IMMEDIATE FAMILY OR HOUSEHOLD; SHALL NOT APPLY FOR A DRUG ENFORCEMENT ADMINISTRATION CONTROLLED SUBSTANCE REGISTRATION CERTIFICATE WITHOUT PRIOR BOARD AUTHORIZATION; SHALL APPEAR BEFORE THE BOARD FOR AN INFORMAL INTERVIEW UPON REASONABLE NOTICE. PRIOR TO REQUESTING REACTIVATION OF HIS LICENSE HE SHALL: COMPLETE 80 HOURS OF CONTINUING MEDICAL EDUCATION IN PHARMACOLOGY OR PRESCRIBING CONTROLLED SUBSTANCES AND 20 HOURS IN MEDICAL RECORD KEEPING, AND SHALL PRESENT SATISFACTORY WRITTEN EVIDENCE TO THE BOARD UPON COMPLETION; MUST TAKE AND PASS THE SPEX EXAMINATION WITH A SCORE OF 75 OR GREATER; SHALL PRESENT EVIDENCE HE IS PHYSICALLY AND MENTALLY ABLE TO SAFELY ENGAGE IN THE PRACTICE OF MEDICINE; SHALL BEAR ALL COSTS OF COMPLIANCE WITH THIS ORDER; SHALL NOT REQUEST MODIFICATION, AMENDMENT OR TERMINATION OF THIS ORDER.

MCCRACKEN, JOHN JR DO, LICENSE NUMBER 0977, WAS DISCIPLINED BY ARIZONA ON DECEMBER 30, 1997
DISCIPLINARY ACTION: 24-MONTH PROBATION; REQUIRED TO TAKE ADDITIONAL MEDICAL EDUCATION
OFFENSE: SUBSTANDARD CARE, INCOMPETENCE OR NEGLIGENCE

NOTES: BOARD RECEIVED NOTICE OF A MALPRACTICE SETTLEMENT WHICH ALLEGED HE FAILED TO DIAGNOSE OR SUSPECT A PATIENT HAD A BOWEL OBSTRUCTION; THE DELAY IN DIAGNOSIS AND APPROPRIATE SURGICAL TREATMENT IN 8/93 CAUSED SIGNIFICANT INJURIES TO THE PATIENT. HE DENIED THE ALLEGATIONS. CONDITIONS OF PROBATION: SHALL OBTAIN 20 HOURS OF CONTINUING MEDICAL EDUCATION IN THE AREAS OF TREATING ACUTE ABDOMINAL PAIN; SHALL PAY ALL COSTS. ON 12/18/99 CONDITIONS WERE SATISFIED IN FULL AND A FULL AND UNRESTRICTED LICENSE WAS ISSUED.

MCCRACKEN, JOHN JR DO, LICENSE NUMBER 30323, WAS DISCIPLINED BY MISSOURI ON OCTOBER 4, 1999
DISCIPLINARY ACTION: 3-MONTH PROBATION; REQUIRED TO TAKE ADDITIONAL MEDICAL EDUCATION
OFFENSE: DISCIPLINARY ACTION BY ANOTHER STATE OR AGENCY

NOTES: ON 12/30/97 ARIZONA LICENSE PLACED ON PROBATION AFTER RECEIVING NOTICE OF A MALPRACTICE SETTLEMENT ALLEGING HE FAILED TO DIAGNOSE OR SUSPECT THE POSSIBILITY OF A BOWEL OBSTRUCTION. PROBATION WITH FOLLOWING TERMS AND CONDITIONS: SHALL OBTAIN 20 HOURS OF CONTINUING MEDICAL EDUCATION IN AREAS DIRECTLY RELATED TO TREATMENT OF ACUTE ABDOMINAL PAIN; SHALL NOTIFY THE BOARD WITHIN 10 DAYS OF ANY CHANGE IN HIS EMPLOYMENT, ADDRESS OR PHONE NUMBERS; SHALL ACCEPT AND COMPLY WITH UNANNOUNCED VISITS TO MONITOR COMPLIANCE; SHALL SUBMIT REPORTS TO BOARD REGARDING COMPLIANCE; SHALL GIVE A COPY OF THIS ORDER TO ANY HEALTH CARE ENTITY WHERE HE HAS PRIVILEGES.

MCCRACKEN, JOHN WILLIS JR DO, LICENSE NUMBER 1657 OF TUCSON, AZ, WAS DISCIPLINED BY OHIO ON AUGUST 26, 1999

DISCIPLINARY ACTION: PROBATION; RESTRICTION PLACED ON LICENSE
OFFENSE: DISCIPLINARY ACTION BY ANOTHER STATE OR AGENCY

NOTES: ACTION WAS TAKEN AGAINST HIS LICENSE BY THE ARIZONA BOARD FOR HIS FAILURE TO FOLLOW UP WITH A PATIENT IN A TIMELY MANNER FOR ACUTE ABDOMINAL PAIN. ACTION AGAINST HIS CLINICAL PRIVILEGES BY EISENHOWER U.S. ARMY MEDICAL CENTER BASED UPON HIS PATTERN OF SUBSTANDARD CARE IN TREATING SERIOUSLY ILL PATIENTS. PROBATIONARY TERMS, CONDITIONS AND LIMITATIONS IMPOSED FOR AT LEAST THREE YEARS.

MCCULLOUGH, JAMES L MD, LICENSE NUMBER 0006177, WAS DISCIPLINED BY ARIZONA ON APRIL 19, 1996
DISCIPLINARY ACTION: RESTRICTION PLACED ON LICENSE

NOTES: INTERVIEWED BY THE BOARD REGARDING HIS CARE AND TREATMENT OF THREE PATIENTS AND MALPRACTICE CASES. SHALL NOT PERFORM ANY MAJOR SURGERY.

MCGAFFIC, WALTER MD, WAS DISCIPLINED BY ARIZONA ON AUGUST 8, 1998
DISCIPLINARY ACTION: LICENSE SUSPENSION

NOTES: PLACED ON INACTIVE STATUS WITH CAUSE AND MUST ENTER INTO LONG TERM TREATMENT WITHIN TWO WEEKS AT SPECIFIED TREATMENT FACILITY.

MCGAREY, WILLIAM C MD, LICENSE NUMBER 0002661 OF PHOENIX, AZ, WAS DISCIPLINED BY ARIZONA ON APRIL 9, 1992
DISCIPLINARY ACTION: RESTRICTION PLACED ON CONTROLLED SUBSTANCE LICENSE; REQUIRED TO TAKE ADDITIONAL MEDICAL EDUCATION
OFFENSE: SUBSTANDARD CARE, INCOMPETENCE OR NEGLIGENCE

NOTES: GAVE INADEQUATE PHYSICAL EXAMINATIONS ON PATIENTS, INADEQUATE MEDICAL RECORDS AND INAPPROPRIATE THERAPY WHEN STANDARD MEDICATION IS CALLED FOR, CONSTITUTING CONDUCT WHICH IS OR MIGHT BE HARMFUL TO THE HEALTH OF THE PATIENT; IN TREATMENT WITH MEDICATIONS, HE FREQUENTLY DID NOT LIST DRUG DOSAGE, AND NEVER LISTED THE NUMBER OF UNITS. CONDITIONS OF STIPULATED AGREEMENT INCLUDE: CEASE USE OF STEROID AND B12 INJECTIONS, OBTAIN 40 HOURS CONTINUING MEDICAL EDUCATION IN GENERAL PHARMACOLOGY, ENROLL IN A COURSE IN PRACTICE MANAGEMENT TECHNIQUES BY 12/31/92, SIT AND PASS THE SPEX EXAM BEFORE 10/92, AND APPEAR BEFORE THE BOARD AS DIRECTED. HE WAS CENSURED. AS OF 4/14/93, HE HAD NOT PASSED THE SPEX EXAM BUT HAD COMPLIED WITH OTHER CONDITIONS OF ORDER; DEADLINE FOR PASSING THE SPEX EXAM WAS EXTENDED TO 6/93. HE FAILED THE SPEX EXAM AND ON 11/11/93 WAS GRANTED HIS REQUEST FOR INACTIVE STATUS.

MCMILLIAN, RICHARD K MD, WAS DISCIPLINED BY ARIZONA ON JANUARY 29, 1999
DISCIPLINARY ACTION: LICENSE REVOCATION

NOTES: CANCELLATION OF LICENSE WITH CAUSE.

MCRAE, BART L MD, LICENSE NUMBER 0020471, WAS DISCIPLINED BY ARIZONA ON APRIL 11, 1992
DISCIPLINARY ACTION: REQUIRED TO ENTER AN IMPAIRED PHYSICIAN PROGRAM OR SUBSTANCE ABUSE TREATMENT; MONITORING OF PHYSICIAN PERFORMANCE

NOTES: MUST IMMEDIATELY PARTICIPATE IN A BOARD-APPROVED MONITORED AFTERCARE TREATMENT PROGRAM WHOSE THERAPIST MUST SUBMIT QUARTERLY REPORTS; MUST PARTICIPATE IN 90 12-STEP MEETINGS APPROPRIATE FOR SUBSTANCE ABUSE WITHIN 90 DAYS; MUST THEN PARTICIPATE IN A 12-STEP RECOVERY PROGRAM AS DETERMINED BY HIS TREATING THERAPIST AND ATTEND AT LEAST 3 WEEKLY MEETINGS; SHALL OBTAIN A BOARD-APPROVED TREATING PHYSICIAN; SHALL ABSTAIN COMPLETELY FROM THE CONSUMPTION OF ALCOHOLIC BEVERAGES AND DRUGS EXCEPT WHEN PRESCRIBED BY HIS TREATING PHYSICIAN; SHALL SUBMIT TO WITNESSED RANDOM BIOLOGICAL FLUID COLLECTION; SHALL MAINTAIN A LOG OF ANY AND ALL MEDICATIONS PRESCRIBED FOR HIM; SHALL SUBMIT TO ANY EXAMINATIONS OR THERAPY ORDERED BY THE BOARD; SHALL APPEAR BEFORE THE BOARD FOR INTERVIEWS UPON REQUEST; SHALL INFORM BOARD OF CHANGE OF ADDRESS OR IF AWAY FOR MORE THAN 5 DAYS. ON 4/17/93 BOARD ORDERED THAT THIS STIPULATION BE CONTINUED AND THAT HE BE ALLOWED TO REPLACE TWO OF HIS WEEKLY GROUP THERAPY MEETINGS EACH MONTH WITH INDIVIDUAL THERAPY. ON 10/16/93 BOARD APPROVED HIS REQUEST TO CHANGE THERAPISTS AND THAT HE MEET WITH THE BOARD IN NINE MONTHS AT THEIR 7/94 MEETING. ORDER TERMINATED ON 4/4/95.

MCRAE, BART L MD, LICENSE NUMBER 0020471, WAS DISCIPLINED BY ARIZONA ON JULY 18, 1996
DISCIPLINARY ACTION: LICENSE SUSPENSION; REQUIRED TO ENTER AN IMPAIRED PHYSICIAN PROGRAM OR SUBSTANCE ABUSE TREATMENT
OFFENSE: SUBSTANCE ABUSE

NOTES: UNABLE TO SAFELY PRACTICE MEDICINE AT THIS TIME DUE TO A RELAPSE IN CHEMICAL SUBSTANCES USE; AGREES TO ENTER TALBOTT-MARSH RECOVERY CAMPUS FOR CHEMICAL DEPENDENCY AND TREATMENT AND TO REMAIN IN TREATMENT UNTIL THERAPEUTICALLY DISCHARGED; AGREES NOT TO PRACTICE MEDICINE IN ANY JURISDICTION WHILE LICENSE IS IN INACTIVE WITH CAUSE STATUS; UNDERSTANDS THAT HE MAY NOT HOLD OR MAINTAIN A CONTROLLED SUBSTANCE CERTIFICATE WITH THE DRUG ENFORCEMENT ADMINISTRATION OR WRITE OR REFILL PRESCRIPTIONS AS LONG AS LICENSE IS CLASSIFIED AS INACTIVE; SHALL NOT REQUEST REACTIVATION OF LICENSE UNTIL HE MEETS WITH THE BOARD AND COMPLIES WITH ALL BOARD REQUESTS. RETROACTIVE TO 5/12/96.

MCRAE, BART L MD, LICENSE NUMBER 20471, WAS DISCIPLINED BY ARIZONA ON JANUARY 25, 1997
DISCIPLINARY ACTION: PROBATION; REQUIRED TO ENTER AN IMPAIRED PHYSICIAN PROGRAM OR SUBSTANCE ABUSE TREATMENT
OFFENSE: SUBSTANCE ABUSE

NOTES: FROM 5/10/96 TO 9/13/96 HE WAS TREATED AT A RECOVERY CENTER FOR A MAJOR DEPRESSIVE EPISODE AND OPIATE AND BENZODIAZEPINE DEPENDENCE; THERE WERE CONCERNS ABOUT HIS ON-GOING RECOVERY WHICH INCLUDED HIS ANXIETY LEVEL, DIFFICULTY WITH EMOTIONAL HONESTY AND RELATIVELY LIMITED INSIGHT INTO HIMSELF AND HIS BEHAVIOR. CONDITIONS OF PROBATION AS FOLLOWS: MUST IMMEDIATELY PARTICIPATE IN A BOARD-APPROVED MONITORED AFTERCARE TREATMENT PROGRAM WHOSE THERAPIST MUST SUBMIT QUARTERLY REPORTS; MUST PARTICIPATE IN A 12-STEP RECOVERY PROGRAM AS DETERMINED BY HIS TREATING THERAPIST AND ATTEND AT LEAST THREE WEEKLY MEETINGS; SHALL OBTAIN A BOARD-

APPROVED TREATING PHYSICIAN; SHALL ABSTAIN COMPLETELY FROM THE CONSUMPTION OF ALCOHOLIC BEVERAGES AND DRUGS EXCEPT WHEN PRESCRIBED BY HIS TREATING PHYSICIAN; MUST SUBMIT TO WITNESSED RANDOM BIOLOGICAL FLUID COLLECTION; MUST KEEP A LOG OF ANY AND ALL MEDICATIONS PRESCRIBED FOR HIM; SHALL SUBMIT TO ANY EXAMINATIONS OR THERAPY ORDERED BY BOARD; SHALL APPEAR BEFORE BOARD FOR INTERVIEWS UPON REQUEST; SHALL INFORM BOARD OF CHANGE OF ADDRESS OR IF AWAY FOR MORE THAN FIVE DAYS; SHALL IMMEDIATELY ORDER A TREATING PSYCHIATRIST APPROVED BY THE BOARD AND REMAIN IN TREATMENT WITH THE PSYCHIATRIST UNTIL FURTHER ORDER OF THE BOARD.

MECOLI, FRANCIS O MD, WAS DISCIPLINED BY ARIZONA ON JULY 15, 1993
DISCIPLINARY ACTION: RESTRICTION PLACED ON LICENSE; MONITORING OF PHYSICIAN PERFORMANCE
OFFENSE: DISCIPLINARY ACTION BY ANOTHER STATE OR AGENCY

NOTES: ON 12/10/84 CALIFORNIA PHYSICIAN'S AND SURGEON'S LICENSE WAS REVOKED AFTER HE WAS FOUND GUILTY OF UNPROFESSIONAL CONDUCT BY PRESCRIBING CLEARLY EXCESSIVE AMOUNTS OF DILAUDID TO TWO PATIENTS AND RETAINING A PORTION FOR SELF-ADMINISTRATION; SELF-ADMINISTERING HEROIN, DILAUDID AND COCAINE; POSSESSING DANGEROUS DRUGS WITHOUT A VALID PRESCRIPTION; BEING UNABLE TO PRACTICE MEDICINE SAFELY DUE TO IMPAIRMENT BY REASON OF MENTAL ILLNESS AFFECTING HIS COMPETENCY. CALIFORNIA DENIED REINSTATING HIS LICENSE IN 8/89; SUCCESSFULLY COMPLETED OUTPATIENT TREATMENT IN 7/88; BIOLOGICAL FLUID COLLECTION WAS NEGATIVE FOR CHEMICAL SUBSTANCES SINCE THEN; APPEARS TO BE MAINTAINING A CHEMICAL-FREE LIFESTYLE. CONDITIONS OF ARIZONA LICENSE: SHALL OBTAIN A BOARD-APPROVED TREATING PHYSICIAN; DR. MECOLI SHALL ADVISE HIS TREATING PHYSICIAN OF HIS REHABILITATION EFFORTS AND PROVIDE A COPY OF THIS DOCUMENT TO HIS APPROVED TREATING PHYSICIAN; SHALL FURTHER ADVISE ANY HEALTH CARE PRACTITIONER PROVIDING MEDICAL CARE AND TREATMENT OF HIS CHEMICAL MISUSE PROBLEM; SHALL ABSTAIN COMPLETELY FROM THE CONSUMPTION OF ALCOHOLIC BEVERAGES AND DRUGS EXCEPT WHEN PRESCRIBED BY HIS TREATING PHYSICIAN; MUST SUBMIT TO WITNESSED RANDOM BIOLOGICAL FLUID COLLECTION; SHALL NOT PRACTICE IN A SOLO PRACTICE SETTING; SHALL CAUSE A PHYSICIAN ASSOCIATED WITH HIM IN PRACTICE TO PROVIDE QUARTERLY REPORTS TO BOARD. ON 7/22/95 ORDER TERMINATED EFFECTIVE IN 90 DAYS DUE TO SUCCESSFUL ONGOING REHABILITATION.

MEES, LEONARD R MD, LICENSE NUMBER 0035582 OF 78 CROWELL RD, CHATHAM, MA, WAS DISCIPLINED BY MASSACHUSETTS ON APRIL 1, 1994
DISCIPLINARY ACTION: LICENSE REVOCATION
OFFENSE: PROFESSIONAL MISCONDUCT

NOTES: SEXUAL RELATIONS.

MEES, LEONARD R MD, LICENSE NUMBER 0017555, WAS DISCIPLINED BY ARIZONA ON OCTOBER 17, 1995
DISCIPLINARY ACTION: 60-MONTH PROBATION; REQUIRED TO TAKE ADDITIONAL MEDICAL EDUCATION
OFFENSE: DISCIPLINARY ACTION BY ANOTHER STATE OR AGENCY

NOTES: LICENSE REVOKED BY MASSACHUSETTS 4/1/94; ENGAGED IN SEXUAL INTIMACIES WITH A PATIENT; MOVED TO ARIZONA IN 1994 AND HAS NOT PRACTICED MEDICINE SINCE 4/1/94. PROBATION WITH TERMS AND CONDITIONS: WITHIN 60 DAYS, SHALL SUBMIT TO PSYCHOLOGICAL AND PSYCHIATRIC EVALUATIONS BY BOARD-DESIGNATED EVALUATORS, WHO SHALL SUBMIT EVALUATION REPORTS TO THE BOARD; SHALL IMMEDIATELY ENGAGE IN THERAPY WITH A BOARD-APPROVED THERAPIST WHO MUST SUBMIT QUARTERLY REPORTS; SHALL ANNUALLY OBTAIN 30 HOURS OF CONTINUING MEDICAL EDUCATION IN FAMILY PRACTICE OR PREVENTIVE MEDICINE; SHALL NOT PRACTICE IN ARIZONA UNTIL HE HAS COMPLETED A BOARD-APPROVED MINI-RESIDENCY OF AT LEAST 100 HOURS IN THE FIELDS OF FAMILY PRACTICE AND/OR PREVENTIVE MEDICINE.

MEHNE, RICHARD G JR MD, WAS DISCIPLINED BY ARIZONA ON APRIL 11, 1991
DISCIPLINARY ACTION: SURRENDER OF LICENSE
OFFENSE: PHYSICAL OR MENTAL ILLNESS INHIBITING THE ABILITY TO PRACTICE WITH SKILL AND SAFETY

NOTES: RECENTLY ARRESTED AND HOSPITALIZED FOR AN UNCONTROLLED MANIC EPISODE.

MERI, BASEM DO, LICENSE NUMBER 3370 OF 5064 HEALTH APT. 201, DEARBORN, MI, WAS DISCIPLINED BY ARIZONA ON SEPTEMBER 15, 1998
DISCIPLINARY ACTION: 24-MONTH PROBATION; MONITORING OF PHYSICIAN PERFORMANCE
OFFENSE: SUBSTANCE ABUSE

NOTES: PRIOR ADDICTION TO A CONTROLLED SUBSTANCE; REVIEWED CURRENT PARTICIPATION IN MICHIGAN'S HEALTH PROFESSIONAL RECOVERY PROGRAM. CONDITIONS OF PROBATION ARE AS FOLLOWS: SHALL OBTAIN PSYCHIATRIC OR PSYCHOLOGICAL TREATMENT BY A BOARD APPROVED THERAPIST WHO IS EITHER A LICENSED PSYCHIATRIST AND/OR PSYCHOLOGIST WHO SHALL PROVIDE MONTHLY REPORTS; SHALL PROVIDE A COPY OF THIS ORDER TO ALL HEALTH CARE FACILITIES WHERE HE HAS PRIVILEGES; SHALL ABSTAIN COMPLETELY FROM THE CONSUMPTION OF ALCOHOLIC BEVERAGES AND SHALL NOT CONSUME ILLICIT DRUGS OR TAKE ANY MEDICATION UNLESS PRESCRIBED FOR HER BY HER TREATING PHYSICIAN; SHALL MAINTAIN A MONTHLY LOG OF ALL MEDICATIONS TAKEN BY HIS AND PROVIDE A COPY TO THE BOARD; SHALL SUBMIT TO ANY EVALUATIONS ORDERED BY BOARD; SHALL APPEAR BEFORE THE BOARD UPON REQUEST; SHALL SUBMIT TO RANDOM BIOLOGICAL FLUID TESTING; SHALL PARTICIPATE IN A MINIMUM OF THREE SELF-HELP MEETINGS PER WEEK AND KEEP A LOG OF ALL MEETINGS ATTENDED; SHALL NOTIFY THE BOARD IF HE CEASES TO RESIDE IN ARIZONA; SHALL PAY COSTS

METZNER, RICHARD J MD, WAS DISCIPLINED BY ARIZONA ON OCTOBER 18, 1996
DISCIPLINARY ACTION: DENIAL OF NEW LICENSE
OFFENSE: PRACTICING WITHOUT A VALID LICENSE

NOTES: WITHOUT AN ARIZONA LICENSE, HE TREATED THREE PATIENTS IN ARIZONA, PRESCRIBED MEDICATION FOR TWO OF THEM WITHOUT PROPER DRUG ENFORCEMENT ADMINISTRATION REGISTRATION, MAINTAINED INADEQUATE RECORDS ON THEM AND ADVERTISED AS A MEDICAL DOCTOR.

METZNER, RICHARD J MD, WAS DISCIPLINED BY ARIZONA ON JANUARY 24, 1997
DISCIPLINARY ACTION: REPRIMAND

OFFENSE: PRACTICING WITHOUT A VALID CONTROLLED SUBSTANCE LICENSE

NOTES: TREATED THREE PATIENTS IN ARIZONA AND PRESCRIBED MEDICATION FOR TWO OF THEM WITHOUT PROPER DRUG ENFORCEMENT ADMINISTRATION REGISTRATION PRIOR TO COMPLETING THE LICENSING PROCESS; HE ALSO ADVERTISED IN A NEWSPAPER AS A MEDICAL DOCTOR WITHOUT BENEFIT OF ARIZONA LICENSURE.

METZNER, RICHARD JOEL MD, LICENSE NUMBER G16504 OF LOS ANGELES, CA, WAS DISCIPLINED BY CALIFORNIA ON DECEMBER 23, 1997
DISCIPLINARY ACTION: 60-MONTH PROBATION
OFFENSE: DISCIPLINARY ACTION BY ANOTHER STATE OR AGENCY

NOTES: DISCIPLINED BY ARIZONA FOR TREATING AND PRESCRIBING TO THREE PATIENTS BEFORE COMPLETING THE LICENSING PROCESS IN THAT STATE.

MEYER, KARL L MD, LICENSE NUMBER 0003789 OF NOGALES, AZ, WAS DISCIPLINED BY ARIZONA ON JULY 12, 1994
DISCIPLINARY ACTION: RESTRICTION PLACED ON CONTROLLED SUBSTANCE LICENSE
OFFENSE: OVERPRESCRIBING OR MISPRESCRIBING DRUGS

NOTES: FROM 2/92 THROUGH 10/12/92 PRESCRIBED CONTROLLED SUBSTANCES TO FAMILY MEMBERS; ALSO PRESCRIBED EXCESSIVE AMOUNTS OF LORTAB AND VICODIN TO A PATIENT HE KNEW SUFFERED FROM ALCOHOLISM. SHALL NOT TREAT ANY MEMBERS OF HIS IMMEDIATE FAMILY; SHALL NOT MAINTAIN IN HIS RESIDENCE ANY MEDICATIONS NOT PRESCRIBED BY ANOTHER LICENSED PHYSICIAN FOR HIM OR MEMBERS OF HIS HOUSEHOLD.

MEYER, LARRY A MD, LICENSE NUMBER 0024696, WAS DISCIPLINED BY ARIZONA ON OCTOBER 29, 1996
DISCIPLINARY ACTION: 60-MONTH RESTRICTION PLACED ON LICENSE; MONITORING OF PHYSICIAN PERFORMANCE

NOTES: APPLICATION FOR LICENSURE TO BE PROCESSED ROUTINELY; EFFECTIVE ON DATE OF LICENSURE HE SHALL REFRAIN FROM TREATING FEMALE PATIENTS WITHOUT A FEMALE CHAPERONE PRESENT; HE SHALL ENTER THE NAME OF THE CHAPERONE IN THE PATIENT'S CHART AT THE TIME OF THE PATIENT CONTACT; FOR 12 MONTHS AFTER DATE OF LICENSURE, SHALL REFRAIN FROM THE CONSUMPTION OF ALCOHOL AND NON-PRESCRIBED MEDICATIONS AND SHALL SUBMIT TO RANDOM BIOLOGICAL FLUID TESTING; SHALL UNDERGO THERAPY BY A BOARD-APPROVED THERAPIST AT A FREQUENCY TO BE DETERMINED BY THE THERAPIST WITH QUARTERLY REPORTS TO THE BOARD.

MICHAELIS, THOMAS WILLIAM MD, DATE OF BIRTH DECEMBER 23, 1944, LICENSE NUMBER 0032590 OF 832 E COUNTRY GABLES DRIVE, PHOENIX, AZ, WAS DISCIPLINED BY OHIO ON MAY 21, 1992
DISCIPLINARY ACTION: LICENSE SUSPENSION; PROBATION
OFFENSE: CRIMINAL CONVICTION OR PLEA OF GUILTY, NOLO CONTENDERE, OR NO CONTEST TO A CRIME

NOTES: CONVICTIONS FOR MISDEMEANORS INVOLVING MORAL TURPITUDE (ATTEMPTED GROSS SEXUAL IMPOSITION, VOYEURISM, AND PUBLIC INDECENCY). PERMANENT REVOCATION STAYED; INDEFINITE SUSPENSION, MINIMUM ONE YEAR, SUCH TIME TO BE CALCULATED FROM 7/1/91; CONDITIONS FOR REINSTATEMENT; SUBSEQUENT PROBATION, MINIMUM OF 5 YEARS. REQUEST FOR REINSTATEMENT APPROVED 7/8/92 SUBJECT TO PROBATIONARY CONDITIONS OF THIS ORDER. ON 9/8/93 BOARD GRANTED HIS REQUEST TO CHANGE APPEARANCE SCHEDULE FROM THREE TO SIX MONTHS BASED ON HIS RELOCATION. BOARD GRANTED HIS REQUEST TO REDUCE REQUIRED BOARD APPEARANCES TO ONCE A YEAR ON 5/11/94. ON 7/10/97 HE WAS RELEASED FROM THE TERMS OF THIS ORDER.

MICHALAK, PETER DO, LICENSE NUMBER 0001505, WAS DISCIPLINED BY ARIZONA ON NOVEMBER 26, 1996
DISCIPLINARY ACTION: MONITORING OF PHYSICIAN PERFORMANCE
OFFENSE: SUBSTANCE ABUSE

NOTES: ATTEMPTING TO ACQUIRE CONTROLLED SUBSTANCES UNDER FRAUDULENT MEASURES FOR PERSONAL USE; ATTEMPTED TO PICK UP PRESCRIPTIONS FOR LORAZEPAM, A SCHEDULE IV SUBSTANCE, FROM THREE PHARMACISTS USING TWO ALIASES. INTERIM ORDER. MUST SUBMIT TO BIOLOGICAL FLUID TESTING; SHALL MAKE SPECIFIED PATIENT RECORDS AVAILABLE. SUBMIT TO PSYCHIATRIC EVALUATION.

MICHALAK, PETER DO, LICENSE NUMBER 0001505 OF 5520 NORTH SUNCREST, TUCSON, AZ, WAS DISCIPLINED BY ARIZONA ON DECEMBER 19, 1996
DISCIPLINARY ACTION: LICENSE SUSPENSION; RESTRICTION PLACED ON CONTROLLED SUBSTANCE LICENSE
OFFENSE: SUBSTANCE ABUSE

NOTES: ON 11/29/96 ACKNOWLEDGED THAT HE WAS CURRENTLY ADDICTED TO CODEINE AND ATIVAN WAS TAKING VARIOUS QUANTITIES ON A DAILY BASIS; ON 12/03/96 VOLUNTARILY ADMITTED HIMSELF FOR INPATIENT REHABILITATION TREATMENT REGARDING HIS SUBSTANCE ABUSE PROBLEM. MINIMUM ONE YEAR SUSPENSION UNDER TERMS AND CONDITIONS: SHALL DELIVER TO THE BOARD ALL DOCUMENTS THAT INDICATE THAT HE IS A LICENSEE OF THE BOARD; FOR A MINIMUM OF ONE YEAR SHALL OBTAIN PSYCHIATRIC OR PSYCHOLOGICAL TREATMENT BY A LICENSED THERAPIST WHO SHALL SUBMIT TO THE BOARD A WRITTEN PROGRESS REPORT EVERY THREE MONTHS; SHALL ABSTAIN FROM THE CONSUMPTION OF ALCOHOL AND SHALL NOT CONSUME ILLICIT DRUGS OR TAKE ANY CONTROLLED SUBSTANCES UNLESS SUCH MEDICATION IS PRESCRIBED FOR HIM BY HIS TREATING PHYSICIAN; SHALL MAINTAIN A LOG OF SUCH PRESCRIPTIONS AND PROVIDE A COPY TO THE BOARD MONTHLY; SHALL SUBMIT TO AND COOPERATE IN ANY INDEPENDENT MEDICAL OR PSYCHOLOGICAL EVALUATION THAT IS ORDERED BY THE BOARD; SHALL APPEAR BEFORE THE BOARD UPON REQUEST; SHALL SUBMIT TO RANDOM BIOLOGICAL FLUID TESTING; SHALL PARTICIPATE IN A MINIMUM OF TWO SELF-HELP MEETINGS PER WEEK THROUGH SUCH ORGANIZATIONS AS AA, NARCOTICS ANONYMOUS AND DOCTOR'S CADUCEUS GROUP WITH MONTHLY REPORTS; SHALL NOTIFY THE BOARD WITHIN 20 DAYS IF HE CEASES TO RESIDE IN ARIZONA; SHALL NOT HAVE PRESCRIPTION AUTHORITY UNTIL THE BOARD APPROVES THE RESUMPTION OF HIS PRESCRIPTION PRIVILEGES.

MICHALAK, PETER DO, LICENSE NUMBER 1505, WAS DISCIPLINED BY ARIZONA ON MAY 27, 1997
DISCIPLINARY ACTION: 60-MONTH PROBATION; RESTRICTION PLACED ON LICENSE
OFFENSE: SUBSTANCE ABUSE

NOTES: ALLEGATIONS IN 11/96 THAT HE WAS ATTEMPTING TO

ACQUIRE CONTROLLED SUBSTANCES FOR PERSONAL USE UNDER FRAUDULENT MEANS; ADMITTED HE WAS ADDICTED TO CODEINE AND ATIVAN; VOLUNTARILY ADMITTED HIMSELF FOR TREATMENT ON 12/3/96. CONDITIONS OF PROBATION: SHALL OBTAIN A BOARD APPROVED THERAPIST WHO SHALL SEND THE BOARD MONTHLY REPORTS FOR SIX MONTHS THEN QUARTERLY REPORTS FOR THE REMAINDER OF PROBATION; SHALL PROVIDE A COPY OF THIS ORDER TO ANY HEALTH CARE FACILITY WHERE HE PRACTICES; SHALL ABSTAIN FROM ALCOHOL AND SHALL NOT CONSUME ANY CONTROLLED SUBSTANCE UNLESS PRESCRIBED FOR HIM BY HIS TREATING PHYSICIAN; SHALL SUBMIT TO ANY EVALUATIONS ORDERED BY THE BOARD; SHALL SUBMIT TO RANDOM BIOLOGICAL FLUID TESTING; SHALL PARTICIPATE IN A MINIMUM OF TWO AA OR NARCOTICS ANONYMOUS MEETINGS PER WEEK; SHALL NOT WORK MORE THAN 36 HOURS A WEEK OR 12 HOURS A DAY; SHALL INFORM THE BOARD OF CHANGE OF ADDRESS WITHIN 20 DAYS. ON 9/30/97 ORDER MODIFIED ALLOWING HIM TO WORK 48 HOURS A WEEK AND NOT MORE THAN ONE 24 HOUR SHIFT.

MICHAUD, ROBERT MERRILL DO OF JUNEAU, AK, WAS DISCIPLINED BY UTAH ON JANUARY 23, 1998
DISCIPLINARY ACTION: 60-MONTH PROBATION; 60-MONTH CONTROLLED SUBSTANCE LICENSE PLACED ON PROBATION
OFFENSE: EXCEEDING PROFESSIONAL LIMITATIONS

NOTES: SOLD SAMPLE DRUGS WHICH HAD BEEN LABELED AS NOT INTENDED FOR RESALE; DISPENSED DRUGS IN THE UNLICENSED PRACTICE OF PHARMACY; AND NEGLIGENTLY RETURNED EXCESS INJECTABLE MEDICATION TO SOURCE VIALS, REPEATEDLY UTILIZED A SINGLE SYRINGE TO ADMINISTER MEDICATIONS TO NUMEROUS PATIENTS AND REUSED EXCESS AND PURPORTEDLY STERILIZED SUTURE MATERIAL. ORDERED TO CEASE AND DESIST FROM THE UNLAWFUL SALE OF PRESCRIPTIVE SAMPLE MEDICATIONS OR OVER THE COUNTER MEDICATIONS AND FROM THE UNAUTHORIZED PRACTICE OF PHARMACY. ON 6/22/98 THE PROBATIONARY CONDITIONS REQUIRING HIM TO PARTICIPATE IN AND SUCCESSFULLY COMPLETE TRAINING THROUGH AN OSHA APPROVED COURSE ON STERILIZATION AND TO COMPLETE FIVE HOURS IN CONTINUING EDUCATION REGARDING PEDIATRIC PRESCRIPTIVE PRACTICE WERE CHANGED TO ALLOW HIM TO HAVE THOSE CONDITIONS MET VIA PERSONAL INSTRUCTION. ON 12/21/98 PROBATIONS TERMINATED AND LICENSES REINSTATED WITH FULL PRIVILEGES.

MICHAUD, ROBERT MERRILL DO, LICENSE NUMBER 3638, WAS DISCIPLINED BY ALASKA ON JUNE 16, 1999
DISCIPLINARY ACTION: SURRENDER OF LICENSE
OFFENSE: NONCOMPLIANCE WITH A PROFESSIONAL RULE

NOTES: LICENSE UNDER INVESTIGATION FOR QUESTIONS REGARDING THE VALIDITY OF ANSWERS TO QUESTIONS IN INITIAL APPLICATION; ALSO UNDER INVESTIGATION FOR ALLEGATIONS REGARDING PATIENT TREATMENT MATTERS. VOLUNTARY SURRENDER.

MICHAUD, ROBERT MERRILL DO, LICENSE NUMBER 2045 OF 3319 E. UNIVERSITY #341, MESA, AZ, WAS DISCIPLINED BY ARIZONA ON JULY 9, 1999
DISCIPLINARY ACTION: LICENSE SUSPENSION; 12-MONTH PROBATION
OFFENSE: DISCIPLINARY ACTION BY ANOTHER STATE OR AGENCY

NOTES: ON 1/23/98 UTAH PLACED HIS LICENSE ON PROBATION FOR THE FOLLOWING: BETWEEN 1992-1995 PERIODICALLY SOLD ROGAINE SAMPLES MARKED NOT FOR RESALE TO VARIOUS PATIENTS; DURING 2/95 PERIODICALLY SOLD CLEOCIN T & RETIN-A PRESCRIPTIVE MEDICATIONS TO CERTAIN PATIENTS; HE OBTAINED THE LATTER DRUG FROM MEXICO; ALSO DURING 2/95 SOLD CERTAIN OVER THE COUNTER MEDICATIONS TO PATIENTS; HE SUBSEQUENTLY CEASED THAT PRACTICE WHEN IT BECAME TOO TIME-CONSUMING AND HE DECIDED IT WAS NO LONGER COST EFFECTIVE; BETWEEN 1992-1995 PERIODICALLY RETURNED EXCESS CORTISONE SOLUTION TO SOURCE VIALS AFTER HE ADMINISTERED INJECTIONS TO VARIOUS PATIENTS; HE RETURNED THE UNUSED MEDICATION TO AVOID THE NEED TO SUBSEQUENTLY REMIX THE SOLUTION FOR LATER USE AT THE GIVEN CONCENTRATION; HE OCCASIONALLY DIRECTED HIS MEDICAL ASSISTANTS TO ALSO RETURN EXCESS CORTISONE SOLUTION TO THE SOURCE VIALS; DURING VARIOUS SURGICAL PROCEDURES, BETWEEN 1992-1995, HE USED A SINGLE SYRINGE FILLED WITH EPINEPHRINE AND XYLOCAINE FOR MULTIPLE PATIENTS; HE DID USE A SEPARATE NEEDLE FOR EACH INJECTION ON EVERY PATIENT, BUT BASED ON CREDIBLE TESTIMONY FROM HIS MEDICAL ASSISTANTS, HE OFTEN ASPIRATED THOSE INJECTIONS AND THUS COULD HAVE CONTAMINATED THE MEDICATION WITH A GIVEN PATIENT'S BLOOD PRIOR TO RETURNING THE UNUSED PORTION OF THE MEDICATION TO THE SOURCE VIAL; HE PERIODICALLY INSTRUCTED HIS MEDICAL ASSISTANTS TO ALSO RETAIN SUCH EXCESS MEDICATION FOR SUBSEQUENT USE; DURING THE SAME TIME PERIOD, HE REUSED EXCESS SUTURE MATERIAL WHICH HAD BEEN PULLED THROUGH THE TISSUE OF A PREVIOUS PATIENT; ON 8/5/95 WHEN A THREE YEAR OLD PATIENT BECAME AGITATED, HE OVER-PRESCRIBED AN ADULT DOSE OF VALIUM AND INSTRUCTED THE MOTHER TO ADMINISTER THAT MEDICATION ONE-HALF HOUR PRIOR TO THE NEXT SCHEDULED PROCEDURE; ON 8/10/95 THE PATIENT HAD AN ADVERSE REACTION TO VALIUM; HE THEN INSTRUCTED THE PATIENT'S MOTHER TO DOUBLE THE VALIUM DOSAGE PRIOR TO THE NEXT SCHEDULED PROCEDURE WHICH SHE DID NOT DO; THE MOTHER ALSO DID NOT INFORM HIM OF THE PREVIOUS ADVERSE REACTION NOR DID HE ASK; WHEN HE APPEARED BEFORE THE BOARD HE TESTIFIED HE HAD DONE NOTHING WRONG AND HIS UTAH PROBATION HAD BEEN TERMINATED. LICENSE PLACED ON PROBATION WITH THE FOLLOWING TERMS AND CONDITIONS: SUSPENSION NOT TO EXCEED SIX MONTHS AND SUSPENSION WILL BE TERMINATED AFTER HE COMPLETES 15 HOURS OF CONTINUING MEDICAL EDUCATION WITH 10 HOURS IN THE AREA OF MEDICAL ETHICS AND FIVE HOURS IN THE APPLICATION OF STERILE TECHNIQUES AND INFECTIOUS DISEASES; SHALL PROVIDE A COPY OF THIS ORDER TO ANY HEALTH CARE ENTITY WHERE HE HAS PRIVILEGES; SHALL INFORM THE BOARD IF HE CEASES TO PRACTICE IN ARIZONA; TIME SPENT OUT OF ARIZONA DOES NOT COUNT TOWARD PROBATION.

MICHAUD, ROBERT MERRILL DO, LICENSE NUMBER 3638, WAS DISCIPLINED BY ALASKA ON AUGUST 5, 1999
DISCIPLINARY ACTION: DENIAL OF LICENSE REINSTATEMENT
OFFENSE: DISCIPLINARY ACTION BY ANOTHER STATE OR AGENCY

NOTES: REQUEST FOR REINSTATEMENT DENIED BASED ON LICENSE SUSPENSION IN ARIZONA.

MILLER, JAMES DO, LICENSE NUMBER 0003432 OF SCOTTSDALE, AZ, WAS DISCIPLINED BY OHIO ON OCTOBER 26, 1995

DISCIPLINARY ACTION: 12-MONTH LICENSE SUSPENSION; PROBATION
OFFENSE: DISCIPLINARY ACTION BY ANOTHER STATE OR AGENCY

NOTES: PRIOR ACTION BY ARIZONA STATE BOARD OF OSTEOPATHIC EXAMINERS STEMMING FROM HIS CARE AND TREATMENT OF A SURGICAL PATIENT. PROBATIONARY TERMS AND CONDITIONS IMPOSED FOR AT LEAST TWO YEARS.

MILLER, JAMES I DO, LICENSE NUMBER 0002264 OF P.O. BOX 55556, PHOENIX, AZ, WAS DISCIPLINED BY ARIZONA ON APRIL 29, 1994
DISCIPLINARY ACTION: PROBATION; RESTRICTION PLACED ON LICENSE
OFFENSE: SUBSTANDARD CARE, INCOMPETENCE OR NEGLIGENCE

NOTES: MALPRACTICE RESULTING IN THE DEATH OF A PATIENT; PATIENT WAS AN 85 YEAR OLD FEMALE WHOM HE ORIGINALLY DIAGNOSED WITH PERFORATED APPENDIX WHEN IT WAS A PERFORATED ULCER; USED A SURGICAL PROCEDURE WHICH IN RETROSPECT WAS NOT APPROPRIATE; AFTER THE FIRST OPERATIVE DAY HE LEFT TOWN AND TURNED PATIENT OVER TO A COLLEAGUE; PATIENT WAS TRANSFERRED TO ANOTHER SURGEON BUT EXPIRED. PROBATION SHALL CONTINUE UNTIL HE HAS SATISFIED ALL OF THE CONDITIONS: IF HE PERFORMS ANY SURGICAL PROCEDURE REQUIRING THE USE OF GENERAL ANESTHESIA, MAY ONLY PERFORM IT WITH THE SUPERVISION OF A BOARD APPROVED "SENIOR SURGEON" WITH THE EXCEPTION OF HEMORRHOIDECTOMY, HERNIA REPAIR, VASCULAR ACCESS DEVICES FOR LONG TERM CHEMOTHERAPY OR HYPERALIMENTATION, BREAST BIOPSIES, AND REMOVAL OF PILONIDAL CYSTS; ALL OF HIS RECORDS REGARDING ANY PARTICIPATION IN ANY MEDICAL TRAINING PROGRAM AND IN THE COLORADO PROFESSIONAL EDUCATION PROGRAM, INCLUDING MEDICAL SKILL ASSESSMENTS, PSYCHOLOGICAL AND MEDICAL REPORTS, SHALL BE MADE AVAILABLE TO THE BOARD UPON REQUEST; WITHIN 45 DAYS SHALL SUBMIT TO A COMPLETE PSYCHOLOGICAL EVALUATION BY A BOARD APPROVED PSYCHOLOGIST; SHALL ATTEND AND PARTICIPATE IN THE EDUCATIONAL PROGRAMS AT SOUTHWESTERN SURGICAL ASSOCIATION ANNUAL MEETING AND SHALL PARTICIPATE IN AND COMPLETE ONE GENERAL SURGERY REVIEW COURSE YEARLY; SHALL ANNUALLY ENROLL IN AND COMPLETE THE AMERICAN COLLEGE OF SURGEONS SURGICAL EDUCATION AND SELF-ASSESSMENT PROGRAM AND SUBMIT PROOF TO THE BOARD; IF HE WANTS TO PERFORM VASCULAR SURGERY SHALL ATTEND A MINIMUM OF 20 HOURS OF CONTINUING MEDICAL EDUCATION DIRECTLY RELATED TO THE SUBJECT OF VASCULAR SURGERY PROCEDURES AND DIAGNOSIS PRIOR TO 1/01/95; SHALL IMPLEMENT THE "SOAP" FORMAT FOR MAINTAINING COMPLETE OFFICE AND PATIENT RECORDS; DURING THE FIRST THREE YEARS OF PROBATION, SHALL BE SUBJECT TO REVIEW PRIMARILY IN THE AREAS OF SURGICAL PRACTICES AND PROCEDURES AND THE MAINTENANCE OF PATIENT RECORDS; A RANDOM REVIEW OF AT LEAST 10 PATIENT RECORDS SHALL BE SELECTED AT THE REVIEWING PHYSICIAN'S DISCRETION EVERY 120 DAYS WITH A REPORT TO THE BOARD; AND SHALL APPEAR BEFORE THE BOARD UPON REQUEST. THIS ORDER MODIFIED ON 10/20/94 SUCH THAT IF HE PERFORMS ANY SURGICAL PROCEDURE THAT REQUIRES THE USE OF GENERAL ANESTHESIA WHILE HE IS PARTICIPATING IN A SURGICAL TRAINING PROGRAM AT THE MARICOPA MEDICAL CENTER, SHALL BE RELIEVED OF THE REQUIREMENT FOR SUPERVISION OF A SENIOR SURGEON AND SHALL COMPLY WITH ALL APPLICABLE PROTOCOLS GOVERNING SURGICAL PROCEDURES AND GOVERNING PHYSICIANS AT MARICOPA MEDICAL CENTER.

MILLER, JAMES I DO, LICENSE NUMBER 0002264 OF P.O. BOX 55556, PHOENIX, AZ, WAS DISCIPLINED BY ARIZONA ON DECEMBER 14, 1995
DISCIPLINARY ACTION: 36-MONTH PROBATION; REQUIRED TO TAKE ADDITIONAL MEDICAL EDUCATION

NOTES: EXPIRED LICENSE REISSUED ON TERMS AND CONDITIONS: ALL INFORMATION AND REPORTS RECEIVED OR RETAINED BY THE HEALTH SERVICES ADVISORY GROUP, INC. (HSAG) SHALL BE MADE AVAILABLE TO THE BOARD; SHALL REMAIN IN COMPLIANCE WITH HSAG CONCERNING HIS MEDICAL PRACTICE ACTIVITY AND PERFORMANCE REQUIREMENTS; FOR THE NEXT FIVE YEARS SHALL ATTEND AND PARTICIPATE IN THE EDUCATIONAL PROGRAMS AT THE SOUTHWESTERN SURGICAL ASSOCIATION ANNUAL MEETING AND SHALL PARTICIPATE IN AND COMPLETE ONE GENERAL SURGERY REVIEW COURSE YEARLY; SHALL ANNUALLY ENROLL IN AND COMPLETE THE AMERICAN COLLEGE OF SURGEONS SURGICAL EDUCATION AND SELF-ASSESSMENT PROGRAM AND SUBMIT PROOF TO THE BOARD; IF HE WANTS TO PERFORM VASCULAR SURGERY SHALL ATTEND A MINIMUM OF 20 HOURS OF CONTINUING MEDICAL EDUCATION DIRECTLY RELATED TO THE SUBJECT OF VASCULAR SURGERY PROCEDURES AND DIAGNOSIS PRIOR TO 1/01/95; SHALL IMPLEMENT THE "SOAP" FORMAT FOR MAINTAINING COMPLETE OFFICE AND PATIENT RECORDS; DURING THE FIRST THREE YEARS OF PROBATION, SHALL BE SUBJECT TO REVIEW PRIMARILY IN THE AREAS OF SURGICAL PRACTICES AND PROCEDURES AND THE MAINTENANCE OF PATIENT RECORDS; A RANDOM REVIEW OF AT LEAST 10 PATIENT RECORDS SHALL BE SELECTED AT THE REVIEWING PHYSICIAN'S DISCRETION EVERY 120 DAYS WITH A REPORT TO THE BOARD; AND SHALL APPEAR BEFORE THE BOARD UPON REQUEST. ON 6/9/97 ORDER AMENDED ALLOWING HIM TO PERFORM VASCULAR SURGERY.

MILLER, KEITH E MD, LICENSE NUMBER 0003955, WAS DISCIPLINED BY ARIZONA ON SEPTEMBER 10, 1992
DISCIPLINARY ACTION: EMERGENCY SUSPENSION
OFFENSE: SEXUAL ABUSE OF OR SEXUAL MISCONDUCT WITH A PATIENT

NOTES: ON AT LEAST FOUR OCCASIONS DISPENSED OR PRESCRIBED CONTROLLED SUBSTANCES FOR NO THERAPEUTIC PURPOSE TO PATIENTS, IN SOME CASES KNOWING THE PATIENT WAS THEN GOING TO SELL THE DRUGS. HAD SEX WITH SOME OF HIS FEMALE PATIENTS IN CONNECTION WITH THE DRUG TRANSACTIONS. ALSO MAINTAINED INADEQUATE OR FALSE MEDICAL RECORDS.

MILLER, KEITH E MD, LICENSE NUMBER 0003955, WAS DISCIPLINED BY ARIZONA ON JANUARY 21, 1993
DISCIPLINARY ACTION: LICENSE REVOCATION

NOTES: CONSENT AGREEMENT TO CANCELLATION OF LICENSE WITH CAUSE. AGREES NOT TO REAPPLY FOR LICENSURE TO PRACTICE MEDICINE IN ARIZONA FOR A PERIOD OF AT LEAST FIVE YEARS.

MILLER, LOUIS M MD, LICENSE NUMBER 23201, WAS DISCIPLINED BY ARIZONA ON NOVEMBER 14, 1997

DISCIPLINARY ACTION: REPRIMAND

NOTES: AFTER PERFORMING MULTIPLE FACIAL AESTHETIC SURGERIES ON A PATIENT BETWEEN 11/95 AND 7/96, HE GAVE PHOTOGRAPHS AND INFORMATION ABOUT THE SURGERIES TO A LOCAL NEWSPAPER, WITHOUT THE PATIENT'S KNOWLEDGE OR CONSENT.

MILLER, LOUIS M MD, LICENSE NUMBER 166391 OF 2435 S AVENUE A, SUITE C, YUMA, AZ, WAS DISCIPLINED BY NEW YORK ON NOVEMBER 24, 1999
DISCIPLINARY ACTION: REPRIMAND
OFFENSE: DISCIPLINARY ACTION BY ANOTHER STATE OR AGENCY

NOTES: DISCIPLINED BY THE ARIZONA BOARD FOR VIOLATING A PRIVILEGED COMMUNICATION.

MILLER, LOUIS MARK MD, WAS DISCIPLINED BY ARIZONA ON JANUARY 20, 1995
DISCIPLINARY ACTION: MONITORING OF PHYSICIAN PERFORMANCE
OFFENSE: PHYSICAL OR MENTAL ILLNESS INHIBITING THE ABILITY TO PRACTICE WITH SKILL AND SAFETY

NOTES: INTERVIEWED BY THE BOARD RELATIVE TO HIS INDICATION ON HIS ARIZONA LICENSE APPLICATION THAT HE HAS A HISTORY OF A DEPRESSIVE CONDITION. SHALL OBTAIN A BOARD-APPROVED TREATING PSYCHIATRIST; SHALL UNDERGO TREATMENT FOR DEPRESSION (INCLUDING, BUT NOT LIMITED TO, MEDICATION MANAGEMENT, IF INDICATED); PSYCHIATRIST SHALL PROVIDE QUARTERLY REPORTS TO THE BOARD REGARDING HIS DIAGNOSIS, PROGNOSIS AND COMPLIANCE WITH THE TREATMENT PROGRAM. ON 3/26/98 ORDER TERMINATED.

MINDELL, ROBERT S MD, LICENSE NUMBER 18971, WAS DISCIPLINED BY ARIZONA ON MARCH 19, 1997
DISCIPLINARY ACTION: RESTRICTION PLACED ON LICENSE

NOTES: ON 5/7/97 ORDER AMENDED PROHIBITING HIM FROM TAKING CALLS BETWEEN 11 P.M. AND 7 A.M.

MINOR, DAVID DO, LICENSE NUMBER 0002321, WAS DISCIPLINED BY ARIZONA ON JUNE 1, 1991
DISCIPLINARY ACTION: 1-MONTH LICENSE SUSPENSION; 36-MONTH PROBATION
OFFENSE: OVERPRESCRIBING OR MISPRESCRIBING DRUGS

NOTES: PRESCRIBED, DISPENSED, OR ADMINISTERED CONTROLLED SUBSTANCES OR PRESCRIPTION-ONLY DRUGS FOR OTHER THAN THERAPEUTIC PURPOSES AND PERFORMED CONDUCT OR PRACTICE CONSTITUTING A DANGER TO THE HEALTH, SAFETY, OR WELFARE OF THE PATIENT OR THE PUBLIC IN THE CASE OF HIS PRESCRIBING TO EIGHT PATIENTS BETWEEN 1/88 AND 3/91. SUSPENSION COMMENCING 6/01/91 UNTIL 7/01/91; PROBATION UNDER TERMS AND CONDITIONS: SHALL PRESCRIBE NO SCHEDULE IV OR SCHEDULE V MEDICATION FOR ONE YEAR; SHALL PRESCRIBE NO SCHEDULE II OR SCHEDULE III MEDICATION FOR THREE YEARS; SHALL APPEAR BEFORE THE BOARD FOR PROBATIONARY INTERVIEWS UPON REQUEST; SHALL COMPLETE 100 HOURS OF CONTINUING MEDICAL EDUCATION IN THE AREAS OF ADDICTION AND APPROPRIATE PRESCRIBING PRACTICES WITHIN ONE YEAR. $2,500 CIVIL PENALTY. PROBATION SATISFIED IN FULL ON 9/18/93.

MISRA, HARA P MD, LICENSE NUMBER 14933, WAS DISCIPLINED BY ARIZONA ON JANUARY 23, 1998
DISCIPLINARY ACTION: REPRIMAND
OFFENSE: LOSS OR RESTRICTION OF HOSPITAL PRIVILEGES

NOTES: ON 5/20/96 HOSPITAL INFORMED THE BOARD HIS PRIVILEGES WERE SUSPENDED FOR 60 DAYS BECAUSE HE FAILED TO RESPOND APPROPRIATELY TO A MEDICAL EMERGENCY AND DEMONSTRATED UNPROFESSIONAL CONDUCT IN THE CASE; ON 6/17/94 AFTER A PATIENT WAS ADMITTED TO THE EMERGENCY ROOM, HE WAS PAGED AT 1:52 AM, AND SAID HE WOULD BE IN ASAP; AT 2:05 AM HE TOLD AN EMERGENCY ROOM NURSE THAT THEY DID NOT NEED TO PREPARE AN OPERATING ROOM FOR THE PATIENT AT THAT TIME AND HE WOULD BE AROUND EARLY IN THE MORNING; DR. MISRA WAS PAGED BUT DID NOT RESPOND TO TWO PAGES AND ANOTHER PHYSICIAN WAS CALLED; THE PATIENT CONSEQUENTLY HAD CARDIAC ARREST AND DIED; DR. MISRA NEVER SAW THE PATIENT.

MITCHELL, LAUREN E DO, DATE OF BIRTH DECEMBER 12, 1915 OF P O BOX 322, RIMROCK, AZ, WAS DISCIPLINED BY MEDICARE ON FEBRUARY 12, 1990
DISCIPLINARY ACTION: EXCLUSION FROM THE MEDICARE AND/OR MEDICAID PROGRAM
OFFENSE: DISCIPLINARY ACTION BY ANOTHER STATE OR AGENCY

NOTES: LICENSE REVOCATION OR SUSPENSION.

MITCHELL, LAUREN E DO, DATE OF BIRTH DECEMBER 12, 1915, LICENSE NUMBER 0010261 OF LONGMONT, CO, WAS DISCIPLINED BY COLORADO ON JULY 6, 1994
DISCIPLINARY ACTION: REPRIMAND
OFFENSE: PROFESSIONAL MISCONDUCT

MOHR, DARRYL J MD, WAS DISCIPLINED BY ARIZONA ON APRIL 10, 1991
DISCIPLINARY ACTION: FINE; RESTRICTION PLACED ON LICENSE
OFFENSE: OVERCHARGING

NOTES: INVESTIGATION INTO THE STATUS OF HIS HOSPITAL PRIVILEGES AND A FEE COMPLAINT OF OVERPAYMENT BY A PATIENT. CONDITIONS OF ORDER: SHALL IMMEDIATELY CEASE PERFORMING OR ASSISTING IN ANY SURGICAL PROCEDURE UNTIL AUTHORIZED BY THE BOARD; SHALL REIMBURSE ONE PATIENT $895 PLUS INTEREST; SHALL INFORM THE BOARD OF CHANGE OF ADDRESS; FINED $50 FOR FAILURE TO PROVIDE SUCH NOTICE PREVIOUSLY. ON 7/14/94 REQUEST TO TERMINATE THIS STIPULATION WAS DENIED.

MOLNAR, EUGENE M MD, LICENSE NUMBER 00D7193 OF NEWPORT BEACH, CA, WAS DISCIPLINED BY TEXAS ON AUGUST 24, 1991
DISCIPLINARY ACTION: 60-MONTH PROBATION
OFFENSE: DISCIPLINARY ACTION BY ANOTHER STATE OR AGENCY

NOTES: REVOCATION STAYED. BEFORE PRACTICING IN TEXAS SHALL APPEAR BEFORE AND RECEIVE APPROVAL FROM THE TEXAS BOARD.

MOLNAR, EUGENE MICHAEL MD, LICENSE NUMBER 0015405, WAS DISCIPLINED BY ARIZONA ON APRIL 12, 1991
DISCIPLINARY ACTION: LICENSE REVOCATION
OFFENSE: DISCIPLINARY ACTION BY ANOTHER STATE OR AGENCY

NOTES: CALIFORNIA LICENSE WAS REVOKED ON 7/28/89 WITH REVOCATION STAYED TO 5 YEARS PROBATION, ALLEGING IMPROPER SURGICAL PROCEDURES AND INSURANCE FRAUD, AIDING THREE PERSONS IN THE UNAUTHORIZED PRACTICE OF NURSING, AND LYING ON A NEVADA REGISTRATION APPLICATION. ON 10/10/91 HIS REQUEST FOR A REHEARING WAS

DENIED.

MOLNAR, EUGENE MICHAEL MD OF NEWPORT BEACH, CA, WAS DISCIPLINED BY ILLINOIS ON SEPTEMBER 1, 1991
DISCIPLINARY ACTION: LICENSE SUSPENSION
OFFENSE: DISCIPLINARY ACTION BY ANOTHER STATE OR AGENCY

NOTES: DISCIPLINED BY CALIFORNIA. INDEFINITE SUSPENSION.

MONSHAW, ROBERT A MD, LICENSE NUMBER 0148349 OF 898 VALLEY ROAD, BLUEBELL, PA, WAS DISCIPLINED BY NEW YORK ON APRIL 2, 1996
DISCIPLINARY ACTION: LICENSE REVOCATION
OFFENSE: SUBSTANDARD CARE, INCOMPETENCE OR NEGLIGENCE

NOTES: GROSS NEGLIGENCE, GROSS INCOMPETENCE, PRACTICING WITH NEGLIGENCE ON MORE THAN ONE OCCASION, PRACTICING THE PROFESSION FRAUDULENTLY, AND FAILURE TO MAINTAIN ACCURATE PATIENT RECORDS.

MONSHAW, ROBERT A MD, WAS DISCIPLINED BY ARIZONA ON SEPTEMBER 25, 1997
OFFENSE: DISCIPLINARY ACTION BY ANOTHER STATE OR AGENCY

NOTES: ACTION TAKEN AGAINST NEW YORK LICENSE. INTERIM ORDER. MAY NOT PRACTICE MEDICINE IN ARIZONA UNTIL FURTHER ORDER OF THE BOARD.

MONSHAW, ROBERT ALLEN MD, LICENSE NUMBER C42046 OF BLUE BELL, PA, WAS DISCIPLINED BY CALIFORNIA ON JANUARY 2, 1998
DISCIPLINARY ACTION: 60-MONTH PROBATION
OFFENSE: DISCIPLINARY ACTION BY ANOTHER STATE OR AGENCY

NOTES: DISCIPLINED BY NEW YORK FOR PRACTICING WITH NEGLIGENCE AND INCOMPETENCE ON MORE THAN ONE OCCASION, GROSS INCOMPETENCE, FRAUD AND FAILURE TO MAINTAIN ACCURATE RECORDS. REVOCATION STAYED.

MONSHAW, ROBERT ALLEN MD, DATE OF BIRTH MARCH 16, 1941 OF REVERE HOUSE, SCARSDALE, NY, WAS DISCIPLINED BY MEDICARE ON JANUARY 20, 1998
DISCIPLINARY ACTION: EXCLUSION FROM THE MEDICARE AND/OR MEDICAID PROGRAM
OFFENSE: DISCIPLINARY ACTION BY ANOTHER STATE OR AGENCY

NOTES: LICENSE REVOKED, SUSPENDED, SURRENDERED OR OTHERWISE LOST FOR REASONS BEARING ON PROFESSIONAL PERFORMANCE, PROFESSIONAL COMPETENCE OR FINANCIAL INTEGRITY.

MONTASIR, ADEL MD, WAS DISCIPLINED BY ARIZONA ON OCTOBER 19, 1995
OFFENSE: LOSS OR RESTRICTION OF HOSPITAL PRIVILEGES

NOTES: INTERVIEWED BY BOARD MEMBERS RELATIVE TO INFORMATION RECEIVED FROM A HOSPITAL INDICATING THAT PHYSICIAN'S PRIVILEGES WERE REDUCED FROM GENERAL SURGERY TO SURGICAL ASSISTING ONLY; INFORMATION RECEIVED INDICATING THAT THE PHYSICIAN'S TRAUMA SURGERY PRIVILEGES WERE RESTRICTED AND PHYSICIAN WAS REQUIRED TO TAKE A MINI-RESIDENCY IN TRAUMA SURGERY AT THE UNIVERSITY OF ARIZONA; AND INFORMATION RECEIVED INDICATING PHYSICIAN'S PRIVILEGES WERE SUMMARILY SUSPENDED AT A MEDICAL CENTER, WITH THE EXCEPTION OF SURGICAL ASSIST PRIVILEGES, BASED ON PATIENT ABANDONMENT. WITHIN THREE MONTHS, SHALL TAKE AND PASS THE SPECIAL PURPOSE EXAMINATION WITH A SCORE OF 75 OR GREATER; WITHIN 30 DAYS, SHALL SUBMIT TO PSYCHOLOGICAL AND PSYCHOMETRIC EVALUATIONS BY A BOARD-DESIGNATED EVALUATOR.

MONTASIR, ADEL MD, LICENSE NUMBER 6798, WAS DISCIPLINED BY ARIZONA ON JANUARY 24, 1997
DISCIPLINARY ACTION: LICENSE REVOCATION
OFFENSE: FAILURE TO COMPLY WITH PREVIOUS BOARD ORDER

NOTES: IN 1995 MADE MISSTATEMENTS ON A REAPPOINTMENT APPLICATION FOR MEDICAL STAFF PRIVILEGES AT A HOSPITAL BY ANSWERING NO TO THE QUESTIONS THAT SOUGHT INFORMATION ABOUT REDUCTION, MODIFICATION OR SUSPENSION OF CLINICAL PRIVILEGES, AND ABOUT BEING THE SUBJECT OF ANY DISCIPLINARY ACTION; IN 2/96 RECEIVED INSUFFICIENT SCORE ON THE SPEX EXAMINATION AND HAS NOT RE-APPLIED TO TAKE THE SPEX TEST; BOARD-ORDERED PSYCHOLOGICAL PROFILE FOUND THAT HIS NEUROPSYCHOLOGICAL SCREENS WERE POSITIVE SUGGESTING COGNITIVE INFLEXIBILITY AND INEFFICIENCY DETERMINING CAUSE AND EFFECT RELATIONSHIPS AND THAT MOST LIKELY HE WAS EXPERIENCING DEPRESSION.

MONTASIR, ADEL MD, LICENSE NUMBER 107376 OF 9515 NORTH 53RD PLACE, SCOTTSDALE, AZ, WAS DISCIPLINED BY NEW YORK ON DECEMBER 8, 1997
DISCIPLINARY ACTION: SURRENDER OF LICENSE
OFFENSE: DISCIPLINARY ACTION BY ANOTHER STATE OR AGENCY

NOTES: FALSE STATEMENTS ON A JOB APPLICATION; FAILURE TO PASS THE SPEX COMPETENCY EXAMS.

MORA, MARIO A MD, LICENSE NUMBER 0015340, WAS DISCIPLINED BY ARIZONA ON OCTOBER 10, 1990
DISCIPLINARY ACTION: LICENSE REVOCATION
OFFENSE: PROVIDING FALSE INFORMATION TO THE BOARD OR OTHER HEALTH AGENCY

NOTES: ON 12/2/87 LICENSE RENEWAL CARD HE ANSWERED THAT HIS LICENSE HAD NOT BEEN DISCIPLINED BY ANOTHER JURISDICTION. HE HAD BEEN FINED AND REPRIMANDED BY THE PENNSYLVANIA BOARD ON 10/30/87, BECAUSE HE ADMITTED FALSIFYING 2 RECOMMENDATIONS IN SUBMITTING AN APPLICATION FOR EMPLOYMENT AS AN EMERGENCY PHYSICIAN.

MORFORD, PAMELA A MD, LICENSE NUMBER 0017926, WAS DISCIPLINED BY ARIZONA ON JULY 17, 1996
DISCIPLINARY ACTION: RESTRICTION PLACED ON LICENSE

NOTES: SHALL NOT PRACTICE OBSTETRICS; SHALL NOT PERFORM GYNECOLOGICAL SURGERY; SHALL, IN THE CONTEXT OF TREATING CANDIDIASIS . HYPERSENSITIVITY SYNDROME, SHALL COMPLY WITH BOARD RULE BY UTILIZING ADEQUATE INFORMED PATIENT CONSENT AND CONFORMING TO GENERALLY ACCEPTED EXPERIMENTAL CRITERIA.

MORFORD, PAMELA ANN DR, LICENSE NUMBER 0020267, WAS DISCIPLINED BY MINNESOTA ON NOVEMBER 13, 1993

NOTES: STAYED SUSPENSION. AMENDED ORDER ON 1/15/94. UNCONDITIONAL LICENSE GRANTED ON 9/14/96.

MORGAN, JEROLD DO, LICENSE NUMBER 2107 OF 3651 E BASELINE #104, GILBERT, AZ, WAS DISCIPLINED BY ARIZONA ON JANUARY 29, 1999
DISCIPLINARY ACTION: LICENSE REVOCATION
OFFENSE: CRIMINAL CONVICTION OR PLEA OF GUILTY, NOLO CONTENDERE, OR NO CONTEST TO A CRIME

NOTES: ON 11/17/97 PLED GUILTY TO ONE COUNT OF ATTEMPTED AGGRAVATED ASSAULT AND WAS SENTENCED TO FOUR YEARS OF PROBATION AND SIX MONTHS INCARCERATION. MAY APPLY FOR REINSTATEMENT AFTER TWO YEARS. ON 3/6/99 MOTION FOR REHEARING WAS DENIED.

MORITZ, TERRELL C MD, DATE OF BIRTH AUGUST 5, 1937, LICENSE NUMBER 16162, WAS DISCIPLINED BY COLORADO ON JULY 10, 1997
DISCIPLINARY ACTION: SURRENDER OF LICENSE

NOTES: NO UNPROFESSIONAL CONDUCT IDENTIFIED.

MORITZ, TERRELL CONWAY MD, LICENSE NUMBER 0020323, WAS DISCIPLINED BY ARIZONA ON OCTOBER 10, 1991
DISCIPLINARY ACTION: 60-MONTH PROBATION; FINE
OFFENSE: PROVIDING FALSE INFORMATION TO THE BOARD OR OTHER HEALTH AGENCY

NOTES: KNOWINGLY MAKING A FALSE OR MISLEADING STATEMENT TO THE BOARD IN THAT IN HIS 2/14/91 APPLICATION FOR HIS ARIZONA LICENSE, HE DENIED HAVING EVER BEEN TREATED FOR THE USE OF OR MISUSE OF ANY CHEMICAL SUBSTANCES, DESPITE THE FACT THAT HE HAD BEEN AN INPATIENT AT A TREATMENT CENTER IN COLORADO IN 8/90 FOR 28 DAYS AND AN INPATIENT AT A RECOVERY CENTER IN GEORGIA FOR THREE MONTHS IN THE FALL OF 1990 BOTH FOR THE TREATMENT OF ALCOHOLISM; ALSO PRIVILEGES AT A MEDICAL CENTER IN COLORADO WERE TEMPORARILY SUSPENDED IN 12/89 DUE TO HIS MISREADING AN EKG AND HE WAS REQUIRED TO GET ADDITIONAL TRAINING; PRIVILEGES WERE RESTORED IN 4/90. PROBATION WITH CONDITIONS: MUST IMMEDIATELY PARTICIPATE IN A BOARD-APPROVED MONITORED AFTERCARE TREATMENT PROGRAM WHOSE THERAPIST MUST SUBMIT QUARTERLY REPORTS; SHALL ATTEND A MINIMUM OF THREE WEEKLY MEETINGS OF AA AND SHALL OBTAIN A SPONSOR IN AA WITH WHOM HE SHALL HAVE CONTACT AT LEAST ONCE A WEEK; SHALL OBTAIN A BOARD-APPROVED TREATING PHYSICIAN; SHALL ABSTAIN COMPLETELY FROM THE CONSUMPTION OF ALCOHOL AND DRUGS EXCEPT WHEN PRESCRIBED BY HIS TREATING PHYSICIAN; MUST SUBMIT TO WITNESSED RANDOM BIOLOGICAL FLUID COLLECTION; SHALL KEEP A LOG OF ANY AND ALL MEDICATIONS PRESCRIBED FOR HIM; SHALL SUBMIT TO ANY EXAMINATIONS OR THERAPY ORDERED BY THE BOARD; SHALL APPEAR BEFORE BOARD FOR INTERVIEWS UPON REQUEST; SHALL INFORM BOARD OF CHANGE OF ADDRESS OR IF AWAY FOR MORE THAN FIVE DAYS; SHALL PAY $2,500 ADMINISTRATIVE PENALTY WITHIN ONE YEAR.

MORITZ, TERRELL CONWAY MD, LICENSE NUMBER 0020323, WAS DISCIPLINED BY ARIZONA ON JANUARY 25, 1992
DISCIPLINARY ACTION: EMERGENCY SUSPENSION
OFFENSE: SUBSTANCE ABUSE

NOTES: IS CURRENTLY IN TREATMENT FOR ALCOHOL ABUSE.

MORITZ, TERRELL CONWAY MD, LICENSE NUMBER 0020323, WAS DISCIPLINED BY ARIZONA ON SEPTEMBER 11, 1992
DISCIPLINARY ACTION: 120-MONTH PROBATION; REQUIRED TO ENTER AN IMPAIRED PHYSICIAN PROGRAM OR SUBSTANCE ABUSE TREATMENT
OFFENSE: FAILURE TO COMPLY WITH PREVIOUS BOARD ORDER

NOTES: VIOLATED A PREVIOUS BOARD ORDER OF 10/10/91 IN THAT HE DID NOT MAINTAIN MEDICATION LOG AS REQUIRED, STATED HE WAS TAKING ONLY ASPIRIN, MULTIVITAMINS AND MINERALS, BUT TESTED POSITIVE ON 11/8/91 FOR PSEUDOEPHEDRINE AND DEXTROMETHORPHAN, ON 12/2/91 FOR TERPIN HYDRATE, ACETAMINOPHEN, DOXYLAMINE, DEXTROMETHORPHAN, AND PSEUDOEPHEDRINE, ON 12/12/91 FOR DOXYLAMINE, PSEUDOEPHEDRINE, DEXTROMETHORPHAN, AND ACETAMINOPHEN. FROM 1/9/92 TO AT LEAST 1/14/92, DRANK ALCOHOL EVERY DAY RESULTING IN SUBSTANTIAL INTOXICATION. BOARD SUMMARILY SUSPENDED LICENSE ON 1/25/92. ADMITTED HIMSELF FOR ALCOHOL ABUSE TREATMENT TO REHABILITATION CENTER IN ARIZONA. FROM 3/16/92 TO 5/8/92, PARTICIPATED IN TREATMENT AT AN OUTPATIENT CENTER FOR ALCOHOLISM AND DEPRESSION. ORDERED TO PAY COSTS OF $500. MUST IMMEDIATELY PARTICIPATE IN A BOARD-APPROVED MONITORED AFTERCARE TREATMENT PROGRAM WHOSE THERAPIST MUST SUBMIT QUARTERLY REPORTS; MUST PARTICIPATE IN 90 12-STEP MEETINGS FOR SUBSTANCE ABUSE WITHIN 90 DAYS; MUST THEN PARTICIPATE IN A 12-STEP RECOVERY PROGRAM AS DETERMINED BY HIS TREATING THERAPIST AND ATTEND AT LEAST 3 WEEKLY MEETINGS; SHALL OBTAIN A BOARD-APPROVED TREATING PHYSICIAN; SHALL ABSTAIN COMPLETELY FROM THE CONSUMPTION OF ALCOHOLIC BEVERAGES AND DRUGS EXCEPT WHEN PRESCRIBED BY HIS TREATING PHYSICIAN; MUST SUBMIT TO WITNESSED RANDOM BIOLOGICAL FLUID COLLECTION; IF BOARD RECEIVES NOTIFICATION OF A POSITIVE SCREEN, LICENSE SHALL BE CANCELED WITH CAUSE WITHIN 15 DAYS. KEEP A LOG OF ANY AND ALL MEDICATIONS PRESCRIBED FOR HIM; SHALL SUBMIT TO ANY EXAMINATIONS OR THERAPY ORDERED BY BOARD; SHALL APPEAR BEFORE BOARD FOR INTERVIEWS UPON REQUEST; SHALL HAVE EMPLOYER SUBMIT QUARTERLY REPORTS TO THE BOARD; SHALL INFORM BOARD OF CHANGE OF ADDRESS OR EMPLOYMENT OR IF AWAY FOR MORE THAN 5 DAYS. ON 2/15/96 PROBATION TERMINATED.

MORTEL, VICENTE MD, LICENSE NUMBER 0011096, WAS DISCIPLINED BY ARIZONA ON JULY 16, 1996
DISCIPLINARY ACTION: LICENSE REVOCATION

NOTES: DESPITE OVERWHELMING EVIDENCE OF HIS COMPETENCY IN HIS SPECIALTY OF COLON/RECTAL SURGERY, HE IS DEFINED BY THE BOARD AS MEDICALLY INCOMPETENT BASED ON HIS FAILURE OF THE SPECIAL PURPOSE EXAMINATION WITH A SCORE OF 49. ON 10/18/96 BOARD DENIED HIS REQUEST FOR REHEARING/REVIEW. ON 11/12/97 REVOCATION STAYED WITH INDEFINITE SUSPENSION OF LICENSE SUPPORTING THE OPPORTUNITY FOR HIM TO TAKE AND PASS THE SPEX AFTER MATTER WAS REMANDED BACK TO THE BOARD BY SUPERIOR COURT TO MAKE FINDINGS AS TO WHY REVOCATION WAS JUSTIFIED.

MOSHREFZADEH, MASHALLA MD, LICENSE NUMBER 0015724, WAS DISCIPLINED BY ARIZONA ON OCTOBER 21, 1994
DISCIPLINARY ACTION: REQUIRED TO TAKE ADDITIONAL MEDICAL EDUCATION; MONITORING OF PHYSICIAN PERFORMANCE
OFFENSE: SUBSTANDARD CARE, INCOMPETENCE OR NEGLIGENCE

NOTES: ALLEGATIONS OF DELAY IN DIAGNOSING CANCER OF THE RECTUM AND FAILURE TO APPROPRIATELY EVALUATE RECTAL BLEEDING IN ONE PATIENT DURING 1989. WITHIN THE NEXT NINE MONTHS DR. MOSHREFZADEH SHALL PERFORM 15 FLEXIBLE SIGMOIDOSCOPICS UNDER THE DIRECT SUPERVISION OF A PHYSICIAN ACCEPTABLE TO THE BOARD; SHALL ALSO OBTAIN 10 HOURS OF CONTINUING MEDICAL EDUCATION IN CANCER SCREENING AND TREATMENT TO SPECIFICALLY INCLUDE COLON CANCER

SCREENING AND TREATMENT; THIS CONTINUING MEDICAL EDUCATION IS TO BE IN ADDITION TO THE REGULAR ANNUAL REQUIREMENTS FOR CONTINUING MEDICAL EDUCATION. ON 1/20/95 ORDER TERMINATED.

MOSHREFZADEH, MASHALLAH MD, LICENSE NUMBER 0A39663 OF SUN CITY, AZ, WAS DISCIPLINED BY CALIFORNIA ON NOVEMBER 16, 1995
DISCIPLINARY ACTION: REPRIMAND
OFFENSE: DISCIPLINARY ACTION BY ANOTHER STATE OR AGENCY

NOTES: ACTION IN ARIZONA WHICH REQUIRED SUPERVISED FLEXIBLE SIGMOIDOSCOPIES AND EDUCATION COURSES ON CANCER AND COLON CANCER SCREENING AND TREATMENT, FOR FAILING TO PROPERLY DIAGNOSE A RECTAL POLYP IN A PATIENT FOUND WITH CANCER OF THE RECTUM.

MOSS, LEE A MD, LICENSE NUMBER 0011674, WAS DISCIPLINED BY ARIZONA ON APRIL 16, 1996
DISCIPLINARY ACTION: RESTRICTION PLACED ON LICENSE; RESTRICTION PLACED ON CONTROLLED SUBSTANCE LICENSE

NOTES: SHALL NOT PRACTICE CLINICAL MEDICINE IN ARIZONA UNTIL FURTHER ORDER OF THE BOARD; BEFORE PERMITTING HIM TO PRACTICE, BOARD MAY REQUIRE HIM TO UNDERGO MENTAL OR PHYSICAL EVALUATIONS AND ORAL OR WRITTEN COMPETENCY EXAMINATIONS.

MURPHY, JEROME P MD OF SCOTTSDALE, AZ, WAS DISCIPLINED BY MISSOURI ON MAY 21, 1990
OFFENSE: DISCIPLINARY ACTION BY ANOTHER STATE OR AGENCY

NOTES: MUST APPEAR BEFORE BOARD BEFORE RETURNING TO PRACTICE IN MISSOURI.

MURPHY, JEROME P MD, LICENSE NUMBER 0019548, WAS DISCIPLINED BY ARIZONA ON JULY 16, 1990
DISCIPLINARY ACTION: RESTRICTION PLACED ON LICENSE; RESTRICTION PLACED ON CONTROLLED SUBSTANCE LICENSE
OFFENSE: LOSS OR RESTRICTION OF HOSPITAL PRIVILEGES

NOTES: UNPROFESSIONAL CONDUCT INCLUDING: VIOLATING A FORMAL ORDER, FAILING OR REFUSING TO MAINTAIN ADEQUATE RECORDS ON A PATIENT, OR FAILING TO MAKE SUCH RECORDS PROMPTLY AVAILABLE TO ANOTHER PHYSICIAN UPON REQUEST; NUMEROUS INSTANCES OF PRESCRIPTION VIOLATIONS, INCLUDING AFTER HIS SCHEDULE II LICENSE HAD BEEN SURRENDERED AND IN VIOLATION OF BOARD ORDERS; SURGICAL PRIVILEGES WERE SUSPENDED OR DENIED AT TWO HOSPITALS. CONDITIONS OF PROBATION INCLUDE: MAY NOT PERFORM GENERAL SURGERY UNTIL AUTHORIZED BY BOARD; IN ACCORDANCE WITH ORDER OF 4/13/88, MUST SURRENDER CONTROLLED SUBSTANCES REGISTRATION FOR SCHEDULE II DRUGS; MUST MAINTAIN A RECORD IN TRIPLICATE OF SCHEDULE III AND IV PRESCRIPTIONS AND SHALL PROVIDE BOARD WITH A COPY OF THIS RECORD. ON 1/27/99 REQUEST TO PRESCRIBE SCHEDULE V CONTROLLED SUBSTANCES GRANTED; 1991 ORDER HAS LAPSED BUT THIS ORDER IN FULL FORCE AND EFFECT.

MYERS, DAVID P MD OF 12220 BRUCE B DOWNS BLVD, TAMPA, FL, WAS DISCIPLINED BY DEA ON JANUARY 10, 1990
DISCIPLINARY ACTION: RESTRICTION PLACED ON CONTROLLED SUBSTANCE LICENSE
OFFENSE: SUBSTANCE ABUSE

NOTES: WAS ON FIVE YEAR PROBATION THAT BEGAN 10/84 UNTIL 10/89 FOR ALCOHOL DEPENDENCY. PROBATION RESTRICTED HIM FROM ADMINISTERING, DISPENSING, PRESCRIBING OR STORING SCHEDULE II CONTROLLED SUBSTANCES.

MYERS, DAVID P DO, LICENSE NUMBER 0001575 OF 750 SOUTH CRAYCROFT, #150, TUCSON, AZ, WAS DISCIPLINED BY ARIZONA ON SEPTEMBER 12, 1994
DISCIPLINARY ACTION: REQUIRED TO ENTER AN IMPAIRED PHYSICIAN PROGRAM OR TREATMENT
OFFENSE: PHYSICAL OR MENTAL ILLNESS INHIBITING THE ABILITY TO PRACTICE WITH SKILL AND SAFETY

NOTES: INFORMATION RECEIVED BY THE BOARD THAT HE MAY BE PHYSICALLY AND/OR PSYCHOLOGICALLY UNABLE TO SAFELY AND SKILLFULLY ENGAGE IN THE PRACTICE OF MEDICINE AND MAY HAVE COMMITTED ONE OR MORE ACTS OF UNPROFESSIONAL CONDUCT. SHALL REFRAIN COMPLETELY FROM THE PRACTICE OF MEDICINE UNTIL HE HAS COMPLETED THE FOLLOWING CONDITIONS: SHALL PARTICIPATE IN AND SUCCESSFULLY COMPLETE AN INITIAL TREATMENT PROGRAM; SHALL BE EVALUATED AND RECEIVE CLEARANCE FROM ALL PHYSICIANS INVOLVED IN/OR CHARGED WITH HIS CARE AND TREATMENT TO RETURN TO THE PRACTICE OF MEDICINE AND PROVIDE PROOF TO THE BOARD; SHALL AUTHORIZE ALL PHYSICIANS, PSYCHOLOGISTS, AND OTHER HEALTH CARE PROVIDERS INVOLVED IN HIS CARE AND TREATMENT TO RELEASE ANY AND ALL INFORMATION ON HIS DIAGNOSIS, CARE, AND TREATMENT TO THE BOARD; SHALL MEET WITH THE BOARD AFTER SUBMITTING WRITTEN REQUEST TO THE BOARD FOR APPROVAL TO RESUME THE PRACTICE OF MEDICINE.

MYERS, DAVID P DO, LICENSE NUMBER 0001575 OF 750 SOUTH CRAYCROFT, #150, TUCSON, AZ, WAS DISCIPLINED BY ARIZONA ON OCTOBER 8, 1994
DISCIPLINARY ACTION: 60-MONTH PROBATION; REQUIRED TO ENTER AN IMPAIRED PHYSICIAN PROGRAM OR SUBSTANCE ABUSE TREATMENT
OFFENSE: PHYSICAL OR MENTAL ILLNESS INHIBITING THE ABILITY TO PRACTICE WITH SKILL AND SAFETY

NOTES: PHYSICALLY AND/OR PSYCHOLOGICALLY UNABLE TO SAFELY AND SKILLFULLY ENGAGE IN THE PRACTICE OF MEDICINE AND MAY HAVE COMMITTED ONE OR MORE ACTS OF UNPROFESSIONAL CONDUCT. AUTHORIZED TO RESUME THE PRACTICE OF MEDICINE. MINIMUM FIVE YEAR PROBATION UNDER TERMS AND CONDITIONS: AGREES TO PROVIDE AUTHORIZATION FOR ALL PHYSICIANS, PSYCHOLOGISTS, AND OTHER HEALTH CARE PROVIDERS INVOLVED IN HIS CARE AND TREATMENT TO RELEASE ANY INFORMATION ON HIS DIAGNOSIS, CARE AND TREATMENT TO THE BOARD; SHALL PARTICIPATE IN AN OUTPATIENT CHEMICAL/ALCOHOL DEPENDENCY TREATMENT PROGRAM INCLUDING AT LEAST THREE MEETINGS PER WEEK UNTIL RELEASED BY THE PROGRAM DIRECTOR; SHALL TAKE ANTABUSE DAILY FOR TWO YEARS OR UNTIL DETERMINED NO LONGER NECESSARY BY HIS TREATING PHYSICIAN; SHALL OBTAIN AN AA SPONSOR; SHALL ATTEND 90 AA MEETINGS DURING THE 90 DAYS IMMEDIATELY FOLLOWING COMPLETION OF THE OUTPATIENT PROGRAM; SHALL PARTICIPATE IN INDIVIDUAL PSYCHOTHERAPY SESSIONS AT LEAST TWO TIMES PER MONTH; SHALL PARTICIPATE IN COUNSELING SESSIONS AT LEAST TWO TIMES PER MONTH; SHALL CONSUME NO ALCOHOL AND WILL NOT USE CONTROLLED SUBSTANCES OR PRESCRIPTION-ONLY MEDICATIONS UNLESS PRESCRIBED BY A LICENSED

HEALTH CARE PRACTITIONER AS PART OF A LAWFUL COURSE OF TREATMENT; SHALL SUPPLY BODY FLUID SPECIMENS UPON REQUEST; SHALL MEET WITH THE BOARD UPON REQUEST. ON 10/16/99 FULL AND UNRESTRICTED LICENSE ISSUED.

MYERS, RONALD A MD, LICENSE NUMBER 0043456 OF PORT ANGELES, WA, WAS DISCIPLINED BY FLORIDA ON FEBRUARY 12, 1992
DISCIPLINARY ACTION: SURRENDER OF LICENSE
NOTES: AGREES NEVER AGAIN TO APPLY FOR LICENSURE AS A PHYSICIAN IN FLORIDA.

MYERS, RONALD A MD, LICENSE NUMBER 0019234, WAS DISCIPLINED BY ARIZONA ON OCTOBER 22, 1994
DISCIPLINARY ACTION: REQUIRED TO ENTER AN IMPAIRED PHYSICIAN PROGRAM OR SUBSTANCE ABUSE TREATMENT; MONITORING OF PHYSICIAN PERFORMANCE
NOTES: MUST IMMEDIATELY PARTICIPATE IN A BOARD-APPROVED MONITORED AFTERCARE TREATMENT PROGRAM, THE ONE SPONSORED BY ARIZONA BOARD IF HE IS IN ARIZONA OR, IF HE RESIDES IN ANOTHER STATE, A BOARD AFFILIATED PROGRAM IN THAT STATE; MUST PARTICIPATE IN A 12-STEP RECOVERY PROGRAM AND ATTEND AT LEAST THREE WEEKLY MEETINGS; SHALL OBTAIN A BOARD-APPROVED TREATING PHYSICIAN; SHALL ABSTAIN COMPLETELY FROM THE CONSUMPTION OF ALCOHOLIC BEVERAGES AND DRUGS EXCEPT WHEN PRESCRIBED BY HIS TREATING PHYSICIAN; MUST SUBMIT TO WITNESSED RANDOM BIOLOGICAL FLUID COLLECTION; KEEP A LOG OF ANY AND ALL MEDICATIONS PRESCRIBED FOR HIM; SHALL SUBMIT TO ANY EXAMINATIONS OR THERAPY ORDERED BY BOARD; SHALL APPEAR BEFORE BOARD FOR INTERVIEWS UPON REQUEST; SHALL INFORM BOARD OF CHANGE OF ADDRESS OR IF AWAY FOR MORE THAN FIVE DAYS.

MYERS, RONALD A MD, WAS DISCIPLINED BY NEVADA ON MAY 5, 1995
DISCIPLINARY ACTION: SURRENDER OF LICENSE
OFFENSE: DISCIPLINARY ACTION BY ANOTHER STATE OR AGENCY
NOTES: CHARGED WITH DISCIPLINARY ACTION AGAINST HIS LICENSES IN FLORIDA AND CALIFORNIA; RENEWING AND ATTEMPTING TO RENEW A LICENSE BY FRAUD OR MISREPRESENTATION OR BY A FALSE, MISLEADING, INACCURATE OR INCOMPLETE STATEMENT; ENGAGING IN CONDUCT WHICH IS INTENDED TO DECEIVE; FAILING TO NOTIFY THE NEVADA BOARD OF THE DISCIPLINARY ACTIONS TAKEN AGAINST HIS LICENSE IN FLORIDA AND CALIFORNIA. VOLUNTARY SURRENDER OF LICENSE WHILE HE IS UNDER INVESTIGATION.

MYERS, RONALD A MD, LICENSE NUMBER 0019234, WAS DISCIPLINED BY ARIZONA ON AUGUST 5, 1996
DISCIPLINARY ACTION: REPRIMAND
OFFENSE: DISCIPLINARY ACTION BY ANOTHER STATE OR AGENCY
NOTES: IN 12/91, HE VOLUNTARILY RELINQUISHED HIS FLORIDA LICENSE AND AGREED NEVER AGAIN TO APPLY FOR LICENSURE IN FLORIDA IN ORDER TO AVOID ADMINISTRATIVE PROSECUTION FOR FAILING TO MAINTAIN AND SUBMIT DOCUMENTATION VERIFYING THE REQUIRED HOURS OF CONTINUING MEDICAL EDUCATION CREDITS FROM 1/1/88 THROUGH 12/31/89; HE RENEWED HIS FLORIDA LICENSE BY FRAUDULENT MISREPRESENTATION BY CERTIFYING HE HAD COMPLETED THESE CONTINUING MEDICAL EDUCATION REQUIREMENTS.

NASH, ROBERT A MD, LICENSE NUMBER 005065A, WAS DISCIPLINED BY WYOMING ON DECEMBER 29, 1993
DISCIPLINARY ACTION: RESTRICTION PLACED ON LICENSE; REQUIRED TO TAKE ADDITIONAL MEDICAL EDUCATION
NOTES: PERMANENTLY ENJOINED FROM PROVIDING OR PERFORMING ANY COUNSELING OR TREATMENT TO ANY FEMALE PATIENTS UNLESS AN ATTENDANT IS PHYSICALLY PRESENT IN THE EXAMINING OR COUNSELING ROOM OR AREA AT ALL TIMES; SHALL PROVIDE TO THE BOARD WITHIN 6 MONTHS WRITTEN CERTIFICATION OF ATTENDANCE AND SUCCESSFUL COMPLETION OF THE "PATIENT-THERAPIST RELATIONSHIPS: CRITICAL ISSUES OF THE 90S" SEMINAR; SHALL APPEAR BEFORE THE INFORMAL INTERVIEWERS IN 10/94 TO DISCUSS HIS MEDICAL PRACTICE; SHALL NOT SEEK MODIFICATION OR TERMINATION OF THE TERMS AND RESTRICTIONS OF THIS DECREE FOR TWO YEARS.

NASH, ROBERT A MD, LICENSE NUMBER 0005955, WAS DISCIPLINED BY ARIZONA ON MARCH 27, 1995
DISCIPLINARY ACTION: RESTRICTION PLACED ON LICENSE
NOTES: PERMANENTLY ENJOINED FROM PROVIDING OR PERFORMING ANY COUNSELING OR TREATMENT TO ANY FEMALE PATIENT UNLESS PHYSICIAN, NURSE OR SOCIAL WORKER IS PHYSICALLY PRESENT IN THE EXAMINING OR COUNSELING ROOM; SHALL COMPLY WITH ALL TERMS OF THE WYOMING CONSENT DECREE OF 12/29/93 AND 1/23/94 ENFORCEMENT ORDER; SHALL APPEAR BEFORE THE BOARD UPON REQUEST; SHALL NOT SEEK TO MODIFY OR TERMINATE THIS ORDER FOR TWO YEARS.

NASH, ROBERT A MD, LICENSE NUMBER 0028684 OF EVANSTON, WY, WAS DISCIPLINED BY WASHINGTON ON OCTOBER 6, 1995
DISCIPLINARY ACTION: RESTRICTION PLACED ON LICENSE
NOTES: CANNOT PROVIDE COUNSELING OR TREATMENT TO ANY FEMALE PATIENT UNLESS AN ATTENDANT IS PHYSICALLY PRESENT IN THE ROOM AT ALL TIMES.

NELSON, DONALD H DO OF TUCSON, AZ, WAS DISCIPLINED BY MISSOURI ON JUNE 22, 1993
DISCIPLINARY ACTION: SURRENDER OF LICENSE
OFFENSE: CRIMINAL CONVICTION OR PLEA OF GUILTY, NOLO CONTENDERE, OR NO CONTEST TO A CRIME
NOTES: VIOLATED TERMS OF A PROBATION AGREEMENT HE SIGNED ON 05/14/86 BY OPERATING A MOTOR VEHICLE WHILE INTOXICATED ON 06/21/89 IN COLUMBIA, MO AND PLEADING GUILTY TO HAVING ABH IN EXCESS OF .10; ALSO ARRESTED ON 07/21/90 FOR DRIVING WHILE INTOXICATED. SURRENDER RETROACTIVE TO 9/10/90.

NELSON, DONALD H DO, LICENSE NUMBER 0002846 OF 3269 STOCKTON HILL ROAD, KINGMAN, AZ, WAS DISCIPLINED BY ARIZONA ON SEPTEMBER 21, 1993
DISCIPLINARY ACTION: 36-MONTH PROBATION; MONITORING OF PHYSICIAN PERFORMANCE
OFFENSE: DISCIPLINARY ACTION BY ANOTHER STATE OR AGENCY
NOTES: ACTION IN MISSOURI ON 6/17/93. VOLUNTARILY SURRENDERED LICENSE IN MISSOURI RETROACTIVE TO 9/10/90 WHEN HE ADMITTED THAT IN 1989 PLED GUILTY TO DRIVING WHILE HAVING A BLOOD ALCOHOL CONTENT IN EXCESS OF .10. PROBATION ON TERMS AND CONDITIONS: SHALL SUBMIT TO RANDOM URINALYSIS TESTING ADMINISTERED BY THE BOARD; SHALL USE NO CONTROLLED SUBSTANCE OR

PRESCRIPTION-ONLY MEDICATION UNLESS PRESCRIBED BY HIS ATTENDING PHYSICIAN; SHALL REFRAIN FROM THE USE OF ALCOHOL; SHALL MEET REGULARLY WITH THE BOARD; SHALL AUTHORIZE ANY ATTENDING PHYSICIAN, PSYCHIATRIST, OR PSYCHOLOGIST TO RELEASE TO THE BOARD ALL RECORDS PERTAINING TO HIS CARE AND TREATMENT; SHALL ATTEND A GROUP THERAPY MEETING, WITH A BOARD APPROVED PSYCHIATRIST OR PSYCHOLOGIST, NO LESS THAN TWO TIMES PER MONTH, WHO SHALL PROVIDE REGULAR REPORTS TO THE BOARD; SHALL ATTEND A PRIVATE COUNSELING SESSION NO LESS THAN ONCE PER WEEK WITH A BOARD APPROVED PSYCHIATRIST OR PSYCHOLOGIST WHO SHALL PROVIDE REGULAR REPORTS TO THE BOARD; SHALL SUBMIT TO A PSYCHOLOGICAL AND/OR MEDICAL EVALUATION BY A BOARD DESIGNATED PSYCHIATRIST AND/OR PSYCHOLOGIST WITHIN 90 DAYS. ORDER MODIFIED ON 10/21/93; ON 9/27/93 UNDERWENT A PSYCHIATRIC EVALUATION AND THE RESULTS WERE CONVEYED TO THE BOARD ALONG WITH RECOMMENDATIONS FOR CONTINUING TREATMENT. BASED ON THIS EVALUATION REQUIRED THAT ON 1/21/95 PROBATION TERMINATED.

NELSON, S ARNOLD MD, LICENSE NUMBER 7590, WAS DISCIPLINED BY ARIZONA ON SEPTEMBER 21, 1999
DISCIPLINARY ACTION: 60-MONTH PROBATION; REQUIRED TO TAKE ADDITIONAL MEDICAL EDUCATION

NOTES: WITHIN SIX MONTHS, SHALL TAKE BOARD-APPROVED COURSES IN PSYCHOPHARMACOLOGY OF NOT LESS THAN 30 HOURS AND IN SUBSTANCE ABUSE OF NOT LESS THAN 15 HOURS; SHALL SUBMIT TO FOLLOW-UP RANDOM RECORDS REVIEW WITHIN ONE YEAR, AND AT A MINIMUM EVERY YEAR THEREAFTER FOR THE LENGTH OF PROBATION. ON 12/9/99 THE BOARD DENIED THE MOTION FOR A REHEARING.

NEVIUS, FRED L DO, LICENSE NUMBER 0002042 OF 3838 NORTH CAMPBELL, TUCSON, AZ, WAS DISCIPLINED BY ARIZONA ON APRIL 19, 1994
DISCIPLINARY ACTION: PROBATION; REQUIRED TO ENTER AN IMPAIRED PHYSICIAN PROGRAM OR SUBSTANCE ABUSE TREATMENT
OFFENSE: SUBSTANCE ABUSE

NOTES: ON 3/14/94 ADMITTED FOR TREATMENT OF A CHEMICAL DEPENDENCY; ADMITTED THAT HE HAD SELF-MEDICATED PLACIDYL FOR AN EXTENDED PERIOD; AT THAT TIME WAS NOT UNDER THE CARE AND TREATMENT OF A PHYSICIAN AS PART OF A RECOGNIZED COURSE OF TREATMENT. PROBATION NOT LESS THAN FIVE YEARS: SHALL SUCCESSFULLY COMPLETE THE EVENING OUTPATIENT TREATMENT PROGRAM; SHALL SECURE AND MAINTAIN A SPONSOR FOR 12 STEP RECOVERY PROGRAM; SHALL ATTEND AT LEAST FOUR 12 STEP MEETINGS PER WEEK FOR THE FIRST 12 MONTHS; SHALL HAVE REGULAR MEETINGS WITH THIS ATTENDING PHYSICIAN OR THERAPIST; SHALL ATTEND NO LESS THAN THREE GROUP THERAPY MEETINGS PER MONTH WITH A BOARD APPROVED COUNSELOR; SHALL SUBMIT TO RANDOM BODY FLUID TESTING; SHALL MEET WITH THE BOARD UPON REQUEST; SHALL NOT USE CONTROLLED SUBSTANCES OR PRESCRIPTION MEDICATION UNLESS PRESCRIBED BY HIS ATTENDING PHYSICIAN; SHALL REFRAIN COMPLETELY FROM THE USE OF ALCOHOL; SHALL AUTHORIZE ALL TREATING PERSONNEL INVOLVED IN HIS CARE TO RELEASE INFORMATION ON HIS PROGRESS AND PROGNOSIS TO THE BOARD UPON REQUEST. ON 9/1/97 ORDER AMENDED AS FOLLOWS: WITHIN THIRTY DAYS SHALL COMPLETE AN OUTPATIENT RELAPSE PREVENTION PROGRAM; SHALL PARTICIPATE IN THREE 12 STEP SELF-HELP MEETINGS PER WEEK AND MAINTAIN A LOG OF THOSE MEETINGS WITH A COPY SUBMITTED TO THE BOARD; HIS TREATING PHYSICIAN SHALL BE RESPONSIBLE FOR ALL MEDICATIONS PRESCRIBED TO HIM; A LOG OF ALL PRESCRIPTIONS SHALL BE MAINTAINED WITH A COPY PROVIDED TO THE BOARD ON A MONTHLY BASIS; SHALL ATTEND WEEKLY GROUP THERAPY SESSIONS AFTER COMPLETION OF HIS OUTPATIENT RELAPSE PREVENTION PROGRAM; SHALL MEET WITH A SPECIFIED DOCTOR AFTER COMPLETION OF HIS OUTPATIENT RELAPSE PREVENTION PROGRAM AND UPON BOARD'S REQUEST. ON 4/10/99 TERMS SATISFIED; UNRESTRICTED LICENSE ISSUED.

NEVIUS, FRED L DO OF TUCSON, AZ, WAS DISCIPLINED BY MISSOURI ON JUNE 6, 1996
DISCIPLINARY ACTION: 60-MONTH PROBATION
OFFENSE: DISCIPLINARY ACTION BY ANOTHER STATE OR AGENCY

NOTES: ACTION IN ARIZONA; AND MEMORANDUM OF UNDERSTANDING WITH THE MISSOURI BUREAU OF NARCOTICS AND DANGEROUS DRUGS AND THE DRUG ENFORCEMENT ADMINISTRATION.

NJEMANZE, JAMES MD, LICENSE NUMBER 19235, WAS DISCIPLINED BY ARIZONA ON NOVEMBER 17, 1999
DISCIPLINARY ACTION: PROBATION; REQUIRED TO TAKE ADDITIONAL MEDICAL EDUCATION

NOTES: WITHIN SIX MONTHS, SHALL TAKE 20 HOURS OF BOARD-APPROVED CONTINUING MEDICAL EDUCATION IN HIGH RISK PREGNANCY, INCLUDING PRE-ECLAMPSIA.

NOCERA, ROGER MD, LICENSE NUMBER 14570, WAS DISCIPLINED BY ARIZONA ON DECEMBER 9, 1999
DISCIPLINARY ACTION: PROBATION; RESTRICTION PLACED ON LICENSE

NOTES: PREVIOUS STIPULATED AGREEMENT WAS TERMINATED AND REPLACED BY A CONSENT AGREEMENT WITH THE FOLLOWING RESTRICTIONS: SHALL LIMIT HIS WORK TO 30 HOURS A WEEK, IN AN OFFICE OR CLINIC SETTING ONLY, WITH NO ANGIOGRAPHY OR OTHER PROLONGED PROCEDURES THAT MAY AGGRAVATE HIS CONDITION.

O'DONNELL, ROBERT DO, LICENSE NUMBER 0000864 OF 1520 WEST WARNER, #106-126, GILBERT, AZ, WAS DISCIPLINED BY ARIZONA ON NOVEMBER 27, 1996
DISCIPLINARY ACTION: MONITORING OF PHYSICIAN PERFORMANCE
OFFENSE: OVERPRESCRIBING OR MISPRESCRIBING DRUGS

NOTES: ALLEGATIONS THAT HE VIOLATED FEDERAL AND STATE STATUTES AND REGULATIONS CONCERNING THE ISSUANCE OF PRESCRIPTIONS FOR CONTROLLED SUBSTANCES FOR FAMILY MEMBERS; ON 11/22/96 ADMITTED TO PRESCRIBING CONTROLLED SUBSTANCES TO HIS WIFE, SISTER AND STEPDAUGHTER. INTERIM ORDER. SHALL SUBMIT TO BIOLOGICAL FLUID TESTING; SHALL APPEAR BEFORE THE BOARD ON 12/07/96; SHALL MAKE AVAILABLE AND BRING WITH HIM THE ORIGINAL PATIENT RECORDS FOR THE INDIVIDUALS LISTED ON THE CONFIDENTIAL PATIENT LISTING; AND SHALL APPEAR FOR AND SUBMIT TO A PSYCHIATRIC EVALUATION BY A BOARD DESIGNATED PSYCHIATRIST.

ODELL, BRUCE LAVON MD, LICENSE NUMBER G054528 OF MESA,

AZ, WAS DISCIPLINED BY CALIFORNIA ON JANUARY 11, 1991
DISCIPLINARY ACTION: SURRENDER OF LICENSE

NOTES: VOLUNTARY SURRENDER WHILE CHARGES PENDING.

OGIN, GARY MD, WAS DISCIPLINED BY ARIZONA ON JANUARY 27, 1999

NOTES: DECREE OF CENSURE.

OH, RICHARD D MD, LICENSE NUMBER 0011500 OF SIERRA VISTA, AZ, WAS DISCIPLINED BY ARIZONA ON JANUARY 17, 1995
DISCIPLINARY ACTION: 60-MONTH PROBATION; MONITORING OF PHYSICIAN PERFORMANCE
OFFENSE: SUBSTANDARD CARE, INCOMPETENCE OR NEGLIGENCE

NOTES: ON 3/12/93, HE PERFORMED WHAT WAS TO HAVE BEEN LAPAROSCOPIC SURGERY ON A 24-YEAR OLD PATIENT WITH A PELVIC MASS AND REMOVED HER RIGHT OVARY AND FALLOPIAN TUBE WITH NO INDICATION FOR THIS PROCEDURE; IN ANOTHER CASE BETWEEN 6/26/90 AND 1/11/91, HE SAW A PATIENT DURING HER PREGNANCY WHICH RESULTED IN THE DELIVERY OF A STILLBORN FEMALE AT 39 WEEKS; REGARDLESS OF THE CAUSE OF THE STILLBIRTH, HE IGNORED THE PATIENT'S TOXEMIA AND FAILED TO INSTITUTE TREATMENT OR EVALUATION FOR PRE-ECLAMPSIA AT TERM. PROBATION WITH CONDITIONS: SHALL PROMPTLY UNDERGO PSYCHOMETRIC, PSYCHOLOGICAL AND PSYCHIATRIC EVALUATIONS BY EVALUATORS DESIGNATED BY BOARD STAFF; SHALL TAKE AND PASS THE 1995 RECERTIFICATION EXAMINATION OF THE AMERICAN BOARD OF OBSTETRICS AND GYNECOLOGY; IF HE IS UNABLE TO REGISTER FOR THE EXAMINATION, HE SHALL TAKE AND PASS THE SPEX WITH A SCORE OF 75 OR GREATER IN ONE SITTING WITHIN THE NEXT SIX MONTHS; BOARD SHALL PROMPTLY CONDUCT A REVIEW OF HIS OFFICE CHARTS AND HOSPITAL CHARTS. ON 7/21/95 REQUEST FOR RECONSIDERATION OF THIS ORDER WAS DENIED. ON 1/19/96 ORDER TERMINATED.

OLSON, MERTON W MD, WAS DISCIPLINED BY ARIZONA ON JANUARY 20, 1995
DISCIPLINARY ACTION: LICENSE REVOCATION

NOTES: APPEARED BEFORE THE BOARD ON 10/21/94 TO DISCUSS A COMPLAINT AND WAS ORDERED TO TAKE AND PASS THE SPECIAL PURPOSE EXAMINATION. SUBMITTED A REQUEST FOR CANCELLATION OF LICENSE WITH CAUSE WHICH WAS APPROVED.

ONGLEY, GLENN M MD, WAS DISCIPLINED BY ARIZONA ON MARCH 25, 1999
DISCIPLINARY ACTION: REPRIMAND
OFFENSE: SUBSTANCE ABUSE

NOTES: ADMITTED TO DIVERTING LORTAB TO HIMSELF, AND TO HAVING A CHEMICAL DEPENDENCY PROBLEM; PRESCRIBED TO A NURSE WHO THEN SHARED IT WITH HIM; USED AN ALTERED DEA NUMBER; CURRENTLY PARTICIPATES IN A CHEMICAL DEPENDENCY TREATMENT PROGRAM.

OSBORNE, ROBERT C MD, LICENSE NUMBER 0009796, WAS DISCIPLINED BY ARIZONA ON OCTOBER 18, 1996

NOTES: INTERVIEWED BY THE BOARD REGARDING A COMPLAINT ALLEGING THAT DURING ANESTHESIA HE BROKE A PATIENT'S TOOTH. WITHIN 21 DAYS, SHALL PAY PATIENT $1,988 AND SHALL PROVIDE SATISFACTORY WRITTEN EVIDENCE TO THE BOARD OF PAYMENT; THIS IS NOT A FINDING OF UNPROFESSIONAL CONDUCT. ON 3/14/97 BOARD ACKNOWLEDGED HIS COMPLIANCE WITH ORDER REQUIREMENT THAT HE PAY RESTITUTION TO A PATIENT.

PAINE, FREDERICK O MD, LICENSE NUMBER 0011707, WAS DISCIPLINED BY ARIZONA ON JANUARY 19, 1996
DISCIPLINARY ACTION: LICENSE SUSPENSION

NOTES: INACTIVE STATUS DUE TO CURRENT HEALTH STATUS; AGREES NOT TO PRACTICE MEDICINE IN ANY JURISDICTION WHILE ARIZONA LICENSE IS IN INACTIVE STATUS; MAY NOT HOLD OR MAINTAIN A CONTROLLED SUBSTANCE CERTIFICATE WITH THE DEA OR WRITE OR REFILL PRESCRIPTIONS AS LONG AS LICENSE IS CLASSIFIED AS INACTIVE; SHALL NOT REQUEST REACTIVATION OF LICENSE UNTIL HE MEETS WITH THE BOARD AND COMPLIES WITH ALL BOARD REQUESTS. LICENSE WILL NOT BE REACTIVATED UNTIL BOARD RECEIVES SATISFACTORY EVIDENCE THAT HE IS MEDICALLY COMPETENT AND MENTALLY AND PHYSICALLY ABLE TO SAFELY PRACTICE MEDICINE.

PANOSIAN, JEFFREY MD, LICENSE NUMBER 0176047 OF 1686 SHEA ROAD, NAPLES, NY, WAS DISCIPLINED BY NEW YORK ON APRIL 29, 1996
DISCIPLINARY ACTION: 60-MONTH PROBATION; RESTRICTION PLACED ON LICENSE
OFFENSE: CRIMINAL CONVICTION OR PLEA OF GUILTY, NOLO CONTENDERE, OR NO CONTEST TO A CRIME

NOTES: PLED GUILTY TO CRIMINAL POSSESSION OF A WEAPON IN THE FOURTH DEGREE. LICENSE LIMITED UNTIL EVALUATED BY A PSYCHIATRIST.

PANOSIAN, JEFFREY O MD, LICENSE NUMBER 176047 OF 350 NORTH MAIN STREET, CANANDAIGUA, NY, WAS DISCIPLINED BY NEW YORK ON APRIL 2, 1998
DISCIPLINARY ACTION: LICENSE REVOCATION
OFFENSE: CRIMINAL CONVICTION OR PLEA OF GUILTY, NOLO CONTENDERE, OR NO CONTEST TO A CRIME

NOTES: PLED GUILTY IN THE NEW YORK STATE SUPREME COURT TO GRAND LARCENY.

PANOSIAN, JEFFREY O MD, LICENSE NUMBER 18972, WAS DISCIPLINED BY ARIZONA ON SEPTEMBER 25, 1998
DISCIPLINARY ACTION: LICENSE REVOCATION

PARDI, EUGENE HANNIBAL DO OF 2201 E CORTEZ ST, PHOENIX, AZ, WAS DISCIPLINED BY DEA ON JANUARY 8, 1990
DISCIPLINARY ACTION: SURRENDER OF CONTROLLED SUBSTANCE LICENSE
OFFENSE: SUBSTANCE ABUSE

NOTES: REPORTEDLY WROTE PRESCRIPTIONS UNDER FALSE NAME FOR ANEXIA WHICH HE USED AND ON PROBATION SINCE 1986 FOR DRUG ABUSE: APPROVAL OF APPLICATION WITH RESTRICTIONS PLACED ON REGISTRATION.

PARDI, EUGENE HANNIBAL DO, LICENSE NUMBER 0002221 OF 4512 NORTH 40TH STREET, PHOENIX, AZ, WAS DISCIPLINED BY ARIZONA ON SEPTEMBER 14, 1994
DISCIPLINARY ACTION: EMERGENCY SUSPENSION
OFFENSE: PROFESSIONAL MISCONDUCT

NOTES: INFORMATION RECEIVED BY THE BOARD THAT HE MAY BE PHYSICALLY AND/OR PSYCHOLOGICALLY UNABLE TO SAFELY AND SKILLFULLY ENGAGE IN THE PRACTICE OF MEDICINE AND MAY HAVE COMMITTED

ONE OR MORE ACTS OF UNPROFESSIONAL CONDUCT. SHALL PROVIDE SIGNED AUTHORIZATION FOR ALL PHYSICIANS, PSYCHOLOGISTS, AND OTHER HEALTH CARE PROVIDERS INVOLVED IN HIS CARE AND TREATMENT TO RELEASE ANY INFORMATION ON HIS DIAGNOSIS, CARE, AND TREATMENT TO THE BOARD; AND SHALL MEET WITH THE BOARD UPON REQUEST.

PARDI, EUGENE HANNIBAL DO OF 2201 EAST CORTEZ STREET, PHOENIX, AZ, WAS DISCIPLINED BY DEA ON FEBRUARY 3, 1995
DISCIPLINARY ACTION: SURRENDER OF CONTROLLED SUBSTANCE LICENSE

NOTES: IN LIEU OF ORDER TO SHOW CAUSE.

PARDI, EUGENE HANNIBAL DO, LICENSE NUMBER 0002221 OF 4512 NORTH 40TH STREET, PHOENIX, AZ, WAS DISCIPLINED BY ARIZONA ON MAY 15, 1995
DISCIPLINARY ACTION: 48-MONTH PROBATION; RESTRICTION PLACED ON CONTROLLED SUBSTANCE LICENSE
OFFENSE: SUBSTANCE ABUSE

NOTES: RECEIVED TREATMENT FROM 10/03/94 TO 2/23/95 AT RUSH BEHAVIORAL HEALTH CENTER; USED CONTROLLED SUBSTANCES OR PRESCRIPTION-ONLY DRUGS NOT PRESCRIBED BY ANOTHER MEDICAL PRACTITIONER. SUSPENSION RETROACTIVE TO THE BOARD'S TEMPORARY SUSPENSION ORDER OF 9/14/94 WHICH SHALL TERMINATE THE DATE OF THIS ORDER. PROBATION TERMS AND CONDITIONS: FOR A MINIMUM OF ONE YEAR SHALL OBTAIN PSYCHIATRIC OR PSYCHOLOGICAL TREATMENT BY A BOARD SELECTED THERAPIST WHO SHALL PROVIDE THE BOARD WITH A WRITTEN PROGRESS REPORT EVERY THREE MONTHS; SHALL ABSTAIN COMPLETELY FROM THE CONSUMPTION OF ALCOHOL AND SHALL NOT CONSUME ILLICIT DRUGS OR TAKE ANY CONTROLLED SUBSTANCES UNLESS PRESCRIBED BY HIS TREATING PHYSICIAN; SHALL MAINTAIN A MONTHLY LOG OF ALL PRESCRIPTION ONLY DRUGS TAKEN BY HIM; SHALL SUBMIT TO AND COOPERATE IN ANY INDEPENDENT MEDICAL OR PSYCHOLOGICAL EVALUATION ORDERED BY THE BOARD; SHALL APPEAR BEFORE THE BOARD UPON REQUEST; SHALL SUBMIT TO RANDOM BIOLOGICAL FLUID TESTING; SHALL PARTICIPATE IN A MINIMUM OF TWO SELF-HELP MEETINGS PER WEEK THROUGH SUCH ORGANIZATIONS AS AA, NARCOTICS ANONYMOUS, AND DOCTORS CADUCEUS GROUP; SHALL NOTIFY THE BOARD WITHIN 20 DAYS IF HE CEASES TO RESIDE IN ARIZONA; AND SHALL NOT PRESCRIBE ANY CONTROLLED SUBSTANCES UNTIL THE BOARD APPROVES RESUMPTION OF HIS PRESCRIPTION PRIVILEGES FOR CONTROLLED SUBSTANCES AND HE OBTAINS RECERTIFICATION OF HIS DEA LICENSE.

PARDI, EUGENE HANNIBAL DO, LICENSE NUMBER 0002221 OF 4512 NORTH 40TH STREET, PHOENIX, AZ, WAS DISCIPLINED BY ARIZONA ON NOVEMBER 29, 1996
DISCIPLINARY ACTION: LICENSE SUSPENSION; RESTRICTION PLACED ON CONTROLLED SUBSTANCE LICENSE
OFFENSE: FAILURE TO COMPLY WITH PREVIOUS BOARD ORDER

NOTES: AFTER SELF-ADMINISTERING THE CONTROLLED SUBSTANCE DEMEROL, VOLUNTARILY ADMITTED HIMSELF FOR TREATMENT ON 11/21/96. MINIMUM ONE YEAR SUSPENSION. SHALL DELIVER TO THE BOARD ALL DOCUMENTS IN HIS POSSESSION OR SUBJECT TO HIS CONTROL THAT INDICATE THAT HE IS A LICENSEE OF THE BOARD; FOR A MINIMUM OF ONE YEAR, SHALL OBTAIN PSYCHIATRIC OR PSYCHOLOGICAL TREATMENT BY A THERAPIST WHO SHALL SEND A WRITTEN PROGRESS REPORT EVERY THREE MONTHS; SHALL ABSTAIN COMPLETELY FROM THE CONSUMPTION OF ALCOHOL AND SHALL NOT CONSUME ILLICIT DRUGS OR TAKE ANY CONTROLLED SUBSTANCES UNLESS PRESCRIBED BY HIS TREATING PHYSICIAN; SHALL MAINTAIN A MONTHLY LOG OF ALL PRESCRIPTION ONLY DRUGS TAKEN BY HIM; SHALL SUBMIT TO AND COOPERATE IN ANY INDEPENDENT MEDICAL OR PSYCHOLOGICAL EVALUATION ORDERED BY THE BOARD; SHALL APPEAR BEFORE THE BOARD UPON REQUEST; SHALL SUBMIT TO RANDOM BIOLOGICAL FLUID TESTING; SHALL PARTICIPATE IN A MINIMUM OF TWO SELF-HELP MEETINGS PER WEEK THROUGH SUCH ORGANIZATIONS SUCH AS AA, NARCOTICS ANONYMOUS, AND DOCTOR'S CADUCEUS GROUP; SHALL NOTIFY THE BOARD WITHIN 20 DAYS IF CEASES TO RESIDE IN ARIZONA; SHALL NOT PRESCRIBE ANY CONTROLLED SUBSTANCES UNTIL THE BOARD APPROVES RESUMPTION OF HIS PRESCRIPTION PRIVILEGES FOR CONTROLLED SUBSTANCE USE AND HE OBTAINS RECERTIFICATION OF HIS DRUG ENFORCEMENT AGENCY LICENSE.

PARDI, EUGENE HANNIBAL DO, LICENSE NUMBER 2221 OF 6980 E SAHUARO DRIVE #1033, SCOTTSDALE, AZ, WAS DISCIPLINED BY ARIZONA ON JULY 24, 1998
DISCIPLINARY ACTION: 60-MONTH PROBATION; MONITORING OF PHYSICIAN PERFORMANCE
OFFENSE: FAILURE TO COMPLY WITH PREVIOUS BOARD ORDER

NOTES: ON 12/10/96 VOLUNTARILY ENTERED A PROGRAM FOR TREATMENT OF SUBSTANCE ABUSE ADDICTION AND WAS IN SOME FORM OF TREATMENT THROUGH 10/25/97. PROBATION WITH FOLLOWING CONDITIONS: SHALL OBTAIN PSYCHIATRIC OR PSYCHOLOGICAL TREATMENT BY A THERAPIST WHO IS A LICENSED PSYCHIATRIST AND/OR PSYCHOLOGIST APPROVED BY THE BOARD WHO SHALL PROVIDE MONTHLY REPORTS; SHALL PROVIDE A COPY OF THIS ORDER TO ALL HEALTH CARE FACILITIES WHERE HE PRACTICES; SHALL ABSTAIN COMPLETELY FROM THE CONSUMPTION OF ALCOHOLIC BEVERAGES AND SHALL NOT CONSUME ILLICIT DRUGS OR TAKE ANY CONTROLLED SUBSTANCES UNLESS PRESCRIBED FOR HIM BY HIS TREATING PHYSICIAN; SHALL MAINTAIN A MONTHLY LOG OF ALL PRESCRIPTION ONLY DRUGS TAKEN BY HIM AND SHALL PROVIDE A COPY TO THE BOARD; SHALL SUBMIT TO ANY EVALUATIONS ORDERED BY THE BOARD; SHALL APPEAR BEFORE THE BOARD UPON REQUEST; SHALL SUBMIT TO RANDOM BIOLOGICAL FLUID TESTING; SHALL OBTAIN A SPONSOR AND PARTICIPATE IN A MINIMUM OF TWO SELF-HELP MEETINGS PER WEEK; SHALL INFORM THE BOARD IF HE CEASES TO RESIDE IN ARIZONA; SHALL PAY COSTS.

PARKIN, DOUGLAS EDWARD MD, DATE OF BIRTH SEPTEMBER 20, 1942, LICENSE NUMBER 0005603, WAS DISCIPLINED BY ARIZONA ON AUGUST 28, 1990
DISCIPLINARY ACTION: REQUIRED TO TAKE ADDITIONAL MEDICAL EDUCATION

NOTES: MUST TAKE 20 HOURS OF CONTINUING MEDICAL EDUCATION IN ADDICTION AND PAIN CONTROL PRIOR TO 1991 LICENSE RENEWAL. EFFECTIVE 10/15/93, THIS ORDER TERMINATED AS HE HAD COMPLETED THE EDUCATION REQUIREMENTS.

PARRY, DARRELL DO, LICENSE NUMBER 2475 OF 1699 E COTTONWOOD, COTTONWOOD, AZ, WAS DISCIPLINED BY ARIZONA ON APRIL 23, 1997
DISCIPLINARY ACTION: EMERGENCY SUSPENSION; MONITORING OF PHYSICIAN PERFORMANCE

OFFENSE: PHYSICAL OR MENTAL ILLNESS INHIBITING THE ABILITY TO PRACTICE WITH SKILL AND SAFETY

NOTES: IN APRIL 1997, HE AGREED TO VOLUNTARILY WITHDRAW FROM THE PRACTICE OF MEDICINE BECAUSE HE WAS NOT CURRENTLY COMPETENT TO PRACTICE MEDICINE DUE TO HIS EXISTING MEDICAL CONDITIONS AS HE HAD A BLOOD AMMONIA LEVEL OF 170 WHEN 11-30 IS NORMAL. MUST OBTAIN AN IME PERFORMED BY AN IME PHYSICIAN TO DETERMINE HIS COMPETENCY TO PRACTICE MEDICINE; MUST SUBMIT TO AND COOPERATE IN ANY INDEPENDENT MEDICAL OR PSYCHOLOGICAL EVALUATION THE BOARD MAY ORDER; APPEAR BEFORE THE BOARD UPON REQUEST.

PARRY, DARRELL BOYD DO, LICENSE NUMBER H3278 OF PRESCOTT, AZ, WAS DISCIPLINED BY TEXAS ON OCTOBER 15, 1999
DISCIPLINARY ACTION: LICENSE SUSPENSION
OFFENSE: DISCIPLINARY ACTION BY ANOTHER STATE OR AGENCY

NOTES: ON 4/14/97 THE ARIZONA BOARD TEMPORARILY SUSPENDED HIS LICENSE DUE TO HIS MEDICAL CONDITION; HE SUFFERS FROM CHRONIC HEPATIC CELLULAR NECROSIS AND IS BEING TREATED BY A PHYSICIAN FOR LIVER NECROSIS CAUSED BY TYLENOL TOXICITY; HE HAS NOT PRACTICED SINCE 4/19/97; ON 4/22/97 HE VOLUNTARILY WITHDREW FROM THE PRACTICE OF MEDICINE DUE TO HIS EXTREME MEDICAL CONDITION. SUSPENSION UNTIL HE REQUESTS TO HAVE HIS SUSPENSION STAYED OR APPEARS BEFORE THE BOARD WITH SUFFICIENT EVIDENCE THAT HE IS PHYSICALLY, MENTALLY AND OTHERWISE COMPETENT TO SAFELY PRACTICE INCLUDING AT A MINIMUM COMPLETE COPIES OF MEDICAL RECORDS AND REPORTS OF MEDICAL EVALUATIONS; SHALL CONTINUE TO RECEIVE CARE AND TREATMENT FROM PRESENT PHYSICIAN WITH QUARTERLY REPORTS; SHALL COOPERATE WITH THE BOARD IN VERIFYING COMPLIANCE INCLUDING PROVIDING COPIES OF MEDICAL RELEASES AND ANY DOCUMENTS SENT TO OR RECEIVED FROM ARIZONA BOARD UPON REQUEST ; SHALL GIVE A COPY OF THIS ORDER TO ANY HEALTH CARE ENTITY WHERE HE HAS PRIVILEGES; SHALL PROVIDE A COPY OF THIS ORDER TO ANYONE REQUESTING IT WITHIN 10 DAYS; TIME SPENT OUT OF TEXAS DOES NOT COUNT TOWARD PROBATION/RESTRICTION; SHALL INFORM THE BOARD OF CHANGE OF ADDRESS WITHIN 10 DAYS OR IF HE LEAVES THE STATE; SHALL NOT SEEK MODIFICATION FOR ONE YEAR.

PATRIDGE, JEROME P DO, LICENSE NUMBER 0002031 OF 2904 COUNTRY CLUB DRIVE, BULLHEAD CITY, AZ, WAS DISCIPLINED BY ARIZONA ON FEBRUARY 8, 1993
DISCIPLINARY ACTION: 12-MONTH PROBATION; MONITORING OF PHYSICIAN PERFORMANCE
OFFENSE: PROFESSIONAL MISCONDUCT

NOTES: ON 10/29/92 PRIOR TO UNDERGOING A HEMORRHOIDECTOMY INSTRUCTED A SURGICAL NURSE TO ADMINISTER 200-300 MG OF DEMEROL TO HIM AS A SEDATING AGENT FOR SURGERY WHICH SHE DID; HE WAS AT THAT TIME NOT FUNCTIONING IN THE CAPACITY OF A PHYSICIAN. PROBATION UNDER TERMS AND CONDITIONS: SHALL UNDERGO INDIVIDUAL AND/OR MARITAL THERAPY FOR A PERIOD OF NO LESS THAN SIX MONTHS OR UNTIL DISCHARGED BY HIS TREATING CLINICIAN; SHALL ATTEND TWO TO THREE AA MEETINGS PER WEEK; SHALL ATTEND AFTERCARE GROUP THERAPY MEETINGS WITH A BOARD APPROVED PSYCHOLOGIST; SHALL SUBMIT TO RANDOM BODY FLUID TESTING; SHALL MEET REGULARLY WITH THE BOARD UPON REQUEST; SHALL USE NO CONTROLLED SUBSTANCE OR PRESCRIPTION-ONLY MEDICATION UNLESS PRESCRIBED BY HIS ATTENDING PHYSICIAN; SHALL REFRAIN FROM THE USE OF ALCOHOL; FOLLOWING PROBATION HE WILL BE RE-EVALUATED BY A BOARD APPROVED PSYCHOLOGIST OR PSYCHIATRIST TO DETERMINE WHETHER OR NOT THIS PROBATION SHALL BE EXTENDED OR TERMINATED; SHALL AUTHORIZE ALL TREATING PERSONNEL INVOLVED IN HIS CARE TO RELEASE INFORMATION ON HIS PROGRESS AND PROGNOSIS TO THE BOARD UPON REQUEST. ON 5/7/93 PROBATION MODIFIED. ON 1/14/94 PROBATION SATISFIED IN FULL.

PATTERSON, JOHN G MD, LICENSE NUMBER 0017572, WAS DISCIPLINED BY ARIZONA ON APRIL 19, 1996
OFFENSE: DISCIPLINARY ACTION BY ANOTHER STATE OR AGENCY

NOTES: ON 3/29/91 KNOWINGLY MADE FALSE STATEMENT WHEN APPLYING FOR PRIVILEGES AT A HEALTH CARE INSTITUTION IN THAT HE APPLIED FOR APPOINTMENT TO THE STAFF OF A HOSPITAL AND FALSELY INDICATED THAT HE HAD NOT HAD DISCIPLINARY ACTION TAKEN AGAINST HIS LICENSE BY ANY JURISDICTION DESPITE THE FACT THAT BETWEEN 1/87 AND 7/88, HE HAD BEEN INVESTIGATED, SUSPENDED AND FINED BY THE BOARD OF BRITISH COLUMBIA; ON APPLICATION, ALSO FALSELY RESPONDED THAT HE HAD COMPLETED REQUIREMENTS NECESSARY TO APPLY FOR THE AMERICAN BOARD OF FAMILY PRACTICE EXAMINATION WHEN IN FACT HE WAS NEITHER BOARD-CERTIFIED NOR BOARD-ELIGIBLE. CENSURED.

PATTON, MARK K MD, LICENSE NUMBER 0023562, WAS DISCIPLINED BY ARIZONA ON FEBRUARY 7, 1996
DISCIPLINARY ACTION: RESTRICTION PLACED ON LICENSE

NOTES: SHALL HAVE AN ADULT FEMALE PRESENT WHEN HE EXAMINES ANY PATIENT UNDER 18 YEARS OLD; SHALL WRITE THE NAME OF THIS PERSON IN THE PATIENT'S CHART AT THE TIME OF EXAMINATION. INTERIM ORDER.

PATTON, MARK K MD, LICENSE NUMBER 23562, WAS DISCIPLINED BY ARIZONA ON JANUARY 29, 1999
DISCIPLINARY ACTION: 60-MONTH PROBATION; RESTRICTION PLACED ON LICENSE
OFFENSE: PROFESSIONAL MISCONDUCT

NOTES: ADMITTED ON 3 OR 4 OCCASIONS HE SEXUALLY MOLESTED HIS SISTER-IN-LAW BETWEEN 1986 AND 1987 WHEN SHE WAS 12 OR 13 AND HE WAS AN ADULT; HAS BEEN IN THERAPY SINCE THEN. TERMS AND CONDITIONS: SHALL ALWAYS HAVE A FEMALE CHAPERONE PRESENT WHEN HE EXAMINES FEMALE PATIENTS AND THE CHAPERONE SHALL INITIAL THE PATIENT'S CHART AT THE TIME OF EXAMINATION; SHALL UNDERGO PSYCHOTHERAPY WITH A BOARD-APPROVED THERAPIST WITH QUARTERLY REPORTS TO THE BOARD; SHALL PRACTICE IN A STRUCTURED SETTING; SHALL NOT EXAMINE THE BREAST AND GENITALIA OF FEMALE PATIENTS 10 YEARS OF AGE AND OLDER.

PAVESE, MARIE MD, LICENSE NUMBER 0015484 OF AVONDALE, AZ, WAS DISCIPLINED BY ARIZONA ON OCTOBER 18, 1994
DISCIPLINARY ACTION: FINE
OFFENSE: OVERCHARGING

NOTES: PATIENT COMPLAINED TO THE BOARD ABOUT WHAT SHE CONSIDERED EXCESSIVE FEES CHARGED BY DR. PAVESE FOR TWO EMERGENCY EYE SURGERIES;

AMOUNT CHARGED WAS SEVEN TIMES THE HIGH END OF A BOARD-CONDUCTED FEE SURVEY; ALSO CHARGES FOR SERVICES NOT PERFORMED IN 8/90. SHALL PAY RESTITUTION TO THE PATIENT INVOLVED IN THE AMOUNT OF $39,352.60 WITHIN ONE WEEK FROM THE DATE OF THIS ORDER; SHALL BE ASSESSED A CIVIL PENALTY OF $5,000 PAYABLE WITHIN SIX MONTHS FROM THE DATE OF THIS ORDER. IS HEREBY CENSURED.

PAVESE, TERESA MD, LICENSE NUMBER 0015485, WAS DISCIPLINED BY ARIZONA ON OCTOBER 18, 1995
DISCIPLINARY ACTION: RESTRICTION PLACED ON LICENSE; REQUIRED TO TAKE ADDITIONAL MEDICAL EDUCATION
OFFENSE: LOSS OR RESTRICTION OF HOSPITAL PRIVILEGES

NOTES: INTERVIEWED BY THE BOARD REGARDING HER CARE AND TREATMENT OF A PATIENT AND A COMPLAINT ALLEGING IMPROPERLY PERFORMED BLEPHAROPLASTY; INQUIRY REGARDING CARE AND TREATMENT OF A SECOND PATIENT; AND INFORMATION RECEIVED BY THE BOARD FROM A MEDICAL CENTER INDICATING THAT HER SURGICAL PRIVILEGES HAD BEEN SUSPENDED AS A RESULT OF TWO CATARACT EXTRACTIONS RESULTING IN COMPLICATIONS AND INJURY. SHALL PERFORM NO SURGERY UNTIL SUCCESSFUL COMPLETION OF ONE YEAR OF TRAINING IN AN APPROVED AND ACCREDITED OPHTHALMOLOGICAL RESIDENCY OR FELLOWSHIP.

PAYNE, DAVID L DO, LICENSE NUMBER 0001640 OF 1050 EAST UNIVERSITY #3, MESA, AZ, WAS DISCIPLINED BY ARIZONA ON SEPTEMBER 26, 1996
DISCIPLINARY ACTION: 60-MONTH PROBATION; REPRIMAND
OFFENSE: SUBSTANDARD CARE, INCOMPETENCE OR NEGLIGENCE

NOTES: MISCONDUCT ARISING FROM THE FOLLOWING CIRCUMSTANCES IN 2/94 RESULTING FROM HIS TREATMENT OF AN HIV POSITIVE PATIENT; NEGLIGENT ACTS BY ACCEPTING AN EXPERIMENTAL SUBSTANCE THAT WAS PURPORTED TO BE OF MEDICINAL VALUE, WITHOUT FIRST TAKING THE ELEMENTARY PRECAUTIONS OF ASSURING HIMSELF OF THE SAFETY AND STERILITY OF THE PRODUCT, REGARDLESS OF ANY EFFICACY THE SUBSTANCE MIGHT HAVE HAD; GAVE HIS PATIENT TWO VIALS OF THE EXPERIMENTAL SUBSTANCE, UNDER CIRCUMSTANCES WHEREBY HE KNEW, OR SHOULD HAVE KNOWN, THAT THE SUBSTANCE WAS MANUFACTURED, PACKAGED, AND STORED UNDER CONDITIONS THAT COULD NOT REASONABLY ASSURE AN ORDINARILY PRUDENT PERSON THAT THE SUBSTANCE WAS FREE FROM CONTAMINATION; NOR DID HE DO ANY TESTS ON THE SUBSTANCE TO DETERMINE THIS; FAILED TO OBTAIN PATIENTS' INFORMED CONSENT; FAILED TO ADVISE HIS PATIENT OF THE RISK OF AN EXPERIMENTAL THERAPY; CONTAMINATION OF THE SUBSTANCE LED TO THE PATIENT GOING INTO A DISTRESSED CONDITION ON 2/12/94 AFTER BEING INFUSED WITH TWO DOSES OF THE EXPERIMENTAL SUBSTANCE, ONE ON 2/8 AND ONE ON 2/12/94, WHICH DISTRESS WAS CAUSED BY SEPIS RELATED TO THE CONTAMINATION OF THE EXPERIMENTAL SUBSTANCE; FAILED TO DOCUMENT IN PATIENT RECORD THE ADMINISTRATION OF AN EXPERIMENTAL SUBSTANCE. PROBATION UNDER TERMS AND CONDITIONS: SHALL USE ONLY THOSE RECOGNIZED EXPERIMENTAL THERAPIES FOR PATIENT TREATMENT AND IN COMPLIANCE WITH RECOGNIZED AND STANDARD PROTOCOLS APPLICABLE TO EXPERIMENTAL THERAPIES; MAY USE FOOD AND DRUG ADMINISTRATION RECOGNIZED EXPERIMENTAL THERAPIES FOR PATIENT TREATMENT IN A MANNER NOT EXPRESSLY APPROVED BY THE FDA IF SUCH TREATMENT IS MEDICALLY JUSTIFIED AND PROVIDED ACCORDING TO CONTEMPORARY MEDICAL STANDARDS OF CARE; SHALL OBTAIN 40 HOURS OF BOARD APPROVED CONTINUING MEDICAL EDUCATION DURING THE NEXT TWO YEARS CONCERNING THE TOPIC OF MEDICAL PROFESSIONAL ETHICS GENERALLY AND PROTOCOLS GOVERNING THE USE OF EXPERIMENTAL THERAPIES AND SUBMIT PROOF TO THE BOARD; SHALL MAINTAIN ALL PATIENT CHARTS ACCORDING TO THE "SOAP" FORMAT; BEFORE PROVIDING EXPERIMENTAL FORMS OF THERAPY TO A PATIENT, SHALL OBTAIN A SIGNED INFORMED CONSENT AGREEMENT FROM THE PATIENT; THE BOARD SHALL CONDUCT A REVIEW OF PATIENT CHARTS; SHALL APPEAR BEFORE THE BOARD UPON REQUEST; SHALL PAY ALL COSTS OF THE INVESTIGATION; EVERY THREE MONTHS SHALL REPORT TO THE BOARD IN EITHER A WRITTEN REPORT OR PERSONAL ORAL PRESENTATION ON THE CURRENT HIV-AIDS RESEARCH AND CURRENT DEVELOPMENTS IN THE FIELD OF HIV-AIDS RESEARCH

PEARL, CONRAD R DO, DATE OF BIRTH DECEMBER 19, 1931, LICENSE NUMBER 0004524 OF 27676 CHERRY HILL ROAD, GARDEN CITY, MI, WAS DISCIPLINED BY MICHIGAN ON NOVEMBER 17, 1993
DISCIPLINARY ACTION: 6-MONTH SUSPENSION OF CONTROLLED SUBSTANCE LICENSE; FINE
OFFENSE: PROFESSIONAL MISCONDUCT

NOTES: DRUG RELATED. DRUG CONTROL LICENSE REVOKED; $2,500 FINE. ON 2/27/95 REINSTATEMENT OF CONTROLLED SUBSTANCE LICENSE DENIED.

PEARL, CONRAD R DO, DATE OF BIRTH DECEMBER 19, 1931, LICENSE NUMBER 0004524 OF 27676 CHERRY HILL ROAD, GARDEN CITY, MI, WAS DISCIPLINED BY MICHIGAN ON DECEMBER 2, 1993
DISCIPLINARY ACTION: 12-MONTH PROBATION; FINE
OFFENSE: SUBSTANDARD CARE, INCOMPETENCE OR NEGLIGENCE

NOTES: NEGLIGENCE/INCOMPETENCE. $2,500 FINE; LICENSE LIMITED.

PEARL, CONRAD R DO, LICENSE NUMBER 0002003 OF GARDEN CITY, MI, WAS DISCIPLINED BY FLORIDA ON JUNE 26, 1996
DISCIPLINARY ACTION: SURRENDER OF LICENSE
OFFENSE: DISCIPLINARY ACTION BY ANOTHER STATE OR AGENCY

NOTES: CHARGED WITH HAVING DISCIPLINARY ACTION TAKEN AGAINST LICENSE BY ANOTHER JURISDICTION. HE ACCEPTED RELINQUISHMENT OF LICENSE AGREEING NEVER AGAIN TO APPLY FOR LICENSURE IN FLORIDA.

PEARL, CONRAD R OF SOUTHFIELD, MI, WAS DISCIPLINED BY MISSOURI ON DECEMBER 3, 1996
DISCIPLINARY ACTION: SURRENDER OF LICENSE
OFFENSE: DISCIPLINARY ACTION BY ANOTHER STATE OR AGENCY

NOTES: BASED ON DISCIPLINE IN MICHIGAN AND VIOLATIONS OF THE DRUG RULES AND REGULATIONS. LICENSE WAS VOLUNTARILY SURRENDERED IN LIEU OF DISCIPLINARY ACTION.

PEARL, CONRAD ROBERT DO, LICENSE NUMBER 00D6842 OF GARDEN CITY, MI, WAS DISCIPLINED BY TEXAS ON JANUARY 6, 1995
DISCIPLINARY ACTION: SURRENDER OF LICENSE

NOTES: IN LIEU OF FURTHER INVESTIGATION OR A HEARING ON ALLEGATIONS THAT HE VIOLATED THE MEDICAL PRACTICE ACT. SHALL NOT PETITION FOR REINSTATEMENT.

PEARL, CONRAD ROBERT DO, LICENSE NUMBER 20A3851 OF GARDEN CITY, MI, WAS DISCIPLINED BY CALIFORNIA ON OCTOBER 6, 1995
DISCIPLINARY ACTION: LICENSE REVOCATION
OFFENSE: DISCIPLINARY ACTION BY ANOTHER STATE OR AGENCY

NOTES: ACTION TAKEN BY ANOTHER STATE.

PEARL, CONRAD ROBERT DO, LICENSE NUMBER 0000904 OF 27676 CHERRY HILL ROAD, GARDEN CITY, MI, WAS DISCIPLINED BY ARIZONA ON JULY 1, 1996
DISCIPLINARY ACTION: SURRENDER OF LICENSE
OFFENSE: DISCIPLINARY ACTION BY ANOTHER STATE OR AGENCY

NOTES: LICENSE REVOCATION IN CALIFORNIA ON 8/15/95 BASED ON ACTION IN MICHIGAN DUE TO NEGLIGENCE, INCOMPETENCE AND VIOLATION OF OR AIDING AND ABETTING A VIOLATION OF THE PUBLIC HEALTH CODE WHICH ON 12/07/93 PLACED HIS LICENSE ON ONE YEAR PROBATION AND HIS CONTROLLED DRUG LICENSE WAS REVOKED FOR A MINIMUM OF THREE YEARS DURING WHICH TIME HE IS UNABLE TO DISPENSE ANY CONTROLLED SUBSTANCES FROM HIS OFFICE; HIS CONTROLLED SUBSTANCE LICENSE WAS SUSPENDED FOR A MINIMUM OF SIX MONTHS AND ONE DAY DURING WHICH TIME HE IS UNABLE TO PRESCRIBE ANY CONTROLLED SUBSTANCES. SHALL DELIVER TO THE ARIZONA BOARD ALL DOCUMENTS THAT INDICATE THAT HE IS A LICENSEE OF THE BOARD.

PECK, SIDNEY J MD OF 3000 N OCEAN DRIVE, SINGER ISLAND, FL, WAS DISCIPLINED BY DEA ON FEBRUARY 24, 1994
DISCIPLINARY ACTION: SURRENDER OF CONTROLLED SUBSTANCE LICENSE
OFFENSE: PRACTICING WITHOUT A VALID LICENSE

NOTES: PRESCRIBING PERCODAN, PERCOCET, DEMEROL, VALIUM, TUSSIONEX SUSPENSION, AND ZANTAC WITH INACTIVE STATE MEDICAL LICENSE.

PECK, SIDNEY J MD, LICENSE NUMBER 0003863 OF SCOTTSDALE, AZ, WAS DISCIPLINED BY FLORIDA ON APRIL 11, 1995
DISCIPLINARY ACTION: SURRENDER OF LICENSE
OFFENSE: PRACTICING WITHOUT A VALID LICENSE

NOTES: CHARGED WITH PRACTICING WITH AN INACTIVE LICENSE; FAILING TO KEEP MEDICAL RECORDS JUSTIFYING THE COURSE OF TREATMENT OF A PATIENT; INAPPROPRIATE PRESCRIBING, DISPENSING, ADMINISTERING, MIXING OR OTHERWISE PREPARING A LEGEND DRUG; PRESCRIBING, DISPENSING OR ADMINISTERING ANY SCHEDULED MEDICINAL DRUG FOR HIMSELF; FAILURE TO PRACTICE MEDICINE WITH AN ACCEPTABLE LEVEL OF CARE AND SKILL. ACCEPTED VOLUNTARY RELINQUISHMENT OF LICENSE TO PRACTICE MEDICINE AND AGREES NEVER AGAIN TO APPLY FOR LICENSURE IN FLORIDA.

PECK, SIDNEY J MD, LICENSE NUMBER 0045871 OF 708 AGUAVE AVENUE, BERMUDA DUNES, CA, WAS DISCIPLINED BY NEW YORK ON OCTOBER 3, 1995
DISCIPLINARY ACTION: SURRENDER OF LICENSE
OFFENSE: DISCIPLINARY ACTION BY ANOTHER STATE OR AGENCY

NOTES: ACTION IN FLORIDA FOR PRESCRIBING CONTROLLED DANGEROUS SUBSTANCES WITHOUT ANY PHYSICAL EXAMINATIONS OR MEDICAL JUSTIFICATION.

PENA, FRANCISCO MD, LICENSE NUMBER 0019877, WAS DISCIPLINED BY ARIZONA ON JANUARY 25, 1991
DISCIPLINARY ACTION: REQUIRED TO ENTER AN IMPAIRED PHYSICIAN PROGRAM OR SUBSTANCE ABUSE TREATMENT; MONITORING OF PHYSICIAN PERFORMANCE
OFFENSE: SUBSTANCE ABUSE

NOTES: LICENSE PROCESSED WITH THE FOLLOWING CONDITIONS: MUST IMMEDIATELY PARTICIPATE IN THE ARIZONA MEDICAL ASSOCIATION'S MONITORED AFTERCARE TREATMENT PROGRAM WITH QUARTERLY REPORTS TO THE BOARD; SHALL PARTICIPATE IN 90 12-STEP MEETINGS APPROPRIATE FOR SUBSTANCE ABUSE AND ACCEPTABLE TO THE BOARD IN 90 DAYS FROM THE EFFECTIVE DATE OF THIS ORDER; MUST THEN ATTEND A MINIMUM OF THREE WEEKLY MEETINGS OF A 12-STEP RECOVERY PROGRAM AS DETERMINED BY HIS TREATING THERAPIST; SHALL OBTAIN A SOLE BOARD-APPROVED TREATING PHYSICIAN; SHALL ABSTAIN FROM ALCOHOL AND TAKE NO DRUGS OR MEDICATIONS WHATEVER, WHETHER CONTROLLED SUBSTANCES, PRESCRIPTION-ONLY DRUGS OR OVER-THE-COUNTER PREPARATIONS, UNLESS SUCH DRUG OR MEDICATION WAS PRESCRIBED FOR HIM BY HIS TREATING PHYSICIAN; SHALL SUBMIT TO WITNESSED RANDOM BIOLOGICAL FLUID COLLECTION; SHALL MAINTAIN A LOG OF ANY AND ALL MEDICATIONS TAKEN AND SHALL MAKE SUCH LOG AVAILABLE TO THE BOARD UPON REQUEST; SHALL SUBMIT TO ANY THERAPY ORDERED BY THE BOARD AND ANY MENTAL, PHYSICAL OR MEDICAL COMPETENCY EXAMINATIONS, OR ANY COMBINATION THEREOF; SHALL APPEAR BEFORE THE BOARD FOR INTERVIEWS UPON REQUEST. ORDER EFFECTIVE AS OF 10/25/91. ON 4/16/94 ORDER TERMINATED AFTER 90 DAYS.

PERA, VICTOR F JR MD, LICENSE NUMBER 0011120, WAS DISCIPLINED BY ARIZONA ON FEBRUARY 1, 1996
DISCIPLINARY ACTION: LICENSE SUSPENSION
OFFENSE: LOSS OR RESTRICTION OF HOSPITAL PRIVILEGES

NOTES: UNDER INVESTIGATION FOLLOWING TERMINATION OF EMPLOYMENT FROM THE DEPARTMENT OF CORRECTIONS, CONCERNS ABOUT HIS SKILLS AND DIAGNOSIS IN THE MANAGEMENT OF A PATIENT WITH SCHIZOPHRENIA; FAILED TO APPEAR FOR A SCHEDULED INVESTIGATIONAL INTERVIEW; HAS MEDICAL CONDITION WHICH PREVENTS HIM FROM ENGAGING IN THE PRACTICE OF MEDICINE. LICENSE PLACED ON INACTIVE STATUS WITH CAUSE; SHALL NOT HOLD A DEA CERTIFICATE; SHALL NOT REQUEST REACTIVATION OF LICENSE IN ARIZONA UNTIL HE MEETS WITH THE BOARD AT A REGULARLY SCHEDULED MEETING AND COMPLIES WITH ALL BOARD REQUESTS; BEFORE REACTIVATION, MUST PROVIDE SATISFACTORY EVIDENCE TO THE BOARD THAT HE IS MEDICALLY COMPETENT AND MENTALLY AND PHYSICALLY ABLE TO SAFELY PRACTICE MEDICINE.

PEREIRA, SELWYN J MD, LICENSE NUMBER 0079774 OF 65 LAUREN AVE, DIX HILLS, NY, WAS DISCIPLINED BY NEW YORK ON APRIL 9, 1992
DISCIPLINARY ACTION: 36-MONTH PROBATION
OFFENSE: SUBSTANDARD CARE, INCOMPETENCE OR NEGLIGENCE

NOTES: PLEADED GUILTY TO PRACTICING WITH GROSS NEGLIGENCE, NEGLIGENCE ON MORE THAN ONE OCCASION AND POOR RECORD KEEPING. FAILED TO MONITOR AND RECORD A PATIENT'S RESPONSE TO LITHIUM, FAILED TO TRACK AND RECORD MEDICATIONS FOR THIS PATIENT FOLLOWING A HALLUCINATORY PERIOD, AND PRESCRIBED DRUGS FOR THIS PATIENT IN SPITE OF HER RECENT DISCHARGE FROM THE HOSPITAL FOR ABUSE OF THESE DRUGS IN A SUICIDE ATTEMPT. THREE-YEAR

SUSPENSION, STAYED.

PEREIRA, SELWYN J MD, LICENSE NUMBER 0013037, WAS DISCIPLINED BY ARIZONA ON NOVEMBER 16, 1995
OFFENSE: DISCIPLINARY ACTION BY ANOTHER STATE OR AGENCY

NOTES: ACTION TAKEN AGAINST NEW YORK LICENSE FOR SEXUAL MISCONDUCT. SHALL NOT PRACTICE MEDICINE IN ARIZONA PRIOR TO MEETING WITH THE BOARD.

PETERSEN, CHARLES DR OF TUCSON, AZ, WAS DISCIPLINED BY ILLINOIS ON JULY 1, 1992
DISCIPLINARY ACTION: REPRIMAND
OFFENSE: DISCIPLINARY ACTION BY ANOTHER STATE OR AGENCY

NOTES: ARIZONA AND FEDERAL CONTROLLED SUBSTANCE LICENSES WERE SURRENDERED FOR IMPROPER RECORDKEEPING AND OHIO LICENSE WAS SUSPENDED FOR 90 DAYS AFTER FAILING TO NOTIFY STATE OF ACTION TAKEN BY ARIZONA.

PETERSEN, RICHARD J MD, LICENSE NUMBER 0016650, WAS DISCIPLINED BY ARIZONA ON AUGUST 27, 1990
DISCIPLINARY ACTION: REQUIRED TO ENTER AN IMPAIRED PHYSICIAN PROGRAM OR SUBSTANCE ABUSE TREATMENT; MONITORING OF PHYSICIAN PERFORMANCE
OFFENSE: SUBSTANCE ABUSE

NOTES: MUST IMMEDIATELY PARTICIPATE IN THE ARIZONA MEDICAL ASSOCIATION'S MONITORED AFTERCARE TREATMENT PROGRAM WITH QUARTERLY REPORTS TO THE BOARD; MUST OBTAIN A BOARD APPROVED TREATING PHYSICIAN; MUST ABSTAIN COMPLETELY FROM ALCOHOL AND ALL OTHER DRUGS; MUST COMPLY WITH REQUESTS FOR RANDOM BIOLOGICAL FLUID TESTS; MUST SUBMIT TO ANY EXAMS OR THERAPY ORDERED BY THE BOARD; MUST PARTICIPATE IN A 12-STEP RECOVERY PROGRAM FOR SUBSTANCE ABUSE AS DETERMINED BY THERAPIST AND ATTEND AT LEAST 3 WEEKLY MEETINGS; MUST APPEAR BEFORE BOARD FOR INTERVIEWS UPON REQUEST; MUST MAINTAIN A LOG OF ALL MEDICATIONS TAKEN; MUST ADVISE BOARD OF CHANGE IN OFFICE OR HOME ADDRESSES OR IF PLANS TO BE AWAY FOR MORE THAN FIVE DAYS.

PETERSON, CHARLES A MD, DATE OF BIRTH JANUARY 28, 1926, LICENSE NUMBER 0016712 OF 9575 E. MORRILL WAY, TUCSON, AZ, WAS DISCIPLINED BY NEW JERSEY ON JANUARY 2, 1990
DISCIPLINARY ACTION: RESTRICTION PLACED ON LICENSE
OFFENSE: DISCIPLINARY ACTION BY ANOTHER STATE OR AGENCY

NOTES: ACTION BASED ON ARIZONA SANCTION FOR ALLEGED INDISCRIMINATE DISPENSING OF CONTROLLED DANGEROUS SUBSTANCES. PRIOR TO COMMENCING ACTIVE PRACTICE SHALL PROVIDE NOTICE OF SUCH INTENTION IN WRITING AND APPEAR BEFORE THE BOARD TO PRESENT EVIDENCE OF COMPLIANCE WITH TERMS OF THIS ORDER.

PETERSON, CHARLES A MD, LICENSE NUMBER 0050273 OF TUCSON, AZ, WAS DISCIPLINED BY OHIO ON JULY 13, 1990
DISCIPLINARY ACTION: 3-MONTH LICENSE SUSPENSION; 36-MONTH PROBATION
OFFENSE: DISCIPLINARY ACTION BY ANOTHER STATE OR AGENCY

NOTES: DISCIPLINED BY ARIZONA, FAILURE TO NOTIFY OHIO BOARD OF ARIZONA ACTION. REVOCATION STAYED, INDEFINITE SUSPENSION, MINIMUM 90 DAYS, CONDITIONS FOR REINSTATEMENT.

PETERSON, CHARLES A MD, LICENSE NUMBER C29059 OF SAN LEANDRO, CA, WAS DISCIPLINED BY CALIFORNIA ON MAY 5, 1997
DISCIPLINARY ACTION: 84-MONTH PROBATION
OFFENSE: SUBSTANDARD CARE, INCOMPETENCE OR NEGLIGENCE

NOTES: COMMITTED ACTS OF NEGLIGENCE AND INCOMPETENCE IN THE CARE AND TREATMENT OF FIVE PATIENTS. REVOCATION STAYED.

PETERSON, CHARLES A MD, LICENSE NUMBER C29059 OF SAN LEANDRO, CA, WAS DISCIPLINED BY CALIFORNIA ON JULY 12, 1999
DISCIPLINARY ACTION: LICENSE REVOCATION
OFFENSE: SUBSTANDARD CARE, INCOMPETENCE OR NEGLIGENCE

NOTES: MENTAL ILLNESS AFFECTING HIS ABILITY TO PRACTICE SAFELY, INCOMPETENCE, NEGLIGENCE AND EXCESSIVE PRESCRIBING IN CONNECTION WITH HIS CARE AND TREATMENT OF A NURSING HOME PATIENT.

PETERSON, MARION G MD, LICENSE NUMBER 0A13817 OF MESA, AZ, WAS DISCIPLINED BY CALIFORNIA ON FEBRUARY 13, 1996
DISCIPLINARY ACTION: SURRENDER OF LICENSE

NOTES: WHILE CHARGES PENDING.

PETERSON, MARION G MD, LICENSE NUMBER C2089 OF MESA, AZ, WAS DISCIPLINED BY TEXAS ON MAY 16, 1998
DISCIPLINARY ACTION: SURRENDER OF LICENSE
OFFENSE: DISCIPLINARY ACTION BY ANOTHER STATE OR AGENCY

NOTES: VOLUNTARY SURRENDER ORDER WITH THE CALIFORNIA BOARD EFFECTIVE 2/13/96. VOLUNTARY AND PERMANENT SURRENDER.

PETERSON, RICHARD I MD, DATE OF BIRTH SEPTEMBER 2, 1947, LICENSE NUMBER 0022904 OF COLORADO SPRINGS, CO, WAS DISCIPLINED BY COLORADO ON AUGUST 13, 1990
DISCIPLINARY ACTION: EMERGENCY SUSPENSION
OFFENSE: SUBSTANDARD CARE, INCOMPETENCE OR NEGLIGENCE

NOTES: SELF-ADMINISTERING A HABIT-FORMING DRUG OR CONTROLLED SUBSTANCE NOT IN THE COURSE OF LEGITIMATE MEDICAL PRACTICE; EXCESSIVE USE OF A HABIT-FORMING DRUG OR CONTROLLED SUBSTANCE; PHYSICAL OR MENTAL DISABILITY WHICH RENDERS HIM UNABLE TO PERFORM MEDICAL SERVICES WITH REASONABLE SKILL AND SAFETY TO PATIENTS; ACTS OR OMISSIONS WHICH CONSTITUTE GROSSLY NEGLIGENT MEDICAL PRACTICE OR WHICH FAIL TO MEET GENERALLY ACCEPTED STANDARDS OF MEDICAL PRACTICE; SELF-ADMINISTERING A CONTROLLED SUBSTANCE NOT ON AN EMERGENCY BASIS. LICENSE SUMMARILY SUSPENDED PENDING COMPLETION OF FORMAL DISCIPLINARY PROCEEDINGS, BASED UPON FINDINGS THAT HE WAS GUILTY OF DELIBERATE AND WILLFUL VIOLATION AND THAT THE PUBLIC HEALTH, SAFETY AND WELFARE IMPERATIVELY REQUIRED EMERGENCY ACTION. FORMAL DISCIPLINARY HEARING CONCLUDED 11/9/90; FINAL DECISION PENDING.

PETERSON, RICHARD I MD, DATE OF BIRTH SEPTEMBER 2, 1947, LICENSE NUMBER 0022904 OF SCOTTSDALE, AZ, WAS DISCIPLINED BY COLORADO ON MAY 10, 1991
DISCIPLINARY ACTION: 12-MONTH LICENSE SUSPENSION; 12-MONTH PROBATION
OFFENSE: SUBSTANDARD CARE, INCOMPETENCE OR NEGLIGENCE

NOTES: SELF-ADMINISTERING A CONTROLLED SUBSTANCE NOT IN THE COURSE OF LEGITIMATE MEDICAL PRACTICE; EXCESSIVE USE OF A CONTROLLED SUBSTANCE; PHYSICAL OR MENTAL DISABILITY WHICH RENDERS HIM UNABLE TO PERFORM MEDICAL

SERVICES WITH REASONABLE SKILL AND SAFETY; ACTS OR OMISSIONS WHICH CONSTITUTE GROSSLY NEGLIGENT MEDICAL PRACTICE. SUSPENSION RETROACTIVE TO 8/15/90. ON 08/16/91 STIPULATION: HE ADMITS FELONY CONVICTION RE: PERSONAL USE OF CONTROLLED SUBSTANCES AND AGREES NOT TO CHALLENGE PREVIOUS ORDER SUSPENDING LICENSE. BOARD AGREES NOT TO IMPOSE FURTHER DISCIPLINE.

PETTY, WENDELL M MD, DATE OF BIRTH DECEMBER 4, 1931, LICENSE NUMBER 0017299 OF 849 25 ROAD, GRAND JUNCTION, CO, WAS DISCIPLINED BY IOWA ON AUGUST 26, 1993
DISCIPLINARY ACTION: SURRENDER OF LICENSE

PETTY, WENDELL M MD, DATE OF BIRTH DECEMBER 4, 1931, LICENSE NUMBER 0015505 OF GRAND JUNCTION, CO, WAS DISCIPLINED BY COLORADO ON SEPTEMBER 16, 1994
DISCIPLINARY ACTION: LICENSE SUSPENSION
OFFENSE: NONCOMPLIANCE WITH A PROFESSIONAL RULE

NOTES: FAILURE TO UNDERGO PHYSICAL/MENTAL EXAMINATIONS ORDERED BY THE BOARD.

PETTY, WENDELL MEARL DR, LICENSE NUMBER 0015367, WAS DISCIPLINED BY ARIZONA ON JULY 15, 1994
DISCIPLINARY ACTION: LICENSE SUSPENSION
OFFENSE: NONCOMPLIANCE WITH A PROFESSIONAL RULE

NOTES: FAILURE TO PAY RENEWAL FEE DURING PENDING INVESTIGATION.

PETTY, WENDELL MEARL MD, LICENSE NUMBER 15367, WAS DISCIPLINED BY ARIZONA ON JANUARY 23, 1998
DISCIPLINARY ACTION: LICENSE REVOCATION
OFFENSE: DISCIPLINARY ACTION BY ANOTHER STATE OR AGENCY

NOTES: IN A PATIENT HE SAW IN 1990 FAILED TO FOLLOW THROUGH ON HIS TREATMENT FOR DEPRESSION AND BLURRING THE BOUNDARIES OF A THERAPEUTIC ALLIANCE BY ENTERING INTO A BUSINESS TRANSACTION WITH HIM; THE DOCTOR MADE A LOAN TO THE PATIENT WHOM HE HAD SIGN A NOTE; WHEN THE LOAN WAS NOT PAID, DR. PETTY RETAINED AN ATTORNEY TO COLLECT THE MONEY; DR. PETTY WAS APPROVED FOR DISABILITY BENEFITS ON 11/7/91 BASED ON HIS SUFFERING "ONGOING ANXIETY, DEPRESSION AND STRESS DISORDER;" VOLUNTARILY SURRENDERED IOWA LICENSE ON 8/3/93.

PICKERING, BRYANT MD, WAS DISCIPLINED BY ARIZONA ON JANUARY 27, 1999
DISCIPLINARY ACTION: REPRIMAND

PICKERING, BRYANT I MD, DATE OF BIRTH JULY 19, 1929 OF 77 E MISSOURI, #38, PHOENIX, AZ, WAS DISCIPLINED BY MEDICARE ON JULY 3, 1997
DISCIPLINARY ACTION: 60-MONTH EXCLUSION FROM THE MEDICARE AND/OR MEDICAID PROGRAM
OFFENSE: CRIMINAL CONVICTION OR PLEA OF GUILTY, NOLO CONTENDERE, OR NO CONTEST TO A CRIME

NOTES: CONVICTED OF A CRIME INVOLVING THE MEDICARE, MEDICAID, MATERNAL AND CHILD HEALTH SERVICES BLOCK GRANT OR BLOCK GRANTS TO STATES FOR SOCIAL SERVICES PROGRAMS.

PIMIENTA, GILBERT MD, WAS DISCIPLINED BY ARIZONA ON NOVEMBER 20, 1998
DISCIPLINARY ACTION: PROBATION

NOTES: REQUIRED NOT TO PRACTICE MEDICINE AND HAVE AN INPATIENT EVALUATION AT A BOARD-APPROVED FACILITY. STIPULATED PROBATIONARY ORDER.

PIMIENTA, GILBERT MD, WAS DISCIPLINED BY ARIZONA ON JANUARY 28, 1999
DISCIPLINARY ACTION: PROBATION; REQUIRED TO ENTER AN IMPAIRED PHYSICIAN PROGRAM OR SUBSTANCE ABUSE TREATMENT
OFFENSE: SUBSTANCE ABUSE

NOTES: INHALANT ABUSE. TERMS OF PROBATION INCLUDE: SHALL NOT PRACTICE MEDICINE UNTIL HE MEETS WITH THE BOARD AND RECEIVES THEIR APPROVAL TO PRACTICE; MUST ENTER, WITHIN 30 DAYS, AND SUCCESSFULLY COMPLETE AN INPATIENT TREATMENT PROGRAM AT A BOARD APPROVED CENTER; TREATMENT FACILITY MUST PROVIDE A WRITTEN EVALUATION REPORT TO THE BOARD. THIS IS AN INTERIM ORDER.

PINERES, EFRAIM MD, LICENSE NUMBER 0012500, WAS DISCIPLINED BY ARIZONA ON OCTOBER 18, 1995
OFFENSE: SUBSTANDARD CARE, INCOMPETENCE OR NEGLIGENCE

NOTES: MEDICAL MALPRACTICE LAWSUIT INSTITUTED RESULTING FROM A PATIENT HE SAW IN APRIL AND MAY 1991; AFTER REVIEWING THIS CASE, THE BOARD CONCLUDED THAT HIS CARE WAS TOTALLY INAPPROPRIATE DUE TO HIS FAILURE TO OBTAIN OLD MEDICAL RECORDS ON THE PATIENT, FAILURE TO OBTAIN AN APPROPRIATE MEDICAL HISTORY OF HER GASTROINTESTINAL PROBLEMS, FAILURE TO EVALUATE HER COMPLAINTS OF NAUSEA, VOMITING, HEARTBURN AND BLOODY DIARRHEA AND FAILURE TO PERFORM A SIGMOIDOSCOPY EXAMINATION OR REFER HER TO AN APPROPRIATE SPECIALIST; THE RESULT WAS THAT ON 6/1/91 THE PATIENT WAS FOUND IN AN EMERGENCY ROOM TO HAVE A CYANOTIC RIGHT FOOT AND LOWER LEG; HER RIGHT LEG WAS AMPUTATED ABOVE THE KNEE. AFTER REVIEWING HIS RECORDS, IT WAS CONCLUDED THAT THERE WERE SOME LAPSES IN HIS HISTORY-TAKING CONCERNING PRIOR DRUGS THAT PATIENTS HAVE BEEN ON AND AS TO WHY THOSE DRUGS WERE INSTITUTED. WITHIN THREE MONTHS, SHALL TAKE AND PASS THE SPECIAL PURPOSE EXAMINATION WITH A SCORE OF 75 OR GREATER.

PINERES, EFRAIM MD, LICENSE NUMBER 0012500, WAS DISCIPLINED BY ARIZONA ON OCTOBER 18, 1996
DISCIPLINARY ACTION: LICENSE REVOCATION
OFFENSE: FAILURE TO COMPLY WITH PREVIOUS BOARD ORDER

NOTES: FAILED TO TAKE SPECIAL PURPOSE EXAMINATION WITHIN THREE MONTHS OF 10/95 ORDER; SAID HE WOULD NOT TAKE IT DUE TO HIS AGE AND THE NATURE OF THE EXAM. ON 1/24/97 HIS MOTION FOR REHEARING OR REVIEW OF REVOCATION ORDER DENIED.

PINNAMANENI, KRISHNA M MD, LICENSE NUMBER 0014173 OF TEMPE, AZ, WAS DISCIPLINED BY ARIZONA ON SEPTEMBER 20, 1995
DISCIPLINARY ACTION: REQUIRED TO TAKE ADDITIONAL MEDICAL EDUCATION

NOTES: MUST UNDERGO BOARD APPROVED TRAINING REGARDING APPROPRIATE PHYSICIAN-PATIENT RELATIONS. ON 4/16/96 ORDER TERMINATED AFTER HE SUBMITTED MATERIAL ON A WORKSHOP HE ATTENDED.

POLSDORFER, J RICKER MD, LICENSE NUMBER 1042093 OF PEACE CORPS,HARARE DEPT OF STATE, WASHINGTON, DC, WAS DISCIPLINED BY INDIANA ON NOVEMBER 3, 1993
DISCIPLINARY ACTION: 18-MONTH PROBATION; RESTRICTION PLACED ON LICENSE
OFFENSE: LOSS OR RESTRICTION OF HOSPITAL PRIVILEGES

NOTES: LICENSE REQUEST DENIED 6/24/93 BASED ON PROBLEMS AT DOMINICAN HOSPITAL, SANTA CRUZ, CALIFORNIA REGARDING HIS TREATMENT AND CARE OF A PATIENT WHO ULTIMATELY DEVELOPED THIGH ABSCESSES LEADING TO LIFE-THREATENING COMPLICATIONS OF SEPSIS, BRAIN ABSCESS, AND AORTIC VALVE ENDOCARDITIS; HE TESTIFIED AT 9/30/93 HEARING THAT HE MADE MISTAKES IN HIS TREATMENT OF THE PATIENT WHICH RESULTED IN HIS HOSPITAL PRIVILEGES BEING PUT ON PROBATION. CONDITIONS OF INDIANA BOARD PROBATION: MAY ONLY PRACTICE IN A BOARD APPROVED ACADEMIC OR OTHER SUPERVISED SETTING; SHALL HAVE SUPERVISOR SUBMIT QUARTERLY REPORTS AND HE SHALL APPEAR BEFORE THE BOARD QUARTERLY; BOARD RESERVES RIGHT TO INSPECT AND/OR REVIEW HIS MEDICAL CHARTS.

POLSDORFER, J RICKER MD, LICENSE NUMBER 0A23365 OF WASHINGTON, DC, WAS DISCIPLINED BY CALIFORNIA ON JUNE 21, 1996
DISCIPLINARY ACTION: 36-MONTH PROBATION
OFFENSE: SUBSTANDARD CARE, INCOMPETENCE OR NEGLIGENCE

NOTES: GROSS NEGLIGENCE, INCOMPETENCE, EXCESSIVE TREATMENT OR PRESCRIBING, AND REPEATED NEGLIGENT ACTS IN THE DIAGNOSIS AND TREATMENT OF ONE PATIENT. REVOCATION, STAYED.

POLSDORFER, J RICKER MD, LICENSE NUMBER 28995 OF PHOENIX, AZ, WAS DISCIPLINED BY WASHINGTON ON MARCH 16, 1998
OFFENSE: DISCIPLINARY ACTION BY ANOTHER STATE OR AGENCY

NOTES: COMMITTED UNPROFESSIONAL CONDUCT. SUSPENSION STAYED ON CONDITION THAT HE COMPLY WITH AN ORDER OF THE CALIFORNIA MEDICAL BOARD, AMONG OTHER CONDITIONS.

POMEROY, KENT L MD, LICENSE NUMBER 0004962, WAS DISCIPLINED BY ARIZONA ON FEBRUARY 14, 1990
DISCIPLINARY ACTION: REQUIRED TO TAKE ADDITIONAL MEDICAL EDUCATION

NOTES: SHALL OBTAIN 40 HOURS OF CONTINUING MEDICAL EDUCATION IN PHARMACOLOGY, CHRONIC PAIN AND/OR DRUG ADDICTION PRIOR TO 1991 LICENSE RENEWAL. ORDER TERMINATED ON 4/10/91.

POMEROY, KENT L MD, LICENSE NUMBER 4962, WAS DISCIPLINED BY ARIZONA ON JANUARY 25, 1997
DISCIPLINARY ACTION: MONITORING OF PHYSICIAN PERFORMANCE

NOTES: IN THE CONTEXT OF PRACTICE OF PROLOTHERAPY/SCLEROTHERAPY, COMPLY WITH AN ARIZONA STATUTE BY UTILIZING ADEQUATE INFORMED PATIENT CONSENT AND CONFORMING TO GENERALLY ACCEPTED EXPERIMENTAL CRITERIA, INCLUDING PROTOCOLS, DETAILED RECORDS, PERIODIC ANALYSIS OF RESULTS AND PERIODIC REVIEW BY A MEDICAL PEER REVIEW COMMITTEE AS APPROVED BY THE FOOD AND DRUG ADMINISTRATION OR ITS SUCCESSOR AGENCY; THE BOARD SHALL CONDUCT A RECORDS REVIEW OF HIS RECORDS IN ONE YEAR TO DETERMINE IF HE IS IN COMPLIANCE WITH THIS STIPULATION AND ORDER.

PONITCH, JERRY A MD OF TEMPE, AZ, WAS DISCIPLINED BY ILLINOIS ON NOVEMBER 1, 1992
DISCIPLINARY ACTION: SUSPENSION OF CONTROLLED SUBSTANCE LICENSE; PROBATION
OFFENSE: DISCIPLINARY ACTION BY ANOTHER STATE OR AGENCY

NOTES: DISCIPLINED IN ARIZONA. SUSPENSION AND PROBATION INDEFINITE.

PONITCH, JERRY ALLEN MD, LICENSE NUMBER 0007979, WAS DISCIPLINED BY ARIZONA ON SEPTEMBER 4, 1990
DISCIPLINARY ACTION: RESTRICTION PLACED ON CONTROLLED SUBSTANCE LICENSE; REQUIRED TO TAKE ADDITIONAL MEDICAL EDUCATION

NOTES: MUST SURRENDER CONTROLLED SUBSTANCE REGISTRATION FOR SCHEDULES II THROUGH V. MUST COMPLETE 30 HOURS OF CONTINUING MEDICAL EDUCATION ON THE SUBJECT OF PHARMACOLOGY.

PORTER, GREGORY MD, WAS DISCIPLINED BY ARIZONA ON NOVEMBER 20, 1998
DISCIPLINARY ACTION: REPRIMAND

PORTER, GREGORY J MD, LICENSE NUMBER 156234 OF 1701 W ST MARY'S ROAD #C117, TUCSON, AZ, WAS DISCIPLINED BY NEW YORK ON AUGUST 3, 1999
DISCIPLINARY ACTION: REPRIMAND
OFFENSE: DISCIPLINARY ACTION BY ANOTHER STATE OR AGENCY

NOTES: DISCIPLINED BY THE ARIZONA BOARD FOR ENGAGING IN CONDUCT OR PRACTICE WHICH IS HARMFUL OR DANGEROUS TO THE HEALTH OF THE PATIENT OR PUBLIC.

PORTER, JOHN C MD, LICENSE NUMBER 0015286, WAS DISCIPLINED BY ARIZONA ON APRIL 26, 1996
DISCIPLINARY ACTION: REQUIRED TO TAKE ADDITIONAL MEDICAL EDUCATION
OFFENSE: OVERPRESCRIBING OR MISPRESCRIBING DRUGS

NOTES: INTERVIEWED BY THE BOARD REGARDING HIS PRACTICE, INCLUDING BUT NOT LIMITED TO HIS PRESCRIBING PRACTICES. WITHIN SIX MONTHS, SHALL SUCCESSFULLY COMPLETE 20 HOURS OF BOARD-APPROVED CONTINUING MEDICAL EDUCATION IN PAIN MANAGEMENT AND RECORD KEEPING; SHALL SUBMIT PROOF OF SUCCESSFUL COMPLETION TO THE BOARD. ON 1/22/97 THIS ORDER WAS TERMINATED.

POWELL, MORRIS EARL MD, WAS DISCIPLINED BY ARIZONA ON JUNE 10, 1996

NOTES: SHALL NOT PRACTICE MEDICINE IN ARIZONA UNTIL FIRST MEETING WITH THE BOARD AND RECEIVING APPROVAL TO DO SO. THIS ORDER WAS TERMINATED ON 1/22/97.

POWELL, TOM MD, LICENSE NUMBER 5378, WAS DISCIPLINED BY ARIZONA ON NOVEMBER 18, 1999
OFFENSE: SUBSTANDARD CARE, INCOMPETENCE OR NEGLIGENCE

NOTES: FAILURE TO TIMELY DIAGNOSE RECTAL CANCER. DECREE OF CENSURE ISSUED.

PREISER, FRANKLIN M MD, LICENSE NUMBER 0005848, WAS DISCIPLINED BY ARIZONA ON APRIL 17, 1996
OFFENSE: SUBSTANDARD CARE, INCOMPETENCE OR NEGLIGENCE

NOTES: DURING THE COURSE OF TREATMENT OF A PATIENT BETWEEN 2/94 AND 8/94, HE MISSED A DIAGNOSIS OF SQUAMOUS CELL CARCINOMA OF THE BASE OF THE

TONGUE AND EPIGLOTTIS WITH LYMPHANGETIC SPREAD WHICH RESULTED IN THE PATIENT UNDERGOING AN EMERGENCY TRACHEOSTOMY AND A TOTAL LARYNGECTOMY; FAILED TO MAINTAIN ADEQUATE RECORDS IN THAT HIS MEDICAL RECORDS ARE UNINTELLIGIBLE AND UNDECIPHERABLE. CENSURED.

PRUITT, CHRISTOPHER R MD, DATE OF BIRTH MARCH 19, 1962 OF 16232 S 32ND PLACE, PHOENIX, AZ, WAS DISCIPLINED BY MEDICARE ON JANUARY 5, 1997
DISCIPLINARY ACTION: EXCLUSION FROM THE MEDICARE AND/OR MEDICAID PROGRAM
OFFENSE: NONCOMPLIANCE WITH A PROFESSIONAL RULE

NOTES: DEFAULTED ON PUBLIC HEALTH SERVICE EDUCATION LOAN.

PUMA, LILLIAN D DO, LICENSE NUMBER 0002836 OF 4045 EAST BELL ROAD #125, PHOENIX, AZ, WAS DISCIPLINED BY ARIZONA ON OCTOBER 7, 1995
DISCIPLINARY ACTION: PROBATION; MONITORING OF PHYSICIAN PERFORMANCE
OFFENSE: SUBSTANCE ABUSE

NOTES: RECEIVED TREATMENT FROM 5/03/95 TO 5/27/95 FOR CHEMICAL DEPENDENCE. ON 6/29/95 ADMITTED TO USING VICODIN, A SCHEDULE III CONTROLLED SUBSTANCE, WITHOUT RECEIVING IT IN THE COURSE OF REGULAR MEDICAL TREATMENT PRESCRIBED BY HER TREATING PHYSICIAN. MINIMUM FOUR YEAR PROBATION UNDER TERMS AND CONDITIONS: SHALL ATTEND AT LEAST ONE INDIVIDUAL COUNSELING SESSION PER WEEK WITH A BOARD APPROVED MENTAL HEALTH THERAPIST WHO SHALL SUBMIT MONTHLY REPORTS TO THE BOARD; HER PARTICIPATION AND ATTENDANCE AT THE PHYSICIAN RECOVERY PROGRAM MAY BE SUBSTITUTED FOR THE WEEKLY MEETING WITH THE MENTAL HEALTH THERAPIST, BUT NOT MORE THAN TWICE IN ANY MONTH; SHALL MAINTAIN AN ACTIVE SPONSOR FOR HER PARTICIPATION IN NARCOTICS ANONYMOUS; SHALL BE SUBJECT TO RANDOM BODILY FLUID TESTING FOR DRUGS AT ANY TIME; SHALL REFRAIN FROM THE CONSUMPTION OF ALCOHOL; SHALL NOT USE ANY ILLICIT SUBSTANCES OR PRESCRIPTION ONLY MEDICATIONS UNLESS SUCH MEDICATIONS ARE PRESCRIBED BY A LICENSED PHYSICIAN; SHALL ATTEND AT LEAST FOUR 12 STEP RECOVERY MEETINGS FOR AT LEAST ONE HOUR PER MEETING THROUGH NARCOTICS ANONYMOUS; SHALL MEET REGULARLY WITH THE BOARD; SHALL NOTIFY THE BOARD WITHIN 20 DAYS IF SHE CEASES TO RESIDE IN ARIZONA; AND SHALL AUTHORIZE ALL OF HER HEALTH CARE PROVIDERS TO RELEASE AND DISCLOSE INFORMATION UPON BOARD REQUEST.

PUMA, LILLIAN D DO, LICENSE NUMBER 0191953 OF 6349 EAST JOAN DEARC, SCOTTSDALE, AZ, WAS DISCIPLINED BY NEW YORK ON NOVEMBER 8, 1996
DISCIPLINARY ACTION: 48-MONTH PROBATION
OFFENSE: DISCIPLINARY ACTION BY ANOTHER STATE OR AGENCY

NOTES: ACTION IN ARIZONA FOR BEING DEPENDENT ON, OR AN HABITUAL USER OF NARCOTICS. PROBATION COMMENCING UPON PRACTICING IN NEW YORK.

PUYANA, ALFONSO JR MD, WAS DISCIPLINED BY ARIZONA ON JANUARY 22, 1998
DISCIPLINARY ACTION: REQUIRED TO TAKE ADDITIONAL MEDICAL EDUCATION

NOTES: MUST OBTAIN 20 HOURS OF TRAINING IN RECORD KEEPING AND RECORD MANAGEMENT TO BE APPROVED BY THE BOARD AND COMPLETED WITHIN 6 MONTHS.

QUIROZ, EDWARD E MD, LICENSE NUMBER 0016323, WAS DISCIPLINED BY ARIZONA ON JANUARY 21, 1992
OFFENSE: SUBSTANDARD CARE, INCOMPETENCE OR NEGLIGENCE

NOTES: INADEQUATE AND INCOMPLETE MANAGEMENT OF A PATIENT, SPECIFICALLY, FAILURE TO EVALUATE PERSISTENT ANEMIA AND PAINFUL PROTRUDING HEMORRHOIDS, LEADING TO AN ADVANCED CARCINOMA OF THE RECTUM WHICH HAD TO BE TREATED BY AN ABDOMINAL PERINEAL RESECTION. DECREE OF CENSURE.

RAIKHELKAR, KRANTINATH MD, DATE OF BIRTH JANUARY 1, 1947 OF 2929 N CENTRAL #2100, PHOENIX, AZ, WAS DISCIPLINED BY MEDICARE ON JANUARY 12, 1997
DISCIPLINARY ACTION: 36-MONTH EXCLUSION FROM THE MEDICARE AND/OR MEDICAID PROGRAM
OFFENSE: CRIMINAL CONVICTION OR PLEA OF GUILTY, NOLO CONTENDERE, OR NO CONTEST TO A CRIME

NOTES: CONVICTED OF A CRIME RELATED TO THE DELIVERY OF HEALTH CARE OR FINANCIAL MISCONDUCT INVOLVING A GOVERNMENT-OPERATED PROGRAM.

RAIKHELKAR, KRANTINATH V MD, LICENSE NUMBER 0014151 OF RIVIERA, AZ, WAS DISCIPLINED BY ARIZONA ON JANUARY 20, 1993
OFFENSE: SUBSTANDARD CARE, INCOMPETENCE OR NEGLIGENCE

NOTES: SEVERAL DEFICIENCIES APPARENT IN TREATMENT OF A PATIENT ON WHOM HE PERFORMED SURGERY 1/6/92. PHYSICIAN'S FIRST FEW LAPAROSCOPIC CHOLECYSTECTOMY SURGERIES ARE SUPPOSED TO BE SUPERVISED OR ASSISTED BY A SURGEON EXPERIENCED IN THIS TYPE OF PROCEDURE WHICH THEY WERE NOT; THIS WAS HIS FIRST SUCH PROCEDURE WITH NO SUPERVISION NOTED; THIS TYPE OF SURGERY IS NOT RECOMMENDED FOR OBESE PATIENTS EARLY IN ONE'S EXPERIENCE YET IT WAS DONE IN THIS CASE; HE INAPPROPRIATELY CLIPPED BILE DUCT DURING THE SURGICAL PROCEDURE AND THEREAFTER FAILED TO PROPERLY DIAGNOSE OR MANAGE THE COMPLICATION WHEN IT AROSE; FAILED TO ENSURE ADEQUATE POSTOPERATIVE TREATMENTS; IMPROPERLY BILLED FOR POSTOPERATIVE VISITS AND IMPROPERLY DELAYED THE DICTATION OF HIS OPERATIVE REPORTS. CENSURED. ON 4/15/93 REQUEST FOR RECONSIDERATION WAS DENIED.

RAIKHELKAR, KRANTINATH V MD, LICENSE NUMBER 0014151, WAS DISCIPLINED BY ARIZONA ON JULY 14, 1994
DISCIPLINARY ACTION: RESTRICTION PLACED ON LICENSE

NOTES: WAS INDICTED BY A GRAND JURY DURING PENDENCY OF THE BOARD'S FORMAL PROCEEDINGS; BOARD HAS GRANTED A CONTINUANCE OF THESE HEARINGS PENDING THE OUTCOME OF THE CRIMINAL MATTER. SHALL NOT PERFORM NEEDLE LOCALIZATIONS OR BIOPSIES OF THE HUMAN BREAST WITHOUT DIRECT SURGICAL ASSISTANCE FROM A BOARD-CERTIFIED AND ARIZONA LICENSED GENERAL SURGEON. ON 10/19/95, THIS ORDER WAS WITHDRAWN BASED ON A CONTINUANCE IN THE CRIMINAL CASE THE MATTER WAS REMANDED TO A FORMAL HEARING BEFORE THE BOARD.

RAIKHELKAR, KRANTINATH V MD, LICENSE NUMBER 0014151, WAS DISCIPLINED BY ARIZONA ON JANUARY 19, 1996

DISCIPLINARY ACTION: LICENSE SUSPENSION; REQUIRED TO TAKE ADDITIONAL MEDICAL EDUCATION
OFFENSE: PROFESSIONAL MISCONDUCT

NOTES: BETWEEN 1991 AND 1992 IN THE CASE OF FOUR PATIENTS DOCUMENTATION WAS INADEQUATE IN THAT HE DID NOT DOCUMENT INTERPRETATION OF POST-BIOPSY FILMS IN ONE CASE, INADEQUATE HISTORY RECORDS IN TWO PATIENTS AND INAPPROPRIATE BILLING IN TWO CASES; IN 1/93, AUDIT OF HIS BILLING AND CODING PRACTICES WAS ORDERED WITH THE FOLLOWING RESULTS: OF 14 CASES IN THE AUDIT, SEVEN CASES REVEALED EXCESSIVE OR INAPPROPRIATE CHARGES FOR PROCEDURES NOT PERFORMED OR DOCUMENTED IN OPERATIVE REPORTS, AND TWO CASES REVEALED PROCEDURES PERFORMED WITHOUT CORRESPONDING PATHOLOGY REPORTS; AS SUPERVISING PHYSICIAN IN HIS OFFICE, HE ACKNOWLEDGES RESPONSIBILITY FOR COMMITTING MISDEMEANORS IN CONNECTION WITH INACCURATE BILLINGS FOR DIAGNOSTIC SERVICES TO PATIENTS ELIGIBLE FOR FEDERAL REIMBURSEMENT. SUSPENSION FOR A MINIMUM PERIOD OF THREE YEARS TO RUN CONCURRENTLY WITH THE THREE-YEAR SUSPENSION FROM MEDICARE AND TO CONTINUE UNTIL HE TAKES AND PASSES THE SPECIAL PURPOSE EXAMINATION WITH A SCORE OF 75 OR BETTER; SHALL SIT FOR THE EXAMINATION ONLY WITHIN THE LAST THREE MONTHS OF HIS SUSPENSION; IN THE EVENT THAT HE PRACTICES MEDICINE FULL-TIME IN ANOTHER JURISDICTION DURING SUSPENSION, HE SHALL SUCCESSFULLY COMPLETE A BOARD-APPROVED MINI-RESIDENCY IN GENERAL SURGERY; IF HE HAS NOT BEEN PRACTICING FULL-TIME IN ANOTHER JURISDICTION DURING SUSPENSION, SHALL SUCCESSFULLY COMPLETE A ONE-YEAR RESIDENCY PROGRAM IN GENERAL SURGERY; FOLLOWING COMPLETION OF SUSPENSION, SHALL BE PLACED ON PROBATION WITH TERMS. ON 11/ 20/98 A SUPERSEDING ORDER WAS IMPOSED. ON 1/27/99 REQUEST FOR REHEARING DENIED.

RANDHAWA, GURCHARAN S MD, LICENSE NUMBER 0022036, WAS DISCIPLINED BY ARIZONA ON OCTOBER 18, 1996

NOTES: SHALL NOT PRACTICE MEDICINE UNTIL FIRST MEETING WITH THE BOARD AND OBTAINING ITS AFFIRMATIVE APPROVAL TO DO SO. INTERIM ORDER. ON 3/26/99 REQUEST TO LIFT RESTRICTION ON LICENSE DENIED.

RANDHAWA, GURCHARAN SINGH MD, DATE OF BIRTH SEPTEMBER 12, 1948, LICENSE NUMBER 0027214 OF MARSHALLTOWN, IA, WAS DISCIPLINED BY IOWA ON OCTOBER 19, 1995
DISCIPLINARY ACTION: PROBATION; RESTRICTION PLACED ON LICENSE
OFFENSE: SUBSTANDARD CARE, INCOMPETENCE OR NEGLIGENCE

NOTES: PROVIDED SUBSTANDARD CARE TO FOUR PATIENTS. RESTRICTIONS ON LICENSE PROHIBIT HIM FROM PRACTICING EMERGENCY MEDICINE UNTIL COMPLETING A BOARD APPROVED TRAINING PROGRAM AND RESTRICT HIM FROM SUPERVISING A PHYSICIAN ASSISTANT. ADDITIONALLY, PRACTICE IS LIMITED TO THE VETERANS HOME IN MARSHALLTOWN AND V.A. HOSPITAL IN KNOXVILLE. INDEFINITE PROBATION.

RANDHAWA, GURCHARAN SINGH MD, DATE OF BIRTH SEPTEMBER 12, 1948, LICENSE NUMBER 0032870 OF P.O. BOX 984, MARSHALLTOWN, IA, WAS DISCIPLINED BY WISCONSIN ON SEPTEMBER 25, 1996
DISCIPLINARY ACTION: MONITORING OF PHYSICIAN PERFORMANCE
OFFENSE: DISCIPLINARY ACTION BY ANOTHER STATE OR AGENCY

NOTES: ON 10/19/95 THE IOWA BOARD IMPOSED DISCIPLINE UPON HIS LICENSE TO PRACTICE MEDICINE. AS LONG AS HE NEITHER RESIDES NOR PRACTICES IN WISCONSIN, HIS WISCONSIN LICENSE IS LIMITED BY REQUIRING HIM TO COMPLY WITH ALL THE CONDITIONS IMPOSED BY IOWA. SHALL CAUSE COPIES OF QUARTERLY REPORTS FROM THE IOWA BOARD TO BE FILED WITH THE WISCONSIN BOARD WHICH DOCUMENT HIS COMPLIANCE WITH THE TERMS AND CONDITIONS; SHALL IMMEDIATELY SURRENDER ALL INDICIA OF WISCONSIN REGISTRATION TO THE DEPARTMENT MONITOR WHO SHALL REISSUE REGISTRATION CREDENTIALS MARKED "LIMITED"; PRIOR TO HIS RESUMPTION OF THE PRACTICE OF MEDICINE SHALL NOTIFY THE BOARD OF HIS DESIRE TO RESUME THE ACTIVE USE OF HIS LICENSE AND PETITION THE BOARD.

RAPPAPORT, WILLIAM DAVID MD, LICENSE NUMBER 0015658, WAS DISCIPLINED BY ARIZONA ON OCTOBER 13, 1991
DISCIPLINARY ACTION: 120-MONTH PROBATION; REQUIRED TO ENTER AN IMPAIRED PHYSICIAN PROGRAM OR SUBSTANCE ABUSE TREATMENT
OFFENSE: SUBSTANCE ABUSE

NOTES: ON OR ABOUT 3/21/86, HE ENTERED INTO A DRUG AND ALCOHOL STIPULATION WITH THE BOARD, WHICH WAS TERMINATED ON 6/30/90 WITH AN ORDER DECLARING HIS SUCCESSFUL REHABILITATION; HIS DRUG USE AND POOR DRUG MANAGEMENT CHOICES FROM 10/90 UNTIL 2/91 REPRESENT A RELAPSE OF HIS ADDICTIVE DISEASE IN THAT IN 4/91, BOARD INVESTIGATORS DISCOVERED THAT HE HAD RECEIVED CONTROLLED AND NON-CONTROLLED DRUGS FROM SEVEN DIFFERENT PHYSICIANS AT SEVEN DIFFERENT PHARMACIES, BETWEEN 10/90 AND 2/91; HE STATED THAT THE DRUG ACTIVITY WAS DUE TO VARIOUS PHYSICAL PROBLEMS BETWEEN 8/90 AND 2/91; IN 2/91, CONTACTED THE DOCTOR'S HEALTH PROGRAM, WHERE HE WAS ADVISED TO HAVE AT MOST ONE TREATING AND ONE SURGICAL PHYSICIAN; THROUGH 4/91, HE DROPPED OUT OF HIS AA PROGRAM AND RESTARTED AND IS CURRENTLY ATTENDING MEETINGS THREE TIMES A WEEK; SINCE 6/91, RANDOM URINE TESTS HAVE PROVED POSITIVE FOR ONLY THOSE DRUGS PRESCRIBED BY HIS ATTENDING PHYSICIAN. MUST IMMEDIATELY PARTICIPATE IN A BOARD-APPROVED MONITORED AFTERCARE TREATMENT PROGRAM WHOSE THERAPIST MUST SUBMIT QUARTERLY REPORTS; MUST PARTICIPATE IN 90 12-STEP MEETINGS FOR SUBSTANCE ABUSE WITHIN 90 DAYS; MUST THEN PARTICIPATE IN A 12-STEP RECOVERY PROGRAM AS DETERMINED BY HIS TREATING THERAPIST AND ATTEND AT LEAST THREE WEEKLY MEETINGS; SHALL OBTAIN A BOARD-APPROVED TREATING PHYSICIAN; SHALL ABSTAIN COMPLETELY FROM THE CONSUMPTION OF ALCOHOLIC BEVERAGES AND DRUGS EXCEPT WHEN PRESCRIBED BY HIS TREATING PHYSICIAN; MUST SUBMIT TO WITNESSED RANDOM BIOLOGICAL FLUID COLLECTION; SHALL KEEP A LOG OF ANY AND ALL MEDICATIONS PRESCRIBED FOR HIM; SHALL SUBMIT TO ANY EXAMINATIONS OR THERAPY ORDERED BY THE BOARD; SHALL APPEAR BEFORE THE BOARD FOR INTERVIEWS UPON REQUEST; SHALL INFORM BOARD OF CHANGE OF ADDRESS OR IF AWAY FOR MORE THAN FIVE DAYS. AS OF 2/15/96 THIS ORDER IS TERMINATED.

RATH, JOGESWAR MD, LICENSE NUMBER 0010077, WAS DISCIPLINED BY ARIZONA ON APRIL 9, 1992
DISCIPLINARY ACTION: REQUIRED TO TAKE ADDITIONAL MEDICAL EDUCATION
OFFENSE: SUBSTANDARD CARE, INCOMPETENCE OR NEGLIGENCE

NOTES: CONCERNS WERE EXPRESSED BY ARIZONA HEALTH CARE COST CONTAINMENT SERVICES ABOUT HIS PATIENT CARE. STAFF SHOULD CONDUCT AN OFFICE SURVEY IN ONE YEAR OF HIS OFFICE CHARTS. SHALL SUCCESSFULLY PARTICIPATE IN AND COMPLETE 40 HOURS OF CATEGORY I CONTINUING MEDICAL EDUCATION IN THE TOPIC OF CARDIOLOGY WITH A SPECIAL EMPHASIS ON E.K.G. READING AND CARDIOVASCULAR DISEASE BEFORE 12/31/92.

RATHER, DANIEL A MD, DATE OF BIRTH APRIL 22, 1934, LICENSE NUMBER 0014885 OF PEORIA, AZ, WAS DISCIPLINED BY COLORADO ON OCTOBER 16, 1991
OFFENSE: SUBSTANCE ABUSE

NOTES: HABITUAL INTEMPERANCE, AND ALCOHOL DEPENDENCE AND ABUSE. STIPULATION AND ORDER IMPOSING CONDITIONS FOR RETURN TO THE PRACTICE OF MEDICINE IN COLORADO.

RAY, LANCE I MD, DATE OF BIRTH MAY 15, 1944, LICENSE NUMBER 0012094, WAS DISCIPLINED BY WASHINGTON ON NOVEMBER 14, 1990
DISCIPLINARY ACTION: EMERGENCY SUSPENSION
OFFENSE: PROFESSIONAL MISCONDUCT

NOTES: ALLEGATIONS INCLUDE UNPROFESSIONAL CONDUCT AND INABILITY TO PRACTICE WITH REASONABLE SKILL AND SAFETY TO CONSUMERS.

RAY, LANCE I MD, DATE OF BIRTH MAY 15, 1944, LICENSE NUMBER 0012094 OF SEATTLE, WA, WAS DISCIPLINED BY WASHINGTON ON MARCH 25, 1991
DISCIPLINARY ACTION: LICENSE REVOCATION
OFFENSE: SUBSTANCE ABUSE

NOTES: LICENSE SUMMARILY SUSPENDED ON 11/14/90. DIVERTED RITALIN, A CONTROLLED SUBSTANCE, FOR HIS OWN NON-THERAPEUTIC USE; BETWEEN 4-6/90 PRESCRIBED FIORINAL WITH CODEINE FOR PATIENT IN NONTHERAPEUTIC AMOUNTS, PATIENT HAD BEEN HOSPITALIZED IN 3/90 AND WITHDRAWN FROM FIORINAL; BETWEEN 4-6/90 OBTAINED $12,635 FROM A PATIENT BUT PRESENTED NO BILLS FOR MEDICAL SERVICES TO THE PATIENT; WAS ALSO PAID $1,354.23 BY MEDICARE FOR HIS TREATMENT OF THE PATIENT FROM 3/30/90 TO 5/17/90; BEGAN TREATMENT FOR MAJOR DEPRESSION IN 7/88; ALLOWED TO VOLUNTARILY RESIGN HIS PRIVILEGES AT PROVIDENCE MEDICAL CENTER IN SEATTLE ON 9/24/90 FOR ADMINISTRATIVE REASONS, INCLUDING INABILITY TO PROVIDE CERTIFICATION OF MALPRACTICE INSURANCE; ON 9/8/90 PERFORMED SURGERY AT PROVIDENCE MEDICAL CENTER WITHOUT QUALIFIED SURGICAL ASSISTANT AS REQUIRED; ON 3/12 AND 3/14/91 WROTE PRESCRIPTIONS FOR PATIENTS WHILE LICENSE WAS SUSPENDED. NO RIGHT TO REAPPLY FOR ONE YEAR; SHALL SUBMIT TO AN IN-PATIENT PSYCHIATRIC AND CHEMICAL DEPENDENCY EVALUATION WITHIN 20 DAYS; SHALL APPEAR WITHIN 60 DAYS FOR DETERMINATION OF ADDITIONAL CONDITIONS, AND SHALL DEVISE A PLAN FOR FINANCIAL RESTITUTION TO THE ESTATE OF THE PATIENT; SHALL CONTINUE CONTINUING MEDICAL EDUCATION AS IF HIS LICENSE WERE ACTIVE.

RAY, LANCE I MD, DATE OF BIRTH MAY 15, 1944, LICENSE NUMBER 0025565 OF 18666 NORTH 72ND AVENUE, GLENDALE, AZ, WAS DISCIPLINED BY NEW JERSEY ON JUNE 7, 1994
DISCIPLINARY ACTION: LICENSE REVOCATION; FINE
OFFENSE: DISCIPLINARY ACTION BY ANOTHER STATE OR AGENCY

NOTES: DISCIPLINARY ACTION TAKEN IN WASHINGTON FOR INAPPROPRIATE DISTRIBUTION OF CONTROLLED DANGEROUS SUBSTANCES FOR OTHER THAN LEGITIMATE MEDICAL PURPOSES. ASSESSED A $1,000 PENALTY. LICENSE REINSTATED ON 3/14/96: SHALL NOT PRACTICE UNTIL HE HAS APPEARED BEFORE THE BOARD TO DEMONSTRATE TO ITS SATISFACTION THAT HIS PRACTICE WOULD NOT ENDANGER THE HEALTH AND WELFARE OF THE PUBLIC.

RAY, LANCE I MD, DATE OF BIRTH MAY 15, 1944, LICENSE NUMBER 0024076, WAS DISCIPLINED BY ARIZONA ON APRIL 20, 1996
DISCIPLINARY ACTION: 60-MONTH PROBATION; REQUIRED TO TAKE ADDITIONAL MEDICAL EDUCATION
OFFENSE: DISCIPLINARY ACTION BY ANOTHER STATE OR AGENCY

NOTES: DISCIPLINARY ACTION TAKEN BY WASHINGTON AND NEW JERSEY; WASHINGTON REVOKED HIS LICENSE IN 3/91; IN 3/95, PASSED SPECIAL PURPOSE EXAMINATION; IN 6/95, WASHINGTON BOARD WITHDREW REVOCATION; SINCE THE SUMMER OF 1995, HAS NOT BEEN IN COMPLIANCE WITH PAYMENT PLAN SET BY WASHINGTON BOARD IN 6/92 TO REPAY $41,500 TO THE ESTATE OF A PATIENT; IN 6/94 NEW JERSEY REVOKED HIS LICENSE BASED ON THE WASHINGTON ORDER; IN 3/96, NEW JERSEY BOARD REINSTATED HIS LICENSE AND ORDERED THAT HE NOT PRACTICE SURGERY UNTIL HE HAD MET WITH THE BOARD AND DEMONSTRATED THAT HIS PRACTICE WOULD NOT ENDANGER THE HEALTH OF THE PUBLIC. EXCEPT FOR RESTITUTION TO PATIENT'S ESTATE, ARIZONA BOARD FINDS HIS CONDUCT HAS BEEN CORRECTED, MONITORED AND RESOLVED. PROBATION WITH TERMS: SHALL REMAIN IN PSYCHIATRIC TREATMENT WITH A BOARD-APPROVED TREATING PSYCHIATRIST WHO SHALL SUBMIT QUARTERLY REPORTS; SHALL CONTINUE MAKING FULL RESTITUTION TO ESTATE OF PATIENT IN WASHINGTON; IN THE EVENT THAT HE IS NOT ACCEPTED INTO HIS INTENDED FELLOWSHIP PROGRAM, SHALL COMPLETE A 30-DAY MINI-RESIDENCY IN SURGERY.

REGER, HARRY L MD, LICENSE NUMBER 0003349, WAS DISCIPLINED BY ARIZONA ON JULY 19, 1996
OFFENSE: SUBSTANDARD CARE, INCOMPETENCE OR NEGLIGENCE

NOTES: ON 2/7/91, HE SAW A 27-YEAR OLD FEMALE COMPLAINING OF A LUMP IN HER BREAST; NO RECORD OF AN APPROPRIATE EXAMINATION AND NO REFERRAL FOR A MAMMOGRAM; ON TWO SUBSEQUENT VISITS IN 6/91, HIS RECORDS INDICATED THAT HE FAILED TO FOLLOW UP THE BREAST LUMP COMPLAINT, PERFORMED NO BREAST EXAMINATION AND DID NOT ORDER A MAMMOGRAM; IN LATTER VISIT, HE NOTED THAT THE PATIENT WAS BETTER; IN 3/92, PATIENT UNDERWENT A BILATERAL BREAST BIOPSY WHICH REVEALED INFILTRATING CARCINOMA OF BOTH THE LEFT AND RIGHT BREASTS; SHE SUBSEQUENTLY HAD INTENSE CHEMOTHERAPY AND EVENTUALLY SUCCUMBED TO THE DISEASE. CENSURED.

REID, E JANET DO, DATE OF BIRTH JULY 21, 1942 OF 246 SOUTH 4TH AVENUE, TUCSON, AZ, WAS DISCIPLINED BY MEDICARE ON APRIL 2, 1997
DISCIPLINARY ACTION: EXCLUSION FROM THE MEDICARE AND/OR

MEDICAID PROGRAM
OFFENSE: NONCOMPLIANCE WITH A PROFESSIONAL RULE

NOTES: DEFAULTED ON PUBLIC HEALTH SERVICE EDUCATION LOAN. REINSTATED ON 6/17/97.

REINMUTH, OSCAR M MD, WAS DISCIPLINED BY ARIZONA ON JANUARY 18, 1995
DISCIPLINARY ACTION: RESTRICTION PLACED ON CONTROLLED SUBSTANCE LICENSE
OFFENSE: DISCIPLINARY ACTION BY ANOTHER STATE OR AGENCY

NOTES: IN 2/83 HE RELINQUISHED FLORIDA LICENSE VOLUNTARILY WHILE NOT ADMITTING TO CHARGES; IN 10/86, PENNSYLVANIA REPRIMANDED HIS LICENSE BASED ON DISCIPLINARY ACTION IN FLORIDA; ARIZONA BOARD DETERMINED THAT HIS CONDUCT WAS CORRECTED, MONITORED AND RESOLVED. HE SHALL NOT APPLY FOR A DEA CONTROLLED SUBSTANCE REGISTRATION PERMIT IN ARIZONA.

REINMUTH, OSCAR MCNAUGHTON MD OF 322 SCAIFE HALL U OF PITTSBURGH, PITTSBURGH, PA, WAS DISCIPLINED BY DEA ON AUGUST 29, 1995
DISCIPLINARY ACTION: RESTRICTION PLACED ON CONTROLLED SUBSTANCE LICENSE
OFFENSE: DISCIPLINARY ACTION BY ANOTHER STATE OR AGENCY

NOTES: STATE BOARD.

REMILONG, ALAN R DO OF MARIONVILLE, MO, WAS DISCIPLINED BY MISSOURI ON JULY 20, 1995
DISCIPLINARY ACTION: 4-MONTH LICENSE SUSPENSION
OFFENSE: PROFESSIONAL MISCONDUCT

NOTES: MISAPPROPRIATING TYLOX AND PERCOCET; SURRENDERING BUREAU OF NARCOTICS AND DANGEROUS DRUGS PERMIT. SUSPENSION BEGINS 8/3/95. UPON SUCCESSFUL COMPLETION OF THIS SUSPENSION, LICENSE WILL BE RETURNED ON SEVEN YEARS PROBATION WITH TERMS AND CONDITIONS.

REMILONG, ALAN R DO, LICENSE NUMBER 0002181 OF #1 NORTH COLLEGE, MARIONVILLE, MO, WAS DISCIPLINED BY ARIZONA ON MAY 16, 1996
DISCIPLINARY ACTION: 60-MONTH PROBATION; RESTRICTION PLACED ON CONTROLLED SUBSTANCE LICENSE
OFFENSE: DISCIPLINARY ACTION BY ANOTHER STATE OR AGENCY

NOTES: MISSOURI LICENSE SUSPENDED FOR 120 DAYS BEGINNING 8/03/95 DUE TO UNAUTHORIZED USE AND ABUSE OF PRESCRIPTION MEDICATIONS CUSTOMARILY USED FOR CONTROL OF PAIN. CURRENTLY ENROLLED IN THE MISSOURI PHYSICIAN'S HEALTH PROGRAM AND IS IN COMPLIANCE WITH THE TERMS AND CONDITIONS OF HIS SUBSTANCE ABUSE RECOVERY PROGRAM IN MISSOURI. PROBATION UNDER TERMS AND CONDITIONS: WHEN RESIDING IN MISSOURI SHALL COMPLY WITH THE MISSOURI ORDER; WHEN RESIDING IN ARIZONA, SHALL OBTAIN PSYCHIATRIC OR PSYCHOLOGICAL TREATMENT BY A BOARD APPROVED THERAPIST WHO SHALL SUBMIT TO THE BOARD A WRITTEN PROGRESS REPORT EVERY MONTH FOR THE FIRST SIX MONTHS AND THEN EVERY THREE MONTHS FOR THE REMAINDER OF PROBATION; SHALL PROVIDE A COPY OF THIS ORDER TO ALL FACILITIES WHERE HE HIS CURRENTLY EMPLOYED AS A PHYSICIAN AND/OR HAS PRIVILEGES TO ENGAGE IN THE PRACTICE OF MEDICINE; WHEN RESIDING AND PRACTICING IN ARIZONA, SHALL ABSTAIN FROM THE CONSUMPTION OF ALCOHOL AND SHALL NOT CONSUME ILLICIT DRUGS OR TAKE ANY CONTROLLED SUBSTANCES UNLESS SUCH MEDICATION IS PRESCRIBED FOR HIM BY HIS TREATING PHYSICIAN; SHALL MAINTAIN A LOG OF THESE PRESCRIPTIONS AND PROVIDE A COPY TO THE BOARD MONTHLY; SHALL SUBMIT TO AND COOPERATE IN ANY INDEPENDENT MEDICAL OR PSYCHOLOGICAL EVALUATION THAT IS ORDERED BY THE BOARD; SHALL APPEAR BEFORE THE BOARD UPON REQUEST; SHALL SUBMIT TO RANDOM BIOLOGICAL FLUID TESTING; SHALL PARTICIPATE IN A MINIMUM OF TWO SELF-HELP MEETINGS PER WEEK THROUGH SUCH ORGANIZATIONS AS AA, NARCOTICS ANONYMOUS, AND DOCTOR'S CADUCEUS GROUP; IF HE CHANGES HIS RESIDENCE OR BUSINESS ADDRESS SHALL SUBMIT WRITTEN NOTICE TO THE BOARD WITHIN 20 DAYS; SHALL COMPLY WITH CONDITIONS IMPOSED BY DEA; MUST USE TRIPLICATE COPIES OF PRESCRIPTION PADS AND SUPPLY COPIES TO THE BOARD; SHALL COMPLY WITH ANY CONDITIONS PLACED ON HOSPITAL PRIVILEGES.

RICHARDSON, ROBERT A MD, LICENSE NUMBER 0A34155 OF NEEDLES, CA, WAS DISCIPLINED BY CALIFORNIA ON MARCH 31, 1993
DISCIPLINARY ACTION: PROBATION

NOTES: REVOCATION STAYED.

RICHARDSON, ROBERT ALAN MD, LICENSE NUMBER 0012436, WAS DISCIPLINED BY ARIZONA ON MARCH 10, 1990
DISCIPLINARY ACTION: 60-MONTH PROBATION; 24-MONTH REQUIRED TO ENTER AN IMPAIRED PHYSICIAN PROGRAM OR SUBSTANCE ABUSE TREATMENT
OFFENSE: SUBSTANCE ABUSE

NOTES: ON 8/2/89 ENTERED TREATMENT FOR SUBSTANCE ABUSE. ON 9/27/89 A BIOLOGICAL FLUID SAMPLE TESTED POSITIVE FOR MEPERIDINE METABOLITES AND FOR LIDOCAINE. ENTERED INTO STIPULATION WITH THE BOARD ON 10/20/89 WHEREIN LICENSE PLACED ON INACTIVE STATUS WITH OTHER CONDITIONS. CURRENT ORDER REACTIVATES LICENSE WITH THE FOLLOWING CONDITIONS OF PROBATION: MUST IMMEDIATELY PARTICIPATE IN ARIZONA MEDICAL ASSOCIATION PHYSICIAN'S HEALTH PROGRAM WITH QUARTERLY REPORTS SUBMITTED TO BOARD; MUST OBTAIN A BOARD-APPROVED TREATING PHYSICIAN; MUST ABSTAIN FROM ALCOHOL AND ALL OTHER DRUGS; MUST COMPLY WITH REQUESTS FOR RANDOM BIOLOGICAL FLUID TESTS; MUST SUBMIT TO ALL EXAMS AND THERAPY ORDERED BY BOARD; MUST PARTICIPATE IN A 12-STEP RECOVERY PROGRAM FOR SUBSTANCE ABUSE AS DETERMINED BY THERAPIST AND ATTEND AT LEAST 3 WEEKLY MEETINGS; MUST APPEAR BEFORE BOARD FOR INTERVIEWS UPON REQUEST; MUST MAINTAIN LOG OF ALL MEDICATIONS TAKEN; MUST ADVISE BOARD OF CHANGE IN OFFICE OR HOME ADDRESSES OR IF HE PLANS TO BE AWAY FOR MORE THAN FIVE DAYS. EFFECTIVE 1/27/94 BOARD ORDER TERMINATED.

RICKE, P SCOTT MD OF 3346 NUGENT BLVD, COLUMBUS, IN, WAS DISCIPLINED BY DEA ON JUNE 21, 1990
DISCIPLINARY ACTION: SURRENDER OF CONTROLLED SUBSTANCE LICENSE
OFFENSE: DISCIPLINARY ACTION BY ANOTHER STATE OR AGENCY

NOTES: REQUIRED TO MEET DIVERSION PROGRAM FOR ALCOHOLISM BEFORE PRACTICING MEDICINE DUE TO REVOCATION OF LICENSE AND FIVE YEARS PROBATION; MEDICAL LICENSE SUSPENDED INDEFINITELY; APPLICATION FOR REGISTRATION; DEA NUMBER ISSUED 05/20/92.

RICKE, P SCOTT MD, LICENSE NUMBER 0012731 OF 3972 N. CAMPBELL AVENUE, TUCSON, AZ, WAS DISCIPLINED BY ARIZONA ON NOVEMBER 12, 1996
DISCIPLINARY ACTION: REPRIMAND
OFFENSE: PROFESSIONAL MISCONDUCT

NOTES: DISPENSING FENFLURAMINE AND PHENTERMINE WITHOUT HAVING FIRST REGISTERED AS A DISPENSING PHYSICIAN AND WITHOUT INDICATING THE FORM OF THE DRUG DISPENSED OR NUMBER OF REFILLS; FAILING TO WRITE A PRESCRIPTION BUT INSTEAD ACCOUNTING FOR THE DRUGS BEING DISPENSED ON THE PATIENT MEDICATION LOG; FAILING TO PROPERLY LABEL THE DRUGS; FAILING TO KEEP AN INDIVIDUAL LOG FOR EACH SCHEDULED DRUG DISPENSED.

RICKE, P SCOTT MD, LICENSE NUMBER 12731, WAS DISCIPLINED BY ARIZONA ON JANUARY 24, 1997
DISCIPLINARY ACTION: REPRIMAND
OFFENSE: PRACTICING WITHOUT A VALID CONTROLLED SUBSTANCE LICENSE

NOTES: WAS DISPENSING FENFLURAMINE AND PHENTERMINE IN VARIOUS STRENGTHS WITHOUT HAVING FIRST REGISTERED WITH THE BOARD AS A DISPENSING PHYSICIAN; WAS NOT INDICATING THE FORM OF THE DRUG DISPENSED OR NUMBER OF REFILLS FOR THAT DRUG; DID NOT WRITE PRESCRIPTIONS BUT INSTEAD ACCOUNTED FOR THE DRUGS BEING DISPENSED ON THE PATIENT MEDICATION LOG; WAS NOT PROPERLY LABELING THE DRUGS; WAS NOT KEEPING AN INDIVIDUAL LOG FOR EACH SCHEDULED DRUG DISPENSED.

RICKE, P SCOTT MD, LICENSE NUMBER C37788 OF TUCSON, AZ, WAS DISCIPLINED BY CALIFORNIA ON SEPTEMBER 5, 1997
DISCIPLINARY ACTION: REPRIMAND
OFFENSE: DISCIPLINARY ACTION BY ANOTHER STATE OR AGENCY

NOTES: DISCIPLINED BY ARIZONA FOR DISPENSING DRUGS WITHOUT FIRST BEING REGISTERED WITH THEIR BOARD AS A DISPENSING PHYSICIAN; FAILING TO KEEP RECORDS WITH REGARD TO THE DISPENSING OF THESE DRUGS.

RICO, DAVID DO, DATE OF BIRTH JUNE 6, 1951 OF C/O UNIVERSITY OF AZ MED CENTER, TUCSON, AZ, WAS DISCIPLINED BY MEDICARE ON NOVEMBER 9, 1994
DISCIPLINARY ACTION: EXCLUSION FROM THE MEDICARE AND/OR MEDICAID PROGRAM
OFFENSE: NONCOMPLIANCE WITH A PROFESSIONAL RULE

NOTES: DEFAULTED ON PUBLIC HEALTH SERVICE EDUCATION LOAN. REINSTATED ON 3/26/97.

RITLAND, STEPHEN MD, LICENSE NUMBER 0012786, WAS DISCIPLINED BY ARIZONA ON OCTOBER 21, 1994

NOTES: INTERVIEWED BY BOARD MEMBERS RELATIVE TO HIS CARE AND TREATMENT OF A PATIENT, RECORD KEEPING AND BILLING PRACTICES AND AN OFFICE SURVEY CONDUCTED BY THE BOARD. SHALL ENGAGE THE SERVICES OF AN OFFICE MANAGEMENT CONSULTANT ACCEPTABLE TO THE BOARD TO ASSIST HIM IN DEVELOPING APPROPRIATE CODING AND RECORDKEEPING PRACTICES AT HIS OWN EXPENSE. ON 10/18/95 ORDER TERMINATED SINCE HE HAS FULFILLED THE CONDITIONS.

RIVERA, ANA MD, WAS DISCIPLINED BY ARIZONA ON JANUARY 20, 1995
DISCIPLINARY ACTION: DENIAL OF NEW LICENSE
OFFENSE: NONCOMPLIANCE WITH A PROFESSIONAL RULE

NOTES: SHE DID NOT MEET BOMEX REQUIREMENTS. ON 10/18/95 THIS ORDER CONFIRMED DUE TO THE FOLLOWING: IN 1990 BASED ON AN INTERVIEW A HOSPITAL FOUND SHE SHOWED POOR JUDGMENT IN ADMITTING PATIENTS TO THE HOSPITAL WITH VERY DIFFICULT CLINICAL CONDITIONS AND UNDERTAKING VERY DIFFICULT SURGICAL PROCEDURES THAT SHOULD HAVE BEEN PERFORMED IN INSTITUTIONS SPECIALIZING IN THE SPECIFIC AREAS OF SURGERY; REJECTED THE ADVICE AND OPINIONS OF HER COLLEAGUES IN SURGERY WHO WERE GASTROENTEROLOGISTS AND INTERNISTS INVOLVED IN HANDLING HER CASES WHICH LED TO GREATER MORBIDITY OF PATIENTS AND GREATER HOSPITAL COSTS; HOSPITAL RESTRICTED HER PRIVILEGES IN 10/90; FAILED SPEX THREE TIMES IN ARIZONA. PASSED SPEX WITH SCORE OF 75 IN NEVADA. HAS TAKEN AMERICAN BOARD OF SURGERY EXAM ABOUT 11 TIMES BUT HAS NOT PASSED. SHE PROVIDED INACCURATE RESPONSES DURING HER SPEX EXAM PORTION RELATING TO CASE PRESENTATIONS.

ROBBINS, RICHARD MD, WAS DISCIPLINED BY ARIZONA ON OCTOBER 18, 1996
OFFENSE: DISCIPLINARY ACTION BY ANOTHER STATE OR AGENCY

NOTES: ACTION TAKEN AGAINST HIS LICENSE IN FLORIDA. BOARD APPROVED HIS REHABILITATION STIPULATION AND ORDER. THIS IS A STANDARD REHABILITATION ORDER. ON 9/21/99 ORDER TERMINATED.

ROBERTS, BERNICE DO, LICENSE NUMBER 0002339, WAS DISCIPLINED BY ARIZONA ON JANUARY 5, 1990
DISCIPLINARY ACTION: 36-MONTH PROBATION; MONITORING OF PHYSICIAN PERFORMANCE
OFFENSE: SUBSTANCE ABUSE

NOTES: ADMITS TO AN ALCOHOL ABUSE PROBLEM; HAS COMPLETED A TREATMENT PROGRAM. PROBATION UNDER TERMS AND CONDITIONS: SHALL REFRAIN FROM THE USE OF ALL ILLICIT DRUGS AND SHALL NOT TAKE PRESCRIPTION DRUGS, EXCEPT UNDER EMERGENCY CIRCUMSTANCES, UNTIL PRIOR NOTIFICATION HAS BEEN GIVEN TO THE BOARD AND ONLY UPON PRESCRIPTION OF A TREATING PHYSICIAN EXCEPT FOR ASPIRIN AND TYLENOL; SHALL NOT CONSUME ALCOHOL; SHALL ATTEND AT LEAST FIVE AA/NARCOTICS ANONYMOUS MEETINGS PER WEEK AND KEEP A LOG OF ATTENDANCE TO BE SIGNED BY THE CHAIR OF EACH MEETING; SHALL CONTINUE IN THE PHYSICIANS' MONITORED AFTERCARE PROGRAM; SHALL SUBMIT TO BIOLOGICAL FLUID TESTING UPON BOARD REQUEST.

RODELAS, RAUL M MD, WAS DISCIPLINED BY ARIZONA ON SEPTEMBER 24, 1998
DISCIPLINARY ACTION: REPRIMAND
OFFENSE: SEXUAL ABUSE OF OR SEXUAL MISCONDUCT WITH A PATIENT

NOTES: SEXUAL INTIMACIES WITH A PATIENT.

RODRIGUEZ, CLARENCE EDWARD MD, LICENSE NUMBER 0014409, WAS DISCIPLINED BY ARIZONA ON APRIL 11, 1992
OFFENSE: FAILURE TO COMPLY WITH PREVIOUS BOARD ORDER

NOTES: VIOLATED A PROVISION ON HIS 3/13/91 PROBATIONARY ORDER BY TAKING PRESCRIPTION ONLY MEDICATION (DARVON-A CONTROLLED SUBSTANCE) WITHOUT CLEAR EVIDENCE OF IT HAVING BEEN PRESCRIBED BY HIS TREATING PHYSICIAN. PROBATIONARY ORDER AMENDED TO

INCLUDE THE FOLLOWING PROVISIONS: SHALL TAKE NO MEDICATION WHATSOEVER, INCLUDING OVER-THE-COUNTER MEDICATIONS, OTHER THAN PLAIN ASPIRIN OR PLAIN ACETAMINOPHEN, WITHOUT THE WRITTEN PRESCRIPTION OF HIS TREATING PHYSICIAN; THAT PRIOR TO OBTAINING ANY MEDICATION FROM ANY PHYSICIAN HE SHALL FORMALLY NOTIFY THE DOCTOR OF HIS STATUS WITH THE BOARD; SHOULD HE TAKE ANY PRESCRIPTION-ONLY DRUG OR CONTROLLED SUBSTANCES SHALL NOTIFY THE BOARD WITHIN 72 HOURS BY TELEPHONE, AND FOLLOW-UP TO THE BOARD WITH AN EXPLANATION IN WRITING.

RODRIGUEZ, CLARENCE EDWARD MD, LICENSE NUMBER 0014409, WAS DISCIPLINED BY ARIZONA ON OCTOBER 22, 1993
DISCIPLINARY ACTION: LICENSE SUSPENSION; REQUIRED TO ENTER AN IMPAIRED PHYSICIAN PROGRAM OR SUBSTANCE ABUSE TREATMENT
OFFENSE: FAILURE TO COMPLY WITH PREVIOUS BOARD ORDER

NOTES: IN SEPTEMBER 1993 HE DRANK ALCOHOL IN VIOLATION OF TERMS OF THE BOARD'S ORDER OF PROBATION DATED 03/13/91. AGREES NOT TO PRACTICE MEDICINE IN ARIZONA OR ANYWHERE ELSE; HE MAY NOT HOLD REGISTRATION WITH THE DRUG ENFORCEMENT ADMINISTRATION OR WRITE PRESCRIPTIONS; AGREES TO SUCCESSFULLY COMPLETE LONG-TERM RESIDENTIAL/IN-PATIENT TREATMENT FOR CHEMICAL DEPENDENCY AND ALCOHOLISM; SHALL NOT REQUEST REACTIVATION OF HIS LICENSE UNTIL HE MEETS WITH THE BOARD AT A REGULARLY SCHEDULED MEETING AND COMPLIES WITH ANY REQUESTS; MUST SHOW SIX MONTHS DOCUMENTED SOBRIETY FOLLOWING SUCCESSFUL COMPLETION OF ALL RECOMMENDED TREATMENT.

RODRIGUEZ, CLARENCE EDWARD MD OF 560 W BROWN RD STE 2012 E VALLEY, MESA, AZ, WAS DISCIPLINED BY DEA ON APRIL 7, 1994
DISCIPLINARY ACTION: SURRENDER OF CONTROLLED SUBSTANCE LICENSE

NOTES: IN LIEU OF PUBLIC INTEREST REVOCATION.

RODRIGUEZ, CLARENCE EDWARD MD, LICENSE NUMBER 0014409, WAS DISCIPLINED BY ARIZONA ON OCTOBER 22, 1994
DISCIPLINARY ACTION: 60-MONTH PROBATION; REQUIRED TO ENTER AN IMPAIRED PHYSICIAN PROGRAM OR SUBSTANCE ABUSE TREATMENT
OFFENSE: FAILURE TO COMPLY WITH PREVIOUS BOARD ORDER

NOTES: LICENSE INACTIVATED WITH CAUSE ON 10/22/93; ENTERED LONG-TERM TREATMENT FOR ALCOHOLISM AND DISCHARGED ON 3/5/94. LICENSE REACTIVATED ON PROBATION. PROBATION INCLUDES THE FOLLOWING: MUST IMMEDIATELY PARTICIPATE IN A BOARD-APPROVED MONITORED AFTERCARE TREATMENT PROGRAM WHOSE THERAPIST MUST SUBMIT QUARTERLY REPORTS; MUST PARTICIPATE IN A 12-STEP RECOVERY PROGRAM AS DETERMINED BY HIS TREATING THERAPIST AND ATTEND AT LEAST THREE WEEKLY MEETINGS; SHALL OBTAIN A BOARD-APPROVED TREATING PHYSICIAN; SHALL ABSTAIN COMPLETELY FROM THE CONSUMPTION OF ALCOHOLIC BEVERAGES AND DRUGS EXCEPT WHEN PRESCRIBED BY HIS TREATING PHYSICIAN; IF PRESCRIPTION-ONLY MEDICATIONS OR CONTROLLED SUBSTANCES ARE TAKEN, SHALL NOTIFY THE BOARD WITHIN 72 HOURS. MUST SUBMIT TO WITNESSED RANDOM BIOLOGICAL FLUID COLLECTION; KEEP A LOG OF ANY AND ALL MEDICATIONS PRESCRIBED FOR HIM; SHALL SUBMIT TO ANY EXAMINATIONS OR THERAPY ORDERED BY BOARD; SHALL APPEAR BEFORE BOARD FOR INTERVIEWS UPON REQUEST; SHALL INFORM BOARD OF CHANGE OF ADDRESS OR IF AWAY FOR MORE THAN FIVE DAYS. ON 5/15/98 ORDER TERMINATED IN 90 DAYS.

ROMANIA, ANTHONY MD, LICENSE NUMBER 0018642, WAS DISCIPLINED BY ARIZONA ON OCTOBER 20, 1995
DISCIPLINARY ACTION: 36-MONTH PROBATION; FINE
OFFENSE: PROFESSIONAL MISCONDUCT

NOTES: IN 12/92, WHEN NOTIFIED THAT THE BOARD HAD RECEIVED A COMPLAINT ABOUT HIM ATTEMPTED TO DETERMINE WHO PROVIDED THE INFORMATION TO THE BOARD BY PRESSURING EMPLOYEES AND THREATENING THEM WITH THEIR JOBS AND CAUSING ONE EMPLOYEE TO FEAR FOR HER PHYSICAL SAFETY ON ONE OCCASION; BETWEEN 12/92 AND 8/93, HE FIRED OR FORCED TO RESIGN MANY OF THE EMPLOYEES WHO WERE EMPLOYED AT HIS OFFICE AT THE TIME THE INVESTIGATION BEGAN; HIRED TWO PRIVATE INVESTIGATORS TO OBTAIN CONFIDENTIAL INFORMATION REGARDING THE BOARD'S INVESTIGATION; ONE PRIVATE INVESTIGATOR OBTAINED CONFIDENTIAL TELEPHONE RECORDS REGARDING THE HOME PHONE OF ONE OF HIS EMPLOYEES, WHICH SHE BELIEVES WAS AN ATTEMPT TO INTIMIDATE HER INTO CONFESSING WHETHER SHE HAD PROVIDED INFORMATION TO THE BOARD; ANOTHER PRIVATE INVESTIGATOR HIRED BY HIS ATTORNEY CONTACTED EX-EMPLOYEES SUSPECTED OF PROVIDING INFORMATION TO THE BOARD AND OTHER INDIVIDUALS REGARDING THE EX-EMPLOYEES; IN 1992 AND EARLY 1993, SOME EMPLOYEES OF HIS OFFICE OBSERVED HIM EXHIBITING WHAT THEY DESCRIBED AS EXTREME MOOD SWINGS, PRIMARILY BETWEEN ANGER AND DESPAIR/DEPRESSION, ALLEGEDLY SITTING IN HIS OFFICE FOR HOURS AT A TIME, UNABLE TO SEE WAITING PATIENTS, AND RAISING HIS VOICE AT EMPLOYEES AND PATIENTS; IN A PSYCHOLOGICAL EVALUATION IN 5/93, IT WAS CONCLUDED THAT IN THE EVENT THAT THE BOARD FINDS EVIDENCE OF POORLY MODULATED EMOTIONALITY OR LASHING OUT, IT WOULD BENEFIT THE PHYSICIAN TO ENTER PSYCHOTHERAPY; IN 10/93, ORDERED BY THE BOARD TO SUBMIT TO PSYCHIATRIC EVALUATION. IN 10/95, CENSURED. PROBATION WITH CONDITIONS: $3,000 FINE WITHIN 90 DAYS; WITHIN 30 DAYS, SHALL ENTER INTO THERAPY WITH A BOARD-APPROVED THERAPIST REGARDING THE ISSUES OF APPROPRIATE MANAGEMENT OF ANGER, IMPULSE CONTROL, APPROPRIATE INTERPERSONAL RELATIONSHIPS WITH OFFICE STAFF AND OTHER AREAS DEEMED APPROPRIATE BY THE THERAPIST FOR AT LEAST ONE YEAR, FOUR HOURS PER MONTH CONTINUE IN THERAPY AT INTERVALS AND FOR A DURATION DEEMED NECESSARY BY THE THERAPIST; THERAPIST SHALL PROVIDE QUARTERLY REPORTS TO THE BOARD; IN ONE YEAR, SHALL SUBMIT TO A FOLLOW-UP PSYCHOLOGICAL EVALUATION; SHALL MEET WITH THE BOARD UPON REQUEST; SHALL NOT THREATEN, HARASS OR INTIMIDATE ANY EMPLOYEE OR FORMER EMPLOYEE; PERIOD OF PROBATION SHALL BE TOLLED FOR ALL PERIODS OF TIME THAT HE PRACTICES OR RESIDES IN ANY OTHER STATE THAN ARIZONA. ON 7/18/96 HIS REQUEST TO MODIFY OR TERMINATE THE COUNSELING REQUIREMENT OF THIS ORDER WAS DENIED AND HIS CURRENT THERAPIST IS DISAPPROVED; HE IS IMMEDIATELY ORDERED TO OBTAIN A NEW THERAPIST ACCEPTABLE TO BOARD STAFF.

ROSEN, BARUCH MD OF 7555 EAST OSBORN ROAD, SCOTTSDALE,

AZ, WAS DISCIPLINED BY NEW MEXICO ON DECEMBER 16, 1994
DISCIPLINARY ACTION: LICENSE REVOCATION
OFFENSE: DISCIPLINARY ACTION BY ANOTHER STATE OR AGENCY

ROSEN, BARUCH D MD, WAS DISCIPLINED BY NEVADA ON AUGUST 24, 1994
DISCIPLINARY ACTION: LICENSE REVOCATION
OFFENSE: DISCIPLINARY ACTION BY ANOTHER STATE OR AGENCY

NOTES: ACTION TAKEN BY THE ARIZONA MEDICAL BOARD AGAINST HIS ARIZONA MEDICAL LICENSE; FAILURE TO REPORT TO NEVADA BOARD WITHIN 30 DAYS OF THE ACTIONS TAKEN AGAINST HIS ARIZONA LICENSE.

ROSEN, BARUCH D MD OF 7555 EAST OSBORN #206, SCOTTSDALE, AZ, WAS DISCIPLINED BY DEA ON APRIL 20, 1995
DISCIPLINARY ACTION: RESTRICTION PLACED ON CONTROLLED SUBSTANCE LICENSE
OFFENSE: PROFESSIONAL MISCONDUCT

NOTES: PRIOR ALLEGED CONTROLLED SUBSTANCE VIOLATIONS.

ROSEN, BARUCH D MD, DATE OF BIRTH JULY 27, 1941 OF 5407 E ELMWOOD STREET, MESA, AZ, WAS DISCIPLINED BY MEDICARE ON DECEMBER 20, 1998
DISCIPLINARY ACTION: EXCLUSION FROM THE MEDICARE AND/OR MEDICAID PROGRAM
OFFENSE: DISCIPLINARY ACTION BY ANOTHER STATE OR AGENCY

NOTES: LICENSE REVOKED, SUSPENDED, SURRENDERED OR OTHERWISE LOST FOR REASONS BEARING ON PROFESSIONAL PERFORMANCE, PROFESSIONAL COMPETENCE OR FINANCIAL INTEGRITY.

ROSEN, BARUCH DANIEL MD, LICENSE NUMBER 0010880 OF 7555 EAST OSBORN RD #206, SCOTTSDALE, AZ, WAS DISCIPLINED BY ARIZONA ON APRIL 8, 1992
DISCIPLINARY ACTION: LICENSE REVOCATION
OFFENSE: PROVIDING FALSE INFORMATION TO THE BOARD OR OTHER HEALTH AGENCY

NOTES: HAD AT HIS PRACTICE A PHYSICIAN WHO WAS UNLICENSED IN ARIZONA, THEN FALSELY INFORMED THE BOARD THAT THIS DOCTOR WAS NOT PERFORMING PROCEDURES; MAINTAINED INADEQUATE AND/OR FALSE MEDICAL RECORDS SOME OF WHICH STATED HE HAD PERFORMED SURGERY WHICH HE HAD NOT PERFORMED; BILLED PATIENT AND/OR HER INSURANCE CARRIER FOR A PROCEDURE ADVERTISED AS FREE; STATED ON 1988 LICENSE RENEWAL FORM AND IN 1990 BOARD INTERVIEW THAT HE WAS BOARD CERTIFIED WHEN IN FACT HIS CERTIFICATION EXPIRED 12/31/86; MADE FALSE CLAIMS ON HIS BUSINESS CARDS; ADMINISTERED CONTROLLED SUBSTANCES IN 1989 AFTER HAVING SURRENDERED IN MAY 1986 HIS DEA CONTROLLED SUBSTANCES REGISTRATION CERTIFICATE FOR SCHEDULES II AND IIN; THEN LIED TO BOARD ABOUT HIS ACTIONS; PERFORMED GROSSLY NEGLIGENT AND SUBSTANDARD COSMETIC SURGERIES WITHOUT PROPER CONSULTATION WITH PATIENTS. PERMANENT REVOCATION, NO OPPORTUNITY FOR REHEARING OR REVIEW. HE APPEALED THIS PERMANENT REVOCATION BY THE ARIZONA BOARD TO THE SUPERIOR COURT AND THE COURT GRANTED A PARTIAL STAY PENDING APPEAL. ON 5/6/93, SUPERIOR COURT AFFIRMED THE BOARD'S ORDER AND SUBSEQUENTLY GRANTED HIS REQUEST FOR STAY OF THE PERMANENT REVOCATION PENDING FURTHER APPEAL. THE STAY LIMITS HIM TO "PRACTICING TRADITIONAL FAMILY MEDICINE" ONLY. ON 1/24/94, THE BOARD REJECTED A SETTLEMENT PROPOSAL PRESENTED BY DR. ROSEN.

ROSEN, BARUCH DANIEL MD, LICENSE NUMBER 0010880, WAS DISCIPLINED BY ARIZONA ON FEBRUARY 23, 1994
DISCIPLINARY ACTION: 12-MONTH LICENSE SUSPENSION; 60-MONTH PROBATION
OFFENSE: PRACTICING WITHOUT A VALID CONTROLLED SUBSTANCE LICENSE

NOTES: DID NOT RECOMMEND OR SUGGEST THAT ONE OF HIS PATIENTS GO TO A HOSPITAL FOR EVALUATION OR TREATMENT FOR SYMPTOMS FOLLOWING A 7 FOOT FALL; PATIENT WENT INTO CARDIAC ARREST AND WAS TRANSPORTED TO A HOSPITAL EMERGENCY ROOM PRIOR TO DEATH; HAD NO RECORDS FOR THIS PATIENT; VIOLATED 10/15/93 ORDER BY REFUSING THE BOARD ACCESS TO HIS MEDICAL RECORDS FOR AN OFFICE PRACTICE SURVEY; PRESCRIBED SCHEDULE II SUBSTANCES TWICE IN 7/93 WITH NO DEA REGISTRATION. SHALL PROMPTLY TRANSFER PATIENT RECORDS TO OTHER HEALTH CARE PROVIDERS IN ORDER TO PROVIDE CONTINUITY OF PATIENT CARE. RECONSIDERATION WAS DENIED 4/15/94. COURT DISMISSED HIS APPEAL FOR LACK OF JURISDICTION; CASE PENDING IN COURT OF APPEALS. SUSPENSION ENDED IN 2/95. HIS MOTION TO CONSOLIDATE TWO CASES GRANTED 4/19/95; HIS MOTION FOR ORAL ARGUMENT DENIED BY COURTS.

ROSEN, BARUCH DANIEL MD OF 7555 E OSBORN SUITE 206, PHOENIX, AZ, WAS DISCIPLINED BY DEA ON JULY 18, 1994
DISCIPLINARY ACTION: SURRENDER OF CONTROLLED SUBSTANCE LICENSE
OFFENSE: DISCIPLINARY ACTION BY ANOTHER STATE OR AGENCY

NOTES: OTHER STATE.

ROSEN, BARUCH DANIEL MD, LICENSE NUMBER 0G22901 OF MESA, AZ, WAS DISCIPLINED BY CALIFORNIA ON DECEMBER 2, 1996
DISCIPLINARY ACTION: LICENSE REVOCATION
OFFENSE: DISCIPLINARY ACTION BY ANOTHER STATE OR AGENCY

NOTES: DISCIPLINED BY ARIZONA FOR MAKING FALSE AND FRAUDULENT STATEMENTS IN CONNECTION WITH HIS PRACTICE OF MEDICINE; ENGAGING IN CONDUCT DANGEROUS TO HIS PATIENTS; AND ASSISTING AN UNLICENSED PRACTITIONER.

ROSS, MERVYN B MD, LICENSE NUMBER 0010557 OF SCOTTSDALE, AZ, WAS DISCIPLINED BY ARIZONA ON JANUARY 17, 1995

NOTES: SHALL NOT PRACTICE MEDICINE UNTIL HE PROVIDES THE BOARD WITH WRITTEN EVALUATIONS BY BOARD-APPROVED EVALUATORS REGARDING HIS PHYSICAL AND PSYCHOLOGICAL CONDITIONS THAT INDICATE THAT HE IS ABLE TO SAFELY PRACTICE MEDICINE, AND UNTIL FURTHER ORDER OF THE BOARD.

ROZACI, JAROMIR MD, LICENSE NUMBER 15935, WAS DISCIPLINED BY ARIZONA ON MAY 20, 1999

NOTES: ISSUED A DECREE OF CENSURE FOR POSTOPERATIVE MANAGEMENT OF A PATIENT.

RUBIN, MARTIN H MD, LICENSE NUMBER 0012996, WAS DISCIPLINED BY ARIZONA ON APRIL 15, 1993
DISCIPLINARY ACTION: 24-MONTH PROBATION; REQUIRED TO TAKE ADDITIONAL MEDICAL EDUCATION
OFFENSE: SUBSTANDARD CARE, INCOMPETENCE OR NEGLIGENCE

NOTES: FAILED TO PROPERLY TREAT A PATIENT WHOM HE HAD BEEN SEEING FOR FOUR YEARS FOR HYPERTENSIVE CARDIOVASCULAR DISEASE; HE

NEVER IN THAT FOUR YEARS OBTAINED A STRESS TEST OR THALLIUM SCAN WHICH "A REASONABLY PRUDENT DOCTOR WOULD STRONGLY CONSIDER" AND WHEN HE SAW THE PATIENT ON 12/13/89 WITH SYMPTOMS STRONGLY SUGGESTIVE OF PERSISTENT ANGINA; PATIENT SHOULD HAVE BEEN HOSPITALIZED; DR. RUBIN SENT HIM HOME WHERE HE EXPIRED LATER THAT DAY. PROBATION WITH FOLLOWING CONDITIONS: SHALL WITHIN ONE YEAR SUCCESSFULLY COMPLETE A ONE MONTH MINI-RESIDENCY APPROVED BY THE BOARD IN THE FIELD OF CARDIOLOGY AND THAT HE SHALL SIGN ANY RELEASES OR WAIVERS NECESSARY FOR THE BOARD TO RECEIVE INFORMATION FROM THE PROGRAM. IN 18 MONTHS, BOARD SHALL PERFORM A SURVEY OF THE DOCTOR'S PRACTICE WITH AN EMPHASIS ON CARDIOLOGY CASES; SHALL APPEAR BEFORE THE BOARD PRIOR TO THE EXPIRATION OF PROBATION. PROBATION TERMINATED ON 4/7/95.

RUBIN, PHILLIP JULES MD OF 5501 NORTH 19TH AVENUE SUITE 210, PHOENIX, AZ, WAS DISCIPLINED BY DEA ON JULY 19, 1994
DISCIPLINARY ACTION: RESTRICTION PLACED ON CONTROLLED SUBSTANCE LICENSE
OFFENSE: PROFESSIONAL MISCONDUCT

NOTES: PERSONAL MISUSE OF CONTROLLED SUBSTANCES.

RUESCH, MCLAREN MD, LICENSE NUMBER 4852, WAS DISCIPLINED BY ARIZONA ON NOVEMBER 14, 1997
DISCIPLINARY ACTION: REPRIMAND
OFFENSE: PRACTICING WITHOUT A VALID CONTROLLED SUBSTANCE LICENSE

NOTES: FROM 12/95 THROUGH 5/96 DISPENSED TERAMINE, A SCHEDULE IV CONTROLLED SUBSTANCE, WHEN HE WAS NOT REGISTERED BY THE BOARD AS A DISPENSING DOCTOR.

RUIZ, ROBERTO MD, DATE OF BIRTH MAY 26, 1957, LICENSE NUMBER 0014478, WAS DISCIPLINED BY ARIZONA ON JULY 15, 1992
DISCIPLINARY ACTION: FINE
OFFENSE: PROFESSIONAL MISCONDUCT

NOTES: CHARGING A FEE FOR SERVICES NOT RENDERED OR DIVIDING A PROFESSIONAL FEE FOR PATIENT REFERRALS AMONG HEALTH CARE PROVIDERS OR HEALTH CARE INSTITUTIONS OR BETWEEN THESE PROVIDERS AND INSTITUTIONS OR A CONTRACTUAL ARRANGEMENT WHICH HAS THE SAME EFFECT. LACK OF OR INAPPROPRIATE DIRECTION, COLLABORATION OR SUPERVISION OF A LICENSED, CERTIFIED OR REGISTERED HEALTH CARE PROVIDER EMPLOYED BY OR ASSIGNED TO THE PHYSICIAN. CENSURED; SHALL PAY $1000 ADMINISTRATIVE FINE WITHIN 60 DAYS; SHALL BE REEVALUATED IN SIX MONTHS TO DETERMINE WHETHER THIS CONDUCT IS REMEDIED.

RUIZ, ROBERTO MD, DATE OF BIRTH MAY 26, 1957, LICENSE NUMBER 0D28330, WAS DISCIPLINED BY MARYLAND ON MARCH 23, 1993
DISCIPLINARY ACTION: REPRIMAND
OFFENSE: DISCIPLINARY ACTION BY ANOTHER STATE OR AGENCY

NOTES: IN 7/92, ARIZONA MEDICAL BOARD CENSURED HIM FOR UNPROFESSIONAL CONDUCT AND REQUIRED PAYMENT OF $1000 FINE. HE WAS ALSO REQUIRED TO BE REEVALUATED IN 6 MONTHS. SHALL APPEAR BEFORE THE BOARD BEFORE PRACTICING IN MARYLAND.

RUSSELL, MELINDA LOU MD, LICENSE NUMBER 21074, WAS DISCIPLINED BY ARIZONA ON MAY 19, 1997
DISCIPLINARY ACTION: EMERGENCY SUSPENSION
OFFENSE: LOSS OR RESTRICTION OF HOSPITAL PRIVILEGES

NOTES: ON 11/6/96 PLACED ON EMERGENCY 30 DAY SUSPENSION BY UNIVERSITY OF ARIZONA COLLEGE OF MEDICINE ON THE GROUNDS SHE MAY HAVE BEEN UNDER THE INFLUENCE OF ALCOHOL WHEN SHE WAS ON CALL TO THE EMERGENCY DEPARTMENT PENDING AN INVESTIGATION. ON 1/8/97 BOARD REQUESTED SHE SUBMIT TO A PHYSICAL EXAM AND RANDOM URINE TESTING FOR 90 DAYS; ON 4/30/97 SHE TESTED POSITIVE FOR METHAMPHETAMINE IN AMOUNTS CONSISTENT WITH ILLICIT METHAMPHETAMINE USE. ON 7/26/97 THIS SUSPENSION WAS TERMINATED.

RUTGARD, JEFFREY J MD, LICENSE NUMBER 0011096, WAS DISCIPLINED BY ARIZONA ON OCTOBER 20, 1994

NOTES: SHALL NOT ENGAGE IN THE PRACTICE OF MEDICINE IN ARIZONA UNTIL: HE FIRST INFORMS THE ARIZONA BOARD OF MEDICAL EXAMINERS IN WRITING OF HIS INTENTION TO DO SO, APPEARS BEFORE THE BOARD FOR AN INTERVIEW AND RECEIVES AUTHORIZATION OF THE BOARD TO PRACTICE MEDICINE IN THE STATE.

RUTGARD, JEFFREY J MD, LICENSE NUMBER 0021130 OF LA JOLLA, CA, WAS DISCIPLINED BY IOWA ON APRIL 17, 1995
DISCIPLINARY ACTION: LICENSE REVOCATION
OFFENSE: DISCIPLINARY ACTION BY ANOTHER STATE OR AGENCY

NOTES: ACTION TAKEN BY THE CALIFORNIA MEDICAL LICENSING AUTHORITIES FOR HIS CONVICTION IN U.S. DISTRICT COURT. HE WAS FOUND GUILTY OF 132 CRIMINAL VIOLATIONS INCLUDING MAIL FRAUD, FALSE CLAIMS, FALSE STATEMENTS, AND ENGAGING IN MONETARY TRANSACTIONS.

RUTGARD, JEFFREY J MD, WAS DISCIPLINED BY HAWAII ON JANUARY 17, 1996
DISCIPLINARY ACTION: LICENSE REVOCATION
OFFENSE: DISCIPLINARY ACTION BY ANOTHER STATE OR AGENCY

NOTES: INCOMPETENCE OR MULTIPLE INSTANCES OF NEGLIGENCE INCLUDING THE CONSISTENT USE OF SERVICE WHICH WAS INAPPROPRIATE OR UNNECESSARY; ACTION TAKEN BY ANOTHER AGENCY AND FAILURE TO REPORT THIS TO THE BOARD; CONVICTION OR GUILTY PLEA TO A CRIME RELATED TO THE PRACTICE OF MEDICINE.

RUTGARD, JEFFREY J MD, LICENSE NUMBER 0011096, WAS DISCIPLINED BY ARIZONA ON JANUARY 19, 1996
DISCIPLINARY ACTION: LICENSE REVOCATION
OFFENSE: DISCIPLINARY ACTION BY ANOTHER STATE OR AGENCY

NOTES: APPLIED FOR LICENSE RENEWAL IN 12/92 AND FAILED TO FULLY RESPOND TO BOARD'S REQUESTS FOR INFORMATION ABOUT LICENSE SUSPENSION IN CALIFORNIA; STATED THAT LICENSE WAS TEMPORARILY SUSPENDED WHILE HE RESPONDED TO ACCUSATIONS MADE AGAINST HIM BY SEVERAL DISGRUNTLED EX-EMPLOYEES, WHEN IN FACT HIS CALIFORNIA LICENSE WAS NOT BEING INVESTIGATED MERELY DUE TO ALLEGATIONS BY EX-EMPLOYEES, BUT FOR OVER 100 ALLEGATIONS OF FRAUD AND FALSE STATEMENTS RELATED TO HIS MEDICAL PRACTICE AND INSURANCE BILLINGS; IN 6/94, LICENSE REVOKED BY CALIFORNIA BOARD FOR PERFORMING UNNECESSARY SURGERIES THAT WERE FRAUDULENTLY BILLED TO INSURANCE CARRIERS; ON 3/15/95, FOUND GUILTY OF ABOUT 132 COUNTS OF MAIL FRAUD, FALSE CLAIMS, FALSE STATEMENTS AND ENGAGING IN MONEY LAUNDERING INVOLVING HIS

PRACTICE AND INSURANCE BILLINGS; SENTENCED TO PRISON FOR 135 MONTHS AT A FEDERAL PRISON FOLLOWED BY THREE YEARS OF SUPERVISED PROBATION; ORDERED TO MAKE RESTITUTION PAYMENTS OF ABOUT $16 MILLION TO INSURANCE CARRIERS, TO FORFEIT ABOUT $7.5 MILLION AND TO PAY A FINE OF $150,000; FAILED TO NOTIFY BOARD OF CHANGE IN RESIDENCE OR OFFICE ADDRESS AND TELEPHONE NUMBER. PERMANENT REVOCATION; FINAL DECISION WITH NO OPPORTUNITY FOR REHEARING OR REVIEW.

RUTGARD, JEFFREY JAY MD, DATE OF BIRTH DECEMBER 18, 1951, WAS DISCIPLINED BY MEDICARE ON DECEMBER 19, 1995
DISCIPLINARY ACTION: 360-MONTH EXCLUSION FROM THE MEDICARE AND/OR MEDICAID PROGRAM
OFFENSE: CRIMINAL CONVICTION OR PLEA OF GUILTY, NOLO CONTENDERE, OR NO CONTEST TO A CRIME

NOTES: CONVICTED OF A CRIME INVOLVING THE MEDICARE, MEDICAID, MATERNAL AND CHILD HEALTH SERVICES BLOCK GRANT OR BLOCK GRANTS TO STATES FOR SOCIAL SERVICES PROGRAMS.

RUTZ, VIRGINIA DO, LICENSE NUMBER 3090 OF 7601 N CALLE SIN ENVIDIA #54, TUCSON, AZ, WAS DISCIPLINED BY ARIZONA ON OCTOBER 24, 1997
DISCIPLINARY ACTION: EMERGENCY SUSPENSION
OFFENSE: OVERPRESCRIBING OR MISPRESCRIBING DRUGS

NOTES: SHE PRESCRIBED VICODIN FOR ANOTHER DOCTOR WITHOUT APPROPRIATE NOTES AS TO THE REASON IN HER MEDICAL CHARTS; SHE BELIEVED THAT THE DOCTOR SHE WAS PRESCRIBING FOR, HAD A SUBSTANCE ABUSE PROBLEM RELATED TO THE VICODIN, BUT CONTINUED TO SIGN OFF ON HIS REMOVAL OF THE VICODIN FOR HIMSELF BECAUSE OF HIS RIGHT WRIST PAIN; SHE ALSO ADMITTED TO SELF-PRESCRIBING VICODIN ES, ACTING AS BOTH A PATIENT AND PHYSICIAN, TAKING 1-2 VICODIN ES TABLETS PER WORK DAY, AND ALLOWING A NURSE PRACTITIONER TO USE HER PRESCRIPTION PAD AND DRUG ENFORCEMENT ADMINISTRATION NUMBER PRIOR TO A NURSE PRACTITIONER'S PRESCRIBING AUTHORIZATION. SHALL SUBMIT HERSELF FOR SUCH MENTAL, PHYSICAL OR ORAL OR WRITTEN MEDICAL COMPETENCY EXAMINATIONS AS DESIGNATED BY THE BOARD.

RYAN, MARGARET A MD, LICENSE NUMBER 0019523, WAS DISCIPLINED BY ARIZONA ON DECEMBER 12, 1990
DISCIPLINARY ACTION: REQUIRED TO ENTER AN IMPAIRED PHYSICIAN PROGRAM OR SUBSTANCE ABUSE TREATMENT; MONITORING OF PHYSICIAN PERFORMANCE
OFFENSE: SUBSTANCE ABUSE

NOTES: MISUSING CHEMICAL SUBSTANCES. MUST IMMEDIATELY PARTICIPATE IN THE ARIZONA MEDICAL ASSOCIATION'S MONITORED AFTERCARE TREATMENT PROGRAM WHOSE THERAPIST MUST SUBMIT QUARTERLY REPORTS; MUST PARTICIPATE IN 90 12-STEP MEETINGS APPROPRIATE FOR SUBSTANCE ABUSE WITHIN 90 DAYS; MUST THEN PARTICIPATE IN A 12-STEP RECOVERY PROGRAM AND ATTEND A MINIMUM OF THREE WEEKLY MEETINGS; MUST OBTAIN A BOARD APPROVED SOLE TREATING PHYSICIAN; MUST ABSTAIN COMPLETELY FROM THE CONSUMPTION OF ALCOHOL OR OTHER DRUGS; MUST SUBMIT TO RANDOM BIOLOGICAL FLUID TESTING; MUST MAINTAIN A LOG OF ANY MEDICATIONS TAKEN; MUST SUBMIT TO MENTAL, PHYSICAL OR MEDICAL COMPETENCY EXAMS UPON BOARD'S REQUEST; MUST SUBMIT TO ANY THERAPY ORDERED BY BOARD; MUST APPEAR BEFORE THE BOARD FOR INTERVIEWS UPON REQUEST; MUST ADVISE THE BOARD OF CHANGE OF ADDRESS OR IF SHE IS AWAY FOR MORE THAN FIVE DAYS.

RYAN, MARGARET A MD, LICENSE NUMBER 0019523, WAS DISCIPLINED BY ARIZONA ON AUGUST 13, 1991
DISCIPLINARY ACTION: LICENSE SUSPENSION; 120-MONTH PROBATION
OFFENSE: FAILURE TO COMPLY WITH PREVIOUS BOARD ORDER

NOTES: VIOLATION OF A 12/90 BOARD ORDER IN THAT ON 4/8/91, 5/17/91, AND 7/29/91, HER URINE SPECIMENS TESTED POSITIVE FOR ETHANOL. SUSPENSION NOT TO EXCEED 12 MONTHS WHICH MAY BE REDUCED OR TERMINATED IF SHE COMPLIES IN A TIMELY MANNER WITH THE REQUIREMENT THAT ON OR BEFORE 10/1/91, SHALL ENTER INTO A BOARD-APPROVED LONG-TERM RESIDENTIAL CHEMICAL DEPENDENCY REHABILITATION PROGRAM, WHICH SHE SHALL SUCCESSFULLY COMPLETE PRIOR TO 8/9/92. MUST IMMEDIATELY PARTICIPATE IN A BOARD-APPROVED MONITORED AFTERCARE TREATMENT PROGRAM WHOSE THERAPIST MUST SUBMIT QUARTERLY REPORTS; MUST PARTICIPATE IN 90 12-STEP MEETINGS FOR SUBSTANCE ABUSE WITHIN 90 DAYS; MUST THEN PARTICIPATE IN A 12-STEP RECOVERY PROGRAM AND ATTEND AT LEAST THREE WEEKLY MEETINGS; SHALL OBTAIN A BOARD-APPROVED TREATING PHYSICIAN; SHALL ABSTAIN COMPLETELY FROM THE CONSUMPTION OF ALCOHOLIC BEVERAGES AND DRUGS EXCEPT WHEN PRESCRIBED BY HER TREATING PHYSICIAN; MUST SUBMIT TO WITNESSED RANDOM BIOLOGICAL FLUID COLLECTION; SHALL KEEP A LOG OF ANY AND ALL MEDICATIONS PRESCRIBED FOR HER; SHALL SUBMIT TO ANY EXAMINATIONS OR THERAPY ORDERED BY BOARD; SHALL APPEAR BEFORE BOARD FOR INTERVIEWS UPON REQUEST; SHALL INFORM BOARD OF CHANGE OF ADDRESS OR IF AWAY FOR MORE THAN FIVE DAYS.

RYAN, MARGARET A MD, LICENSE NUMBER 0019523, WAS DISCIPLINED BY ARIZONA ON JULY 18, 1992
DISCIPLINARY ACTION: 120-MONTH PROBATION; REQUIRED TO ENTER AN IMPAIRED PHYSICIAN PROGRAM OR SUBSTANCE ABUSE TREATMENT
OFFENSE: FAILURE TO COMPLY WITH PREVIOUS BOARD ORDER

NOTES: VIOLATED PREVIOUS BOARD ORDER DATED 12/18/90 REQUIRING HER TO ABSTAIN FROM THE CONSUMPTION OF ALCOHOL. TESTED POSITIVE FOR ALCOHOL IN HER URINE ON 4/8/91, 5/17/91, AND 7/29/91. AN 8/9/91 PROBATION ORDER REQUIRED HER TO ENTER LONG-TERM TREATMENT FOR CHEMICAL DEPENDENCY BEFORE 10/1/91. LICENSE EXPIRED ON 5/1/92 DUE TO NON-PAYMENT OF RENEWAL FEES; WAS REISSUED LICENSE WHEN APPLIED. ALSO ON 5/1/92 ENTERED LONG-TERM TREATMENT FOR ALCOHOL ADDICTION WHICH WAS COMPLETED 7/92. MUST IMMEDIATELY PARTICIPATE IN A BOARD-APPROVED MONITORED AFTERCARE TREATMENT PROGRAM WHOSE THERAPIST MUST SUBMIT QUARTERLY REPORTS; MUST PARTICIPATE IN 90 12-STEP MEETINGS FOR SUBSTANCE ABUSE WITHIN 90 DAYS; MUST THEN PARTICIPATE IN A 12-STEP RECOVERY PROGRAM AS DETERMINED BY HER TREATING THERAPIST AND ATTEND AT LEAST THREE WEEKLY MEETINGS; SHALL OBTAIN A BOARD-APPROVED TREATING PHYSICIAN; SHALL ABSTAIN COMPLETELY FROM THE CONSUMPTION OF ALCOHOLIC BEVERAGES AND DRUGS EXCEPT WHEN PRESCRIBED BY HER TREATING PHYSICIAN; MUST

SUBMIT TO WITNESSED RANDOM BIOLOGICAL FLUID COLLECTION; KEEP A LOG OF ANY AND ALL MEDICATIONS PRESCRIBED FOR HER; SHALL SUBMIT TO ANY EXAMINATIONS OR THERAPY ORDERED BY BOARD; SHALL APPEAR BEFORE BOARD FOR INTERVIEWS UPON REQUEST; SHALL INFORM BOARD OF CHANGE OF ADDRESS OR IF AWAY FOR MORE THAN 5 DAYS.

SACKS, ALAN CHASBY MD, LICENSE NUMBER 0009475 OF PHOENIX, AZ, WAS DISCIPLINED BY ARIZONA ON JANUARY 19, 1993
OFFENSE: SUBSTANDARD CARE, INCOMPETENCE OR NEGLIGENCE

NOTES: FAILED TO MAINTAIN ADEQUATE MEDICAL RECORDS AND FAILED TO ORDER TESTS IN RESPONSE TO MEDICAL FINDING OF POSSIBLE CANCER AFTER A 06/01/82 MAMMOGRAM. THIS CONSTITUTED NEGLIGENCE. PATIENT LATER UNDERWENT A MODIFIED RADICAL MASTECTOMY WHICH COULD HAVE BEEN AVOIDED. CENSURED. ON 04/15/93 HIS REQUEST FOR RECONSIDERATION WAS DENIED. ON 1/27/94 BOARD WAS INFORMED THAT THE SUPERIOR COURT AFFIRMED THIS ACTION.

SACKS, ALAN CHASBY MD, LICENSE NUMBER 0009475, WAS DISCIPLINED BY ARIZONA ON JULY 20, 1995
DISCIPLINARY ACTION: RESTRICTION PLACED ON LICENSE
OFFENSE: PROFESSIONAL MISCONDUCT

NOTES: INTERVIEWED BY BOARD RELATIVE TO MALPRACTICE CLAIM ALLEGING UNSATISFACTORY RESULT FOLLOWING A RHINOPLASTY. SHALL NOT PERFORM NASAL COSMETIC SURGERY UNTIL FURTHER ORDER 0F THE BOARD.

SAIKEWICZ, JARROWLAW R MD, WAS DISCIPLINED BY ARIZONA ON NOVEMBER 20, 1998
DISCIPLINARY ACTION: RESTRICTION PLACED ON LICENSE

NOTES: LIMITED LICENSE GRANTED, AS LONG AS HE STIPULATES THAT HE WILL NOT PRACTICE OUTSIDE OF HIS SPECIALTY. ON 1/27/99 BOARD GRANTED STATE'S MOTION FOR REHEARING.

SAINZ, GILBERT R MD, LICENSE NUMBER 0C31264 OF SACRAMENTO, CA, WAS DISCIPLINED BY CALIFORNIA ON DECEMBER 31, 1993
DISCIPLINARY ACTION: 84-MONTH PROBATION
OFFENSE: SEXUAL ABUSE OF OR SEXUAL MISCONDUCT WITH A PATIENT

NOTES: SEXUAL RELATIONS WITH A PATIENT. REVOCATION STAYED.

SAINZ, GILBERT RAY MD, LICENSE NUMBER 0004651, WAS DISCIPLINED BY ARIZONA ON APRIL 16, 1996
DISCIPLINARY ACTION: LICENSE REVOCATION
OFFENSE: PROVIDING FALSE INFORMATION TO THE BOARD OR OTHER HEALTH AGENCY

NOTES: IN 12/91, IN AN APPLICATION FOR A MEDICAL STAFF APPOINTMENT, HE ANSWERED "NO" TO A QUESTION REGARDING WHETHER HE WAS CURRENTLY UNDER INVESTIGATION OR WHETHER HE HAD EVER BEEN SUBJECT TO DISCIPLINARY ACTION, DESPITE HIS AWARENESS THAT HE WAS UNDER INVESTIGATION AT THE TIME BY THE CALIFORNIA BOARD; ON THE APPLICATION, HE ALSO ANSWERED "NO" TO A QUESTION ABOUT WHETHER HE HAD EVER WITHDRAWN HIS APPLICATION OR RESIGNED FROM EMPLOYMENT IN LIEU OF BEING DENIED MEMBERSHIP OR PRIVILEGES OR SUBJECT TO DISCIPLINARY ACTION, DESPITE THE FACT THAT HE HAD BEEN ASKED TO RESIGN FROM A POSITION IN CALIFORNIA IN 10/91 DUE TO HIS ROMANTIC INVOLVEMENT WITH A FEMALE PATIENT BEGINNING IN 1983 AND LASTING BETWEEN ONE AND TWO YEARS. SHALL SURRENDER LICENSE FOR CANCELLATION WITH CAUSE.

SAINZ, GILBERT RAY MD, LICENSE NUMBER C31264 OF IONE, CA, WAS DISCIPLINED BY CALIFORNIA ON MARCH 19, 1999
DISCIPLINARY ACTION: PROBATION
OFFENSE: DISCIPLINARY ACTION BY ANOTHER STATE OR AGENCY

NOTES: DISCIPLINED BY ARIZONA FOR MAKING FALSE STATEMENTS IN AN APPLICATION FOR PRACTICE PRIVILEGES, AND VIOLATED THE TERMS AND CONDITIONS OF CALIFORNIA PROBATIONARY ORDER BY FAILING TO REPORT THE ARIZONA ACTION TO THE CALIFORNIA BOARD. ADDITIONAL TERMS AND CONDITIONS ADDED TO CURRENT PROBATIONARY ORDER.

SALAZAR, ROBERTO GONZALES DR, LICENSE NUMBER 0016337, WAS DISCIPLINED BY ARIZONA ON JULY 15, 1994
DISCIPLINARY ACTION: LICENSE SUSPENSION
OFFENSE: NONCOMPLIANCE WITH A PROFESSIONAL RULE

NOTES: FAILURE TO PAY RENEWAL FEE DURING PENDING INVESTIGATION.

SAMPAT, JULI N MD, WAS DISCIPLINED BY ARIZONA ON SEPTEMBER 24, 1998
DISCIPLINARY ACTION: REQUIRED TO TAKE ADDITIONAL MEDICAL EDUCATION
OFFENSE: NONCOMPLIANCE WITH A PROFESSIONAL RULE

NOTES: LACK OF DOCUMENTATION OF PATIENT CARE IN THE EMERGENCY ROOM. MUST UNDERTAKE AN ON-SITE MINI RESIDENCY, APPROVED BY THE BOARD, IN EMERGENCY MEDICAL CARE AND TRAUMA CARE MANAGEMENT OF AT LEAST 40 HOURS OF CONTINUING MEDICAL EDUCATION WITHIN SIX MONTHS.

SAMPAT, SUSHILA J MD, LICENSE NUMBER 0013380, WAS DISCIPLINED BY ARIZONA ON MAY 1, 1996
DISCIPLINARY ACTION: LICENSE SUSPENSION
OFFENSE: PHYSICAL OR MENTAL ILLNESS INHIBITING THE ABILITY TO PRACTICE WITH SKILL AND SAFETY

NOTES: UNABLE TO COMPLY WITH 10/18/95 BOARD ORDER IN THAT SUFFERS FROM SEVERE MIGRAINE AND ATYPICAL BIPOLAR DISORDER. LICENSE PLACED IN INACTIVE STATUS; AGREES NOT TO PRACTICE MEDICINE IN ARIZONA OR ANY OTHER JURISDICTION WHILE LICENSE IS INACTIVE; UNDERSTANDS MAY NOT HOLD OR MAINTAIN A CONTROLLED SUBSTANCE CERTIFICATE WITH THE DRUG ENFORCEMENT ADMINISTRATION OR WRITE OR REFILL PRESCRIPTIONS WHILE LICENSE IS INACTIVE; SHALL NOT REQUEST REACTIVATION OF LICENSE UNTIL MEETS WITH THE BOARD AND COMPLIES WITH ALL REQUESTS; BOARD WILL NOT REACTIVATE LICENSE UNTIL SHE PRESENTS TO THE BOARD THAT SHE IS MEDICALLY COMPETENT AND MENTALLY AND PHYSICALLY ABLE TO SAFELY PRACTICE MEDICINE, THAT SHE HAS PASSED THE SPECIAL PURPOSE EXAMINATION AND AN ORAL COMPETENCY EXAMINATION WITH THE BOARD.

SANDERS, MARC R MD, LICENSE NUMBER 11039, WAS DISCIPLINED BY ARIZONA ON MAY 15, 1998
DISCIPLINARY ACTION: LICENSE SUSPENSION
OFFENSE: FAILURE TO COMPLY WITH PREVIOUS BOARD ORDER

NOTES: VIOLATED THE TERMS OF HIS REHABILITATION AND STIPULATION ORDER OF 2/12/98. AGREES NOT TO PRACTICE MEDICINE IN ARIZONA OR ANY OTHER STATE WHILE HIS ARIZONA LICENSE IS IN INACTIVE STATUS; MAY NOT HOLD OR MAINTAIN A CONTROLLED SUBSTANCE CERTIFICATE WITH THE DRUG ENFORCEMENT ADMINISTRATION OR WRITE OR REFILL PRESCRIPTIONS AS LONG AS LICENSE IS CLASSIFIED AS INACTIVE; PRIOR TO HIS LICENSE BEING PLACED ON INACTIVE STATUS, HE AGREES THAT HE SHALL HAVE PAID ALL FEES REQUIRED BY THE MEDICAL PRACTICE ACT; SHALL NOT REQUEST REACTIVATION OF HIS LICENSE TO PRACTICE MEDICINE IN ARIZONA UNTIL HE MEETS WITH THE BOARD AT A REGULARLY SCHEDULED MEETING AND COMPLIES WITH ALL REQUESTS OF THE BOARD WHICH MAY INCLUDE INPATIENT TREATMENT, PSYCHIATRIC AND PSYCHOMETRIC EVALUATION, PHYSICAL EXAMINATION AND TESTING AND WRITTEN AND/OR ORAL COMPETENCY EXAMINATIONS; THE BOARD WILL NOT REACTIVATE HIS LICENSE UNTIL HE PRESENTS EVIDENCE SATISFACTORY TO THE BOARD THAT HE IS MEDICALLY COMPETENT AND MENTALLY AND PHYSICALLY ABLE TO SAFELY PRACTICE MEDICINE.

SANDERS, MARC R MD, DATE OF BIRTH AUGUST 26, 1946 OF 5402 E PARADISE DRIVE, SCOTTSDALE, AZ, WAS DISCIPLINED BY MEDICARE ON APRIL 20, 1999
DISCIPLINARY ACTION: EXCLUSION FROM THE MEDICARE AND/OR MEDICAID PROGRAM
OFFENSE: DISCIPLINARY ACTION BY ANOTHER STATE OR AGENCY

NOTES: LICENSE REVOKED, SUSPENDED, SURRENDERED OR OTHERWISE LOST FOR REASONS BEARING ON PROFESSIONAL PERFORMANCE, PROFESSIONAL COMPETENCE OR FINANCIAL INTEGRITY.

SANTIAGO, OSVALDO JOSE DR, LICENSE NUMBER 0017855, WAS DISCIPLINED BY ARIZONA ON JULY 15, 1994
DISCIPLINARY ACTION: LICENSE SUSPENSION
OFFENSE: NONCOMPLIANCE WITH A PROFESSIONAL RULE

NOTES: FAILURE TO PAY RENEWAL FEE DURING PENDING INVESTIGATION.

SANTINI, JUDITH J MD, LICENSE NUMBER 0019946 OF PHOENIX, AZ, WAS DISCIPLINED BY ARIZONA ON JANUARY 26, 1994
DISCIPLINARY ACTION: MONITORING OF PHYSICIAN PERFORMANCE

NOTES: SHALL CONTINUE IN GROUP OR INDIVIDUAL THERAPY WITH THERAPIST APPROVED BY BOARD WITH QUARTERLY REPORTS REGARDING HER COMPLIANCE WITH MEDICATION PROTOCOL, HER MENTAL HEALTH STATUS, AND HER ABILITY TO SAFELY PRACTICE MEDICINE. ON 10/20/95 ORDER TERMINATED.

SAULTS, CHARLES J MD, LICENSE NUMBER 3175, WAS DISCIPLINED BY ARIZONA ON MAY 8, 1997
DISCIPLINARY ACTION: REPRIMAND
OFFENSE: SUBSTANDARD CARE, INCOMPETENCE OR NEGLIGENCE

NOTES: IN SEVEN OF HIS PATIENTS DURING 1995 WHEN A PHARMACY SURVEY WAS DONE THE FOLLOWING DEFICIENCIES WERE FOUND: FAILED TO NOTE OBJECTIVE FINDINGS ON THE MAJORITY OF EXAMINATIONS CONDUCTED ON ALL THESE PATIENTS; GAVE KENALOG INJECTIONS TO A PATIENT ON SEVERAL OCCASIONS WITHOUT MAKING ANY ATTEMPT TO USE MORE STANDARD THERAPY; FAILED TO DETERMINE WHAT SIDE A PATIENT'S NEURALGIA WAS ON, FAILED TO NOTE MEDICATIONS SHE HAD TAKEN PREVIOUSLY FOR IT AND FAILED TO NOTE WHAT PRECIPITATING FACTORS MAY HAVE BEEN PRESENT; IN ANOTHER PATIENT FAILED TO PROVIDE NON STEROIDAL ANTI-INFLAMMATORY DRUGS PRIOR TO EMBARKING ON A COURSE OF TREATMENT INVOLVING NARCOTICS.

SAVAJIYANI, RAJENDRAKUMAR D MD, LICENSE NUMBER 0011928 OF GLENDALE, AZ, WAS DISCIPLINED BY ARIZONA ON JANUARY 17, 1995
OFFENSE: SUBSTANDARD CARE, INCOMPETENCE OR NEGLIGENCE

NOTES: MALPRACTICE CLAIM ALLEGING THAT HE MADE AN INACCURATE DIAGNOSIS; UNPROFESSIONAL CONDUCT; CONDUCT THAT IS GROSS NEGLIGENCE, REPEATED NEGLIGENCE OR NEGLIGENCE RESULTING IN HARM TO OR THE DEATH OF A PATIENT IN THAT ON 8/6/89 HE DID NOT INITIATE AN INVESTIGATION OF THE CAUSE OF INCREASED SYMPTOMS IN A PATIENT, WHOM HE HAD BEEN TREATING IN THE HOSPITAL, WHO LATER DIED OF RESPIRATORY ARREST. CENSURED.

SAVAJIYANT, RAJ DHIRAJLAL MD, LICENSE NUMBER 0139460 OF 5620 W THUNDERBIRD ROAD, GLENDALE, AZ, WAS DISCIPLINED BY NEW YORK ON DECEMBER 22, 1995
DISCIPLINARY ACTION: REPRIMAND
OFFENSE: DISCIPLINARY ACTION BY ANOTHER STATE OR AGENCY

NOTES: ACTION IN ARIZONA FOR HIS NEGLIGENCE AND INCOMPETENCE IN NOT INVESTIGATING THE INCREASED SYMPTOMS OF A PATIENT WHO LATER DIED DUE TO CARDIAC ARREST.

SAVETAMAL, CHAROEN MD, LICENSE NUMBER 0012858 OF AVONDALE, AZ, WAS DISCIPLINED BY ARIZONA ON OCTOBER 19, 1994
DISCIPLINARY ACTION: RESTRICTION PLACED ON LICENSE

NOTES: SHALL NOT PROVIDE CARE OR TREATMENT TO ANY INFANT IN THE HOSPITAL OR AT HIS OFFICE WITHIN THE FIRST ONE-MONTH OF THE INFANT'S LIFE. SHALL TAKE AND PASS THE SPECIAL PURPOSE EXAMINATION IN 12/94 WITH A SCORE OF 75 OR GREATER. HIS REQUEST FOR RECONSIDERATION DENIED ON 4/07/95.

SAVETAMAL, CHAROEN MD, LICENSE NUMBER 0012858, WAS DISCIPLINED BY ARIZONA ON APRIL 19, 1996
DISCIPLINARY ACTION: RESTRICTION PLACED ON LICENSE

NOTES: MEDICAL PRACTICE SHALL CLOSE BY 7/31/96; SHALL PROVIDE NOTICE TO ALL PATIENTS AT LEAST 60 DAYS IN ADVANCE AND SHALL PROVIDE FOR THE TRANSFER OF PATIENT MEDICAL RECORDS; SHALL LIMIT HIS PRACTICE TO ASSISTING IN SURGERY UNDER THE DIRECT SUPERVISION OF A PRIMARY SURGEON LICENSED IN ARIZONA; SHALL NOT ENGAGE OR ASSIST IN ANY SORT OF EXPERIMENTAL SURGERY; SHALL NOT PERFORM ANY SURGERY BY HIMSELF; LICENSE WILL BE INACTIVATED ON 5/10/98, WHEN HE CERTIFIES THAT HE WILL BE RETIRED FROM MEDICINE.

SAVETAMAL, NGAMPEN B MD, LICENSE NUMBER 0015866, WAS DISCIPLINED BY ARIZONA ON APRIL 9, 1990
DISCIPLINARY ACTION: RESTRICTION PLACED ON LICENSE

NOTES: MUST NOT PROVIDE NEONATAL CARE, INCLUSIVE OF NORMAL NEWBORNS, OR NEWBORNS DELIVERED BY CESAREANS. ON 4/16/93 BOARD ADDED THE FOLLOWING CONDITION TO CLARIFY ORDER: SHALL NOT PROVIDE CARE OR TREATMENT TO ANY INFANT IN THE HOSPITAL OR AT HER OFFICE WITHIN THE

FIRST 28 DAYS OF THE INFANT'S LIFE; SHALL WITHIN ONE YEAR SUCCESSFULLY COMPLETE A ONE MONTH MINI-RESIDENCY ACCEPTABLE TO THE BOARD IN THE CARE AND TREATMENT OF INFANTS UP TO ONE YEAR OLD WHICH SHALL INCLUDE SUCCESSFUL COMPLETION OF ADVANCED LIFE SUPPORT TRAINING; SHALL MEET WITH THE BOARD UPON COMPLETION OF THE MINI-RESIDENCY PROGRAM. ON 1/20/95 ORDER WAS TERMINATED.

SAYEGH, ABRAHAM MD, WAS DISCIPLINED BY ARIZONA ON JANUARY 27, 1999
DISCIPLINARY ACTION: 60-MONTH PROBATION; RESTRICTION PLACED ON CONTROLLED SUBSTANCE LICENSE

NOTES: SHALL TAKE AND PASS THE SPEX EXAM WITHIN 90 DAYS AT HIS EXPENSE, AFTER WHICH HIS LICENSE WILL BE REACTIVATED ON PROBATION WITH THE FOLLOWING TERMS AND CONDITIONS: SHALL PARTICIPATE IN THE MONITORED AFTER CARE PROGRAM; SHALL NOT PRESCRIBE, ADMINISTER, DISPENSE, ORDER OR POSSESS ANY CONTROLLED SUBSTANCES EXCEPT FOR THOSE LISTED IN SCHEDULE IV AND V; MAY NOT REAPPLY FOR SCHEDULES II AND III WITHOUT BOARD PERMISSION BUT MAY ISSUE HOSPITAL ORDERS FOR THEM; EACH YEAR FOR TWO YEARS, HE SHALL OBTAIN 30 HOURS OF CONTINUING MEDICAL EDUCATION IN PRESCRIBING CONTROLLED SUBSTANCES; SHALL SUBMIT QUARTERLY DECLARATIONS SHOWING HIS COMPLIANCE WITH ALL THE CONDITIONS OF THE PROBATION; SHALL KEEP THE BOARD INFORMED OF HIS ADDRESS; IF HE LEAVES ARIZONA HE SHALL NOTIFY THE BOARD IN WRITING WITHIN 10 DAYS; SHALL APPEAR BEFORE THE BOARD UPON REQUEST.

SAYEGH, ABRAHAM MD OF 18404 NORTH TATUM BLVD. #201, PHOENIX, AZ, WAS DISCIPLINED BY DEA ON OCTOBER 6, 1999
DISCIPLINARY ACTION: SURRENDER OF CONTROLLED SUBSTANCE LICENSE
OFFENSE: PROFESSIONAL MISCONDUCT

NOTES: ARRESTED FOR OBTAINING CONTROLLED SUBSTANCES BY FRAUD AND DECEIT.

SAYEGH, ABRAHAM J MD, LICENSE NUMBER 0018816, WAS DISCIPLINED BY ARIZONA ON NOVEMBER 19, 1990
DISCIPLINARY ACTION: REQUIRED TO ENTER AN IMPAIRED PHYSICIAN PROGRAM OR SUBSTANCE ABUSE TREATMENT; MONITORING OF PHYSICIAN PERFORMANCE
OFFENSE: SUBSTANCE ABUSE

NOTES: MUST IMMEDIATELY PARTICIPATE IN ARIZONA MEDICAL ASSOCIATION'S MONITORED AFTERCARE TREATMENT PROGRAM WITH QUARTERLY REPORTS TO THE BOARD; MUST PARTICIPATE IN 90 12-STEP MEETINGS APPROPRIATE FOR SUBSTANCE ABUSE WITHIN 90 DAYS; MUST THEN PARTICIPATE IN A 12-STEP RECOVERY PROGRAM DETERMINED BY THERAPIST AND ATTEND AT LEAST 3 WEEKLY MEETINGS; MUST OBTAIN A BOARD APPROVED TREATING PHYSICIAN; MUST ABSTAIN COMPLETELY FROM ALCOHOL AND ALL OTHER DRUGS; MUST COMPLY WITH REQUESTS FOR RANDOM BIOLOGICAL FLUID TESTS; MUST MAINTAIN A LOG OF ALL MEDICATIONS TAKEN; MUST SUBMIT TO ANY EXAMS OR THERAPY ORDERED BY BOARD; MUST APPEAR BEFORE BOARD FOR INTERVIEWS UPON REQUEST; MUST ADVISE BOARD OF CHANGE IN OFFICE OR HOME ADDRESSES OR IF PLANS TO BE AWAY FOR MORE THAN FIVE DAYS. ON 10/16/93 ORDER TERMINATED AFTER 90 DAYS.

SAYEGH, ABRAHAM J MD, LICENSE NUMBER 18816, WAS DISCIPLINED BY ARIZONA ON MARCH 13, 1997
DISCIPLINARY ACTION: 60-MONTH PROBATION; RESTRICTION PLACED ON CONTROLLED SUBSTANCE LICENSE
OFFENSE: OVERPRESCRIBING OR MISPRESCRIBING DRUGS

NOTES: BETWEEN 11/94 ND 12/96 PRESCRIBED LARGE AMOUNTS OF CONTROLLED SUBSTANCES MAINLY VICODIN OR OXYCODONE TO THREE PATIENTS; IN ONE CASE, HIS MEDICAL RECORDS DO NOT SHOW THAT HE OBTAINED ANY CONSULTATION TO SUBSTANTIATE THE NEED FOR 95 PRESCRIPTIONS OF CONTROLLED SUBSTANCES; MANY OF THE PRESCRIPTIONS WERE NOT DOCUMENTED IN THE PATIENTS' CHART AND MANY WERE MADE BY PHONE WITHOUT SEEING THE PATIENTS; WHEN AN INVESTIGATOR MADE AN UNANNOUNCED VISIT TO HIS CLINIC, IN 1/97 HE SAID HE DID NOT MAINTAIN RECORDS OF THE PRESCRIPTIONS IN QUESTION AS THE PATIENTS WERE FRIENDS OF HIS. CONDITIONS OF PROBATION ARE AS FOLLOWS: WITHIN SEVEN DAYS, HE SHALL SURRENDER CONTROLLED SUBSTANCE REGISTRATION CERTIFICATE FOR SCHEDULES II AND III AND PROVIDE WRITTEN EVIDENCE OF THE SURRENDER TO THE BOARD; SHALL NOT REAPPLY FOR THESE REGISTRATIONS FOR ONE YEAR; HE MAY, HOWEVER, ISSUE HOSPITAL ORDERS FOR SCHEDULES II OR III SUBSTANCES FOR HOSPITALIZED PATIENTS, USING THE HOSPITAL'S DEA NUMBER AS PERMITTED BY LAW; SHALL COMPLY WITH REQUESTS FROM BOARD TO SUBMIT TO WITNESSED BIOLOGICAL FLUID COLLECTION; EACH YEAR FOR TWO YEARS SHALL OBTAIN 30 HOURS OF CONTINUING MEDICAL EDUCATION IN PRESCRIBING CONTROLLED SUBSTANCES; SHALL IMMEDIATELY OBTAIN A THERAPIST APPROVED BY THE BOARD AND SHALL REMAIN IN TREATMENT WITH THE THERAPIST UNTIL FURTHER ORDER OF THE BOARD WITH QUARTERLY REPORTS; ISSUED A DECREE OF CENSURE. ON 3/28/98 THIS ORDER WAS CONTINUED, WITH EIGHT HOURS OF CONTINUING MEDICAL EDUCATION REQUIREMENTS WAIVED.

SAYEGH, ABRAHAM J MD, LICENSE NUMBER 18816, WAS DISCIPLINED BY ARIZONA ON MAY 15, 1998
DISCIPLINARY ACTION: LICENSE SUSPENSION
OFFENSE: SUBSTANCE ABUSE

NOTES: IMPAIRED BY ALCOHOL OR DRUG ABUSE. AGREES NOT TO PRACTICE MEDICINE IN ARIZONA OR ANY OTHER STATE WHILE HIS ARIZONA LICENSE IS IN INACTIVE STATUS; MAY NOT HOLD OR MAINTAIN A CONTROLLED SUBSTANCE CERTIFICATE WITH THE DRUG ENFORCEMENT ADMINISTRATION OR WRITE OR REFILL PRESCRIPTIONS AS LONG AS LICENSE IS CLASSIFIED AS INACTIVE; SHALL PAY ALL FEES REQUIRED BY THE MEDICAL PRACTICE ACT, PRIOR TO HIS LICENSE BEING PLACED ON INACTIVE STATUS; SHALL NOT REQUEST REACTIVATION OF HIS LICENSE TO PRACTICE UNTIL HE MEETS WITH THE BOARD AND COMPLIES WITH ALL REQUESTS WHICH MAY INCLUDE INPATIENT TREATMENT, PSYCHIATRIC AND PSYCHOMETRIC EVALUATION, PHYSICAL EXAMINATION AND TESTING AND WRITTEN AND/OR ORAL COMPETENCY EXAMINATIONS. PLACED ON INACTIVE STATUS.

SAYEGH, ABRAHAM JOSEPH MD, LICENSE NUMBER 173788 OF 14018 NORTH 30TH STREET, PHOENIX, AZ, WAS DISCIPLINED BY NEW YORK ON NOVEMBER 19, 1997
DISCIPLINARY ACTION: SURRENDER OF LICENSE
OFFENSE: DISCIPLINARY ACTION BY ANOTHER STATE OR AGENCY

NOTES: DISCIPLINED BY THE ARIZONA BOARD FOR

PRESCRIBING AND/OR DISPENSING A CONTROLLED SUBSTANCE FOR OTHER THAN THERAPEUTIC PURPOSES; FAILING TO MAINTAIN ADEQUATE PATIENT RECORDS.

SCALICI, TONY F DO, DATE OF BIRTH OCTOBER 14, 1951 OF 6864 MAPLECREST SE, GRAND RAPIDS, MI, WAS DISCIPLINED BY MEDICARE ON DECEMBER 3, 1990
DISCIPLINARY ACTION: 60-MONTH EXCLUSION FROM THE MEDICARE AND/OR MEDICAID PROGRAM
OFFENSE: CRIMINAL CONVICTION OR PLEA OF GUILTY, NOLO CONTENDERE, OR NO CONTEST TO A CRIME

NOTES: CONVICTION RELATING TO CONTROLLED SUBSTANCES.

SCALICI, TONY F DO, DATE OF BIRTH OCTOBER 14, 1951, LICENSE NUMBER 0007093 OF 5491 S DIVISION, WYOMING, MI, WAS DISCIPLINED BY MICHIGAN ON JUNE 3, 1993
DISCIPLINARY ACTION: SURRENDER OF LICENSE

NOTES: VOLUNTARY SURRENDER OF LICENSE PENDING CONCLUSION OF PROCEEDINGS PENDING IN U.S. DISTRICT COURT -- WESTERN DISTRICT.

SCALICI, TONY F DO, DATE OF BIRTH OCTOBER 14, 1951, LICENSE NUMBER 0007093 OF 5491 S DIVISION, WYOMING, MI, WAS DISCIPLINED BY MICHIGAN ON DECEMBER 2, 1993
DISCIPLINARY ACTION: LICENSE REVOCATION
OFFENSE: CRIMINAL CONVICTION OR PLEA OF GUILTY, NOLO CONTENDERE, OR NO CONTEST TO A CRIME

NOTES: CONVICTION/DRUG RELATED.

SCALICI, TONY F DO, DATE OF BIRTH OCTOBER 14, 1951 OF 6864 MAPLECREST SE, GRAND RAPIDS, MI, WAS DISCIPLINED BY MEDICARE ON MAY 5, 1994
DISCIPLINARY ACTION: 60-MONTH EXCLUSION FROM THE MEDICARE AND/OR MEDICAID PROGRAM
OFFENSE: CRIMINAL CONVICTION OR PLEA OF GUILTY, NOLO CONTENDERE, OR NO CONTEST TO A CRIME

NOTES: CONVICTED OF A CRIME RELATED TO THE UNLAWFUL MANUFACTURE OF A CONTROLLED SUBSTANCE.

SCALICI, TONY F DO, LICENSE NUMBER 1537 OF 330 E. FULTON STREET, GRAND RAPIDS, MI, WAS DISCIPLINED BY ARIZONA ON NOVEMBER 4, 1999
DISCIPLINARY ACTION: LICENSE REVOCATION
OFFENSE: DISCIPLINARY ACTION BY ANOTHER STATE OR AGENCY

NOTES: IN 12/93 MICHIGAN LICENSE REVOKED DUE TO FELONY CONVICTION FOR USING, DELIVERING, AND/OR DISTRIBUTING CONTROLLED SUBSTANCES FOR OTHER THAN LEGITIMATE PURPOSES IN 1990.

SCHAUT, DAVID JOHN DR, LICENSE NUMBER 0019236, WAS DISCIPLINED BY ARIZONA ON JULY 15, 1994
DISCIPLINARY ACTION: LICENSE SUSPENSION
OFFENSE: NONCOMPLIANCE WITH A PROFESSIONAL RULE

NOTES: FAILURE TO PAY RENEWAL FEE DURING PENDING INVESTIGATION.

SCHIEVE, DONALD R MD, DATE OF BIRTH FEBRUARY 23, 1933 OF 1800 HWY 95, #4, BULLHEAD CITY, AZ, WAS DISCIPLINED BY MEDICARE ON JUNE 18, 1998
DISCIPLINARY ACTION: EXCLUSION FROM THE MEDICARE AND/OR MEDICAID PROGRAM
OFFENSE: DISCIPLINARY ACTION BY ANOTHER STATE OR AGENCY

NOTES: LICENSE REVOKED, SUSPENDED, SURRENDERED OR OTHERWISE LOST FOR REASONS BEARING ON PROFESSIONAL PERFORMANCE, PROFESSIONAL COMPETENCE OR FINANCIAL INTEGRITY.

SCHIEVE, DONALD R MD, LICENSE NUMBER C21402 OF BULLHEAD CITY, AZ, WAS DISCIPLINED BY CALIFORNIA ON DECEMBER 16, 1998
DISCIPLINARY ACTION: LICENSE REVOCATION
OFFENSE: DISCIPLINARY ACTION BY ANOTHER STATE OR AGENCY

NOTES: DISCIPLINED BY NEVADA FOR PERFORMING PHENOL FACE PEELS WITH AN UNLICENSED INDIVIDUAL.

SCHIEVE, DONALD REYNOLDS MD, DATE OF BIRTH FEBRUARY 23, 1933, LICENSE NUMBER 0002056 OF 1800 HIGHWAY 95 #4, BULLHEAD CITY, AZ, WAS DISCIPLINED BY NEVADA ON DECEMBER 7, 1996
DISCIPLINARY ACTION: 60-MONTH PROBATION; REPRIMAND
OFFENSE: PROFESSIONAL MISCONDUCT

NOTES: CHARGED WITH 4 COUNTS OF SIGNING A BLANK PRESCRIPTION FORM; 9 COUNTS OF ENGAGING IN ANY CONDUCT WHICH IS INTENDED TO DECEIVE; 2 COUNTS OF FAILURE TO MAINTAIN MEDICAL RECORDS RELATING TO THE DIAGNOSIS, TREATMENT AND CARE OF A PATIENT; 7 COUNTS OF ALTERING MEDICAL RECORDS OF A PATIENT; 4 COUNTS OF ENGAGING IN ANY CONDUCT WHICH THE BOARD HAS DETERMINED IS A VIOLATION OF THE STANDARDS OF PRACTICE ESTABLISHED BY REGULATION OF THE BOARD; 2 COUNTS OF WRITING A PRESCRIPTION FOR CONTROLLED SUBSTANCES FOR ANY PERSON WITHOUT AN APPROPRIATE EXAMINATION WHICH CONFIRMS THE MEDICAL NECESSITY FOR THE CONTROLLED SUBSTANCES; 2 COUNTS OF ACQUIRING ANY CONTROLLED SUBSTANCES FROM ANY PHARMACY OR OTHER SOURCE BY MISREPRESENTATION, FRAUD, DECEPTION OR SUBTERFUGE; 9 COUNTS OF AIDING, ASSISTING, EMPLOYING OR ADVISING, DIRECTLY OR INDIRECTLY, ANY UNLICENSED PERSON TO ENGAGE IN THE PRACTICE OF MEDICINE CONTRARY TO THE PROVISION OR THE REGULATIONS OF THE BOARD; AND 1 COUNT OF PERFORMING SERVICES WHICH HE KNOWS OR HAS REASON TO KNOW THAT HE IS NOT COMPETENT TO PERFORM; ENGAGED IN THE MEDICAL PRACTICE OF PERFORMING "PHENOL FACE PEELS" TOGETHER WITH AN INDIVIDUAL NOT LICENSED TO PRACTICE MEDICINE IN NEVADA; ACTION HAD NO RELATIONSHIP TO HIS PRACTICE OF OPHTHALMOLOGY. LICENSE REVOCATION, STAYED, PROBATION UNDER TERMS AND CONDITIONS: SHALL NOT PRACTICE IN NEVADA DURING HIS PROBATIONARY PERIOD; SHALL, AT THE NEXT BI-ENNIAL LICENSING, ON 7/01/97, REQUEST TO BE PLACED ON INACTIVE STATUS IN NEVADA AND REMAIN ON INACTIVE STATUS DURING THE TERM OF HIS PROBATION. PUBLIC REPRIMAND. $7,500 FINE.

SCHIEVE, DONALD REYNOLDS MD, DATE OF BIRTH FEBRUARY 23, 1933, LICENSE NUMBER 028226E OF 1195 PINEVIEW DRIVE, MORGANTOWN, WV, WAS DISCIPLINED BY PENNSYLVANIA ON NOVEMBER 17, 1997
DISCIPLINARY ACTION: LICENSE REVOCATION
OFFENSE: DISCIPLINARY ACTION BY ANOTHER STATE OR AGENCY

NOTES: DISCIPLINARY ACTION TAKEN BY NEVADA.

SCHMUTZER, GENE D DO OF TUCSON, AZ, WAS DISCIPLINED BY MISSOURI ON FEBRUARY 9, 1990
OFFENSE: DISCIPLINARY ACTION BY ANOTHER STATE OR AGENCY

NOTES: MUST APPEAR BEFORE BOARD BEFORE RETURNING TO PRACTICE IN MISSOURI.

SCHNEIDER, MARVIN C MD, LICENSE NUMBER C28612 OF PHOENIX, AZ, WAS DISCIPLINED BY CALIFORNIA ON SEPTEMBER 29, 1997
DISCIPLINARY ACTION: REPRIMAND
OFFENSE: OVERPRESCRIBING OR MISPRESCRIBING DRUGS

NOTES: TWICE FAILED TO LIMIT A PRESCRIPTION ORDER FOR A CONTROLLED SUBSTANCE TO ONE DRUG ORDER PER PRESCRIPTION BLANK.

SCHNEIDER, MARVIN CHARLES MD, LICENSE NUMBER 4036, WAS DISCIPLINED BY ARIZONA ON JANUARY 22, 1997
DISCIPLINARY ACTION: REPRIMAND
OFFENSE: NONCOMPLIANCE WITH A PROFESSIONAL RULE

NOTES: ON 12/22/93 AND 11/6/95 HE FAILED TO LIMIT A PRESCRIPTION ORDER FOR A CONTROLLED SUBSTANCE DRUG TO ONE DRUG ORDER PER PRESCRIPTION BLANK; ON 11/20/95 WROTE A PRESCRIPTION ORDER FOR TWO DRUGS ON ONE SINGLE PRESCRIPTION BLANK WHEN BOTH OF THE MEDICATIONS SHOULD HAVE BEEN ORDERED UTILIZING SEPARATE PRESCRIPTION BLANKS.

SCHOENHALS, MICHAEL R MD, LICENSE NUMBER 8501, WAS DISCIPLINED BY ARIZONA ON NOVEMBER 14, 1997
DISCIPLINARY ACTION: PROBATION; REQUIRED TO ENTER AN IMPAIRED PHYSICIAN PROGRAM OR SUBSTANCE ABUSE TREATMENT
OFFENSE: SUBSTANCE ABUSE

NOTES: ON 6/30/97 HE REPORTED TO BOARD THAT HE HAD RELAPSED IN THE USE OF ALCOHOL AND WAS ADMITTED TO THE HOSPITAL; TREATED FROM 7/2/97 TO 9/27/97. ON 10/16/97 ENTERED INTO A REHABILITATION ORDER WITH THE BOARD. CONDITIONS OF PROBATION: MUST IMMEDIATELY PARTICIPATE IN A BOARD-APPROVED MONITORED AFTERCARE TREATMENT PROGRAM WHOSE THERAPIST MUST SUBMIT MONTHLY REPORTS; MUST PARTICIPATE IN A 12-STEP RECOVERY PROGRAM AS DETERMINED BY HIS TREATING THERAPIST AND ATTEND AT LEAST THREE WEEKLY MEETINGS; SHALL OBTAIN A BOARD-APPROVED TREATING PHYSICIAN; SHALL ABSTAIN COMPLETELY FROM THE CONSUMPTION OF ALCOHOLIC BEVERAGES AND DRUGS EXCEPT WHEN PRESCRIBED BY HIS TREATING PHYSICIAN; SHALL NOT CONSUME FOOD OR SUBSTANCES CONTAINING POPPYSEEDS; MUST SUBMIT TO WITNESSED RANDOM BIOLOGICAL FLUID COLLECTION; MUST KEEP A LOG OF ANY AND ALL MEDICATIONS PRESCRIBED FOR HIM; SHALL SUBMIT TO ANY EXAMINATIONS OR THERAPY ORDERED BY BOARD; SHALL APPEAR BEFORE BOARD FOR INTERVIEWS UPON REQUEST; SHALL INFORM BOARD OF CHANGE OF ADDRESS OR IF AWAY FOR MORE THAN FIVE DAYS.

SCHROEDER, W GENE MD, DATE OF BIRTH NOVEMBER 30, 1934, LICENSE NUMBER 1024360 OF 2063 THUMB BUTTE RD, PRESCOTT, AZ, WAS DISCIPLINED BY MICHIGAN ON APRIL 12, 1996
DISCIPLINARY ACTION: FINE; REPRIMAND
OFFENSE: DISCIPLINARY ACTION BY ANOTHER STATE OR AGENCY

NOTES: FAILURE TO REPORT. $500 FINE.

SCHROEDER, W GENE MD, DATE OF BIRTH NOVEMBER 30, 1934, LICENSE NUMBER 1024360 OF 3021 CHEYENNE CIRCLE, PRESCOTT, AZ, WAS DISCIPLINED BY MICHIGAN ON NOVEMBER 19, 1999
DISCIPLINARY ACTION: SURRENDER OF LICENSE
OFFENSE: DISCIPLINARY ACTION BY ANOTHER STATE OR AGENCY

NOTES: SISTER STATE DISCIPLINARY ACTION; FAILURE TO REPORT/COMPLY. VOLUNTARY SURRENDER. ALSO KNOW AS WALTER G. SCHROEDER.

SCHROEDER, WALTER G MD, WAS DISCIPLINED BY ARIZONA ON MARCH 26, 1990
DISCIPLINARY ACTION: REQUIRED TO TAKE ADDITIONAL MEDICAL EDUCATION; MONITORING OF PHYSICIAN PERFORMANCE
OFFENSE: OVERPRESCRIBING OR MISPRESCRIBING DRUGS

NOTES: ACTION BASED ON PRESCRIBING PRACTICES. MATTER FILED WITH LETTER OF CONCERN FOR HIS PRESCRIBING AS RELATES TO PATIENTS OUTLINED IN STAFF SURVEY; HE MUST OBTAIN WITHIN SIX MONTHS 20 HOURS OF CONTINUING MEDICAL EDUCATION IN CHRONIC PAIN MANAGEMENT; STAFF CONDUCT A FOLLOW-UP PHARMACY SURVEY IN SIX MONTHS TO ENSURE THAT HE HAS MADE APPROPRIATE MODIFICATIONS IN HIS PRESCRIBING PRACTICES. ON 1/23/92 BOARD ACCEPTED THE CONTINUING MEDICAL EDUCATION SUBMITTED BY DR. SCHROEDER AS FULFILLMENT OF THE BOARD ORDER AND TERMINATED THE STIPULATION AND ORDER. STAFF WILL CONDUCT A PHARMACY SURVEY IN SIX MONTHS TO DETERMINE IF HE IS APPROPRIATELY PRESCRIBING PAIN MEDICATIONS.

SCHROEDER, WALTER G MD, LICENSE NUMBER 0013043 OF PRESCOTT, AZ, WAS DISCIPLINED BY ARIZONA ON JANUARY 25, 1994
DISCIPLINARY ACTION: RESTRICTION PLACED ON LICENSE
OFFENSE: FAILURE TO COMPLY WITH PREVIOUS BOARD ORDER

NOTES: ON 7/12/93 BOARD ORDERED THAT HE TAKE AND PASS THE SPEX EXAM BY 12/31/93. HE DID NOT TAKE THE EXAM AS ORDERED. TERMS OF ORDER: SHALL NOT USE HERBVEIL 8 CREAM ON SKIN LESIONS; SHALL TAKE PASS THE SPEX EXAM ON 3/17/94; AND SHALL APPEAR BEFORE THE BOARD AT ITS 7/94 MEETING. HE PASSED THE EXAM AND ON 7/13/94 HE ENTERED INTO AN ORDER WITH THE BOARD WHICH REQUIRED THAT HE NOT USE HERBVEIL 8 CREAM ON SKIN LESIONS NOR VITAMIN B-12 OR COLCHICINE FOR OTHER THAN ACCEPTED THERAPEUTIC PURPOSES.

SCHROEDER, WALTER GENE MD OF 3012 CHEYENNE CIRCLE, PRESCOTT, AZ, WAS DISCIPLINED BY IDAHO ON JUNE 14, 1995
DISCIPLINARY ACTION: DENIAL OF NEW LICENSE
OFFENSE: PROVIDING FALSE INFORMATION TO THE BOARD OR OTHER HEALTH AGENCY

NOTES: LIED IN RESPONSE TO A QUESTION ON HIS APPLICATION BY FAILING TO REPORT ACTIONS BY THE ARIZONA BOARD AND A HOSPITAL IN ARIZONA; HAD NUMEROUS LAWSUITS WITHIN A SHORT PERIOD OF TIME.

SCHULER, CALVIN MD, LICENSE NUMBER 0011229, WAS DISCIPLINED BY ARIZONA ON JULY 17, 1996
DISCIPLINARY ACTION: PROBATION; REQUIRED TO TAKE ADDITIONAL MEDICAL EDUCATION
OFFENSE: SUBSTANDARD CARE, INCOMPETENCE OR NEGLIGENCE

NOTES: IN 9/93, HE FAILED TO ADMIT A THREE-MONTH OLD PATIENT TO THE HOSPITAL WHOSE CONDITION HAD BEEN DETERIORATING FOR THREE DAYS AND FAILED TO PROCEED WITH A SEPTIC WORKUP; PRESCRIBED ANTIBIOTICS FOR HER ALLEGED CASE OF PNEUMONIA, DESPITE A NEGATIVE X-RAY, AND SENT HER HOME TO BE FOLLOWED UP BY A PRIMARY CARE PHYSICIAN; LESS THAN 48 HOURS AFTER HE HAD SEEN HER, SHE WAS BROUGHT TO THE EMERGENCY ROOM IN RESPIRATORY DISTRESS AND DIED AFTER UNSUCCESSFUL CARDIAC ARREST RESUSCITATIVE EFFORTS WERE PERFORMED; IN 3/94, HE FAILED TO

PUT A 17-MONTH CHILD ON PULSE OXIMETRY UNTIL ALMOST THREE HOURS AFTER HE ARRIVED AT THE EMERGENCY ROOM, WHEN THE READING RAN BETWEEN 50 AND 55%; UNSUCCESSFULLY ATTEMPTED TO INTUBATE THE CHILD; WHEN THE CHILD CONTINUED TO DETERIORATE, CPR WAS PERFORMED UNTIL IT BECAME EVIDENT THAT CHILD HAD SUSTAINED SIGNIFICANT BRAIN STEM DAMAGE AND RESUSCITATION EFFORTS WERE STOPPED. CENSURED; PROBATION WITH TERMS: WITHIN ONE YEAR, SHALL BECOME RECERTIFIED IN PEDIATRIC ADVANCED LIFE SUPPORT; WITHIN NINE MONTHS, SHALL OBTAIN 30 HOURS OF CONTINUING MEDICAL EDUCATION IN PEDIATRIC CRITICAL CARE; SHALL PROVIDE EVIDENCE OF COMPLETION OF THE HOURS TO THE BOARD. ON 5/8/97 PROBATION TERMINATED; UPON FULFILLMENT OF CONDITIONS THE ORDER FOR DECREE OF CENSURE REMAINS IN EFFECT.

SCHUMACHER, JAMES MD, LICENSE NUMBER 0004598, WAS DISCIPLINED BY ARIZONA ON APRIL 5, 1995
OFFENSE: NONCOMPLIANCE WITH A PROFESSIONAL RULE

NOTES: FAILED TO INFORM A PATIENT OF THE RESULTS OF NUMEROUS STUDIES, INCLUDING A CAROTID DOPPLER EXAM AND SEQUENTIAL ARTERIAL EXAM OF BOTH LOWER EXTREMITIES AS WELL AS A URINALYSIS AND CULTURE; BETWEEN 10/93 AND 2/94 FAILED TO FURNISH INFORMATION IN A TIMELY MANNER TO THE BOARD REGARDING THIS MATTER AFTER THREE REQUESTS; DID PROVIDE INFORMATION ON 3/2/94 BUT FAILED TO APPEAR AT THE BOARD'S OFFICES IN RESPONSE TO A SUBPOENA; FAILED TO ADDRESS HIS DELAY IN RESPONDING TO BOARD'S REQUESTS. HAS PREVIOUSLY RECEIVED TWO LETTERS OF CONCERN: ON 4/11/91 FOR FAILING TO PROVIDE TEST RESULTS AND FORWARD MEDICAL RECORDS AND ON 10/17/89 FOR FAILING OR REFUSING TO HONOR AN APPROPRIATE REQUEST BY A PATIENT TO FORWARD MEDICAL RECORDS TO AN INSURANCE COMPANY AND FAILING TO FURNISH INFORMATION IN A TIMELY MANNER TO THE BOARD. CENSURED. ON 10/18/96 HIS MOTION FOR RECONSIDERATION WAS DENIED ON THE GROUNDS THAT IT WAS UNTIMELY.

SCHWARK, WILLIAM G MD, WAS DISCIPLINED BY ARIZONA ON OCTOBER 21, 1994
OFFENSE: LOSS OR RESTRICTION OF HOSPITAL PRIVILEGES

NOTES: ANESTHETIC PRIVILEGES AT ONE HOSPITAL SUSPENDED RESULTING FROM CARE AND TREATMENT OF PATIENTS. SHALL TAKE AND PASS THE ANESTHESIA EXAMINATION OF THE JOINT COUNCIL OF IN-SERVICE TRAINING IN ANESTHESIA IN JULY 1995.

SCOTT, MICHAEL E MD, LICENSE NUMBER 14234, WAS DISCIPLINED BY ARIZONA ON NOVEMBER 14, 1997
DISCIPLINARY ACTION: LICENSE SUSPENSION
OFFENSE: FAILURE TO COMPLY WITH PREVIOUS BOARD ORDER

NOTES: HE WAS PREVIOUSLY UNDER A BOARD STIPULATION FOR SUBSTANCE ABUSE AND RELAPSED WITH THE USE OF CHEMICAL SUBSTANCES. REQUESTED LICENSE TO BE PLACED ON INACTIVE STATUS WITH CAUSE. AGREES NOT TO PRACTICE IN ARIZONA OR ANY OTHER STATE AND MAY NOT HOLD A CONTROLLED SUBSTANCE CERTIFICATE WITH THE DRUG ENFORCEMENT ADMINISTRATION OR WRITE OR REFILL PRESCRIPTIONS AS LONG AS HIS LICENSE IS INACTIVE; MUST PAY ALL FEES REQUIRED PRIOR TO LICENSE BEING PLACED ON INACTIVE STATUS; SHALL NOT REQUEST REACTIVATION OF HIS LICENSE UNTIL HE MEETS WITH THE BOARD AND COMPLIES WITH ALL REQUESTS OF THE BOARD WHICH MAY INCLUDE INPATIENT TREATMENT, PSYCHIATRIC AND PSYCHOMETRIC EVALUATION, PHYSICAL EXAMINATION AND TESTING AND WRITTEN AND/OR ORAL COMPETENCY EXAMINATIONS. LICENSE PLACED ON INACTIVE STATUS.

SCOTT, MICHAEL E MD, LICENSE NUMBER 14234, WAS DISCIPLINED BY ARIZONA ON JANUARY 23, 1998
DISCIPLINARY ACTION: PROBATION; RESTRICTION PLACED ON LICENSE
OFFENSE: SUBSTANCE ABUSE

NOTES: RELAPSED IN THE USE OF DRUGS OR ALCOHOL IN THE SUMMER OF 1997; IN TREATMENT DURING 9/97 AND 10/97. PROBATION FOR NOT LESS THAN FIVE YEARS ON THE FOLLOWING TERMS AND CONDITIONS: MUST IMMEDIATELY PARTICIPATE IN A BOARD-APPROVED MONITORED AFTERCARE TREATMENT PROGRAM WHOSE THERAPIST MUST SUBMIT MONTHLY REPORTS; MUST PARTICIPATE IN 90 12-STEP MEETINGS FOR SUBSTANCE ABUSE WITHIN 90 DAYS; SHALL OBTAIN A BOARD-APPROVED TREATING PHYSICIAN; SHALL ABSTAIN COMPLETELY FROM THE CONSUMPTION OF ALCOHOLIC BEVERAGES AND DRUGS EXCEPT WHEN PRESCRIBED BY HIS TREATING PHYSICIAN; SHALL NOT CONSUME FOOD OR SUBSTANCES CONTAINING POPPYSEEDS; MUST SUBMIT TO WITNESSED RANDOM BIOLOGICAL FLUID COLLECTION; MUST KEEP A LOG OF ANY AND ALL MEDICATIONS PRESCRIBED FOR HIM; SHALL SUBMIT TO ANY EXAMINATIONS OR THERAPY ORDERED BY BOARD; SHALL APPEAR BEFORE BOARD FOR INTERVIEWS UPON REQUEST; SHALL INFORM BOARD OF CHANGE OF ADDRESS OR IF AWAY FOR MORE THAN FIVE DAYS. SHALL CONTINUE IN THERAPY WITH A TREATING PSYCHIATRIST APPROVED BY THE BOARD UNTIL FURTHER ORDER OF THE BOARD WITH QUARTERLY REPORTS; HE SHALL LIMIT HIS PRACTICE TO NON-CLINICAL MEDICINE. ON 3/28/98 THIS LAST RESTRICTION WAS DELETED.

SCOTT, ROGER D DO, LICENSE NUMBER 20A3520 OF PARKER, AZ, WAS DISCIPLINED BY CALIFORNIA ON OCTOBER 6, 1994
DISCIPLINARY ACTION: LICENSE REVOCATION
OFFENSE: DISCIPLINARY ACTION BY ANOTHER STATE OR AGENCY

NOTES: ACTION IN ARIZONA FOR SUBSTANCE ABUSE.

SCOTT, ROGER DAVID DO, LICENSE NUMBER 0001318 OF P.O. BOX AV, PARKER, AZ, WAS DISCIPLINED BY ARIZONA ON AUGUST 3, 1993
DISCIPLINARY ACTION: 12-MONTH LICENSE SUSPENSION; REQUIRED TO TAKE ADDITIONAL MEDICAL EDUCATION
OFFENSE: PROFESSIONAL MISCONDUCT

NOTES: FAILED TO CREATE PATIENT RECORDS TO ONE PATIENT AFTER REMOVING A MOLE AND ADMINISTERING AN INJECTION OF A DRUG ON ONE OCCASION; FAILED TO CREATE PATIENT RECORDS FOR ANOTHER PATIENT AFTER REMOVING A WART AND ADMINISTERING AN INJECTION OF DEMEROL AND/OR VERSED AFTER THAT PATIENT HAD BEEN DRINKING ALCOHOL; IN OCTOBER AND NOVEMBER 1991 ADMINISTERED AN INJECTION OF DEMEROL AND/OR VERSED TO PATIENT FOR OTHER THAN ACCEPTED THERAPEUTIC PURPOSES; FAILED TO CREATE A PATIENT RECORD FOR HIS WIFE FOR WHOM HE INJECTED DEMEROL AND/OR VERSED IN 12/91, ADMINISTERED DEMEROL ON NUMEROUS OCCASIONS IN 1992, TELEPHONED IN A VALIUM PRESCRIPTION FOR HER IN 5/92 WHEN OTHER

PHYSICIANS WERE AVAILABLE; ALSO ADMINISTERED DEMEROL AND/OR VERSED TO HIS WIFE FROM 12/26/91 THROUGH 5/2/92 TO ENHANCE SEXUAL RELATIONS WHICH WAS FOR OTHER THAN THERAPEUTIC PURPOSES. DIAGNOSED WITH AXIS II PERSONALITY DISORDER, CHARACTERIZED BY NARCISSISM AND ANTI-SOCIAL BEHAVIOR WHICH MIGHT IMPAIR HIS ABILITY TO SAFELY PRACTICE MEDICINE. SUSPENDED FOR NO LESS THAN ONE YEAR UNDER TERMS AND CONDITIONS: SHALL DELIVER WITHIN 10 DAYS ALL DOCUMENTS REFLECTING HE IS LICENSED; SHALL CONTINUE TO SATISFY ALL CONTINUING EDUCATION REQUIREMENTS, PLUS AN ADDITIONAL 20 HOURS PER YEAR IN THE AREA OF SUBSTANCE ABUSE AND PRESCRIBING OF CONTROLLED SUBSTANCES; SHALL PAY COSTS ASSOCIATED WITH THE BOARD'S ADMINISTRATIVE HEARING; WITHIN 30 DAYS SHALL UNDERTAKE PSYCHOTHERAPY UNDER THE SUPERVISION OF A BOARD APPROVED LICENSED PSYCHIATRIST OR PSYCHOLOGIST WHO SHALL PROVIDE A QUARTERLY REPORT TO THE BOARD; MAY PETITION FOR REINSTATEMENT AFTER THE MINIMUM PERIOD OF SUSPENSION. ON 11/29/93 THE BOARD DENIED A MOTION FOR REHEARING.

SEEMAN, ROY D MD, WAS DISCIPLINED BY ARIZONA ON OCTOBER 17, 1995
DISCIPLINARY ACTION: RESTRICTION PLACED ON LICENSE
OFFENSE: PROFESSIONAL MISCONDUCT

NOTES: ALLEGATIONS RELATIVE TO CARE AND TREATMENT OF TWO PATIENTS INCLUDING UNNECESSARY TESTS AND WRONGFULLY PRESCRIBING CARDIZEM; ANOTHER PATIENT ALLEGED A CONTRACT SIGNED WITH HIM MISREPRESENTED BENEFITS. INTERIM BOARD ORDER: SHALL NOT INTERPRET ANY ULTRASOUND OR ECHOCARDIOGRAM.

SEEMAN, ROY D MD, WAS DISCIPLINED BY ARIZONA ON APRIL 1, 1997
DISCIPLINARY ACTION: RESTRICTION PLACED ON LICENSE; REQUIRED TO TAKE ADDITIONAL MEDICAL EDUCATION

NOTES: CAN NOT PERFORM ULTRASOUND STROKE SCREENING, DOPPLER CIRCULATION SCREENING, ULTRASOUND ANEURYSM SCREENING, ULTRASOUND THYROID SCREENING, HEART SCREENING BY CARDIOINTEROGRAPH MACHINE; SHALL NOT PERFORM GLAUCOMA SCREENING BY METHODS OTHER THAN AIR PUFF, SLITLAMP AND TONOMETRY AND SHALL NOT PERFORM, SPONSOR, MARKET OR LEND HIS NAME TO THE MARKETING OF HEALTH SCREENINGS; CANNOT PERFORM ULTRASOUND INTERPRETATIONS UNTIL HE HAS COMPLETED 20 HOURS OF CONTINUING MEDICAL EDUCATION IN VASCULAR ULTRASONOGRAPHY AND 2O HOURS IN INTERPRETATION OF ECHOCARDIOGRAPHY; HE MUST PROVIDE SATISFACTORY COMPLETION OF THIS EDUCATION. ON 9/26/97 HE HAD COMPLETED REQUIREMENTS AND ORDER WAS TERMINATED.

SENA, JAMES DO OF P.O. BOX 1990, BULLHEAD CITY, AZ, WAS DISCIPLINED BY DEA ON FEBRUARY 6, 1992
DISCIPLINARY ACTION: SURRENDER OF CONTROLLED SUBSTANCE LICENSE
OFFENSE: DISCIPLINARY ACTION BY ANOTHER STATE OR AGENCY

NOTES: 11 OF 13 PATIENT RECORDS REVIEWED BY ARIZONA BOARD FAILED TO SUPPORT USE OF CONTROLLED SUBSTANCES. ARIZONA BOARD OF OSTEOPATHIC EXAMINERS ORDERED DR. SENA TO DISCONTINUE PRESCRIBING SCHEDULES II-IV CONTROLLED SUBSTANCES. SURRENDER OF REGISTRATION SCHEDULES II THROUGH IV.

SEPTER, MICHAEL J DO OF TUCSON, AZ, WAS DISCIPLINED BY DEA ON NOVEMBER 14, 1996
DISCIPLINARY ACTION: 36-MONTH RESTRICTION PLACED ON CONTROLLED SUBSTANCE LICENSE; MONITORING OF PHYSICIAN PERFORMANCE
OFFENSE: FAILURE TO COMPLY WITH PREVIOUS BOARD ORDER

NOTES: DEA ENTERED AN AGREEMENT WITH HIM IN 1992 RESTRICTING HIS CONTROLLED SUBSTANCE REGISTRATION SUBJECT TO TERMS AND CONDITIONS BASED ON A 5/4/81 CONVICTION OF MAIL FRAUD, A 10/21/81 PROBATION ON HIS LICENSE BY THE ARIZONA BOARD, AND A 12/09/81 EXCLUSION FROM THE MEDICARE PROGRAM; ON 10/08/92 HE SOUGHT MEDICAL LICENSURE IN MISSISSIPPI AND DENIED ON HIS APPLICATION OF EVER HAVING HIS DEA REGISTRATION RESTRICTED; IN VIOLATION OF THE PREVIOUS MEMO OF AGREEMENT WITH THE DEA , FAILED TO NOTIFY DEA OF HIS CHANGE OF ADDRESS TO MICHIGAN, AND ALLOWED CONTROLLED SUBSTANCES TO BE DISPENSED FROM HIS ARIZONA OFFICE WITHOUT A PHYSICIAN PRESENT AND FOR NO LONGER THAN EIGHT WEEKS; FAILED TO OBTAIN A MODIFICATION OF HIS REGISTRATION TO CHANGE THE ADDRESS TO MICHIGAN BEFORE WRITING OR AUTHORIZING PRESCRIPTIONS; FALSIFIED TWO OF HIS APPLICATIONS FILED WITH THE DEA. DEA REGISTRATION RESTRICTED UNDER THE FOLLOWING TERMS AND CONDITIONS FOR THREE YEARS: HIS CONTROLLED SUBSTANCE HANDLING AUTHORITY SHALL BE LIMITED TO THE WRITING OF PRESCRIPTIONS FOR SCHEDULE III, IV, AND V CONTROLLED SUBSTANCES ONLY; HE SHALL NOT DISPENSE, ADMINISTER, POSSESS, OR STORE ANY CONTROLLED SUBSTANCES EXCEPT THOSE MEDICALLY NECESSARY FOR HIS OWN USE AND WHICH HE HAS OBTAINED LAWFULLY FROM ANOTHER AUTHORIZED PHYSICIAN; SHALL MAINTAIN A LOG OF ALL PRESCRIPTIONS THAT HE ISSUES; SHALL SUBMIT THIS LOG TO THE DEA UPON REQUEST; SHALL NOTIFY THE DEA OF HIS PLACE OF EMPLOYMENT AND ANY SUBSEQUENT CHANGES IN EMPLOYMENT.

SEPTER, MICHAEL J DO, DATE OF BIRTH AUGUST 21, 1950, LICENSE NUMBER 1009470 OF PO BOX 5038, NORTH MUSKEGON, MI, WAS DISCIPLINED BY MICHIGAN ON AUGUST 17, 1997
DISCIPLINARY ACTION: 6-MONTH LICENSE SUSPENSION; FINE
OFFENSE: DISCIPLINARY ACTION BY ANOTHER STATE OR AGENCY

NOTES: $10,000 FINE. ON 11/15/98 REINSTATEMENT DENIED.

SEPTER, MICHAEL J DO OF GRAND RAPIDS, MI, WAS DISCIPLINED BY DEA ON SEPTEMBER 17, 1998
DISCIPLINARY ACTION: REVOCATION OF CONTROLLED SUBSTANCE LICENSE
OFFENSE: DISCIPLINARY ACTION BY ANOTHER STATE OR AGENCY

NOTES: ON 8/18/97 THE MICHIGAN BOARD SUSPENDED HIS LICENSE FOR AT LEAST SIX MONTHS; HE CHALLENGED THIS ACTION AND AN ARIZONA REVOCATION BUT DID NOT DENY THAT HE WAS NOT AUTHORIZED TO HANDLE CONTROLLED SUBSTANCES; HAS NOT SUBMITTED EVIDENCE THAT HE HAS SOUGHT TO HAVE LICENSE REINSTATED.

SETTLES, RICHARD DO, LICENSE NUMBER 2686 OF 10752 N 89TH PLACE #218, SCOTTSDALE, AZ, WAS DISCIPLINED BY ARIZONA ON JULY 14, 1997
DISCIPLINARY ACTION: REQUIRED TO TAKE ADDITIONAL MEDICAL EDUCATION; MONITORING OF PHYSICIAN PERFORMANCE

OFFENSE: OVERPRESCRIBING OR MISPRESCRIBING DRUGS

NOTES: IN 6/96 THE BOARD RECEIVED A COMPLAINT ALLEGING THAT HE WAS OVER PRESCRIBING NARCOTIC MEDICATION. SHALL COMPLETE 20 HOURS OF CONTINUING MEDICAL EDUCATION WITHIN ONE YEAR IN THE AREA OF APPROPRIATE PRESCRIBING OF NARCOTIC AND CONTROLLED SUBSTANCES; WILL BE SUBJECT TO REVIEW OF ALL ASPECTS OF HIS MEDICAL PRACTICE BUT PRIMARILY IN DIAGNOSIS AND TREATMENT OF PATIENTS AND MAINTENANCE OF PATIENT RECORDS; THERE WILL BE A RANDOM REVIEW OF AT LEAST 10 PATIENT RECORDS CONDUCTED EVERY 120 DAYS FOR ONE YEAR. CONDITIONS OF THIS ORDER WERE MET AND ON 6/26/99 REINSTATED TO A FULL AND UNRESTRICTED LICENSE.

SHAH, DAULAT MD, LICENSE NUMBER 13432, WAS DISCIPLINED BY ARIZONA ON JANUARY 22, 1998
DISCIPLINARY ACTION: REPRIMAND
OFFENSE: DISCIPLINARY ACTION BY ANOTHER STATE OR AGENCY

NOTES: IN 1994 TEXAS HAD TAKEN ACTION AGAINST HIS LICENSE BASED ON: IN 2/94 HE LIED STATING HE HAD NEVER HAD MEDICAL PRIVILEGES MONITORED, REVOKED, SUSPENDED, LIMITED OR DENIED BY ANY ORGANIZATION OR HEALTH CARE FACILITY WHEN HE IN FACT WAS DENIED PRIVILEGES AT ONE HOSPITAL FOR FAILURE TO REVEAL THAT HIS PRIVILEGES AT ANOTHER HOSPITAL WERE DENIED DUE TO HIS FAILURE TO ATTEND SURGERY COMMITTEE MEETINGS; HE WAS SUSPENDED FROM EMERGENCY ROOM CALL IN GENERAL SURGERY AT A MEDICAL CENTER SINCE HE HAD SHOWED POOR JUDGMENT WITH REGARD TO TREATMENT IN A CASE AND AN INDEPENDENT REVIEW OF RECORDS INDICATED THAT HE DEVIATED FROM THE ACCEPTED STANDARD OF CARE. IN 8/95 THE TEXAS BOARD SUSPENDED HIS LICENSE PURSUANT TO THIS ORDER.

SHAMOS, RAYMOND F MD, LICENSE NUMBER 0013612 OF PHOENIX, AZ, WAS DISCIPLINED BY ARIZONA ON JANUARY 18, 1995
OFFENSE: SUBSTANDARD CARE, INCOMPETENCE OR NEGLIGENCE

NOTES: IN 10/90 INADEQUATELY DOCUMENTED A HISTORY AND PHYSICAL EXAMINATION OF A PATIENT PRIOR TO SURGICAL REMOVAL OF HER ADRENAL GLAND; HE THEN FAILED TO REVIEW A CT SCAN TO CONFIRM THE CORRECT PROCEDURE INDICATED AND REMOVED THE PATIENT'S HEALTHY LEFT ADRENAL GLAND, INSTEAD OF THE RIGHT ADRENAL GLAND; PRIOR TO SURGERY, PATIENT WAS ASKED TO EXECUTE A SURGICAL CONSENT FORM WHICH IMPROPERLY DENOTED THE SURGERY AS A LEFT ADRENALECTOMY. PATIENT POINTED OUT THE DISCREPANCY TO STAFF AND WAS ASSURED THAT IT WOULD BE CORRECTED PRIOR TO SURGERY; SHE NOW REQUIRES PERMANENT DRUG REPLACEMENT THERAPY FOR THE REST OF HER LIFE. CENSURED.

SHAMOS, RAYMOND F MD, LICENSE NUMBER 0136333 OF 222 WEST THOMAS ROAD SUITE 201, PHOENIX, AZ, WAS DISCIPLINED BY NEW YORK ON MARCH 11, 1996
DISCIPLINARY ACTION: SURRENDER OF LICENSE
OFFENSE: DISCIPLINARY ACTION BY ANOTHER STATE OR AGENCY

NOTES: ACTION IN ARIZONA FOR PERFORMING A LEFT ADRENALECTOMY ON A HEALTHY ADRENAL GLAND WHEN IT WAS THE RIGHT ADRENAL GLAND WHICH NEEDED SURGICAL INTERVENTION.

SHARP, JEFFREY A MD, LICENSE NUMBER 0008664, WAS DISCIPLINED BY ARIZONA ON JANUARY 23, 1992
DISCIPLINARY ACTION: 60-MONTH PROBATION; RESTRICTION PLACED ON LICENSE
OFFENSE: SEXUAL ABUSE OF OR SEXUAL MISCONDUCT WITH A PATIENT

NOTES: SEXUAL RELATIONSHIPS WITH A NUMBER OF PATIENTS OVER A TEN YEAR PERIOD; HAS BEEN TREATED FOR DEPRESSION AND PSYCHOSEXUAL DISORDER. MAY PETITION FOR MODIFICATION OR TERMINATION OF PROBATION AFTER THREE YEARS. TERMS AND CONDITIONS: SHALL IMMEDIATELY ENTER INTO OUTPATIENT THERAPY WITH BOARD-APPROVED THERAPIST WHO SHALL RELEASE RECORDS TO BOARD AND SUBMIT QUARTERLY REPORTS; SHALL SUBMIT TO MENTAL OR PHYSICAL EXAMS REQUESTED BY BOARD; SHALL LIMIT PRACTICE TO ADULT MALES, AND WOMEN OVER AGE 55; SHALL APPEAR BEFORE THE BOARD FOR INTERVIEWS UPON REQUEST; SHALL INFORM BOARD OF CHANGE OF ADDRESS OR IF AWAY FOR MORE THAN FIVE DAYS. ISSUED A DECREE OF CENSURE. ON 8/8/98 PROBATION TERMINATED.

SHARP, JEFFREY ALAN MD OF SEDONA, AZ, WAS DISCIPLINED BY UTAH ON FEBRUARY 8, 1993
DISCIPLINARY ACTION: PROBATION; REPRIMAND
OFFENSE: DISCIPLINARY ACTION BY ANOTHER STATE OR AGENCY

NOTES: INAPPROPRIATE CONDUCT WITH A FEMALE PATIENT RESULTING IN DISCIPLINARY ACTION AGAINST HIS MEDICAL LICENSE IN ARIZONA. PROBATION CONSISTENT WITH TERMS OF THE ARIZONA ORDER.

SHAUT, CHRISTOPHER ALDERSON MD, LICENSE NUMBER 0010963, WAS DISCIPLINED BY ARIZONA ON OCTOBER 11, 1991
DISCIPLINARY ACTION: RESTRICTION PLACED ON LICENSE
OFFENSE: SUBSTANDARD CARE, INCOMPETENCE OR NEGLIGENCE

NOTES: COMPLAINT ALLEGING INAPPROPRIATE TREATMENT IN PERFORMANCE OF A D&C AND PELVIC LAPAROTOMY OF PATIENT. SHALL NOT PERFORM ELECTIVE GYNECOLOGIC SURGERY AND SHALL NOT PRACTICE GYNECOLOGY IN ARIZONA IN ANY FORM, UNLESS AND UNTIL APPROVED BY THE BOARD; IF HE PERFORMS ANY EMERGENCY GYNECOLOGIC SURGERY OR PROCEDURES, HE SHALL INFORM THE BOARD FOR ITS REVIEW.

SHAW, GERALD P MD, LICENSE NUMBER 0010342, WAS DISCIPLINED BY ARIZONA ON JANUARY 17, 1990
DISCIPLINARY ACTION: 24-MONTH PROBATION; 24-MONTH REQUIRED TO TAKE ADDITIONAL MEDICAL EDUCATION
OFFENSE: SUBSTANDARD CARE, INCOMPETENCE OR NEGLIGENCE

NOTES: IN JULY 1986 TREATED PATIENT FOR CHEMICAL DEPENDENCY; PATIENT HAD A LONG-STANDING HISTORY OF OPIATE DEPENDENCY AND POLYSUBSTANCE ABUSE, AND ALSO SUFFERED FROM DEPRESSION AND BACK PAIN. ON 9/19/86 PATIENT RELAPSED AND WAS GETTING NARCOTICS FROM ANOTHER PHYSICIAN. DR. SHAW ASSESSED NARCOTIC ADDICTION AND MADE ARRANGEMENTS FOR PATIENT TO ENTER A METHADONE MAINTENANCE CLINIC. GAVE PATIENT PRESCRIPTION FOR METHADONE WITHOUT PERFORMING A PHYSICAL EXAM AND WITHOUT WARNING PATIENT NOT TO COMBINE OTHER CENTRAL NERVOUS SYSTEM DEPRESSANTS WITH METHADONE. PATIENT WAS FOUND DEAD DUE TO THE COMBINED EFFECTS OF BARBITURATES AND METHADONE. MUST OBTAIN 20 HOURS OF CONTINUING EDUCATION IN NARCOTIC ADDICTION AND PRESCRIBING PER YEAR FOR TWO YEARS.

SHERMAN, SCOTT J MD, LICENSE NUMBER 0019692, WAS DISCIPLINED BY ARIZONA ON OCTOBER 19, 1990
DISCIPLINARY ACTION: 60-MONTH PROBATION; REQUIRED TO ENTER AN IMPAIRED PHYSICIAN PROGRAM OR SUBSTANCE ABUSE TREATMENT
OFFENSE: SUBSTANCE ABUSE

NOTES: LICENSED TO PRACTICE IN WASHINGTON 7/86. BECAME ADDICTED TO NARCOTICS DURING RESIDENCY IN ANESTHESIOLOGY IN 1987; UNDERWENT INPATIENT TREATMENT AND RESIGNED FROM RESIDENCY PROGRAM IN 5/87. REENTERED PROGRAM IN 1/88. RELAPSED IN 9/88 WHEN HE USED FENTANYL ONCE. IN 7/89, DURING RESIDENCY TRAINING, ATTENDING PHYSICIANS BELIEVED HE HAD RELAPSED, WHICH HE DENIED. IN 1/90 RECOMMENDATION MADE TO TERMINATE HIM FROM PROGRAM, WHICH IS STILL PENDING. CEASED CLINICAL DUTIES IN 8/89 AND LEFT PROGRAM IN 1/90. CONDITIONS OF PROBATION: MUST IMMEDIATELY PARTICIPATE IN ARIZONA MEDICAL ASSOCIATION'S MONITORED AFTERCARE TREATMENT PROGRAM WITH QUARTERLY REPORTS SUBMITTED TO THE BOARD; MUST OBTAIN A BOARD-APPROVED TREATING PHYSICIAN; MUST ABSTAIN FROM ALCOHOL AND ALL OTHER DRUGS; MUST COMPLY WITH REQUESTS FOR RANDOM BIOLOGICAL FLUID TESTS; MUST SUBMIT TO ANY EXAMS AND THERAPY ORDERED BY THE BOARD; MUST PARTICIPATE IN A 12-STEP RECOVERY PROGRAM FOR SUBSTANCE ABUSE AND ATTEND A MINIMUM OF THREE WEEKLY MEETINGS; MUST APPEAR BEFORE BOARD FOR INTERVIEWS UPON REQUEST; MUST MAINTAIN A LOG OF ALL MEDICATION TAKEN; MUST ADVISE BOARD OF CHANGE IN OFFICE OR HOME ADDRESSES OR IF HE PLANS TO BE AWAY FOR MORE THAN FIVE DAYS.

SHERMAN, SCOTT J MD, LICENSE NUMBER 0019692, WAS DISCIPLINED BY ARIZONA ON APRIL 11, 1992
DISCIPLINARY ACTION: REQUIRED TO ENTER AN IMPAIRED PHYSICIAN PROGRAM OR SUBSTANCE ABUSE TREATMENT; MONITORING OF PHYSICIAN PERFORMANCE

NOTES: PROBATION TERMINATED; HE AGREED TO ENTER INTO THE FOLLOWING ORDER: MUST PARTICIPATE IN THE ARIZONA MEDICAL ASSOCIATION'S MONITORED AFTERCARE TREATMENT PROGRAM WITH QUARTERLY REPORTS FROM THERAPIST; SHALL OBTAIN A BOARD-APPROVED TREATING PHYSICIAN; SHALL ABSTAIN COMPLETELY FROM THE CONSUMPTION OF ALCOHOLIC BEVERAGES AND DRUGS EXCEPT WHEN PRESCRIBED BY HIS TREATING PHYSICIAN; SHALL SUBMIT TO WITNESSED RANDOM BIOLOGICAL FLUID COLLECTION; SHALL SUBMIT TO ANY EXAMINATIONS OR THERAPY ORDERED BY THE BOARD; SHALL MAINTAIN A LOG OF ANY AND ALL MEDICATIONS PRESCRIBED FOR HIM; SHALL PARTICIPATE IN A 12-STEP RECOVERY PROGRAM APPROPRIATE FOR SUBSTANCE ABUSE AS DETERMINED BY HIS THERAPIST AND ATTEND A MINIMUM OF THREE WEEKLY MEETINGS; SHALL APPEAR BEFORE THE BOARD FOR INTERVIEWS UPON REQUEST; SHALL INFORM THE BOARD OF CHANGE OF ADDRESS OR IF AWAY FOR MORE THAN 5 DAYS. ON 10/23/92, FOLLOWING DISCUSSION OF HIS SUCCESSFUL COMPLETION OF THE BOARD'S REHABILITATION ORDER, THE BOARD ORDERED HIS PROBATION TERMINATED TO BECOME EFFECTIVE IN 90 DAYS.

SHERMETA, DENNIS WILLIAM DR, LICENSE NUMBER 0017441, WAS DISCIPLINED BY ARIZONA ON JULY 15, 1994
DISCIPLINARY ACTION: LICENSE SUSPENSION
OFFENSE: NONCOMPLIANCE WITH A PROFESSIONAL RULE

NOTES: FAILURE TO PAY RENEWAL FEE DURING PENDING INVESTIGATION.

SHOEMAKER, LESTER MD, WAS DISCIPLINED BY ARIZONA ON OCTOBER 16, 1993
DISCIPLINARY ACTION: LICENSE SUSPENSION
OFFENSE: PHYSICAL OR MENTAL ILLNESS INHIBITING THE ABILITY TO PRACTICE WITH SKILL AND SAFETY

NOTES: HE IS SUFFERING FROM A NEUROLOGICAL DEFICIT.

SIEGEL, BERTON DO, DATE OF BIRTH JUNE 19, 1933 OF 10642 CAMINO DEL SOL #22, YUMA, AZ, WAS DISCIPLINED BY MEDICARE ON APRIL 12, 1993
DISCIPLINARY ACTION: 60-MONTH EXCLUSION FROM THE MEDICARE AND/OR MEDICAID PROGRAM
OFFENSE: CRIMINAL CONVICTION OR PLEA OF GUILTY, NOLO CONTENDERE, OR NO CONTEST TO A CRIME

NOTES: CONVICTED OF THREE COUNTS OF FACILITATION OF THEFT OF MEDICAID PROGRAM FUNDS.

SIEGEL, BERTON DO, LICENSE NUMBER 0000726 OF 4225 WEST GLENDALE, #119, PHOENIX, AZ, WAS DISCIPLINED BY ARIZONA ON JULY 21, 1994
DISCIPLINARY ACTION: LICENSE SUSPENSION
OFFENSE: CRIMINAL CONVICTION OR PLEA OF GUILTY, NOLO CONTENDERE, OR NO CONTEST TO A CRIME

NOTES: ON 7/03/92 FOUND GUILTY OF THREE UNDESIGNATED CLASS VI OFFENSES STEMMING FROM HIS ORDERING EQUIPMENT TO PERFORM COSMETIC TREATMENTS USING FUNDS PROVIDED TO THE HEALTH CARE PROVIDERS OF ARIZONA WHICH CONSTITUTED FACILITATION OF THEFT AND WAS PLACED ON THREE YEAR SUPERVISED PROBATION, REQUIRED TO MAKE REIMBURSEMENT, AND FINED; ON 10/19/92 ACKNOWLEDGED TO THE BOARD THESE CONVICTIONS; ON 4/27/94 SENTENCED TO A TERM OF INCARCERATION FOR 1 AND 1/2 YEARS, ORDERED TO COMPLETE 1000 HOURS OF COMMUNITY SERVICE, AND THE FINANCIAL TERMS WERE REAFFIRMED FOR NONCOMPLIANCE WITH THE FINANCIAL TERMS OF HIS PROBATION. MINIMUM TWO YEAR SUSPENSION ON MEDICAL LICENSE OR THE DURATION OF HIS INCARCERATION, WHICHEVER PERIOD IS LONGER; MAY SUBMIT AN APPLICATION FOR REINSTATEMENT, BUT AS A CONDITION FOR REINSTATEMENT MUST TAKE AND PASS THE SPEX WITH A SCORE OF AT LEAST 75%; AND SHALL NOTIFY THE BOARD WITHIN 10 DAYS OF ANY CHANGE IN THE STATUS AND/OR CONDITIONS OF HIS COURT ORDERED PROBATION, INCARCERATION, OR PAROLE.

SIEGEL, BERTON DO, LICENSE NUMBER 20A3430 OF PHOENIX, AZ, WAS DISCIPLINED BY CALIFORNIA ON MAY 11, 1995
DISCIPLINARY ACTION: LICENSE REVOCATION
OFFENSE: DISCIPLINARY ACTION BY ANOTHER STATE OR AGENCY

NOTES: ACTION IN ARIZONA FOR CONVICTION OF A CRIME.

SIEGEL, BERTON DO, LICENSE NUMBER 2000302 OF 3801 WEST ROSE LANE, PHOENIX, AZ, WAS DISCIPLINED BY INDIANA ON AUGUST 12, 1997
DISCIPLINARY ACTION: SURRENDER OF LICENSE

NOTES: AGREED TO SUBMIT HIS CERTIFICATE OF LICENSURE IN LIEU OF CONTESTING THE DISCIPLINARY CHARGES PENDING AGAINST HIM.

SIEGEL, PHILIP MD, LICENSE NUMBER 0004742, WAS DISCIPLINED BY ARIZONA ON MAY 1, 1995

NOTES: SHALL NOT ENGAGE IN THE PRACTICE OF MEDICINE UNTIL HE HAS FIRST INFORMED THE ARIZONA BOARD OF HIS INTENTION TO DO SO.

SILVA, ROMULO MD, LICENSE NUMBER 100129 OF 177 WEST COTTONWOOD LANE SUITE 1, CASA GRANDE, AZ, WAS DISCIPLINED BY NEW YORK ON FEBRUARY 13, 1997
DISCIPLINARY ACTION: SURRENDER OF LICENSE
OFFENSE: DISCIPLINARY ACTION BY ANOTHER STATE OR AGENCY

NOTES: DISCIPLINED BY THE ARIZONA BOARD FOR FALSELY STATING HE WAS BOARD CERTIFIED IN OCCUPATIONAL MEDICINE BY THE AMERICAN BOARD OF PREVENTATIVE MEDICINE.

SILVA, ROMULO MD, DATE OF BIRTH SEPTEMBER 5, 1930, LICENSE NUMBER 1029792 OF 9209 E EMERALD DRIVE, SUN LAKES, AZ, WAS DISCIPLINED BY MICHIGAN ON JULY 18, 1997
DISCIPLINARY ACTION: 1-MONTH LICENSE SUSPENSION; FINE
OFFENSE: DISCIPLINARY ACTION BY ANOTHER STATE OR AGENCY

NOTES: FAILURE TO REPORT/COMPLY. $1000 FINE; REPRIMAND.

SILVA, ROMULO E MD, LICENSE NUMBER 0008687, WAS DISCIPLINED BY ARIZONA ON JANUARY 17, 1996
DISCIPLINARY ACTION: FINE
OFFENSE: PROVIDING FALSE INFORMATION TO THE BOARD OR OTHER HEALTH AGENCY

NOTES: IN 2/94, NOTIFIED BY THE AMERICAN BOARD OF PREVENTIVE MEDICINE THAT HE HAD FAILED THE EXAMINATION FOR CERTIFICATION IN OCCUPATIONAL MEDICINE FOR THE SECOND TIME; IN THE SUMMER OF 1994, APPLIED FOR THE POSITION OF OCCUPATIONAL MEDICINE PHYSICIAN AT A HOSPITAL MEDICAL CENTER; IN SUPPORT OF HIS APPLICATION, SUBMITTED A CERTIFICATE OF BOARD CERTIFICATION IN OCCUPATIONAL MEDICINE OF THE AMERICAN BOARD OF PREVENTIVE MEDICINE DATED 1/92 AND BEARING HIS NAME; HE FORGED THE CERTIFICATE BY ALTERING ANOTHER PHYSICIAN'S CERTIFICATE AND ADDED HIS NAME TO IT; IN 8/94, BOARD REQUESTED AN EXPLANATION FROM HIM REGARDING HIS CONDUCT AND HE RESPONDED IN 9/94, EXTENDING HIS APOLOGIES TO THE BOARD. CENSURED; $2,500 FINE.

SILVER, RICHARD A MD, WAS DISCIPLINED BY ARIZONA ON JULY 19, 1996
DISCIPLINARY ACTION: MONITORING OF PHYSICIAN PERFORMANCE

NOTES: INTERVIEWED BY THE BOARD REGARDING HIS CARE AND TREATMENT OF A PATIENT AND THE MALPRACTICE CLAIM ALLEGING AN UNSATISFACTORY RESULT FOLLOWING KNEE SURGERY. SHALL EMPLOY THE SERVICES OF A CONSULTANT TO WORK WITH HIM AND HIS OFFICE ON PROPER CODING AND BILLING AND ADDRESS OFFICE MANAGEMENT AND RECORD-KEEPING. ON 5/8/97 ORDER TERMINATED BASED ON CONSULTANT'S REVIEW.

SIMONS, MORTON MD, LICENSE NUMBER 0006616, WAS DISCIPLINED BY ARIZONA ON MAY 8, 1992
DISCIPLINARY ACTION: RESTRICTION PLACED ON CONTROLLED SUBSTANCE LICENSE; MONITORING OF PHYSICIAN PERFORMANCE
OFFENSE: OVERPRESCRIBING OR MISPRESCRIBING DRUGS

NOTES: OVERPRESCRIBING SCHEDULE II AND IV DRUGS. SHALL CANCEL HIS DEA CERTIFICATE FOR ALL SCHEDULE II, III, AND IV CONTROLLED SUBSTANCES; SHALL CEASE PRESCRIBING, DISPENSING, OR ADMINISTERING B-12 INJECTIONS EXCEPT FOR ACCEPTABLE THERAPEUTIC REASONS. STAFF WILL CONDUCT A FOLLOW-UP PHARMACY SURVEY WITHIN SIX TO NINE MONTHS TO ENSURE HIS COMPLIANCE WITH BOARD'S STIPULATION AND ORDER.

SINGH, BALDEV D MD, LICENSE NUMBER 0C40540 OF YUMA, AZ, WAS DISCIPLINED BY CALIFORNIA ON SEPTEMBER 29, 1994
DISCIPLINARY ACTION: 60-MONTH PROBATION
OFFENSE: DISCIPLINARY ACTION BY ANOTHER STATE OR AGENCY

NOTES: RESTRICTION BY ARIZONA BOARD DUE TO DRINKING PROBLEM AND HIGH STRESS. REVOCATION STAYED.

SINGH, BALDEV D MD, LICENSE NUMBER 0016824, WAS DISCIPLINED BY ARIZONA ON JULY 18, 1996

NOTES: SHALL NOT PRACTICE MEDICINE IN ARIZONA UNTIL HE HAS MET WITH THE BOARD AND OBTAINED ITS APPROVAL TO DO SO.

SINGH, SAGGOO H MD, LICENSE NUMBER 0013697, WAS DISCIPLINED BY ARIZONA ON APRIL 8, 1992
DISCIPLINARY ACTION: FINE
OFFENSE: LOSS OR RESTRICTION OF HOSPITAL PRIVILEGES

NOTES: PRIVILEGES TO PRACTICE AT DESERT SAMARITAN HOSPITAL WERE SUSPENDED FOR DELINQUENCY IN PREPARING MEDICAL RECORDS FOR MORE THAN 60 DAYS. ASSESSED AN ADMINISTRATIVE PENALTY OF $3,000 PAYABLE WITHIN 45 DAYS FROM THE DATE THIS ORDER IS SERVED. SHALL COMPLETE ALL HOSPITAL RECORD DICTATIONS AND SIGNATURES WITHIN AT LEAST 20 DAYS FROM THE DATE THEY ARE TO BE DONE. IN 11/92 HE REQUESTED THAT STIPULATION BE TERMINATED. ON 11/10/92 BOARD RECEIVED INFORMATION THAT HE HAD BEEN SUSPENDED FOR DELINQUENT MEDICAL RECORDS AT THE SAME TIME HE WAS UNDER BOARD STIPULATION SO ORDER CONTINUED AS OF 1/20/93.

SINGH, SAGGOO H MD, LICENSE NUMBER 0013697, WAS DISCIPLINED BY ARIZONA ON APRIL 13, 1993
DISCIPLINARY ACTION: 60-MONTH PROBATION
OFFENSE: FAILURE TO COMPLY WITH PREVIOUS BOARD ORDER

NOTES: IN 12 CASES DOCTOR SINGH FAILED TO COMPLETE HOSPITAL RECORDS WITHIN 20 DAYS FROM THE DATE THE RECORDS WERE TO BE DONE. THIS CONSTITUTES 12 VIOLATIONS OF THE BOARD'S ORDER DATED 06/08/92. CONDITIONS OF PROBATION INCLUDE: SHALL COMPLETE ALL HOSPITAL RECORD DICTATIONS WITHIN AT LEAST 20 DAYS FROM THE DATE THEY ARE TO BE DONE AND COMPLETE ALL HOSPITAL RECORD SIGNATURES WITHIN AT LEAST 30 DAYS FROM THE DATE THEY ARE TO BE DONE. THE HISTORY AND PHYSICAL ON PATIENT SHALL BE DICTATED WITHIN 20 DAYS OF THE PATIENT'S ADMISSION AND SIGNED WITHIN 30 DAYS OF THE PATIENT'S ADMISSION. AN OPERATIVE NOTE SHALL BE DICTATED WITHIN 20 DAYS OF THE OPERATION AND SIGNED WITHIN 30 DAYS OF THE OPERATION. THE DISCHARGE SUMMARY SHALL BE DICTATED WITHIN 20 DAYS FROM THE DATE OF DISCHARGE AND SIGNED WITHIN 30 DAYS FROM THE DATE OF DISCHARGE. DR. SINGH SHALL PAY THE BOARD A $1,000 ADMINISTRATIVE PENALTY FOR EVERY FUTURE VIOLATION OF THIS ORDER OF PROBATION. ON 7/13/94 THIS ORDER TERMINATED.

SINGH, SAGGOO H MD, DATE OF BIRTH MARCH 19, 1947, LICENSE

NUMBER 0033647 OF 485 SOUTH DOBSON ROAD, STE 202, CHANDLER, AZ, WAS DISCIPLINED BY NEW JERSEY ON SEPTEMBER 14, 1994
DISCIPLINARY ACTION: LICENSE SUSPENSION
OFFENSE: DISCIPLINARY ACTION BY ANOTHER STATE OR AGENCY

NOTES: LEAVE GRANTED TO SEEK REINSTATEMENT UPON PROOF OF SATISFACTORY COMPLETION OF THE TERMS OF ARIZONA SANCTION.

SKINNER, JAMES R DO, LICENSE NUMBER 0001643, WAS DISCIPLINED BY ARIZONA ON JANUARY 11, 1991
DISCIPLINARY ACTION: PROBATION; MONITORING OF PHYSICIAN PERFORMANCE
OFFENSE: FAILURE TO COMPLY WITH PREVIOUS BOARD ORDER

NOTES: NONCOMPLIANCE TO PREVIOUS ORDERS: ON 4/09/88 HIS URINE SAMPLE TESTED POSITIVE FOR THE PRESENCE OF ALCOHOL; ON 7/22/88 THE BOARD COULD NOT LOCATE HIM FOR HIS RANDOM URINE SAMPLES; ON 12/08/88 HIS URINE SAMPLE TESTED POSITIVE FOR THE PRESENCE OF COCAINE; ON 12/14/88 HE ADMITTED THAT HE HAD PREVIOUSLY USED COCAINE; ON 7/21/89 HE TOLD THE BOARD HE WOULD REFRAIN FROM THE USE OF ILLICIT DRUGS AND ALCOHOLIC BEVERAGES, ATTEND AT LEAST FIVE "12-STEP" MEETINGS PER WEEK, AND SUBMIT TO RANDOM URINE SAMPLES; ON 11/14/90 HIS URINE SAMPLE TESTED POSITIVE FOR THE PRESENCE OF ETHANOL. PROBATION UNDER TERMS AND CONDITIONS: SHALL SUBMIT TO RANDOM URINALYSIS TESTING; SHALL USE NO CONTROLLED SUBSTANCES OR PRESCRIPTION-ONLY MEDICATION UNLESS PRESCRIBED BY HIS ATTENDING PHYSICIAN; SHALL REFRAIN FROM THE CONSUMPTION OF ALCOHOL; SHALL MEET WITH THE BOARD REGULARLY TO REVIEW HIS COMPLIANCE WITH THIS ORDER; SHALL AUTHORIZE ANY ATTENDING PHYSICIAN, PSYCHIATRIST, OR PSYCHOLOGIST TO RELEASE TO THE BOARD ALL RECORDS PERTAINING TO HIS CARE AND TREATMENT; SHALL IMMEDIATELY ENROLL IN THE MONITORED PHYSICIANS AFTER-CARE PROGRAM; SHALL ATTEND NO FEWER THAN FIVE AA MEETINGS PER WEEK, NO FEWER THAN ONE OF THESE MEETINGS SHALL TAKE PLACE WITH THE CADUCEUS CLUB. ORDER MODIFIED ON 7/24/92 LIFTING REQUIREMENT THAT HE ENROLL IN THE MONITORED PHYSICIANS AFTERCARE PROGRAM; SHALL PROVIDE THE BOARD WITHIN 30 DAYS AN AFTERCARE TREATMENT PLAN CONTAINING PROVISIONS FOR PSYCHIATRIC TREATMENT, ATTENDANCE AT GROUP THERAPY SESSIONS, ATTENDANCE AT 12 STEP PROGRAM MEETINGS, SPONSORSHIP IN A 12 STEP PROGRAM, AND REPORTING OF HIS COMPLIANCE, ATTENDANCE, AND PROGRESS IN THE TREATMENT PLAN TO THE BOARD; SHALL PROVIDE THE BOARD WITH OBSERVED BODY FLUID SAMPLES UPON REQUEST. ON 9/18/93 PROBATION SATISFIED IN FULL.

SKLAR, ROBERT MD, LICENSE NUMBER 22986, WAS DISCIPLINED BY ARIZONA ON NOVEMBER 18, 1999
DISCIPLINARY ACTION: REPRIMAND
OFFENSE: NONCOMPLIANCE WITH A PROFESSIONAL RULE

NOTES: INADEQUATE RECORD KEEPING; AND, FAILURE TO REMAIN CURRENT IN OBSTETRICAL/GYNECOLOGICAL PROCEDURES.

SLATER, ROGER C MD, LICENSE NUMBER C18017 OF PRESCOTT, AZ, WAS DISCIPLINED BY CALIFORNIA ON AUGUST 1, 1999
DISCIPLINARY ACTION: 24-MONTH PROBATION

NOTES: REVOCATION STAYED.

SMITH, DIANA J MD, LICENSE NUMBER 0015141, WAS DISCIPLINED BY ARIZONA ON OCTOBER 15, 1993
DISCIPLINARY ACTION: LICENSE REVOCATION
OFFENSE: OVERPRESCRIBING OR MISPRESCRIBING DRUGS

NOTES: HAS A MEDICAL CONDITION WHICH PREVENTS HER FROM SAFELY ENGAGING IN THE PRACTICE OF MEDICINE AT THIS TIME; PRESCRIBED DEMEROL ON 05/08/93 AND 12/3/91 FOR HER HUSBAND; REFUSED TO PRODUCE PATIENT RECORDS FOR INSPECTION BY THE BOARD ON ANY PATIENT FOR WHOM SHE CLAIMED TO HAVE PRESCRIBED OR DISPENSED CONTROLLED SUBSTANCES; HAD LARGE QUANTITIES OF CONTROLLED SUBSTANCES DELIVERED TO HER RESIDENCE, INCLUDING A PACKAGE DELIVERED 07/07/93 CONTAINING 4 500-UNIT DOSE CONTAINERS OF HYDROCODONE WITH APAP AND ONE VIAL DIAZEPAM AND OTHER ASSORTED PHARMACEUTICALS WHICH WERE NOT PROPERLY STORED OR CONTROLLED. SHALL NOT BE ALLOWED TO APPLY FOR A LICENSE TO PRACTICE MEDICINE IN ARIZONA FOR ONE YEAR FROM THE EFFECTIVE DATE OF THIS ORDER; IN ADDITION TO THE ONE-YEAR PERIOD SET FORTH ABOVE, PRIOR TO APPLYING FOR LICENSURE IN ARIZONA, SHE MUST FIRST DEMONSTRATE TO THE SATISFACTION OF THE BOARD THAT SHE IS PHYSICALLY, MENTALLY AND MEDICALLY COMPETENT TO SAFELY ENGAGE IN THE PRACTICE OF MEDICINE, AND PROVIDE PROOF THAT SHE HAS NOT MISUSED ALCOHOL AND/OR LICIT OR ILLICIT DRUGS OR SUBSTANCES OR HAS SUCCESSFULLY COMPLETED LONG-TERM TREATMENT FOR SUBSTANCE ABUSE AND HAS AT LEAST 18 MONTHS DOCUMENTED SOBRIETY FOLLOWING TREATMENT.

SMITH, DIANA J MD OF WA, WAS DISCIPLINED BY DEA ON AUGUST 12, 1994
DISCIPLINARY ACTION: REVOCATION OF CONTROLLED SUBSTANCE LICENSE
OFFENSE: DISCIPLINARY ACTION BY ANOTHER STATE OR AGENCY

NOTES: ON 10/14/93 VOLUNTARILY RELINQUISHED HER LICENSE IN ARIZONA.

SMITH, RICHARD L MD, WAS DISCIPLINED BY ARIZONA ON JULY 17, 1992
DISCIPLINARY ACTION: REQUIRED TO TAKE ADDITIONAL MEDICAL EDUCATION
OFFENSE: OVERPRESCRIBING OR MISPRESCRIBING DRUGS

NOTES: EXCESSIVE PRESCRIBING OF SCHEDULE II DRUGS. MUST ATTEND A ONE MONTH MINI-RESIDENCY IN THE PHARMACOLOGY OF PAIN MANAGEMENT WITHIN SIX MONTHS. ON 1/21/93 HIS REQUEST TO EXTEND THE DEADLINE FOR COMPLETION OF THIS STIPULATION WAS GRANTED; DEADLINE EXTENDED TO 3/93.

SMITH, RODNEY LESTER MD, LICENSE NUMBER 16325, WAS DISCIPLINED BY ARIZONA ON MAY 19, 1999
DISCIPLINARY ACTION: 60-MONTH PROBATION; RESTRICTION PLACED ON LICENSE

NOTES: MAY NOT PRACTICE EMERGENCY MEDICINE EXCEPT IN A SITUATION IN WHICH HE HAS ON SITE CONCURRENT SUPERVISION BY AN APPROPRIATE SUPERVISING PHYSICIAN; ALSO ISSUED A DECREE OF CENSURE. ON 7/30/99, MOTION FOR REHEARING DENIED.

SMITH, STANLEY A MD, LICENSE NUMBER 0003783 OF PHOENIX, AZ, WAS DISCIPLINED BY ARIZONA ON OCTOBER 31, 1994
DISCIPLINARY ACTION: RESTRICTION PLACED ON LICENSE;

MONITORING OF PHYSICIAN PERFORMANCE

NOTES: RELATIVE TO ACTION TAKEN BY ST. JOSEPH'S HOSPITAL REGARDING HIS PRIVILEGES; CARE AND TREATMENT OF ONE PATIENT; AND BOARD ORDERED EVALUATIONS. SHALL NOT PRACTICE MEDICINE IN ARIZONA AS A SOLE PRACTITIONER BUT SHALL PRACTICE ONLY IN A GROUP SETTING WHERE THERE IS AT LEAST ONE OTHER PHYSICIAN OF THE SAME AREA OF SPECIALTY AVAILABLE ONSITE TO SUPERVISE OR ASSIST HIM IN HIS MEDICAL PRACTICE; MENTAL AND PHYSICAL CONDITION SHALL BE PERIODICALLY REEVALUATED AT THE REQUEST OF THE BOARD.

SMITH, STANLEY A MD, LICENSE NUMBER 3783, WAS DISCIPLINED BY ARIZONA ON JANUARY 22, 1997
DISCIPLINARY ACTION: REPRIMAND

NOTES: VIOLATED 7/18/94 ORDER BY PRACTICING SOLO RATHER THAN IN A GROUP SETTING AS WAS ORDERED.

SMITH, SUSAN M DO, LICENSE NUMBER 0002606 OF P.O. BOX 40502, MESA, AZ, WAS DISCIPLINED BY ARIZONA ON FEBRUARY 13, 1992
DISCIPLINARY ACTION: REQUIRED TO TAKE ADDITIONAL MEDICAL EDUCATION; MONITORING OF PHYSICIAN PERFORMANCE
OFFENSE: OVERPRESCRIBING OR MISPRESCRIBING DRUGS

NOTES: ALLEGED INAPPROPRIATE PRESCRIBING OF CONTROLLED SUBSTANCES AND FAILURE TO MAINTAIN MEDICAL RECORDS ON A PATIENT. SHALL MAINTAIN A LOG OF ALL PRESCRIPTIONS WRITTEN BY HER WITH COPIES SUBMITTED TO THE BOARD; THE BOARD MAY REQUEST THAT SHE MAKE HER MEDICAL RECORDS AVAILABLE FOR REVIEW UPON DEMAND TO VERIFY THE ACCURACY OF HER PRESCRIPTION LOG; SHALL ATTEND NO LESS THAN 30 HOURS OF CONTINUING MEDICAL EDUCATION IN THE FIELDS OF ADDICTIONOLOGY AND PRESCRIBING OF NARCOTICS AND OTHER MEDICATIONS WITHIN TWO YEARS AND SUBMIT EVIDENCE TO THE BOARD.

SMITH, SUSAN M DO, LICENSE NUMBER 0002606 OF P.O. BOX 40502, MESA, AZ, WAS DISCIPLINED BY ARIZONA ON DECEMBER 13, 1992
DISCIPLINARY ACTION: PROBATION; MONITORING OF PHYSICIAN PERFORMANCE
OFFENSE: SUBSTANCE ABUSE

NOTES: ON 10/15/92 ATTEMPTED TO PROCURE, BY MEANS OF A FRAUDULENT PRESCRIPTION, A QUANTITY OF THE CONTROLLED, PRESCRIPTION ONLY MEDICATION, XANAX AND BUSPAR AND WAS ARRESTED ON SUSPICION OF ATTEMPTING TO ILLEGALLY OBTAIN CONTROLLED AND PRESCRIPTION-ONLY DRUGS AND AT WHICH SHE TIME SHE ADMITTED TO USING XANAX FOR AT LEAST SIX MONTHS PRIOR TO THIS INCIDENT; AT THE TIME WAS NOT UNDER THE CARE AND TREATMENT OF A PHYSICIAN AS PART OF A RECOGNIZED COURSE OF TREATMENT FOR THE MEDICATION SHE ATTEMPTED TO PROCURE. PROBATION WITH TERMS AND CONDITIONS: SHALL SECURE AND MAINTAIN A SPONSOR FOR A 12 STEP RECOVERY PROGRAM; SHALL ATTEND AT LEAST FOUR 12 STEP MEETINGS PER WEEK FOR THE FIRST 12 MONTHS OF THIS ORDER; SHALL ATTEND REGULAR MEETINGS WITH HER ATTENDING PHYSICIAN PER HER CONTINUING CARE PLAN; SHALL ATTEND NO LESS THAN THREE GROUP THERAPY MEETINGS PER MONTH WITH A BOARD APPROVED COUNSELOR; SHALL SUBMIT TO RANDOM BODY FLUID TESTING; SHALL MEET WITH THE BOARD REGULARLY AND UPON REQUEST; SHALL USE NO CONTROLLED SUBSTANCE OR PRESCRIPTION-ONLY MEDICATION UNLESS PRESCRIBED BY HER ATTENDING PHYSICIAN; SHALL REFRAIN FROM THE USE OF ALCOHOL; SHALL AUTHORIZE ALL TREATING PERSONNEL INVOLVED IN HER CARE TO RELEASE INFORMATION ON HER PROGRESS AND PROGNOSIS UPON BOARD REQUEST.

SMITH, SUSAN M DO, DATE OF BIRTH MAY 10, 1958 OF 7800 E LINCOLN WAY #1031, SCOTTSDALE, AZ, WAS DISCIPLINED BY MEDICARE ON MAY 12, 1994
DISCIPLINARY ACTION: EXCLUSION FROM THE MEDICARE AND/OR MEDICAID PROGRAM
OFFENSE: NONCOMPLIANCE WITH A PROFESSIONAL RULE

NOTES: DEFAULTED ON PUBLIC HEALTH SERVICE EDUCATION LOAN. REINSTATED ON 7/7/94.

SMITH, SUSAN M DO, LICENSE NUMBER 0002606 OF P.O. BOX 40502, MESA, AZ, WAS DISCIPLINED BY ARIZONA ON DECEMBER 6, 1994
DISCIPLINARY ACTION: EMERGENCY SUSPENSION
OFFENSE: FAILURE TO COMPLY WITH PREVIOUS BOARD ORDER

NOTES: NONCOMPLIANCE TO HER ORDER DATED 12/31/92 IN THAT ON 11/08/94 AN ANALYSIS OF A URINE DRUG SCREEN INDICATED THE PRESENCE OF HYDROCODONE (LORTAB) AND CARISOPRODOL (SOMA); AS OF 11/30/94 THE BOARD HAD NOT BEEN NOTIFIED BY EITHER HER OR HER TREATING PHYSICIAN THAT SHE HAS BEEN PRESCRIBED EITHER DRUG; AS OF 11/30/94 HAS NOT SUBMITTED PRESCRIBING LOGS FOR THE PERIOD OF 9/19/92 THROUGH 11/30/94 TO THE BOARD; ON 3/31/94 THE BOARD RECEIVED INFORMATION FROM CIGNA HEALTH CARE OF ARIZONA INDICATING THAT SHE WAS PROVIDED THE OPPORTUNITY TO RESIGN HER POSITION WITH THE ORGANIZATION, IN LIEU OF BEING DISCHARGED FOR VARIOUS ASPECTS OF MEDICAL PRACTICE DEEMED TO BE BELOW THE STANDARD OF CARE INCLUDING: FAILURE TO MAINTAIN APPROPRIATE RECORDS ON PATIENTS; AND PERFORMING A VASECTOMY ON A PATIENT WITHOUT APPROPRIATE TRAINING AND/OR SUPERVISION.

SMITH, SUSAN M DO, DATE OF BIRTH MAY 10, 1958 OF 7800 E LINCOLN WAY, SCOTTSDALE, AZ, WAS DISCIPLINED BY MEDICARE ON MARCH 22, 1995
DISCIPLINARY ACTION: EXCLUSION FROM THE MEDICARE AND/OR MEDICAID PROGRAM
OFFENSE: NONCOMPLIANCE WITH A PROFESSIONAL RULE

NOTES: DEFAULTED ON PUBLIC HEALTH SERVICE EDUCATION LOAN.

SMITH, SUSAN M DO, LICENSE NUMBER 0002606 OF P.O. BOX 40502, MESA, AZ, WAS DISCIPLINED BY ARIZONA ON MAY 17, 1995
DISCIPLINARY ACTION: 48-MONTH PROBATION; MONITORING OF PHYSICIAN PERFORMANCE
OFFENSE: FAILURE TO COMPLY WITH PREVIOUS BOARD ORDER

NOTES: SUSPENSION RETROACTIVE TO THE SUMMARY SUSPENSION ORDER DATED 12/06/94 WHICH TERMINATES THE DATE OF THIS ORDER. PROBATION WITH TERMS AND CONDITIONS: FOR A MINIMUM OF ONE YEAR SHALL OBTAIN PSYCHIATRIC OR PSYCHOLOGICAL TREATMENT WITH A WRITTEN PROGRESS REPORT TO THE BOARD EVERY TWO MONTHS; SHALL ABSTAIN FROM THE CONSUMPTION OF ALCOHOL AND SHALL NOT CONSUME ILLICIT DRUGS OR TAKE ANY CONTROLLED SUBSTANCES UNLESS SUCH MEDICATION WAS PRESCRIBED BY A TREATING PHYSICIAN; SHALL MAINTAIN A MONTHLY

LOG OF ALL PRESCRIPTION ONLY DRUGS TAKEN BY HER WHICH SHALL BE SUBMITTED TO THE BOARD MONTHLY; SHALL SUBMIT TO AND COOPERATE IN ANY INDEPENDENT EVALUATION THAT IS ORDERED BY THE BOARD; SHALL APPEAR BEFORE THE BOARD UPON REQUEST; SHALL SUBMIT TO RANDOM BIOLOGICAL FLUID TESTING; SHALL NOTIFY THE BOARD WITHIN 20 DAYS IF SHE CEASES TO RESIDE IN ARIZONA.

SMITH, SUSAN M DO, DATE OF BIRTH MAY 10, 1958, LICENSE NUMBER 02180 OF PO BOX 40502, MESA, AZ, WAS DISCIPLINED BY IOWA ON JANUARY 23, 1997
DISCIPLINARY ACTION: LICENSE REVOCATION
OFFENSE: DISCIPLINARY ACTION BY ANOTHER STATE OR AGENCY

NOTES: ACTION BY ARIZONA BOARD.

SMITH, SUSAN MARGARET DO, LICENSE NUMBER 2606 OF PO BOX 40502, MESA, AZ, WAS DISCIPLINED BY ARIZONA ON APRIL 28, 1997
DISCIPLINARY ACTION: 60-MONTH PROBATION; REQUIRED TO TAKE ADDITIONAL MEDICAL EDUCATION
OFFENSE: FAILURE TO COMPLY WITH PREVIOUS BOARD ORDER

NOTES: FROM 3/4/96 TO 5/22/96 AT THE MEDICAL CENTER WHERE SHE WAS EMPLOYED SHE REGULARLY FAILED TO COMPLETE APPROPRIATE NOTATIONS AND DICTATION FOR PATIENT FILES IN A TIMELY FASHION; FAILED TO TIMELY AND COMPLETELY PREPARE PATIENT CHARTS FOR PATIENTS SHE TREATED; AS REQUIRED BY 5/28/96 CONSENT ORDER SHE FAILED TO PROVIDE A URINE SAMPLE FOR DRUG TESTING. CENSURED FOR UNPROFESSIONAL CONDUCT; TERMS OF PROBATION ARE AS FOLLOWS: ALL TERMS AND CONDITIONS OF 5/17/95 PROBATION IN EFFECT; SHE WILL CHANGE HER TREATING PSYCHIATRIST WITHIN 20 DAYS TO A NEW TREATING PSYCHIATRIST APPROVED BY THE BOARD WITH MONTHLY REPORTS; SHALL REIMBURSE THE BOARD FOR COSTS RELATED TO HER EXAMINATIONS; SHALL ALSO SUBMIT TO ANY EVALUATIONS ORDERED BY THE BOARD; SHALL OBTAIN 20 HOURS OF CONTINUING MEDICAL EDUCATION APPROVED BY THE BOARD; EACH YEAR FOR THE NEXT TWO YEARS IN PROPER CHARTING; SHALL IMPLEMENT PROCEDURES FOR MAINTAINING COMPLETE OFFICE AND PATIENT RECORDS THAT FOLLOW THE "SOAP" FORMAT; SHALL CONTACT THE BOARD OFFICE DAILY AND IF TOLD TO REPORT TO THAT OFFICE OR ANOTHER DESIGNATED LOCATION FOR BODILY FLUID TESTING, SHALL REPORT WITHIN 60 MINUTES OF NOTIFICATION; SHALL COMPLY WITH ALL TERMS IMPOSED BY ANY ARIZONA HOSPITAL AT WHICH SHE OBTAINS PRIVILEGES TO PRACTICE.

SMITH, SUSAN MARGARET DO, LICENSE NUMBER 2606 OF 219 S. MOUNTAIN AVENUE, SPRINGERVILLE, AZ, WAS DISCIPLINED BY ARIZONA ON OCTOBER 16, 1999
DISCIPLINARY ACTION: 60-MONTH PROBATION

NOTES: ISSUED A LICENSE WITH FOLLOWING CONDITIONS: SHALL IMMEDIATELY OBTAIN A TREATING THERAPIST APPROVED BY THE BOARD AND SHALL REMAIN IN TREATMENT UNTIL FURTHER ORDER OF THE BOARD; THE THERAPIST SHALL PROVIDE MONTHLY REPORTS TO THE BOARD FOR THE FIRST SIX MONTHS THEN EVERY THREE MONTHS FOR THE REMAINDER OF THE PROBATION; SHALL PROVIDE A COPY OF THIS ORDER TO ANY HEALTH CARE ENTITY WHERE SHE HAS PRIVILEGES; SHALL ABSTAIN COMPLETELY FROM THE CONSUMPTION OF ALCOHOLIC BEVERAGES AND DRUGS EXCEPT WHEN PRESCRIBED BY HER TREATING PHYSICIAN; SHALL SUBMIT TO ANY EXAMINATIONS ORDERED BY BOARD; SHALL APPEAR BEFORE BOARD UPON REQUEST; SHALL SUBMIT TO RANDOM BIOLOGICAL FLUID COLLECTION; SHALL PARTICIPATE IN A MINIMUM OF TWO SELF-HELP MEETINGS PER WEEK THROUGH SUCH ORGANIZATIONS SUCH AS AA OR NARCOTICS ANONYMOUS; THIS ORDER SUPERSEDES ALL PRIOR ORDERS; SHALL INFORM THE BOARD IF SHE CEASES TO PRACTICE IN ARIZONA; SHALL PAY COSTS.

SMOLEV, BARRY A MD, LICENSE NUMBER 0145867 OF 2885 NICADA DRIVE, LOS ANGELES, CA, WAS DISCIPLINED BY NEW YORK ON MAY 9, 1996
DISCIPLINARY ACTION: 6-MONTH LICENSE SUSPENSION; 84-MONTH PROBATION
OFFENSE: DISCIPLINARY ACTION BY ANOTHER STATE OR AGENCY

NOTES: ACTION IN CALIFORNIA. CONVICTED OF MAIL FRAUD AND ASSISTING IN THE PREPARATION AND PRESENTATION OF A FALSE INCOME TAX RETURN. DISCIPLINED BY CALIFORNIA BOARD FOR PARTICIPATING IN A FRAUDULENT SCHEME BY MISREPRESENTING TO INSURANCE COMPANIES WEIGHT LOSS PATIENTS' SYMPTOMS IN ORDER TO QUALIFY THE PATIENTS FOR INSURANCE BENEFITS. SUSPENSION WITH PROBATION UPON COMMENCEMENT OF NEW YORK PRACTICE.

SMOLEV, BARRY ALAN MD, LICENSE NUMBER 0G23299 OF LOS ANGELES, CA, WAS DISCIPLINED BY CALIFORNIA ON APRIL 5, 1995
DISCIPLINARY ACTION: LICENSE SUSPENSION; 83-MONTH PROBATION
OFFENSE: INSURANCE, MEDICARE OR MEDICAID FRAUD

NOTES: ENGAGED IN A DISHONEST SCHEME TO DEFRAUD INSURANCE BY CREATING PHONY PSYCHIATRIC REPORTS STATING FALSELY THAT PATIENTS (FOR WEIGHT LOSS) HAD PSYCHIATRIC DISORDERS TO JUSTIFY INSURANCE PAYMENTS FOR $35,000-29 DAY STAY IN AN ACUTE CARE FACILITY WHERE HE WAS A TREATING PSYCHIATRIST. ALSO, DISHONESTY FOR TAX FRAUD. REVOCATION STAYED. 7 YEARS PROBATION, INCLUDING 21 DAYS ACTUAL SUSPENSION.

SMOLEV, BARRY ALAN MD, DATE OF BIRTH MAY 8, 1946 OF 2885 NICADA DRIVE, LOS ANGELES, CA, WAS DISCIPLINED BY MEDICARE ON JULY 18, 1996
DISCIPLINARY ACTION: 36-MONTH EXCLUSION FROM THE MEDICARE AND/OR MEDICAID PROGRAM
OFFENSE: CRIMINAL CONVICTION OR PLEA OF GUILTY, NOLO CONTENDERE, OR NO CONTEST TO A CRIME

NOTES: CONVICTED OF A CRIME RELATED TO THE DELIVERY OF HEALTH CARE OR FINANCIAL MISCONDUCT INVOLVING A GOVERNMENT-OPERATED PROGRAM.

SMOLEV, BARRY ALAN MD, LICENSE NUMBER 0015914, WAS DISCIPLINED BY ARIZONA ON NOVEMBER 12, 1996
DISCIPLINARY ACTION: LICENSE REVOCATION
OFFENSE: DISCIPLINARY ACTION BY ANOTHER STATE OR AGENCY

NOTES: ON 4/5/95 CALIFORNIA BOARD PLACED HIS LICENSE ON PROBATION FOR SEVEN YEARS WITH CONDITIONS; CONVICTED IN 1995 OF ONE FELONY COUNT OF MAIL FRAUD AND ONE FELONY COUNT OF TAX FRAUD; IN 1986 ATTENDED A THREE MONTH CHEMICAL DEPENDENCY PROGRAM FOR DRUG ADDICTION; LIED ABOUT ALL THREE OF THESE ON HIS 12/95 ARIZONA RENEWAL APPLICATION AND ALSO LIED ABOUT CHEMICAL DEPENDENCY ON 12/93 AND 12/94 RENEWAL APPLICATIONS. SINCE 5/93 HAS BEEN UNDERGOING THERAPY FOR SEVERE AND RECURRENT DEPRESSION, LOW SELF-ESTEEM AND

CHEMICAL DEPENDENCY. SHALL NOT PRACTICE IN ARIZONA WITHOUT FIRST MEETING WITH THE BOARD.

SNYDER, DONALD ELWOOD DO, DATE OF BIRTH MARCH 10, 1918 OF 7910 E CAMELBACK ROAD #401, SCOTTSDALE, AZ, WAS DISCIPLINED BY MEDICARE ON NOVEMBER 16, 1995
DISCIPLINARY ACTION: 60-MONTH EXCLUSION FROM THE MEDICARE AND/OR MEDICAID PROGRAM
OFFENSE: CRIMINAL CONVICTION OR PLEA OF GUILTY, NOLO CONTENDERE, OR NO CONTEST TO A CRIME

NOTES: CONVICTED OF A CRIME INVOLVING THE MEDICARE, MEDICAID, MATERNAL AND CHILD HEALTH SERVICES BLOCK GRANT OR BLOCK GRANTS TO STATES FOR SOCIAL SERVICES PROGRAMS.

SOBEL, LARRY MD, LICENSE NUMBER 12792, WAS DISCIPLINED BY ARIZONA ON DECEMBER 9, 1999
DISCIPLINARY ACTION: PROBATION

SOBOTKA, JOSEPH J MD OF 7617 S CENTRAL AVENUE, PHOENIX, AZ, WAS DISCIPLINED BY MEDICARE ON MARCH 16, 1995
DISCIPLINARY ACTION: 60-MONTH EXCLUSION FROM THE MEDICARE AND/OR MEDICAID PROGRAM
OFFENSE: CRIMINAL CONVICTION OR PLEA OF GUILTY, NOLO CONTENDERE, OR NO CONTEST TO A CRIME

NOTES: CONVICTED OF A CRIME INVOLVING THE MEDICARE, MEDICAID, MATERNAL AND CHILD HEALTH SERVICES BLOCK GRANT OR BLOCK GRANTS TO STATES FOR SOCIAL SERVICES PROGRAMS.

SOMOSHEGYI-SZOKOL, ATTILA MD, LICENSE NUMBER 0007970, WAS DISCIPLINED BY ARIZONA ON SEPTEMBER 10, 1992
DISCIPLINARY ACTION: LICENSE REVOCATION
OFFENSE: FAILURE TO COMPLY WITH PREVIOUS BOARD ORDER

NOTES: IN 12/87 BOARD RECEIVED INFORMATION HE MAY BE MISUSING ALCOHOL; IN EARLY 1988 COMPLETED A SIX WEEK OUTPATIENT PROGRAM; 8/1/88 BOARD ORDER PROVIDED HE ABSTAIN FROM ALCOHOL; DID NOT COMPLY WITH THIS ORDER; BOARD ORDERED HIM TO ENTER A DESIGNATED INPATIENT TREATMENT CENTER FOR EVALUATION IN 4/92; BASED ON THIS WAS ORDERED TO UNDERGO INTENSIVE PSYCHOTHERAPY; VIOLATED PREVIOUS BOARD ORDERS. ON 8/23/92, CALLED TO ASSIST IN SURGERY. ARRIVED OBVIOUSLY INTOXICATED, BUT STILL ASSISTED IN THE OPERATING ROOM. ARRESTED ON HIS WAY HOME AND CHARGED WITH TWO COUNTS OF DRIVING WHILE INTOXICATED. ALCOHOL LEVELS MEASURED AT .26 PERCENT AND .25 PERCENT. ON 8/24/92, THE HOSPITAL AT WHICH HE PRACTICED INFORMED THE BOARD THAT HIS HOSPITAL PRIVILEGES WERE SUMMARILY SUSPENDED. HE ENTERED A TREATMENT PROGRAM FOR CHEMICAL DEPENDENCY. LICENSE SURRENDERED FOR CANCELLATION WITH CAUSE.

SOMOSHEGYI-SZOKOL, ATTILA MD, WAS DISCIPLINED BY ARIZONA ON JULY 16, 1993
DISCIPLINARY ACTION: REQUIRED TO ENTER AN IMPAIRED PHYSICIAN PROGRAM OR SUBSTANCE ABUSE TREATMENT
OFFENSE: FAILURE TO COMPLY WITH PREVIOUS BOARD ORDER

NOTES: PASSED SPEX EXAM; POSITIVE URINE TEST FOR ALCOHOL. MUST ATTEND ADDITIONAL EXTENDED TREATMENT FOR CHEMICAL DEPENDENCY; MUST SHOW AT LEAST 3 YEARS SOBRIETY BEFORE HE CAN REAPPLY.

SORGEN, ROBERT MD, WAS DISCIPLINED BY ARIZONA ON JANUARY 17, 1996
DISCIPLINARY ACTION: LICENSE SUSPENSION

NOTES: LICENSE PLACED ON INACTIVE STATUS WITH CAUSE.

SORGEN, ROBERT W MD OF 3326 EAST SWEETWATER, PHOENIX, AZ, WAS DISCIPLINED BY DEA ON SEPTEMBER 12, 1995
DISCIPLINARY ACTION: SURRENDER OF CONTROLLED SUBSTANCE LICENSE

NOTES: IN LIEU OF ORDER TO SHOW CAUSE.

SORGEN, ROBERT WILLIAM MD, LICENSE NUMBER 0012567, WAS DISCIPLINED BY ARIZONA ON JUNE 19, 1991
DISCIPLINARY ACTION: 60-MONTH PROBATION; RESTRICTION PLACED ON CONTROLLED SUBSTANCE LICENSE
OFFENSE: SUBSTANCE ABUSE

NOTES: ON 12/3/82 BOARD FOUND HE DEMONSTRATED HABITUAL INTEMPERANCE IN THE USE OF ALCOHOL AND PLACED HIM ON PROBATION FOR FIVE YEARS WITH CONDITIONS. HE UNDERWENT OUTPATIENT TREATMENT FOR ALCOHOLISM IN 1983. A 4/1/85 ORDER REQUIRED THAT HE CONTINUE TREATMENT FOR ALCOHOL MISUSE; ABSTAIN FROM THE USE OF ALCOHOL, TAKE NO DRUGS, ATTEND AA, AND APPEAR BEFORE THE BOARD WHEN REQUESTED; THIS ORDER WAS TERMINATED 12/7/85. ON 2/7/86 BOARD ISSUED LETTER OF CONCERN FOR INAPPROPRIATE BILLING PRACTICES. ON 1/28/87 ISSUED LETTER OF CONCERN FOR DELAY IN TRANSMITTING PATIENT RECORDS. BETWEEN 2/85 AND 8/88 HE PRESCRIBED DRUGS TO THREE PATIENTS WITHOUT APPROPRIATE DOCUMENTATION IN CHART OR A PROPER EXAMINATION. IN EARLY 1989 HE RESUMED DRINKING. IN 12/89 THE BOARD REQUESTED A PHYSICAL AND PSYCHOLOGICAL EVALUATION, AND IN 1/90 HE UNDERWENT AN ORAL COMPETENCY EXAM. ON 1/17/90 HE REQUESTED THAT BOARD PLACE HIS LICENSE IN INACTIVE STATUS. FROM 1/90 TO 4/90 HE UNDERWENT INPATIENT TREATMENT FOR CHEMICAL DEPENDENCY. ON 4/30/90 HE ASKED BOARD TO RETURN LICENSE TO ACTIVE STATUS. AFTER TAKING THE SPEX EXAM TWICE, HE PASSED. CONDITIONS OF PROBATION INCLUDE: MUST ONLY PRACTICE IN A GROUP SETTING WITH QUARTERLY REPORTS TO THE BOARD; MUST SURRENDER HIS DEA REGISTRATION FOR SCHEDULE II DRUGS AND MAY NOT REAPPLY WITHOUT BOARD AUTHORIZATION; MUST PARTICIPATE IN THE ARIZONA MEDICAL ASSOCIATION'S MONITORED AFTERCARE TREATMENT PROGRAM; MUST INSTRUCT THERAPIST TO RELEASE RECORDS TO THE BOARD WITH QUARTERLY REPORTS; MUST ATTEND A MINIMUM OF 3 AA MEETINGS PER WEEK; MUST OBTAIN ONE BOARD-APPROVED TREATING PHYSICIAN; MUST ABSTAIN COMPLETELY FROM ALCOHOL AND OTHER DRUGS; MUST SUBMIT TO RANDOM TESTS OF BODILY FLUIDS; MUST MAINTAIN A LOG OF ALL MEDICATIONS TAKEN; SHALL SUBMIT TO MENTAL, PHYSICAL OR MEDICAL COMPETENCY EXAMS OR THERAPY WHICH THE BOARD REQUESTS; MUST APPEAR BEFORE THE BOARD UPON REQUEST AND INFORM THEM IF HE'S AWAY FOR MORE THAN FIVE DAYS. ON 1/25/92 HE REQUESTED PERMISSION TO PRACTICE IN A SOLO SETTING TO DO LOCUM TENENS AND ACT AS A MEDICAL DIRECTOR/ADMINISTRATOR WITH OR WITHOUT CLINICAL PRIVILEGES, IN A SINGLE OR GROUP POSITION. BOARD REAFFIRMED ITS POSITION THAT HE NOT ENGAGE IN CLINICAL PRACTICE, EXCEPT IN A GROUP SETTING. ALSO AMENDED PROBATION TO ALLOW HIM TO PRACTICE IN AN ADMINISTRATIVE ROLE ONLY AS AN INDIVIDUAL

PHYSICIAN, AND TO REQUEST QUARTERLY REPORTS FROM PEER REVIEW PROGRAM OR EMPLOYER. ON 4/17/93 BOARD CONTINUED PROBATION ORDER WITH CONDITION THAT HIS GROUP THERAPY REQUIREMENT BE DROPPED. ON 4/16/94 HIS REQUEST TO TERMINATE ORDER AND ENTER INTO THE BOARD'S STANDARD REHABILITATION STIPULATION UNDER THE SAME TERMS AS HIS PROBATIONARY ORDER DENIED. HE MUST MEET WITH THE BOARD IN ONE YEAR AT THE 4/95 MEETING.

SORGEN, ROBERT WILLIAM MD OF 3326 E SWEETWATER, PHOENIX, AZ, WAS DISCIPLINED BY DEA ON JANUARY 26, 1994
DISCIPLINARY ACTION: RESTRICTION PLACED ON CONTROLLED SUBSTANCE LICENSE

NOTES: VOLUNTARY SURRENDER OF REGISTRATION 03/01/90. PLACED ON PROBATION 06/19/91. APPROVAL OF REGISTRATION. RESTRICTED TO SCHEDULE III, IV AND V CONTROLLED SUBSTANCES. ALIAS ROBERT SORGIN.

SOTELO-GARZA, DANILO H MD, LICENSE NUMBER 0013879 OF TUCSON, AZ, WAS DISCIPLINED BY ARIZONA ON JANUARY 17, 1995
DISCIPLINARY ACTION: REQUIRED TO TAKE ADDITIONAL MEDICAL EDUCATION; MONITORING OF PHYSICIAN PERFORMANCE
OFFENSE: PROFESSIONAL MISCONDUCT

NOTES: BOARD HAD INFORMATION THAT THE AMERICAN ACADEMY OF ORTHOPEDIC SURGEONS DENIED HIS MEMBERSHIP, AND A MALPRACTICE CASE ALLEGING UNSATISFACTORY TREATMENT OF A LEG FRACTURE. SHALL OBTAIN 20 HOURS OF CONTINUING MEDICAL EDUCATION IN THE DIAGNOSIS AND MANAGEMENT OF POST-OPERATIVE WOUND INFECTION WITHIN ONE YEAR. BOARD WILL CONDUCT A REVIEW OF 10 OF HIS OFFICE OR HOSPITAL CASES WITHIN A YEAR.

SOTELO-GARZA, DANILO H MD, LICENSE NUMBER 0013879, WAS DISCIPLINED BY ARIZONA ON OCTOBER 16, 1996

NOTES: INTERIM STIPULATION AND ORDER; VOLUNTARY AGREEMENT NOT TO PRACTICE MEDICINE IN ARIZONA UNTIL FIRST MEETING WITH THE BOARD.

SPINAZZOLA, VICTORIA MD, WAS DISCIPLINED BY ARIZONA ON JANUARY 29, 1999
DISCIPLINARY ACTION: LICENSE SUSPENSION
OFFENSE: SUBSTANCE ABUSE

NOTES: STIPULATED REHABILITATION AGREEMENT. REQUEST FOR INACTIVE STATUS WITH CAUSE GRANTED.

SPRINGER, GREGG E MD, DATE OF BIRTH MARCH 7, 1945, LICENSE NUMBER 0017915 OF COLORADO SPRINGS, CO, WAS DISCIPLINED BY COLORADO ON DECEMBER 10, 1993
DISCIPLINARY ACTION: 60-MONTH PROBATION; MONITORING OF PHYSICIAN PERFORMANCE
OFFENSE: SUBSTANCE ABUSE

NOTES: ALLEGATIONS OF EXCESSIVE USE OF A CONTROLLED SUBSTANCE. PROBATIONARY PERIOD INCLUDES TREATMENT AND PRACTICE MONITORING.

SPRINGER, GREGG E MD, DATE OF BIRTH MARCH 7, 1945, LICENSE NUMBER 0017915, WAS DISCIPLINED BY COLORADO ON OCTOBER 10, 1996
DISCIPLINARY ACTION: EMERGENCY SUSPENSION

SPRINGER, GREGG E MD, DATE OF BIRTH MARCH 7, 1945, LICENSE NUMBER 17915, WAS DISCIPLINED BY COLORADO ON JANUARY 9, 1997
DISCIPLINARY ACTION: MONITORING OF PHYSICIAN PERFORMANCE
OFFENSE: FAILURE TO COMPLY WITH PREVIOUS BOARD ORDER

NOTES: VIOLATION OF A VALID BOARD ORDER AND GIVING A SCHEDULE II SUBSTANCE TO SELF OR A FAMILY MEMBER. REVOCATION STAYED FOR AN INDEFINITE PERIOD. HE MAY NOT PRACTICE UNTIL TREATERS STATE THAT HE IS SAFE TO RESUME PRACTICE; SHALL BE SUBJECT TO TREATMENT AND PRACTICE MONITORING PROVISIONS.

SPRINGER, GREGG E MD, DATE OF BIRTH MARCH 7, 1945, LICENSE NUMBER 1048010 OF 509 BEAR PAW LANE, COLORADO SPRINGS, CO, WAS DISCIPLINED BY MICHIGAN ON AUGUST 15, 1997
DISCIPLINARY ACTION: PROBATION; FINE
OFFENSE: DISCIPLINARY ACTION BY ANOTHER STATE OR AGENCY

NOTES: FAILURE TO REPORT/COMPLY. $2000 FINE.

SPRINGER, GREGG EDWARD MD, LICENSE NUMBER 0017379, WAS DISCIPLINED BY ARIZONA ON MAY 4, 1995

NOTES: 90 DAYS PRIOR TO PRACTICING MEDICINE IN ARIZONA, SHALL NOTIFY THE ARIZONA BOARD OF HIS INTENT TO DO SO.

SRINARAYANA, HANUMAIAH MD, WAS DISCIPLINED BY ARIZONA ON MARCH 14, 1997

NOTES: WITHIN 60 DAYS, HE SHALL SUBMIT TO PSYCHIATRIC AND PSYCHOLOGICAL/PSYCHOMETRIC EVALUATIONS BY EVALUATORS APPROVED BY THE BOARD, WHO SHALL SUBMIT WRITTEN REPORTS TO THE BOARD.

STAVROS, GEORGE E MD, LICENSE NUMBER 0004409, WAS DISCIPLINED BY ARIZONA ON JUNE 20, 1991
DISCIPLINARY ACTION: FINE
OFFENSE: LOSS OR RESTRICTION OF HOSPITAL PRIVILEGES

NOTES: ON 3/14/90 THE BOARD WAS TOLD THAT THE EXECUTIVE COMMITTEE OF A LOCAL HOSPITAL HAD REQUESTED THAT HE OBTAIN A MANDATORY CONSULTATION ON EVERY PATIENT HE ADMITTED TO THE HOSPITAL. THE HOSPITAL COMMITTEE CONCLUDED HE HAD PROVIDED INADEQUATE PATIENT CARE, PATIENT VISITS, PATIENT COVERAGE, CONSULTATION ORDERS AND/OR RECORDKEEPING WITH RESPECT TO 12 PATIENTS. ON 10/15/90 THE BOARD WAS NOTIFIED THAT A SECOND HOSPITAL HAD DENIED HIM STAFF PRIVILEGES. $2,5OO FINE. ON 1/23/92 THE BOARD DENIED HIS MOTION FOR A REHEARING.

STAVROS, GEORGE E MD, LICENSE NUMBER 0005304, WAS DISCIPLINED BY HAWAII ON MARCH 17, 1993
DISCIPLINARY ACTION: 24-MONTH SURRENDER OF LICENSE; FINE

NOTES: FINE OF $100.

STEIN, ELIZABETH D MD, LICENSE NUMBER 0011424 OF PHOENIX, AZ, WAS DISCIPLINED BY ARIZONA ON JULY 14, 1993
DISCIPLINARY ACTION: PROBATION; REQUIRED TO TAKE ADDITIONAL MEDICAL EDUCATION
OFFENSE: LOSS OR RESTRICTION OF HOSPITAL PRIVILEGES

NOTES: ON 5/20/91 PRIVILEGES HAD BEEN SUSPENDED AT ONE HOSPITAL AND ON 9/12/91 AT ANOTHER BASED ON A REVIEW OF ANESTHESIA CASES WHICH WERE MISMANAGED; BOARD CONSULTANT WHO REVIEWED THE CASES CAME TO THE CONCLUSION THAT SHE "CONSISTENTLY FELL BELOW REASONABLE PRACTICE STANDARDS ON A NUMBER OF AREAS, MOST NOTABLY AIRWAY MANAGEMENT, MONITORING

FOR DEVELOPMENT OF CARDIAC AND RESPIRATORY PROBLEMS AND AGGRESSIVE THERAPEUTIC INTERVENTION...JUDGMENT IS CONSISTENTLY POOR IN ASSESSING AND DEALING WITH SEVERELY ILL PATIENTS"; PRIVILEGES REINSTATED ON 4/14/92; HASN'T PRACTICED CLINICAL ANESTHESIA SINCE THEN. CONDITIONS OF PROBATION ARE AS FOLLOWS: SHALL NOT PRACTICE MEDICINE FOR ONE YEAR; SHALL, WITHIN ONE YEAR, SUCCESSFULLY COMPLETE A MINI-RESIDENCY OF AT LEAST SIX MONTHS DURATION IN AN ANESTHESIA PROGRAM APPROVED BY THE BOARD AND SHALL MEET WITH THE BOARD PRIOR TO RESUMING HER PRACTICE OF MEDICINE IN ARIZONA. A REQUEST FOR RECONSIDERATION WAS DENIED ON 10/13/93.

STEIN, ELIZABETH D MD OF 5201 NORTH 19TH AVENUE SUITE 113, PHOENIX, AZ, WAS DISCIPLINED BY DEA ON NOVEMBER 16, 1993
DISCIPLINARY ACTION: SURRENDER OF CONTROLLED SUBSTANCE LICENSE
OFFENSE: SUBSTANDARD CARE, INCOMPETENCE OR NEGLIGENCE

NOTES: FOUND GUILTY 07/22/93 OF GROSS AND REPEATED NEGLIGENCE RESULTING IN THE HARM OR DEATH OF A PATIENT. PLACED ON PROBATION.

STEIN, ELIZABETH D KINNIE MD, LICENSE NUMBER 0106859 OF 7320 NORTH BROOKVIEW WAY, SCOTTSDALE, AZ, WAS DISCIPLINED BY NEW YORK ON NOVEMBER 20, 1995
DISCIPLINARY ACTION: SURRENDER OF LICENSE
OFFENSE: DISCIPLINARY ACTION BY ANOTHER STATE OR AGENCY

NOTES: ACTION IN ARIZONA FOR NEGLIGENCE AND GROSS NEGLIGENCE DURING HER PRACTICE OF ANESTHESIOLOGY.

STEINHOFF, NEIL MD, LICENSE NUMBER 0008290, WAS DISCIPLINED BY ARIZONA ON OCTOBER 16, 1993
DISCIPLINARY ACTION: MONITORING OF PHYSICIAN PERFORMANCE

NOTES: RELATIVE TO EVALUATIONS BY TALBOTT RECOVERY SYSTEMS, INC. SHALL OBTAIN A BOARD-APPROVED TREATING PHYSICIAN; SHALL ABSTAIN COMPLETELY FROM THE CONSUMPTION OF ALCOHOLIC BEVERAGES AND DRUGS EXCEPT WHEN PRESCRIBED BY HIS TREATING PHYSICIAN; MUST SUBMIT TO WITNESSED RANDOM BIOLOGICAL FLUID COLLECTION; SHALL AUTHORIZE AND REQUEST ALL TREATMENT CENTERS WHERE HE RECEIVED TREATMENT OR EVALUATION TO RELEASE ALL RECORDS. SHALL COMPLY WITH ORDER WHETHER OR NOT HE IS IN ARIZONA. ON 1/17/95 THIS ORDER TERMINATED.

STEINHOFF, NEIL GEORGE MD, DATE OF BIRTH JULY 19, 1941, LICENSE NUMBER 0026536 OF 1300 NORTH 12TH STREET, #613, PHOENIX, AZ, WAS DISCIPLINED BY NEW JERSEY ON NOVEMBER 18, 1994
OFFENSE: DISCIPLINARY ACTION BY ANOTHER STATE OR AGENCY

NOTES: SHALL CONTINUE TO COMPLY WITH ALL THE REQUIREMENTS OF AN ORDER DATED 04/17/93 ISSUED BY THE ARIZONA BOARD. SHALL PROVIDE NOTICE TO THE NEW JERSEY BOARD OF ANY CHANGE IN ANY OF THE TERMS OF THE ARIZONA AGREEMENT. PRIOR TO ENGAGING IN ANY ACTIVE PRACTICE IN NEW JERSEY, SHALL APPEAR BEFORE THE BOARD TO RESPOND TO QUESTIONS CONCERNING THE STATUS OF HIS HEALTH AND HIS COMPLIANCE WITH THE ARIZONA AGREEMENT.

STEINKE, KURT DO, LICENSE NUMBER 1977 OF 1631 E. GUADALUPE ROAD #104, TEMPE, AZ, WAS DISCIPLINED BY ARIZONA ON JULY 29, 1999
DISCIPLINARY ACTION: 18-MONTH PROBATION; FINE
OFFENSE: FALSIFYING OR ALTERING PATIENT RECORDS

NOTES: ON OR ABOUT 2/6/98 WHILE EXAMINING A PATIENT, THE PATIENT COMPLAINED THAT HE TESTED POSITIVE FOR AMPHETAMINES DURING A DRUG SCREEN THAT WAS FURNISHED FOR THE U.S. POSTAL SERVICE; THE PATIENT ADAMANTLY DENIED ANY USE OF AMPHETAMINES, AND THE DOCTOR THEN WROTE THE PATIENT A NOTE ON A PRESCRIPTION PAD STATING THAT HE HAD GIVEN THE PATIENT A DIET PILL PHENTERMINE; HE THEN ALTERED THE MEDICAL RECORD TO SHOW THAT HE HAD PRESCRIBED PHENTERMINE ON 1/5/98; AT THE PATIENT'S REQUEST, HE PROVIDED ANOTHER NOTE STATING THAT HE HAD INDEED GIVEN THE PATIENT PHENTERMINE ON 1/5/98. LICENSE LIMITED AS FOLLOWS: SHALL OBTAIN THIRTY HOURS OF CONTINUING MEDICAL EDUCATION IN THE AREAS OF MALPRACTICE PREVENTION, MEDICAL ETHICS, AND A MEDICAL REVIEW OFFICER-TRAINING COURSE; $1500 FINE. ON 11/20/99 PROBATION TERMINATED; FULL AND UNRESTRICTED LICENSE.

STEINKE, KURT H DO, DATE OF BIRTH MARCH 6, 1951, LICENSE NUMBER 1007338 OF 1631 E. GUADALUPE, SUITE 104, TEMPE, AZ, WAS DISCIPLINED BY MICHIGAN ON NOVEMBER 6, 1999
DISCIPLINARY ACTION: PROBATION; FINE
OFFENSE: DISCIPLINARY ACTION BY ANOTHER STATE OR AGENCY

NOTES: SISTER STATE DISCIPLINARY ACTION. $1,000 FINE.

STERN, DARRYL R MD, LICENSE NUMBER 0007513 OF TEMPE, AZ, WAS DISCIPLINED BY ARIZONA ON OCTOBER 22, 1992
DISCIPLINARY ACTION: REQUIRED TO TAKE ADDITIONAL MEDICAL EDUCATION; MONITORING OF PHYSICIAN PERFORMANCE

NOTES: SHALL COMPLETE 20 HOURS OF CONTINUING MEDICAL EDUCATION IN THE PRESCRIBING OF PSYCHOACTIVE MEDICATIONS, WITH CONCENTRATION IN THE EFFECTS OF CHANGING MEDICATIONS RAPIDLY AND/OR REPEATEDLY; SHALL OBTAIN COUNSELING BY A THERAPIST IN THE AREAS OF UNDUE FAMILIARITY WITH PATIENTS, AND MAINTAINING AN APPROPRIATE THERAPEUTIC RELATIONSHIP WITH PATIENTS, AS WELL AS GENERAL ISSUES OF TRANSFERENCE IN A THERAPEUTIC RELATIONSHIP; THERAPIST SHALL SUBMIT QUARTERLY REPORTS TO BOARD; SHALL UNDERGO PERIODIC REVIEW OF CASES, AT LEAST EVERY SIX MONTHS, WHICH WILL INCLUDE CHART STIMULATED RECALL AS TO THE AREAS OF DEFINITION OF THERAPEUTIC RELATIONSHIP AND MAINTENANCE OF APPROPRIATE BOUNDARIES. EFFECTIVE 7/16/93, HIS STIPULATIONS AND ORDERS WILL CONTINUE WITH THE BOARD; A CHART REVIEW WILL BE DONE BY SOMEONE OTHER THAN HIS TREATING PSYCHIATRIST; AND HE WILL MEET WITH THE BOARD AT ITS 10/93 MEETING. ON 7/22/95 ORDER TERMINATED. STAFF WILL CONDUCT A RECORDS SURVEY OF HIS RECORDS IN ONE YEAR. ON 11/14/97 ORDER TERMINATED EFFECTIVE IN 90 DAYS.

STERN, DARRYL R MD, DATE OF BIRTH JUNE 6, 1942, LICENSE NUMBER 0016733 OF 2034 EAST SOUTHERN AVENUE, TEMPE, AZ, WAS DISCIPLINED BY WISCONSIN ON JULY 24, 1996
DISCIPLINARY ACTION: REQUIRED TO ENTER AN IMPAIRED PHYSICIAN PROGRAM OR SUBSTANCE ABUSE TREATMENT; MONITORING OF PHYSICIAN PERFORMANCE
OFFENSE: DISCIPLINARY ACTION BY ANOTHER STATE OR AGENCY

NOTES: ON 3/10/93 HIS LICENSE TO PRACTICE MEDICINE AND SURGERY WAS MADE SUBJECT TO COMPLIANCE WITH

A REHABILITATION ORDER FOR AN INDEFINITE PERIOD BY THE ARIZONA BOARD ON THE GROUNDS THAT HE IS RECOVERING FROM ALCOHOL DEPENDENCE. AT THAT TIME HE ENTERED TREATMENT AND IS FULLY COOPERATING WITH ALL TREATMENT RECOMMENDED BY HIS TREATING PROFESSIONALS AND HAS BEEN FREE OF ALCOHOL AND UNPRESCRIBED DRUGS SINCE 11/92. HIS LICENSE TO PRACTICE MEDICINE IN WISCONSIN IS LIMITED UNDER THE FOLLOWING TERMS AND CONDITIONS: SHALL REMAIN IN COMPLIANCE WITH ALL OF THE TERMS AND CONDITIONS OF THE ARIZONA BOARD ORDER; SHALL ABSTAIN FROM ALL PERSONAL USE OF ALCOHOL AND CONTROLLED SUBSTANCES UNLESS APPROVED BY HIS HEALTH CARE PROVIDED FOR A LEGITIMATE MEDICAL NEED; SHALL PROVIDE TO HIS TREATING PHYSICIAN AND ALL TREATMENT FACILITIES CURRENT RELEASES AUTHORIZING RELEASE OF HIS MEDICAL AND TREATMENT RECORDS TO THE WISCONSIN BOARD AND SHALL CAUSE COPIES OF THE RELEASES TO FILED WITH THE BOARD MONITOR; SHALL CAUSE COPIES OF ALL REQUIRED REPORTS UNDER THE 3/93 ARIZONA ORDER TO BE FILED WITH THE WISCONSIN DEPARTMENT MONITOR; SHALL NOT ENGAGE IN THE PRACTICE OF MEDICINE AND SURGERY IN WISCONSIN UNTIL HE HAS SUBMITTED A PETITION TO THE BOARD INDICATING HIS INTENT TO PRACTICE AND SHALL PROVIDE EVIDENCE OF HIS CONTINUING SOBRIETY AND THE ABSENCE OF A NEED FOR MONITORING AND TREATMENT, OR, IN THE ALTERNATIVE, OF HIS ENROLLMENT AND SUCCESSFUL PARTICIPATION IN ALL COMPONENTS OF A DRUG AND ALCOHOL TREATMENT PROGRAM. SHALL REPORT TO THE BOARD ANY CHANGE OF EMPLOYMENT STATUS, RESIDENCE, ADDRESS, OR TELEPHONE NUMBER WITHIN FIVE DAYS OF THE DATE OF CHANGE.

STEVENS, ROBERT E MD, LICENSE NUMBER 0002423 OF PHOENIX, AZ, WAS DISCIPLINED BY ARIZONA ON JANUARY 25, 1994
DISCIPLINARY ACTION: REQUIRED TO TAKE ADDITIONAL MEDICAL EDUCATION
OFFENSE: OVERPRESCRIBING OR MISPRESCRIBING DRUGS

NOTES: ALLEGATIONS OF EXCESSIVE NUMBER OF NARCOTICS PROVIDED TO A PATIENT; POOR RECORD KEEPING. SHALL COMPLETE 20 HOURS OF CONTINUING MEDICAL EDUCATION IN PHARMACOLOGY, INCLUDING BUT NOT LIMITED TO PAIN MANAGEMENT. IN ADDITION TO THE HOURS REQUIRED BY LAW FOR ANNUAL RENEWAL OF AN ARIZONA MEDICAL LICENSE. THE DOCTOR FULFILLED THE TERMS OF THE ORDER AND THE ORDER TERMINATED ON 10/20/94.

STONE, RICHARD MD, LICENSE NUMBER 25893, WAS DISCIPLINED BY ARIZONA ON JULY 30, 1999

NOTES: PROHIBITED FROM THE PRACTICE OF CLINICAL MEDICINE UNTIL HE RECEIVES AFFIRMATIVE APPROVAL FROM THE BOARD TO DO SO. ORDERED TO PARTICIPATE IN URINE MONITORING. PREVIOUS ORDER RESCINDED.

STONE, RICHARD MD, LICENSE NUMBER 25893, WAS DISCIPLINED BY ARIZONA ON SEPTEMBER 23, 1999
DISCIPLINARY ACTION: LICENSE REVOCATION

NOTES: CANCELLATION OF LICENSE FOR CAUSE.

STONE, RICHARD B MD, LICENSE NUMBER 006400, WAS DISCIPLINED BY ARIZONA ON AUGUST 23, 1990
DISCIPLINARY ACTION: 24-MONTH LICENSE SUSPENSION; REQUIRED TO ENTER AN IMPAIRED PHYSICIAN PROGRAM OR SUBSTANCE ABUSE TREATMENT
OFFENSE: FAILURE TO COMPLY WITH PREVIOUS BOARD ORDER

NOTES: CONTINUED MISUSE OF CHEMICAL SUBSTANCES IN VIOLATION OF PAST BOARD REHABILITATION ORDERS. PRIOR TO OBTAINING REINSTATEMENT: MUST PROVE HE IS PHYSICALLY, MENTALLY AND MEDICALLY COMPETENT TO PRACTICE; MUST NOTIFY BOARD 4 MONTHS IN ADVANCE OF REINSTATEMENT REQUEST AND THEN SUBMIT URINE TESTS FOR 90 CONSECUTIVE DAYS; SUCCESSFULLY TAKE AND PASS THE SPEX EXAM; DEMONSTRATE HE HAS BEEN PARTICIPATING IN A TREATMENT PROGRAM FOR DRUG ABUSE AT LEAST THREE TIMES PER WEEK. LICENSE PREVIOUSLY PLACED ON PROBATION 8/3/89 AND 1/30/90.

STONE, RICHARD B MD, LICENSE NUMBER 0006400, WAS DISCIPLINED BY ARIZONA ON JANUARY 26, 1994
DISCIPLINARY ACTION: LICENSE REVOCATION; REQUIRED TO ENTER AN IMPAIRED PHYSICIAN PROGRAM OR SUBSTANCE ABUSE TREATMENT
OFFENSE: FAILURE TO COMPLY WITH PREVIOUS BOARD ORDER

NOTES: FAILED TO COMPLY WITH PREVIOUS RESTRICTIONS/CONDITIONS PUT ON HIS LICENSE. REPEATEDLY OUT OF COMPLIANCE WITH PREVIOUS BOARD ORDER STARTING WITH 11/29/85 WHEN HE ENTERED A MONITORING AGREEMENT BASED ON COCAINE USE WHICH HE VIOLATED BY USING CHEMICAL SUBSTANCES; CONVICTED IN 1987 OF OBTAINING PRESCRIPTION-ONLY DRUGS BY FRAUD; LICENSE PLACED ON PROBATION WITH MONITORING CONDITIONS IN 1/87 WHICH HE VIOLATED; LICENSE SUSPENDED IN 1/88 AND PLACED ON PROBATION AGAIN IN 6/89; VIOLATED THIS ORDER BY FAILING TO DELIVER COPIES OF CONTROLLED SUBSTANCES PRESCRIPTIONS FOR NUMEROUS PATIENTS AND SUBMITTING A URINE TEST WHICH TESTED POSITIVE FOR CODEINE; LICENSE SUSPENDED IN 8/90 AND DEA REGISTRATION PERMANENTLY SURRENDERED IN 11/90; LICENSE REMAINS SUSPENDED. ENTERED A GUILTY PLEA ON 8/27/91 TO ONE COUNT OF OBTAINING NARCOTIC DRUGS BY FRAUD AND ONE ON 8/11/93 TO ATTEMPTED ACQUISITION OF PRESCRIPTION DRUGS. SHALL NOT REAPPLY FOR LICENSURE FOR TWO YEARS. CONDITIONS DURING CANCELLATION: SHALL OBTAIN A BOARD-APPROVED THERAPIST WITH QUARTERLY REPORTS; MUST IMMEDIATELY PARTICIPATE IN A BOARD-APPROVED MONITORED AFTERCARE TREATMENT PROGRAM WHOSE THERAPIST MUST SUBMIT QUARTERLY REPORTS; MUST PARTICIPATE IN A 12-STEP RECOVERY PROGRAM AS DETERMINED BY HIS TREATING THERAPIST AND ATTEND AT LEAST THREE WEEKLY MEETINGS; SHALL OBTAIN A BOARD-APPROVED TREATING PHYSICIAN; SHALL ABSTAIN COMPLETELY FROM THE CONSUMPTION OF ALCOHOLIC BEVERAGES AND DRUGS EXCEPT WHEN PRESCRIBED BY HIS TREATING PHYSICIAN; MUST SUBMIT TO WITNESSED RANDOM BIOLOGICAL FLUID COLLECTION; KEEP A LOG OF ANY AND ALL MEDICATIONS PRESCRIBED FOR HIM; SHALL SUBMIT TO ANY EXAMINATIONS OR THERAPY ORDERED BY BOARD; SHALL OBEY ALL TERMS OF COURT ORDERED PROBATION. SIX MONTHS PRIOR TO RE-APPLICATION FOR LICENSURE, HE SHALL NOTIFY THE BOARD THAT HE INTENDS TO REAPPLY AND WILL SUBMIT TO RANDOM BIOLOGICAL FLUID TESTING. ON 1/25/97 REQUEST THAT THE BOARD APPROVE A SPECIFIED PHYSICIAN AS HIS THERAPIST AND ADDICTIONOLOGIST GRANTED.

STONE, RICHARD B MD OF PO BOX 1388, SCOTTSDALE, AZ, WAS

DISCIPLINED BY MEDICARE ON SEPTEMBER 1, 1994
DISCIPLINARY ACTION: EXCLUSION FROM THE MEDICARE AND/OR MEDICAID PROGRAM
OFFENSE: DISCIPLINARY ACTION BY ANOTHER STATE OR AGENCY

NOTES: LICENSE REVOKED FOR REASONS BEARING ON PROFESSIONAL COMPETENCE.

STONE, RICHARD B MD, WAS DISCIPLINED BY ARIZONA ON NOVEMBER 14, 1997
DISCIPLINARY ACTION: LICENSE REINSTATEMENT; 120-MONTH PROBATION

NOTES: IS IN COMPLIANCE WITH THE TERMS OF 1/26/94 ORDER. CONDITIONS OF REINSTATEMENT: MUST IMMEDIATELY PARTICIPATE IN A BOARD-APPROVED MONITORED AFTERCARE TREATMENT PROGRAM WHOSE THERAPIST MUST SUBMIT MONTHLY REPORTS; MUST PARTICIPATE IN 90 12-STEP MEETINGS FOR SUBSTANCE ABUSE WITHIN 90 DAYS; MUST THEN PARTICIPATE IN A 12-STEP RECOVERY PROGRAM AS DETERMINED BY HIS TREATING THERAPIST AND ATTEND AT LEAST THREE WEEKLY MEETINGS; SHALL OBTAIN A BOARD-APPROVED TREATING PHYSICIAN; SHALL ABSTAIN COMPLETELY FROM THE CONSUMPTION OF ALCOHOLIC BEVERAGES AND DRUGS EXCEPT WHEN PRESCRIBED BY HIS TREATING PHYSICIAN; SHALL NOT CONSUME FOOD OR SUBSTANCES CONTAINING POPPYSEEDS; MUST SUBMIT TO WITNESSED RANDOM BIOLOGICAL FLUID COLLECTION; MUST KEEP A LOG OF ANY AND ALL MEDICATIONS PRESCRIBED FOR HIM; SHALL SUBMIT TO ANY EXAMINATIONS OR THERAPY ORDERED BY BOARD; SHALL APPEAR BEFORE BOARD FOR INTERVIEWS UPON REQUEST; SHALL INFORM BOARD OF CHANGE OF ADDRESS OR IF AWAY FOR MORE THAN FIVE DAYS. SHALL CONTINUE IN THERAPY WITH A TREATING PSYCHIATRIST APPROVED BY THE BOARD AND SHALL REMAIN IN TREATMENT WITH THE PSYCHIATRIST UNTIL FURTHER ORDER OF THE BOARD WITH QUARTERLY REPORTS; SHALL NOT REQUEST TERMINATION OF THIS ORDER FOR A PERIOD OF AT LEAST FIVE YEARS. ON 5/21/99, ORDER MODIFIED AS FOLLOWS: WILL JOINTLY SELECT OUTPATIENT EVALUATORS AND EXPERTS WITH THE BOARD; MODIFICATIONS TO BIOLOGICAL FLUID COLLECTION REQUIREMENTS AND PRESCRIBING BY HEALTH CARE PROVIDER; SHALL SUBMIT QUARTERLY REPORTS TO THE BOARD; SHOULD BE ALLOWED TO APPLY FOR A DEA LICENSE THAT SHOULD BE REGULATED TO NOT INCLUDE SCHEDULE II AND III DRUGS AND SHALL NOT PRACTICE IN A SITUATION WHERE HE WILL BE THE SOLE PROVIDER; ALL OTHER TERMS OF THIS ORDER STILL APPLY; A SUPPLEMENTAL ORDER OF PROBATION IS ALSO OFFERED TO NOT REQUIRE PARTICIPATION IN THE MONITORED AFTERCARE PROGRAM.

STONE, RICHARD B MD, WAS DISCIPLINED BY ARIZONA ON MAY 13, 1998
OFFENSE: FAILURE TO COMPLY WITH PREVIOUS BOARD ORDER

NOTES: SHALL NOT PRACTICE UNTIL HE COMPLETES A MEDICAL EVALUATION PERFORMED BY A BOARD APPROVED EVALUATOR WHICH HAS BEEN REVIEWED BY THE BOARD.

STONE, RICHARD BRUCE MD OF 8710 E CLYDESDALE, SCOTTSDALE, AZ, WAS DISCIPLINED BY DEA ON DECEMBER 17, 1990
DISCIPLINARY ACTION: SURRENDER OF CONTROLLED SUBSTANCE LICENSE
OFFENSE: CRIMINAL CONVICTION OR PLEA OF GUILTY, NOLO CONTENDERE, OR NO CONTEST TO A CRIME

NOTES: ARRESTED 11/06/86 IN SCOTTSDALE ARIZONA FOR OBTAINING HALCION AND TYLENOL III BY FRAUD; CONVICTED AND SENTENCED AROUND 01/31/87 TO FIVE YEARS PROBATION; TESTED POSITIVE FOR COCAINE AROUND 11/14/88; SURRENDER OF REGISTRATION 03/04/89; REGISTRATION REINSTATED 06/22/89.

STRUG, BURT S MD OF TUCSON, AZ, WAS DISCIPLINED BY LOUISIANA ON SEPTEMBER 21, 1995
DISCIPLINARY ACTION: 24-MONTH PROBATION; RESTRICTION PLACED ON LICENSE
OFFENSE: DISCIPLINARY ACTION BY ANOTHER STATE OR AGENCY

NOTES: DISCIPLINARY ACTION BY ARIZONA; FRAUD, DECEIT OR PERJURY IN OBTAINING RENEWAL OF LICENSURE. CONDITIONS OF PROBATION: PRACTICE PROHIBITED IN LOUISIANA DURING PROBATIONARY TERM; MUST COMPLY WITH TERMS AND CONDITIONS OF ARIZONA ORDER AND GIVE PRIOR NOTICE TO LOUISIANA BOARD BEFORE RELOCATING THERE.

SUFFECOOL, STEVEN L MD, LICENSE NUMBER 0011240, WAS DISCIPLINED BY ARIZONA ON OCTOBER 12, 1991
DISCIPLINARY ACTION: 60-MONTH PROBATION; REQUIRED TO ENTER AN IMPAIRED PHYSICIAN PROGRAM OR SUBSTANCE ABUSE TREATMENT
OFFENSE: SUBSTANCE ABUSE

NOTES: HOSPITALIZED FOR CHEMICAL DEPENDENCY FROM 11/6/85 UNTIL 12/6/85; ON 3/17/86 BOARD ENTERED AN ORDER THAT HE CONTINUE CARE AND TREATMENT WITH A THERAPIST FOR ALCOHOL MISUSE, ABSTAIN FROM CONSUMPTION OF ALCOHOL, TAKE NO DRUGS UNLESS PRESCRIBED, SUBMIT TO RANDOM BIOLOGICAL FLUID TESTING, PARTICIPATE IN AA, OBEY ALL LAWS AND APPEAR FOR INTERVIEWS UPON REQUEST. THE STIPULATION AND ORDER WERE TERMINATED 1/20/90; ON 8/9/91, HOSPITAL WHERE HE HAD ANESTHESIA PRIVILEGES REPORTED THAT HIS CLINICAL PRACTICE PRIVILEGES WERE SUMMARILY SUSPENDED FOLLOWING HIS BEING APPARENTLY SELF-ANESTHETIZED WHILE RESPONSIBLE FOR ADMINISTERING ANESTHESIA TO A PATIENT. PROBATION WITH CONDITIONS: MUST IMMEDIATELY PARTICIPATE IN A BOARD-APPROVED MONITORED AFTERCARE TREATMENT PROGRAM WHOSE THERAPIST MUST SUBMIT QUARTERLY REPORTS; MUST ATTEND AT LEAST THREE WEEKLY MEETINGS OF AA OR OTHER PROGRAM PERTAINING TO SUBSTANCE ABUSE FOR THE TERM OF PROBATION; SHALL OBTAIN A BOARD-APPROVED TREATING PHYSICIAN; SHALL ABSTAIN COMPLETELY FROM THE CONSUMPTION OF ALCOHOLIC BEVERAGES AND DRUGS EXCEPT WHEN PRESCRIBED BY HIS TREATING PHYSICIAN; MUST SUBMIT TO WITNESSED RANDOM BIOLOGICAL FLUID COLLECTION; SHALL KEEP A LOG OF ANY AND ALL MEDICATIONS PRESCRIBED FOR HIM; SHALL SUBMIT TO ANY EXAMINATIONS OR THERAPY ORDERED BY THE BOARD; SHALL APPEAR BEFORE THE BOARD FOR INTERVIEWS UPON REQUEST; SHALL INFORM BOARD OF CHANGE OF ADDRESS OR IF AWAY FOR MORE THAN FIVE DAYS.

SUFFECOOL, STEVEN L MD, LICENSE NUMBER 11240, WAS DISCIPLINED BY ARIZONA ON JANUARY 25, 1997
DISCIPLINARY ACTION: LICENSE REVOCATION
OFFENSE: SUBSTANCE ABUSE

NOTES: FOLLOWING TERMINATION OF HIS REHABILITATION ORDER HE RELAPSED REGARDING HIS DRUG

ADDICTION. CANCELLATION WITH CAUSE. HE SHALL NOT APPLY FOR A MEDICAL LICENSE OF ANY KIND IN ARIZONA PRIOR TO 1/25/00.

SWEENEY, MICHAEL W MD, LICENSE NUMBER 0022866, WAS DISCIPLINED BY ARIZONA ON OCTOBER 21, 1995
OFFENSE: SUBSTANCE ABUSE

NOTES: INTERVIEWED BY THE BOARD REGARDING HIS ALLEGED USE OF CHEMICAL SUBSTANCES AND HIS ASSESSMENT AT A RECOVERY CENTER; VIOLATION OF FEDERAL LAWS AND COMMISSION OF A FELONY BY POSSESSION AND USE OF A NARCOTIC DRUG IN THAT IN 7/95, HE AND A HOUSE GUEST SNORTED OR OTHERWISE CONSUMED A COMPOUND THAT WAS LATER REVEALED UPON AUTOPSY OF THE HOUSE GUEST TO BE A MORPHINE DERIVATIVE AND AT THE TIME OF USE ASSUMED TO BE HEROIN; THE COMPOUND WAS INGESTED BY HIM TWICE IN THE SAME EVENING AND CONCURRENT WITH THE USE OF ALCOHOL; HE HAS A PAST HISTORY OF SELF-PRESCRIBING CONTROLLED SUBSTANCES IN THAT HE PRESCRIBED PERCOCET #20 TO HIS THEN WIFE FOR HIS OWN SELF USE FOLLOWING A LAMINECTOMY IN 1990. CENSURED; SHALL NOT PRACTICE MEDICINE IN ARIZONA UNTIL FURTHER ORDER OF THE BOARD.

SWENSON, E J MD OF 60 SOUTH 58TH STREET, MESA, AZ, WAS DISCIPLINED BY DEA ON MAY 16, 1995
DISCIPLINARY ACTION: SURRENDER OF CONTROLLED SUBSTANCE LICENSE
OFFENSE: DISCIPLINARY ACTION BY ANOTHER STATE OR AGENCY

NOTES: STATE BOARD.

SWENSON, EUGENE J MD, LICENSE NUMBER 0003005 OF MESA, AZ, WAS DISCIPLINED BY ARIZONA ON OCTOBER 18, 1994
DISCIPLINARY ACTION: RESTRICTION PLACED ON LICENSE
OFFENSE: SUBSTANDARD CARE, INCOMPETENCE OR NEGLIGENCE

NOTES: ALLEGATIONS OF UNSATISFACTORY SURGICAL TREATMENT AND POSTOPERATIVE CARE OF A PATIENT WITH CARPAL TUNNEL SYNDROME. SHALL NOT INVOLVE HIMSELF IN ANY ACTIVE PATIENT CARE OR SURGERY.

TAM, LETTO KINSU MD, LICENSE NUMBER 0014069, WAS DISCIPLINED BY ARIZONA ON APRIL 12, 1991
DISCIPLINARY ACTION: LICENSE REVOCATION
OFFENSE: DISCIPLINARY ACTION BY ANOTHER STATE OR AGENCY

NOTES: ON 10/17/88 DR. TAM PLED GUILTY IN THE SUPERIOR COURT OF NEWTON COUNTY, GEORGIA TO FOUR COUNTS OF PRESCRIBING A CONTROLLED SUBSTANCE; HE WAS SENTENCED ON EACH COUNT TO FIVE YEARS IN PRISON, TO BE SERVED ON PROBATION, AND A $500 FINE. ENTERED INTO A CONSENT ORDER WITH GEORGIA ON 12/8/88, WHICH SUSPENDED HIS LICENSE FOR 45 DAYS AND PLACED HIM ON PROBATION WITH TERMS AND CONDITIONS FOR AN ADDITIONAL FIVE YEARS. ON 03/13/90 DR. TAM WAS INDICTED BY THE NEWTON COUNTY GRAND JURY IN GEORGIA FOR THE FRAUDULENT SUBMISSION OF CLAIMS AND RECEIPT OF PAYMENT FOR MEDICAL ASSISTANCE PAYMENTS IN THIRTEEN SEPARATE INDICTMENTS. ON 5/09/90 GEORGIA REVOKED HIS LICENSE. ARIZONA LICENSE PERMANENTLY REVOKED.

TANGELOS, JANIS L MD, LICENSE NUMBER 0019667, WAS DISCIPLINED BY ARIZONA ON APRIL 16, 1993
DISCIPLINARY ACTION: RESTRICTION PLACED ON LICENSE; MONITORING OF PHYSICIAN PERFORMANCE

NOTES: AMENDMENT TO 8/29/90 STIPULATION AND ORDER. SHALL PARTICIPATE IN ONGOING PSYCHIATRIC THERAPY WITH A BOARD APPROVED THERAPIST WITH MONTHLY REPORTS; SHALL PRACTICE IN A SUPERVISED SETTING EXCEPT IF SHE'S NOT INVOLVED IN PATIENT CARE IN WHICH CASE SHE WILL MAKE PATIENT RECORDS AVAILABLE; EMPLOYER WILL PROVIDE MONTHLY REPORTS. THIS ORDER IS NOT DISCIPLINARY IN NATURE; RETROACTIVE TO 4/11/92.

TANNER, RICHARD D MD, DATE OF BIRTH JUNE 9, 1952, LICENSE NUMBER 0G46810 OF 2824 EAST SIERRA VISTA ROAD, TUCSON, AZ, WAS DISCIPLINED BY CALIFORNIA ON FEBRUARY 26, 1992
OFFENSE: DISCIPLINARY ACTION BY ANOTHER STATE OR AGENCY

NOTES: ARIZONA PUT CONDITIONS ON HIS LICENSE 1/5/89. SHALL COMPLY WITH THE TERMS OF THIS ORDER; ARIZONA TO RELEASE INFORMATION TO CALIFORNIA ON HIS PROGRESS AND PARTICIPATION IN THEIR ALCOHOL REHABILITATION PROGRAM, OR OTHER PROGRESS WITH THE TERMS OF THE ARIZONA ORDER; SHALL PROVIDE CALIFORNIA WITH 30 DAYS NOTICE OF INTENT TO PRACTICE IN THE STATE.

TAYLOR, JOHN S DO, LICENSE NUMBER 0002775 OF 155 CALLE PORTAL, SIERRA VISTA, AZ, WAS DISCIPLINED BY ARIZONA ON JANUARY 29, 1996
DISCIPLINARY ACTION: 60-MONTH PROBATION; RESTRICTION PLACED ON CONTROLLED SUBSTANCE LICENSE
OFFENSE: PROFESSIONAL MISCONDUCT

NOTES: ILLEGALLY OBTAINED DEMEROL; ENGAGED IN UNPROFESSIONAL CONDUCT: USING CONTROLLED SUBSTANCES OR PRESCRIPTION ONLY DRUGS NOT PROVIDED BY A MEDICAL PRACTITIONER; PRESCRIBING, DISPENSING, OR ADMINISTERING CONTROLLED SUBSTANCES PRESCRIPTION ONLY DRUGS FOR OTHER THAN ACCEPTED THERAPEUTIC PURPOSES. PROBATION UNDER TERMS AND CONDITIONS: CENSURED; SHALL OBTAIN PSYCHIATRIC OR PSYCHOLOGICAL TREATMENT BY A BOARD APPROVED THERAPIST WHO SHALL SUBMIT TO THE BOARD A WRITTEN PROGRESS REPORT EVERY MONTH FOR THE FIRST SIX MONTHS AND THEN EVERY THREE MONTHS FOR THE REMAINDER OF THE PROBATION; SHALL PROVIDE A COPY OF THIS ORDER TO ALL FACILITIES WHERE HE IS EMPLOYED AS A PHYSICIAN AND/OR HAS PRIVILEGES TO ENGAGE IN THE PRACTICE OF MEDICINE; SHALL ABSTAIN FROM THE CONSUMPTION OF ALCOHOL AND SHALL NOT CONSUME ILLICIT DRUGS OR TAKE ANY CONTROLLED SUBSTANCES UNLESS SUCH MEDICATION IS PRESCRIBED FOR HIM BY HIS TREATING PHYSICIAN; SHALL MAINTAIN A LOG OF SUCH PRESCRIPTIONS AND PROVIDE A COPY TO THE BOARD MONTHLY; SHALL SUBMIT TO AND COOPERATE IN ANY INDEPENDENT MEDICAL OR PSYCHOLOGICAL EVALUATION THAT IS ORDERED BY THE BOARD; SHALL APPEAR BEFORE THE BOARD UPON REQUEST; SHALL SUBMIT TO RANDOM BIOLOGICAL FLUID TESTING; SHALL PARTICIPATE IN A MINIMUM OF TWO SELF-HELP MEETINGS PER WEEK THROUGH SUCH ORGANIZATIONS AS AA, NARCOTICS ANONYMOUS AND DOCTOR'S CADUCEUS GROUP WITH MONTHLY REPORTS; SHALL NOTIFY THE BOARD WITHIN 20 DAYS IF HE CEASES TO RESIDE IN ARIZONA; MAY ONLY PRESCRIBE CONTROLLED SUBSTANCES PURSUANT TO THE TERMS AND CONDITIONS IMPOSED BY THE DEA AND PROVIDE THE BOARD WITH A COPY OF ALL DEA ORDERS; UPON APPROVAL OF PRESCRIPTION PRIVILEGES, MUST USE TRIPLICATE COPIES OF PRESCRIPTION PADS AND SUPPLY THE BOARD WITH

COPIES; SHALL COMPLY WITH ANY CONDITIONS PLACED ON HOSPITAL PRIVILEGES; WHILE EMPLOYED OR OTHERWISE CONTRACTS WITH THE U.S. GOVERNMENT, SHALL DISCLOSE A COPY OF THIS ORDER TO HIS IMMEDIATE SUPERVISOR.

TAYLOR, JOHN S DO, LICENSE NUMBER 0002775 OF 155 CALLE PORTAL, SIERRA VISTA, AZ, WAS DISCIPLINED BY ARIZONA ON APRIL 5, 1996
DISCIPLINARY ACTION: EMERGENCY SUSPENSION
OFFENSE: FAILURE TO COMPLY WITH PREVIOUS BOARD ORDER

NOTES: NONCOMPLIANCE TO PROBATION ORDER DATED 1/29/96: FAILED TO APPEAR DIRECTLY FOR THE BOARD'S PUBLIC MEETING ON 3/30/96; FAILED TO INFORM BOARD OF NAME OF PSYCHIATRIST TO SUPPLY THEM WITH HIS MONTHLY PRESCRIPTION LOG, TO PAY COSTS AND TO SUBMIT MONTHLY REPORTS REGARDING SELF-HELP MEETINGS. ON 5/20/96 RELEASED FROM SUMMARY SUSPENSION AND PLACED ON THE REMAINDER OF THE PROBATION OF 1/29/96. SHALL COMPLY WITH ORDER FOR PSYCHOLOGICAL EXAMINATION AND EVALUATION.

TAYLOR, JOHN S DO, LICENSE NUMBER 0002775 OF 155 CALLE PORTAL, SIERRA VISTA, AZ, WAS DISCIPLINED BY ARIZONA ON MAY 28, 1996
DISCIPLINARY ACTION: MONITORING OF PHYSICIAN PERFORMANCE

NOTES: WITHIN THREE DAYS SHALL SCHEDULE A COMPREHENSIVE PSYCHOLOGICAL EVALUATION AND ANY OTHER SUCH EXAMINATION OR TESTING AS THERAPIST DEEMS NECESSARY; SHALL AUTHORIZE THE THERAPIST TO TRANSMIT THE RESULTS DIRECTLY TO THE BOARD WITHIN 10 DAYS.

TAYLOR, JOHN S DO, DATE OF BIRTH MAY 19, 1948 OF 155 CALLE PROTAL, SIERRA VISTA, AZ, WAS DISCIPLINED BY MEDICARE ON APRIL 13, 1997
DISCIPLINARY ACTION: EXCLUSION FROM THE MEDICARE AND/OR MEDICAID PROGRAM
OFFENSE: NONCOMPLIANCE WITH A PROFESSIONAL RULE

NOTES: DEFAULTED ON PUBLIC HEALTH SERVICE EDUCATION LOAN.

TAYLOR, LOREN MD, LICENSE NUMBER 0003556, WAS DISCIPLINED BY ARIZONA ON APRIL 13, 1994

NOTES: SHALL NOT PRACTICE IN ARIZONA PRIOR TO NOTIFYING THE BOARD AND MEETING WITH THEM.

TEAGUE, ROBERT C MD, LICENSE NUMBER 0003925, WAS DISCIPLINED BY ARIZONA ON JULY 18, 1996
DISCIPLINARY ACTION: SURRENDER OF CONTROLLED SUBSTANCE LICENSE; 120-MONTH PROBATION
OFFENSE: OVERPRESCRIBING OR MISPRESCRIBING DRUGS

NOTES: PRESCRIBING, DISPENSING OR ADMINISTERING ANY CONTROLLED SUBSTANCE OR PRESCRIPTION-ONLY DRUG FOR OTHER THAN ACCEPTED THERAPEUTIC PURPOSES; BETWEEN 6/9/92 AND 11/4/92, HE PRESCRIBED A TOTAL OF 2,530 OF THE 15 MG SERAX, A SCHEDULE IV CONTROLLED SUBSTANCE, TO A 62-YEAR OLD PATIENT FOR AN AVERAGE DOSE OF MORE THAN 210 MG PER DAY, WHEN THE RECOMMENDED DOSE FOR ELDERLY PATIENTS IS NOT TO EXCEED 60 MG PER DAY; AS A CONSEQUENCE OF THE ABOVE FINDINGS, A PHARMACY SURVEY WAS UNDERTAKEN BY THE BOARD AND FROM PHARMACY PRINTOUTS BETWEEN 12/23/91 AND 1/6/93, IT WAS DETERMINED THAT ONE PATIENT RECEIVED 52 PRESCRIPTIONS OF PERCOCET FOR A TOTAL OF 1,956 DOSAGE UNITS AND ONE PRESCRIPTION OF ROXICET FOR 30 DOSAGE UNITS; A SECOND PATIENT RECEIVED 28 PRESCRIPTIONS OF ROXICET FOR A TOTAL OF 1,265 DOSAGE UNITS; PHYSICIAN WAS UNABLE TO ARTICULATE THE SPECIFIC USE FOR THE MEDICATIONS, BOTH OF WHICH ARE SCHEDULE II CONTROLLED SUBSTANCES. WITHIN 10 DAYS, SHALL SURRENDER HIS DRUG ENFORCEMENT ADMINISTRATION CERTIFICATE TO THE BOARD AND NOT PRESCRIBE ANY CONTROLLED SUBSTANCES THEREAFTER. ON 5/7/97 REQUEST TO TERMINATE ORDER DENIED. ON 11/19/98 REQUEST TO OBTAIN DEA CERTIFICATE DENIED. ON 7/29/99 REQUEST TO REINSTATE HIS DEA LICENSE UPON COMPLETION OF ADDITIONAL CONTINUING MEDICAL EDUCATION IN THE AREA OF PHARMACOLOGY GRANTED AS RESOLUTION OF SUPERIOR COURT CASE.

TEAGUE, ROBERT COLE MD, LICENSE NUMBER C5261 OF PHOENIX, AZ, WAS DISCIPLINED BY TEXAS ON APRIL 8, 1999
DISCIPLINARY ACTION: LICENSE REVOCATION; FINE
OFFENSE: DISCIPLINARY ACTION BY ANOTHER STATE OR AGENCY

NOTES: ON OR ABOUT 7/96 HE WAS PLACED ON 10 YEARS PROBATION BY THE ARIZONA BOARD FOR NON-THERAPEUTIC PRESCRIBING OF CONTROLLED SUBSTANCES IN 3 PATIENT CASES; IN 3/98 HE FAILED TO RESPOND TO THE TEXAS BOARD'S WRITTEN REQUEST FOR MEDICAL RECORDS AND HAD NOT DONE SO AS OF THE DATE OF THE ORDER. $50,000 FINE.

TEKELL, GORDON SILAS MD, LICENSE NUMBER 0007235 OF YUMA, AZ, WAS DISCIPLINED BY ARIZONA ON JANUARY 21, 1993
DISCIPLINARY ACTION: RESTRICTION PLACED ON CONTROLLED SUBSTANCE LICENSE; REQUIRED TO TAKE ADDITIONAL MEDICAL EDUCATION
OFFENSE: OVERPRESCRIBING OR MISPRESCRIBING DRUGS

NOTES: ALLEGATIONS THAT HE HAD BEEN PRESCRIBING LARGE AMOUNTS OF SCHEDULED DRUGS. SHALL SUCCESSFULLY COMPLETE 40 HOURS OF CONTINUING MEDICAL EDUCATION ACCEPTABLE TO THE BOARD WITHIN SIX MONTHS OF THE EFFECTIVE DATE OF THIS ORDER IN THE SUBJECT OF THE USE OF NARCOTICS FOR PAIN CONTROL AND CHRONIC PAIN MANAGEMENT; CONSULT WITH AN INDEPENDENT ORGANIZATION ACCEPTABLE TO THE BOARD REGARDING THE PROPER CREATION, MANAGEMENT AND MAINTENANCE OF MEDICAL RECORDS; EFFECTIVE TWO WEEKS FROM 01/21/93, CEASE ANY AND ALL PRESCRIBING, DISPENSING, OR ADMINISTRATION OF ALL SCHEDULE II AND III CONTROLLED SUBSTANCES, EXCEPT FOR THOSE PATIENTS IN A RECOGNIZED HOSPICE PROGRAM. SUCCESSFULLY FULFILLED THE TERMS OF THIS STIPULATION AND ORDER, SO AS OF 07/15/93 THIS STIPULATION AND ORDER IS TERMINATED.

TEKELL, GORDON SILAS MD, LICENSE NUMBER 00C9159 OF YUMA, AZ, WAS DISCIPLINED BY TEXAS ON NOVEMBER 3, 1994
DISCIPLINARY ACTION: SURRENDER OF CONTROLLED SUBSTANCE LICENSE; LICENSE SUSPENSION
OFFENSE: DISCIPLINARY ACTION BY ANOTHER STATE OR AGENCY

NOTES: ARIZONA BOARD INITIATED DISCIPLINARY ACTION BASED ON ALLEGATIONS THAT HE HAD OVERPRESCRIBED VARIOUS PRESCRIPTION MEDICATIONS INCLUDING CONTROLLED SUBSTANCES; ENTERED INTO A WRITTEN STIPULATION WITH ARIZONA ON 3/18/93 WHICH REQUIRED HIM TO CEASE ANY PRESCRIBING OF SCHEDULE II AND III CONTROLLED SUBSTANCES

EXCEPT IN A RECOGNIZED HOSPICE PROGRAM; THIS ORDER WAS TERMINATED ON 7/15/93. SUSPENSION UNTIL HE APPEARS BEFORE THE BOARD AND PROVIDES SUFFICIENT EVIDENCE THAT HE IS PHYSICALLY, MENTALLY AND OTHERWISE COMPETENT TO SAFELY PRACTICE; SHALL GIVE A COPY OF THIS ORDER TO ANY HEALTH CARE ENTITY WHERE HE HAS PRIVILEGES; SHALL COOPERATE WITH THE BOARD IN VERIFYING COMPLIANCE; SHALL INFORM BOARD OF CHANGE OF ADDRESS WITHIN 10 DAYS; SHALL SURRENDER TEXAS CONTROLLED SUBSTANCES CERTIFICATE AND ALL UNUSED TRIPLICATE PRESCRIPTION FORMS; SHALL NOT ATTEMPT TO REREGISTER WITHOUT PERMISSION.

TEMPLETON, FLOYD L MD, LICENSE NUMBER 2984, WAS DISCIPLINED BY ARIZONA ON MARCH 14, 1997
DISCIPLINARY ACTION: REPRIMAND
OFFENSE: INSURANCE, MEDICARE OR MEDICAID FRAUD

NOTES: ALTHOUGH HE DID NOT PROVIDE ANY PSYCHOTHERAPY SERVICES, HIS SIGNATURE APPEARED ON THE BOTTOM OF TWO CLAIM FORMS WHICH STATED HE PROVIDED 45-50 MINUTES OF INDIVIDUAL MEDICAL PSYCHOTHERAPY BY A PHYSICIAN WITH CONTINUING MEDICAL DIAGNOSTIC EVALUATION AND DRUG MANAGEMENT ON THREE OCCASIONS FOR EACH FORM; IT APPEARED TO THE BOARD THAT WHEN HIS SIGNATURE WAS SUPERIMPOSED THAT HE HAD SIGNED A BLANK FORM.

TEMPLETON, FLOYD L MD, LICENSE NUMBER A17001 OF PHOENIX, AZ, WAS DISCIPLINED BY CALIFORNIA ON OCTOBER 27, 1997
DISCIPLINARY ACTION: REPRIMAND
OFFENSE: DISCIPLINARY ACTION BY ANOTHER STATE OR AGENCY

NOTES: DISCIPLINED BY ARIZONA FOR SIGNING A BLANK MEDICAL CLAIM FORM WHICH WAS SUBMITTED TWO TIMES FOR PAYMENT OF PSYCHOTHERAPY SERVICES EVEN THOUGH NO SERVICES WERE PROVIDED ON THE DATE CLAIMED.

TEMPLETON, FLOYD LUTHER MD, LICENSE NUMBER 0002984, WAS DISCIPLINED BY ARIZONA ON APRIL 4, 1995
DISCIPLINARY ACTION: RESTRICTION PLACED ON LICENSE
OFFENSE: PROFESSIONAL MISCONDUCT

NOTES: ALLEGEDLY SUBMITTED CLAIMS TO AN INSURANCE COMPANY WITH HIS SIGNATURE FOR THERAPY THAT WAS PERFORMED BY A SOCIAL WORKER. INTERIM ORDER WHILE INVESTIGATION CONTINUES. SHALL NOT SUPERVISE SOCIAL WORKERS.

TENORIO, PAUL A MD, LICENSE NUMBER 0013311, WAS DISCIPLINED BY ARIZONA ON APRIL 6, 1990
DISCIPLINARY ACTION: REQUIRED TO ENTER AN IMPAIRED PHYSICIAN PROGRAM OR SUBSTANCE ABUSE TREATMENT; MONITORING OF PHYSICIAN PERFORMANCE
OFFENSE: SUBSTANCE ABUSE

NOTES: MUST IMMEDIATELY PARTICIPATE IN THE ARIZONA MEDICAL ASSOCIATION PHYSICIAN'S HEALTH COMMITTEE PROGRAM WITH QUARTERLY REPORTS TO THE BOARD; MUST OBTAIN BOARD APPROVED TREATING PHYSICIAN; MUST ABSTAIN FROM ALCOHOL AND ALL OTHER DRUGS; MUST COMPLY WITH REQUESTS FOR RANDOM BIOLOGICAL FLUID TESTS; MUST SUBMIT TO ANY TESTS OR THERAPY ORDERED BY BOARD; MUST PARTICIPATE IN 12-STEP RECOVERY PROGRAM FOR SUBSTANCE ABUSE AS DETERMINED BY THERAPIST AND ATTEND AT LEAST 3 WEEKLY MEETINGS; MUST APPEAR BEFORE BOARD FOR INTERVIEWS UPON REQUEST; MUST MAINTAIN A LOG OF ALL MEDICATIONS TAKEN; MUST ADVISE BOARD OF CHANGE IN OFFICE OR HOME ADDRESSES OR IF PLANS TO BE AWAY FOR MORE THAN FIVE DAYS. ORDER TERMINATED 1/23/93.

TENORIO, PAUL A MD, LICENSE NUMBER 0013311, WAS DISCIPLINED BY ARIZONA ON JANUARY 23, 1993
DISCIPLINARY ACTION: 60-MONTH PROBATION; REQUIRED TO ENTER AN IMPAIRED PHYSICIAN PROGRAM OR SUBSTANCE ABUSE TREATMENT
OFFENSE: FAILURE TO COMPLY WITH PREVIOUS BOARD ORDER

NOTES: ON 7/20/92 CONSUMED ALCOHOL IN VIOLATION OF 4/6/90 ORDER; ENTERED RESIDENTIAL TREATMENT FOR CHEMICAL DEPENDENCY WHICH HE COMPLETED 11/25/92. STIPULATION OF 4/6/90 TERMINATED. CONDITIONS OF PROBATION: MUST IMMEDIATELY PARTICIPATE IN A BOARD-APPROVED MONITORED AFTERCARE TREATMENT PROGRAM WHOSE THERAPIST MUST SUBMIT QUARTERLY REPORTS; MUST PARTICIPATE IN 90 12-STEP MEETINGS FOR SUBSTANCE ABUSE WITHIN 90 DAYS; MUST THEN PARTICIPATE IN A 12-STEP RECOVERY PROGRAM AS DETERMINED BY HIS TREATING THERAPIST AND ATTEND AT LEAST THREE WEEKLY MEETINGS; SHALL OBTAIN A BOARD-APPROVED TREATING PHYSICIAN; SHALL ABSTAIN COMPLETELY FROM THE CONSUMPTION OF ALCOHOLIC BEVERAGES AND DRUGS EXCEPT WHEN PRESCRIBED BY HIS TREATING PHYSICIAN; MUST SUBMIT TO WITNESSED RANDOM BIOLOGICAL FLUID COLLECTION; KEEP A LOG OF ANY AND ALL MEDICATIONS PRESCRIBED FOR HIM; SHALL SUBMIT TO ANY EXAMINATIONS OR THERAPY ORDERED BY BOARD; SHALL APPEAR BEFORE BOARD FOR INTERVIEWS UPON REQUEST; SHALL INFORM BOARD OF CHANGE OF ADDRESS OF IF AWAY FOR MORE THAN 5 DAYS. ON 4/16/94 PROBATION TERMINATED. OTHERWISE TERMS REMAIN THE SAME. ON 2/15/96 THE BOARD ORDERED THAT HIS REHABILITATION STIPULATION AND ORDER BE TERMINATED IN SIX MONTHS.

THOMPSON, LARRY W MD, WAS DISCIPLINED BY NEVADA ON APRIL 9, 1992
DISCIPLINARY ACTION: LICENSE REVOCATION
OFFENSE: PROFESSIONAL MISCONDUCT

NOTES: CHARGED WITH LACK OF CARE OF A PATIENT TO THE POINT OF CONSCIOUS INDIFFERENCE TO THE SAFETY AND WELFARE OF SAID PATIENT CONSTITUTING GROSS MALPRACTICE.

THOMPSON, LARRY W MD, LICENSE NUMBER 0011653, WAS DISCIPLINED BY ARIZONA ON JULY 15, 1993
DISCIPLINARY ACTION: RESTRICTION PLACED ON LICENSE

NOTES: HE SHALL NOT PERFORM ANY PREGNANCY TERMINATION, SURGERY, OR INVASIVE PROCEDURE EXCEPT AT A LICENSED HEALTH CARE FACILITY. ON 1/25/94 BOARD ACCEPTED HIS REQUEST FOR INACTIVE STATUS.

THOMPSON, VINSON C MD, LICENSE NUMBER 0013010, WAS DISCIPLINED BY ARIZONA ON APRIL 5, 1995
DISCIPLINARY ACTION: RESTRICTION PLACED ON LICENSE; RESTRICTION PLACED ON CONTROLLED SUBSTANCE LICENSE

NOTES: SHALL NOT PRESCRIBE ANY ANTI-COAGULATION THERAPY NOR MONITOR PATIENTS WITH ANY ANTI-COAGULATION THERAPY OTHER THAN FOR PROPHYLAXIS.

THORPE, DAVID MD, LICENSE NUMBER 14023, WAS DISCIPLINED BY ARIZONA ON NOVEMBER 18, 1999
DISCIPLINARY ACTION: REPRIMAND
OFFENSE: SUBSTANDARD CARE, INCOMPETENCE OR NEGLIGENCE

NOTES: INADEQUATE PRE-EPIDURAL WORK-UP AND A DELAY IN OBTAINING A CT SCAN AND A NEUROLOGY CONSULTATION.

TINSLEY, MARK S MD, LICENSE NUMBER 0014907, WAS DISCIPLINED BY ARIZONA ON JUNE 8, 1990
OFFENSE: FAILURE TO COMPLY WITH PREVIOUS BOARD ORDER

NOTES: VIOLATED BOARD ORDER OF 10/7/88 BY USING ILLICIT DRUGS AND FAILING TO RESPOND TO A REQUEST FOR A URINE SPECIMEN. LICENSE PLACED ON INACTIVE STATUS IN ORDER FOR HIM TO ENTER A LONG-TERM DRUG DEPENDENCY PROGRAM.

TINSLEY, MARK S MD, LICENSE NUMBER 0014907, WAS DISCIPLINED BY ARIZONA ON JUNE 19, 1991
DISCIPLINARY ACTION: 60-MONTH PROBATION; RESTRICTION PLACED ON CONTROLLED SUBSTANCE LICENSE
OFFENSE: SUBSTANCE ABUSE

NOTES: ON 1/15/88 BOARD RECEIVED INFORMATION HE HAD BEEN TERMINATED FROM HIS SURGICAL RESIDENCY FOR FAILURE TO PERFORM IN ACCORDANCE WITH HIS CONTRACT AND FOR CONCERNS REGARDING HIS CLINICAL ABILITIES. ON 6/9/88 HE ENTERED AN INPATIENT CHEMICAL DEPENDENCY TREATMENT PROGRAM WHICH HE SUCCESSFULLY COMPLETED ON 09/29/88. ON 4/13/89 THE BOARD ISSUED A LETTER OF CONCERN REGARDING A MALPRACTICE COMPLAINT FOR FAILURE TO CORRECTLY DIAGNOSE TORSION OF THE PATIENT'S TESTICLE. IN EARLY 1990 HE WAS FIRED FROM HIS POSITION AS AN EMERGENCY ROOM PHYSICIAN. IN MAY 1990 HE ACKNOWLEDGED MISUSING DRUGS BETWEEN 4/7/90 AND 5/17/90. IN JUNE 1990 HE REQUESTED THE BOARD PLACE HIS LICENSE ON INACTIVE STATUS. ENTERED INPATIENT CHEMICAL DEPENDENCY TREATMENT ON 7/15/90 AND COMPLETED THE PROGRAM ON 8/17/90. ENTERED A SECOND INPATIENT CHEMICAL DEPENDENCY TREATMENT PROGRAM ON 8/29/90 AND WAS DISCHARGED ON 3/30/91. ON 6/19/91 HE ASKED THE BOARD TO RETURN HIS LICENSE TO ACTIVE STATUS. CONDITIONS OF PROBATION: SHALL SURRENDER HIS DEA REGISTRATION FOR SCHEDULE II SUBSTANCES AND SHALL NOT APPLY FOR REINSTATEMENT WITHOUT BOARD APPROVAL; SHALL PARTICIPATE IN THE ARIZONA MEDICAL ASSOCIATION'S MONITORED AFTERCARE TREATMENT PROGRAM; MUST HAVE THERAPIST SUBMIT QUARTERLY REPORTS TO THE BOARD AND OPEN HIS RECORDS TO THE BOARD; MUST ATTEND A MINIMUM OF 90 MEETINGS OF A 12 STEP RECOVERY PROGRAM WITHIN 90 DAYS AND THREE MEETINGS PER WEEK AFTER THAT; MUST OBTAIN ONE BOARD-APPROVED TREATING PHYSICIAN; MUST ABSTAIN FROM ALCOHOL AND OTHER DRUGS; MUST COMPLY WITH REQUESTS FOR RANDOM SCREENING OF BODILY FLUIDS; MUST MAINTAIN A LOG OF ALL MEDICATION; MUST SUBMIT TO MENTAL, PHYSICAL OR MEDICAL COMPETENCY EXAMS AS REQUESTED BY BOARD; MUST SUBMIT TO ANY THERAPY ORDERED BY BOARD; MUST APPEAR BEFORE BOARD FOR INTERVIEWS UPON REQUEST AND INFORM THE BOARD IF HE CHANGES ADDRESS OR WILL BE AWAY FOR MORE THAN FIVE DAYS. ON 1/25/92 BOARD GAVE WRITTEN PERMISSION FOR HIM TO REAPPLY FOR DEA CONTROLLED SUBSTANCES REGISTRATION FOR SCHEDULE II NARCOTICS DUE TO HIS ONGOING REHABILITATION EFFORTS. EFFECTIVE 10/16/93 HIS REQUEST TO CHANGE SUPPORT GROUPS WAS APPROVED. EFFECTIVE 4/16/94 PROBATION TERMINATED AND HE MUST ENTER INTO A STIPULATION WITH THE SAME TERMS AS HIS PROBATIONARY ORDER. ON 4/8/95 ORDER TERMINATED.

TINSLEY, MARK STANLY MD, LICENSE NUMBER 00G5693 OF PHOENIX, AZ, WAS DISCIPLINED BY TEXAS ON MARCH 6, 1992
DISCIPLINARY ACTION: 60-MONTH PROBATION
OFFENSE: DISCIPLINARY ACTION BY ANOTHER STATE OR AGENCY

NOTES: DISCIPLINARY ACTION TAKEN BY ANOTHER STATE BOARD FOR INTEMPERATE USE OF ALCOHOL OR DRUGS. LICENSE SUSPENDED, SUSPENSION STAYED; PROBATION UNDER TERMS AND CONDITIONS.

TIZARD, GARY T MD, LICENSE NUMBER 0012551 OF 394 WEST MAIN STREET, HENDERSONVILLE, TN, WAS DISCIPLINED BY TENNESSEE ON JULY 17, 1990
DISCIPLINARY ACTION: EMERGENCY SUSPENSION; RESTRICTION PLACED ON LICENSE
OFFENSE: PROFESSIONAL MISCONDUCT

NOTES: ALLEGED SEXUAL MISCONDUCT, PERSON UNSPECIFIED. ON 6/2/95 THIS ORDER SHALL REMAIN IN FULL FORCE AND EFFECT; HE DOES NOT WISH TO PURSUE THE MATTER AND THE CASE IS RETIRED FOR ADMINISTRATIVE PURPOSES ONLY.

TIZARD, GARY T MD, LICENSE NUMBER 00D7334 OF HENDERSONVILLE, TN, WAS DISCIPLINED BY TEXAS ON OCTOBER 26, 1990
DISCIPLINARY ACTION: LICENSE SUSPENSION
OFFENSE: DISCIPLINARY ACTION BY ANOTHER STATE OR AGENCY

NOTES: SUSPENDED PENDING OUTCOME OF FINAL HEARING BEFORE TENNESSEE BOARD; MUST AUTHORIZE TENNESSEE BOARD TO RELEASE INFORMATION TO TEXAS AS TO STATUS AND COMPLIANCE WITH PROBATION; RECEIVE APPROVAL OF TEXAS BOARD PRIOR TO PRACTICING MEDICINE IN TEXAS.

TIZARD, GARY T MD, WAS DISCIPLINED BY ARIZONA ON JANUARY 23, 1992
DISCIPLINARY ACTION: LICENSE REVOCATION
OFFENSE: DISCIPLINARY ACTION BY ANOTHER STATE OR AGENCY

NOTES: LICENSE WAS SUSPENDED IN TENNESSEE FOR UNPROFESSIONAL CONDUCT. TEXAS ENTERED INTO AN AGREED ORDER WITH DOCTOR TIZARD'S SURRENDERING HIS TEXAS LICENSE AS A RESULT OF ACTIONS TAKEN IN TENNESSEE. DR. TIZARD SIGNED A CANCELLATION OF HIS ARIZONA LICENSE WITH CAUSE WHICH REQUIRES BOARD ACTION.

TIZARD, GARY TIFFANY MD, DATE OF BIRTH JUNE 17, 1944 OF 111 WILLIAM SHY DR, HENDERSONVILLE, TN, WAS DISCIPLINED BY MEDICARE ON AUGUST 18, 1991
DISCIPLINARY ACTION: EXCLUSION FROM THE MEDICARE AND/OR MEDICAID PROGRAM
OFFENSE: DISCIPLINARY ACTION BY ANOTHER STATE OR AGENCY

NOTES: LICENSE REVOCATION OR SUSPENSION.

TOUR, ROBERT L MD OF PHOENIX, AZ, WAS DISCIPLINED BY OHIO ON MARCH 9, 1990
DISCIPLINARY ACTION: RESTRICTION PLACED ON LICENSE
OFFENSE: DISCIPLINARY ACTION BY ANOTHER STATE OR AGENCY

NOTES: PRIOR ACTION BY ARIZONA BOARD. CONSENT AGREEMENT UNSPECIFIED, CONDITIONS AND LIMITATIONS IMPOSED ON LICENSE .

TOUR, ROBERT L MD, LICENSE NUMBER C013632 OF PHOENIX, AZ, WAS DISCIPLINED BY CALIFORNIA ON MAY 10, 1991
DISCIPLINARY ACTION: 60-MONTH PROBATION
OFFENSE: DISCIPLINARY ACTION BY ANOTHER STATE OR AGENCY

NOTES: DISCIPLINED BY ARIZONA BOARD FOR EXCESSIVE USE OF ALCOHOL. REVOCATION STAYED.

TOUR, ROBERT LOUIS MD, LICENSE NUMBER 0011609, WAS DISCIPLINED BY ARIZONA ON JANUARY 16, 1996
DISCIPLINARY ACTION: 60-MONTH PROBATION; REQUIRED TO ENTER AN IMPAIRED PHYSICIAN PROGRAM OR SUBSTANCE ABUSE TREATMENT
OFFENSE: SUBSTANCE ABUSE

NOTES: IN 1988 COMPLETED A ONE-MONTH REHABILITATION PROGRAM AND IN 1/89, ENTERED INTO A STIPULATION WITH THE BOARD REGARDING AN ORDER FOR REHABILITATION FOR SUBSTANCE ABUSE WHICH WAS TERMINATED ON 4/11/92; IN 2/95, BOARD RECEIVED INFORMATION THAT BETWEEN 1/94 AND 2/95, HE PRESCRIBED LORCET, HYDROCODONE, ALPRAZOLAM, TEMAZEPAM, AND PLACIDYL IN THE NAME OF A MEMBER OF HIS IMMEDIATE FAMILY FOR HIS OWN USE; IN A BOARD INTERVIEW ON 6/29/95, ADMITTED PRESCRIBING DALMANE, LORTABS, VICODIN, AND TYLENOL #3 FOR HIS USE IN THE NAME OF THE FAMILY MEMBER; IN 4/95, CAUSED A MOTOR VEHICLE ACCIDENT WHILE DRIVING UNDER THE INFLUENCE OF CONTROLLED SUBSTANCES AND/OR ALCOHOL; ON 7/31/95, LICENSE PLACED ON INACTIVE STATUS WITH CAUSE AT HIS REQUEST; TREATED FOR SUBSTANCE ABUSE AS AN INPATIENT FROM 7/31/95 TO 10/6/95; AFTER SUCCESSFULLY COMPLETING TREATMENT, HE WAS DISCHARGED WITH A DIAGNOSIS OF SEDATIVE-HYPNOTIC DEPENDENCE AND HISTORY OF OPIATE AND ALCOHOL DEPENDENCE. LICENSE REACTIVATED TO PROBATION WITH TERMS: MUST IMMEDIATELY PARTICIPATE IN A BOARD-APPROVED MONITORED AFTERCARE TREATMENT PROGRAM WHOSE THERAPIST MUST SUBMIT QUARTERLY REPORTS; MUST PARTICIPATE IN A 12-STEP RECOVERY PROGRAM AS DETERMINED BY HIS TREATING THERAPIST AND ATTEND AT LEAST THREE WEEKLY MEETINGS; SHALL OBTAIN A BOARD-APPROVED TREATING PHYSICIAN; SHALL ABSTAIN COMPLETELY FROM THE CONSUMPTION OF ALCOHOLIC BEVERAGES AND DRUGS EXCEPT WHEN PRESCRIBED BY HIS TREATING PHYSICIAN; SHALL NOT CONSUME ANY FOOD OR SUBSTANCE CONTAINING POPPYSEEDS; MUST SUBMIT TO WITNESSED RANDOM BIOLOGICAL FLUID COLLECTION; MUST KEEP A LOG OF ANY AND ALL MEDICATIONS PRESCRIBED FOR HIM; SHALL SUBMIT TO ANY EXAMINATIONS OR THERAPY ORDERED BY THE BOARD; SHALL APPEAR BEFORE BOARD FOR INTERVIEWS UPON REQUEST; SHALL INFORM BOARD OF CHANGE OF ADDRESS OR IF AWAY FOR MORE THAN FIVE DAYS. IF HE DOES RESIDE IN ANOTHER STATE, SHALL PARTICIPATE IN THAT STATE'S PHYSICIAN REHABILITATION PROGRAM WITH REPORTS TO ARIZONA TWICE YEARLY; TIME SPENT OUT OF ARIZONA MAY BE TOLLED FOR THIS ORDER.

TREVELLINE, ERIC MD, WAS DISCIPLINED BY ARIZONA ON FEBRUARY 15, 1996
DISCIPLINARY ACTION: LICENSE SUSPENSION
OFFENSE: FAILURE TO COMPLY WITH PREVIOUS BOARD ORDER

NOTES: IN VIOLATION OF HIS REHABILITATION STIPULATION AND ORDER AND CURRENTLY AT TREATMENT CENTER. BOARD ACCEPTED HIS REQUEST FOR INACTIVE STATUS WITH CAUSE.

TREVELLINE, ERIC E MD, LICENSE NUMBER 21213, WAS DISCIPLINED BY ARIZONA ON FEBRUARY 11, 1997
DISCIPLINARY ACTION: 120-MONTH PROBATION; RESTRICTION PLACED ON LICENSE
OFFENSE: FAILURE TO COMPLY WITH PREVIOUS BOARD ORDER

NOTES: ON 10/18/96 ADULTERATED HIS URINE SPECIMEN BY ADDING WATER WHICH VIOLATED PREVIOUS ORDER. CONDITIONS OF REACTIVATED LICENSE ARE AS FOLLOWS: MUST IMMEDIATELY PARTICIPATE IN A BOARD-APPROVED MONITORED AFTERCARE TREATMENT PROGRAM WHOSE THERAPIST MUST SUBMIT QUARTERLY REPORTS; MUST PARTICIPATE IN A 12-STEP RECOVERY PROGRAM AS DETERMINED BY HIS TREATING THERAPIST AND ATTEND AT LEAST THREE WEEKLY MEETINGS; SHALL OBTAIN A BOARD-APPROVED TREATING PHYSICIAN; SHALL ABSTAIN COMPLETELY FROM THE CONSUMPTION OF ALCOHOLIC BEVERAGES AND DRUGS EXCEPT WHEN PRESCRIBED BY HIS TREATING PHYSICIAN; MUST SUBMIT TO WITNESSED RANDOM BIOLOGICAL FLUID COLLECTION; MUST KEEP A LOG OF ANY AND ALL MEDICATIONS PRESCRIBED FOR HIM/HER; SHALL SUBMIT TO ANY EXAMINATIONS OR THERAPY ORDERED BY BOARD; SHALL APPEAR BEFORE BOARD FOR INTERVIEWS UPON REQUEST; SHALL INFORM BOARD OF CHANGE OF ADDRESS OR IF AWAY FOR MORE THAN FIVE DAYS; SHALL IMMEDIATELY OBTAIN A TREATING PSYCHIATRIST APPROVED BY THE BOARD AND SHALL REMAIN IN TREATMENT WITH THE PSYCHIATRIST UNTIL FURTHER ORDER OF THE BOARD WITH QUARTERLY REPORTS; SHALL ONLY PRACTICE WHEN ANOTHER PHYSICIAN IS ON THE PREMISES OR IN A GROUP SETTING. ON 3/26/98 ORDER MODIFIED TO ALLOW HIM TO APPLY FOR A FEDERAL CONTROLLED SUBSTANCE REGISTRATION CERTIFICATE STATING HE SHALL NOT PRESCRIBE, DISPENSE, OR ADMINISTER CONTROLLED SUBSTANCES UNDER THIS REGISTRATION UNTIL FURTHER ORDER OF THE BOARD.

TURGUT, HASAN MD, LICENSE NUMBER 0016658, WAS DISCIPLINED BY ARIZONA ON JANUARY 23, 1992
DISCIPLINARY ACTION: LICENSE REVOCATION
OFFENSE: FAILURE TO COMPLY WITH PREVIOUS BOARD ORDER

NOTES: DR. TURGUT IS REQUESTING AND HAS SIGNED A CANCELLATION OF HIS LICENSE WITH CAUSE FOR FAILURE TO SIT FOR EITHER THE BOARD ORDERED ORAL COMPETENCY EXAM OR THE SPEX EXAM.

TURLEY, LOREN M DO, LICENSE NUMBER 0002638, WAS DISCIPLINED BY ARIZONA ON SEPTEMBER 14, 1992
DISCIPLINARY ACTION: LICENSE SUSPENSION; MONITORING OF PHYSICIAN PERFORMANCE
OFFENSE: PROFESSIONAL MISCONDUCT

NOTES: ON 9/10/92 ADMITTED TO THE BOARD THAT HE HAD SELF-MEDICATED WITH CONTROLLED AND/OR PRESCRIPTION ONLY MEDICATIONS (FLEXERIL) ON ONE OR MORE OCCASIONS PRIOR TO THAT DATE WHILE NOT UNDER THE CARE AND TREATMENT OF A PHYSICIAN AND NOT PRESCRIBED AS PART OF A RECOGNIZED COURSE OF TREATMENT. SHALL UNDERGO AN IN-PATIENT EVALUATION PROGRAM FOR SUSPECTED ALCOHOL AND SUBSTANCE ABUSE AND CHEMICAL DEPENDENCE FOR NOT LESS THAN FIVE DAYS; SHALL AUTHORIZE TREATING PERSONNEL AT THE IN-PATIENT EVALUATION PROGRAM TO RELEASE TO THE BOARD FINDINGS OF HIS EVALUATION AND ANY NECESSARY RECOMMENDATIONS FOR TREATMENT; SHALL MEET WITH THE BOARD FOLLOWING THE COMPLETION OF THE EVALUATION

PROGRAM TO DETERMINE WHETHER OR NOT ANY ADDITIONAL ACTIONS ARE REQUIRED; SHALL USE NO CONTROLLED SUBSTANCES OR PRESCRIPTION-ONLY MEDICATIONS UNLESS PRESCRIBED BY HIS ATTENDING PHYSICIAN; SHALL REFRAIN FROM THE USE OF ALCOHOL.

TURLEY, LOREN M DO, LICENSE NUMBER 0002638, WAS DISCIPLINED BY ARIZONA ON SEPTEMBER 19, 1992
DISCIPLINARY ACTION: PROBATION; RESTRICTION PLACED ON LICENSE
OFFENSE: PROFESSIONAL MISCONDUCT

NOTES: SUBMITTED DOCUMENTATION OF COMPLIANCE WITH TERMS OF 9/14/92 ORDER. REINSTATED WITH MINIMUM THREE YEAR PROBATION UNDER TERMS AND CONDITIONS: SHALL COMPLETE AN INTENSIVE OUTPATIENT CHEMICAL DEPENDENCE PROGRAM; SHALL SECURE AND MAINTAIN A SPONSOR FOR 12 STEP RECOVERY PROGRAM; SHALL ATTEND AT LEAST FOUR 12 STEP MEETINGS PER WEEK FOR THE FIRST 12 MONTHS; SHALL MEET REGULARLY WITH HIS ATTENDING PHYSICIAN; SHALL ATTEND NO LESS THAN THREE GROUP THERAPY MEETINGS PER MONTH WITH A BOARD APPROVED COUNSELOR; SHALL SUBMIT TO RANDOM BODY FLUID TESTING UPON BOARD REQUEST; SHALL MEET WITH THE BOARD REGULARLY UPON REQUEST; SHALL USE NO CONTROLLED SUBSTANCE OR PRESCRIPTION-ONLY MEDICATION UNLESS PRESCRIBED BY HIS ATTENDING PHYSICIAN; SHALL REFRAIN FROM THE USE OF ALCOHOL; SHALL WORK NO MORE THAN 14 EMERGENCY DEPARTMENT SHIFTS PER MONTH UNLESS AUTHORIZED BY THE BOARD; SHALL AUTHORIZE ALL TREATING PERSONNEL INVOLVED IN HIS CARE TO RELEASE INFORMATION ON HIS PROGRESS AND PROGNOSIS TO THE BOARD UPON REQUEST. ORDER AMENDED ON 1/14/94 ALLOWING HIM TO WORK 17 RATHER THAN 14 EMERGENCY DEPARTMENT SHIFTS PER MONTH. OTHER PROVISIONS REMAIN IN FULL FORCE AND EFFECT.

TURLEY, LOREN M DO, LICENSE NUMBER 0002331 OF 19155 NORTH 94TH PLACE, SCOTTSDALE, AZ, WAS DISCIPLINED BY OKLAHOMA ON MARCH 12, 1993
DISCIPLINARY ACTION: 60-MONTH PROBATION
OFFENSE: DISCIPLINARY ACTION BY ANOTHER STATE OR AGENCY

NOTES: LICENSE SUSPENSION IN ARIZONA ON 9/14/92 WHICH WAS REINSTATED SUBJECT TO TERMS AND CONDITIONS. CONDITIONS OF PROBATION: SHALL REMAIN IN STRICT COMPLIANCE WITH THE ARIZONA ORDER; SHALL APPEAR BEFORE THE BOARD UPON REQUEST AND BEFORE HE REENTERS PRACTICE IN OKLAHOMA.

TURLEY, LOREN M MD, DATE OF BIRTH MARCH 7, 1945, LICENSE NUMBER 0028104 OF SCOTTSDALE, AZ, WAS DISCIPLINED BY COLORADO ON NOVEMBER 19, 1993
DISCIPLINARY ACTION: 60-MONTH PROBATION; MONITORING OF PHYSICIAN PERFORMANCE
OFFENSE: SUBSTANCE ABUSE

NOTES: EXCESSIVE USE OF A CONTROLLED SUBSTANCE AND HABITUAL INTEMPERANCE. PROBATIONARY PERIOD INCLUDES TREATMENT AND PRACTICE MONITORING.

TURNER, HARVEY A MD, DATE OF BIRTH JUNE 9, 1932, LICENSE NUMBER 0025732 OF 7920 EAST CORONADO RD, SCOTTSDALE, AZ, WAS DISCIPLINED BY WISCONSIN ON JUNE 20, 1991
DISCIPLINARY ACTION: RESTRICTION PLACED ON LICENSE; REPRIMAND
OFFENSE: DISCIPLINARY ACTION BY ANOTHER STATE OR AGENCY

NOTES: HAS BEEN PRACTICING IN ARIZONA AS AN ASSISTANT SURGEON SINCE 6/88. IN 3/89 THE ARIZONA BOARD CENSURED AND FINED HIM AFTER FINDING HIM GUILTY OF UNPROFESSIONAL CONDUCT FOR PROCURING OR ATTEMPTING TO PROCURE A LICENSE OR LICENSE RENEWAL BY FRAUD, MISREPRESENTATION, OR BY KNOWINGLY TAKING ADVANTAGE OF THE MISTAKE OF ANOTHER PERSON OR AGENCY AND FOR MAKING A FALSE OR MISLEADING STATEMENT ON APPLICATION FORM; ARIZONA LICENSE RESTRICTED ON 5/8/89 TO ONLY PRACTICING AS AN ASSISTANT SURGEON; THIS LIMITATION WAS REMOVED 6/28/90. SHALL ONLY PRACTICE AS AN ASSISTANT SURGEON IN WISCONSIN.

TURNER, HARVEY A MD, LICENSE NUMBER 0086744 OF 7920 E CORONADO RD, SCOTTSDALE, AZ, WAS DISCIPLINED BY NEW YORK ON APRIL 24, 1992
DISCIPLINARY ACTION: 12-MONTH PROBATION; RESTRICTION PLACED ON LICENSE
OFFENSE: DISCIPLINARY ACTION BY ANOTHER STATE OR AGENCY

NOTES: DISCIPLINED IN ARIZONA FOR KNOWINGLY MAKING FALSE AND MISLEADING STATEMENTS IN HIS ARIZONA LICENSE APPLICATION AND IN A PRELIMINARY QUESTIONNAIRE, AN ACT TO WHICH HE PLEADED GUILTY WHICH WOULD ALSO CONSTITUTE MISCONDUCT IN NEW YORK STATE. ONE-YEAR SUSPENSION, STAYED. PROBATION WITH SPECIAL CONDITION THAT PRACTICE BE LIMITED TO THE ROLE OF ASSISTANT SURGEON.

TUTT, MICHAEL L MD, LICENSE NUMBER 0020226, WAS DISCIPLINED BY ARIZONA ON AUGUST 9, 1991
DISCIPLINARY ACTION: REQUIRED TO ENTER AN IMPAIRED PHYSICIAN PROGRAM OR SUBSTANCE ABUSE TREATMENT; MONITORING OF PHYSICIAN PERFORMANCE
OFFENSE: SUBSTANCE ABUSE

NOTES: INFORMATION RECEIVED THAT HE HAD VOLUNTARILY ADMITTED HIMSELF FOR INPATIENT TREATMENT FOR SUBSTANCE ABUSE. MUST IMMEDIATELY PARTICIPATE IN A BOARD-APPROVED MONITORED AFTERCARE TREATMENT PROGRAM WHOSE THERAPIST MUST SUBMIT QUARTERLY REPORTS; MUST PARTICIPATE IN 90 12-STEP MEETINGS FOR SUBSTANCE ABUSE WITHIN 90 DAYS; MUST THEN PARTICIPATE IN A 12-STEP RECOVERY PROGRAM AS DETERMINED BY HIS TREATING THERAPIST AND ATTEND AT LEAST THREE WEEKLY MEETING; SHALL OBTAIN A BOARD-APPROVED TREATING PHYSICIAN; SHALL ABSTAIN COMPLETELY FROM THE CONSUMPTION OF DRUGS EXCEPT WHEN PRESCRIBED BY HIS TREATING PHYSICIAN; MUST SUBMIT TO WITNESSED RANDOM BIOLOGICAL FLUID COLLECTION; MUST KEEP A LOG OF ANY AND ALL MEDICATIONS PRESCRIBED FOR HIM; SHALL SUBMIT TO ANY EXAMINATIONS OR THERAPY ORDERED BY THE BOARD; SHALL APPEAR BEFORE THE BOARD FOR INTERVIEWS UPON REQUEST; SHALL INFORM THE BOARD OF CHANGE OF ADDRESS OR IF AWAY FOR MORE THAN FIVE DAYS.

UDALL, COLLIN MD, LICENSE NUMBER 0015439 OF GILBERT, AZ, WAS DISCIPLINED BY ARIZONA ON OCTOBER 19, 1994
DISCIPLINARY ACTION: REQUIRED TO TAKE ADDITIONAL MEDICAL EDUCATION; MONITORING OF PHYSICIAN PERFORMANCE

NOTES: REGARDING FOLLOW-UP OFFICE RECORD REVIEW. WITHIN 9 MONTHS SHALL OBTAIN 30 HOURS OF CATEGORY I CONTINUING MEDICAL EDUCATION IN ADDITION TO THE 20 HOURS REQUIRED FOR THE RENEWAL OF MEDICAL LICENSE; 15 HOURS SHALL BE

IN THE MANAGEMENT OF ATTENTION DEFICIT DISORDER AND 15 HOURS SHALL BE IN THE MANAGEMENT OF PAIN; WITHIN 60 DAYS AND AT ONE YEAR INTERVALS THEREAFTER SHALL HAVE A PEDIATRICIAN APPROVED BY THE BOARD EVALUATE THE MANAGEMENT OF ALL PATIENTS HE TREATS FOR ATTENTION DEFICIT DISORDER BY REVIEWING CHARTS FOR THOSE PATIENTS; SHALL CONSULT WITH PEDIATRICIAN REGARDING HIS MANAGEMENT OF EACH ATTENTION DEFICIT DISORDER PATIENT; THE PEDIATRICIAN SHALL PROVIDE A WRITTEN REPORT TO THE BOARD EVALUATING THE QUALITY OF HIS CARE OF EACH PATIENT. ON 10/19/95 ORDER AMENDED TO EXTEND TIME FOR COMPLIANCE WITH EDUCATION REQUIREMENTS UNTIL 12/31/95.

UDALL, COLLIN MD, LICENSE NUMBER 0015439, WAS DISCIPLINED BY ARIZONA ON JULY 17, 1996
DISCIPLINARY ACTION: 60-MONTH PROBATION; MONITORING OF PHYSICIAN PERFORMANCE
OFFENSE: FAILURE TO COMPLY WITH PREVIOUS BOARD ORDER

NOTES: VIOLATED PREVIOUS BOARD ORDER OF 10/94 IN THAT HE FAILED TO COMPLETE ANY CONTINUING MEDICAL EDUCATION HOURS IN THE MANAGEMENT OF ATTENTION DISORDER AND DID NOT RECEIVE REPORTS FROM THE PEDIATRIC CONSULTANT AS REQUIRED; IN 3/96, BOARD REVIEWED THE CHARTS FOR 19 PATIENTS HE SAW FOR ATTENTION DEFICIT DISORDER (ADD) IN 1994 AND 1995, 15 FOR WHICH HE HAD PRESCRIBED RITALIN; FAILED TO MAINTAIN ADEQUATE RECORDS ON PATIENTS IN THAT OF THE 12 REVIEWED CHARTS FOR PATIENTS SEEN IN 1995, MOST FAILED TO INDICATE THAT HE DISCUSSED THE BENEFITS AND RISKS OF RITALIN AND FAILED TO DOCUMENT THE ATTRIBUTES OF ADD; FOR MANY OF THE PATIENTS, DIAGNOSES WERE MADE ON THE BASIS OF REPORTS THAT OTHER FAMILY MEMBERS HAD THE DISORDER OR THAT A PSYCHOLOGIST HAD DIAGNOSED THE DISORDER; OTHER THAN FOR ONE PATIENT WHO HAD BEEN TO AN EMERGENCY ROOM, THERE WERE NO LABORATORY STUDIES OR EKG'S; THERE IS NO INDICATION THAT HE ASKED THE ADULT PATIENTS WHO RECEIVED RITALIN AND DEXEDRINE ABOUT ANY HISTORY OF SUBSTANCE ABUSE; FEW OF THE CHARTS INDICATED THAT HE PERFORMED PHYSICAL EXAMINATIONS ON THE PATIENTS; BETWEEN 11/88 AND 8/91, REPEATEDLY PRESCRIBED NARCOTICS TO A PATIENT WHOM HE SUSPECTED TO HAVE NARCOTIC SEEKING BEHAVIOR; GAVE THIS PATIENT OVER 100 INJECTIONS OF DEMEROL AND PHENERGAN, MOST OF WHICH WERE GIVEN AT HIS AUTHORIZATION, WITHOUT HIS SEEING THE PATIENT; BETWEEN 1/10/90 AND 1/19/90, DECREASED PATIENT'S DEMEROL IN FIVE INJECTIONS AND BETWEEN 1/22/90 AND 3/9/90, GAVE THE PATIENT PLACEBO INJECTIONS EVERY TWO TO THREE DAYS; DID NOT DISCUSS CHANGE TO PLACEBO IN CHART UNTIL 3/9/90, ON WHICH DATE HE NOTED THAT HE COULD NOT ETHICALLY GIVE PATIENT NARCOTICS SINCE HE DID AS WELL WITH THE PLACEBO; DESPITE THIS, GAVE PATIENT NARCOTICS FROM 5/90 UNTIL 8/91; DURING THE TIME PATIENT WAS RECEIVING DEMEROL INJECTIONS FROM PHYSICIAN, WAS ALSO RECEIVING DEMEROL AT AT LEAST THREE LOCAL HOSPITALS; PATIENT SUBSEQUENTLY UNDERWENT SEVERAL INPATIENT AND OUTPATIENT CHEMICAL DEPENDENCY PROGRAMS AND IN 1993, PATIENT WAS HOSPITALIZED IN INTENSIVE CARE FOR A MONTH DUE TO HIS ADDICTION PROBLEM. CENSURED; PROBATION WITH TERMS: WITHIN 60 DAYS AND AT YEARLY INTERVALS THEREAFTER, MANAGEMENT OF HIS PATIENTS WITH ADD WILL BE EVALUATED BY A CHART REVIEW BY A BOARD-APPROVED PEDIATRICIAN, WHO SHALL SUBMIT A REPORT TO THE BOARD; SHALL CONSULT WITH THE PEDIATRICIAN REGARDING HIS MANAGEMENT OF EACH PATIENT. ON 11/14/97 ORDER OF PROBATION WAS TERMINATED.

URUCHURTA-VALDIVIA, RICHARD DO, LICENSE NUMBER 0005123 OF 10684 HENSLEY BLVD., YUMA, AZ, WAS DISCIPLINED BY FLORIDA ON NOVEMBER 11, 1999
DISCIPLINARY ACTION: LICENSE SUSPENSION
OFFENSE: DISCIPLINARY ACTION BY ANOTHER STATE OR AGENCY

NOTES: ARIZONA LICENSE SUSPENDED ON 10/23/97 FOR AN INDEFINITE PERIOD OF TIME DUE TO POSSESSION AND ABUSE OF CONTROLLED SUBSTANCES; THIS WAS BASED UPON HIS NOTIFYING THE ARIZONA BOARD THAT HE TESTED POSITIVE FOR AMPHETAMINES, BENZODIAZEPINES AND OPIATE METABOLITES; ALSO FAILED TO NOTIFY THE FLORIDA BOARD OF AN ADDRESS CHANGE. LICENSE SUSPENDED UNTIL HE APPEARS BEFORE THE BOARD AND DEMONSTRATES THAT HE IS ABLE TO PRACTICE WITH REASONABLE SKILL AND SAFETY.

URUCHURTU, RICHARD DO, LICENSE NUMBER 2720 OF 2001 CRESTVIEW DRIVE, NEWBERG, OR, WAS DISCIPLINED BY ARIZONA ON OCTOBER 23, 1997
DISCIPLINARY ACTION: REQUIRED TO ENTER AN IMPAIRED PHYSICIAN PROGRAM OR SUBSTANCE ABUSE TREATMENT; MONITORING OF PHYSICIAN PERFORMANCE
OFFENSE: SUBSTANCE ABUSE

NOTES: HE ADMITTED TESTING POSITIVE FOR AMPHETAMINES, BENZODIAZEPINES, AND OPIATE METABOLITES ON 9/25/97; HE WAS EVALUATED AT A TREATMENT CENTER WHERE HIS DIAGNOSES INCLUDED OPIATE DEPENDENCE, PHENTERMINE ABUSE, AND AMBIEN ABUSE; SHALL REFRAIN FROM THE PRACTICE OF OSTEOPATHIC MEDICINE AND SURGERY UNTIL COMPLYING THE THESE CONDITIONS: WILL SUCCESSFULLY COMPLETE THE IN-PATIENT PROGRAM FOR CHEMICAL DEPENDENCY; WILL DEVELOP A PLAN FOR AFTERCARE TREATMENT AND MONITORING THAT SHALL INCLUDE, BUT MAY NOT BE LIMITED TO, INDIVIDUAL AND/OR GROUP COUNSELING SESSIONS, RANDOM BODY FLUID TESTING, AGREEMENT FOR RELEASE OF TREATMENT RECORDS AND REPORTS TO THE BOARD, PROHIBITION OF THE USE OF ALCOHOL AND CONTROLLED SUBSTANCES UNLESS PRESCRIBED BY HIS TREATING PHYSICIAN AND REGULAR MEETINGS WITH THE BOARD. SHALL INFORM BOARD OF CHANGE OF ADDRESS IF HE LEAVES ARIZONA; WILL REIMBURSE THE BOARD FOR ALL EXPENSES ASSOCIATED WITH THIS MATTER.

URUCHURTU, RICHARD DO, LICENSE NUMBER 2720 OF 1322 W. RIDGEVIEW DRIVE, YUMA, AZ, WAS DISCIPLINED BY ARIZONA ON JULY 15, 1998
DISCIPLINARY ACTION: 60-MONTH PROBATION; RESTRICTION PLACED ON LICENSE
OFFENSE: FAILURE TO COMPLY WITH PREVIOUS BOARD ORDER

NOTES: ON 10/7/97 HE ADMITTED TESTING POSITIVE FOR AMPHETAMINES, BENZODIAZEPINES AND OPIATE METABOLITES; ENTERED INTO AN EVALUATION AND TREATMENT PROGRAM ON 10/13/97 AND ON 11/11/97 HE LEFT THE PROGRAM WITHOUT FINISHING HIS TREATMENT; ON 12/8/97 HE WAS RELEASED FROM ANOTHER TREATMENT PROGRAM FOR NONCOMPLIANCE OF HIS EXISTING STIPULATED CONSENT ORDER AND VIOLATING FEDERAL DRUG LAWS; ON 4/16/98 HE COMPLETED INPATIENT TREATMENT. CONDITIONS AND TERMS OF HIS PROBATION ARE AS FOLLOWS: SHALL OBTAIN

PSYCHIATRIC OR PSYCHOLOGICAL TREATMENT BY A LICENSED PSYCHIATRIST AND/OR PSYCHOLOGIST APPROVED BY THE BOARD WHO SHALL PROVIDE MONTHLY REPORTS; SHALL PROVIDE A COPY OF THIS ORDER TO ALL HEALTH CARE FACILITIES WHERE HE PRACTICES; SHALL ABSTAIN COMPLETELY FROM THE CONSUMPTION OF ALCOHOLIC BEVERAGES AND SHALL NOT CONSUME ILLICIT DRUGS OR TAKE ANY CONTROLLED SUBSTANCES UNLESS PRESCRIBED FOR HIM BY HIS TREATING PHYSICIAN; SHALL MAINTAIN A MONTHLY LOG OF ALL PRESCRIPTION ONLY DRUGS TAKEN BY HIM AND SHALL PROVIDE A COPY TO THE BOARD; SHALL SUBMIT TO RANDOM BIOLOGICAL FLUID TESTING; SHALL OBTAIN A SPONSOR AND PARTICIPATE IN A MINIMUM OF TWO SELF-HELP MEETINGS PER WEEK; SHALL NOT ENGAGE IN THE PRACTICE OF MEDICINE FOR MORE THAN 20 HOURS PER WEEK UNLESS BOARD APPROVED; SHALL ATTEND 90 AA MEETINGS IN 90 DAYS; SHALL INFORM THE BOARD IF HE CEASES TO RESIDE IN ARIZONA; SHALL PAY COSTS.

URUCHURTU, RICHARD DO, LICENSE NUMBER 2720 OF 1322 E RIDGEVIEW DRIVE, YUMA, AZ, WAS DISCIPLINED BY ARIZONA ON NOVEMBER 14, 1998
DISCIPLINARY ACTION: EMERGENCY SUSPENSION
OFFENSE: FAILURE TO COMPLY WITH PREVIOUS BOARD ORDER

NOTES: HE VIOLATED THE 5/20/96 BOARD PROBATIONARY ORDER BY CONSUMING ALCOHOL, MARIJUANA AND COCAINE, SPECIFICALLY OPIATES/MORPHINE FOR WHICH DRUG SCREENS TESTED POSITIVE ON 11/3/98 & 11/10/98. HE DENIED USE OR KNOWLEDGE OF HOW MORPHINE WAS FOUND IN THE URINE DRUG SCREEN.

URUCHURTU, RICHARD DO, LICENSE NUMBER 2720 OF 1322 W RIDGEVIEW DIRVE, YUMA, AZ, WAS DISCIPLINED BY ARIZONA ON JANUARY 22, 1999
DISCIPLINARY ACTION: LICENSE REVOCATION
OFFENSE: PRACTICING WITHOUT A VALID LICENSE

NOTES: IN 11/98 TESTED POSITIVE FOR OPIATES/MORPHINE IN VIOLATION OF PRIOR BOARD ORDER; PRACTICED MEDICINE THE WEEK OF 11/16-20, 1998 AFTER LICENSE WAS SUSPENDED; WROTE A PRESCRIPTION FOR HIS GIRLFRIEND FOR ROXANOL WHICH WAS FILLED ON 12/2/97; HE CLAIMED HE WROTE IT BEFORE LICENSE WAS SUMMARILY SUSPENDED; LIED ABOUT THE PRESCRIPTION ON 12/12/98. HE MAY APPLY FOR A LICENSE TWO YEARS FROM THE DATE OF THIS ORDER.

URUCHURTU, RICHARD DO OF 1150 W 24TH STREET SUITE F, YUMA, AZ, WAS DISCIPLINED BY DEA ON JUNE 15, 1999
DISCIPLINARY ACTION: SURRENDER OF CONTROLLED SUBSTANCE LICENSE

URUCHURTU, RICHARD A DO, LICENSE NUMBER 20A6372 OF YUMA, AZ, WAS DISCIPLINED BY CALIFORNIA ON JUNE 25, 1998
DISCIPLINARY ACTION: LICENSE REVOCATION
OFFENSE: DISCIPLINARY ACTION BY ANOTHER STATE OR AGENCY

NOTES: ACTION TAKEN BY ANOTHER STATE.

URUCHURTU, RICHARD A DO, DATE OF BIRTH DECEMBER 30, 1951 OF 1322 W RIDGEVIEW DRIVE, YUMA, AZ, WAS DISCIPLINED BY MEDICARE ON JULY 20, 1999
DISCIPLINARY ACTION: EXCLUSION FROM THE MEDICARE AND/OR MEDICAID PROGRAM
OFFENSE: DISCIPLINARY ACTION BY ANOTHER STATE OR AGENCY

NOTES: LICENSE REVOKED, SUSPENDED, SURRENDERED OR OTHERWISE LOST FOR REASONS BEARING ON PROFESSIONAL PERFORMANCE, PROFESSIONAL COMPETENCE OR FINANCIAL INTEGRITY.

UTZ, JOHN MD OF 6402 EAST SHEPHERD HILLS DRIVE, TUCSON, AZ, WAS DISCIPLINED BY DEA ON JULY 6, 1999
DISCIPLINARY ACTION: SURRENDER OF CONTROLLED SUBSTANCE LICENSE
OFFENSE: PROFESSIONAL MISCONDUCT

NOTES: ILLEGALLY OBTAINING PRESCRIPTIONS FOR CONTROLLED SUBSTANCES.

VALEROS, QUIRINO MD, LICENSE NUMBER 9962, WAS DISCIPLINED BY ARIZONA ON JULY 28, 1999
DISCIPLINARY ACTION: 12-MONTH PROBATION; REPRIMAND
OFFENSE: SUBSTANDARD CARE, INCOMPETENCE OR NEGLIGENCE

NOTES: FAILURE TO ADEQUATELY ASSESS THE SYMPTOMS OF CARDIAC ISCHEMIA. SHALL OBTAIN 40 HOURS OF BOARD APPROVED CONTINUING MEDICAL EDUCATION IN CARDIOVASCULAR DISEASE IN AN OUTPATIENT SETTING.

VALLEY, GEORGE N DO, DATE OF BIRTH MAY 2, 1938 OF 3247-B CORRINE DRIVE, PRESCOTT VALLEY, AZ, WAS DISCIPLINED BY MEDICARE ON AUGUST 1, 1990
DISCIPLINARY ACTION: EXCLUSION FROM THE MEDICARE AND/OR MEDICAID PROGRAM
OFFENSE: DISCIPLINARY ACTION BY ANOTHER STATE OR AGENCY

NOTES: LICENSE REVOCATION OR SUSPENSION.

VAN BUREN, DAVID DO, LICENSE NUMBER 0002675 OF ROUTE 1, BOX 269, LAKESIDE, AZ, WAS DISCIPLINED BY ARIZONA ON DECEMBER 13, 1994
DISCIPLINARY ACTION: MONITORING OF PHYSICIAN PERFORMANCE
OFFENSE: PROFESSIONAL MISCONDUCT

NOTES: INFORMATION RECEIVED BY THE BOARD THAT HE MAY BE PHYSICALLY AND/OR PSYCHOLOGICALLY UNABLE TO SAFELY AND SKILLFULLY ENGAGE IN THE PRACTICE OF MEDICINE AND/OR MAY HAVE COMMITTED ONE OR MORE ACTS OF UNPROFESSIONAL CONDUCT. THIS ORDER PENDING FINAL DECISION ON THESE ALLEGATIONS. COMPLETELY RESTRICTED FROM PROVIDING ANY MEDICAL SERVICES OF ANY TYPE WHATSOEVER UNTIL 2/15/95; SHALL SUBMIT TO A MEDICAL AND/OR PSYCHOLOGICAL EVALUATION BY A BOARD APPROVED PHYSICIAN AND/OR PSYCHOLOGIST BY 12/30/94 AND/OR PSYCHOLOGIST AND SUBMIT COPIES OF THE REPORT TO THE BOARD. ORDER AMENDED ON 12/23/94 SUCH THAT HE SHALL INDEFINITELY REFRAIN FROM THE PRACTICE OF OSTEOPATHIC MEDICINE PENDING A HEARING AND ENTRY OF A FINAL BOARD ORDER; THE DEADLINE TO COMPLETE THE PSYCHIATRIC AND PSYCHOLOGICAL EXAMINATION EXTENDED TO 1/31/95; HIS CURRENT TREATING PSYCHIATRIST SHALL DELIVER COPIES OF ALL HIS PATIENT TEST REPORTS AND NOTES OF ALL TYPES TO THE DESIGNATED PSYCHIATRIST AND PSYCHOLOGIST; SHALL PROVIDE THE BOARD WITH ALL OTHER RECORDS OF HIS PRIOR TREATMENT BY PSYCHOLOGISTS OR PHYSICIANS FOR A BEHAVIORAL DISORDER.

VAN BUREN, DAVID DO, LICENSE NUMBER 0002675 OF ROUTE 1, BOX 269, LAKESIDE, AZ, WAS DISCIPLINED BY ARIZONA ON APRIL 4, 1995
DISCIPLINARY ACTION: LICENSE SUSPENSION; MONITORING OF PHYSICIAN PERFORMANCE

OFFENSE: PHYSICAL OR MENTAL ILLNESS INHIBITING THE ABILITY TO PRACTICE WITH SKILL AND SAFETY

NOTES: PROCURING OR ATTEMPTING TO PROCURE A LICENSE TO PRACTICE BY MISREPRESENTATION; MENTALLY UNABLE TO SAFELY ENGAGE IN THE PRACTICE OF MEDICINE. MINIMUM ONE YEAR SUSPENSION. DURING THE FIRST YEAR SHALL OBTAIN PSYCHIATRIC OR PSYCHOLOGICAL TREATMENT BY A THERAPIST INVOLVING AT LEAST 15 HOURS PER MONTH OF DIRECT PERSONAL THERAPY SESSIONS; THE TREATING THERAPIST SHALL SUBMIT A PROGRESS REPORT TO THE BOARD EVERY TWO MONTHS; AFTER SIX MONTHS OF THERAPY MAY SUBMIT A WRITTEN REQUEST TO THE BOARD SEEKING MODIFICATION OF THE MINIMUM NUMBER OF HOURS OF THERAPY.

VAN BUREN, DAVID DO, LICENSE NUMBER 0002675 OF ROUTE 1, BOX 269, LAKESIDE, AZ, WAS DISCIPLINED BY ARIZONA ON DECEMBER 21, 1995
DISCIPLINARY ACTION: PROBATION; RESTRICTION PLACED ON LICENSE

NOTES: RELEASED FROM SUSPENSION. MINIMUM THREE YEAR PROBATION. SHALL CONTINUE WITH PSYCHIATRIC OR PSYCHOLOGICAL TREATMENT AT LEAST ONCE A MONTH BY A THERAPIST WHO SHALL SEND WRITTEN PROGRESS REPORTS TO THE BOARD EVERY TWO MONTHS; SHALL HAVE A NURSE PRESENT AT ALL TIMES DURING THE EXAMINATION OF A FEMALE PATIENT; SHALL MEET WITH THE BOARD UPON REQUEST. ON 11/4/98 TERMS SATISFIED; FULL AND UNRESTRICTED LICENSE.

VAN NOSTRAND, WILLARD R III MD, LICENSE NUMBER 0007028 OF TUCSON, AZ, WAS DISCIPLINED BY ARIZONA ON JANUARY 28, 1994
DISCIPLINARY ACTION: FINE
OFFENSE: OVERCHARGING

NOTES: TREATMENT OF PATIENTS WAS DEEMED EXPERIMENTAL AND DID NOT CONFORM TO GENERALLY ACCEPTED EXPERIMENTAL CRITERIA, INCLUDING PROTOCOLS, DETAILED RECORDS, PERIODIC ANALYSIS OF RESULTS AND PERIODIC REVIEW BY A MEDICAL PEER REVIEW COMMITTEE AS APPROVED BY THE FOOD AND DRUG ADMINISTRATION; SEVERAL PATIENTS WERE CHARGED FOR TREATMENTS AND/OR CONSULTATIONS NOT RENDERED; IN SOME CASES RECORDS WERE SCANTY, INCOMPLETE OR ILLEGIBLE. WAS CENSURED AND MUST PAY A $2,000 PENALTY.

VAN NOSTRAND, WILLIAM R III MD, LICENSE NUMBER 0126342 OF 3737 CALLE CORTEZ, TUCSON, AZ, WAS DISCIPLINED BY NEW YORK ON MARCH 24, 1995
DISCIPLINARY ACTION: LICENSE REVOCATION
OFFENSE: DISCIPLINARY ACTION BY ANOTHER STATE OR AGENCY

NOTES: ACTION IN ARIZONA FOR FRAUDULENTLY BILLING FOR SERVICES NOT PROVIDED TO PATIENTS, FAILURE TO MAINTAIN ADEQUATE PATIENT RECORDS AND GIVING EXPERIMENTAL TREATMENT WITHOUT ADHERING TO GENERALLY ACCEPTED EXPERIMENTAL CRITERIA AND STANDARDS.

VAN PATTEN, MERRILL D DO, DATE OF BIRTH MAY 15, 1952 OF 1241 N ALLEN STREET, MESA, AZ, WAS DISCIPLINED BY MEDICARE ON DECEMBER 9, 1996
DISCIPLINARY ACTION: EXCLUSION FROM THE MEDICARE AND/OR MEDICAID PROGRAM
OFFENSE: NONCOMPLIANCE WITH A PROFESSIONAL RULE

NOTES: DEFAULTED ON PUBLIC HEALTH SERVICE EDUCATION LOAN. INDEFINITE EXCLUSION.

VAN PATTEN, MERRILL D DO OF 210 NORTH CENTER #103, MESA, AZ, WAS DISCIPLINED BY DEA ON APRIL 29, 1997
DISCIPLINARY ACTION: SURRENDER OF CONTROLLED SUBSTANCE LICENSE

VAN PATTEN, MERRILL D DO, LICENSE NUMBER 01179 OF PHOENIX, AZ, WAS DISCIPLINED BY IOWA ON APRIL 23, 1998
DISCIPLINARY ACTION: SURRENDER OF LICENSE
OFFENSE: DISCIPLINARY ACTION BY ANOTHER STATE OR AGENCY

NOTES: DISCIPLINARY ACTION TAKEN IN ARIZONA. VOLUNTARY SURRENDER.

VAN PATTEN, MERRILL DEAN DO, LICENSE NUMBER 1550 OF 1241 N ALLEN, MESA, AZ, WAS DISCIPLINED BY ARIZONA ON DECEMBER 7, 1996
DISCIPLINARY ACTION: EMERGENCY SUSPENSION

VAN PATTEN, MERRILL DEAN DO, LICENSE NUMBER 1550 OF 1241 N ALLEN, MESA, AZ, WAS DISCIPLINED BY ARIZONA ON JANUARY 30, 1997
DISCIPLINARY ACTION: LICENSE REVOCATION
OFFENSE: DISCIPLINARY ACTION BY ANOTHER STATE OR AGENCY

NOTES: IN 6/90 CONVICTED OF TWO COUNTS OF FRAUDULENT PRACTICES OF FILING FALSE CERTIFICATIONS RELATED TO MEDICAID CLAIMS; BASED UPON THIS CONVICTION, THE IOWA BOARD SUSPENDED HIS LICENSE FOR 90 DAYS ON 4/19/91 WHICH LICENSE HE ALLOWED TO EXPIRE; ON 10/10/96 AFTER BEING EXAMINED BY A PSYCHOLOGIST AND PSYCHIATRIST, IT WAS FOUND THAT HE SUFFERS FROM A MENTAL DISORDER THAT SIGNIFICANTLY IMPAIRS HIS ABILITY TO PRACTICE; LIED ABOUT THE CONVICTION AND SUSPENSION ON SUBSEQUENT RENEWALS OF HIS ARIZONA LICENSE; HE ADMITTED TO THE BOARD THAT HE HAD CONTINUED TO SEE AND TREAT PATIENTS AFTER RECEIVING AN ORDER WHICH SUMMARILY SUSPENDED HIS LICENSE.

VANCE, MICHAEL V MD, LICENSE NUMBER 0007616, WAS DISCIPLINED BY ARIZONA ON SEPTEMBER 18, 1996
OFFENSE: FAILURE TO COMPLY WITH PREVIOUS BOARD ORDER

NOTES: BIOLOGICAL FLUID SPECIMEN COLLECTED 8/20/96 TESTED POSITIVE FOR ETHANOL; INFORMED HOSPITALS IN WRITING THAT HE HAD RELAPSED. LICENSE WAS INACTIVATED. MAY NOT PRACTICE MEDICINE IN ARIZONA OR ANY OTHER STATE; MAY NOT HOLD OR MAINTAIN A DEA CONTROLLED SUBSTANCE CERTIFICATE OR WRITE OR REFILL PRESCRIPTIONS.

VANDERWAL, CALVIN H MD, LICENSE NUMBER 0010625 OF SCOTTSDALE, AZ, WAS DISCIPLINED BY ARIZONA ON APRIL 13, 1993
DISCIPLINARY ACTION: 60-MONTH PROBATION; FINE
OFFENSE: OVERCHARGING

NOTES: CENSURED BY THE BOARD IN 5/84 FOR EXCESSIVE FEES. IN 7/92 CHARGED ONE PATIENT EXCESSIVE AND UNCUSTOMARY FEES FOR A C-SECTION DELIVERY; IN ANOTHER CASE FEES WERE NOT JUSTIFIED IN MEDICAL RECORD. CONDITIONS OF PROBATION: $5,000 FINE; CENSURED; SHALL ENGAGE THE SERVICES OF A BOARD-APPROVED MONITOR TO CONSULT WITH ON HIS PRACTICE MANAGEMENT AND BILLING PROCEDURES WITH WRITTEN REPORTS TO THE BOARD; SHALL APPEAR BEFORE THE BOARD IN SIX MONTHS. ON 7/12/94 BOARD RECONSIDERED AND

WITHDREW THE CENSURE.

VANPATTEN, MERRILL D DO, DATE OF BIRTH MARCH 20, 1928 OF 3623 CHEYENNE BLVD, SIOUX CITY, IA, WAS DISCIPLINED BY MEDICARE ON JULY 22, 1991
DISCIPLINARY ACTION: 60-MONTH EXCLUSION FROM THE MEDICARE AND/OR MEDICAID PROGRAM
OFFENSE: CRIMINAL CONVICTION OR PLEA OF GUILTY, NOLO CONTENDERE, OR NO CONTEST TO A CRIME

NOTES: PROGRAM-RELATED CONVICTION.

VANPATTEN, MERRILL D DO, DATE OF BIRTH MARCH 20, 1928, LICENSE NUMBER 0S01179 OF 2038 SOUTH ST AUBIN, SIOUX CITY, IA, WAS DISCIPLINED BY IOWA ON AUGUST 16, 1991
DISCIPLINARY ACTION: LICENSE SUSPENSION

NOTES: MEDICAL LICENSE INDEFINITELY SUSPENDED; MINIMUM OF 90 DAYS MUST PASS BEFORE SEEKING REINSTATEMENT.

VANPATTEN, MERRILL D DO, DATE OF BIRTH MARCH 20, 1928, LICENSE NUMBER 0S01179 OF 210 N. CENTER, SUITE 103, MESA, AZ, WAS DISCIPLINED BY IOWA ON OCTOBER 8, 1992
DISCIPLINARY ACTION: 36-MONTH PROBATION

NOTES: SUSPENDED LICENSE IS REINSTATED.

VANPATTEN, MERRILL D DO OF SIOUX CITY, IA, WAS DISCIPLINED BY MISSOURI ON AUGUST 16, 1993
DISCIPLINARY ACTION: 3-MONTH LICENSE SUSPENSION
OFFENSE: DISCIPLINARY ACTION BY ANOTHER STATE OR AGENCY

NOTES: BASED ON ACTION TAKEN BY IOWA BOARD OF MEDICAL EXAMINERS, HE WAS CONVICTED ON 2 COUNTS OF FRAUDULENT PRACTICE IN THE THIRD DEGREE IN IOWA DISTRICT COURT.

VARGAS, JAIME C MD, LICENSE NUMBER 0004330, WAS DISCIPLINED BY ARIZONA ON JANUARY 21, 1993
DISCIPLINARY ACTION: RESTRICTION PLACED ON LICENSE

NOTES: LICENSE REACTIVATED ON CONDITION THAT ACTIVITIES IN THE PRACTICE OF MEDICINE BE LIMITED TO SURGICAL ASSISTANCE.

VELAZQUEZ-TORRES, MANUEL R MD OF PHOENIX, AZ, WAS DISCIPLINED BY ARIZONA ON JANUARY 19, 1995

NOTES: INFORMATION RECEIVED THAT HE WAS CHARGED WITH DRIVING UNDER THE INFLUENCE. SHALL SUBMIT HIMSELF TO AND COMPLETE INPATIENT EVALUATION FOR CHEMICAL DEPENDENCY AT A RECOVERY CENTER BY 3/10/95.

VESPE, JOHN ROBERT MD, LICENSE NUMBER G72675 OF PHOENIX, AZ, WAS DISCIPLINED BY CALIFORNIA ON NOVEMBER 30, 1998
DISCIPLINARY ACTION: 60-MONTH PROBATION
OFFENSE: CRIMINAL CONVICTION OR PLEA OF GUILTY, NOLO CONTENDERE, OR NO CONTEST TO A CRIME

NOTES: USE OF ALCOHOLIC BEVERAGES TO THE EXTENT DANGEROUS TO HIMSELF OR THE PUBLIC; TWO CRIMINAL CONVICTIONS FOR DRIVING UNDER THE INFLUENCE OF ALCOHOL. REVOCATION STAYED.

VITO, REYNALDO L MD, LICENSE NUMBER 13850, WAS DISCIPLINED BY ARIZONA ON MAY 15, 1998
DISCIPLINARY ACTION: LICENSE SUSPENSION
OFFENSE: FAILURE TO COMPLY WITH PREVIOUS BOARD ORDER

NOTES: ON 5/21/96, BOARD ORDERED HIM TO TAKE AND PASS THE SPEX WITH A SCORE OF 75; HE TOOK THE SPEX EXAM AND DID NOT RECEIVE A SCORE OF 75. LICENSE PLACED ON INACTIVE STATUS WITH CAUSE; MAY NOT HOLD OR MAINTAIN A CONTROLLED SUBSTANCE CERTIFICATE WITH THE DEA OR WRITE OR REFILL PRESCRIPTIONS; AND AUTHORIZED BY THE BOARD TO CONTINUE TO TAKE THE SPEX EXAM UPON HIS APPLICATION TO DO SO. SHALL NOT REQUEST REACTIVATION OF HIS LICENSE UNTIL HE SUCCESSFULLY PASSES THE SPEX EXAM, MEETS WITH THE BOARD AT A REGULARLY SCHEDULED MEETING, AND COMPLIES WITH ALL BOARD REQUESTS.

WADE, MICHAEL G MD, LICENSE NUMBER 0015797 OF SCOTTSDALE, AZ, WAS DISCIPLINED BY ARIZONA ON APRIL 14, 1994
DISCIPLINARY ACTION: REQUIRED TO TAKE ADDITIONAL MEDICAL EDUCATION
OFFENSE: OVERPRESCRIBING OR MISPRESCRIBING DRUGS

NOTES: ALLEGED PRESCRIBING OF LARGE AMOUNTS OF SCHEDULED DRUGS TO A PATIENT. SHALL OBTAIN 40 HOURS OF CONTINUING MEDICAL EDUCATION REGARDING THE MANAGEMENT OF BACK PAIN, HEADACHE, NECK PAIN AND/OR CHRONIC PAIN OTHER THAN CHRONIC PAIN RELATED TO TERMINAL ILLNESS. ON 4/5/95 ORDER TERMINATED DUE TO COMPLIANCE WITH EDUCATIONAL REQUIREMENTS.

WAGNER, MITCHELL S MD, WAS DISCIPLINED BY ARIZONA ON JANUARY 28, 1999

NOTES: LICENSE GRANTED WITH THE CAVEAT THAT HE AGREE NOT TO PRACTICE UNTIL AN EVALUATION BY A BOARD-APPROVED ADDICTIONOLOGIST COULD BE CONDUCTED AND SENT TO THE BOARD FOR REVIEW AND POSSIBLE ISSUANCE OF ADDITIONAL PROBATIONARY TERMS.

WAKEFIELD, RONALD DEAN MD, LICENSE NUMBER 0016032, WAS DISCIPLINED BY ARIZONA ON JULY 31, 1990
DISCIPLINARY ACTION: SURRENDER OF LICENSE
OFFENSE: FAILURE TO COMPLY WITH PREVIOUS BOARD ORDER

NOTES: IN 7/86 THE BOARD RECEIVED INFORMATION INDICATING THAT THERE WAS A DISCREPANCY IN NARCOTICS HE DISTRIBUTED. BOARD DETERMINED TO MONITOR HIM FOR SUBSTANCE ABUSE WITH RANDOM URINE SAMPLES. ON 11/17/86 A SAMPLE TESTED POSITIVE FOR COCAINE, CANNABINOIDS, AND FENTANYL. ENTERED SUBSTANCE ABUSE TREATMENT ON 12/28/86 AND COMPLETED THE PROGRAM ON 1/27/87. ON 1/31/87 ENTERED INTO AGREEMENT WITH BOARD, WHICH HE VIOLATED 1/16/88 WHEN A URINE TEST WAS POSITIVE FOR COCAINE AND PHENYLPROPANOLAMINE. BOARD PLACED LICENSE ON INACTIVE STATUS 2/5/88 AND REQUIRED HIM TO ENTER A SUBSTANCE ABUSE TREATMENT PROGRAM. HE ENTERED SUCH A PROGRAM ON 2/8/88 AND COMPLETED THE PROGRAM ON 5/14/88. ON 7/18/88 A URINE SAMPLE TESTED POSITIVE FOR COCAINE. IN 12/88 HE COMPLETED OUTPATIENT SUBSTANCE ABUSE TREATMENT AND ON 4/14/89 THE BOARD REACTIVATED HIS LICENSE SUBJECT TO THE CONDITIONS OF THE 1/3/87 ORDER. ON 5/20/89 THE BOARD ORDERED THAT THE 1/31/87 ORDER BE TERMINATED, AND HE VOLUNTARILY ENTERED INTO AN ORDER THAT REQUIRED, IN PART, THAT HE ABSTAIN FROM ALCOHOL AND TAKE NO DRUGS UNLESS PRESCRIBED FOR HIM BY HIS TREATING PHYSICIAN, AND THAT HE IMMEDIATELY COMPLY WITH REQUESTS FOR RANDOM BIOLOGICAL FLUID TESTS. HE VIOLATED THESE PROVISIONS BY FAILING TO UNDERGO REQUIRED PHYSICAL

EXAMINATIONS AND BY PROVIDING A URINE SAMPLE THAT TESTED POSITIVE FOR FENTANYL. BOARD SUMMARILY SUSPENDED LICENSE 6/8/90.

WALDRIP, ROBERT C MD, LICENSE NUMBER 0013525 OF SUN CITY, AZ, WAS DISCIPLINED BY ARIZONA ON OCTOBER 20, 1995
DISCIPLINARY ACTION: REPRIMAND
OFFENSE: OVERPRESCRIBING OR MISPRESCRIBING DRUGS

NOTES: BETWEEN 1/93 AND 4/94, PRESCRIBED CONTROLLED SUBSTANCES TO A MEMBER OF HIS IMMEDIATE FAMILY: XANAX, ATIVAN, LORTABS, DARVOCET AND SOMA CPD/CODEINE.

WALGREN, HAROLD MD, LICENSE NUMBER 15798, WAS DISCIPLINED BY ARIZONA ON NOVEMBER 18, 1999
DISCIPLINARY ACTION: PROBATION; REQUIRED TO TAKE ADDITIONAL MEDICAL EDUCATION

NOTES: WITHIN SIX MONTHS, SHALL OBTAIN 15 HOURS OF BOARD-APPROVED CONTINUING MEDICAL EDUCATION IN THE AREA OF THORACIC CT INTERPRETATION; PROBATION UNTIL THE CONTINUING MEDICAL EDUCATION IS COMPLETED..

WALINSKI, THOMAS N MD, LICENSE NUMBER 0002308 OF 9125 EAST PURDUE NO 114, SCOTTSDALE, AZ, WAS DISCIPLINED BY HAWAII ON OCTOBER 2, 1992
DISCIPLINARY ACTION: NONRENEWAL OF LICENSE
OFFENSE: NONCOMPLIANCE WITH A PROFESSIONAL RULE

NOTES: ALLEGED TO HAVE ENGAGED IN INAPPROPRIATE SEXUAL CONTACTS WITH FEMALE MINOR PATIENTS BETWEEN 1980 AND 1988. LICENSE TERMINATED FOR FAILURE TO RENEW BETWEEN 1/31/90 AND 1/31/92. ENTERED INTO SETTLEMENT AGREEMENT ON THAT HE WILL NOT ATTEMPT TO REACTIVATE OR REAPPLY FOR HIS HAWAII LICENSE NOR RETURN AT ANY FUTURE DATE TO PRACTICE MEDICINE IN HAWAII.

WALINSKI, THOMAS N MD, LICENSE NUMBER 0G17996 OF SCOTTSDALE, AZ, WAS DISCIPLINED BY CALIFORNIA ON SEPTEMBER 29, 1994
DISCIPLINARY ACTION: SURRENDER OF LICENSE

NOTES: VOLUNTARY SURRENDER OF LICENSE WHILE CHARGES PENDING.

WALINSKI, THOMAS N MD, LICENSE NUMBER 0005977, WAS DISCIPLINED BY ARIZONA ON JULY 22, 1995
DISCIPLINARY ACTION: LICENSE REVOCATION
OFFENSE: DISCIPLINARY ACTION BY ANOTHER STATE OR AGENCY

NOTES: SURRENDER FOR CANCELLATION WITH CAUSE BASED ON DISCIPLINARY ACTIONS BY HAWAII ON 10/2/92 FOR INAPPROPRIATE TOUCHING OF FEMALE PATIENTS AND BY CALIFORNIA ON 9/30/94 BASED ON THE HAWAII ACTION.

WALKER, GREGORY T MD, LICENSE NUMBER 0021091 OF PHOENIX, AZ, WAS DISCIPLINED BY ARIZONA ON OCTOBER 15, 1993
DISCIPLINARY ACTION: MONITORING OF PHYSICIAN PERFORMANCE
OFFENSE: NONCOMPLIANCE WITH A PROFESSIONAL RULE

NOTES: UNAVAILABILITY FOR BIOLOGICAL FLUID COLLECTION AS DIRECTED BY THE BOARD. SHALL SUBMIT TO RANDOM WITNESSED BIOLOGICAL FLUID COLLECTION UPON REQUEST BY BOARD STAFF; SHALL CONSUME NO ALCOHOL. IT WAS ALSO DECIDED THAT A PRACTICE SURVEY WAS TO BE CONDUCTED IN 6 MONTHS OF DR. WALKER'S RETURNING TO PRACTICE.

WALKER, GREGORY TRENT MD, DATE OF BIRTH JANUARY 20, 1959, LICENSE NUMBER 0014444 OF 403 GETWELL DRIVE, SUITE B, SENATOBIA, MS, WAS DISCIPLINED BY MISSISSIPPI ON JULY 20, 1995

NOTES: INITIAL LICENSURE, SUBJECT TO CERTAIN CONDITIONS.

WALKER, GREGORY TRENT MD, DATE OF BIRTH JANUARY 20, 1959, LICENSE NUMBER 0014444 OF 403 GETWELL DRIVE SUITE B, SENATOBIA, MS, WAS DISCIPLINED BY MISSISSIPPI ON OCTOBER 28, 1996

NOTES: HE IS PROHIBITED FROM PRACTICING MEDICINE UNTIL SUCH TIME AS THE BOARD HAS MADE A DETERMINATION THAT HE IS ABLE TO RETURN TO THE PRACTICE OF MEDICINE WITH REASONABLE SKILL AND SAFETY TO PATIENTS. ON 11/04/96 THE ORDER OF PROHIBITION WAS REMOVED. HE IS AUTHORIZED TO RETURN TO THE PRACTICE OF MEDICINE SUBJECT TO ANY OTHER PROCEEDINGS WHICH THE BOARD MAY DEEM NECESSARY.

WALKER, GREGORY TRENT MD, DATE OF BIRTH JANUARY 20, 1959, LICENSE NUMBER 14444 OF 403 GETWELL DRIVE SUITE B, SENATOBIA, MS, WAS DISCIPLINED BY MISSISSIPPI ON MARCH 20, 1997
DISCIPLINARY ACTION: RESTRICTION PLACED ON LICENSE

WALKER, GREGORY TRENT MD, DATE OF BIRTH JANUARY 20, 1959, LICENSE NUMBER 14444 OF 403 GETWELL DRIVE SUITE B, SENATOBIA, MS, WAS DISCIPLINED BY MISSISSIPPI ON FEBRUARY 12, 1998

NOTES: PROHIBITED FROM PRACTICING MEDICINE.

WALKER, GREGORY TRENT MD, DATE OF BIRTH JANUARY 20, 1959, LICENSE NUMBER 14444 OF 403 GETWELL DRIVE SUITE B, SENATOBIA, MS, WAS DISCIPLINED BY MISSISSIPPI ON FEBRUARY 19, 1998
DISCIPLINARY ACTION: 6-MONTH LICENSE SUSPENSION

NOTES: SUSPENSION SHALL BE STAYED AFTER THE EXPIRATION OF SIX MONTHS, WHEREUPON HE MAY APPEAR BEFORE THE BOARD AND REQUEST REINSTATEMENT, PROVIDED CERTAIN PREREQUISITES HAVE BEEN MET.

WALKER, GREGORY TRENT MD, DATE OF BIRTH JANUARY 20, 1959 OF 403 GETWELL DRIVE SUITE B, SENATOBIA, MS, WAS DISCIPLINED BY MEDICARE ON DECEMBER 20, 1998
DISCIPLINARY ACTION: EXCLUSION FROM THE MEDICARE AND/OR MEDICAID PROGRAM
OFFENSE: DISCIPLINARY ACTION BY ANOTHER STATE OR AGENCY

NOTES: LICENSE REVOKED, SUSPENDED, SURRENDERED OR OTHERWISE LOST FOR REASONS BEARING ON PROFESSIONAL PERFORMANCE, PROFESSIONAL COMPETENCE OR FINANCIAL INTEGRITY.

WANG, JOHN T K MD, LICENSE NUMBER 0009301 OF PHOENIX, AZ, WAS DISCIPLINED BY ARIZONA ON JANUARY 21, 1992
DISCIPLINARY ACTION: RESTRICTION PLACED ON CONTROLLED SUBSTANCE LICENSE; REQUIRED TO TAKE ADDITIONAL MEDICAL EDUCATION
OFFENSE: PROFESSIONAL MISCONDUCT

NOTES: GIVING INJECTIONS OF MEDICATIONS FOR WHICH THERE IS NO MEDICAL BASIS OR JUSTIFICATION, SPECIFICALLY COMBINATIONS OF STEROIDS AND ANTIBIOTICS, AND LIVER AND VITAMIN INJECTIONS. SHALL TAKE AND PASS SPEX PRIOR TO 7/1/92; SHALL ATTEND 30 HOURS CONTINUING MEDICAL EDUCATION

IN PHARMACOLOGY PRIOR TO 12/31/92, IN ADDITION TO THE 20 HOURS ALREADY REQUIRED BY BOARD RULES; SHALL DISCONTINUE PRESCRIBING, DISPENSING OR ADMINISTERING INJECTABLE STEROIDS UNTIL FURTHER ORDER OF THE BOARD; SHALL MEET WITH BOARD FOLLOWING COMPLETION OF SPEX.

WANG, JOHN T K MD, LICENSE NUMBER 0009301, WAS DISCIPLINED BY ARIZONA ON JANUARY 27, 1993
OFFENSE: FAILURE TO COMPLY WITH PREVIOUS BOARD ORDER

NOTES: SHALL TAKE AND PASS THE SPECIAL PURPOSE EXAMINATION (SPEX) ON ONE ATTEMPT PRIOR TO 07/01/93; ALL PROVISIONS OF THE STIPULATION DATED 02/28/92 REMAIN IN FULL FORCE AND EFFECT. FAILED THE SPEX EXAM FOR THE THIRD TIME SO THE BOARD GRANTED HIS REQUEST FOR INACTIVE STATUS EFFECTIVE 11/10/93.

WEBB, DALE F MD, LICENSE NUMBER 0003492, WAS DISCIPLINED BY ARIZONA ON APRIL 18, 1996
OFFENSE: SUBSTANDARD CARE, INCOMPETENCE OR NEGLIGENCE

NOTES: IN 2/94, WHEN TREATING A PATIENT FOR A PAINFUL, ENLARGED LYMPH NODE ON TWO OCCASIONS, NO EVIDENCE SHOWS THAT HE TOOK A BIOPSY OR CULTURE WHEN HE PERFORMED INCISION AND DRAINAGE OF THE WOUND WHICH SPONTANEOUSLY CLOSED AFTER FIVE DAYS; SAW PATIENT TWO MORE TIMES DURING 2/94, WHEN PATIENT WAS EXPERIENCING SEVERE PAIN AND A RE-EXCISION OF AREA; HE DID NOT EXAMINE THE PATIENT FOR A SOURCE OF LOBE ENLARGEMENT BUT ADVISED HER TO RETURN IN ONE WEEK TO CHECK FOR IMPROVEMENT; PATIENT DID NOT RETURN; ON 5/17/94, PATIENT WENT TO A CLINIC WITH COMPLAINT OF THE SAME MASS AND RECTAL BLEEDING AND WAS DIAGNOSED AS HAVING SQUAMOUS CELL CARCINOMA OF THE ANUS WITH METASTASIS TO THE INGUINAL NODES; UNDERWENT RADIATION AND CHEMOTHERAPY AND PROGNOSIS WAS POOR. CENSURED. ON 7/18/96 HIS REQUEST FOR REVIEW/REHEARING WAS DENIED. ON 9/23/98 APPEALED TO THE ARIZONA COURT OF APPEALS.

WEICH, MARTIN MD OF 1601 N TUCSON BLVD MED SQUARE, TUCSON, AZ, WAS DISCIPLINED BY DEA ON SEPTEMBER 20, 1994
DISCIPLINARY ACTION: SURRENDER OF CONTROLLED SUBSTANCE LICENSE

NOTES: IN LIEU OF PUBLIC INTEREST REVOCATION.

WEICH, MARTIN L MD, LICENSE NUMBER 0005145 OF TUCSON, AZ, WAS DISCIPLINED BY ARIZONA ON JULY 15, 1993
DISCIPLINARY ACTION: EMERGENCY SUSPENSION
OFFENSE: PHYSICAL OR MENTAL ILLNESS INHIBITING THE ABILITY TO PRACTICE WITH SKILL AND SAFETY

NOTES: INADEQUATELY MAINTAINED PATIENT RECORDS; LARGE AMOUNTS OF MULTIDOSE BOTTLES OF DRUGS FOR INJECTION, SOME OF WHICH OUTDATED IN 1975, WERE KEPT IN CABINETS AND SOME MEDICINES NOT LABELED; ON 09/21/91 INFORMED THE BOARD THAT BECAUSE OF SIGNIFICANT PROGRESSION OF DEGENERATIVE OSTEOARTHRITIS INVOLVING HIS LEFT KNEE AND SPINE, HE WAS UNABLE TO WORK SINCE 1/5/91. LATER, DID NOT APPEAR FOR INFORMAL INTERVIEW REGARDING HIS CONDITION. ON 7/14/93 BOARD INVESTIGATORS DISCOVERED THAT STAFF AT HIS OFFICE WERE ADMINISTERING ALLERGY SHOTS ALTHOUGH HE HAD NOT BEEN IN OFFICE SINCE 1991 STATING OTHER PHYSICIANS WERE "ON CALL" BUT NOT IN THE OFFICE. WITHIN TWO WEEKS SHALL ARRANGE FOR THE ORDERLY TRANSFER OF HIS MEDICAL RECORDS FOR ALL ACTIVE PATIENTS.

WEICH, MARTIN L MD, LICENSE NUMBER 0005145, WAS DISCIPLINED BY ARIZONA ON OCTOBER 15, 1993
DISCIPLINARY ACTION: LICENSE SUSPENSION
OFFENSE: PHYSICAL OR MENTAL ILLNESS INHIBITING THE ABILITY TO PRACTICE WITH SKILL AND SAFETY

NOTES: HE REQUESTED THAT THE ARIZONA BOARD OF MEDICAL EXAMINERS PLACE HIS MEDICAL LICENSE IN INACTIVE STATUS WITH CAUSE BECAUSE HE IS PHYSICALLY AND MENTALLY UNABLE TO SAFELY ENGAGE IN THE PRACTICE OF MEDICINE; HE CERTIFIES THAT HE HAS TOTALLY RETIRED FROM THE PRACTICE OF MEDICINE IN ARIZONA AND ELSEWHERE; DURING THE TIME THAT HE HOLDS AN INACTIVE LICENSE, HE SHALL NOT CONTINUE TO HOLD OR MAINTAIN A DRUG ENFORCEMENT ADMINISTRATION CONTROLLED SUBSTANCE REGISTRATION CERTIFICATE.

WEISER, RICHARD A MD, DATE OF BIRTH OCTOBER 27, 1942, LICENSE NUMBER 1028681 OF 21216 HAYMEADOW DR, SARATOGA, CA, WAS DISCIPLINED BY MICHIGAN ON JULY 3, 1996
DISCIPLINARY ACTION: LICENSE REVOCATION; FINE
OFFENSE: DISCIPLINARY ACTION BY ANOTHER STATE OR AGENCY

NOTES: FAILURE TO REPORT/COMPLY. $5,000 FINE.

WEISER, RICHARD A MD, LICENSE NUMBER 0020478, WAS DISCIPLINED BY ARIZONA ON OCTOBER 28, 1996

NOTES: SHALL NOT PRACTICE MEDICINE IN ARIZONA WITHOUT FIRST MEETING WITH THE BOARD AND RECEIVING APPROVAL.

WEISER, RICHARD ALLEN MD, LICENSE NUMBER 0C31874 OF LOS GATOS, CA, WAS DISCIPLINED BY CALIFORNIA ON SEPTEMBER 18, 1995
DISCIPLINARY ACTION: 24-MONTH PROBATION
OFFENSE: PROFESSIONAL MISCONDUCT

NOTES: REFERRED PATIENTS FOR PSYCHOTHERAPY TO HIS WIFE WHO WAS NOT LICENSED IN ANY CATEGORY TO PROVIDE AND BILL FOR PSYCHOTHERAPEUTIC SERVICES. REVOCATION, STAYED.

WEISS, SCOTT S MD, LICENSE NUMBER 0020073, WAS DISCIPLINED BY ARIZONA ON MAY 6, 1996
DISCIPLINARY ACTION: REQUIRED TO TAKE ADDITIONAL MEDICAL EDUCATION

NOTES: WITHIN SIX MONTHS, HE SHALL OBTAIN 30 HOURS OF CONTINUING MEDICAL EDUCATION IN THE EVALUATION AND TREATMENT OF PAIN. ON 10/16/96 ORDER TERMINATED AFTER HE SUBMITTED DOCUMENTATION INDICATING HIS COMPLIANCE WITH THE ORDER.

WELLS, MARILYN DO, LICENSE NUMBER 2111, WAS DISCIPLINED BY ARIZONA ON NOVEMBER 23, 1998
DISCIPLINARY ACTION: LICENSE SUSPENSION; REQUIRED TO ENTER AN IMPAIRED PHYSICIAN PROGRAM OR SUBSTANCE ABUSE TREATMENT
OFFENSE: PROFESSIONAL MISCONDUCT

NOTES: IN 11/98 BOARD RECEIVED INFORMATION FROM A PHARMACIST ALLEGING THAT SHE ATTEMPTED TO ACQUIRE DEMEROL INJECTIBLE UNDER A FALSE IDENTITY WITH A PRESCRIPTION SHE HAD WRITTEN; A PRESCRIBING HISTORY REVEALED SHE WAS

PRESCRIBING DEMEROL TO SEVERAL OF HER PATIENTS; ADMITTED TO FORGING PRESCRIPTIONS OF HER ASSOCIATES AND PRESCRIBING UNDER ASSUMED NAME; CLAIMED SHE WAS PRESCRIBING DUE TO PHYSICAL INJURIES CAUSING CHRONIC PAIN. SHALL REFRAIN FROM PRACTICE UNTIL SHE HAS MET THE FOLLOWING TERMS AND CONDITIONS: WILL SUCCESSFULLY COMPLETE INPATIENT EVALUATION FOR CHEMICAL DEPENDENCY AND DEVELOP A PLAN FOR AFTERCARE TREATMENT AND MONITORING; SHALL SIGN A RELEASE ALLOWING TREATMENT PERSONNEL TO RELEASE HER MEDICAL RECORDS; SHALL MEET WITH THE BOARD UPON COMPLIANCE WITH THESE CONDITIONS; SHALL PROVIDE A COPY OF THE ORDER TO ANY HEALTH CARE ENTITY WHERE SHE PRACTICES; SHALL INFORM BOARD OF CHANGE OF ADDRESS WITHIN 20 DAYS..

WELLS, MARILYN DO, LICENSE NUMBER 2111 OF 2138 E. GELDING DRIVE, PHOENIX, AZ, WAS DISCIPLINED BY ARIZONA ON AUGUST 7, 1999
DISCIPLINARY ACTION: 60-MONTH PROBATION; RESTRICTION PLACED ON LICENSE
OFFENSE: SUBSTANCE ABUSE

NOTES: ON 11/23/98 LICENSE WAS SUSPENDED AFTER INFORMATION RECEIVED THAT SHE MAY BE UNABLE TO SAFELY PRACTICE; IN 3/99 SHE COMPLETED A TREATMENT PROGRAM FOR SUBSTANCE ABUSE ADDICTION. LICENSE LIMITED AS FOLLOWS: SHALL IMMEDIATELY OBTAIN A TREATING THERAPIST APPROVED BY THE BOARD AND SHALL REMAIN IN TREATMENT UNTIL FURTHER ORDER OF THE BOARD; THE THERAPIST WILL PROVIDE MONTHLY REPORTS TO THE BOARD; SHALL PROVIDE A COPY OF THIS ORDER TO ANY HEALTH CARE ENTITY WHERE SHE HAS PRIVILEGES; SHALL ONLY ENGAGE IN OSTEOPATHIC MEDICINE FOR TWENTY HOURS PER WEEK; SHALL NOT PRESCRIBE ANY CONTROLLED SUBSTANCES FOR A MINIMUM OF ONE YEAR; SHALL ABSTAIN COMPLETELY FROM THE CONSUMPTION OF ALCOHOLIC BEVERAGES AND DRUGS EXCEPT WHEN PRESCRIBED BY HER TREATING PHYSICIAN; SHALL SUBMIT TO ANY EXAMINATIONS ORDERED BY BOARD; SHALL APPEAR BEFORE BOARD UPON REQUEST; SHALL SUBMIT TO RANDOM BIOLOGICAL FLUID COLLECTION; SHALL OBTAIN A MINIMUM OF TWO SELF-HELP MEETINGS PER WEEK THROUGH SUCH ORGANIZATIONS AS AA OR NARCOTICS ANONYMOUS; SHALL INFORM THE BOARD IF SHE CEASES TO PRACTICE IN ARIZONA; SHALL PAY COSTS. THIS ORDER SUPERSEDES PREVIOUS ORDERS..

WESTERVELT, MARK MD, LICENSE NUMBER 4320, WAS DISCIPLINED BY ARIZONA ON NOVEMBER 14, 1997
DISCIPLINARY ACTION: 12-MONTH PROBATION; REQUIRED TO TAKE ADDITIONAL MEDICAL EDUCATION
OFFENSE: SUBSTANDARD CARE, INCOMPETENCE OR NEGLIGENCE

NOTES: IN SEVERAL CASES, DID NOT PROPERLY EXAMINE PATIENTS AND GAVE PATIENTS STEROIDS INAPPROPRIATELY; WHEN AN OFFICE SURVEY WAS CONDUCTED, IN ACCORDANCE WITH A PRIOR ORDER, SEVERAL DEFICIENCIES WERE FOUND IN HIS CARE OF PATIENTS HE HAD SEEN BETWEEN 10/88 AND 7/96: ALL OF THE PROGRESS NOTES, LAB SLIPS, HOSPITAL DATA, INSURANCE DATA AND CONSULTATIONS WERE LOOSELY HELD IN A MANILA FOLDER WITHOUT DIVIDERS; NOTABLY ABSENT FROM THE DOCTOR'S CHARTS WERE A MEDICATION LIST, A PROBLEM LIST AND IMMUNIZATION LIST: AFTER PATIENT CAME IN WITH A COUGH, THERE WAS NO FURTHER HISTORIC EVALUATION OF THIS COUGH PROBLEM, NOR WAS ANY EXAM CONDUCTED; IN THIS CASE THERE WAS ALSO NO EVIDENCE THAT AN EXAM OF THE LUNGS OR HEART WAS CONDUCTED DURING THE PERIOD OF TIME THE PATIENT WAS UNDER THE DOCTOR'S CARE, NOR ANY WORK-UP INSTIGATED TO EVALUATE THE PATIENT'S CHRONIC COUGH; ANOTHER PATIENT CAME IN WITH REFRACTORY UPPER RESPIRATORY ALLERGIES AND NO EXAM WAS CONDUCTED NOR WERE THERE ANY HISTORICAL DETAILS TAKEN CONCERNING THE PATIENT'S RESPIRATORY SYMPTOMS; ANOTHER PATIENT WAS GIVEN KENALOG WHEN THE INDICATION FOR INTRAMUSCULAR KENALOG WAS NOT SUPPORTED IN THE CASE; CARE HE GAVE TO A PATIENT WITH DIABETES WAS SUBSTANDARD IN THAT NO EXAM WAS GIVEN TO EVALUATE AN ORGAN DAMAGED FROM THE DIABETES AND HE GAVE A STEROID WHICH MAY HAVE AGGRAVATED THE DIABETES. CONDITIONS OF THE PROBATION ARE AS FOLLOWS: WITHIN 12 MONTHS, HE SHALL COMPLETE A TWO WEEK MINI-RESIDENCY IN INTERNAL MEDICINE AND PEDIATRICS IN A BOARD APPROVED FACILITY; WITHIN 90 DAYS HE SHALL ENGAGE THE SERVICES OF A BOARD-APPROVED OFFICE MANAGEMENT CONSULTANT WHO SHALL SUBMIT A WRITTEN PLAN REGARDING PATIENT INFORMATION AND BILLING PRACTICES TO THE BOARD; WITHIN 6 MONTHS, HE SHALL COMPLETE 20 HOURS OF CONTINUING MEDICAL EDUCATION IN RECORD-KEEPING AND DOCUMENTATION; IN NINE MONTHS, AN OFFICE SURVEY OF HIS PRACTICE WILL BE CONDUCTED.

WESTERVELT, MARK JUSTIN MD, LICENSE NUMBER 0004320, WAS DISCIPLINED BY ARIZONA ON APRIL 9, 1992
DISCIPLINARY ACTION: REQUIRED TO TAKE ADDITIONAL MEDICAL EDUCATION
OFFENSE: SUBSTANDARD CARE, INCOMPETENCE OR NEGLIGENCE

NOTES: INADEQUATE RECORDKEEPING AND USE OF INTRAMUSCULAR STEROIDS ON PEDIATRIC PATIENTS. SHALL COMPLETE 20 HOURS OF CONTINUING MEDICAL EDUCATION IN THE TOPIC OF PEDIATRIC PULMONARY DISEASE OR ALLERGY BEFORE 12/31/92. THIS REQUIREMENT SHALL BE IN ADDITION TO THE 20 HOURS OF CONTINUING MEDICAL EDUCATION REQUIRED ANNUALLY IN BOARD'S RULES FOR RENEWAL OF LICENSURE. SHALL OBTAIN A PRACTICE MANAGEMENT AUDIT BY A BOARD-APPROVED OFFICE PRACTICE CONSULTANT, WITH SPECIAL INTEREST IN RECORDKEEPING. ON 10/18/95 ORDER TERMINATED; STAFF TO CONDUCT A FOLLOW-UP SURVEY IN 8 MONTHS TO DETERMINE IF HE IS IN COMPLIANCE WITH RECOMMENDATIONS MADE BY OFFICE MANAGEMENT CONSULTANT.

WESTMAN, LINCOLN H MD, LICENSE NUMBER 0003138, WAS DISCIPLINED BY ARIZONA ON SEPTEMBER 11, 1992
DISCIPLINARY ACTION: EMERGENCY SUSPENSION
OFFENSE: SEXUAL ABUSE OF OR SEXUAL MISCONDUCT WITH A PATIENT

NOTES: PLACED HIS HAND ON THE CROTCH OF A MALE PSYCHIATRIC PATIENT OF HIS AND SAID "YOU'VE GOT BIG BALLS." ORIGINALLY DENIED HIS ACTIONS TO THE BOARD, THEN LATER STATED THEY WERE INTENDED AS THERAPY TO SHOCK THE PATIENT OUT OF HIS DEPRESSION.

WESTMAN, LINCOLN H MD, LICENSE NUMBER 0003138, WAS DISCIPLINED BY ARIZONA ON APRIL 16, 1993
DISCIPLINARY ACTION: LICENSE REVOCATION

NOTES: SHALL NOT REAPPLY FOR FIVE YEARS.

WESTMAN, LINCOLN H MD OF 7330 N 16TH STREET, PHOENIX, AZ, WAS DISCIPLINED BY DEA ON SEPTEMBER 9, 1993
DISCIPLINARY ACTION: SURRENDER OF CONTROLLED SUBSTANCE LICENSE
OFFENSE: DISCIPLINARY ACTION BY ANOTHER STATE OR AGENCY

NOTES: SURRENDER OF ARIZONA STATE MEDICAL LICENSE FOR UNPROFESSIONAL CONDUCT AND MEDICAL INCOMPETENCY.

WHITLOW, FRANCIS DO, LICENSE NUMBER 0001569, WAS DISCIPLINED BY ARIZONA ON JANUARY 8, 1990
DISCIPLINARY ACTION: LICENSE REVOCATION; FINE
OFFENSE: OVERPRESCRIBING OR MISPRESCRIBING DRUGS

NOTES: BETWEEN 5/79 AND 5/88 PRESCRIBED CONTROLLED SUBSTANCES AND PRESCRIPTION ONLY DRUGS TO FIVE PATIENTS IN AMOUNTS AND FREQUENCY THAT CANNOT BE JUSTIFIED BASED ON DIAGNOSIS SET FORTH IN PATIENT RECORDS. $2500 ADMINISTRATIVE PENALTY; $598 INVESTIGATION COSTS.

WICO, ANTONIO R JR MD, DATE OF BIRTH JUNE 21, 1942, LICENSE NUMBER 0020674, WAS DISCIPLINED BY ARIZONA ON APRIL 10, 1992
DISCIPLINARY ACTION: RESTRICTION PLACED ON LICENSE; REQUIRED TO TAKE ADDITIONAL MEDICAL EDUCATION

NOTES: GRANTED LICENSURE WITH THE RESTRICTION THAT HE SHALL NOT PERFORM OR SUPERVISE THE PERFORMANCE OF ANESTHESIOLOGY ON ANY CHILD 23 MONTHS OR YOUNGER EXCEPT IN EMERGENCY CASES INVOLVING NEONATAL RESUSCITATION OR EMERGENCY CESAREAN SECTIONS; RESTRICTION LIFTED ONLY WITH PROOF OF COMPLETION OF AN 8-WEEK BOARD-APPROVED HOSPITAL-BASED MINI-RESIDENCY IN NEONATAL AND INFANT ANESTHESIOLOGY. ON 1/19/95 ORDER TERMINATED AS HE HAD COMPLETED THIS REQUIREMENT.

WICO, ANTONIO R JR MD, DATE OF BIRTH JUNE 21, 1942, LICENSE NUMBER 0018998 OF 1834 SOUTHFORK DRIVE, PHOENIX, AZ, WAS DISCIPLINED BY WISCONSIN ON JANUARY 21, 1993
DISCIPLINARY ACTION: RESTRICTION PLACED ON LICENSE
OFFENSE: DISCIPLINARY ACTION BY ANOTHER STATE OR AGENCY

NOTES: ON 4/10/92 LICENSE RESTRICTED IN ARIZONA BASED UPON PROVISION OF CARE TO AN INFANT AT SAINT ELIZABETH'S HOSPITAL IN APPLETON, WISCONSIN WHICH FELL BELOW MINIMALLY ACCEPTABLE STANDARDS FOR THE PRACTICE OF ANESTHESIOLOGY. SHALL NOT PERFORM OR SUPERVISE THE PERFORMANCE OF ANESTHESIOLOGY ON ANY CHILD TWENTY-THREE MONTHS OR YOUNGER EXCEPT IN EMERGENCY CASES INVOLVING NEONATAL RESUSCITATION OR EMERGENCY CESAREAN SECTIONS; UPON SUBMISSION OF PROOF THAT HE HAS SATISFIED THE TERMS AND CONDITIONS FOR A RETURN TO UNRESTRICTED PRACTICE IN ARIZONA, MAY PETITION FOR REMOVAL OF THIS RESTRICTION ON HIS LICENSE.

WICO, ANTONIO R JR MD, LICENSE NUMBER 0C42887 OF PHOENIX, AZ, WAS DISCIPLINED BY CALIFORNIA ON MAY 22, 1995
OFFENSE: DISCIPLINARY ACTION BY ANOTHER STATE OR AGENCY

NOTES: DISCIPLINE BY WISCONSIN AND ARIZONA BOARDS BASED ON SHORTCOMINGS IN NEONATAL AND PEDIATRIC ANESTHESIOLOGY. IF HE RETURNS TO PRACTICE IN CALIFORNIA, HE MUST FIRST PASS AN ORAL CLINICAL EXAM IN HIS FIELD TO PROVE COMPETENCY.

WILBIRT, DAVID A MD, LICENSE NUMBER 0009920, WAS DISCIPLINED BY ARIZONA ON JULY 17, 1996
DISCIPLINARY ACTION: REPRIMAND

NOTES: IN 4/96, BOARD DISCUSSED COMPLAINT AND VOTED TO OFFER HIM AN OPPORTUNITY TO ENTER INTO A CONSENT AGREEMENT TO A LETTER OF REPRIMAND; SIGNED CONSENT AGREEMENT WHICH IS PRESENTED TO THE BOARD FOR APPROVAL.

WILCOX, MELINDA J MD, LICENSE NUMBER 0012951, WAS DISCIPLINED BY ARIZONA ON JANUARY 25, 1991
DISCIPLINARY ACTION: REQUIRED TO ENTER AN IMPAIRED PHYSICIAN PROGRAM OR SUBSTANCE ABUSE TREATMENT; MONITORING OF PHYSICIAN PERFORMANCE
OFFENSE: SUBSTANCE ABUSE

NOTES: MISUSING CHEMICAL SUBSTANCES. MUST IMMEDIATELY PARTICIPATE IN THE ARIZONA MEDICAL ASSOCIATION'S MONITORED AFTERCARE TREATMENT PROGRAM WHOSE THERAPIST MUST SUBMIT QUARTERLY REPORTS; MUST PARTICIPATE IN 90 12-STEP MEETINGS APPROPRIATE FOR SUBSTANCE ABUSE WITHIN 90 DAYS, MUST THEN PARTICIPATE IN A 12-STEP RECOVERY PROGRAM AND ATTEND A MINIMUM OF 3 WEEKLY MEETINGS; MUST OBTAIN A BOARD APPROVED TREATING PHYSICIAN; MUST ABSTAIN COMPLETELY FROM THE CONSUMPTION OF ALCOHOLIC BEVERAGES AND OTHER DRUGS; MUST SUBMIT TO RANDOM TESTS OF BIOLOGICAL FLUID; MUST MAINTAIN A LOG OF ALL MEDICATIONS PRESCRIBED BY TREATING PHYSICIAN WHICH WILL BE OPEN TO THE BOARD; MUST SUBMIT TO MENTAL, PHYSICAL OR MEDICAL COMPETENCY EXAMS UPON THE BOARD'S REQUEST; MUST SUBMIT TO ANY THERAPY ORDERED BY THE BOARD; MUST APPEAR IN PERSON BEFORE THE BOARD UPON REQUEST; MUST INFORM THE BOARD OF CHANGE OF ADDRESS OR IF SHE PLANS TO BE AWAY FROM HER OFFICE OR HOME FOR MORE THAN FIVE DAYS. EFFECTIVE 1/29/94 ORDER TERMINATED.

WILDEMAN, LEONARD MD, WAS DISCIPLINED BY ARIZONA ON JANUARY 17, 1996
OFFENSE: PROFESSIONAL MISCONDUCT

NOTES: INFORMAL INTERVIEW WITH THE BOARD TO DISCUSS COMPLAINT REGARDING HIS ADVERTISEMENT WHICH APPEARED TO BE PROMOTING THE USE OF PROZAC; INTERIM ORDER. WITHIN 60 DAYS, SHALL UNDERGO A PSYCHIATRIC AND PSYCHOMETRIC EVALUATION BY EVALUATORS SELECTED BY THE BOARD; WITHIN 60 DAYS SHALL TAKE AND PASS THE SPECIAL PURPOSE EXAMINATION WITH A SCORE OF 75 OR GREATER.

WILDEMAN, LEONARD MD, LICENSE NUMBER 13979, WAS DISCIPLINED BY ARIZONA ON SEPTEMBER 26, 1997
DISCIPLINARY ACTION: LICENSE SUSPENSION
OFFENSE: FAILURE TO COMPLY WITH PREVIOUS BOARD ORDER

NOTES: BETWEEN 10/94 AND 5/95 THE BOARD RECEIVED COMPLAINTS AGAINST HIM; HE FAILED TO CONFIRM IN WRITING THAT HE WOULD APPEAR FOR A BOARD INTERVIEW AND THEN FAILED TO APPEAR TO MORE THAN ONE INTERVIEW; INAPPROPRIATELY DISCLOSED THE NATURE OF ONE OF THE COMPLAINTS AGAINST HIM TO HIS PSYCHIATRIC PATIENTS AND A COMPLAINAINTS ADDRESS WHICH LED PATIENTS TO TAKE ACTION AGAINST THE PERSON COMPLAINING IN THE FORM OF LETTERS AND NOTES LEFT AT HER HOME; DID NOT FULFILL REQUIREMENTS OF 2/96 ORDER THAT HE OBTAIN A PSYCHIATRIC EVALUATION AND PASS THE SPEX EXAM; EXHIBITED

INAPPROPRIATE BEHAVIOR IN RESPONDING AND REACTING TO THE BOARD'S INVESTIGATION INCLUDING NOT SUPPLYING REQUESTED INFORMATION. LICENSE SHALL REMAIN SUSPENDED UNTIL HE SUBMITS TO PSYCHIATRIC AND PSYCHOMETRIC EVALUATIONS, TAKES AND PASSES THE SPEX EXAM AND DEMONSTRATES HIS FITNESS AND COMPETENCE TO PRACTICE MEDICINE.

WILDEMAN, LEONARD H MD, LICENSE NUMBER 17401 OF TUCSON, AZ, WAS DISCIPLINED BY WASHINGTON ON SEPTEMBER 23, 1997
DISCIPLINARY ACTION: LICENSE REVOCATION
OFFENSE: NONCOMPLIANCE WITH A PROFESSIONAL RULE

NOTES: FAILING TO RESPOND TO A STATEMENT OF CHARGES.

WILDEMAN, LEONARD H MD, DATE OF BIRTH DECEMBER 21, 1949 OF 2600 IRONWOOD HILL DR. #1, TUCSON, AZ, WAS DISCIPLINED BY MEDICARE ON APRIL 20, 1999
DISCIPLINARY ACTION: EXCLUSION FROM THE MEDICARE AND/OR MEDICAID PROGRAM
OFFENSE: DISCIPLINARY ACTION BY ANOTHER STATE OR AGENCY

NOTES: LICENSE REVOKED, SUSPENDED, SURRENDERED OR OTHERWISE LOST FOR REASONS BEARING ON PROFESSIONAL PERFORMANCE, PROFESSIONAL COMPETENCE OR FINANCIAL INTEGRITY.

WILLIAMS, HARVEY E DO, DATE OF BIRTH APRIL 5, 1945, LICENSE NUMBER 0001258, WAS DISCIPLINED BY ARIZONA ON JANUARY 6, 1992
OFFENSE: PROFESSIONAL MISCONDUCT

NOTES: ADVERTISED IN A FALSE, DECEPTIVE, OR MISLEADING MANNER IN THAT A 100% GUARANTEE IN HIS ADVERTISEMENT OF 4/24/91 REGARDING BREAST AUGMENTATION WAS NOT EVER MEANT TO BE 100% MONEY BACK. CENSURED.

WILLIAMS, HARVEY E DO, DATE OF BIRTH APRIL 5, 1945, LICENSE NUMBER 0001258, WAS DISCIPLINED BY ARIZONA ON JULY 25, 1992
DISCIPLINARY ACTION: RESTRICTION PLACED ON LICENSE; REPRIMAND
OFFENSE: SUBSTANDARD CARE, INCOMPETENCE OR NEGLIGENCE

NOTES: SIX COMPLAINTS CONCERNING HIS INABILITY TO APPROPRIATELY PERFORM COSMETIC SURGERY PROCEDURES ON THE BREASTS OF FEMALE PATIENTS. PERMANENTLY RESTRICTED FROM PERFORMING ANY BREAST SURGERY MEANING ALL BREAST IMPLANTS, LIFTS, RECONSTRUCTION, OR OTHER SURGERIES RELATED TO THE BREAST AND PERFORMED EITHER ENTIRELY OR PARTIALLY FOR COSMETIC PURPOSES.

WILLIAMS, HARVEY E DO, DATE OF BIRTH APRIL 5, 1945, LICENSE NUMBER 00E5643 OF PO BOX 5673, SCOTTSDALE, AZ, WAS DISCIPLINED BY TEXAS ON JANUARY 29, 1993
DISCIPLINARY ACTION: RESTRICTION PLACED ON LICENSE
OFFENSE: DISCIPLINARY ACTION BY ANOTHER STATE OR AGENCY

NOTES: ON 7/25/92 ARIZONA BOARD RESTRICTED HIM FROM PERFORMING ANY BREAST SURGERY DEFINED AS ALL BREAST IMPLANTS, LIFTS, RECONSTRUCTION, OR OTHER SURGERIES RELATED TO THE BREAST AND PERFORMED EITHER ENTIRELY OR PARTIALLY FOR COSMETIC PURPOSES BASED ON HIS INABILITY TO APPROPRIATELY PERFORM SUCH SURGERY BASED ON SIX COMPLAINTS. HE IS PERMANENTLY RESTRICTED FROM PERFORMING SUCH SURGERY IN TEXAS; PRIOR TO PRACTICING IN TEXAS SHALL APPEAR BEFORE THE BOARD. SHALL NOT SEEK MODIFICATION FOR ONE YEAR.

WILLIAMS, HARVEY E D0, DATE OF BIRTH APRIL 5, 1945, LICENSE NUMBER 0001258, WAS DISCIPLINED BY ARIZONA ON MAY 12, 1993
DISCIPLINARY ACTION: PROBATION; REPRIMAND
OFFENSE: SUBSTANDARD CARE, INCOMPETENCE OR NEGLIGENCE

NOTES: ON 3/29/89 PERFORMED A BREAST IMPLANT PROCEDURE; FAILED TO MAINTAIN ADEQUATE RECORDS ON THE PATIENT; ON 8/5/89 A BACTERIAL CULTURE WAS OBTAINED WHICH WAS NOTED IN RECORDS; ALTHOUGH HE SHOULD HAVE BEEN AWARE OF IT, IMPLANT WAS NOT REMOVED UNTIL 4/24/90. MINIMUM TWO YEAR PROBATION UNDER TERMS AND CONDITIONS: SHALL COMPLETE A MINIMUM OF 10 HOURS OF BOARD APPROVED CONTINUING MEDICAL EDUCATION IN THE AREA OF RECORD KEEPING WITHIN ONE YEAR; SHALL MAKE HIS RECORDS OPEN FOR INSPECTION BY THE BOARD; SHALL MEET WITH THE BOARD UPON REQUEST TO REVIEW COMPLIANCE WITH THIS ORDER. ON 3/10/95 PROBATION SATISFIED IN FULL.

WILLIAMS, HARVEY E DO, DATE OF BIRTH APRIL 5, 1945, LICENSE NUMBER 00E5643 OF SCOTTSDALE, AZ, WAS DISCIPLINED BY TEXAS ON SEPTEMBER 30, 1994
DISCIPLINARY ACTION: SURRENDER OF LICENSE
OFFENSE: NONCOMPLIANCE WITH A PROFESSIONAL RULE

NOTES: ALLEGATIONS CONCERNING POSSIBLE VIOLATIONS OF THE MEDICAL PRACTICE ACT; DID NOT ADMIT ALLEGATIONS. SURRENDER IN LIEU OF FURTHER INVESTIGATION. SHALL NOT PETITION FOR REINSTATEMENT OF LICENSE.

WILLIAMS, HARVEY E DO, LICENSE NUMBER 20A3800 OF TUCSON, AZ, WAS DISCIPLINED BY CALIFORNIA ON MAY 13, 1996
DISCIPLINARY ACTION: LICENSE REVOCATION
OFFENSE: DISCIPLINARY ACTION BY ANOTHER STATE OR AGENCY

NOTES: ACTION IN ARIZONA FOR UNPROFESSIONAL CONDUCT

WILLIAMS, KIRK G MD, LICENSE NUMBER 0013691, WAS DISCIPLINED BY ARIZONA ON DECEMBER 7, 1990
DISCIPLINARY ACTION: 60-MONTH PROBATION; RESTRICTION PLACED ON LICENSE
OFFENSE: CRIMINAL CONVICTION OR PLEA OF GUILTY, NOLO CONTENDERE, OR NO CONTEST TO A CRIME

NOTES: PLED GUILTY TO 6 COUNTS IN U.S. DISTRICT COURT ON 5/7/90. PRIOR TO 12/1/87 HE JOINED A CONSPIRACY TO PROCURE ALIEN REGISTRATIONS THROUGH SUBMISSION OF FRAUDULENT MEDICAL CERTIFICATIONS TO THE IMMIGRATION SERVICE; OBTAINED FEES FOR PREPARING MEDICAL CERTIFICATIONS FOR ALIENS WITHOUT EXAMS AND WITHOUT DETERMINING LAB TEST RESULTS; AUTHORIZED TWO EMPLOYEES TO SIGN HIS NAME TO MEDICAL EXAM FORMS; FRAUDULENTLY CERTIFIED THAT AT LEAST 4 APPLICANTS MET THE MEDICAL REQUIREMENTS FOR IMMIGRATION STATUS WHEN MEDICAL EXAMS WERE NOT PERFORMED. WHILE ON PROBATION MUST NOT COLLABORATE WITH, SUPERVISE OR HIRE A NURSE PRACTITIONER OR PHYSICIAN'S ASSISTANT. SHALL APPEAR BEFORE THE BOARD AS REQUESTED. ON 12/7/95 PROBATION TERMINATED.

WILLIAMS, KIRK GILBERT MD, LICENSE NUMBER 0023004 OF 5 N 12TH ST STE 201, PHOENIX, AZ, WAS DISCIPLINED BY GEORGIA ON JULY 8, 1991
DISCIPLINARY ACTION: NONRENEWAL OF LICENSE
OFFENSE: DISCIPLINARY ACTION BY ANOTHER STATE OR AGENCY

NOTES: DISCIPLINARY ACTION IN ARIZONA. ADMINISTRATIVE

REVOCATION FOR FAILURE TO RENEW.

WILLIAMS, PAUL C MD, LICENSE NUMBER 0014868, WAS DISCIPLINED BY ARIZONA ON JANUARY 19, 1990
DISCIPLINARY ACTION: 60-MONTH PROBATION; REQUIRED TO ENTER AN IMPAIRED PHYSICIAN PROGRAM OR SUBSTANCE ABUSE TREATMENT
OFFENSE: FAILURE TO COMPLY WITH PREVIOUS BOARD ORDER
NOTES: VIOLATED 5/24/89 ORDER IN THE FOLLOWING WAYS: IN 10/89 A BLOOD SAMPLE TESTED POSITIVE FOR ALCOHOL; ALSO FAILED TO OBTAIN A BOARD-APPROVED TREATING PHYSICIAN AND MAINTAIN A LOG OF ALL MEDICATIONS TAKEN. CONDITIONS OF PROBATION: MUST IMMEDIATELY ENROLL IN THE LEVEL III AFTERCARE PROGRAM OF NAVAL HOSPITAL AND ATTEND 4 12-STEP AA WEEKLY MEETINGS; WEEKLY MEETINGS WITH AFTERCARE PROGRAM MANAGER; MANDATORY URINALYSIS TWICE WEEKLY; MANDATORY USE OF ANTABUSE. MUST CONTINUE TO PARTICIPATE IN A SUBSTANCE ABUSE TREATMENT PROGRAM EVEN WHEN FORMAL REGIMEN ENDS ON 12/11/90. QUARTERLY REPORTS MUST BE SUBMITTED TO BOARD BY PROGRAM OR THERAPIST; WILL ALSO ABIDE BY TERMS OF 5/24/89 ORDER.

WILLIAMS, PAUL C MD, DATE OF BIRTH DECEMBER 4, 1942, LICENSE NUMBER 0017317 OF LAKE OSWEGO, OR, WAS DISCIPLINED BY COLORADO ON JULY 12, 1991
DISCIPLINARY ACTION: 60-MONTH PROBATION; REQUIRED TO ENTER AN IMPAIRED PHYSICIAN PROGRAM OR SUBSTANCE ABUSE TREATMENT
OFFENSE: SUBSTANCE ABUSE
NOTES: HABITUAL INTEMPERANCE, ALCOHOL ABUSE AND ALCOHOL DEPENDENCE. ALCOHOL TREATMENT AND MONITORING AND PRACTICE MONITORING. IN ABEYANCE.

WILLIAMS, PAUL CARROLL MD, LICENSE NUMBER 0017419 OF PORTLAND, OR, WAS DISCIPLINED BY OREGON ON AUGUST 15, 1991
DISCIPLINARY ACTION: 120-MONTH PROBATION
OFFENSE: SUBSTANCE ABUSE
NOTES: ALLEGED PERSONAL SUBSTANCE ABUSE. REVOCATION STAYED. AS OF 2/22/95 NO LONGER LISTED AS ON PROBATION.

WILLIAMS, PAUL CARROLL MD, LICENSE NUMBER 0C34650 OF LAKE OSWEGO, OR, WAS DISCIPLINED BY CALIFORNIA ON JUNE 18, 1992
DISCIPLINARY ACTION: 60-MONTH PROBATION
OFFENSE: DISCIPLINARY ACTION BY ANOTHER STATE OR AGENCY
NOTES: DISCIPLINED BY ARIZONA BOARD RELATED TO ALCOHOL ABUSE. REVOCATION, STAYED. PROBATION WITH TERMS AND CONDITIONS.

WILLIAMS, ROBERT A MD, LICENSE NUMBER 0012287, WAS DISCIPLINED BY ARIZONA ON APRIL 6, 1990
DISCIPLINARY ACTION: REQUIRED TO ENTER AN IMPAIRED PHYSICIAN PROGRAM OR SUBSTANCE ABUSE TREATMENT; MONITORING OF PHYSICIAN PERFORMANCE
OFFENSE: SUBSTANCE ABUSE
NOTES: MUST IMMEDIATELY PARTICIPATE IN THE ARIZONA MEDICAL ASSOCIATION PHYSICIAN'S HEALTH COMMITTEE PROGRAM WITH QUARTERLY REPORTS TO THE BOARD; MUST OBTAIN A BOARD APPROVED TREATING PHYSICIAN; MUST ABSTAIN COMPLETELY FROM ALCOHOL AND ALL OTHER DRUGS; MUST COMPLY WITH REQUESTS FOR RANDOM BIOLOGICAL FLUID TESTS; MUST SUBMIT TO ANY EXAMS OR THERAPY ORDERED BY THE BOARD; MUST PARTICIPATE IN A 12-STEP RECOVERY PROGRAM FOR SUBSTANCE ABUSE AS DETERMINED BY THERAPIST AND ATTEND AT LEAST 3 WEEKLY MEETINGS; MUST APPEAR BEFORE BOARD FOR INTERVIEWS UPON REQUEST; MUST ADVISE THE BOARD OF CHANGE IN OFFICE OR HOME ADDRESSES OR IF AWAY FOR MORE THAN FIVE DAYS; MUST MAINTAIN A LOG OF ALL MEDICATIONS TAKEN. ON 10/16/93 ORDER TERMINATED AFTER 90 DAYS.

WILLIAMS, ROBERT A MD OF JACKSON, OH, WAS DISCIPLINED BY OHIO ON JUNE 11, 1990
DISCIPLINARY ACTION: LICENSE REVOCATION
OFFENSE: CRIMINAL CONVICTION OR PLEA OF GUILTY, NOLO CONTENDERE, OR NO CONTEST TO A CRIME
NOTES: FOUND GUILTY OF FELONY COUNTS (ILLEGAL PROCESSING OF DRUG DOCUMENTS). THE FRANKLIN COUNTY COURT OF COMMON PLEAS COURT DECISION OF 9/17/91 AFFIRMING THE REVOCATION WAS REVERSED AND REMANDED TO THE COMMON PLEAS COURT BY THE TENTH DISTRICT COURT OF APPEALS ON 3/20/92. THE COMMON PLEAS COURT WAS INSTRUCTED TO REMAND THE MATTER TO THE BOARD FOR RECONSIDERATION OF ITS ACTION IN LIGHT OF THE REVERSAL OF HIS CRIMINAL CONVICTIONS. THE CASE WAS REMANDED TO THE MEDICAL BOARD ON 5/27/92. ON 1/23/94 ORDER ON REMAND; PERMANENT REVOCATION, STAYED. PROBATION FOR AT LEAST THREE YEARS. ON 1/12/94 SUSPENSION STAYED BY FRANKLIN COUNTY COURT OF COMMON PLEAS DURING PENDENCY OF APPEAL. ON 2/9/95 FRANKLIN COUNTY COURT OF COMMON PLEAS AFFIRMED THIS SUSPENSION ORDER. ON 3/13/95 THE COURT GRANTED STAY OF SUSPENSION UNTIL 4/3/95. SUSPENSION EFFECTIVE 4/4/95 TO 10/4/95. ON 4/25/95 10TH DISTRICT COURT OF APPEALS DISMISSED HIS APPEAL OF BOARD'S REPORT AND RECOMMENDATION ON REMAND FILED 11/01/93; SUSPENSION EFFECTIVE 4/03/95.

WILLIAMS, ROBERT ARTHUR MD, LICENSE NUMBER 22129 OF JACKSON, OH, WAS DISCIPLINED BY OHIO ON NOVEMBER 16, 1998
DISCIPLINARY ACTION: LICENSE REVOCATION
OFFENSE: FAILURE TO COMPLY WITH PREVIOUS BOARD ORDER
NOTES: VIOLATION OF CONDITIONS OF LIMITATION IMPOSED ON LICENSE BY 12/8/93 BOARD ORDER AND OF MEDICAL BOARD RULES DUE TO HIS FAILURE TO MAINTAIN ADEQUATE PATIENT RECORDS; AND HIS FAILURE TO COMPLY WITH MEDICAL BOARD RULES GOVERNING THE USE OF CONTROLLED SUBSTANCES FOR WEIGHT LOSS. PERMANENT REVOCATION. NOTICE OF APPEAL OF ORDER FILED BY DOCTOR IN FRANKLIN COUNTY COURT OF COMMON PLEAS ON 10/27/98. ON 11/18/98, THE COURT OVERRULED DOCTOR'S MOTION FOR STAY OF ORDER.

WILLIAMS, ROBERT DEAN DR, LICENSE NUMBER 0017756, WAS DISCIPLINED BY ARIZONA ON JULY 15, 1994
DISCIPLINARY ACTION: LICENSE SUSPENSION
OFFENSE: NONCOMPLIANCE WITH A PROFESSIONAL RULE
NOTES: FAILURE TO PAY RENEWAL FEE DURING A PENDING INVESTIGATION.

WILLIAMSON, THOMAS MD, WAS DISCIPLINED BY ARIZONA ON AUGUST 8, 1998
DISCIPLINARY ACTION: PROBATION; 60-MONTH RESTRICTION PLACED ON LICENSE
NOTES: MUST PARTICIPATE IN THE MONITORED AFTERCARE

PROGRAM AND LIMIT HIS WORK SCHEDULE TO AN AVERAGE OF 36 HOURS PER WEEK WITH NO NIGHTCALL.

WILLIAMSON, THOMAS LEE MD, LICENSE NUMBER 21101, WAS DISCIPLINED BY ARIZONA ON JULY 26, 1997
DISCIPLINARY ACTION: LICENSE SUSPENSION
OFFENSE: FAILURE TO COMPLY WITH PREVIOUS BOARD ORDER

NOTES: HE VIOLATED THE TERMS OF THE REHABILITATION AND STIPULATION ORDER OF 1/31/97 BY RELAPSING WITH THE USE OF CHEMICAL SUBSTANCES. MAY NOT PRACTICE MEDICINE IN ARIZONA WHILE HIS LICENSE IS IN INACTIVE STATUS; MUST PAY ALL FEES PRIOR TO HIS LICENSE BEING PLACED ON INACTIVE STATUS; SHALL NOT REQUEST REACTIVATION OF HIS LICENSE UNTIL HE MEETS WITH THE BOARD AND COMPLIES WITH ALL REQUESTS OF THE BOARD WHICH MAY INCLUDE INPATIENT TREATMENT, PSYCHIATRIC AND PSYCHOMETRIC EVALUATION, PHYSICAL EXAMINATION AND TESTING, AND WRITTEN AND/OR ORAL COMPETENCY EXAMINATIONS. LICENSE PLACED ON INACTIVE STATUS.

WILLIAMSON, THOMAS LEE MD, LICENSE NUMBER H7105 OF PHOENIX, AZ, WAS DISCIPLINED BY TEXAS ON MAY 14, 1999
OFFENSE: DISCIPLINARY ACTION BY ANOTHER STATE OR AGENCY

NOTES: ON 1/31/97 HE WAS PLACED ON A NON-DISCIPLINARY REHABILITATION STIPULATION AND ORDER BY THE ARIZONA BOARD BASED UPON HIS HISTORY OF SUBSTANCE ABUSE; IN 6/97 HE RELAPSED; ON 7/26/97 HIS ARIZONA MEDICAL LICENSE WAS PLACED ON INACTIVE STATUS AFTER HE RELAPSED; ARIZONA MEDICAL LICENSE IS CURRENTLY ACTIVE; HE ADMITS THAT HE VIOLATED THE TERMS OF HIS REHABILITATION ORDER; HE STATES THAT AFTER A YEAR OF SOBRIETY HE FEELS HE CAN SAFELY RETURN TO THE PRACTICE OF MEDICINE AND PLANS TO PRACTICE IN PHOENIX; HE STATES THAT HE WILL CONTINUE TO BE MONITORED BY THE ARIZONA BOARD FOR 3-5 YEARS, INCLUDING RANDOM URINE DRUG SCREENS, REGULAR AA MEETINGS, AND THERAPY GROUPS. TEXAS LICENSE LIMITED AS FOLLOWS: SHALL NOT PRACTICE UNTIL HE APPEARS BEFORE THE BOARD TO ORALLY PETITION FOR PERMISSION TO RESUME PRACTICE AND PROVIDES EVIDENCE THAT HE IS PHYSICALLY, MENTALLY AND OTHERWISE COMPETENT TO PRACTICE SAFELY INCLUDING AT A MINIMUM: SHALL COMPLY WITH OR COMPLETE THE ARIZONA BOARD ORDER; SHALL HAVE DOCUMENTED SOBRIETY; SHALL COOPERATE WITH THE BOARD IN VERIFYING COMPLIANCE INCLUDING PROVIDING COPIES OF MEDICAL RELEASES UPON REQUEST; SHALL INFORM THE BOARD OF CHANGE OF ADDRESS WITHIN 10 DAYS; SHALL NOT SEEK MODIFICATION FOR ONE YEAR.

WILSON, JACK HERBERT MD, LICENSE NUMBER 0003904 OF PHOENIX, AZ, WAS DISCIPLINED BY ARIZONA ON JANUARY 21, 1993
DISCIPLINARY ACTION: RESTRICTION PLACED ON LICENSE
OFFENSE: SUBSTANDARD CARE, INCOMPETENCE OR NEGLIGENCE

NOTES: COMPLAINT ALLEGES THAT HE CAUSED EXCESSIVE DAMAGE BY LASER TREATMENT. SHALL NOT PERFORM LASER THERAPY OF THE CERVIX, VAGINA, OR LOWER GENITAL TRACT.

WODKA, RICHARD M MD OF 1850 SOUTH AZUSA SUITE 111, HACIENDA HEIGHTS, CA, WAS DISCIPLINED BY DEA ON AUGUST 1, 1990
DISCIPLINARY ACTION: SURRENDER OF CONTROLLED SUBSTANCE LICENSE
OFFENSE: OVERPRESCRIBING OR MISPRESCRIBING DRUGS

NOTES: AS A RESULT OF ILLEGAL PRESCRIBING AND USE OF HYCOTUSS SYRUP.

WODKA, RICHARD M MD OF TUCSON, AZ, WAS DISCIPLINED BY DEA ON SEPTEMBER 7, 1999
DISCIPLINARY ACTION: REVOCATION OF CONTROLLED SUBSTANCE LICENSE
OFFENSE: DISCIPLINARY ACTION BY ANOTHER STATE OR AGENCY

NOTES: ON 7/17/96 ARIZONA BOARD PLACED HIS LICENSE IN INACTIVE STATUS AND REVOKED HIS PRESCRIBING PRIVILEGES.

WODKA, RICHARD MARK MD, LICENSE NUMBER 0018531, WAS DISCIPLINED BY ARIZONA ON JULY 18, 1996
DISCIPLINARY ACTION: LICENSE SUSPENSION

NOTES: REQUESTS THAT LICENSE BE PLACED IN INACTIVE WITH CAUSE STATUS BECAUSE HE IS UNABLE TO SAFELY ENGAGE IN THE PRACTICE OF MEDICINE AND IS IN TREATMENT AT TIMBERLAWN MENTAL HEALTH SYSTEMS; AGREES NOT TO PRACTICE MEDICINE IN ANY JURISDICTION WHILE LICENSE IS INACTIVE; UNDERSTANDS THAT HE MAY NOT HOLD OR MAINTAIN A CONTROLLED SUBSTANCE CERTIFICATE WITH THE DRUG ENFORCEMENT ADMINISTRATION OR WRITE OR REFILL PRESCRIPTIONS AS LONG AS LICENSE IS CLASSIFIED INACTIVE; SHALL NOT REQUEST REACTIVATION OF LICENSE UNTIL HE MEETS WITH THE BOARD AND COMPLIES WITH ALL BOARD REQUESTS; BOARD WILL NOT REACTIVATE LICENSE UNTIL PRESENTS SATISFACTORY EVIDENCE THAT HE IS MEDICALLY COMPETENT AND MENTALLY AND PHYSICALLY ABLE TO SAFELY PRACTICE MEDICINE. RETROACTIVE TO 5/3/96.

WODKA, RICHARD MARK MD, LICENSE NUMBER A44022 OF MARANA, AZ, WAS DISCIPLINED BY CALIFORNIA ON FEBRUARY 17, 1998
DISCIPLINARY ACTION: LICENSE REVOCATION
OFFENSE: DISCIPLINARY ACTION BY ANOTHER STATE OR AGENCY

NOTES: DISCIPLINED BY ARIZONA DUE TO MENTAL ILLNESS AFFECTING HIS ABILITY TO PRACTICE MEDICINE SAFELY.

WODKA, RICHARD MARK MD, DATE OF BIRTH MARCH 20, 1959 OF 7655 N BLANCO WASH TRAIL, MARANA, AZ, WAS DISCIPLINED BY MEDICARE ON MARCH 18, 1999
DISCIPLINARY ACTION: EXCLUSION FROM THE MEDICARE AND/OR MEDICAID PROGRAM
OFFENSE: DISCIPLINARY ACTION BY ANOTHER STATE OR AGENCY

NOTES: LICENSE REVOKED, SUSPENDED, SURRENDERED OR OTHERWISE LOST FOR REASONS BEARING ON PROFESSIONAL PERFORMANCE, PROFESSIONAL COMPETENCE OR FINANCIAL INTEGRITY.

WOO, FRANCIS J JR MD, LICENSE NUMBER 0010705, WAS DISCIPLINED BY ARIZONA ON NOVEMBER 6, 1990
OFFENSE: PROFESSIONAL MISCONDUCT

NOTES: PERFORMED CHELATION THERAPY ON 50 TO 100 PATIENTS PRIMARILY FOR THE TREATMENT OF ARTERIOSCLEROSIS WITHOUT ADEQUATE INFORMED CONSENT AND WITHOUT FOLLOWING PROPER PROTOCOL REGARDING THIS EXPERIMENTAL TREATMENT. CENSURED FOR UNPROFESSIONAL CONDUCT.

WOO, FRANCIS J JR MD, LICENSE NUMBER 0010705, WAS

DISCIPLINED BY ARIZONA ON OCTOBER 20, 1994
DISCIPLINARY ACTION: PROBATION; RESTRICTION PLACED ON LICENSE
OFFENSE: SUBSTANDARD CARE, INCOMPETENCE OR NEGLIGENCE

NOTES: ALLEGATIONS OF NEGLIGENT CARE RENDERED BY DR. WOO AND HIS PHYSICIANS ASSISTANT FOR A TWO WEEK OLD INFANT FOR WHOM HE DID NOT OBTAIN A BIRTH HISTORY OR ADEQUATELY EXAMINE THE HEART; FOLLOW-UP WAS DONE BY HIS PHYSICIANS ASSISTANT WHO DID NOT INFORM HIM OF THE BABY'S WEIGHT LOSS; BABY DIED OF CARDIAC ARREST. PLACED ON INDEFINITE PROBATION, AND CAN PROVIDE NO MEDICAL CARE TO PATIENTS FIVE YEARS AND UNDER EXCEPT IN THE CASE OF TRUE LIFE AND LIMB EMERGENCY; SHALL TAKE AND PASS THE SPECIAL PURPOSE EXAMINATION IN 12/94 WITH A SCORE OF 75 OR GREATER.

WOO, FRANCIS J JR MD, LICENSE NUMBER 0010705 OF LAKE HAVASU CITY, AZ, WAS DISCIPLINED BY ARIZONA ON JANUARY 17, 1995
DISCIPLINARY ACTION: FINE; RESTRICTION PLACED ON LICENSE
OFFENSE: FAILURE TO COMPLY WITH PREVIOUS BOARD ORDER

NOTES: FAILED TO TAKE THE 12/94 SPECIAL PURPOSE EXAMINATION AS ORDERED IN 10/20/94 BOARD ORDER. $1,000 FINE TO BE PAID WITHIN 90 DAYS. THIS ORDER AMENDED: INDEFINITE PROBATION SHALL PROVIDE NO MEDICAL CARE TO PATIENTS UNDER TWO YEARS OF AGE EXCEPT IN THE CASE OF TRUE LIFE AND LIMB EMERGENCY; SHALL OBTAIN AN ADDITIONAL 20 HOURS PER YEAR OF CONTINUING MEDICAL EDUCATION IN PEDIATRICS; SHALL TAKE AND PASS THE SPECIAL PURPOSE EXAMINATION IN 3/95 WITH A SCORE OF 75 OR GREATER. ON 4/16/96 BOARD RESCINDED THIS ORDER AS HE HAD PASSED THE SPEX EXAM AND COMPLETED THE REQUIRED CONTINUING MEDICAL EDUCATION. ON 1/24/97 PROBATION TERMINATED.

WOODS, CHARLES J MD, DATE OF BIRTH APRIL 17, 1939, LICENSE NUMBER 1028751 OF 4771 ENDEAVOR LANE, CARLSBAD, CA, WAS DISCIPLINED BY MICHIGAN ON JULY 16, 1997
DISCIPLINARY ACTION: 24-MONTH PROBATION
OFFENSE: DISCIPLINARY ACTION BY ANOTHER STATE OR AGENCY

NOTES: FAILURE TO REPORT/COMPLY.

WOODS, CHARLES J MD, DATE OF BIRTH APRIL 17, 1939, LICENSE NUMBER 1028751 OF 4771 ENDEAVOR LANE, CARLSBAD, CA, WAS DISCIPLINED BY MICHIGAN ON MAY 29, 1998
DISCIPLINARY ACTION: EMERGENCY SUSPENSION
OFFENSE: FAILURE TO COMPLY WITH PREVIOUS BOARD ORDER

NOTES: PROBATION VIOLATION.

WOODS, CHARLES J MD, DATE OF BIRTH APRIL 17, 1939, LICENSE NUMBER 1028751 OF 4771 ENDEAVOR LANE, CARLSBAD, CA, WAS DISCIPLINED BY MICHIGAN ON OCTOBER 7, 1998
DISCIPLINARY ACTION: LICENSE REVOCATION
OFFENSE: FAILURE TO COMPLY WITH PREVIOUS BOARD ORDER

NOTES: PROBATION VIOLATION.

WOODS, CHARLES J MD, DATE OF BIRTH APRIL 17, 1939 OF 6822 E BROWNSTONE, TUCSON, AZ, WAS DISCIPLINED BY MEDICARE ON APRIL 20, 1999
DISCIPLINARY ACTION: EXCLUSION FROM THE MEDICARE AND/OR MEDICAID PROGRAM
OFFENSE: DISCIPLINARY ACTION BY ANOTHER STATE OR AGENCY

NOTES: LICENSE REVOKED, SUSPENDED, SURRENDERED OR OTHERWISE LOST FOR REASONS BEARING ON PROFESSIONAL PERFORMANCE, PROFESSIONAL COMPETENCE OR FINANCIAL INTEGRITY.

WRIGHT, WILLIAM C MD, LICENSE NUMBER 0012732 OF P.O. BOX 493, GLOBE, AZ, WAS DISCIPLINED BY ARIZONA ON SEPTEMBER 26, 1996
DISCIPLINARY ACTION: REQUIRED TO TAKE ADDITIONAL MEDICAL EDUCATION

NOTES: SHALL SUCCESSFULLY COMPLETE 12 HOURS CONTINUING MEDICAL EDUCATION ON FETAL MONITORING. ON 5/7/97 ORDER WAS TERMINATED AS HE COMPLETED THE REQUIRED EDUCATION.

WRY, ORLIN V JR MD, LICENSE NUMBER 0005411, WAS DISCIPLINED BY ARIZONA ON JANUARY 3, 1991
DISCIPLINARY ACTION: REQUIRED TO ENTER AN IMPAIRED PHYSICIAN PROGRAM OR SUBSTANCE ABUSE TREATMENT; MONITORING OF PHYSICIAN PERFORMANCE
OFFENSE: SUBSTANCE ABUSE

NOTES: VOLUNTARILY ENTERED AN INPATIENT TREATMENT PROGRAM FOR MISUSE OF CHEMICAL SUBSTANCES. MUST IMMEDIATELY PARTICIPATE IN THE ARIZONA MEDICAL ASSOCIATION'S MONITORED AFTERCARE TREATMENT PROGRAM WHOSE THERAPIST MUST SUBMIT QUARTERLY REPORTS; MUST PARTICIPATE IN 90 12-STEP MEETINGS APPROPRIATE FOR SUBSTANCE ABUSE WITHIN 90 DAYS; MUST THEN PARTICIPATE IN A 12-STEP RECOVERY PROGRAM AND ATTEND A MINIMUM OF 3 WEEKLY MEETINGS; MUST OBTAIN A BOARD APPROVED TREATING PHYSICIAN; MUST ABSTAIN COMPLETELY FROM THE CONSUMPTION OF ALCOHOL OR OTHER DRUGS; MUST COMPLY WITH REQUESTS FOR RANDOM BIOLOGICAL FLUID TESTS; MUST MAINTAIN A LOG OF ALL MEDICATIONS; MUST SUBMIT TO MENTAL, PHYSICAL OR MEDICAL COMPETENCY EXAMS AT THE BOARD'S REQUEST; MUST SUBMIT TO ANY THERAPY ORDERED BY THE BOARD; MUST APPEAR BEFORE BOARD FOR INTERVIEWS UPON REQUEST; MUST ADVISE THE BOARD OF CHANGE OF ADDRESS OR IF HE IS AWAY FOR MORE THAN FIVE DAYS. ON 10/15/93 THIS ORDER WAS TERMINATED.

YEE, DENNIS W MD, LICENSE NUMBER 0013472, WAS DISCIPLINED BY ARIZONA ON OCTOBER 19, 1996
DISCIPLINARY ACTION: 120-MONTH PROBATION; RESTRICTION PLACED ON LICENSE
OFFENSE: SEXUAL ABUSE OF OR SEXUAL MISCONDUCT WITH A PATIENT

NOTES: IN 1995, FONDLED THE BREASTS OF ONE PATIENT ON FOUR OCCASIONS; BETWEEN 1994 AND 1996, FONDLED THE BREASTS OF THREE ADDITIONAL PATIENTS, TWO PATIENTS ON ONE OCCASION EACH AND ONE PATIENT ON FOUR OCCASIONS. PROBATION WITH TERMS: SHALL HAVE A FEMALE CHAPERONE PRESENT FOR ALL PHYSICAL EXAMINATIONS HE PERFORMS ON FEMALE PATIENTS AND HAVE HER SIGN THE PATIENT CHART THAT SHE WAS PRESENT; SHALL PROMPTLY ENTER PSYCHOTHERAPY WITH A BOARD-APPROVED TREATING PSYCHIATRIST WHO SHALL SUBMIT QUARTERLY REPORTS; SHALL REMAIN IN THERAPY UNTIL FURTHER ORDER OF THE BOARD; SHALL SUBMIT TO ANY EXAMINATIONS OR ADDITIONAL THERAPY ORDERED BY THE BOARD; SHALL APPEAR BEFORE BOARD FOR INTERVIEWS UPON REQUEST; SHALL INFORM BOARD OF CHANGE OF ADDRESS.

YELLEN, ROSS MD, LICENSE NUMBER 0010271, WAS DISCIPLINED BY ARIZONA ON DECEMBER 20, 1990
DISCIPLINARY ACTION: MONITORING OF PHYSICIAN PERFORMANCE

OFFENSE: PROFESSIONAL MISCONDUCT

NOTES: PRESCRIBED A CONTROLLED SUBSTANCE FOR HIMSELF, DALMANE. MUST CONTINUE RECEIVING TREATMENT FOR SLEEP DISORDER THERAPY WITH QUARTERLY REPORTS SUBMITTED TO THE BOARD; SHALL OBTAIN TREATMENT FROM BOARD APPROVED THERAPIST FOR DIAGNOSIS AND TREATMENT OF ANY AFFECTIVE DISORDER WITH QUARTERLY REPORTS SUBMITTED TO BOARD; SHALL NOT TAKE ANY DRUGS UNLESS PRESCRIBED; SHALL APPEAR BEFORE BOARD AND SUBMIT TO RANDOM BODILY FLUID TESTS UPON REQUEST.

YELLEN, ROSS MD, LICENSE NUMBER 0010271, WAS DISCIPLINED BY ARIZONA ON JULY 13, 1991
DISCIPLINARY ACTION: 60-MONTH PROBATION; REQUIRED TO TAKE ADDITIONAL MEDICAL EDUCATION
OFFENSE: PROFESSIONAL MISCONDUCT

NOTES: UNPROFESSIONAL CONDUCT AND FAILURE TO MAINTAIN ADEQUATE LEVEL OF MEDICAL COMPETENCY. FOR PERFORMING LARYNGOSCOPIES AND COLONOSCOPIES THAT WERE INDICATED, ASSESSING EXTRA FEES AND FAILING TO TRANSFER PATIENT RECORDS, ARIZONA ISSUED HIM A DECREE OF CENSURE ON 9/13/83, A LETTER OF CONCERN ON 12/1/83, ENTERED INTO A STIPULATION AND ORDER ON 6/8/84, AND A LETTER OF CONCERN ON 1/25/89. HOSPITAL PRIVILEGES SUMMARILY SUSPENDED ON 9/14/90 AT PHOENIX BAPTIST HOSPITAL AND MEDICAL CENTER, AND ON 10/17/90 AT ARROWHEAD COMMUNITY HOSPITAL AND MEDICAL CENTER. ALSO FAILED THE SPECIAL EDUCATION PURPOSE EXAM (SPEX). CONDITIONS OF PROBATION ARE AS FOLLOWS: SHALL NOT ENGAGE IN THE PRACTICE OF MEDICINE FROM 04/01/91 TO 07/12/91; LICENSE SHALL BE PLACED ON INACTIVE STATUS BEGINNING 07/13/91. PRIOR TO REQUESTING REACTIVATION, OF HIS MEDICAL LICENSE, HE MUST SUCCESSFULLY COMPLETE AN APPROVED POSTGRADUATE MEDICAL TRAINING PROGRAM OF NOT LESS THAN TWELVE MONTHS, AND SUCH PROGRAM MUST HAVE BEEN APPROVED BY THE ACCREDITATION COUNCIL FOR GRADUATE MEDICAL EDUCATION; PASS THE SPEX EXAM; MUST SUBMIT TO PHYSICAL, PSYCHIATRIC AND PSYCHOMETRIC EVALUATIONS. IF REACTIVATED, THE BOARD MAY RESTRICT HIS LICENSE HOWEVER IT FEELS NECESSARY. EFFECTIVE 10/15/93 THE BOARD APPROVED THE COLORADO PHYSICIANS EDUCATION PROGRAM FOR DR. YELLEN'S EVALUATION AND PARTICIPATION. ON 1/20/95 HIS REQUEST TO ACCEPT AN ALTERNATE EDUCATION PLAN IN LIEU OF A RESIDENCY WAS DENIED.

YELLEN, ROSS MD, DATE OF BIRTH MAY 2, 1941, LICENSE NUMBER 0020417 OF 7613 N 40TH DRIVE, PHOENIX, AZ, WAS DISCIPLINED BY IOWA ON JULY 1, 1993
DISCIPLINARY ACTION: LICENSE SUSPENSION
OFFENSE: DISCIPLINARY ACTION BY ANOTHER STATE OR AGENCY

NOTES: BASED ON SETTLEMENT TO ALLEGATIONS OF A DISCIPLINARY ACTION TAKEN IN ANOTHER STATE. INDEFINITE SUSPENSION.

ZAKALA, MARINA LISA MD, LICENSE NUMBER 18863, WAS DISCIPLINED BY ARIZONA ON MARCH 14, 1997
DISCIPLINARY ACTION: REQUIRED TO TAKE ADDITIONAL MEDICAL EDUCATION

NOTES: SHE AGREES NOT TO PRACTICE MEDICINE IN ARIZONA UNTIL SHE MEETS WITH THE BOARD AND RECEIVES ITS AFFIRMATIVE APPROVAL; SHALL PROVIDE 60 DAYS WRITTEN NOTIFICATION TO EACH OF HER CURRENT PATIENTS REGARDING HER DISCONTINUATION OF MEDICAL PRACTICE AND SHALL ALLOW FOR THE ORDERLY TRANSFER OF ALL MEDICAL RECORDS IN HER POSSESSION; PRIOR TO REQUESTING APPROVAL BY THE BOARD TO RESUME PRACTICE, SHE WILL SUBMIT TO 10 HOURS OF EDUCATION IN THE AREA OF BOUNDARY ISSUES AND WILL OBTAIN 30 HOURS OF CONTINUING MEDICAL EDUCATION IN INADEQUATE RECORDS AND DOCUMENTATION; IF SHE REMAINS OUT OF CLINICAL PRACTICE FOR MORE THAN 12 MONTHS WITHIN 60 TO 90 DAYS PRIOR TO HER REQUESTING TO RESUME THE PRACTICE OF MEDICINE SHALL TAKE AND PASS THE SPEX EXAMINATION AND SUBMIT TO OTHER BOARD EVALUATIONS AS NECESSARY.

ZAKRZEWSKI, TADEUSZ MD, LICENSE NUMBER 0A25638 OF PHOENIX, AZ, WAS DISCIPLINED BY CALIFORNIA ON NOVEMBER 18, 1993
DISCIPLINARY ACTION: LICENSE REVOCATION
OFFENSE: DISCIPLINARY ACTION BY ANOTHER STATE OR AGENCY

NOTES: DISCIPLINED BY ARIZONA FOR EXCESSIVE DIAGNOSTIC PROCEDURES WITH NO SCIENTIFIC OR MEDICAL JUSTIFICATION; FOR CHARGING EXCESSIVE FEES AND FOR FRAUD. DEFAULT DECISION.

ZAKRZEWSKI, TADEUSZ MD, LICENSE NUMBER 0007433, WAS DISCIPLINED BY ARIZONA ON AUGUST 21, 1995
DISCIPLINARY ACTION: LICENSE REVOCATION
OFFENSE: FAILURE TO COMPLY WITH PREVIOUS BOARD ORDER

NOTES: IN 11/89, LICENSE SUSPENDED FOR SIX MONTHS AND CONCURRENTLY PLACED ON PROBATION FOR FIVE YEARS AND WAS ORDERED TO PAY A FINE OF $5,000 TO THE BOARD AND RESTITUTION TO A PATIENT OF $4,463. HE HAS NOT PAID THE FINE NOR MADE RESTITUTION. IN RESPONSE TO PATIENT COMPLAINTS IN 7/94 DURING HIS PROBATION, BOARD ORDERED HIM TO TAKE AND PASS THE 9/94 SPECIAL PURPOSE EXAMINATION AND AT HIS REQUEST WAS GIVEN AN EXTENSION TO TAKE THE 12/94 EXAMINATION. HE FAILED TO TAKE THE EXAMINATION, ALLEGEDLY ON ACCOUNT OF ILLNESS. DUE TO A COMPLAINT ABOUT HIS PRACTICES AT A CLINIC IN 8/93, THE BOARD SUBPOENAED ALL INFORMATION RELATING TO ALL HIS PATIENTS AT THE CLINIC; BOARD WAS PROVIDED 25 REPRESENTATIVE RECORDS FROM 1992 AND 1993 TO FURTHER ANALYZE; THEY REVEALED SUBSTANTIAL OMISSIONS AND INACCURACIES: GROSS NEGLIGENCE REGARDING RECORD KEEPING AND BILLING PRACTICES IN THAT FOR 19 PATIENTS, HE CHARGED FOR COMPREHENSIVE HISTORY AND EXAMINATION AS WELL AS MEDICAL DECISIONS OF HIGH COMPLEXITY WHICH WERE NOT DOCUMENTED; CHARGED ONE PATIENT FOR VISIT WHICH WAS NOT DOCUMENTED. FAILED TO MAINTAIN ADEQUATE RECORDS ON PATIENTS IN THAT RECORDS WERE ILLEGIBLE; FAILED TO RECORD LAB RESULTS; FAILED TO RECORD TREATMENT AND SCHEDULED PROCEDURES; MEDICATIONS WERE NOT DOCUMENTED; FAILED TO DOCUMENT SYMPTOMS AND DESCRIPTIONS OF PATIENTS' CONDITIONS; ENGAGED IN CONDUCT OR PRACTICE WHICH IS OR MIGHT BE HARMFUL OR DANGEROUS TO THE HEALTH OF PATIENTS IN THAT HE FAILED TO PERFORM ADEQUATE PHYSICAL EXAMINATIONS; FAILED TO TAKE HISTORY; FAILED TO ORDER X-RAYS AND LABORATORY TESTS WHEN APPROPRIATE; FAILED TO PERFORM A NECESSARY NEUROLOGICAL EXAMINATION; PRESCRIBED MEDICATIONS WITHOUT PHYSICAL EXAMINATION; GAVE PATIENTS MOTRIN, WHICH COULD HAVE AGGRAVATED EXISTING

GASTROINTESTINAL PROBLEMS; FAILED TO PROVIDE FOLLOW-UP CARE AND DIAGNOSED CONDITIONS WITHOUT SUPPORT FOR DIAGNOSIS THROUGH HISTORY, RECORDS, OR FINDINGS. FAILED TO FURNISH INFORMATION IN A TIMELY MANNER TO THE BOARD. ON 10/20/95 HIS MOTION FOR REHEARING WAS DENIED.

ZALES, MICHAEL R MD, DATE OF BIRTH APRIL 26, 1937, LICENSE NUMBER 0014235 OF 6925 N CHAPARRAL PLACE, TUCSON, AZ, WAS DISCIPLINED BY CONNECTICUT ON AUGUST 21, 1990
DISCIPLINARY ACTION: 36-MONTH LICENSE SUSPENSION
OFFENSE: PROFESSIONAL MISCONDUCT

NOTES: SEXUAL OFFENSE. SUSPENSION RETROACTIVE TO 10-28-89; UNDERGO PSYCHOTHERAPY UNTIL 10/28/93, MINIMUM OF ONE VISIT A MONTH WITH MONTHLY REPORTS.

ZALES, MICHAEL R MD, DATE OF BIRTH APRIL 26, 1937, LICENSE NUMBER 0013842, WAS DISCIPLINED BY ARIZONA ON JANUARY 25, 1991
DISCIPLINARY ACTION: 60-MONTH PROBATION; RESTRICTION PLACED ON LICENSE
OFFENSE: DISCIPLINARY ACTION BY ANOTHER STATE OR AGENCY

NOTES: ON 8/20/90 CONNECTICUT LICENSE WAS SUSPENDED FOR 3 YEARS RETROACTIVE TO 10/28/89 AND HE WAS REQUIRED TO UNDERGO PSYCHOTHERAPY UNTIL 10/28/93 FOR PROFESSIONAL MISCONDUCT WITH A PATIENT. CONDITIONS OF PROBATION: MUST UNDERGO PHYSICAL, PSYCHOLOGICAL AND PSYCHIATRIC EXAMS BY PHYSICIAN DESIGNATED BY BOARD WHO WILL DETERMINE WHETHER OR NOT HE CAN SAFELY PRACTICE AND SUBMIT WRITTEN REPORTS TO THE BOARD; FROM 2/1/91 ONWARDS AND DURING THE PERIOD OF THESE EXAMINATIONS MAY NOT PROVIDE MEDICAL OR PSYCHIATRIC CARE OR THERAPY TO ANY PATIENT; MUST OBTAIN A TREATING PSYCHOTHERAPIST WHO MUST SUBMIT QUARTERLY REPORTS TO THE BOARD; MUST APPEAR BEFORE THE BOARD FOR INTERVIEWS UPON REQUEST; MUST INFORM THE BOARD OF A CHANGE IN OFFICE OR HOME ADDRESS.

ZALES, MICHAEL R MD, DATE OF BIRTH APRIL 26, 1937, LICENSE NUMBER 0013842, WAS DISCIPLINED BY ARIZONA ON OCTOBER 9, 1991
DISCIPLINARY ACTION: 60-MONTH PROBATION; FINE
OFFENSE: SUBSTANCE ABUSE

NOTES: UNPROFESSIONAL CONDUCT; HABITUAL INTEMPERANCE IN THE USE OF ALCOHOL; ABUSE WAS DIAGNOSED BY BOARD EVALUATORS; SOUGHT TREATMENT IN 3/91 AND 4/91; FAILING TO FURNISH INFORMATION IN A TIMELY MANNER TO THE BOARD IN THAT HE LIED CONCERNING HIS ALCOHOL ABUSE. PROBATION WITH CONDITIONS: SHALL LIMIT HIS PRACTICE TO NO MORE THAN 40 HOURS PER WEEK; SHALL OBTAIN A PSYCHIATRIST APPROVED BY THE BOARD TO REVIEW HIS CASES AT RANDOM FOUR TIMES A YEAR AND REPORT TO THE BOARD ON THE APPROPRIATENESS OF THE TREATMENT AND MAINTENANCE OF PROFESSIONAL BOUNDARIES; MUST IMMEDIATELY PARTICIPATE IN A BOARD-APPROVED MONITORED AFTERCARE TREATMENT PROGRAM WHOSE THERAPIST MUST SUBMIT QUARTERLY REPORTS; MUST PARTICIPATE IN 90 12-STEP MEETINGS FOR SUBSTANCE ABUSE WITHIN 90 DAYS; MUST THEN PARTICIPATE IN A 12-STEP RECOVERY PROGRAM AS DETERMINED BY HIS TREATING THERAPIST AND ATTEND AT LEAST THREE WEEKLY MEETINGS; SHALL OBTAIN A BOARD-APPROVED TREATING PHYSICIAN; SHALL ABSTAIN COMPLETELY FROM THE CONSUMPTION OF ALCOHOLIC BEVERAGES AND DRUGS EXCEPT WHEN PRESCRIBED BY HIS TREATING PHYSICIAN; MUST SUBMIT TO WITNESSED RANDOM BIOLOGICAL FLUID COLLECTION; SHALL KEEP A LOG OF ANY AND ALL MEDICATIONS PRESCRIBED FOR HIM; SHALL SUBMIT TO ANY EXAMINATIONS OR THERAPY ORDERED BY THE BOARD; SHALL APPEAR BEFORE THE BOARD FOR INTERVIEWS UPON REQUEST; SHALL INFORM BOARD OF CHANGE OF ADDRESS OR IF AWAY FOR MORE THAN FIVE DAYS; SHALL PAY ADMINISTRATIVE PENALTY OF $2,000 WITHIN THREE MONTHS. THIS ORDER SUPERSEDES ALL PREVIOUS ORDERS. ON 10/23/92 THE BOARD AMENDED THIS ORDER DROPPING THE REQUIREMENT THAT HE OBTAIN A BOARD-APPROVED PSYCHIATRIST TO REVIEW HIS CASES AT RANDOM AND REPORT TO BOARD QUARTERLY ON APPROPRIATENESS OF TREATMENT AND MAINTENANCE OF APPROPRIATE PROFESSIONAL BOUNDARIES. ALL OTHER TERMS REMAIN IN EFFECT. AS OF 10/16/93 THE PROBATION PORTION OF THIS ORDER WAS TERMINATED.

ZALES, MICHAEL R MD, DATE OF BIRTH APRIL 26, 1937, LICENSE NUMBER 0427581 OF TUCSON, AZ, WAS DISCIPLINED BY VERMONT ON AUGUST 5, 1992
DISCIPLINARY ACTION: 36-MONTH LICENSE SUSPENSION; 47-MONTH PROBATION
OFFENSE: DISCIPLINARY ACTION BY ANOTHER STATE OR AGENCY

NOTES: ON AUGUST 20, 1990, CONNECTICUT LICENSE SUSPENDED FOR THREE YEARS RETROACTIVE TO OCTOBER 28, 1989, FOR INAPPROPRIATE SOCIAL AND SEXUAL RELATIONSHIPS WITH PATIENTS AND FOR BREACH OF PATIENT CONFIDENTIALITY. ON OCTOBER 28, 1991, ARIZONA LICENSE WAS PLACED ON PROBATION FOR FIVE YEARS EFFECTIVE OCTOBER 8, 1991, FOR ALCOHOL ABUSE. VERMONT SUSPENSION RETROACTIVE TO START OF SUSPENSION BY AMERICAN PSYCHIATRIC ASSOCIATION ON OCTOBER 28, 1989. PROBATION UNTIL OCTOBER 9, 1996, FOLLOWS SUSPENSION. MONTHLY THERAPY WITH A BOARD-APPROVED THERAPIST UNTIL OCTOBER 28, 1993 WITH MONTHLY REPORTS TO THE BOARD. LIMIT PRACTICE TO NO MORE THAN 40 HOURS/WEEK. REVIEW OF CASES QUARTERLY. MONITORED AFTERCARE TREATMENT PROGRAM ADMINISTERED BY CONTRACT WITH ARIZONA BOARD WITH QUARTERLY REPORTS. WITHIN 30 DAYS PROOF OF NINETY 12-STEP MEETINGS FOR SUBSTANCE ABUSE AND 12-STEP RECOVERY PROGRAM. ABSTAIN FROM ALCOHOL. OBTAIN ONE BOARD APPROVED TREATING PHYSICIAN; NO MEDICATIONS UNLESS PRESCRIBED BY SAID PHYSICIAN; LOG KEPT OF ALL MEDICATIONS TAKEN. WITNESSED RANDOM BIOLOGICAL FLUID COLLECTION; SHALL SUBMIT TO ANY COMPETENCY EXAMS OR THERAPY ORDERED BY BOARD; SHALL APPEAR BEFORE BOARD UPON REQUEST; SHALL INFORM THE BOARD IF HE MOVES OR WILL BE AWAY FOR MORE THAN FIVE DAYS. ON 10/28/92 SUSPENSION TERMINATED. ON 8/6/93 DECISION EFFECTIVE MODIFYING ORDER AND STATING THAT HE SHALL CONTINUE TO BE RESPONSIBLE FOR THE PERIODIC REPORTS REQUIRED BY THIS ORDER AND THIS SHALL REMAIN IN EFFECT UNTIL AT LEAST 1/1/94. ON 7/10/95 PROBATION TERMINATED BASED ON THE FACT THAT ARIZONA PROBATION WAS TERMINATED ON 1/18/95 AND CONDITIONS WERE SATISFIED IN CONNECTICUT.

ZALES, MICHAEL R MD, LICENSE NUMBER 0095317 OF 6925 NORTH CHAPARRAL PLACE, TUCSON, AZ, WAS DISCIPLINED BY NEW

YORK ON JULY 19, 1994
DISCIPLINARY ACTION: SURRENDER OF LICENSE
OFFENSE: DISCIPLINARY ACTION BY ANOTHER STATE OR AGENCY

NOTES: COULD NOT SUCCESSFULLY DEFEND AGAINST CHARGES THAT HE WAS FOUND GUILTY OF PROFESSIONAL MISCONDUCT AND DISCIPLINED BY THE CONNECTICUT BOARD.

ZALES, MICHAEL R MD, WAS DISCIPLINED BY ARIZONA ON MARCH 26, 1999
DISCIPLINARY ACTION: LICENSE SUSPENSION

NOTES: ORDER GRANTING INACTIVE STATUS WITH CAUSE.

ZALES, MICHAEL R MD, LICENSE NUMBER 0007581 OF TUCSON, AZ, WAS DISCIPLINED BY VERMONT ON MAY 6, 1999
DISCIPLINARY ACTION: SURRENDER OF LICENSE

NOTES: NO DISCIPLINARY CHARGES PENDING. SURRENDER SHALL BE A PERMANENT AND IRREVOCABLE ACT, AND HE SHALL NOT SEEK MEDICAL LICENSURE IN VERMONT AT ANY TIME IN THE FUTURE. VOLUNTARY SURRENDER.

ZALES, MICHAEL ROBERT MD, WAS DISCIPLINED BY NEW HAMPSHIRE ON JULY 17, 1991

NOTES: ALLOWED HIS LICENSE TO LAPSE DURING PENDING INVESTIGATION.

ZAMUDIO-MILLAN, ROBERTO MD, LICENSE NUMBER 0014156 OF TUCSON, AZ, WAS DISCIPLINED BY ARIZONA ON JANUARY 27, 1994
DISCIPLINARY ACTION: MONITORING OF PHYSICIAN PERFORMANCE
OFFENSE: NONCOMPLIANCE WITH A PROFESSIONAL RULE

NOTES: REGARDING CARE AND TREATMENT OF ONE PATIENT AND ALLEGATIONS THAT HE REFUSED TO BILL MEDICARE; CARE AND TREATMENT OF THREE PATIENTS AND ALLEGATIONS THAT HE REFUSED TO FORWARD THEIR MEDICAL RECORDS TO THEIR ATTORNEY; LICENSED UNDER HYPHENATED NAME BUT USES JUST ZAMUDIO. SHALL WITHIN THE NEXT 30 DAYS EMPLOY THE SERVICES OF A BOARD-APPROVED PRACTICE MANAGEMENT CONSULTANT FOR PURPOSES OF EVALUATION OF HIS MEDICAL PRACTICE IN ALL ASPECTS; SHALL COMPLY FULLY WITH THE RECOMMENDATIONS OF THE PRACTICE MANAGEMENT CONSULTANT; SHALL BEAR ALL EXPENSES RELATED TO THE EMPLOYMENT OF THE PRACTICE MANAGEMENT CONSULTANT; SHALL BE RE-EVALUATED BY THE PRACTICE MANAGEMENT CONSULTANT AFTER THE PASSAGE OF ONE YEAR; SHALL ENSURE THAT ALL REPORTS AND RECOMMENDATIONS OF THE PRACTICE MANAGEMENT CONSULTANT ARE MADE AVAILABLE TO THE BOARD; WILL USE THE HYPHENATED VERSION OF HIS NAME. ON 7/21/95 ORDER TERMINATED.

ZEBRANEK, JAMES D JR DO, LICENSE NUMBER 0005033 OF ELM SPRINGS, AZ, WAS DISCIPLINED BY FLORIDA ON APRIL 1, 1992
DISCIPLINARY ACTION: LICENSE REVOCATION
OFFENSE: PRACTICING WITHOUT A VALID CONTROLLED SUBSTANCE LICENSE

NOTES: IN 7/90 WHILE WORKING AT A UNIVERSITY HEALTH CLINIC WROTE PRESCRIPTIONS AND SIGNED THE NAME OF THE MEDICAL DIRECTOR ON ONE OCCASION AND USED HIS EXPIRED DEA REGISTRATION ON TWO OTHERS; THIS CONSTITUTED PRACTICING WITHOUT A LICENSE WHILE LICENSE WAS STILL UNDER SUSPENSION.

ZIMMERMAN, MARC H MD, WAS DISCIPLINED BY ARIZONA ON OCTOBER 20, 1995
DISCIPLINARY ACTION: REQUIRED TO TAKE ADDITIONAL MEDICAL EDUCATION
OFFENSE: SUBSTANDARD CARE, INCOMPETENCE OR NEGLIGENCE

NOTES: INAPPROPRIATE MANAGEMENT OF A PELVIC FRACTURE. WITHIN ONE YEAR SHALL OBTAIN 30 HOURS OF CONTINUING MEDICAL EDUCATION IN PELVIC/ACETABULAR FRACTURES. ON 3/13/97 ORDER AMENDED EXTENDING THE TIME TO COMPLETE THE TERMS OF HIS STIPULATION TO 7/1/97. ON 5/9/97 ORDER TERMINATED.

ZMYSLINSKI, RONALD MD, LICENSE NUMBER 0012843, WAS DISCIPLINED BY ARIZONA ON APRIL 4, 1995
DISCIPLINARY ACTION: RESTRICTION PLACED ON LICENSE
OFFENSE: LOSS OR RESTRICTION OF HOSPITAL PRIVILEGES

NOTES: INTERVIEWED BY BOARD MEMBERS RELATIVE TO INFORMATION RECEIVED THAT HIS ABLATION PRIVILEGES, EXCEPT FOR AV NODE ABLATION, HAVE BEEN REVOKED BY A HOSPITAL AND HIS CARE AND TREATMENT OF ONE PATIENT. SHALL NOT PERFORM RADIO FREQUENCY ABLATION PROCEDURES OF THE HEART.

ZONIS, JULIO MD OF URUGUAY, WAS DISCIPLINED BY ARIZONA ON JANUARY 19, 1993
DISCIPLINARY ACTION: MONITORING OF PHYSICIAN PERFORMANCE

NOTES: MAY RESUME THE PRACTICE OF MEDICINE UPON THE FOLLOWING CONDITIONS: FOR A SIX MONTH PERIOD SHALL COMPLY IMMEDIATELY WITH REQUESTS FROM BOARD STAFF TO SUBMIT TO WITNESSED RANDOM BIOLOGICAL FLUID COLLECTION, AND AUTHORIZE ANY PERSON OR ORGANIZATION CONDUCTING TESTS TO PROVIDE TESTING RESULTS TO THE BOARD; WILL OBTAIN A SOLE TREATING PHYSICIAN AND SHALL TAKE NO DRUGS OR MEDICATIONS WHATEVER (EXCEPT FOR PLAIN ASPIRIN AND/OR ACETAMINOPHEN) UNLESS SUCH DRUG OR MEDICATION WAS PRESCRIBED FOR HIM BY THE SOLE TREATING PHYSICIAN; SHALL ABSTAIN COMPLETELY FROM THE CONSUMPTION OF ALCOHOLIC BEVERAGES; SHALL OBTAIN A THERAPIST APPROVED BY THE BOARD (PRIOR TO PRACTICING MEDICINE IN ARIZONA) AND SHALL ENGAGE IN THERAPY ON A FREQUENCY TO BE DETERMINED BY THE THERAPIST; THERAPIST SHALL SUPPLY MONTHLY REPORTS TO THE BOARD. ORDER TERMINATED ON 10/17/96.

ZUERLEIN, KEVIN MD, LICENSE NUMBER 0019620 OF GLENDALE, AZ, WAS DISCIPLINED BY ARIZONA ON JANUARY 19, 1995
OFFENSE: SUBSTANCE ABUSE

NOTES: FAILED TO APPEAR BEFORE THE BOARD FOR AN INFORMAL INTERVIEW. SHALL, WITHIN 15 DAYS, SUBMIT HIMSELF TO AND COMPLETE AN INPATIENT EVALUATION FOR CHEMICAL DEPENDENCY AT A BOARD-DESIGNATED INPATIENT FACILITY.

ZUERLEIN, KEVIN MD, LICENSE NUMBER 0019620, WAS DISCIPLINED BY ARIZONA ON JANUARY 19, 1996
DISCIPLINARY ACTION: LICENSE REVOCATION
OFFENSE: CRIMINAL CONVICTION OR PLEA OF GUILTY, NOLO CONTENDERE, OR NO CONTEST TO A CRIME

NOTES: INVITED BY THE BOARD TO MEET ON 10/13/94 REGARDING ALLEGATIONS OF SUBSTANCE ABUSE; DID NOT ATTEND MEETING AND INVESTIGATIONAL INTERVIEW WAS SET FOR 10/25/94; BOARD LEARNED THAT ON 10/21/94, WHEN HE WAS ALREADY ON PROBATION FOR DOMESTIC VIOLENCE, HE WAS

ARRESTED FOR UNLAWFUL IMPRISONMENT AND ASSAULT FOR ACTIONS TAKEN AGAINST HIS GIRLFRIEND; AT 10/25 INTERVIEW, HE DENIED BEING IMPAIRED IN HIS FUNCTIONING AS A PHYSICIAN BUT ADMITTED THAT HE WAS USING MARIJUANA AND HAD USED AMPHETAMINES IN THE PAST, WITH THE MOST RECENT USE OCCURRING THE WEEK BEFORE THE INTERVIEW; INDICATED A DESIRE TO ENTER INTO ANY STIPULATION WITH THE BOARD THAT WAS NECESSARY; BOARD RECOMMENDED THAT HE BE EVALUATED DURING A FOUR-DAY INPATIENT EVALUATION BEGINNING ON 10/28/94; ON 10/25, SUBMITTED A URINE SAMPLE WHICH WAS POSITIVE FOR CANNABINOIDS; AS OF 10/31, HAD NOT APPEARED FOR EVALUATION; IN 1/95, FAILED TO APPEAR FOR AN INTERVIEW WITH THE BOARD AND DID NOT COMPLY WITH A SECOND ORDER BY THE BOARD TO COMPLETE INPATIENT EVALUATION FOR CHEMICAL DEPENDENCY; NO EVIDENCE THAT SINCE 10/94 HE HAS BEEN EVALUATED OR UNDERGONE TREATMENT FOR CHEMICAL DEPENDENCY; PERMANENT REVOCATION; FINAL DECISION OF THE BOARD WITH NO OPPORTUNITY FOR REHEARING OR REVIEW.

Physicians Placed on Rehabilitation Contracts

The physicians listed below voluntarily entered into a contract with the Arizona Board to monitor substance abuse treatment. The Board does not view these actions as "disciplinary." These listings may represent the sole action these physicians have with a board or there may be sanctions imposed by Arizona, another state medical board, the Medicare/Medicaid programs, the FDA or the DEA that are included in the main listings.

ADICKMAN, MICHAEL D MD, LICENSE NUMBER 0010376, HAD ACTION TAKEN BY ARIZONA ON AUGUST 2, 1992

NOTES: MUST IMMEDIATELY PARTICIPATE IN A BOARD-APPROVED MONITORED AFTERCARE TREATMENT PROGRAM WHOSE THERAPIST MUST SUBMIT QUARTERLY REPORTS; MUST PARTICIPATE IN 90 12-STEP MEETINGS FOR SUBSTANCE ABUSE WITHIN 90 DAYS; MUST THEN PARTICIPATE IN A 12-STEP RECOVERY PROGRAM AS DETERMINED BY HIS TREATING THERAPIST AND ATTEND AT LEAST THREE WEEKLY MEETINGS; SHALL OBTAIN A BOARD-APPROVED TREATING PHYSICIAN; SHALL ABSTAIN COMPLETELY FROM THE CONSUMPTION OF ALCOHOLIC BEVERAGES AND DRUGS EXCEPT WHEN PRESCRIBED BY HIS TREATING PHYSICIAN; MUST SUBMIT TO WITNESSED RANDOM BIOLOGICAL FLUID COLLECTION; KEEP A LOG OF ANY AND ALL MEDICATIONS PRESCRIBED FOR HIM; SHALL SUBMIT TO ANY EXAMINATIONS OR THERAPY ORDERED BY BOARD; SHALL APPEAR BEFORE BOARD FOR INTERVIEWS UPON REQUEST; SHALL INFORM BOARD OF CHANGE OF ADDRESS OR IF AWAY FOR MORE THAN 5 DAYS. ARIZONA, IN COMPLIANCE WITH THE AMERICANS WITH DISABILITIES ACT, PROCLAIMS THIS IS NOT A DISCIPLINARY ACTION BUT MERELY A MONITORING PROCEDURE WHICH HE VOLUNTARILY ENTERED INTO. ON 10/19/96 ORDER TERMINATED EFFECTIVE IN 90 DAYS.

AREBALO, RONALD E MD, HAD ACTION TAKEN BY ARIZONA ON APRIL 8, 1995

NOTES: INTERVIEWED BY BOARD RELATIVE TO HIS TREATMENT AND PARTICIPATION IN BOARD'S MONITORED AFTERCARE PROGRAM. MUST IMMEDIATELY PARTICIPATE IN A BOARD-APPROVED MONITORED AFTERCARE TREATMENT PROGRAM WHOSE THERAPIST MUST SUBMIT QUARTERLY REPORTS; MUST PARTICIPATE IN 90 12-STEP MEETINGS FOR SUBSTANCE ABUSE WITHIN 90 DAYS; MUST THEN PARTICIPATE IN A 12-STEP RECOVERY PROGRAM AS DETERMINED BY HIS TREATING THERAPIST AND ATTEND AT LEAST THREE WEEKLY MEETINGS; SHALL OBTAIN A BOARD-APPROVED TREATING PHYSICIAN; SHALL ABSTAIN COMPLETELY FROM THE CONSUMPTION OF ALCOHOLIC BEVERAGES AND DRUGS EXCEPT WHEN PRESCRIBED BY HIS TREATING PHYSICIAN; MUST SUBMIT TO WITNESSED RANDOM BIOLOGICAL FLUID COLLECTION; MUST KEEP A LOG OF ANY AND ALL MEDICATIONS PRESCRIBED FOR HIM; SHALL SUBMIT TO ANY EXAMINATIONS OR THERAPY ORDERED BY THE BOARD; SHALL APPEAR BEFORE THE BOARD FOR INTERVIEWS UPON REQUEST; SHALL INFORM BOARD OF CHANGE OF ADDRESS OR IF AWAY FOR MORE THAN FIVE DAYS. ARIZONA, IN COMPLIANCE WITH THE AMERICANS WITH DISABILITIES ACT, PROCLAIMS THAT THIS IS NOT A DISCIPLINARY ACTION BUT MERELY A MONITORING PROCEDURE WHICH HE ENTERED INTO VOLUNTARILY.

ARTHUR, FORREST C MD, LICENSE NUMBER 21812, HAD ACTION TAKEN BY ARIZONA ON JANUARY 23, 1997

NOTES: MUST IMMEDIATELY PARTICIPATE IN A BOARD-APPROVED MONITORED AFTERCARE TREATMENT PROGRAM WHOSE THERAPIST MUST SUBMIT QUARTERLY REPORTS; MUST PARTICIPATE IN 90 12-STEP MEETINGS FOR SUBSTANCE ABUSE WITHIN 90 DAYS; MUST THEN PARTICIPATE IN A 12-STEP RECOVERY PROGRAM AS DETERMINED BY HIS/HER TREATING THERAPIST AND ATTEND AT LEAST THREE WEEKLY MEETINGS; SHALL OBTAIN A BOARD-APPROVED TREATING PHYSICIAN; SHALL ABSTAIN COMPLETELY FROM THE CONSUMPTION OF ALCOHOLIC BEVERAGES AND DRUGS EXCEPT WHEN PRESCRIBED BY HIS/HER TREATING PHYSICIAN; SHALL NOT CONSUME FOOD OR SUBSTANCES CONTAINING POPPYSEEDS; MUST SUBMIT TO WITNESSED RANDOM BIOLOGICAL FLUID COLLECTION; MUST KEEP A LOG OF ANY AND ALL MEDICATIONS PRESCRIBED FOR HIM/HER; SHALL SUBMIT TO ANY EXAMINATIONS OR THERAPY ORDERED BY BOARD; SHALL APPEAR BEFORE BOARD FOR INTERVIEWS UPON REQUEST; SHALL INFORM BOARD OF CHANGE OF ADDRESS OR IF AWAY FOR MORE THAN FIVE DAYS. ARIZONA, IN COMPLIANCE WITH THE AMERICANS WITH DISABILITIES ACT, PROCLAIMS THIS IS NOT A DISCIPLINARY ACTION BUT MERELY A MONITORING PROCEDURE WHICH HE VOLUNTARILY ENTERED INTO.

ASHBY, RALPH MD, LICENSE NUMBER 0013504, HAD ACTION TAKEN BY ARIZONA ON JANUARY 21, 1995

NOTES: RECENT TREATMENT AT TALBOTT RECOVERY SYSTEMS. MUST IMMEDIATELY PARTICIPATE IN A BOARD-APPROVED MONITORED AFTERCARE TREATMENT PROGRAM WHOSE THERAPIST MUST SUBMIT QUARTERLY REPORTS; MUST PARTICIPATE IN 90 12-STEP MEETINGS FOR SUBSTANCE ABUSE WITHIN 90 DAYS; MUST THEN PARTICIPATE IN A 12-STEP RECOVERY PROGRAM AS DETERMINED BY HIS TREATING THERAPIST AND ATTEND AT LEAST THREE WEEKLY MEETINGS; SHALL OBTAIN A BOARD-APPROVED TREATING PHYSICIAN; SHALL ABSTAIN COMPLETELY FROM THE CONSUMPTION OF ALCOHOLIC BEVERAGES AND DRUGS EXCEPT WHEN PRESCRIBED BY HIS TREATING PHYSICIAN; MUST SUBMIT TO WITNESSED RANDOM BIOLOGICAL FLUID COLLECTION; SHALL KEEP A LOG OF ANY AND ALL MEDICATIONS PRESCRIBED FOR HIM; AGREES TO PAY CHARGES FOR BIOLOGICAL FLUID TESTING AND THERAPY; SHALL SUBMIT TO ANY EXAMINATIONS OR THERAPY ORDERED BY THE BOARD; SHALL APPEAR BEFORE THE BOARD FOR INTERVIEWS UPON REQUEST; SHALL INFORM BOARD OF CHANGE OF ADDRESS OR IF AWAY FOR MORE THAN FIVE DAYS. ARIZONA IN COMPLIANCE WITH THE AMERICANS WITH DISABILITIES ACT, PROCLAIMS THIS IS NOT A DISCIPLINARY ACTION BUT MERELY A MONITORING PROCEDURE WHICH HE ENTERED INTO VOLUNTARILY. ON 7/30/99 ORDER TERMINATED.

BAKER, GREGORY LONSDALE MD, HAD ACTION TAKEN BY ARIZONA ON OCTOBER 23, 1992

NOTES: LICENSE ISSUED ON CONDITIONS: MUST IMMEDIATELY PARTICIPATE IN A BOARD-APPROVED MONITORED AFTERCARE TREATMENT PROGRAM WHOSE THERAPIST MUST SUBMIT QUARTERLY REPORTS; MUST THEN PARTICIPATE IN A 12-STEP RECOVERY PROGRAM AS DETERMINED BY HIS TREATING THERAPIST AND ATTEND AT LEAST 3 WEEKLY MEETINGS; SHALL OBTAIN A BOARD-APPROVED TREATING PHYSICIAN; SHALL ABSTAIN COMPLETELY FROM THE CONSUMPTION OF ALCOHOLIC BEVERAGES AND DRUGS EXCEPT WHEN PRESCRIBED BY HIS TREATING PHYSICIAN; MUST SUBMIT TO WITNESSED RANDOM BIOLOGICAL FLUID COLLECTION; KEEP A LOG OF ANY AND ALL MEDICATIONS PRESCRIBED FOR HIM; SHALL SUBMIT TO ANY EXAMINATIONS OR THERAPY ORDERED BY BOARD; SHALL APPEAR BEFORE BOARD FOR INTERVIEWS UPON REQUEST; SHALL INFORM BOARD OF CHANGE OF ADDRESS OR IF AWAY FOR MORE THAN 5 DAYS. IN COMPLIANCE WITH THE AMERICANS WITH DISABILITIES ACT, THE ORDER AS IT STANDS IS NOT A DISCIPLINARY ACTION. ORDER TERMINATED ON 7/17/96.

BAST, RICHIE P MD, LICENSE NUMBER 0014854, HAD ACTION TAKEN BY ARIZONA ON OCTOBER 21, 1995

NOTES: INTERVIEWED BY BOARD REGARDING TREATMENT AND PARTICIPATION IN THE MONITORED AFTERCARE PROGRAM. MUST IMMEDIATELY PARTICIPATE IN A BOARD-APPROVED MONITORED AFTERCARE TREATMENT PROGRAM AT LEAST ONCE A WEEK WHOSE THERAPIST MUST SUBMIT QUARTERLY REPORTS; MUST PARTICIPATE IN 90 12-STEP MEETINGS FOR SUBSTANCE ABUSE WITHIN 90 DAYS; MUST THEN PARTICIPATE IN A 12-STEP RECOVERY PROGRAM AS DETERMINED BY TREATING THERAPIST AND ATTEND AT LEAST THREE WEEKLY MEETINGS; SHALL OBTAIN A BOARD-APPROVED TREATING PHYSICIAN; SHALL ABSTAIN COMPLETELY FROM THE CONSUMPTION OF ALCOHOLIC BEVERAGES AND ANY FOODS OR SUBSTANCES CONTAINING POPPYSEEDS; SHALL ABSTAIN FROM THE CONSUMPTION OF ANY DRUGS EXCEPT WHEN PRESCRIBED BY TREATING PHYSICIAN; MUST SUBMIT TO WITNESSED RANDOM BIOLOGICAL FLUID COLLECTION; MUST KEEP A LOG OF ANY AND ALL MEDICATIONS PRESCRIBED; SHALL SUBMIT TO ANY EXAMINATIONS OR THERAPY ORDERED BY THE BOARD; SHALL APPEAR BEFORE BOARD FOR INTERVIEWS UPON REQUEST; SHALL INFORM BOARD OF CHANGE OF ADDRESS OR IF AWAY FOR MORE THAN FIVE DAYS; REQUIREMENTS OF THIS ORDER SHALL BE TOLLED FOR ALL PERIOD OF TIME THAT HE RESIDES OR PRACTICES MEDICINE IN ANY OTHER STATE; IF HE RESIDES OR PRACTICES OUTSIDE ARIZONA SHALL PARTICIPATE IN A PHYSICIANS REHABILITATION PROGRAM WITH REPORTS EVERY SIX MONTHS; SHALL IMMEDIATELY NOTIFY BOARD IF LEAVES ARIZONA; PRIOR TO RETURNING, SHALL PROVIDE 90 DAYS ADVANCE NOTICE TO THE BOARD WITH INTENTION TO PRACTICE MEDICINE IN ARIZONA; UPON RETURN, TIME PERIOD TOLLED BY PHYSICIAN'S DEPARTURE SHALL CONTINUE UNTIL ORDER IS TERMINATED BY THE BOARD; SHALL PRACTICE MEDICINE ONLY IN A GROUP SETTING; SHALL NOT ENGAGE IN THE PRACTICE OF ANESTHESIOLOGY UNTIL FURTHER ORDER OF THE BOARD. IN COMPLIANCE WITH AMERICANS WITH DISABILITIES ACT THIS REHABILITATION STIPULATION AND ORDER IS NOT A DISCIPLINARY ACTION BUT MERELY A VOLUNTARY MONITORING PROGRAM TO REHABILITATE THE PHYSICIAN AND ENSURE PHYSICIAN'S ABILITY TO SAFELY PRACTICE MEDICINE.

BAUDER, MARC A MD, LICENSE NUMBER 15235, HAD ACTION TAKEN BY ARIZONA ON SEPTEMBER 26, 1997

NOTES: INTERVIEWED BY THE BOARD REGARDING HIS TREATMENT FOR SUBSTANCE ABUSE AND PARTICIPATION IN THE PHYSICIAN'S RECOVERY NETWORK IN IDAHO. WITHIN 30 DAYS SHALL UNDERGO PSYCHO SEXUAL EVALUATION BY THE BOARD, PAY THE COST OF THE EVALUATION AND EXECUTE A RELEASE OF ALL RECORDS AND REPORT CONCERNING THE EVALUATION TO THE BOARD. MUST IMMEDIATELY PARTICIPATE IN A BOARD-APPROVED MONITORED AFTERCARE TREATMENT PROGRAM WHOSE THERAPIST MUST SUBMIT MONTHLY REPORTS; MUST PARTICIPATE IN 90 12-STEP MEETINGS FOR SUBSTANCE ABUSE WITHIN 90 DAYS; MUST THEN PARTICIPATE IN A 12-STEP RECOVERY PROGRAM AS DETERMINED BY HIS TREATING THERAPIST AND ATTEND AT LEAST THREE WEEKLY MEETINGS; SHALL OBTAIN A BOARD-APPROVED TREATING PHYSICIAN; SHALL ABSTAIN COMPLETELY FROM THE CONSUMPTION OF ALCOHOLIC BEVERAGES AND DRUGS EXCEPT WHEN PRESCRIBED BY HIS TREATING PHYSICIAN; SHALL NOT CONSUME FOOD OR SUBSTANCES CONTAINING POPPYSEEDS; MUST SUBMIT TO WITNESSED RANDOM BIOLOGICAL FLUID COLLECTION; MUST KEEP A LOG OF ANY AND ALL MEDICATIONS PRESCRIBED FOR HIM; SHALL SUBMIT TO ANY EXAMINATIONS OR THERAPY ORDERED BY BOARD; SHALL APPEAR BEFORE BOARD FOR INTERVIEWS UPON REQUEST; SHALL INFORM BOARD OF CHANGE OF ADDRESS OR IF AWAY FOR MORE THAN FIVE DAYS; ARIZONA, IN COMPLIANCE WITH THE AMERICANS WITH DISABILITIES ACT, PROCLAIMS THIS IS NOT A DISCIPLINARY ACTION BUT MERELY A MONITORING PROCEDURE WHICH HE VOLUNTARILY ENTERED INTO; SHALL IMMEDIATELY OBTAIN A TREATING PSYCHIATRIST APPROVED BY THE BOARD AND SHALL REMAIN IN TREATMENT WITH THE PSYCHIATRIST UNTIL FURTHER ORDER OF THE BOARD WITH QUARTERLY REPORTS. ORDER TERMINATED ON 1/22/98.

BERNDT, JACK EDWARD MD, LICENSE NUMBER 0024306, HAD ACTION TAKEN BY ARIZONA ON APRIL 20, 1996

NOTES: IN 6/87 AND 8/88, ENTERED REHABILITATION AGREEMENT WITH TEXAS BOARD; IN 9/87 AND 6/94, RELAPSED IN THE USE OF DRUGS, SPECIFICALLY FENTANYL; IN 8/94, REQUESTED THAT SOUTH DAKOTA BOARD ACCEPT HIS VOLUNTARY SURRENDER; IN 6/95, LICENSE SUSPENDED, STAYED AND PUT ON PROBATION BY TEXAS BOARD; IN 3/96, SOUTH DAKOTA BOARD REINSTATED LICENSE AND SUSPENDED IT INDEFINITELY WHICH WAS THEN STAYED TO PROBATION; AGREED NOT TO PRACTICE MEDICINE IN SOUTH DAKOTA; IN 2/95, PLED GUILTY TO A CHARGE OF OBTAINING POSSESSION OF A CONTROLLED SUBSTANCE BY THEFT, MISREPRESENTATION, FORGERY OR FRAUD; IN 5/95, EXCLUDED BY THE DEPARTMENT OF HEALTH AND HUMAN SERVICES FROM THE MEDICARE PROGRAM. PROBATION WITH TERMS: SHALL NOT PRACTICE ANESTHESIOLOGY UNTIL FURTHER ORDER OF THE BOARD AND NOT FOR AT LEAST TWO YEARS; PRIOR TO PRACTICING IN ARIZONA, SHALL ENROLL IN AND SUCCESSFULLY COMPLETE FORMAL TRAINING AT A BOARD-APPROVED INSTITUTION FOR AT LEAST 90 DAYS IN AN AREA OF MEDICINE OTHER THAN ANESTHESIOLOGY; SHALL NOT APPLY FOR A DRUG ENFORCEMENT ADMINISTRATION CONTROLLED SUBSTANCE REGISTRATION CERTIFICATE WITHOUT PRIOR WRITTEN APPROVAL; SHALL SUBMIT TO THE MONITORED ADMINISTRATION OF NALTREXONE; SHALL COMPLY WITH ALL TERMS OF PROBATION

RELATING TO CONVICTION; SHALL ENTER REHABILITATION STIPULATION AND ORDER: MUST IMMEDIATELY PARTICIPATE IN A BOARD-APPROVED MONITORED AFTERCARE TREATMENT PROGRAM WHOSE THERAPIST MUST SUBMIT QUARTERLY REPORTS; SHALL PARTICIPATE IN A 12-STEP RECOVERY PROGRAM AS DETERMINED BY HIS TREATING THERAPIST; SHALL OBTAIN A BOARD-APPROVED TREATING PHYSICIAN; SHALL ABSTAIN COMPLETELY FROM THE CONSUMPTION OF ALCOHOLIC BEVERAGES AND DRUGS EXCEPT WHEN PRESCRIBED BY HIS TREATING PHYSICIAN; SHALL NOT CONSUME FOOD OR SUBSTANCES CONTAINING POPPYSEEDS; MUST SUBMIT TO WITNESSED RANDOM BIOLOGICAL FLUID COLLECTION; MUST KEEP A LOG OF ANY AND ALL MEDICATIONS PRESCRIBED FOR HIM; SHALL SUBMIT TO ANY EXAMINATIONS OR THERAPY ORDERED BY THE BOARD; SHALL APPEAR BEFORE BOARD FOR INTERVIEWS UPON REQUEST; SHALL INFORM BOARD OF CHANGE OF ADDRESS OR IF AWAY FOR MORE THAN FIVE DAYS. IF HE DOES RESIDE IN ANOTHER STATE, SHALL PARTICIPATE IN THAT STATE'S PHYSICIAN REHABILITATION PROGRAM WITH REPORTS TO ARIZONA TWICE YEARLY; TIME SPENT OUT OF ARIZONA MAY BE TOLLED FOR THIS ORDER. ARIZONA, IN COMPLIANCE WITH THE AMERICANS WITH DISABILITIES ACT, PROCLAIMS THIS IS NOT A DISCIPLINARY ACTION BUT MERELY A MONITORING PROCEDURE WHICH HE VOLUNTARILY ENTERED INTO. ON 10/19/96 ORDER AMENDED AS FOLLOWS: HE MAY APPLY TO THE DEA FOR CONTROLLED SUBSTANCE REGISTRATION PERMIT BUT SHALL NOT APPLY TO OBTAIN DEA ORDER FORMS FOR CONTROLLED SUBSTANCES WITHOUT PRIOR WRITTEN APPROVAL OF THE BOARD; HE MAY PERFORM HISTORIES AND PHYSICALS PRIOR TO ENROLLING TRAINING SPECIFIED IN THIS ORDER. ON 11/14/97 ORDER AMENDED DELETING PROHIBITION THAT HE NOT PRACTICE ANESTHESIOLOGY AND PERFORM HISTORIES AND PHYSICALS, AND ADDING REQUIREMENT THAT HE SUBMIT TO THE DAILY, MONITORED ADMINISTRATION OF NALTREXONE. ON 3/26/98 REQUEST TO MODIFY PROBATION GRANTED.

BEYMER, CHARLES H MD, HAD ACTION TAKEN BY ARIZONA ON JANUARY 23, 1998

NOTES: MUST IMMEDIATELY PARTICIPATE IN A BOARD-APPROVED MONITORED AFTERCARE TREATMENT PROGRAM WHOSE THERAPIST MUST SUBMIT MONTHLY REPORTS; MUST PARTICIPATE IN 90 12-STEP MEETINGS FOR SUBSTANCE ABUSE WITHIN 90 DAYS; MUST THEN PARTICIPATE IN A 12-STEP RECOVERY PROGRAM AS DETERMINED BY HIS TREATING THERAPIST AND ATTEND AT LEAST THREE WEEKLY MEETINGS; SHALL OBTAIN A BOARD-APPROVED TREATING PHYSICIAN; SHALL ABSTAIN COMPLETELY FROM THE CONSUMPTION OF ALCOHOLIC BEVERAGES AND DRUGS EXCEPT WHEN PRESCRIBED BY HIS TREATING PHYSICIAN; SHALL NOT CONSUME FOOD OR SUBSTANCES CONTAINING POPPYSEEDS; MUST SUBMIT TO WITNESSED RANDOM BIOLOGICAL FLUID COLLECTION; MUST KEEP A LOG OF ANY AND ALL MEDICATIONS PRESCRIBED FOR HIM; SHALL SUBMIT TO ANY EXAMINATIONS OR THERAPY ORDERED BY BOARD; SHALL APPEAR BEFORE BOARD FOR INTERVIEWS UPON REQUEST; SHALL INFORM BOARD OF CHANGE OF ADDRESS OR IF AWAY FOR MORE THAN FIVE DAYS. ARIZONA, IN COMPLIANCE WITH THE AMERICANS WITH DISABILITIES ACT, PROCLAIMS THIS IS NOT A DISCIPLINARY ACTION BUT MERELY A MONITORING PROCEDURE WHICH HE VOLUNTARILY ENTERED INTO. ON 1/29/99, ORDER TERMINATED.

BINETTE, MARK J MD, LICENSE NUMBER 0020392 OF PHOENIX, AZ, HAD ACTION TAKEN BY ARIZONA ON APRIL 15, 1994

NOTES: ALLEGATIONS OF CHEMICAL ABUSE. MUST IMMEDIATELY PARTICIPATE IN A BOARD-APPROVED MONITORED AFTERCARE TREATMENT PROGRAM WHOSE THERAPIST MUST SUBMIT QUARTERLY REPORTS; MUST PARTICIPATE IN 90 12-STEP MEETINGS FOR SUBSTANCE ABUSE WITHIN 90 DAYS; MUST THEN PARTICIPATE IN A 12-STEP RECOVERY PROGRAM AS DETERMINED BY HIS TREATING THERAPIST AND ATTEND AT LEAST THREE WEEKLY MEETINGS; SHALL OBTAIN A BOARD-APPROVED TREATING PHYSICIAN; SHALL ABSTAIN COMPLETELY FROM THE CONSUMPTION OF ALCOHOLIC BEVERAGES AND DRUGS EXCEPT WHEN PRESCRIBED BY HIS TREATING PHYSICIAN; MUST SUBMIT TO WITNESSED RANDOM BIOLOGICAL FLUID COLLECTION; KEEP A LOG OF ANY AND ALL MEDICATIONS PRESCRIBED FOR HIM; SHALL SUBMIT TO ANY EXAMINATIONS OR THERAPY ORDERED BY BOARD; SHALL APPEAR BEFORE BOARD FOR INTERVIEWS UPON REQUEST; SHALL INFORM BOARD OF CHANGE OF ADDRESS OR IF AWAY FOR MORE THAN FIVE DAYS; AGREED NOT TO PRACTICE UNTIL HE FINISHES INPATIENT TREATMENT AND MEETS WITH BOARD IN JULY 1994. ARIZONA, IN COMPLIANCE WITH THE AMERICANS WITH DISABILITIES ACT, PROCLAIMS THIS IS NOT A DISCIPLINARY ACTION BUT MERELY A MONITORING PROCEDURE WHICH HE VOLUNTARILY ENTERED INTO.

BINETTE, MARK J MD, LICENSE NUMBER 0020392, HAD ACTION TAKEN BY ARIZONA ON JANUARY 18, 1996

NOTES: ON 2/6/95, HE WAS CONVICTED OF SIMPLE POSSESSION OF CONTROLLED SUBSTANCES AND USE OF A COMMUNICATION FACILITY TO FACILITATE THE DISTRIBUTION OF A CONTROLLED SUBSTANCE; ON 3/20/95, TRANSFERRED TO A TREATMENT CENTER TO COMPLETE HIS SENTENCE; ON 5/18/95, RELEASED FROM CUSTODY AND IS ON FEDERAL PROBATION UNTIL 5/18/96; IN 8/95, REQUESTED THAT HIS LICENSE BE REACTIVATED. REACTIVATION TO PROBATION WITH CONDITIONS: SHALL PERFORM 150 HOURS OF BOARD-APPROVED COMMUNITY SERVICE EACH YEAR FOR THE TERM OF PROBATION; SHALL SUBMIT EVIDENCE OF COMPLETION OF SERVICE TO THE BOARD. IN RECOGNITION OF THE AMERICANS WITH DISABILITIES ACT, THE FOLLOWING REHABILITATION STIPULATION AND ORDER IS NOT A DISCIPLINARY ACTION BUT A MONITORING PROGRAM WHICH HE VOLUNTARILY ENTERED INTO: MUST IMMEDIATELY PARTICIPATE IN A BOARD-APPROVED MONITORED AFTERCARE TREATMENT PROGRAM WHOSE THERAPIST MUST SUBMIT QUARTERLY REPORTS; MUST PARTICIPATE IN A 12-STEP RECOVERY PROGRAM AS DETERMINED BY HIS TREATING THERAPIST AND ATTEND AT LEAST THREE WEEKLY MEETINGS; SHALL OBTAIN A BOARD-APPROVED TREATING PHYSICIAN; SHALL NOT CONSUME FOOD OR ANY SUBSTANCES WHICH CONTAIN POPPY SEEDS; SHALL ABSTAIN COMPLETELY FROM THE CONSUMPTION OF ALCOHOLIC BEVERAGES AND DRUGS EXCEPT WHEN PRESCRIBED BY HIS TREATING PHYSICIAN; MUST SUBMIT TO WITNESSED RANDOM BIOLOGICAL FLUID COLLECTION; MUST KEEP A LOG OF ANY AND ALL MEDICATIONS PRESCRIBED FOR HIM; SHALL SUBMIT TO ANY EXAMINATIONS OR THERAPY ORDERED BY THE BOARD; SHALL APPEAR BEFORE BOARD FOR INTERVIEWS UPON REQUEST; SHALL INFORM BOARD OF CHANGE OF ADDRESS OR IF AWAY FOR MORE THAN FIVE DAYS. IF HE DOES RESIDE IN ANOTHER STATE, SHALL PARTICIPATE IN THAT STATE'S PHYSICIAN REHABILITATION PROGRAM WITH REPORTS TO ARIZONA TWICE YEARLY; TIME SPENT

OUT OF ARIZONA MAY BE TOLLED FOR THIS ORDER. ON 3/15/97 PROBATION TERMINATED. ON 3/24/99 ORDER TERMINATED.

BLANCK, EUGENE C MD, LICENSE NUMBER 11485, HAD ACTION TAKEN BY ARIZONA ON NOVEMBER 14, 1997

NOTES: INTERVIEWED BY BOARD REGARDING HIS TREATMENT FOR SUBSTANCE ABUSE. MUST IMMEDIATELY PARTICIPATE IN A BOARD-APPROVED MONITORED AFTERCARE TREATMENT PROGRAM WHOSE THERAPIST MUST SUBMIT MONTHLY REPORTS; MUST PARTICIPATE IN 90 12-STEP MEETINGS FOR SUBSTANCE ABUSE WITHIN 90 DAYS; MUST THEN PARTICIPATE IN A 12-STEP RECOVERY PROGRAM AS DETERMINED BY HIS TREATING THERAPIST AND ATTEND AT LEAST THREE WEEKLY MEETINGS; SHALL OBTAIN A BOARD-APPROVED TREATING PHYSICIAN; SHALL ABSTAIN COMPLETELY FROM THE CONSUMPTION OF ALCOHOLIC BEVERAGES AND DRUGS EXCEPT WHEN PRESCRIBED BY HIS TREATING PHYSICIAN; SHALL NOT CONSUME FOOD OR SUBSTANCES CONTAINING POPPYSEEDS; MUST SUBMIT TO WITNESSED RANDOM BIOLOGICAL FLUID COLLECTION; MUST KEEP A LOG OF ANY AND ALL MEDICATIONS PRESCRIBED FOR HIM; SHALL SUBMIT TO ANY EXAMINATIONS OR THERAPY ORDERED BY BOARD; SHALL APPEAR BEFORE BOARD FOR INTERVIEWS UPON REQUEST; SHALL INFORM BOARD OF CHANGE OF ADDRESS OR IF AWAY FOR MORE THAN FIVE DAYS; ARIZONA, IN COMPLIANCE WITH THE AMERICANS WITH DISABILITIES ACT, PROCLAIMS THIS IS NOT A DISCIPLINARY ACTION BUT MERELY A MONITORING PROCEDURE WHICH HE VOLUNTARILY ENTERED INTO; SHALL IMMEDIATELY OBTAIN A TREATING PSYCHIATRIST APPROVED BY THE BOARD AND SHALL REMAIN IN TREATMENT WITH THE PSYCHIATRIST UNTIL FURTHER ORDER OF THE BOARD WITH QUARTERLY REPORTS.

BLOCHER, JOHN D MD, LICENSE NUMBER 0007065, HAD ACTION TAKEN BY ARIZONA ON APRIL 8, 1995

NOTES: INTERVIEWED BY BOARD RELATIVE TO HIS TREATMENT FOR SUBSTANCE ABUSE. MUST IMMEDIATELY PARTICIPATE IN A BOARD-APPROVED MONITORED AFTERCARE TREATMENT PROGRAM WHOSE THERAPIST MUST SUBMIT QUARTERLY REPORTS; MUST PARTICIPATE IN 90 12-STEP MEETINGS FOR SUBSTANCE ABUSE WITHIN 90 DAYS; MUST THEN PARTICIPATE IN A 12-STEP RECOVERY PROGRAM AS DETERMINED BY HIS TREATING THERAPIST AND ATTEND AT LEAST THREE WEEKLY MEETINGS; SHALL OBTAIN A BOARD-APPROVED TREATING PHYSICIAN; SHALL ABSTAIN COMPLETELY FROM THE CONSUMPTION OF ALCOHOLIC BEVERAGES AND DRUGS EXCEPT WHEN PRESCRIBED BY HIS TREATING PHYSICIAN; MUST SUBMIT TO WITNESSED RANDOM BIOLOGICAL FLUID COLLECTION; MUST KEEP A LOG OF ANY AND ALL MEDICATIONS PRESCRIBED FOR HIM; SHALL SUBMIT TO ANY EXAMINATIONS OR THERAPY ORDERED BY THE BOARD; SHALL APPEAR BEFORE THE BOARD FOR INTERVIEWS UPON REQUEST; SHALL INFORM BOARD OF CHANGE OF ADDRESS OR IF AWAY FOR MORE THAN FIVE DAYS. ARIZONA IN COMPLIANCE WITH THE AMERICANS WITH DISABILITIES ACT, PROCLAIMS THIS IS NOT A DISCIPLINARY ACTION BUT MERELY A MONITORING PROCEDURE WHICH HE ENTERED INTO VOLUNTARILY. ON 11/19/99 ORDER TERMINATED IN 90 DAYS.

BOBE, RICHARD R MD, LICENSE NUMBER 0022894, HAD ACTION TAKEN BY ARIZONA ON APRIL 20, 1996

NOTES: MUST IMMEDIATELY PARTICIPATE IN A BOARD-APPROVED MONITORED AFTERCARE TREATMENT PROGRAM WHOSE THERAPIST MUST SUBMIT QUARTERLY REPORTS; MUST PARTICIPATE IN 90 12-STEP MEETINGS FOR SUBSTANCE ABUSE WITHIN 90 DAYS; MUST THEN PARTICIPATE IN A 12-STEP RECOVERY PROGRAM AS DETERMINED BY HIS TREATING THERAPIST AND ATTEND AT LEAST THREE WEEKLY MEETINGS; SHALL OBTAIN A BOARD-APPROVED TREATING PHYSICIAN; SHALL ABSTAIN COMPLETELY FROM THE CONSUMPTION OF ALCOHOLIC BEVERAGES AND DRUGS EXCEPT WHEN PRESCRIBED BY HIS TREATING PHYSICIAN; SHALL NOT CONSUME FOODS OR SUBSTANCES CONTAINING POPPYSEEDS; MUST SUBMIT TO WITNESSED RANDOM BIOLOGICAL FLUID COLLECTION; MUST KEEP A LOG OF ANY AND ALL MEDICATIONS PRESCRIBED FOR HIM; SHALL SUBMIT TO ANY EXAMINATIONS OR THERAPY ORDERED BY THE BOARD; SHALL APPEAR BEFORE BOARD FOR INTERVIEWS UPON REQUEST; SHALL INFORM BOARD OF CHANGE OF ADDRESS OR IF AWAY FOR MORE THAN FIVE DAYS. IF HE DOES RESIDE IN ANOTHER STATE, SHALL PARTICIPATE IN THAT STATE'S PHYSICIAN REHABILITATION PROGRAM WITH REPORTS TO ARIZONA TWICE YEARLY; TIME SPENT OUT OF ARIZONA MAY BE TOLLED FOR THIS ORDER. IN COMPLIANCE WITH THE AMERICANS WITH DISABILITIES ACT, ARIZONA PROCLAIMS THIS IS NOT A DISCIPLINARY ACTION BUT MERELY A MONITORING PROCEDURE WHICH HE ENTERED INTO VOLUNTARILY. ON 1/24/97 ORDER AMENDED ADDING REQUIREMENT THAT HE OBTAIN A TREATING PSYCHIATRIST WHO WILL RELEASE ALL RECORDS UPON BOARD'S REQUEST, AND SUBMIT QUARTERLY REPORTS. ON 3/26/98 ORDER TERMINATED.

BOBER, ARTHUR P MD, LICENSE NUMBER 0015442 OF PHOENIX, AZ, HAD ACTION TAKEN BY ARIZONA ON JANUARY 27, 1994

NOTES: MUST IMMEDIATELY PARTICIPATE IN A BOARD-APPROVED MONITORED AFTERCARE TREATMENT PROGRAM WHOSE THERAPIST MUST SUBMIT QUARTERLY REPORTS; MUST PARTICIPATE IN 90 12-STEP MEETINGS FOR SUBSTANCE ABUSE WITHIN 90 DAYS; MUST THEN PARTICIPATE IN A 12-STEP RECOVERY PROGRAM AS DETERMINED BY HIS TREATING THERAPIST AND ATTEND AT LEAST THREE WEEKLY MEETINGS; SHALL OBTAIN A BOARD-APPROVED TREATING PHYSICIAN; SHALL ABSTAIN COMPLETELY FROM THE CONSUMPTION OF ALCOHOLIC BEVERAGES AND DRUGS EXCEPT WHEN PRESCRIBED BY HIS TREATING PHYSICIAN; MUST SUBMIT TO WITNESSED RANDOM BIOLOGICAL FLUID COLLECTION; KEEP A LOG OF ANY AND ALL MEDICATIONS PRESCRIBED FOR HIM; SHALL SUBMIT TO ANY EXAMINATIONS OR THERAPY ORDERED BY BOARD; SHALL APPEAR BEFORE BOARD FOR INTERVIEWS UPON REQUEST; SHALL INFORM BOARD OF CHANGE OF ADDRESS OR IF AWAY FOR MORE THAN FIVE DAYS. ARIZONA, IN COMPLIANCE WITH THE AMERICANS WITH DISABILITIES ACT, PROCLAIMS THIS IS NOT A DISCIPLINARY ACTION BUT MERELY A MONITORING PROCEDURE WHICH HE VOLUNTARILY ENTERED INTO.

BOUCHER, VICTOR B MD, HAD ACTION TAKEN BY ARIZONA ON AUGUST 8, 1998

NOTES: MUST IMMEDIATELY PARTICIPATE IN A BOARD-APPROVED MONITORED AFTERCARE TREATMENT PROGRAM WHOSE THERAPIST MUST SUBMIT QUARTERLY REPORTS; MUST PARTICIPATE IN 90 12-STEP MEETINGS FOR SUBSTANCE ABUSE WITHIN 90 DAYS; MUST THEN PARTICIPATE IN A 12-STEP RECOVERY PROGRAM AS DETERMINED BY HIS/HER TREATING THERAPIST AND ATTEND AT LEAST THREE

WEEKLY MEETINGS; SHALL OBTAIN A BOARD-APPROVED TREATING PHYSICIAN; SHALL ABSTAIN COMPLETELY FROM THE CONSUMPTION OF ALCOHOLIC BEVERAGES AND DRUGS EXCEPT WHEN PRESCRIBED BY HIS/HER TREATING PHYSICIAN; SHALL NOT CONSUME FOOD OR SUBSTANCES CONTAINING POPPYSEEDS; MUST SUBMIT TO WITNESSED RANDOM BIOLOGICAL FLUID COLLECTION; MUST KEEP A LOG OF ANY AND ALL MEDICATIONS PRESCRIBED FOR HIM/HER; SHALL SUBMIT TO ANY EXAMINATIONS OR THERAPY ORDERED BY BOARD; SHALL APPEAR BEFORE BOARD FOR INTERVIEWS UPON REQUEST; SHALL INFORM BOARD OF CHANGE OF ADDRESS OR IF AWAY FOR MORE THAN FIVE DAYS. ARIZONA, IN COMPLIANCE WITH THE AMERICANS WITH DISABILITIES ACT, PROCLAIMS THIS IS NOT A DISCIPLINARY ACTION BUT MERELY A MONITORING PROCEDURE WHICH HE VOLUNTARILY ENTERED INTO.

BROWN, THOMAS J MD, LICENSE NUMBER 0020063 OF TX, HAD ACTION TAKEN BY ARIZONA ON OCTOBER 13, 1993

NOTES: INFORMATION RECEIVED ALLEGING THAT HE REQUIRES CONTINUED MEDICAL CARE. SHALL OBTAIN A SOLE TREATING PSYCHIATRIST APPROVED BY THE BOARD AND TAKE ONLY THOSE MEDICATIONS PRESCRIBED BY HIM WITH QUARTERLY REPORTS TO THE BOARD, INDICATING DIAGNOSIS, PROGNOSIS, COMPLIANCE WITH MEDICATIONS, RESULTS OF LABORATORY TESTS AND DATE OF VISITS. THE BOARD WILL GET WRITTEN FEEDBACK AT LEAST QUARTERLY FROM EACH OF HIS EMPLOYERS FOR THE PAST QUARTER INDICATING HIS ABILITY TO COMPETENTLY PRACTICE MEDICINE AS WELL AS THE NUMBER OF HOURS WORKED IN THE PREVIOUS QUARTER AND THE TYPE OF WORK DONE; ORDER IS NOT DISCIPLINARY IN NATURE BUT IS DESIGNATED FOR PERSONAL REHABILITATIVE PURPOSES. ORDER TERMINATED ON 4/16/96.

BUDD, SCOTT C MD, LICENSE NUMBER 19880, HAD ACTION TAKEN BY ARIZONA ON JANUARY 23, 1998

NOTES: MUST IMMEDIATELY PARTICIPATE IN A BOARD-APPROVED MONITORED AFTERCARE TREATMENT PROGRAM WHOSE THERAPIST MUST SUBMIT MONTHLY REPORTS; MUST PARTICIPATE IN 90 12-STEP MEETINGS FOR SUBSTANCE ABUSE WITHIN 90 DAYS; MUST THEN PARTICIPATE IN A 12-STEP RECOVERY PROGRAM AS DETERMINED BY HIS TREATING THERAPIST AND ATTEND AT LEAST THREE WEEKLY MEETINGS; SHALL OBTAIN A BOARD-APPROVED TREATING PHYSICIAN; SHALL ABSTAIN COMPLETELY FROM THE CONSUMPTION OF ALCOHOLIC BEVERAGES AND DRUGS EXCEPT WHEN PRESCRIBED BY HIS TREATING PHYSICIAN; SHALL NOT CONSUME FOOD OR SUBSTANCES CONTAINING POPPYSEEDS; MUST SUBMIT TO WITNESSED RANDOM BIOLOGICAL FLUID COLLECTION; MUST KEEP A LOG OF ANY AND ALL MEDICATIONS PRESCRIBED FOR HIM; SHALL SUBMIT TO ANY EXAMINATIONS OR THERAPY ORDERED BY BOARD; SHALL APPEAR BEFORE BOARD FOR INTERVIEWS UPON REQUEST; SHALL INFORM BOARD OF CHANGE OF ADDRESS OR IF AWAY FOR MORE THAN FIVE DAYS. ARIZONA, IN COMPLIANCE WITH THE AMERICANS WITH DISABILITIES ACT, PROCLAIMS THIS IS NOT A DISCIPLINARY ACTION BUT MERELY A MONITORING PROCEDURE WHICH HE VOLUNTARILY ENTERED INTO.

BURWELL, BEVERLY A MD, LICENSE NUMBER 0019548, HAD ACTION TAKEN BY ARIZONA ON OCTOBER 21, 1995

NOTES: SHE PROVIDED THE BOARD INFORMATION REGARDING HER CHEMICAL DEPENDENCY. MUST IMMEDIATELY PARTICIPATE IN A BOARD-APPROVED MONITORED AFTERCARE TREATMENT PROGRAM AT LEAST ONCE A WEEK WHOSE THERAPIST MUST SUBMIT QUARTERLY REPORTS; MUST PARTICIPATE IN 90 12-STEP MEETINGS FOR SUBSTANCE ABUSE WITHIN 90 DAYS; MUST THEN PARTICIPATE IN A 12-STEP RECOVERY PROGRAM AS DETERMINED BY HER TREATING THERAPIST AND ATTEND AT LEAST THREE WEEKLY MEETINGS; SHALL OBTAIN A BOARD-APPROVED TREATING PHYSICIAN; SHALL ABSTAIN COMPLETELY FROM THE CONSUMPTION OF ALCOHOLIC BEVERAGES AND DRUGS EXCEPT WHEN PRESCRIBED BY HER TREATING PHYSICIAN; MUST SUBMIT TO WITNESSED RANDOM BIOLOGICAL FLUID COLLECTION; MUST KEEP A LOG OF ANY AND ALL MEDICATIONS PRESCRIBED FOR HER; SHALL SUBMIT TO ANY EXAMINATIONS OR THERAPY ORDERED BY BOARD; SHALL APPEAR BEFORE BOARD FOR INTERVIEWS UPON REQUEST; SHALL INFORM BOARD OF CHANGE OF ADDRESS OR IF AWAY FOR MORE THAN FIVE DAYS; REQUIREMENTS OF ORDER SHALL BE TOLLED FOR ALL PERIOD OF TIME THAT SHE RESIDES OR PRACTICES IN ANY OTHER STATE; IF SHE RESIDES OR PRACTICES OUTSIDE ARIZONA SHALL PARTICIPATE IN A PHYSICIANS REHABILITATION PROGRAM WITH REPORTS EVERY SIX MONTHS; SHALL IMMEDIATELY NOTIFY THE BOARD IF SHE LEAVES ARIZONA; PRIOR TO RETURNING SHE SHALL PROVIDE 90 DAYS ADVANCE NOTICE TO THE BOARD THAT SHE INTENDS TO PRACTICE IN ARIZONA; UPON RETURN, TIME TOLLED BY HER DEPARTURE SHALL CONTINUE UNTIL ORDER IS TERMINATED BY THE BOARD; SHALL IMMEDIATELY OBTAIN A TREATING PSYCHIATRIST AND PSYCHOTHERAPIST APPROVED BY THE BOARD, BOTH OF WHOM WILL SUBMIT QUARTERLY REPORTS TO THE BOARD; SHALL NOT PRACTICE PHARMACY. IN COMPLIANCE WITH THE AMERICANS WITH DISABILITIES ACT THIS REHABILITATION STIPULATION AND ORDER IS NOT A DISCIPLINARY ACTION, BUT MERELY A VOLUNTARY MONITORING PROGRAM TO REHABILITATE PHYSICIAN AND ENSURE HER ABILITY TO SAFELY PRACTICE MEDICINE.

CAMAZINE, BRIAN M MD, LICENSE NUMBER 17537, HAD ACTION TAKEN BY ARIZONA ON MAY 8, 1997

NOTES: MUST IMMEDIATELY PARTICIPATE IN A BOARD-APPROVED MONITORED AFTERCARE TREATMENT PROGRAM WHOSE THERAPIST MUST SUBMIT QUARTERLY REPORTS; MUST PARTICIPATE IN 90 12-STEP MEETINGS FOR SUBSTANCE ABUSE WITHIN 90 DAYS; MUST THEN PARTICIPATE IN A 12-STEP RECOVERY PROGRAM AS DETERMINED BY HIS TREATING THERAPIST AND ATTEND AT LEAST THREE WEEKLY MEETINGS; SHALL OBTAIN A BOARD-APPROVED TREATING PHYSICIAN; SHALL ABSTAIN COMPLETELY FROM THE CONSUMPTION OF ALCOHOLIC BEVERAGES AND DRUGS EXCEPT WHEN PRESCRIBED BY HIS TREATING PHYSICIAN; SHALL NOT CONSUME FOOD OR SUBSTANCES CONTAINING POPPYSEEDS; MUST SUBMIT TO WITNESSED RANDOM BIOLOGICAL FLUID COLLECTION; MUST KEEP A LOG OF ANY AND ALL MEDICATIONS PRESCRIBED FOR HIM; SHALL SUBMIT TO ANY EXAMINATIONS OR THERAPY ORDERED BY BOARD; SHALL APPEAR BEFORE BOARD FOR INTERVIEWS UPON REQUEST; SHALL INFORM BOARD OF CHANGE OF ADDRESS OR IF AWAY FOR MORE THAN FIVE DAYS. ARIZONA, IN COMPLIANCE WITH THE AMERICANS WITH DISABILITIES ACT, PROCLAIMS THIS IS NOT A DISCIPLINARY ACTION BUT MERELY A MONITORING PROCEDURE WHICH HE VOLUNTARILY ENTERED INTO.

CANAVAN, JAMES T MD, LICENSE NUMBER 19964, HAD ACTION TAKEN BY ARIZONA ON MAY 9, 1997

NOTES: INTERVIEWED BY THE BOARD REGARDING HIS TREATMENT FOR SUBSTANCE ABUSE. MUST IMMEDIATELY PARTICIPATE IN A BOARD-APPROVED MONITORED AFTERCARE TREATMENT PROGRAM WHOSE THERAPIST MUST SUBMIT QUARTERLY REPORTS; MUST PARTICIPATE IN 90 12-STEP MEETINGS FOR SUBSTANCE ABUSE WITHIN 90 DAYS; MUST THEN PARTICIPATE IN A 12-STEP RECOVERY PROGRAM AS DETERMINED BY HIS TREATING THERAPIST AND ATTEND AT LEAST THREE WEEKLY MEETINGS; SHALL OBTAIN A BOARD-APPROVED TREATING PHYSICIAN; SHALL ABSTAIN COMPLETELY FROM THE CONSUMPTION OF ALCOHOLIC BEVERAGES AND DRUGS EXCEPT WHEN PRESCRIBED BY HIS TREATING PHYSICIAN; SHALL NOT CONSUME FOOD OR SUBSTANCES CONTAINING POPPYSEEDS; MUST SUBMIT TO WITNESSED RANDOM BIOLOGICAL FLUID COLLECTION; MUST KEEP A LOG OF ANY AND ALL MEDICATIONS PRESCRIBED FOR HIM; SHALL SUBMIT TO ANY EXAMINATIONS OR THERAPY ORDERED BY BOARD; SHALL APPEAR BEFORE BOARD FOR INTERVIEWS UPON REQUEST; SHALL INFORM BOARD OF CHANGE OF ADDRESS OR IF AWAY FOR MORE THAN FIVE DAYS; ARIZONA, IN COMPLIANCE WITH THE AMERICANS WITH DISABILITIES ACT, PROCLAIMS THIS IS NOT A DISCIPLINARY ACTION BUT MERELY A MONITORING PROCEDURE WHICH HE VOLUNTARILY ENTERED INTO; SHALL SUBMIT TO DAILY WITNESSED ADMINISTRATION OF NALTREXONE BY A PERSON OR PERSONS APPROVED BY THE BOARD.

CHERVENAK, JOHN MD, LICENSE NUMBER 0009926, HAD ACTION TAKEN BY ARIZONA ON FEBRUARY 19, 1996

NOTES: SHALL OBTAIN A BOARD-APPROVED MENTAL HEALTH THERAPIST WHO SHALL SUBMIT REPORTS TWICE A YEAR; SHALL ABSTAIN COMPLETELY FROM THE CONSUMPTION OF ALCOHOLIC BEVERAGES AND DRUGS EXCEPT WHEN PRESCRIBED BY HIS TREATING PHYSICIAN; FOR SIX MONTHS, SHALL SUBMIT TO WITNESSED RANDOM BIOLOGICAL FLUID COLLECTION; SHALL SUBMIT TO ANY EXAMINATIONS OR THERAPY ORDERED BY THE BOARD; SHALL APPEAR BEFORE BOARD FOR INTERVIEWS UPON REQUEST; SHALL INFORM THE BOARD OF CHANGE OF ADDRESS OR IF AWAY FOR MORE THAN FIVE DAYS. ARIZONA, IN COMPLIANCE WITH THE AMERICANS WITH DISABILITIES ACT, PROCLAIMS THIS IS NOT A DISCIPLINARY ACTION BUT MERELY A MONITORING PROCEDURE WHICH HE ENTERED INTO VOLUNTARILY. ON 3/26/98 ORDER TERMINATED.

CHILIAN, RICHARD L MD, HAD ACTION TAKEN BY ARIZONA ON MARCH 27, 1998

NOTES: MUST IMMEDIATELY PARTICIPATE IN A BOARD-APPROVED MONITORED AFTERCARE TREATMENT PROGRAM WHOSE THERAPIST MUST SUBMIT QUARTERLY REPORTS; MUST PARTICIPATE IN 90 12-STEP MEETINGS FOR SUBSTANCE ABUSE WITHIN 90 DAYS; MUST THEN PARTICIPATE IN A 12-STEP RECOVERY PROGRAM AS DETERMINED BY HIS/HER TREATING THERAPIST AND ATTEND AT LEAST THREE WEEKLY MEETINGS; SHALL OBTAIN A BOARD-APPROVED TREATING PHYSICIAN; SHALL ABSTAIN COMPLETELY FROM THE CONSUMPTION OF ALCOHOLIC BEVERAGES AND DRUGS EXCEPT WHEN PRESCRIBED BY HIS/HER TREATING PHYSICIAN; SHALL NOT CONSUME FOOD OR SUBSTANCES CONTAINING POPPYSEEDS; MUST SUBMIT TO WITNESSED RANDOM BIOLOGICAL FLUID COLLECTION; MUST KEEP A LOG OF ANY AND ALL MEDICATIONS PRESCRIBED FOR HIM/HER; SHALL SUBMIT TO ANY EXAMINATIONS OR THERAPY ORDERED BY BOARD; SHALL APPEAR BEFORE BOARD FOR INTERVIEWS UPON REQUEST; SHALL INFORM BOARD OF CHANGE OF ADDRESS OR IF AWAY FOR MORE THAN FIVE DAYS. ARIZONA, IN COMPLIANCE WITH THE AMERICANS WITH DISABILITIES ACT, PROCLAIMS THIS IS NOT A DISCIPLINARY ACTION BUT MERELY A MONITORING PROCEDURE WHICH HE VOLUNTARILY ENTERED INTO.

CLAYTON, DEANNA L MD, HAD ACTION TAKEN BY ARIZONA ON OCTOBER 21, 1995

NOTES: ALLEGATIONS OF CHEMICAL SUBSTANCE ABUSE. MUST IMMEDIATELY PARTICIPATE IN A BOARD-APPROVED MONITORED AFTERCARE TREATMENT PROGRAM WHOSE THERAPIST MUST SUBMIT QUARTERLY REPORTS; MUST PARTICIPATE IN 90 12-STEP MEETINGS FOR SUBSTANCE ABUSE WITHIN 90 DAYS; MUST THEN PARTICIPATE IN A 12-STEP RECOVERY PROGRAM AS DETERMINED BY HER TREATING THERAPIST AND ATTEND AT LEAST THREE WEEKLY MEETINGS; SHALL OBTAIN A BOARD-APPROVED TREATING PHYSICIAN; SHALL ABSTAIN COMPLETELY FROM THE CONSUMPTION OF ALCOHOLIC BEVERAGES AND DRUGS EXCEPT WHEN PRESCRIBED BY HER TREATING PHYSICIAN; MUST SUBMIT TO WITNESSED RANDOM BIOLOGICAL FLUID COLLECTION; MUST KEEP A LOG OF ANY AND ALL MEDICATIONS PRESCRIBED FOR HER; SHALL SUBMIT TO ANY EXAMINATIONS OR THERAPY ORDERED BY THE BOARD; SHALL APPEAR BEFORE BOARD FOR INTERVIEWS UPON REQUEST; SHALL INFORM BOARD OF CHANGE OF ADDRESS OR IF AWAY FOR MORE THAN FIVE DAYS. ARIZONA, IN COMPLIANCE WITH THE AMERICANS WITH DISABILITIES ACT, PROCLAIMS THIS IS NOT A DISCIPLINARY ACTION BUT MERELY A MONITORING PROCEDURE WHICH SHE ENTERED INTO VOLUNTARILY. AS OF 2/15/96, THIS ORDER TERMINATED, ALTHOUGH ABOVE CONDITIONS STILL APPLY AND SHE SHALL MEET WITH THE MONITORED AFTERCARE COMMITTEE IN 3 MONTHS.

COCHRAN, WILLIAM M MD, LICENSE NUMBER 0015469, HAD ACTION TAKEN BY ARIZONA ON JANUARY 29, 1994

NOTES: RELATIVE TO MISUSE OF CHEMICAL SUBSTANCES, HIS SUBSEQUENT TREATMENT AND EARLY RECOVERY PROGRAM. MUST IMMEDIATELY PARTICIPATE IN A BOARD-APPROVED MONITORED AFTERCARE PROGRAM WHOSE THERAPIST MUST SUBMIT QUARTERLY REPORTS; MUST PARTICIPATE IN 90 12-STEP MEETINGS FOR SUBSTANCE ABUSE WITHIN 90 DAYS; MUST THEN PARTICIPATE IN A 12-STEP RECOVERY PROGRAM AS DETERMINED BY HIS TREATING THERAPIST AND ATTEND AT LEAST THREE WEEKLY MEETINGS; SHALL OBTAIN A BOARD-APPROVED TREATING PHYSICIAN; SHALL ABSTAIN COMPLETELY FROM THE CONSUMPTION OF ALCOHOLIC BEVERAGES AND DRUGS EXCEPT WHEN PRESCRIBED BY HIS TREATING PHYSICIAN; MUST SUBMIT TO WITNESSED RANDOM BIOLOGICAL FLUID COLLECTION; KEEP A LOG OF ANY AND ALL MEDICATIONS PRESCRIBED FOR HIM; SHALL SUBMIT TO ANY EXAMINATIONS OR THERAPY ORDERED BY BOARD; SHALL APPEAR BEFORE BOARD FOR INTERVIEWS UPON REQUEST; SHALL INFORM BOARD OF CHANGE OF ADDRESS OR IF AWAY FOR MORE THAN FIVE DAYS. ARIZONA, IN COMPLIANCE WITH THE AMERICANS WITH DISABILITIES ACT, PROCLAIMS THIS IS NOT A DISCIPLINARY ACTION BUT MERELY A MONITORING PROCEDURE WHICH HE VOLUNTARILY ENTERED INTO.

COE, BARRY J MD, LICENSE NUMBER 0012537, HAD ACTION TAKEN BY ARIZONA ON OCTOBER 22, 1994

NOTES: SUBSTANCE ABUSE AND INPATIENT TREATMENT. MUST IMMEDIATELY PARTICIPATE IN A BOARD-APPROVED MONITORED AFTERCARE TREATMENT PROGRAM WHOSE THERAPIST MUST SUBMIT QUARTERLY REPORTS; MUST PARTICIPATE IN 90 12-STEP MEETINGS FOR SUBSTANCE ABUSE WITHIN 90 DAYS; MUST THEN PARTICIPATE IN A 12-STEP RECOVERY PROGRAM AS DETERMINED BY HIS TREATING THERAPIST AND ATTEND AT LEAST THREE WEEKLY MEETINGS; SHALL OBTAIN A BOARD-APPROVED TREATING PHYSICIAN; SHALL ABSTAIN COMPLETELY FROM THE CONSUMPTION OF ALCOHOLIC BEVERAGES AND DRUGS EXCEPT WHEN PRESCRIBED BY HIS TREATING PHYSICIAN; MUST SUBMIT TO WITNESSED RANDOM BIOLOGICAL FLUID COLLECTION; KEEP A LOG OF ANY AND ALL MEDICATIONS PRESCRIBED FOR HIM; SHALL SUBMIT TO ANY EXAMINATIONS OR THERAPY ORDERED BY BOARD; SHALL APPEAR BEFORE BOARD FOR INTERVIEWS UPON REQUEST; SHALL INFORM BOARD OF CHANGE OF ADDRESS OR IF AWAY FOR MORE THAN FIVE DAYS. ARIZONA, IN COMPLIANCE WITH THE AMERICANS WITH DISABILITIES ACT, PROCLAIMS THIS IS NOT A DISCIPLINARY ACTION BUT MERELY A MONITORING PROCEDURE WHICH HE VOLUNTARILY ENTERED INTO. ON 7/26/97 ORDER TERMINATED EFFECTIVE IN 90 DAYS.

CRONISTER, LESLIE MD, HAD ACTION TAKEN BY ARIZONA ON JANUARY 23, 1998

NOTES: MUST IMMEDIATELY PARTICIPATE IN A BOARD-APPROVED MONITORED AFTERCARE TREATMENT PROGRAM WHOSE THERAPIST MUST SUBMIT MONTHLY REPORTS; MUST PARTICIPATE IN 90 12-STEP MEETINGS FOR SUBSTANCE ABUSE WITHIN 90 DAYS; MUST THEN PARTICIPATE IN A 12-STEP RECOVERY PROGRAM AS DETERMINED BY DR. CRONISTER'S TREATING THERAPIST AND ATTEND AT LEAST THREE WEEKLY MEETINGS; SHALL OBTAIN A BOARD-APPROVED TREATING PHYSICIAN; SHALL ABSTAIN COMPLETELY FROM THE CONSUMPTION OF ALCOHOLIC BEVERAGES AND DRUGS EXCEPT WHEN PRESCRIBED BY DR. CRONISTER'S TREATING PHYSICIAN; SHALL NOT CONSUME FOOD OR SUBSTANCES CONTAINING POPPYSEEDS; MUST SUBMIT TO WITNESSED RANDOM BIOLOGICAL FLUID COLLECTION; MUST KEEP A LOG OF ANY AND ALL MEDICATIONS PRESCRIBED FOR HIM; SHALL SUBMIT TO ANY EXAMINATIONS OR THERAPY ORDERED BY BOARD; SHALL APPEAR BEFORE BOARD FOR INTERVIEWS UPON REQUEST; SHALL INFORM BOARD OF CHANGE OF ADDRESS OR IF AWAY FOR MORE THAN FIVE DAYS; ARIZONA, IN COMPLIANCE WITH THE AMERICANS WITH DISABILITIES ACT, PROCLAIMS THIS IS NOT A DISCIPLINARY ACTION BUT MERELY A MONITORING PROCEDURE WHICH DR. CRONISTER VOLUNTARILY ENTERED INTO; SHALL IMMEDIATELY OBTAIN A TREATING PSYCHIATRIST APPROVED BY THE BOARD AND SHALL REMAIN IN TREATMENT WITH THE PSYCHIATRIST UNTIL FURTHER ORDER OF THE BOARD WITH QUARTERLY REPORTS.

DELDEO, VITO RICHARD MD, LICENSE NUMBER 0007634, HAD ACTION TAKEN BY ARIZONA ON APRIL 10, 1992

NOTES: INVESTIGATION CONCERNING HIS ABILITY TO SAFELY PRACTICE; BOARD ORDERED PSYCHOLOGICAL AND PSYCHIATRIC EVALUATIONS. ORDER IS NOT DISCIPLINARY BUT PRECAUTIONED AND REHABILITATIVE. SHALL OBTAIN COUNSELING, AT HIS OWN EXPENSE, FROM A THERAPIST ACCEPTABLE TO THE BOARD WITH QUARTERLY REPORTS TO THE BOARD; SHALL OBTAIN A SOLE BOARD APPROVED TREATING PHYSICIAN; SHALL TAKE NO DRUGS OR MEDICATIONS WHATSOEVER UNLESS PRESCRIBED FOR HIM BY HIS TREATING PHYSICIAN; SHALL COMPLY WITH REQUESTS FROM THE BOARD TO SUBMIT TO WITNESSED RANDOM BIOLOGICAL FLUID COLLECTION. ON 4/23/93 THIS ORDER TERMINATED.

DESCH, MARY M MD, HAD ACTION TAKEN BY ARIZONA ON SEPTEMBER 26, 1997

NOTES: INTERVIEWED BY BOARD REGARDING HER TREATMENT FOR SUBSTANCE ABUSE AND PARTICIPATION IN THE MINNESOTA PROFESSIONAL RECOVERY ASSISTANCE PROGRAM. MUST IMMEDIATELY PARTICIPATE IN A BOARD-APPROVED MONITORED AFTERCARE TREATMENT PROGRAM WHOSE THERAPIST MUST SUBMIT MONTHLY REPORTS; MUST PARTICIPATE IN 90 12-STEP MEETINGS FOR SUBSTANCE ABUSE WITHIN 90 DAYS; MUST THEN PARTICIPATE IN A 12-STEP RECOVERY PROGRAM AS DETERMINED BY HER TREATING THERAPIST AND ATTEND AT LEAST THREE WEEKLY MEETINGS; SHALL OBTAIN A BOARD-APPROVED TREATING PHYSICIAN; SHALL ABSTAIN COMPLETELY FROM THE CONSUMPTION OF ALCOHOLIC BEVERAGES AND DRUGS EXCEPT WHEN PRESCRIBED BY HER TREATING PHYSICIAN; SHALL NOT CONSUME FOOD OR SUBSTANCES CONTAINING POPPYSEEDS; MUST SUBMIT TO WITNESSED RANDOM BIOLOGICAL FLUID COLLECTION; MUST KEEP A LOG OF ANY AND ALL MEDICATIONS PRESCRIBED FOR HER; SHALL SUBMIT TO ANY EXAMINATIONS OR THERAPY ORDERED BY BOARD; SHALL APPEAR BEFORE BOARD FOR INTERVIEWS UPON REQUEST; SHALL INFORM BOARD OF CHANGE OF ADDRESS OR IF AWAY FOR MORE THAN FIVE DAYS; ARIZONA, IN COMPLIANCE WITH THE AMERICANS WITH DISABILITIES ACT, PROCLAIMS THIS IS NOT A DISCIPLINARY ACTION BUT MERELY A MONITORING PROCEDURE WHICH SHE VOLUNTARILY ENTERED INTO; SHALL IMMEDIATELY OBTAIN A TREATING PSYCHIATRIST APPROVED BY THE BOARD AND SHALL REMAIN IN TREATMENT WITH THE PSYCHIATRIST UNTIL FURTHER ORDER OF THE BOARD WITH QUARTERLY REPORTS. ON 1/29/99 ORDER TERMINATED.

DIEHL, CRAIG D MD, LICENSE NUMBER 0016313, HAD ACTION TAKEN BY ARIZONA ON JULY 17, 1993

NOTES: MUST IMMEDIATELY PARTICIPATE IN A BOARD-APPROVED MONITORED AFTERCARE TREATMENT PROGRAM WHOSE THERAPIST MUST SUBMIT QUARTERLY REPORTS; MUST PARTICIPATE IN 90 12-STEP MEETINGS FOR SUBSTANCE ABUSE WITHIN 90 DAYS; MUST THEN PARTICIPATE IN A 12-STEP RECOVERY PROGRAM AS DETERMINED BY HIS TREATING THERAPIST AND ATTEND AT LEAST THREE WEEKLY MEETINGS; SHALL OBTAIN A BOARD-APPROVED TREATING PHYSICIAN; SHALL ABSTAIN COMPLETELY FROM THE CONSUMPTION OF ALCOHOLIC BEVERAGES AND DRUGS EXCEPT WHEN PRESCRIBED BY HIS TREATING PHYSICIAN; MUST SUBMIT TO WITNESSED RANDOM BIOLOGICAL FLUID COLLECTION; KEEP A LOG OF ANY AND ALL MEDICATIONS PRESCRIBED FOR HIM; SHALL SUBMIT TO ANY EXAMINATIONS OR THERAPY ORDERED BY BOARD; SHALL APPEAR BEFORE BOARD FOR INTERVIEWS UPON REQUEST; SHALL INFORM BOARD OF CHANGE OF ADDRESS OR IF AWAY FOR MORE THAN FIVE DAYS. ARIZONA, IN COMPLIANCE WITH THE AMERICANS WITH DISABILITIES ACT, PROCLAIMS THIS IS NOT A DISCIPLINARY ACTION BUT MERELY A MONITORING PROCEDURE WHICH HE VOLUNTARILY ENTERED INTO. ON 1/25/97 ORDER TERMINATED.

DRIES, CHARLES P JR MD, HAD ACTION TAKEN BY ARIZONA ON JANUARY 29, 1999

NOTES: MUST IMMEDIATELY PARTICIPATE IN A BOARD-APPROVED MONITORED AFTERCARE TREATMENT PROGRAM WHOSE THERAPIST MUST SUBMIT QUARTERLY REPORTS; MUST PARTICIPATE IN 90 12-STEP MEETINGS FOR SUBSTANCE ABUSE WITHIN 90 DAYS; MUST THEN PARTICIPATE IN A 12-STEP RECOVERY PROGRAM AS DETERMINED BY HIS/HER TREATING THERAPIST AND ATTEND AT LEAST THREE WEEKLY MEETINGS; SHALL OBTAIN A BOARD-APPROVED TREATING PHYSICIAN; SHALL ABSTAIN COMPLETELY FROM THE CONSUMPTION OF ALCOHOLIC BEVERAGES AND DRUGS EXCEPT WHEN PRESCRIBED BY HIS/HER TREATING PHYSICIAN; SHALL NOT CONSUME FOOD OR SUBSTANCES CONTAINING POPPYSEEDS; MUST SUBMIT TO WITNESSED RANDOM BIOLOGICAL FLUID COLLECTION; MUST KEEP A LOG OF ANY AND ALL MEDICATIONS PRESCRIBED FOR HIM/HER; SHALL SUBMIT TO ANY EXAMINATIONS OR THERAPY ORDERED BY BOARD; SHALL APPEAR BEFORE BOARD FOR INTERVIEWS UPON REQUEST; SHALL INFORM BOARD OF CHANGE OF ADDRESS OR IF AWAY FOR MORE THAN FIVE DAYS; ARIZONA, IN COMPLIANCE WITH THE AMERICANS WITH DISABILITIES ACT, PROCLAIMS THIS IS NOT A DISCIPLINARY ACTION BUT MERELY A MONITORING PROCEDURE WHICH HE VOLUNTARILY ENTERED INTO.

DURAN, ROBERT MD, LICENSE NUMBER 0018870, HAD ACTION TAKEN BY ARIZONA ON JULY 17, 1993

NOTES: RELATIVE TO PARTICIPATION IN AFTERCARE PROGRAM AND ACTION TAKEN BY TWO HOSPITALS REGARDING PRIVILEGES. MUST IMMEDIATELY PARTICIPATE IN A BOARD-APPROVED MONITORING AFTERCARE TREATMENT PROGRAM WHOSE THERAPIST MUST SUBMIT QUARTERLY REPORTS; MUST PARTICIPATE IN 90 12-STEP MEETINGS FOR SUBSTANCE ABUSE WITHIN 90 DAYS; MUST THEN PARTICIPATE IN A 12-STEP RECOVERY PROGRAM AS DETERMINED BY HIS TREATING PHYSICIAN AND ATTEND AT LEAST THREE WEEKLY MEETINGS; SHALL OBTAIN A BOARD-APPROVED SOLE TREATING PHYSICIAN; SHALL ABSTAIN COMPLETELY FROM THE CONSUMPTION OF ALCOHOLIC BEVERAGES AND DRUGS EXCEPT WHEN PRESCRIBED BY HIS TREATING PHYSICIAN; MUST SUBMIT TO WITNESSED RANDOM BIOLOGICAL FLUID COLLECTION; SHALL KEEP A LOG OF ANY AND ALL MEDICATIONS PRESCRIBED FOR HIM; SHALL SUBMIT TO ANY EXAMINATIONS OR THERAPY ORDERED BY BOARD; SHALL APPEAR BEFORE BOARD FOR INTERVIEWS UPON REQUEST; SHALL INFORM BOARD OF CHANGE OF ADDRESS OR IF AWAY FOR MORE THAN FIVE DAYS. ARIZONA, IN COMPLIANCE WITH THE AMERICANS WITH DISABILITIES ACT, PROCLAIMS THIS IS NOT A DISCIPLINARY ACTION BUT MERELY A MONITORING PROCEDURE WHICH HE VOLUNTARILY ENTERED INTO. ON 11/14/97 ORDER TERMINATED; SHALL PAY HIS OUTSTANDING MONITORED AFTERCARE FEES IN FULL ON OR BEFORE 2/12/98.

FELMUS, MARK T MD, LICENSE NUMBER 0010912, HAD ACTION TAKEN BY ARIZONA ON JANUARY 18, 1996

NOTES: MUST IMMEDIATELY PARTICIPATE IN A BOARD-APPROVED MONITORED AFTERCARE TREATMENT PROGRAM WHOSE THERAPIST MUST SUBMIT QUARTERLY REPORTS; MUST PARTICIPATE IN 90 12-STEP MEETINGS FOR SUBSTANCE ABUSE WITHIN 90 DAYS; MUST THEN PARTICIPATE IN A 12-STEP RECOVERY PROGRAM AS DETERMINED BY HIS TREATING THERAPIST AND ATTEND AT LEAST THREE WEEKLY MEETINGS; SHALL OBTAIN A BOARD-APPROVED TREATING PHYSICIAN; SHALL NOT CONSUMER ANY FOOD OR OTHER SUBSTANCE CONTAINING POPPY SEEDS; SHALL ABSTAIN COMPLETELY FROM THE CONSUMPTION OF ALCOHOLIC BEVERAGES AND DRUGS EXCEPT WHEN PRESCRIBED BY HIS TREATING PHYSICIAN; MUST SUBMIT TO WITNESSED RANDOM BIOLOGICAL FLUID COLLECTION; SHALL KEEP A LOG OF ANY AND ALL MEDICATIONS PRESCRIBED FOR HIM; SHALL SUBMIT TO ANY EXAMINATIONS OR THERAPY ORDERED BY BOARD; SHALL APPEAR BEFORE BOARD FOR INTERVIEWS UPON REQUEST; SHALL INFORM BOARD OF CHANGE OF ADDRESS OR IF AWAY FOR MORE THAN FIVE DAYS. IF HE DOES RESIDE IN ANOTHER STATE, SHALL PARTICIPATE IN THAT STATE'S PHYSICIAN REHABILITATION PROGRAM WITH REPORTS TO ARIZONA TWICE YEARLY; TIME SPENT OUT OF ARIZONA MAY BE TOLLED FOR THIS ORDER. THIS ORDER IS NOT A DISCIPLINARY ACTION BUT A VOLUNTARY MONITORING PROGRAM FOR REHABILITATION. ON 3/24/99 ORDER TERMINATED.

FELTER, JEFFREY S MD, LICENSE NUMBER 19572, HAD ACTION TAKEN BY ARIZONA ON JULY 26, 1997

NOTES: INTERVIEWED BY BOARD REGARDING TREATMENT FOR SUBSTANCE ABUSE. MUST IMMEDIATELY PARTICIPATE IN A BOARD-APPROVED MONITORED AFTERCARE TREATMENT PROGRAM WHOSE THERAPIST MUST SUBMIT QUARTERLY REPORTS; MUST PARTICIPATE IN 90 12-STEP MEETINGS FOR SUBSTANCE ABUSE WITHIN 90 DAYS; MUST THEN PARTICIPATE IN A 12-STEP RECOVERY PROGRAM AS DETERMINED BY HIS TREATING THERAPIST AND ATTEND AT LEAST THREE WEEKLY MEETINGS; SHALL OBTAIN A BOARD-APPROVED TREATING PHYSICIAN; SHALL ABSTAIN COMPLETELY FROM THE CONSUMPTION OF ALCOHOLIC BEVERAGES AND DRUGS EXCEPT WHEN PRESCRIBED BY HIS TREATING PHYSICIAN; SHALL NOT CONSUME FOOD OR SUBSTANCES CONTAINING POPPYSEEDS; MUST SUBMIT TO WITNESSED RANDOM BIOLOGICAL FLUID COLLECTION; MUST KEEP A LOG OF ANY AND ALL MEDICATIONS PRESCRIBED FOR HIM; SHALL SUBMIT TO ANY EXAMINATIONS OR THERAPY ORDERED BY BOARD; SHALL APPEAR BEFORE BOARD FOR INTERVIEWS UPON REQUEST; SHALL INFORM BOARD OF CHANGE OF ADDRESS OR IF AWAY FOR MORE THAN FIVE DAYS. ARIZONA, IN COMPLIANCE WITH THE AMERICANS WITH DISABILITIES ACT, PROCLAIMS THIS IS NOT A DISCIPLINARY ACTION BUT MERELY A MONITORING PROCEDURE WHICH HE VOLUNTARILY ENTERED INTO.

FOWLER, TIMOTHY J MD, LICENSE NUMBER 13001, HAD ACTION TAKEN BY ARIZONA ON JANUARY 23, 1998

NOTES: MUST IMMEDIATELY PARTICIPATE IN A BOARD-APPROVED MONITORED AFTERCARE TREATMENT PROGRAM WHOSE THERAPIST MUST SUBMIT MONTHLY REPORTS; MUST PARTICIPATE IN 90 12-STEP MEETINGS FOR SUBSTANCE ABUSE WITHIN 90 DAYS; MUST THEN PARTICIPATE IN A 12-STEP RECOVERY PROGRAM AS DETERMINED BY HIS TREATING THERAPIST AND ATTEND AT LEAST THREE WEEKLY MEETINGS; SHALL OBTAIN A BOARD-APPROVED TREATING PHYSICIAN; SHALL ABSTAIN COMPLETELY FROM THE CONSUMPTION OF ALCOHOLIC BEVERAGES AND DRUGS EXCEPT WHEN PRESCRIBED BY HIS TREATING PHYSICIAN; SHALL NOT CONSUME FOOD OR SUBSTANCES CONTAINING POPPYSEEDS; MUST SUBMIT TO WITNESSED RANDOM BIOLOGICAL FLUID COLLECTION; MUST KEEP A LOG OF ANY AND ALL MEDICATIONS PRESCRIBED FOR HIM;

SHALL SUBMIT TO ANY EXAMINATIONS OR THERAPY ORDERED BY BOARD; SHALL APPEAR BEFORE BOARD FOR INTERVIEWS UPON REQUEST; SHALL INFORM BOARD OF CHANGE OF ADDRESS OR IF AWAY FOR MORE THAN FIVE DAYS. ARIZONA, IN COMPLIANCE WITH THE AMERICANS WITH DISABILITIES ACT, PROCLAIMS THIS IS NOT A DISCIPLINARY ACTION BUT MERELY A MONITORING PROCEDURE WHICH HE VOLUNTARILY ENTERED INTO. THIS REHABILITATION ORDER SUPERSEDES ALL PREVIOUS SUCH ORDERS.

FOX, WILLIAM W MD, LICENSE NUMBER 6811, HAD ACTION TAKEN BY ARIZONA ON JULY 26, 1997

NOTES: MUST IMMEDIATELY PARTICIPATE IN A BOARD-APPROVED MONITORED AFTERCARE TREATMENT PROGRAM WHOSE THERAPIST MUST SUBMIT QUARTERLY REPORTS; MUST PARTICIPATE IN 90 12-STEP MEETINGS FOR SUBSTANCE ABUSE WITHIN 90 DAYS; MUST THEN PARTICIPATE IN A 12-STEP RECOVERY PROGRAM AS DETERMINED BY HIS TREATING THERAPIST AND ATTEND AT LEAST THREE WEEKLY MEETINGS; SHALL OBTAIN A BOARD-APPROVED TREATING PHYSICIAN; SHALL ABSTAIN COMPLETELY FROM THE CONSUMPTION OF ALCOHOLIC BEVERAGES AND DRUGS EXCEPT WHEN PRESCRIBED BY HIS TREATING PHYSICIAN; SHALL NOT CONSUME FOOD OR SUBSTANCES CONTAINING POPPYSEEDS; MUST SUBMIT TO WITNESSED RANDOM BIOLOGICAL FLUID COLLECTION; MUST KEEP A LOG OF ANY AND ALL MEDICATIONS PRESCRIBED FOR HIM; SHALL SUBMIT TO ANY EXAMINATIONS OR THERAPY ORDERED BY BOARD; SHALL APPEAR BEFORE BOARD FOR INTERVIEWS UPON REQUEST; ARIZONA, IN COMPLIANCE WITH THE AMERICANS WITH DISABILITIES ACT, PROCLAIMS THIS IS NOT A DISCIPLINARY ACTION BUT MERELY A MONITORING PROCEDURE WHICH HE VOLUNTARILY ENTERED INTO.

GARRETT, ROBERT LYNDEL MD, LICENSE NUMBER 0010927, HAD ACTION TAKEN BY ARIZONA ON APRIL 12, 1991

NOTES: VIOLATION OF BOARD ORDER DATED 10/24/88; ACTION BASED ON ENTERING INTO A REHABILITATION TREATMENT PROGRAM DUE TO RESUMED DRINKING OF ALCOHOLIC BEVERAGES. PROBATION ORDER ISSUED WITH FOLLOWING CONDITIONS: MUST IMMEDIATELY PARTICIPATE IN THE ARIZONA MEDICAL ASSOCIATION'S MONITORED AFTERCARE TREATMENT PROGRAM WHOSE THERAPIST MUST SUBMIT QUARTERLY REPORTS; SHALL PARTICIPATE IN 90 12-STEP MEETINGS APPROPRIATE FOR SUBSTANCE ABUSE AND ACCEPTABLE TO THE BOARD IN 90 DAYS FROM THE EFFECTIVE DATE OF THIS ORDER; SHALL THEN PARTICIPATE IN A 12-STEP RECOVERY PROGRAM AS DETERMINED BY HIS TREATING THERAPIST AND ATTEND AT LEAST THREE WEEKLY MEETINGS; SHALL OBTAIN A SOLE TREATING PHYSICIAN WHO SHALL BE APPROVED BY THE BOARD; SHALL ABSTAIN COMPLETELY FROM THE CONSUMPTION OF ALCOHOLIC BEVERAGES; SHALL TAKE NO DRUGS OR MEDICATIONS WHATEVER UNLESS PRESCRIBED FOR HIM BY HIS TREATING PHYSICIAN; SHALL SUBMIT TO RANDOM BIOLOGICAL FLUID TESTS; SHALL MAINTAIN A LOG OF ANY AND ALL MEDICATIONS PRESCRIBED FOR HIM BY HIS TREATING PHYSICIAN; SHALL SUBMIT TO ANY EXAMS OR THERAPY ORDERED BY THE BOARD; SHALL APPEAR BEFORE BOARD FOR INTERVIEWS UPON REQUEST AND INFORM THE BOARD IF HE'S AWAY FOR MORE THAN FIVE DAYS. ON 10/16/93 THIS ORDER TERMINATED. MUST IMMEDIATELY PARTICIPATE IN A BOARD-APPROVED MONITORED AFTERCARE TREATMENT PROGRAM WHOSE THERAPIST MUST SUBMIT QUARTERLY REPORTS; MUST THEN PARTICIPATE IN A 12-STEP RECOVERY PROGRAM AS DETERMINED BY HIS TREATING THERAPIST AND ATTEND AT LEAST THREE WEEKLY MEETINGS; SHALL OBTAIN A BOARD-APPROVED TREATING PHYSICIAN; SHALL ABSTAIN COMPLETELY FROM THE CONSUMPTION OF ALCOHOLIC BEVERAGES AND DRUGS EXCEPT WHEN PRESCRIBED BY HIS TREATING PHYSICIAN; MUST SUBMIT TO WITNESSED RANDOM BIOLOGICAL FLUID COLLECTION; KEEP A LOG OF ANY AND ALL MEDICATIONS PRESCRIBED FOR HIM; SHALL SUBMIT TO ANY EXAMINATIONS OR THERAPY ORDERED BY BOARD; SHALL APPEAR BEFORE BOARD FOR INTERVIEWS UPON REQUEST; SHALL INFORM BOARD OF CHANGE OF ADDRESS OR IF AWAY FOR MORE THAN 5 DAYS. ARIZONA, IN COMPLIANCE WITH THE AMERICANS WITH DISABILITIES ACT, PROCLAIMS THIS IS NOT A DISCIPLINARY ACTION BUT MERELY A MONITORING PROCEDURE WHICH HE VOLUNTARILY ENTERED INTO.

GERMAINE, RANDI M MD, LICENSE NUMBER 0021308 OF MESA, AZ, HAD ACTION TAKEN BY ARIZONA ON JULY 16, 1993

NOTES: MUST IMMEDIATELY PARTICIPATE IN A BOARD-APPROVED MONITORED AFTERCARE TREATMENT PROGRAM WHOSE THERAPIST MUST SUBMIT QUARTERLY REPORTS; MUST PARTICIPATE IN 90 12-STEP MEETINGS FOR SUBSTANCE ABUSE WITHIN 90 DAYS; MUST THEN PARTICIPATE IN A 12-STEP RECOVERY PROGRAM AS DETERMINED BY A TREATING THERAPIST AND ATTEND AT LEAST THREE WEEKLY MEETINGS; SHALL OBTAIN A BOARD-APPROVED TREATING PHYSICIAN; SHALL ABSTAIN COMPLETELY FROM THE CONSUMPTION OF ALCOHOLIC BEVERAGES AND DRUGS EXCEPT WHEN PRESCRIBED BY HIS TREATING PHYSICIAN; MUST SUBMIT TO WITNESSED RANDOM BIOLOGICAL FLUID COLLECTION; KEEP A LOG OF ANY AND ALL MEDICATIONS PRESCRIBED FOR HIM; SHALL SUBMIT TO ANY EXAMINATIONS OR THERAPY ORDERED BY BOARD; SHALL APPEAR BEFORE BOARD FOR INTERVIEWS UPON REQUEST; SHALL INFORM BOARD OF CHANGE OF ADDRESS OR IF AWAY FOR MORE THAN FIVE DAYS. ARIZONA, IN COMPLIANCE WITH THE AMERICANS WITH DISABILITIES ACT, PROCLAIMS THIS IS NOT A DISCIPLINARY ACTION BUT MERELY A MONITORING PROCEDURE WHICH SHE VOLUNTARILY ENTERED INTO. ON 5/15/98 ORDER TERMINATED.

GIERKE, KLAUS DETLEV MD, LICENSE NUMBER 0013305, HAD ACTION TAKEN BY ARIZONA ON OCTOBER 21, 1995

NOTES: INTERVIEWED BY BOARD REGARDING INFORMATION RECEIVED ALLEGING HE WAS ABUSING ALCOHOL. MUST IMMEDIATELY PARTICIPATE IN A BOARD-APPROVED MONITORED AFTERCARE TREATMENT PROGRAM WHOSE THERAPIST MUST SUBMIT QUARTERLY REPORTS; MUST PARTICIPATE IN 90 12-STEP MEETINGS FOR SUBSTANCE ABUSE WITHIN 90 DAYS; MUST THEN PARTICIPATE IN A 12-STEP RECOVERY PROGRAM AS DETERMINED BY HIS TREATING THERAPIST AND ATTEND AT LEAST THREE WEEKLY MEETINGS; SHALL OBTAIN A BOARD-APPROVED TREATING PHYSICIAN; SHALL ABSTAIN COMPLETELY FROM THE CONSUMPTION OF ALCOHOLIC BEVERAGES AND DRUGS EXCEPT WHEN PRESCRIBED BY HIS TREATING PHYSICIAN; MUST SUBMIT TO WITNESSED RANDOM BIOLOGICAL FLUID COLLECTION; MUST KEEP A LOG OF ANY AND ALL MEDICATIONS PRESCRIBED FOR HIM; SHALL SUBMIT TO ANY EXAMINATIONS OR THERAPY ORDERED BY BOARD; SHALL APPEAR BEFORE BOARD FOR INTERVIEWS UPON REQUEST; SHALL INFORM BOARD OF CHANGE OF ADDRESS OR IF AWAY FOR MORE THAN FIVE DAYS. ARIZONA, IN COMPLIANCE WITH THE AMERICANS WITH DISABILITIES ACT, PROCLAIMS THIS IS NOT A DISCIPLINARY ACTION BUT MERELY A

MONITORING PROCEDURE WHICH HE ENTERED INTO VOLUNTARILY.

GREENWOOD, FREDERICK MD, LICENSE NUMBER 0013827, HAD ACTION TAKEN BY ARIZONA ON JULY 20, 1992

NOTES: MUST IMMEDIATELY PARTICIPATE IN A BOARD-APPROVED MONITORED AFTERCARE TREATMENT PROGRAM WHOSE THERAPIST MUST SUBMIT QUARTERLY REPORTS; MUST PARTICIPATE IN 90 12-STEP MEETINGS FOR SUBSTANCE ABUSE WITHIN 90 DAYS; MUST THEN PARTICIPATE IN A 12-STEP RECOVERY PROGRAM AS DETERMINED BY HIS TREATING THERAPIST AND ATTEND AT LEAST 3 WEEKLY MEETINGS; SHALL OBTAIN A BOARD-APPROVED TREATING PHYSICIAN; SHALL ABSTAIN COMPLETELY FROM THE CONSUMPTION OF ALCOHOLIC BEVERAGES AND DRUGS EXCEPT WHEN PRESCRIBED BY HIS TREATING PHYSICIAN; MUST SUBMIT TO WITNESSED RANDOM BIOLOGICAL FLUID COLLECTION; KEEP A LOG OF ANY AND ALL MEDICATIONS PRESCRIBED FOR HIM; SHALL SUBMIT TO ANY EXAMINATIONS OR THERAPY ORDERED BY BOARD; SHALL APPEAR BEFORE BOARD FOR INTERVIEWS UPON REQUEST; SHALL INFORM BOARD OF CHANGE OF ADDRESS OR IF AWAY FOR MORE THAN 5 DAYS. ARIZONA, IN COMPLIANCE WITH THE AMERICANS WITH DISABILITIES ACT, PROCLAIMS THIS IS NOT A DISCIPLINARY ACTION BUT MERELY A MONITORING PROCEDURE WHICH HE VOLUNTARILY ENTERED INTO. AS OF 7/22/95 ORDER TO BE TERMINATED IN 90 DAYS.

HADE, RALPH DOUGLAS MD, LICENSE NUMBER 0018114, HAD ACTION TAKEN BY ARIZONA ON OCTOBER 19, 1994

NOTES: MUST IMMEDIATELY PARTICIPATE IN A BOARD-APPROVED MONITORED AFTERCARE TREATMENT PROGRAM WHOSE THERAPIST MUST SUBMIT QUARTERLY REPORTS; MUST PARTICIPATE IN 90 12-STEP MEETINGS FOR SUBSTANCE ABUSE WITHIN 90 DAYS; MUST THEN PARTICIPATE IN A 12-STEP RECOVERY PROGRAM AS DETERMINED BY HIS TREATING THERAPIST AND ATTEND AT LEAST THREE WEEKLY MEETINGS; SHALL OBTAIN A BOARD-APPROVED TREATING PHYSICIAN; SHALL ABSTAIN COMPLETELY FROM THE CONSUMPTION OF ALCOHOLIC BEVERAGES AND DRUGS EXCEPT WHEN PRESCRIBED BY HIS TREATING PHYSICIAN; MUST SUBMIT TO WITNESSED RANDOM BIOLOGICAL FLUID COLLECTION; KEEP A LOG OF ANY AND ALL MEDICATIONS PRESCRIBED FOR HIM; SHALL SUBMIT TO ANY EXAMINATIONS OR THERAPY ORDERED BY BOARD; SHALL APPEAR BEFORE BOARD FOR INTERVIEWS UPON REQUEST; SHALL INFORM BOARD OF CHANGE OF ADDRESS OR IF AWAY FOR MORE THAN FIVE DAYS. ARIZONA, IN COMPLIANCE WITH THE AMERICANS WITH DISABILITIES ACT, PROCLAIMS THIS IS NOT A DISCIPLINARY ACTION BUT MERELY A MONITORING PROCEDURE WHICH HE VOLUNTARILY ENTERED INTO.

HARPER, CHARLES R MD, LICENSE NUMBER 0003597, HAD ACTION TAKEN BY ARIZONA ON JANUARY 18, 1996

NOTES: ACTION IN GEORGIA. MUST IMMEDIATELY PARTICIPATE IN A BOARD-APPROVED MONITORED AFTERCARE TREATMENT PROGRAM WHOSE THERAPIST MUST SUBMIT QUARTERLY REPORTS; MUST PARTICIPATE IN 90 12-STEP MEETINGS FOR SUBSTANCE ABUSE WITHIN 90 DAYS; MUST THEN PARTICIPATE IN A 12-STEP RECOVERY PROGRAM AS DETERMINED BY HIS TREATING THERAPIST AND ATTEND AT LEAST THREE WEEKLY MEETINGS; SHALL OBTAIN A BOARD-APPROVED TREATING PHYSICIAN; SHALL ABSTAIN COMPLETELY FROM THE CONSUMPTION OF ALCOHOLIC BEVERAGES AND DRUGS EXCEPT WHEN PRESCRIBED BY HIS TREATING PHYSICIAN; SHALL NOT CONSUME ANY FOOD OR OTHER SUBSTANCE CONTAINING POPPYSEEDS; MUST SUBMIT TO WITNESSED RANDOM BIOLOGICAL FLUID COLLECTION; SHALL KEEP A LOG OF ANY AND ALL MEDICATIONS PRESCRIBED FOR HIM; SHALL SUBMIT TO ANY EXAMINATIONS OR THERAPY ORDERED BY THE BOARD; SHALL APPEAR BEFORE BOARD FOR INTERVIEWS UPON REQUEST; SHALL INFORM BOARD OF CHANGE OF ADDRESS OR IF AWAY FOR MORE THAN FIVE DAYS; IF HE DOES RESIDE IN ANOTHER STATE, SHALL PARTICIPATE IN THAT STATE'S PHYSICIAN REHABILITATION PROGRAM WITH REPORTS TO ARIZONA TWICE YEARLY; TIME SPENT OUT OF ARIZONA MAY BE TOLLED FOR THIS ORDER. THIS ORDER IS NOT A DISCIPLINARY ACTION BUT A VOLUNTARY MONITORING PROGRAM FOR REHABILITATION.

HEISLER, MARK W MD, LICENSE NUMBER 12212, HAD ACTION TAKEN BY ARIZONA ON JANUARY 25, 1997

NOTES: MUST IMMEDIATELY PARTICIPATE IN A BOARD-APPROVED MONITORED AFTERCARE TREATMENT PROGRAM WHOSE THERAPIST MUST SUBMIT QUARTERLY REPORTS; MUST PARTICIPATE IN 90 12-STEP MEETINGS FOR SUBSTANCE ABUSE WITHIN 90 DAYS; MUST THEN PARTICIPATE IN A 12-STEP RECOVERY PROGRAM AS DETERMINED BY HIS TREATING THERAPIST AND ATTEND AT LEAST THREE WEEKLY MEETINGS; SHALL OBTAIN A BOARD-APPROVED TREATING PHYSICIAN; SHALL ABSTAIN COMPLETELY FROM THE CONSUMPTION OF ALCOHOLIC BEVERAGES AND DRUGS EXCEPT WHEN PRESCRIBED BY HIS TREATING PHYSICIAN; SHALL NOT CONSUME FOOD OR SUBSTANCES CONTAINING POPPYSEEDS; MUST SUBMIT TO WITNESSED RANDOM BIOLOGICAL FLUID COLLECTION; MUST KEEP A LOG OF ANY AND ALL MEDICATIONS PRESCRIBED FOR HIM; SHALL SUBMIT TO ANY EXAMINATIONS OR THERAPY ORDERED BY BOARD; SHALL APPEAR BEFORE BOARD FOR INTERVIEWS UPON REQUEST; SHALL INFORM BOARD OF CHANGE OF ADDRESS OR IF AWAY FOR MORE THAN FIVE DAYS. ARIZONA, IN COMPLIANCE WITH THE AMERICANS WITH DISABILITIES ACT, PROCLAIMS THIS IS NOT A DISCIPLINARY ACTION BUT MERELY A MONITORING PROCEDURE WHICH HE VOLUNTARILY ENTERED INTO.

HERNANDEZ, JULIO MD, HAD ACTION TAKEN BY ARIZONA ON JANUARY 28, 1994

NOTES: MUST IMMEDIATELY PARTICIPATE IN A BOARD-APPROVED MONITORED AFTERCARE TREATMENT PROGRAM WHOSE THERAPIST MUST SUBMIT QUARTERLY REPORTS; MUST PARTICIPATE IN A 12-STEP RECOVERY PROGRAM AS DETERMINED BY HIS TREATING THERAPIST AND ATTEND AT LEAST THREE WEEKLY MEETINGS; SHALL OBTAIN A BOARD-APPROVED TREATING PHYSICIAN; SHALL ABSTAIN COMPLETELY FROM THE CONSUMPTION OF ALCOHOLIC BEVERAGES AND DRUGS EXCEPT WHEN PRESCRIBED BY HIS TREATING PHYSICIAN; MUST SUBMIT TO WITNESSED RANDOM BIOLOGICAL FLUID COLLECTION; KEEP A LOG OF ANY AND ALL MEDICATIONS PRESCRIBED FOR HIM; SHALL SUBMIT TO ANY EXAMINATIONS OR THERAPY ORDERED BY BOARD; SHALL APPEAR BEFORE BOARD FOR INTERVIEWS UPON REQUEST; SHALL INFORM BOARD OF CHANGE OF ADDRESS OR IF AWAY FOR MORE THAN FIVE DAYS. ARIZONA, IN COMPLIANCE WITH THE AMERICANS WITH DISABILITIES ACT, PROCLAIMS THIS IS NOT A DISCIPLINARY ACTION BUT MERELY A MONITORING PROCEDURE WHICH HE VOLUNTARILY

ENTERED INTO.

HERZER, FRED E III MD, LICENSE NUMBER 0016964, HAD ACTION TAKEN BY ARIZONA ON OCTOBER 18, 1996

NOTES: IN 8/94, PROBATION AND RESTRICTION OF HIS LICENSE TO ADMINISTER AND PRESCRIBE CONTROLLED SUBSTANCES BY UTAH FOR ABUSE OF OXYCODONE, A SCHEDULE II CONTROLLED SUBSTANCE AND ALCOHOL, BEGINNING IN 5/93; PRESCRIBED CONTROLLED SUBSTANCES TO TWO PEOPLE FOR HIS OWN USE. MUST IMMEDIATELY PARTICIPATE IN A BOARD-APPROVED MONITORED AFTERCARE TREATMENT PROGRAM WHOSE THERAPIST MUST SUBMIT QUARTERLY REPORTS; MUST PARTICIPATE IN 90 12-STEP MEETINGS FOR SUBSTANCE ABUSE WITHIN 90 DAYS; MUST THEN PARTICIPATE IN A 12-STEP RECOVERY PROGRAM AS DETERMINED BY HIS TREATING THERAPIST AND ATTEND AT LEAST THREE WEEKLY MEETINGS; SHALL OBTAIN A BOARD-APPROVED TREATING PHYSICIAN; SHALL ABSTAIN COMPLETELY FROM THE CONSUMPTION OF ALCOHOLIC BEVERAGES AND DRUGS EXCEPT WHEN PRESCRIBED BY HIS TREATING PHYSICIAN; SHALL NOT CONSUME ANY FOOD OR SUBSTANCE CONTAINING POPPYSEEDS; MUST SUBMIT TO WITNESSED RANDOM BIOLOGICAL FLUID COLLECTION; MUST KEEP A LOG OF ANY AND ALL MEDICATIONS PRESCRIBED FOR HIM; SHALL SUBMIT TO ANY EXAMINATIONS OR THERAPY ORDERED BY THE BOARD; SHALL APPEAR BEFORE BOARD FOR INTERVIEWS UPON REQUEST; SHALL INFORM BOARD OF CHANGE OF ADDRESS OR IF AWAY FOR MORE THAN FIVE DAYS. ARIZONA, IN COMPLIANCE WITH THE AMERICANS WITH DISABILITIES ACT, PROCLAIMS THIS IS NOT A DISCIPLINARY ACTION BUT MERELY A MONITORING PROCEDURE WHICH HE ENTERED INTO VOLUNTARILY. ON 11/19/99 ORDER TERMINATED.

HICKS, WILLIAM R MD, LICENSE NUMBER 0014516, HAD ACTION TAKEN BY ARIZONA ON APRIL 15, 1994

NOTES: INFORMATION RECEIVED THAT HE MAY HAVE A PROBLEM WITH ALCOHOL ABUSE. MUST IMMEDIATELY PARTICIPATE IN A BOARD-APPROVED MONITORED AFTERCARE TREATMENT PROGRAM WHOSE THERAPIST MUST SUBMIT QUARTERLY REPORTS; MUST PARTICIPATE IN 90 12-STEP MEETINGS FOR SUBSTANCE ABUSE WITHIN 90 DAYS; MUST THEN PARTICIPATE IN A 12-STEP RECOVERY PROGRAM AS DETERMINED BY HIS TREATING THERAPIST AND ATTEND AT LEAST THREE WEEKLY MEETINGS; SHALL OBTAIN A BOARD-APPROVED TREATING PHYSICIAN; SHALL ABSTAIN COMPLETELY FROM THE CONSUMPTION OF ALCOHOLIC BEVERAGES AND DRUGS EXCEPT WHEN PRESCRIBED BY HIS TREATING PHYSICIAN; MUST SUBMIT TO WITNESSED RANDOM BIOLOGICAL FLUID COLLECTION; KEEP A LOG OF ANY AND ALL MEDICATIONS PRESCRIBED FOR HIM; SHALL SUBMIT TO ANY EXAMINATIONS OR THERAPY ORDERED BY BOARD; SHALL APPEAR BEFORE BOARD FOR INTERVIEWS UPON REQUEST; SHALL INFORM BOARD OF CHANGE OF ADDRESS OR IF AWAY FOR MORE THAN FIVE DAYS. ARIZONA, IN COMPLIANCE WITH THE AMERICANS WITH DISABILITIES ACT, PROCLAIMS THIS IS NOT A DISCIPLINARY ACTION BUT MERELY A MONITORING PROCEDURE WHICH HE VOLUNTARILY ENTERED INTO.

HILDING, RONALD MD, LICENSE NUMBER 0006043, HAD ACTION TAKEN BY ARIZONA ON OCTOBER 15, 1993

NOTES: LICENSE REACTIVATED ON CONDITIONS: SHALL CONTINUE IN THERAPY WITH A THERAPIST APPROVED BY BOARD WITH QUARTERLY REPORTS TO THE BOARD; THE BOARD OR ITS REPRESENTATIVE SHALL CONDUCT A QUARTERLY REVIEW OF HIS CLINICAL CHARTS FOR ONE YEAR IN COMPLIANCE WITH THE FEDERAL AMERICANS WITH DISABILITIES ACT THIS ORDER IS NOT CONSIDERED A DISCIPLINARY ACTION.

HILDING, RONALD MD, LICENSE NUMBER 0006043, HAD ACTION TAKEN BY ARIZONA ON JANUARY 17, 1996

NOTES: WITHIN NINE MONTHS, SHALL COMPLETE 20 HOURS OF CONTINUING MEDICAL EDUCATION IN THE SUBJECT OF PRESCRIBING PSYCHOACTIVE SUBSTANCES AND SHALL SUBMIT SATISFACTORY EVIDENCE OF COMPLETION TO THE BOARD; WITHIN 60 DAYS, SHALL HAVE A BOARD-APPROVED PRACTICE MANAGEMENT CONSULTANT REVIEW AND PROVIDE RECOMMENDATIONS REGARDING HIS PROCEDURES FOR OFFICE MANAGEMENT AND RECORD KEEPING. IN COMPLIANCE WITH THE AMERICANS WITH DISABILITIES ACT, THE ORDER IS NOT CONSIDERED A DISCIPLINARY ACTION. ON 7/25/97 ORDER TERMINATED AS HE COMPLIED WITH CONDITIONS.

HOLTORF, KENT A MD, LICENSE NUMBER 0024704, HAD ACTION TAKEN BY ARIZONA ON OCTOBER 19, 1996

NOTES: MUST IMMEDIATELY PARTICIPATE IN A BOARD-APPROVED MONITORED AFTERCARE TREATMENT PROGRAM WHOSE THERAPIST MUST SUBMIT QUARTERLY REPORTS; MUST PARTICIPATE IN 90 12-STEP MEETINGS FOR SUBSTANCE ABUSE WITHIN 90 DAYS; MUST THEN PARTICIPATE IN A 12-STEP RECOVERY PROGRAM AS DETERMINED BY HIS TREATING THERAPIST AND ATTEND AT LEAST THREE WEEKLY MEETINGS; SHALL OBTAIN A BOARD-APPROVED TREATING PHYSICIAN; SHALL ABSTAIN COMPLETELY FROM THE CONSUMPTION OF ALCOHOLIC BEVERAGES AND DRUGS EXCEPT WHEN PRESCRIBED BY HIS TREATING PHYSICIAN; SHALL NOT CONSUME FOOD OR SUBSTANCES CONTAINING POPPYSEEDS; MUST SUBMIT TO WITNESSED RANDOM BIOLOGICAL FLUID COLLECTION; MUST KEEP A LOG OF ANY AND ALL MEDICATIONS PRESCRIBED FOR HIM; SHALL SUBMIT TO ANY EXAMINATIONS OR THERAPY ORDERED BY THE BOARD; SHALL APPEAR BEFORE BOARD FOR INTERVIEWS UPON REQUEST; SHALL INFORM BOARD OF CHANGE OF ADDRESS OR IF AWAY FOR MORE THAN FIVE DAYS; IF HE DOES RESIDE IN ANOTHER STATE, SHALL PARTICIPATE IN THAT STATE'S PHYSICIAN REHABILITATION PROGRAM WITH REPORTS TO ARIZONA TWICE YEARLY; TIME SPENT OUT OF ARIZONA MAY BE TOLLED FOR THIS ORDER. ARIZONA, IN COMPLIANCE WITH THE AMERICANS WITH DISABILITIES ACT, PROCLAIMS THIS IS NOT A DISCIPLINARY ACTION BUT MERELY A MONITORING PROCEDURE WHICH HE ENTERED INTO VOLUNTARILY.

JEAL, DAVID E MD, HAD ACTION TAKEN BY ARIZONA ON MARCH 24, 1999

NOTES: MUST IMMEDIATELY PARTICIPATE IN A BOARD-APPROVED MONITORED AFTERCARE TREATMENT PROGRAM WHOSE THERAPIST MUST SUBMIT QUARTERLY REPORTS; MUST PARTICIPATE IN 90 12-STEP MEETINGS FOR SUBSTANCE ABUSE WITHIN 90 DAYS; MUST THEN PARTICIPATE IN A 12-STEP RECOVERY PROGRAM AS DETERMINED BY HIS/HER TREATING THERAPIST AND ATTEND AT LEAST THREE WEEKLY MEETINGS; SHALL OBTAIN A BOARD-APPROVED TREATING PHYSICIAN; SHALL ABSTAIN COMPLETELY FROM THE CONSUMPTION OF ALCOHOLIC BEVERAGES AND DRUGS EXCEPT WHEN PRESCRIBED BY HIS/HER TREATING PHYSICIAN; SHALL NOT CONSUME FOOD OR SUBSTANCES

CONTAINING POPPYSEEDS; MUST SUBMIT TO WITNESSED RANDOM BIOLOGICAL FLUID COLLECTION; MUST KEEP A LOG OF ANY AND ALL MEDICATIONS PRESCRIBED FOR HIM/HER; SHALL SUBMIT TO ANY EXAMINATIONS OR THERAPY ORDERED BY BOARD; SHALL APPEAR BEFORE BOARD FOR INTERVIEWS UPON REQUEST; SHALL INFORM BOARD OF CHANGE OF ADDRESS OR IF AWAY FOR MORE THAN FIVE DAYS; ARIZONA, IN COMPLIANCE WITH THE AMERICANS WITH DISABILITIES ACT, PROCLAIMS THIS IS NOT A DISCIPLINARY ACTION BUT MERELY A MONITORING PROCEDURE WHICH HE VOLUNTARILY ENTERED INTO.

JOHNSON, BRENT E MD, LICENSE NUMBER 0020366 OF PHOENIX, AZ, HAD ACTION TAKEN BY ARIZONA ON JULY 15, 1993

NOTES: ALLEGATIONS THAT HE IS BEING TREATED FOR CHEMICAL DEPENDENCY; ACTIONS TAKEN AGAINST PRIVILEGES AT YAVAPAI REGIONAL MEDICAL CENTER. MUST IMMEDIATELY PARTICIPATE IN A BOARD-APPROVED MONITORED AFTERCARE TREATMENT PROGRAM WHOSE THERAPIST MUST SUBMIT QUARTERLY REPORTS; MUST PARTICIPATE IN 90 12-STEP MEETINGS FOR SUBSTANCE ABUSE WITHIN 90 DAYS; MUST THEN PARTICIPATE IN A 12-STEP RECOVERY PROGRAM AS DETERMINED BY HIS TREATING THERAPIST AND ATTEND AT LEAST THREE WEEKLY MEETINGS; SHALL OBTAIN A BOARD-APPROVED TREATING PHYSICIAN; SHALL ABSTAIN COMPLETELY FROM THE CONSUMPTION OF ALCOHOLIC BEVERAGES AND DRUGS EXCEPT WHEN PRESCRIBED BY HIS TREATING PHYSICIAN; MUST SUBMIT TO WITNESSED RANDOM BIOLOGICAL FLUID COLLECTION; KEEP A LOG OF ANY AND ALL MEDICATIONS PRESCRIBED FOR HIM; SHALL SUBMIT TO ANY EXAMINATIONS OR THERAPY ORDERED BY BOARD; SHALL APPEAR BEFORE BOARD FOR INTERVIEWS UPON REQUEST; SHALL INFORM BOARD OF CHANGE OF ADDRESS OR IF AWAY FOR MORE THAN FIVE DAYS. ARIZONA, IN COMPLIANCE WITH THE AMERICANS WITH DISABILITIES ACT, PROCLAIMS THIS IS NOT A DISCIPLINARY ACTION BUT MERELY A MONITORING PROCEDURE WHICH HE VOLUNTARILY ENTERED INTO. ON 7/26/97 ORDER TERMINATED EFFECTIVE IN 90 DAYS.

JOHNSON, PETER C MD, LICENSE NUMBER 0008760, HAD ACTION TAKEN BY ARIZONA ON OCTOBER 19, 1996

NOTES: MUST IMMEDIATELY PARTICIPATE IN A BOARD-APPROVED MONITORED AFTERCARE TREATMENT PROGRAM WHOSE THERAPIST MUST SUBMIT QUARTERLY REPORTS; MUST PARTICIPATE IN 90 12-STEP MEETINGS FOR SUBSTANCE ABUSE WITHIN 90 DAYS; MUST THEN PARTICIPATE IN A 12-STEP RECOVERY PROGRAM AS DETERMINED BY HIS TREATING THERAPIST AND ATTEND AT LEAST THREE WEEKLY MEETINGS; SHALL OBTAIN A BOARD-APPROVED TREATING PHYSICIAN; SHALL ABSTAIN COMPLETELY FROM THE CONSUMPTION OF ALCOHOLIC BEVERAGES AND DRUGS EXCEPT WHEN PRESCRIBED BY HIS TREATING PHYSICIAN; SHALL NOT CONSUME FOOD OR SUBSTANCES CONTAINING POPPYSEEDS; MUST SUBMIT TO WITNESSED RANDOM BIOLOGICAL FLUID COLLECTION; MUST KEEP A LOG OF ANY AND ALL MEDICATIONS PRESCRIBED FOR HIM; SHALL SUBMIT TO ANY EXAMINATIONS OR THERAPY ORDERED BY THE BOARD; SHALL APPEAR BEFORE BOARD FOR INTERVIEWS UPON REQUEST; SHALL INFORM BOARD OF CHANGE OF ADDRESS OR IF AWAY FOR MORE THAN FIVE DAYS; IF HE DOES RESIDE IN ANOTHER STATE, SHALL PARTICIPATE IN THAT STATE'S PHYSICIAN REHABILITATION PROGRAM WITH REPORTS TO ARIZONA TWICE YEARLY; TIME SPENT OUT OF ARIZONA MAY BE TOLLED FOR THIS ORDER. ARIZONA, IN COMPLIANCE WITH THE AMERICANS WITH DISABILITIES ACT, PROCLAIMS THIS IS NOT A DISCIPLINARY ACTION BUT MERELY A MONITORING PROCEDURE WHICH HE ENTERED INTO VOLUNTARILY. IN 5/98 THE BOARD CONFIRMED THAT HIS FIRST AMENDMENT TO REHABILITATION STIPULATION ON 11/14/97 IS VALID WITHOUT SIGNATURE; HE VERBALLY AGREED TO THE FIRST AMENDMENT DURING AN INFORMAL INTERVIEW. ON 11/14/97 ORDER AMENDED ALLOWING NO MORE THAN SEVEN EXCUSED URINE COLLECTIONS AND NO MORE THAN SEVEN MISSED GROUP MEETINGS WITHIN A 12-MONTH CALENDAR PERIOD BEGINNING 11/14/97.

JOHNSON, ROBERT K JR MD, LICENSE NUMBER 0022407, HAD ACTION TAKEN BY ARIZONA ON JULY 17, 1996

NOTES: INTERVIEWED BY THE BOARD REGARDING HIS PSYCHIATRIC EVALUATION AND INFORMATION THE BOARD RECEIVED ALLEGING THAT HE ORDERED LARGE AMOUNTS OF CONTROLLED SUBSTANCES AND HAD THEM DELIVERED TO HIS HOME. SHALL OBTAIN A BOARD-APPROVED TREATING THERAPIST WHO SHALL SUBMIT QUARTERLY REPORTS; SHALL NOT CONSUME ANY FOOD OR ANY SUBSTANCE CONTAINING POPPYSEEDS; SHALL ABSTAIN COMPLETELY FROM THE CONSUMPTION OF ALCOHOL OR DRUGS EXCEPT WHEN PRESCRIBED BY HIS TREATING PHYSICIAN; MUST SUBMIT TO WITNESSED RANDOM BIOLOGICAL FLUID COLLECTION; MUST KEEP A LOG OF ANY AND ALL MEDICATIONS PRESCRIBED FOR HIM; SHALL APPEAR BEFORE BOARD FOR INTERVIEWS UPON REQUEST; SHALL INFORM BOARD OF CHANGE OF ADDRESS OR IF AWAY FOR MORE THAN FIVE DAYS. ARIZONA, IN COMPLIANCE WITH THE AMERICANS WITH DISABILITIES ACT, PROCLAIMS THIS IS NOT A DISCIPLINARY ACTION BUT MERELY A MONITORING PROCEDURE WHICH HE ENTERED INTO VOLUNTARILY. ON 5/7/97 ORDER AMENDED AND SEVERAL CONDITIONS DELETED. ON 3/26/98 ORDER TERMINATED.

KANAS, RONNIE J MD, LICENSE NUMBER 22902, HAD ACTION TAKEN BY ARIZONA ON JULY 30, 1999

NOTES: LICENSE REACTIVATED WITH STIPULATED REHABILITATION AGREEMENT. UST IMMEDIATELY PARTICIPATE IN A BOARD-APPROVED MONITORED AFTERCARE TREATMENT PROGRAM WHOSE THERAPIST MUST SUBMIT QUARTERLY REPORTS; MUST PARTICIPATE IN 90 12-STEP MEETINGS FOR SUBSTANCE ABUSE WITHIN 90 DAYS; MUST THEN PARTICIPATE IN A 12-STEP RECOVERY PROGRAM AS DETERMINED BY HIS/HER TREATING THERAPIST AND ATTEND AT LEAST THREE WEEKLY MEETINGS; SHALL OBTAIN A BOARD-APPROVED TREATING PHYSICIAN; SHALL ABSTAIN COMPLETELY FROM THE CONSUMPTION OF ALCOHOLIC BEVERAGES AND DRUGS EXCEPT WHEN PRESCRIBED BY HIS/HER TREATING PHYSICIAN; SHALL NOT CONSUME FOOD OR SUBSTANCES CONTAINING POPPYSEEDS; MUST SUBMIT TO WITNESSED RANDOM BIOLOGICAL FLUID COLLECTION; MUST KEEP A LOG OF ANY AND ALL MEDICATIONS PRESCRIBED FOR HIM/HER; SHALL SUBMIT TO ANY EXAMINATIONS OR THERAPY ORDERED BY BOARD; SHALL APPEAR BEFORE BOARD FOR INTERVIEWS UPON REQUEST; SHALL INFORM BOARD OF CHANGE OF ADDRESS OR IF AWAY FOR MORE THAN FIVE DAYS. ARIZONA, IN COMPLIANCE WITH THE AMERICANS WITH DISABILITIES ACT, PROCLAIMS THIS IS NOT A DISCIPLINARY ACTION BUT MERELY A MONITORING PROCEDURE WHICH HE VOLUNTARILY ENTERED INTO.

KASA, ROBERT FRANCIS MD, LICENSE NUMBER 0014790, HAD

ACTION TAKEN BY ARIZONA ON FEBRUARY 15, 1996

NOTES: MUST IMMEDIATELY PARTICIPATE IN A BOARD-APPROVED MONITORED AFTERCARE TREATMENT PROGRAM WHOSE THERAPIST MUST SUBMIT QUARTERLY REPORTS; MUST PARTICIPATE IN 90 12-STEP MEETINGS FOR SUBSTANCE ABUSE WITHIN 90 DAYS; MUST THEN PARTICIPATE IN A 12-STEP RECOVERY PROGRAM AS DETERMINED BY HIS TREATING THERAPIST AND ATTEND AT LEAST THREE WEEKLY MEETINGS; SHALL OBTAIN A BOARD-APPROVED TREATING PHYSICIAN; SHALL NOT CONSUME ANY FOOD OR OTHER SUBSTANCES CONTAINING POPPYSEEDS; SHALL ABSTAIN COMPLETELY FROM THE CONSUMPTION OF ALCOHOLIC BEVERAGES AND DRUGS EXCEPT WHEN PRESCRIBED BY HIS TREATING PHYSICIAN; MUST SUBMIT TO WITNESSED RANDOM BIOLOGICAL FLUID COLLECTION; MUST KEEP A LOG OF ANY AND ALL MEDICATIONS PRESCRIBED FOR HIM; SHALL SUBMIT TO ANY EXAMINATIONS OR THERAPY ORDERED BY BOARD; SHALL APPEAR BEFORE BOARD FOR INTERVIEWS UPON REQUEST; SHALL INFORM BOARD OF CHANGE OF ADDRESS OR IF AWAY FOR MORE THAN FIVE DAYS. IF HE DOES RESIDE IN ANOTHER STATE, SHALL PARTICIPATE IN THAT STATE'S PHYSICIAN REHABILITATION PROGRAM WITH REPORTS TO ARIZONA TWICE YEARLY; TIME SPENT OUT OF ARIZONA MAY BE TOLLED FOR THIS ORDER. HE AGREED TO THE TERMS OF THE STIPULATION AND NOT PERFORMING SURGERY WAS ADDED TO HIS LIST OF CONDITIONS. THIS IS NOT A DISCIPLINARY ACTION BUT MERELY A MONITORING PROCEDURE WHICH HE VOLUNTARILY ENTERED INTO. HE ALSO AGREED IN A SEPARATE ORDER NOT TO PERFORM SURGERY.

KAST, JOHN M MD, LICENSE NUMBER 0023805, HAD ACTION TAKEN BY ARIZONA ON JANUARY 16, 1996

NOTES: IN 10/91, SIGNED A TREATMENT PROGRAM AGREEMENT WITH A PHYSICIAN HEALTH COMMITTEE FOR A TREATMENT CONTRACT FROM 10/91 UNTIL 9/96; IN 12/91, COMPLETED A 28-DAY REHABILITATION PROGRAM FOR CHEMICAL DEPENDENCY IN NEW HAMPSHIRE; SUSPENDED FROM HIS CLINICAL TRAINING PROGRAM IN NEUROSURGERY IN WASHINGTON, D.C. FROM 7/91 THROUGH 6/30/92 AND IN 5/93, WAS LICENSED TO PRACTICE MEDICINE IN THE DISTRICT OF COLUMBIA; ADMITTED USING DARVOCET, TYLENOL #3, IV DRUGS, DEMEROL AND OCCASIONALLY DILAUDID; ON 7/21/95, HE APPEARED BEFORE BOARD FOR AN APPLICATION INTERVIEW, AT WHICH TIME HE ADMITTED SIGNING HIS OWN NAME AND OTHER PHYSICIANS' NAMES TO PRESCRIPTIONS FOR CONTROLLED SUBSTANCES WHICH HE AND WIFE USED; ON 12/20/95, ENTERED A PLEA OF GUILTY WITH THE GOVERNMENT TO FIVE COUNTS OF SIMPLE POSSESSION OF A CONTROLLED SUBSTANCE. PROBATION WITH TERMS: SHALL PERFORM 150 HOURS OF BOARD-APPROVED COMMUNITY SERVICE EACH YEAR DURING PROBATION, FOR WHICH HE SHALL SUBMIT EVIDENCE OF COMPLETION EACH YEAR. SHALL ENTER THE FOLLOWING MONITORING CONTRACT WHICH ARIZONA PROCLAIMS, IN COMPLIANCE WITH THE AMERICANS WITH DISABILITIES ACT, IS NOT A DISCIPLINARY ACTION BUT MERELY A MONITORING PROCEDURE WHICH HE ENTERED INTO VOLUNTARILY. MUST IMMEDIATELY PARTICIPATE IN A BOARD-APPROVED MONITORED AFTERCARE TREATMENT PROGRAM WHOSE THERAPIST MUST SUBMIT QUARTERLY REPORTS; MUST PARTICIPATE IN A 12-STEP RECOVERY PROGRAM AS DETERMINED BY HIS TREATING THERAPIST AND ATTEND AT LEAST THREE WEEKLY MEETINGS; SHALL OBTAIN A BOARD- APPROVED TREATING PHYSICIAN; SHALL ABSTAIN FROM THE CONSUMPTION OF FOOD OR OTHER SUBSTANCES CONTAINING POPPYSEEDS; SHALL ABSTAIN COMPLETELY FROM THE CONSUMPTION OF ALCOHOLIC BEVERAGES AND DRUGS EXCEPT WHEN PRESCRIBED BY HIS TREATING PHYSICIAN; MUST SUBMIT TO WITNESSED RANDOM BIOLOGICAL FLUID COLLECTION; MUST KEEP A LOG OF ANY AND ALL MEDICATIONS PRESCRIBED FOR HIM; SHALL SUBMIT TO ANY EXAMINATIONS OR THERAPY ORDERED BY THE BOARD; SHALL APPEAR BEFORE THE BOARD FOR INTERVIEWS UPON REQUEST; SHALL INFORM BOARD OF CHANGE OF ADDRESS OR IF AWAY FOR MORE THAN FIVE DAYS; IF HE DOES RESIDE IN ANOTHER STATE, SHALL PARTICIPATE IN THAT STATE'S PHYSICIAN REHABILITATION PROGRAM WITH REPORTS TO ARIZONA TWICE YEARLY; TIME SPENT OUT OF ARIZONA MAY BE TOLLED FOR THIS ORDER. ON 3/15/97 ORDER AMENDED: SHALL IMMEDIATELY PARTICIPATE IN THE BOARD-APPROVED AND SPONSORED AFTERCARE TREATMENT PROGRAM; SHALL MEET WITH THE AFTERCARE COMMITTEE IN 9/97. ON 3/24/99 ORDER TERMINATED.

KENNEDY, JAMES J MD, LICENSE NUMBER 9790, HAD ACTION TAKEN BY ARIZONA ON MAY 9, 1997

NOTES: INTERVIEWED BY THE BOARD REGARDING HIS TREATMENT FOR SUBSTANCE ABUSE. MUST IMMEDIATELY PARTICIPATE IN A BOARD-APPROVED MONITORED AFTERCARE TREATMENT PROGRAM WHOSE THERAPIST MUST SUBMIT QUARTERLY REPORTS; MUST PARTICIPATE IN 90 12-STEP MEETINGS FOR SUBSTANCE ABUSE WITHIN 90 DAYS; MUST THEN PARTICIPATE IN A 12-STEP RECOVERY PROGRAM AS DETERMINED BY HIS TREATING THERAPIST AND ATTEND AT LEAST THREE WEEKLY MEETINGS; SHALL OBTAIN A BOARD-APPROVED TREATING PHYSICIAN; SHALL ABSTAIN COMPLETELY FROM THE CONSUMPTION OF ALCOHOLIC BEVERAGES AND DRUGS EXCEPT WHEN PRESCRIBED BY HIS TREATING PHYSICIAN; SHALL NOT CONSUME FOOD OR SUBSTANCES CONTAINING POPPYSEEDS; MUST SUBMIT TO WITNESSED RANDOM BIOLOGICAL FLUID COLLECTION; MUST KEEP A LOG OF ANY AND ALL MEDICATIONS PRESCRIBED FOR HIM; SHALL SUBMIT TO ANY EXAMINATIONS OR THERAPY ORDERED BY BOARD; SHALL APPEAR BEFORE BOARD FOR INTERVIEWS UPON REQUEST; SHALL INFORM BOARD OF CHANGE OF ADDRESS OR IF AWAY FOR MORE THAN FIVE DAYS; ARIZONA, IN COMPLIANCE WITH THE AMERICANS WITH DISABILITIES ACT, PROCLAIMS THIS IS NOT A DISCIPLINARY ACTION BUT MERELY A MONITORING PROCEDURE WHICH HE VOLUNTARILY ENTERED INTO; SHALL IMMEDIATELY OBTAIN A TREATING PSYCHIATRIST APPROVED BY THE BOARD AND SHALL REMAIN IN TREATMENT WITH THE PSYCHIATRIST UNTIL FURTHER ORDER OF THE BOARD WITH QUARTERLY REPORTS. ON 7/30/99 AGREEMENT WAS MODIFIED.

KOENEN, H PETER JR MD, LICENSE NUMBER 0020165, HAD ACTION TAKEN BY ARIZONA ON JULY 15, 1993

NOTES: HAS BEEN PRESCRIBING PRESCRIPTION-ONLY MEDICATIONS WITHOUT PERFORMING EVALUATIONS AND DOCUMENTATION OF WHY THE PRESCRIPTIONS WERE WRITTEN. SHALL NOT PRESCRIBE OR ORDER REFILL OF ANY PRESCRIPTION FOR ANY PRESCRIPTION-ONLY MEDICATION OR CONTROLLED SUBSTANCE WITHOUT FIRST PERFORMING AN EVALUATION OF THE PATIENT AND THE PATIENT'S NEED FOR THE MEDICATION WHICH SHALL BE FULLY DOCUMENTED IN THE PATIENT'S MEDICAL RECORD; SHALL RETAIN THE MEDICAL RECORDS FOR AN INDEFINITE PERIOD AND SHALL MAKE THEM AVAILABLE TO THE BOARD UPON REQUEST; SHALL

NOT PRESCRIBE, ADMINISTER, OR DISPENSE CONTROLLED SUBSTANCES TO HIMSELF, ANY MEMBER OF HIS FAMILY, ANY SIGNIFICANT OTHER OR MEMBER OF HIS HOUSEHOLD; SHALL IMMEDIATELY ENGAGE IN THERAPY WITH A PSYCHOLOGIST OR PSYCHIATRIST ACCEPTABLE TO THE BOARD, AND SHALL INSTRUCT SUCH PERSON TO SUBMIT REPORTS TO THE BOARD ON A QUARTERLY BASIS, OR MORE FREQUENTLY AS THE BOARD MAY REQUEST; SHALL SUBMIT HIMSELF AND HIS PRACTICE OF MEDICINE TO REVIEWS BY A MEDICAL CONSULTANT CHOSEN BY THE BOARD; LICENSE WILL BE ALLOWED TO EXPIRE FOR NONPAYMENT. IN COMPLIANCE WITH THE AMERICANS WITH DISABILITIES ACT, THIS ORDER IS NOT CONSIDERED A DISCIPLINARY ACTION. ON 10/19/94 REQUEST FOR RECONSIDERATION DENIED.

LAFLEUR, MELANIE KOHOUT MD, LICENSE NUMBER 0020339, HAD ACTION TAKEN BY ARIZONA ON JULY 17, 1993

NOTES: MUST IMMEDIATELY PARTICIPATE IN A BOARD-APPROVED MONITORED AFTERCARE TREATMENT PROGRAM WHOSE THERAPIST MUST SUBMIT QUARTERLY REPORTS; MUST PARTICIPATE IN 90 12-STEP MEETINGS FOR SUBSTANCE ABUSE WITHIN 90 DAYS; MUST THEN PARTICIPATE IN A 12-STEP RECOVERY PROGRAM AS DETERMINED BY HER TREATING THERAPIST AND ATTEND AT LEAST THREE WEEKLY MEETINGS; SHALL OBTAIN A BOARD-APPROVED TREATING PHYSICIAN; SHALL ABSTAIN COMPLETELY FROM THE CONSUMPTION OF ALCOHOLIC BEVERAGES AND DRUGS EXCEPT WHEN PRESCRIBED BY HER TREATING PHYSICIAN; MUST SUBMIT TO WITNESSED RANDOM BIOLOGICAL FLUID COLLECTION; KEEP A LOG OF ANY AND ALL MEDICATIONS PRESCRIBED FOR HER; SHALL SUBMIT TO ANY EXAMINATIONS OR THERAPY ORDERED BY BOARD; SHALL APPEAR BEFORE BOARD FOR INTERVIEWS UPON REQUEST; SHALL INFORM BOARD OF CHANGE OF ADDRESS OR IF AWAY FOR MORE THAN FIVE DAYS. ARIZONA, IN COMPLIANCE WITH THE AMERICANS WITH DISABILITIES ACT, PROCLAIMS THIS IS NOT A DISCIPLINARY ACTION BUT MERELY A MONITORING PROCEDURE WHICH SHE VOLUNTARILY ENTERED INTO. ON 3/15/97 ORDER TERMINATED EFFECTIVE IN 90 DAYS.

LEVISON, JEFFREY A MD, LICENSE NUMBER 0020369, HAD ACTION TAKEN BY ARIZONA ON JULY 15, 1994

NOTES: MUST IMMEDIATELY PARTICIPATE IN A BOARD-APPROVED MONITORED AFTERCARE TREATMENT PROGRAM WHOSE THERAPIST MUST SUBMIT QUARTERLY REPORTS; MUST PARTICIPATE IN 90 12-STEP MEETINGS FOR SUBSTANCE ABUSE WITHIN 90 DAYS; MUST THEN PARTICIPATE IN A 12-STEP RECOVERY PROGRAM AS DETERMINED BY HIS TREATING THERAPIST AND ATTEND AT LEAST THREE WEEKLY MEETINGS; SHALL OBTAIN A BOARD-APPROVED TREATING PHYSICIAN; SHALL ABSTAIN COMPLETELY FROM THE CONSUMPTION OF ALCOHOLIC BEVERAGES AND DRUGS EXCEPT WHEN PRESCRIBED BY HIS TREATING PHYSICIAN; MUST SUBMIT TO WITNESSED RANDOM BIOLOGICAL FLUID COLLECTION; KEEP A LOG OF ANY AND ALL MEDICATIONS PRESCRIBED FOR HIM; SHALL SUBMIT TO ANY EXAMINATIONS OR THERAPY ORDERED BY BOARD; SHALL APPEAR BEFORE BOARD FOR INTERVIEWS UPON REQUEST; SHALL INFORM BOARD OF CHANGE OF ADDRESS OR IF AWAY FOR MORE THAN FIVE DAYS. ARIZONA, IN COMPLIANCE WITH THE AMERICANS WITH DISABILITIES ACT, PROCLAIMS THIS IS NOT A DISCIPLINARY ACTION BUT MERELY A MONITORING PROCEDURE WHICH HE VOLUNTARILY ENTERED INTO. ON 3/24/99 ORDER TERMINATED.

LEVITT, KEITH N MD, LICENSE NUMBER 11-39, HAD ACTION TAKEN BY ARIZONA ON MARCH 28, 1998

NOTES: MUST IMMEDIATELY PARTICIPATE IN A BOARD-APPROVED MONITORED AFTERCARE TREATMENT PROGRAM WHOSE THERAPIST MUST SUBMIT MONTHLY REPORTS; MUST PARTICIPATE IN 90 12-STEP MEETINGS FOR SUBSTANCE ABUSE WITHIN 90 DAYS; MUST THEN PARTICIPATE IN A 12-STEP RECOVERY PROGRAM AS DETERMINED BY HIS TREATING THERAPIST AND ATTEND AT LEAST THREE WEEKLY MEETINGS; SHALL OBTAIN A BOARD-APPROVED TREATING PHYSICIAN; SHALL ABSTAIN COMPLETELY FROM THE CONSUMPTION OF ALCOHOLIC BEVERAGES AND DRUGS EXCEPT WHEN PRESCRIBED BY HIS TREATING PHYSICIAN; SHALL NOT CONSUME FOOD OR SUBSTANCES CONTAINING POPPYSEEDS; MUST SUBMIT TO WITNESSED RANDOM BIOLOGICAL FLUID COLLECTION; MUST KEEP A LOG OF ANY AND ALL MEDICATIONS PRESCRIBED FOR HIM; SHALL SUBMIT TO ANY EXAMINATIONS OR THERAPY ORDERED BY BOARD; SHALL APPEAR BEFORE BOARD FOR INTERVIEWS UPON REQUEST; SHALL INFORM BOARD OF CHANGE OF ADDRESS OR IF AWAY FOR MORE THAN FIVE DAYS. ARIZONA, IN COMPLIANCE WITH THE AMERICANS WITH DISABILITIES ACT, PROCLAIMS THIS IS NOT A DISCIPLINARY ACTION BUT MERELY A MONITORING PROCEDURE WHICH HE VOLUNTARILY ENTERED INTO. THIS REHABILITATION ORDER SUPERSEDES ANY PREVIOUS ORDERS.

LITTLE, TRACY L MD, LICENSE NUMBER 0021516, HAD ACTION TAKEN BY ARIZONA ON APRIL 20, 1996

NOTES: MUST IMMEDIATELY PARTICIPATE IN A BOARD-APPROVED MONITORED AFTERCARE TREATMENT PROGRAM WHOSE THERAPIST MUST SUBMIT QUARTERLY REPORTS; MUST PARTICIPATE IN 90 12-STEP MEETINGS FOR SUBSTANCE ABUSE WITHIN 90 DAYS; MUST THEN PARTICIPATE IN A 12-STEP RECOVERY PROGRAM AS DETERMINED BY TREATING THERAPIST AND ATTEND AT LEAST THREE WEEKLY MEETINGS; SHALL OBTAIN A BOARD-APPROVED TREATING PHYSICIAN; SHALL ABSTAIN COMPLETELY FROM THE CONSUMPTION OF ALCOHOLIC BEVERAGES AND DRUGS EXCEPT WHEN PRESCRIBED BY TREATING PHYSICIAN; SHALL NOT CONSUME FOODS OR SUBSTANCES CONTAINING POPPYSEEDS; MUST SUBMIT TO WITNESSED RANDOM BIOLOGICAL FLUID COLLECTION; MUST KEEP A LOG OF ANY AND ALL MEDICATIONS PRESCRIBED BY PHYSICIAN; SHALL SUBMIT TO ANY EXAMINATIONS OR THERAPY ORDERED BY THE BOARD; SHALL APPEAR BEFORE BOARD FOR INTERVIEWS UPON REQUEST; SHALL INFORM BOARD OF CHANGE OF ADDRESS OR IF AWAY FOR MORE THAN FIVE DAYS; IF SHE DOES NOT RESIDE IN ANOTHER STATE, SHALL PARTICIPATE IN THAT STATE'S PHYSICIAN REHABILITATION PROGRAM WITH REPORTS TO ARIZONA TWICE YEARLY; TIME SPENT OUT OF ARIZONA MAY BE TOLLED FOR THIS ORDER. ARIZONA, IN COMPLIANCE WITH THE AMERICANS WITH DISABILITIES ACT, PROCLAIMS THIS IS NOT A DISCIPLINARY ACTION BUT MERELY A MONITORING PROCEDURE WHICH PHYSICIAN ENTERED INTO VOLUNTARILY. ON 1/24/97 ORDER AMENDED ADDING REQUIREMENT THAT SHE OBTAIN A BOARD-APPROVED TREATING PSYCHIATRIST WHO WILL RELEASE ALL RECORDS UPON REQUEST BY THE BOARD, AND SUBMIT QUARTERLY REPORTS.

LOGAN, MARK E MD, LICENSE NUMBER 0022621, HAD ACTION TAKEN BY ARIZONA ON OCTOBER 19, 1996

NOTES: LICENSE REACTIVATED. SHALL NOT PRACTICE MEDICINE MORE THAN 40 HOURS PER WEEK. MUST

IMMEDIATELY PARTICIPATE IN A BOARD-APPROVED MONITORED AFTERCARE TREATMENT PROGRAM WHOSE THERAPIST MUST SUBMIT QUARTERLY REPORTS; MUST PARTICIPATE IN 90 12-STEP MEETINGS FOR SUBSTANCE ABUSE WITHIN 90 DAYS; MUST THEN PARTICIPATE IN A 12-STEP RECOVERY PROGRAM AS DETERMINED BY HIS TREATING THERAPIST AND ATTEND AT LEAST THREE WEEKLY MEETINGS; SHALL OBTAIN A BOARD-APPROVED TREATING PHYSICIAN; SHALL ABSTAIN COMPLETELY FROM THE CONSUMPTION OF ALCOHOLIC BEVERAGES AND DRUGS EXCEPT WHEN PRESCRIBED BY HIS TREATING PHYSICIAN; SHALL NOT CONSUME FOODS OR SUBSTANCES CONTAINING POPPYSEEDS; MUST SUBMIT TO WITNESSED RANDOM BIOLOGICAL FLUID COLLECTION; MUST KEEP A LOG OF ANY AND ALL MEDICATIONS PRESCRIBED FOR HIM; SHALL SUBMIT TO ANY EXAMINATIONS OR THERAPY ORDERED BY BOARD; SHALL APPEAR BEFORE BOARD FOR INTERVIEWS UPON REQUEST; SHALL INFORM BOARD OF CHANGE OF ADDRESS OR IF AWAY FOR MORE THAN FIVE DAYS. IF HE DOES RESIDE IN ANOTHER STATE, SHALL PARTICIPATE IN THAT STATE'S PHYSICIAN REHABILITATION PROGRAM WITH REPORTS TO ARIZONA TWICE YEARLY; TIME SPENT OUT OF ARIZONA MAY BE TOLLED FOR THIS ORDER; ARIZONA, IN COMPLIANCE WITH THE AMERICANS WITH DISABILITIES ACT, PROCLAIMS THIS IS NOT A DISCIPLINARY ACTION BUT MERELY A MONITORING PROCEDURE WHICH HE ENTERED INTO VOLUNTARILY. ON 11/23/98 ORDER AMENDED TERMINATING REQUIREMENT THAT HE WORK NO MORE THAN 40 HOURS PER WEEK.

LUNDSTROM, PAUL E MD, LICENSE NUMBER 0008740 OF FLAGSTAFF, AZ, HAD ACTION TAKEN BY ARIZONA ON JULY 16, 1993

NOTES: MUST IMMEDIATELY PARTICIPATE IN A BOARD-APPROVED MONITORED AFTERCARE TREATMENT PROGRAM WHOSE THERAPIST MUST SUBMIT QUARTERLY REPORTS; MUST PARTICIPATE IN 90 12-STEP MEETINGS FOR SUBSTANCE ABUSE WITHIN 90 DAYS; MUST THEN PARTICIPATE IN A 12-STEP RECOVERY PROGRAM AS DETERMINED BY HIS TREATING THERAPIST AND ATTEND AT LEAST THREE WEEKLY MEETINGS; SHALL OBTAIN A BOARD-APPROVED TREATING PHYSICIAN; SHALL ABSTAIN COMPLETELY FROM THE CONSUMPTION OF ALCOHOLIC BEVERAGES AND DRUGS EXCEPT WHEN PRESCRIBED BY HIS TREATING PHYSICIAN; KEEP A LOG OF ANY AND ALL MEDICATIONS PRESCRIBED FOR HIM; SHALL SUBMIT TO ANY EXAMINATIONS OR THERAPY ORDERED BY BOARD; SHALL APPEAR BEFORE BOARD FOR INTERVIEWS UPON REQUEST; SHALL INFORM BOARD OF CHANGE OF ADDRESS OR IF AWAY FOR MORE THAN FIVE DAYS. ARIZONA, IN COMPLIANCE WITH THE AMERICANS WITH DISABILITIES ACT, PROCLAIMS THIS IS NOT A DISCIPLINARY ACTION BUT MERELY A MONITORING PROCEDURE WHICH HE VOLUNTARILY ENTERED INTO.

MACLACHLAN, ROBERT T MD, LICENSE NUMBER 0012776, HAD ACTION TAKEN BY ARIZONA ON OCTOBER 19, 1996

NOTES: LICENSE REACTIVATED. MUST IMMEDIATELY PARTICIPATE IN A BOARD-APPROVED MONITORED AFTERCARE TREATMENT PROGRAM WHOSE THERAPIST MUST SUBMIT QUARTERLY REPORTS; MUST PARTICIPATE IN 90 12-STEP MEETINGS FOR SUBSTANCE ABUSE WITHIN 90 DAYS; MUST THEN PARTICIPATE IN A 12-STEP RECOVERY PROGRAM AS DETERMINED BY HIS TREATING THERAPIST AND ATTEND AT LEAST THREE WEEKLY MEETINGS; SHALL OBTAIN A BOARD-APPROVED TREATING PHYSICIAN; SHALL ABSTAIN COMPLETELY FROM THE CONSUMPTION OF ALCOHOLIC BEVERAGES AND DRUGS EXCEPT WHEN PRESCRIBED BY HIS TREATING PHYSICIAN; SHALL NOT CONSUME FOOD OR SUBSTANCES CONTAINING POPPYSEEDS; MUST SUBMIT TO WITNESSED RANDOM BIOLOGICAL FLUID COLLECTION; MUST KEEP A LOG OF ANY AND ALL MEDICATIONS PRESCRIBED FOR HIM; SHALL SUBMIT TO ANY EXAMINATIONS OR THERAPY ORDERED BY THE BOARD; SHALL APPEAR BEFORE BOARD FOR INTERVIEWS UPON REQUEST; SHALL INFORM BOARD OF CHANGE OF ADDRESS OR IF AWAY FOR MORE THAN FIVE DAYS; IF HE DOES RESIDE IN ANOTHER STATE, SHALL PARTICIPATE IN THAT STATE'S PHYSICIAN REHABILITATION PROGRAM WITH REPORTS TO ARIZONA TWICE YEARLY; TIME SPENT OUT OF ARIZONA MAY BE TOLLED FOR THIS ORDER. ARIZONA, IN COMPLIANCE WITH THE AMERICANS WITH DISABILITIES ACT, PROCLAIMS THIS IS NOT A DISCIPLINARY ACTION BUT MERELY A MONITORING PROCEDURE WHICH HE ENTERED INTO VOLUNTARILY.

MARCELLO, RICHARD MD, LICENSE NUMBER 0011166, HAD ACTION TAKEN BY ARIZONA ON OCTOBER 21, 1995

NOTES: INTERVIEWED BY BOARD REGARDING HIS TREATMENT AND HIS PARTICIPATION IN THE BOARD'S MONITORED AFTERCARE PROGRAM. MUST IMMEDIATELY PARTICIPATE IN A BOARD-APPROVED MONITORED AFTERCARE TREATMENT PROGRAM WHOSE THERAPIST MUST SUBMIT QUARTERLY REPORTS; MUST PARTICIPATE IN 90 12-STEP MEETINGS FOR SUBSTANCE ABUSE WITHIN 90 DAYS; MUST THEN PARTICIPATE IN A 12-STEP RECOVERY PROGRAM AS DETERMINED BY HIS TREATING THERAPIST AND ATTEND AT LEAST THREE WEEKLY MEETINGS; SHALL OBTAIN A BOARD-APPROVED TREATING PHYSICIAN; SHALL ABSTAIN COMPLETELY FROM THE CONSUMPTION OF ALCOHOLIC BEVERAGES AND DRUGS EXCEPT WHEN PRESCRIBED BY HIS TREATING PHYSICIAN; MUST SUBMIT TO WITNESSED RANDOM BIOLOGICAL FLUID COLLECTION; MUST KEEP A LOG OF ANY AND ALL MEDICATIONS PRESCRIBED FOR HIM; SHALL SUBMIT TO ANY EXAMINATIONS OR THERAPY ORDERED BY THE BOARD; SHALL APPEAR BEFORE BOARD FOR INTERVIEWS UPON REQUEST; SHALL INFORM BOARD OF CHANGE OF ADDRESS OR IF AWAY FOR MORE THAN FIVE DAYS. ARIZONA, IN COMPLIANCE WITH THE AMERICANS WITH DISABILITIES ACT, PROCLAIMS THIS IS NOT A DISCIPLINARY ACTION BUT MERELY A MONITORING PROCEDURE WHICH HE VOLUNTARILY ENTERED INTO.

MARTIN, STEPHEN H MD, LICENSE NUMBER 0022084, HAD ACTION TAKEN BY ARIZONA ON JULY 19, 1995

NOTES: INFORMATION RECEIVED BY THE BOARD THAT HE MAY HAVE A SUBSTANCE ABUSE PROBLEM. MUST IMMEDIATELY PARTICIPATE IN A BOARD-APPROVED MONITORED AFTERCARE TREATMENT PROGRAM WHOSE THERAPIST MUST SUBMIT QUARTERLY REPORTS; MUST PARTICIPATE IN 90 12-STEP MEETINGS FOR SUBSTANCE ABUSE WITHIN 90 DAYS; MUST THEN PARTICIPATE IN A 12-STEP RECOVERY PROGRAM AS DETERMINED BY HIS TREATING THERAPIST AND ATTEND AT LEAST THREE WEEKLY MEETINGS; SHALL OBTAIN A BOARD-APPROVED TREATING PHYSICIAN; SHALL ABSTAIN COMPLETELY FROM THE CONSUMPTION OF ALCOHOLIC BEVERAGES AND DRUGS EXCEPT WHEN PRESCRIBED BY HIS TREATING PHYSICIAN; MUST SUBMIT TO WITNESSED RANDOM BIOLOGICAL FLUID COLLECTION; MUST KEEP A LOG OF ANY AND ALL MEDICATIONS PRESCRIBED FOR HIM; SHALL SUBMIT TO ANY EXAMINATIONS OR THERAPY ORDERED BY THE BOARD; SHALL APPEAR BEFORE BOARD FOR INTERVIEWS UPON REQUEST; SHALL INFORM BOARD

OF CHANGE OF ADDRESS OR IF AWAY FOR MORE THAN FIVE DAYS. ARIZONA, IN COMPLIANCE WITH THE AMERICANS WITH DISABILITIES ACT, PROCLAIMS THIS IS NOT A DISCIPLINARY ACTION BUT MERELY A MONITORING PROCEDURE WHICH HE ENTERED INTO VOLUNTARILY. ON 2/15/96 ORDER CONTINUED; SHALL MEET WITH MONITORED AFTERCARE COMMITTEE IN THREE MONTHS.

MARTINEZ, ALICIA MD, LICENSE NUMBER 0015059, HAD ACTION TAKEN BY ARIZONA ON APRIL 8, 1995

NOTES: INTERVIEWED BY BOARD RELATIVE TO HER TREATMENT FOR SUBSTANCE ABUSE. MUST IMMEDIATELY PARTICIPATE IN A BOARD-APPROVED MONITORED AFTERCARE TREATMENT PROGRAM WHOSE THERAPIST MUST SUBMIT QUARTERLY REPORTS; SHALL ENTER INTO PSYCHOTHERAPY WITH A BOARD-APPROVED PSYCHIATRIST, WHO SHALL SUBMIT QUARTERLY REPORTS TO THE BOARD REGARDING DIAGNOSIS, PROGNOSIS AND RECOMMENDATION FOR CONTINUING CARE AND TREATMENT; MUST PARTICIPATE IN 90 12-STEP MEETINGS FOR SUBSTANCE ABUSE WITHIN 90 DAYS; MUST THEN PARTICIPATE IN A 12-STEP RECOVERY PROGRAM AS DETERMINED BY HER TREATING THERAPIST AND ATTEND AT LEAST THREE WEEKLY MEETINGS; SHALL OBTAIN A BOARD-APPROVED TREATING PHYSICIAN; SHALL ABSTAIN COMPLETELY FROM THE CONSUMPTION OF ALCOHOLIC BEVERAGES AND DRUGS EXCEPT WHEN PRESCRIBED BY HER TREATING PHYSICIAN; MUST SUBMIT TO WITNESSED RANDOM BIOLOGICAL FLUID COLLECTION; MUST KEEP A LOG OF ANY AND ALL MEDICATIONS PRESCRIBED FOR HER; SHALL SUBMIT TO ANY EXAMINATIONS OR THERAPY ORDERED BY BOARD; SHALL APPEAR BEFORE BOARD FOR INTERVIEWS UPON REQUEST; SHALL INFORM BOARD OF CHANGE OF ADDRESS OR IF AWAY FOR MORE THAN FIVE DAYS. ARIZONA IN COMPLIANCE WITH THE AMERICANS WITH DISABILITIES ACT, PROCLAIMS THIS IS NOT A DISCIPLINARY ACTION BUT MERELY A MONITORING PROCEDURE WHICH SHE ENTERED INTO VOLUNTARILY.

MCDONALD, MICHELLE MD, HAD ACTION TAKEN BY ARIZONA ON AUGUST 8, 1998

NOTES: MUST IMMEDIATELY PARTICIPATE IN A BOARD-APPROVED MONITORED AFTERCARE TREATMENT PROGRAM WHOSE THERAPIST MUST SUBMIT QUARTERLY REPORTS; MUST PARTICIPATE IN 90 12-STEP MEETINGS FOR SUBSTANCE ABUSE WITHIN 90 DAYS; MUST THEN PARTICIPATE IN A 12-STEP RECOVERY PROGRAM AS DETERMINED BY HIS/HER TREATING THERAPIST AND ATTEND AT LEAST THREE WEEKLY MEETINGS; SHALL OBTAIN A BOARD-APPROVED TREATING PHYSICIAN; SHALL ABSTAIN COMPLETELY FROM THE CONSUMPTION OF ALCOHOLIC BEVERAGES AND DRUGS EXCEPT WHEN PRESCRIBED BY HIS/HER TREATING PHYSICIAN; SHALL NOT CONSUME FOOD OR SUBSTANCES CONTAINING POPPYSEEDS; MUST SUBMIT TO WITNESSED RANDOM BIOLOGICAL FLUID COLLECTION; MUST KEEP A LOG OF ANY AND ALL MEDICATIONS PRESCRIBED FOR HIM/HER; SHALL SUBMIT TO ANY EXAMINATIONS OR THERAPY ORDERED BY BOARD; SHALL APPEAR BEFORE BOARD FOR INTERVIEWS UPON REQUEST; SHALL INFORM BOARD OF CHANGE OF ADDRESS OR IF AWAY FOR MORE THAN FIVE DAYS. ARIZONA, IN COMPLIANCE WITH THE AMERICANS WITH DISABILITIES ACT, PROCLAIMS THIS IS NOT A DISCIPLINARY ACTION BUT MERELY A MONITORING PROCEDURE WHICH HE VOLUNTARILY ENTERED INTO.

MCKINNEY, MICHAEL MD, HAD ACTION TAKEN BY ARIZONA ON JANUARY 29, 1999

NOTES: MUST IMMEDIATELY PARTICIPATE IN A BOARD-APPROVED MONITORED AFTERCARE TREATMENT PROGRAM WHOSE THERAPIST MUST SUBMIT QUARTERLY REPORTS; MUST PARTICIPATE IN 90 12-STEP MEETINGS FOR SUBSTANCE ABUSE WITHIN 90 DAYS; MUST THEN PARTICIPATE IN A 12-STEP RECOVERY PROGRAM AS DETERMINED BY HIS/HER TREATING THERAPIST AND ATTEND AT LEAST THREE WEEKLY MEETINGS; SHALL OBTAIN A BOARD-APPROVED TREATING PHYSICIAN; SHALL ABSTAIN COMPLETELY FROM THE CONSUMPTION OF ALCOHOLIC BEVERAGES AND DRUGS EXCEPT WHEN PRESCRIBED BY HIS/HER TREATING PHYSICIAN; SHALL NOT CONSUME FOOD OR SUBSTANCES CONTAINING POPPYSEEDS; MUST SUBMIT TO WITNESSED RANDOM BIOLOGICAL FLUID COLLECTION; MUST KEEP A LOG OF ANY AND ALL MEDICATIONS PRESCRIBED FOR HIM/HER; SHALL SUBMIT TO ANY EXAMINATIONS OR THERAPY ORDERED BY BOARD; SHALL APPEAR BEFORE BOARD FOR INTERVIEWS UPON REQUEST; SHALL INFORM BOARD OF CHANGE OF ADDRESS OR IF AWAY FOR MORE THAN FIVE DAYS; ARIZONA, IN COMPLIANCE WITH THE AMERICANS WITH DISABILITIES ACT, PROCLAIMS THIS IS NOT A DISCIPLINARY ACTION BUT MERELY A MONITORING PROCEDURE WHICH HE VOLUNTARILY ENTERED INTO.

MORFORD, PAMELA A MD, LICENSE NUMBER 0017926 OF TUCSON, AZ, HAD ACTION TAKEN BY ARIZONA ON APRIL 16, 1993

NOTES: POSSIBLE SUBSTANCE ABUSE PROBLEM. MUST IMMEDIATELY PARTICIPATE IN A BOARD-APPROVED MONITORED AFTERCARE TREATMENT PROGRAM WHOSE THERAPIST MUST SUBMIT QUARTERLY REPORTS; MUST PARTICIPATE IN 90 12-STEP MEETINGS FOR SUBSTANCE ABUSE WITHIN 90 DAYS; MUST THEN PARTICIPATE IN A 12-STEP RECOVERY PROGRAM AS DETERMINED BY HER TREATING THERAPIST AND ATTEND AT LEAST THREE WEEKLY MEETINGS; SHALL OBTAIN A BOARD-APPROVED TREATING PHYSICIAN; SHALL ABSTAIN COMPLETELY FROM THE CONSUMPTION OF ALCOHOLIC BEVERAGES AND DRUGS EXCEPT WHEN PRESCRIBED BY HER TREATING PHYSICIAN; MUST SUBMIT TO WITNESSED RANDOM BIOLOGICAL FLUID COLLECTION; KEEP A LOG OF ANY AND ALL MEDICATIONS PRESCRIBED FOR HER; SHALL SUBMIT TO ANY EXAMINATIONS OR THERAPY ORDERED BY BOARD; SHALL APPEAR BEFORE BOARD FOR INTERVIEWS UPON REQUEST; SHALL INFORM BOARD OF CHANGE OF ADDRESS OR IF AWAY FOR MORE THAN 5 DAYS. ARIZONA, IN COMPLIANCE WITH THE AMERICANS WITH DISABILITIES ACT, PROCLAIMS THIS IS NOT A DISCIPLINARY ACTION BUT MERELY A MONITORING PROCEDURE WHICH SHE VOLUNTARILY ENTERED INTO. ON 07/17/93, BOARD ORDERED THAT SHE UNDERGO A THOROUGH EVALUATION WITH A CHRONIC PAIN EXPERT AND AUTHORIZE RELEASE OF THESE REPORTS TO THE BOARD. ON 10/15/93 THIS ORDER MODIFIED SUCH THAT THE FIRST 3 PROVISIONS REQUIRING TREATMENT AND RECOVERY PROGRAMS WERE ELIMINATED. ON 7/15/94 STIPULATION WAS TERMINATED.

MORITZ, TERRELL CONWAY MD, LICENSE NUMBER 0020323, HAD ACTION TAKEN BY ARIZONA ON FEBRUARY 15, 1996

NOTES: PROBATION TERMINATED. CONDITIONS OF STIPULATION ARE AS FOLLOWS: MUST IMMEDIATELY PARTICIPATE IN A BOARD-APPROVED MONITORED AFTERCARE TREATMENT PROGRAM WHOSE

THERAPIST MUST SUBMIT QUARTERLY REPORTS; MUST PARTICIPATE IN 90 12-STEP MEETINGS FOR SUBSTANCE ABUSE WITHIN 90 DAYS; MUST THEN PARTICIPATE IN A 12-STEP RECOVERY PROGRAM AS DETERMINED BY HIS TREATING THERAPIST AND ATTEND AT LEAST THREE WEEKLY MEETINGS; SHALL OBTAIN A BOARD-APPROVED TREATING PHYSICIAN; SHALL NOT CONSUME ANY FOOD OR OTHER SUBSTANCES CONTAINING POPPYSEEDS; SHALL ABSTAIN COMPLETELY FROM THE CONSUMPTION OF ALCOHOLIC BEVERAGES AND DRUGS EXCEPT WHEN PRESCRIBED BY HIS TREATING PHYSICIAN; MUST SUBMIT TO WITNESSED RANDOM BIOLOGICAL FLUID COLLECTION; MUST KEEP A LOG OF ANY AND ALL MEDICATIONS PRESCRIBED FOR HIM; SHALL SUBMIT TO ANY EXAMINATIONS OR THERAPY ORDERED BY BOARD; SHALL APPEAR BEFORE BOARD FOR INTERVIEWS UPON REQUEST; SHALL INFORM BOARD OF CHANGE OF ADDRESS OR IF AWAY FOR MORE THAN FIVE DAYS; IF HE DOES RESIDE IN ANOTHER STATE, SHALL PARTICIPATE IN THAT STATE'S PHYSICIAN REHABILITATION PROGRAM WITH REPORTS TO ARIZONA TWICE YEARLY; TIME SPENT OUT OF ARIZONA MAY BE TOLLED FOR THIS ORDER. ARIZONA, IN COMPLIANCE WITH THE AMERICANS WITH DISABILITIES ACT, PROCLAIMS THIS IS NOT A DISCIPLINARY ACTION BUT MERELY A MONITORING PROCEDURE WHICH HE VOLUNTARILY ENTERED INTO. ON 5/9/97 ORDER TERMINATED EFFECTIVE IN 90 DAYS.

MYERS, KENT W MD, LICENSE NUMBER 19597, HAD ACTION TAKEN BY ARIZONA ON JANUARY 23, 1998

NOTES: MUST IMMEDIATELY PARTICIPATE IN A BOARD-APPROVED MONITORED AFTERCARE TREATMENT PROGRAM WHOSE THERAPIST MUST SUBMIT MONTHLY REPORTS; MUST PARTICIPATE IN 90 12-STEP MEETINGS FOR SUBSTANCE ABUSE WITHIN 90 DAYS; MUST THEN PARTICIPATE IN A 12-STEP RECOVERY PROGRAM AS DETERMINED BY HIS TREATING THERAPIST AND ATTEND AT LEAST THREE WEEKLY MEETINGS; SHALL OBTAIN A BOARD-APPROVED TREATING PHYSICIAN; SHALL ABSTAIN COMPLETELY FROM THE CONSUMPTION OF ALCOHOLIC BEVERAGES AND DRUGS EXCEPT WHEN PRESCRIBED BY HIS TREATING PHYSICIAN; SHALL NOT CONSUME FOOD OR SUBSTANCES CONTAINING POPPYSEEDS; MUST SUBMIT TO WITNESSED RANDOM BIOLOGICAL FLUID COLLECTION; MUST KEEP A LOG OF ANY AND ALL MEDICATIONS PRESCRIBED FOR HIM; SHALL SUBMIT TO ANY EXAMINATIONS OR THERAPY ORDERED BY BOARD; SHALL APPEAR BEFORE BOARD FOR INTERVIEWS UPON REQUEST; SHALL INFORM BOARD OF CHANGE OF ADDRESS OR IF AWAY FOR MORE THAN FIVE DAYS. ARIZONA, IN COMPLIANCE WITH THE AMERICANS WITH DISABILITIES ACT, PROCLAIMS THIS IS NOT A DISCIPLINARY ACTION BUT MERELY A MONITORING PROCEDURE WHICH HE VOLUNTARILY ENTERED INTO.

MYERS, RONALD A MD, LICENSE NUMBER 0019234, HAD ACTION TAKEN BY ARIZONA ON APRIL 17, 1996

NOTES: INDICATED ON 1993 RENEWAL FORM HAD BEEN TREATED FOR SUBSTANCE ABUSE. MUST IMMEDIATELY PARTICIPATE IN A BOARD-APPROVED MONITORED AFTERCARE TREATMENT PROGRAM WHOSE THERAPIST MUST SUBMIT QUARTERLY REPORTS; MUST PARTICIPATE IN 90 12-STEP MEETINGS FOR SUBSTANCE ABUSE WITHIN 90 DAYS; MUST THEN PARTICIPATE IN A 12-STEP RECOVERY PROGRAM AS DETERMINED BY HIS TREATING THERAPIST AND ATTEND AT LEAST THREE WEEKLY MEETINGS; SHALL OBTAIN A BOARD-APPROVED TREATING PHYSICIAN; SHALL ABSTAIN COMPLETELY FROM THE CONSUMPTION OF ALCOHOLIC BEVERAGES AND DRUGS EXCEPT WHEN PRESCRIBED BY HIS TREATING PHYSICIAN; SHALL NOT CONSUME ANY FOODS OR SUBSTANCES CONTAINING POPPYSEEDS; MUST SUBMIT TO WITNESSED RANDOM BIOLOGICAL FLUID COLLECTION; SHALL KEEP A LOG OF ANY AND ALL MEDICATIONS PRESCRIBED FOR HIM; SHALL SUBMIT TO ANY EXAMINATIONS OR THERAPY ORDERED BY THE BOARD; SHALL APPEAR BEFORE BOARD FOR INTERVIEWS UPON REQUEST; SHALL INFORM BOARD OF CHANGE OF ADDRESS OR IF AWAY FOR MORE THAN FIVE DAYS. IF HE DOES RESIDE IN ANOTHER STATE, SHALL PARTICIPATE IN THAT STATE'S PHYSICIAN REHABILITATION PROGRAM WITH REPORTS TO ARIZONA TWICE YEARLY; TIME SPENT OUT OF ARIZONA MAY BE TOLLED FOR THIS ORDER. ARIZONA, IN COMPLIANCE WITH THE AMERICANS WITH DISABILITIES ACT PROCLAIMS THIS IS NOT A DISCIPLINARY ACTION, BUT MERELY A MONITORING PROCEDURE WHICH HE VOLUNTARILY ENTERED INTO.

NITKA, ALFRED C MD, LICENSE NUMBER 14902, HAD ACTION TAKEN BY ARIZONA ON MAY 8, 1997

NOTES: MUST IMMEDIATELY PARTICIPATE IN A BOARD-APPROVED MONITORED AFTERCARE TREATMENT PROGRAM WHOSE THERAPIST MUST SUBMIT QUARTERLY REPORTS; MUST PARTICIPATE IN 90 12-STEP MEETINGS FOR SUBSTANCE ABUSE WITHIN 90 DAYS; MUST THEN PARTICIPATE IN A 12-STEP RECOVERY PROGRAM AS DETERMINED BY HIS TREATING THERAPIST AND ATTEND AT LEAST THREE WEEKLY MEETINGS; SHALL OBTAIN A BOARD-APPROVED TREATING PHYSICIAN; SHALL ABSTAIN COMPLETELY FROM THE CONSUMPTION OF ALCOHOLIC BEVERAGES AND DRUGS EXCEPT WHEN PRESCRIBED BY HIS TREATING PHYSICIAN; SHALL NOT CONSUME FOOD OR SUBSTANCES CONTAINING POPPYSEEDS; MUST SUBMIT TO WITNESSED RANDOM BIOLOGICAL FLUID COLLECTION; MUST KEEP A LOG OF ANY AND ALL MEDICATIONS PRESCRIBED FOR HIM; SHALL SUBMIT TO ANY EXAMINATIONS OR THERAPY ORDERED BY BOARD; SHALL APPEAR BEFORE BOARD FOR INTERVIEWS UPON REQUEST; SHALL INFORM BOARD OF CHANGE OF ADDRESS OR IF AWAY FOR MORE THAN FIVE DAYS. ARIZONA, IN COMPLIANCE WITH THE AMERICANS WITH DISABILITIES ACT, PROCLAIMS THIS IS NOT A DISCIPLINARY ACTION BUT MERELY A MONITORING PROCEDURE WHICH HE VOLUNTARILY ENTERED INTO.

ORGAN, PAUL G MD, LICENSE NUMBER 0021890, HAD ACTION TAKEN BY ARIZONA ON OCTOBER 16, 1996

NOTES: WITHIN TWO WEEKS, SHALL ENTER INTO A 30-DAY INPATIENT TREATMENT PROGRAM FOR SUBSTANCE ABUSE AT A BOARD-APPROVED FACILITY AND REMAIN IN TREATMENT UNTIL THERAPEUTICALLY DISCHARGED; MUST IMMEDIATELY PARTICIPATE IN A BOARD-APPROVED MONITORED AFTERCARE TREATMENT PROGRAM WHOSE THERAPIST MUST SUBMIT QUARTERLY REPORTS; MUST PARTICIPATE IN 90 12-STEP MEETINGS FOR SUBSTANCE ABUSE WITHIN 90 DAYS; MUST THEN PARTICIPATE IN A 12-STEP RECOVERY PROGRAM AS DETERMINED BY HIS TREATING THERAPIST AND ATTEND AT LEAST THREE WEEKLY MEETINGS; SHALL OBTAIN A BOARD-APPROVED TREATING PHYSICIAN; SHALL ABSTAIN COMPLETELY FROM THE CONSUMPTION OF ALCOHOLIC BEVERAGES AND DRUGS EXCEPT WHEN PRESCRIBED BY HIS TREATING PHYSICIAN; SHALL NOT CONSUME FOOD OR SUBSTANCES CONTAINING POPPYSEEDS; MUST SUBMIT TO WITNESSED RANDOM BIOLOGICAL FLUID COLLECTION; MUST KEEP A LOG OF ANY AND ALL MEDICATIONS PRESCRIBED FOR HIM; SHALL SUBMIT TO ANY EXAMINATIONS OR THERAPY

ORDERED BY THE BOARD; SHALL APPEAR BEFORE BOARD FOR INTERVIEWS UPON REQUEST; SHALL INFORM BOARD OF CHANGE OF ADDRESS OR IF AWAY FOR MORE THAN FIVE DAYS; IF HE DOES RESIDE IN ANOTHER STATE, SHALL PARTICIPATE IN THAT STATE'S PHYSICIAN REHABILITATION PROGRAM WITH REPORTS TO ARIZONA TWICE YEARLY; TIME SPENT OUT OF ARIZONA MAY BE TOLLED FOR THIS ORDER. ARIZONA, IN COMPLIANCE WITH THE AMERICANS WITH DISABILITIES ACT, PROCLAIMS THIS IS NOT A DISCIPLINARY ACTION BUT MERELY A MONITORING PROCEDURE WHICH HE ENTERED INTO VOLUNTARILY.

OSTERHOLTZ, ROGER L MD, LICENSE NUMBER 0017559, HAD ACTION TAKEN BY ARIZONA ON JUNE 20, 1991

NOTES: MUST IMMEDIATELY PARTICIPATE IN THE ARIZONA MEDICAL ASSOCIATION'S MONITORED AFTERCARE TREATMENT PROGRAM WHOSE THERAPIST MUST SUBMIT QUARTERLY REPORTS; SHALL PARTICIPATE IN 90 12-STEP MEETINGS APPROPRIATE FOR SUBSTANCE ABUSE AND ACCEPTABLE TO THE BOARD IN 90 DAYS FROM THE DATE OF THIS ORDER; MUST THEN PARTICIPATE IN A 12-STEP RECOVERY PROGRAM APPROPRIATE FOR SUBSTANCE ABUSE AS DETERMINED BY HIS TREATING THERAPIST AND ATTEND AT LEAST 3 WEEKLY MEETINGS; SHALL OBTAIN A BOARD-APPROVED TREATING PHYSICIAN; SHALL ABSTAIN COMPLETELY FROM THE CONSUMPTION OF ALCOHOLIC BEVERAGES AND TAKE NO DRUGS OR MEDICATIONS WHATEVER UNLESS PRESCRIBED BY HIS TREATING PHYSICIAN; SHALL COMPLY WITH REQUESTS FOR RANDOM BIOLOGICAL FLUID TESTS; SHALL MAINTAIN A LOG OF ALL MEDICATIONS TAKEN; SHALL SUBMIT TO MENTAL, PHYSICAL OR MEDICAL COMPETENCY EXAMINATIONS AND TO ANY RECOMMENDED THERAPY ORDERED BY BOARD; SHALL APPEAR BEFORE BOARD FOR INTERVIEWS UPON REQUEST; SHALL INFORM THE BOARD OF CHANGE OF ADDRESS OR IF AWAY FOR MORE THAN FIVE DAYS. ON 1/17/96 THE ORDER WAS REPLACED WITH THE SAME CONDITIONS, THE STATEMENT THAT THE REHABILITATION STIPULATION AND ORDER IS NOT A DISCIPLINARY ACTION, BUT A VOLUNTARY MONITORING PROGRAM; IF HE RESIDES OR PRACTICES OUT OF ARIZONA MAY PARTICIPATE IN THAT STATE'S MONITORING AND AFTERCARE PROGRAM WITH SEMI-ANNUAL REPORTS TO THE ARIZONA BOARD. THE REQUIREMENTS OF THIS ORDER SHALL BE TOLLED FOR ALL PERIOD OF TIME HE RESIDES OR PRACTICES MEDICINE IN ANY OTHER STATE THAN ARIZONA; SHALL NOTIFY THE BOARD OF DEPARTURE AND RETURN DATES FROM ARIZONA; SHALL PROVIDE THE BOARD WITH 90 DAYS ADVANCE WRITTEN NOTICE THAT HE INTENDS TO PRACTICE MEDICINE IN ARIZONA. ORDER TERMINATED ON 4/19/96.

PETERS, THOMAS J MD, LICENSE NUMBER 0009582 OF COTTONWOOD, AZ, HAD ACTION TAKEN BY ARIZONA ON APRIL 15, 1993

NOTES: ALLEGATIONS OF POSSIBLE ALCOHOL MISUSE. MUST IMMEDIATELY PARTICIPATE IN A BOARD-APPROVED MONITORED AFTERCARE TREATMENT PROGRAM WHOSE THERAPIST MUST SUBMIT QUARTERLY REPORTS; HE HAS COMPLETED 90 12-STEP MEETINGS FOR SUBSTANCE ABUSE; MUST PARTICIPATE IN A 12-STEP RECOVERY PROGRAM AS DETERMINED BY HIS TREATING THERAPIST AND ATTEND AT LEAST THREE WEEKLY MEETINGS; SHALL OBTAIN A BOARD-APPROVED TREATING PHYSICIAN; SHALL ABSTAIN COMPLETELY FROM THE CONSUMPTION OF ALCOHOLIC BEVERAGES AND DRUGS EXCEPT WHEN PRESCRIBED BY HIS TREATING PHYSICIAN; MUST SUBMIT TO WITNESSED RANDOM BIOLOGICAL FLUID COLLECTION; KEEP A LOG OF ANY AND ALL MEDICATIONS PRESCRIBED FOR HIM; SHALL SUBMIT TO ANY EXAMINATIONS OR THERAPY ORDERED BY BOARD; SHALL APPEAR BEFORE BOARD FOR INTERVIEWS UPON REQUEST; SHALL INFORM BOARD OF CHANGE OF ADDRESS OR IF AWAY FOR MORE THAN FIVE DAYS. ARIZONA, IN COMPLIANCE WITH THE AMERICANS WITH DISABILITIES ACT, PROCLAIMS THIS IS NOT A DISCIPLINARY ACTION BUT MERELY A MONITORING PROCEDURE WHICH HE VOLUNTARILY ENTERED INTO. ON 04/16/94, DR. PETERS' STIPULATION WITH BOARD IS TERMINATED EFFECTIVE IMMEDIATELY.

RAPPAPORT, WILLIAM DAVID MD, LICENSE NUMBER 0015658, HAD ACTION TAKEN BY ARIZONA ON JULY 16, 1994

NOTES: ORDER OF PROBATION TERMINATED. MUST IMMEDIATELY PARTICIPATE IN A BOARD-APPROVED MONITORED AFTERCARE TREATMENT PROGRAM WHOSE THERAPIST MUST SUBMIT QUARTERLY REPORTS; MUST PARTICIPATE IN A 12-STEP RECOVERY PROGRAM AS DETERMINED BY HIS TREATING THERAPIST AND ATTEND AT LEAST THREE WEEKLY MEETINGS; SHALL OBTAIN A BOARD-APPROVED TREATING PHYSICIAN; SHALL ABSTAIN COMPLETELY FROM THE CONSUMPTION OF ALCOHOLIC BEVERAGES AND DRUGS EXCEPT WHEN PRESCRIBED BY HIS TREATING PHYSICIAN; MUST SUBMIT TO WITNESSED RANDOM BIOLOGICAL FLUID COLLECTION; KEEP A LOG OF ANY AND ALL MEDICATIONS PRESCRIBED FOR HIM; SHALL SUBMIT TO ANY EXAMINATIONS OR THERAPY ORDERED BY BOARD; SHALL APPEAR BEFORE BOARD FOR INTERVIEWS UPON REQUEST; SHALL INFORM BOARD OF CHANGE OF ADDRESS OR IF AWAY FOR MORE THAN FIVE DAYS. ARIZONA, IN COMPLIANCE WITH THE AMERICANS WITH DISABILITIES ACT, PROCLAIMS THIS IS NOT A DISCIPLINARY ACTION BUT MERELY A MONITORING PROCEDURE WHICH HE VOLUNTARILY ENTERED INTO.

RITCHIE, THOMAS ALLAN MD, LICENSE NUMBER 16675, HAD ACTION TAKEN BY ARIZONA ON NOVEMBER 14, 1997

NOTES: INTERVIEWED BY BOARD REGARDING HIS TREATMENT FOR SUBSTANCE ABUSE. MUST IMMEDIATELY PARTICIPATE IN A BOARD-APPROVED MONITORED AFTERCARE TREATMENT PROGRAM WHOSE THERAPIST MUST SUBMIT MONTHLY REPORTS; MUST PARTICIPATE IN 90 12-STEP MEETINGS FOR SUBSTANCE ABUSE WITHIN 90 DAYS; MUST THEN PARTICIPATE IN A 12-STEP RECOVERY PROGRAM AS DETERMINED BY HIS TREATING THERAPIST AND ATTEND AT LEAST THREE WEEKLY MEETINGS; SHALL OBTAIN A BOARD-APPROVED TREATING PHYSICIAN; SHALL ABSTAIN COMPLETELY FROM THE CONSUMPTION OF ALCOHOLIC BEVERAGES AND DRUGS EXCEPT WHEN PRESCRIBED BY HIS TREATING PHYSICIAN; SHALL NOT CONSUME FOOD OR SUBSTANCES CONTAINING POPPYSEEDS; MUST SUBMIT TO WITNESSED RANDOM BIOLOGICAL FLUID COLLECTION; MUST KEEP A LOG OF ANY AND ALL MEDICATIONS PRESCRIBED FOR HIM; SHALL SUBMIT TO ANY EXAMINATIONS OR THERAPY ORDERED BY BOARD; SHALL APPEAR BEFORE BOARD FOR INTERVIEWS UPON REQUEST; SHALL INFORM BOARD OF CHANGE OF ADDRESS OR IF AWAY FOR MORE THAN FIVE DAYS. ARIZONA, IN COMPLIANCE WITH THE AMERICANS WITH DISABILITIES ACT, PROCLAIMS THIS IS NOT A DISCIPLINARY ACTION BUT MERELY A MONITORING PROCEDURE WHICH HE VOLUNTARILY ENTERED INTO. ALSO AGREED TO AN ORDER NOT TO PRACTICE ANESTHESIA WITHOUT THE WITNESSED ADMINISTRATION OF NALTREXONE.

RODRIGUEZ, MIGUEL L MD, LICENSE NUMBER 0020139, HAD ACTION TAKEN BY ARIZONA ON AUGUST 19, 1992

NOTES: MUST IMMEDIATELY PARTICIPATE IN A BOARD-APPROVED MONITORED AFTERCARE TREATMENT PROGRAM WHOSE THERAPIST MUST SUBMIT QUARTERLY REPORTS; MUST PARTICIPATE IN 90 12-STEP MEETINGS FOR SUBSTANCE ABUSE WITHIN 90 DAYS; MUST THEN PARTICIPATE IN A 12-STEP RECOVERY PROGRAM AS DETERMINED BY HIS TREATING THERAPIST AND ATTEND AT LEAST 3 WEEKLY MEETINGS; SHALL OBTAIN A BOARD-APPROVED TREATING PHYSICIAN; SHALL ABSTAIN COMPLETELY FROM THE CONSUMPTION OF ALCOHOLIC BEVERAGES AND DRUGS EXCEPT WHEN PRESCRIBED BY HIS TREATING PHYSICIAN; MUST SUBMIT TO WITNESSED RANDOM BIOLOGICAL FLUID COLLECTION; KEEP A LOG OF ANY AND ALL MEDICATIONS PRESCRIBED FOR HIM; SHALL SUBMIT TO ANY EXAMINATIONS OR THERAPY ORDERED BY BOARD; SHALL APPEAR BEFORE BOARD FOR INTERVIEWS UPON REQUEST; SHALL INFORM BOARD OF CHANGE OF ADDRESS OR IF AWAY FOR MORE THAN 5 DAYS. ARIZONA, IN COMPLIANCE WITH THE AMERICANS WITH DISABILITIES ACT, PROCLAIMS THIS IS NOT A DISCIPLINARY ACTION BUT MERELY A MONITORING PROCEDURE WHICH HE VOLUNTARILY ENTERED INTO. ON 7/22/95 ORDER WAS TERMINATED EFFECTIVE IN 90 DAYS.

ROSS, DOUGLAS MD, HAD ACTION TAKEN BY ARIZONA ON AUGUST 6, 1998

NOTES: MUST IMMEDIATELY PARTICIPATE IN A BOARD-APPROVED MONITORED AFTERCARE TREATMENT PROGRAM WHOSE THERAPIST MUST SUBMIT QUARTERLY REPORTS; MUST PARTICIPATE IN 90 12-STEP MEETINGS FOR SUBSTANCE ABUSE WITHIN 90 DAYS; MUST THEN PARTICIPATE IN A 12-STEP RECOVERY PROGRAM AS DETERMINED BY HIS/HER TREATING THERAPIST AND ATTEND AT LEAST THREE WEEKLY MEETINGS; SHALL OBTAIN A BOARD-APPROVED TREATING PHYSICIAN; SHALL ABSTAIN COMPLETELY FROM THE CONSUMPTION OF ALCOHOLIC BEVERAGES AND DRUGS EXCEPT WHEN PRESCRIBED BY HIS/HER TREATING PHYSICIAN; SHALL NOT CONSUME FOOD OR SUBSTANCES CONTAINING POPPYSEEDS; MUST SUBMIT TO WITNESSED RANDOM BIOLOGICAL FLUID COLLECTION; MUST KEEP A LOG OF ANY AND ALL MEDICATIONS PRESCRIBED FOR HIM/HER; SHALL SUBMIT TO ANY EXAMINATIONS OR THERAPY ORDERED BY BOARD; SHALL APPEAR BEFORE BOARD FOR INTERVIEWS UPON REQUEST; SHALL INFORM BOARD OF CHANGE OF ADDRESS OR IF AWAY FOR MORE THAN FIVE DAYS. ARIZONA, IN COMPLIANCE WITH THE AMERICANS WITH DISABILITIES ACT, PROCLAIMS THIS IS NOT A DISCIPLINARY ACTION BUT MERELY A MONITORING PROCEDURE WHICH HE VOLUNTARILY ENTERED INTO.

ROSS, DOUGLAS B MD, LICENSE NUMBER 22056, HAD ACTION TAKEN BY ARIZONA ON SEPTEMBER 24, 1997

NOTES: MUST IMMEDIATELY PARTICIPATE IN A BOARD-APPROVED MONITORED AFTERCARE TREATMENT PROGRAM WHOSE THERAPIST MUST SUBMIT QUARTERLY REPORTS; MUST PARTICIPATE IN 90 12-STEP MEETINGS FOR SUBSTANCE ABUSE WITHIN 90 DAYS; MUST THEN PARTICIPATE IN A 12-STEP RECOVERY PROGRAM AS DETERMINED BY HIS TREATING THERAPIST AND ATTEND AT LEAST THREE WEEKLY MEETINGS; SHALL OBTAIN A BOARD-APPROVED TREATING PHYSICIAN; SHALL ABSTAIN COMPLETELY FROM THE CONSUMPTION OF ALCOHOLIC BEVERAGES AND DRUGS EXCEPT WHEN PRESCRIBED BY HIS TREATING PHYSICIAN; SHALL NOT CONSUME FOOD OR SUBSTANCES CONTAINING POPPYSEEDS; MUST SUBMIT TO WITNESSED RANDOM BIOLOGICAL FLUID COLLECTION; MUST KEEP A LOG OF ANY AND ALL MEDICATIONS PRESCRIBED FOR HIM; SHALL SUBMIT TO ANY EXAMINATIONS OR THERAPY ORDERED BY BOARD; SHALL APPEAR BEFORE BOARD FOR INTERVIEWS UPON REQUEST; SHALL INFORM BOARD OF CHANGE OF ADDRESS OR IF AWAY FOR MORE THAN FIVE DAYS. ARIZONA, IN COMPLIANCE WITH THE AMERICANS WITH DISABILITIES ACT, PROCLAIMS THIS IS NOT A DISCIPLINARY ACTION BUT MERELY A MONITORING PROCEDURE WHICH HE VOLUNTARILY ENTERED INTO. ON 11/19/99 THE REHABILITATION AGREEMENT WAS TERMINATED.

RYAN, MARGARET A MD, LICENSE NUMBER 0019523, HAD ACTION TAKEN BY ARIZONA ON APRIL 15, 1994

NOTES: ON 1/29/94 DURING A COMPLIANCE HEARING BOARD ORDERED SHE SUBMIT HERSELF TO AN INPATIENT CHEMICAL DEPENDENCY EVALUATION ON OR BEFORE 2/22/94. ON 3/18/94 FAILED TO RESPOND PROMPTLY OR AT ALL TO REPEATED PAGES FROM A BOARD INVESTIGATOR WHICH WERE MADE FOR THE PURPOSE OF REQUESTING HER TO SUBMIT TO RANDOM BIOLOGICAL FLUID COLLECTION AS AGREED IN ORDER OF PROBATION OF 8/21/92. PROBATION UPON FOLLOWING TERMS AND CONDITIONS: SUSPENDED FOR A PERIOD NOT TO EXCEED ONE YEAR; WITHIN 10 DAYS SHALL OBTAIN A SOLE TREATING PSYCHIATRIST WHO IS ACCEPTABLE TO BOARD AND SHALL ENTER INTO PSYCHOTHERAPY WITH THE PSYCHIATRIST ON A FREQUENCY TO BE DETERMINED BY THE PSYCHIATRIST; SHALL DIRECT THE PSYCHIATRIST TO SUBMIT WRITTEN REPORTS TO THE BOARD QUARTERLY REGARDING HIS CARE AND TREATMENT. THIS ORDER OF PROBATION DOES NOT SUPERSEDE THE BOARD'S ORDER OF PROBATION DATED 08/21/92 WHICH SHALL REMAIN IN FULL FORCE AND EFFECT. MUST SUBMIT TO AN INPATIENT CHEMICAL DEPENDENCY EVALUATION BY 2/22/94. ON 7/13/94 SUSPENSION TERMINATED; ALL OTHER PROVISIONS REMAIN IN EFFECT. ON 4/20/96 PROBATION AND SUSPENSION TERMINATED AND THE FOLLOWING CONDITIONS WERE PLACED ON LICENSE: MUST IMMEDIATELY PARTICIPATE IN A BOARD-APPROVED MONITORED AFTERCARE TREATMENT PROGRAM WHOSE THERAPIST MUST SUBMIT QUARTERLY REPORTS; MUST OBTAIN A BOARD APPROVED TREATING PHYSICIAN; MUST ABSTAIN COMPLETELY FROM ALCOHOL AND ALL OTHER DRUGS; MUST COMPLY WITH REQUESTS FOR RANDOM BIOLOGICAL FLUID TESTS; MUST MAINTAIN A LOG OF ALL MEDICATIONS TAKEN; MUST SUBMIT TO ANY EXAMS OR THERAPY ORDERED BY BOARD; MUST APPEAR BEFORE BOARD FOR INTERVIEWS UPON REQUEST; MUST ADVISE BOARD OF CHANGE IN OFFICE OR HOME ADDRESSES OR IF PLANS TO BE AWAY FOR MORE THAN FIVE DAYS. ARIZONA, IN COMPLIANCE WITH THE AMERICANS WITH DISABILITIES ACT, PROCLAIMS THIS IS NOT A DISCIPLINARY ACTION BUT MERELY A MONITORING PROCEDURE WHICH SHE VOLUNTARILY ENTERED INTO.

RYCHLIK, NORMAN MD, HAD ACTION TAKEN BY ARIZONA ON JANUARY 29, 1999

NOTES: MUST IMMEDIATELY PARTICIPATE IN A BOARD-APPROVED MONITORED AFTERCARE TREATMENT PROGRAM WHOSE THERAPIST MUST SUBMIT QUARTERLY REPORTS; MUST PARTICIPATE IN 90 12-STEP MEETINGS FOR SUBSTANCE ABUSE WITHIN 90 DAYS; MUST THEN PARTICIPATE IN A 12-STEP

RECOVERY PROGRAM AS DETERMINED BY HIS/HER TREATING THERAPIST AND ATTEND AT LEAST THREE WEEKLY MEETINGS; SHALL OBTAIN A BOARD-APPROVED TREATING PHYSICIAN; SHALL ABSTAIN COMPLETELY FROM THE CONSUMPTION OF ALCOHOLIC BEVERAGES AND DRUGS EXCEPT WHEN PRESCRIBED BY HIS/HER TREATING PHYSICIAN; SHALL NOT CONSUME FOOD OR SUBSTANCES CONTAINING POPPYSEEDS; MUST SUBMIT TO WITNESSED RANDOM BIOLOGICAL FLUID COLLECTION; MUST KEEP A LOG OF ANY AND ALL MEDICATIONS PRESCRIBED FOR HIM/HER; SHALL SUBMIT TO ANY EXAMINATIONS OR THERAPY ORDERED BY BOARD; SHALL APPEAR BEFORE BOARD FOR INTERVIEWS UPON REQUEST; SHALL INFORM BOARD OF CHANGE OF ADDRESS OR IF AWAY FOR MORE THAN FIVE DAYS; ARIZONA, IN COMPLIANCE WITH THE AMERICANS WITH DISABILITIES ACT, PROCLAIMS THIS IS NOT A DISCIPLINARY ACTION BUT MERELY A MONITORING PROCEDURE WHICH HE VOLUNTARILY ENTERED INTO.

SANDERS, MARC R MD, LICENSE NUMBER 11039, HAD ACTION TAKEN BY ARIZONA ON MARCH 28, 1998

NOTES: MAY ONLY WORK AN AVERAGE OF 40 HOURS WEEKLY; MUST IMMEDIATELY PARTICIPATE IN A BOARD-APPROVED MONITORED AFTERCARE TREATMENT PROGRAM WHOSE THERAPIST MUST SUBMIT MONTHLY REPORTS; MUST PARTICIPATE IN 90 12-STEP MEETINGS FOR SUBSTANCE ABUSE WITHIN 90 DAYS; MUST THEN PARTICIPATE IN A 12-STEP RECOVERY PROGRAM AS DETERMINED BY HIS TREATING THERAPIST AND ATTEND AT LEAST THREE WEEKLY MEETINGS; SHALL OBTAIN A BOARD-APPROVED TREATING PHYSICIAN; SHALL ABSTAIN COMPLETELY FROM THE CONSUMPTION OF ALCOHOLIC BEVERAGES AND DRUGS EXCEPT WHEN PRESCRIBED BY HIS TREATING PHYSICIAN; SHALL NOT CONSUME FOOD OR SUBSTANCES CONTAINING POPPYSEEDS; MUST SUBMIT TO WITNESSED RANDOM BIOLOGICAL FLUID COLLECTION; MUST KEEP A LOG OF ANY AND ALL MEDICATIONS PRESCRIBED FOR HIM; SHALL SUBMIT TO ANY EXAMINATIONS OR THERAPY ORDERED BY BOARD; SHALL APPEAR BEFORE BOARD FOR INTERVIEWS UPON REQUEST; SHALL INFORM BOARD OF CHANGE OF ADDRESS OR IF AWAY FOR MORE THAN FIVE DAYS; ARIZONA, IN COMPLIANCE WITH THE AMERICANS WITH DISABILITIES ACT, PROCLAIMS THIS IS NOT A DISCIPLINARY ACTION BUT MERELY A MONITORING PROCEDURE WHICH HE VOLUNTARILY ENTERED INTO; SHALL IMMEDIATELY OBTAIN A TREATING PSYCHIATRIST APPROVED BY THE BOARD AND SHALL REMAIN IN TREATMENT WITH THE PSYCHIATRIST UNTIL FURTHER ORDER OF THE BOARD WITH QUARTERLY REPORTS.

SHEEHY, MARTIN C MD, HAD ACTION TAKEN BY ARIZONA ON MAY 1, 1999

NOTES: MUST IMMEDIATELY PARTICIPATE IN A BOARD-APPROVED MONITORED AFTERCARE TREATMENT PROGRAM WHOSE THERAPIST MUST SUBMIT QUARTERLY REPORTS; MUST PARTICIPATE IN 90 12-STEP MEETINGS FOR SUBSTANCE ABUSE WITHIN 90 DAYS; MUST THEN PARTICIPATE IN A 12-STEP RECOVERY PROGRAM AS DETERMINED BY HIS/HER TREATING THERAPIST AND ATTEND AT LEAST THREE WEEKLY MEETINGS; SHALL OBTAIN A BOARD-APPROVED TREATING PHYSICIAN; SHALL ABSTAIN COMPLETELY FROM THE CONSUMPTION OF ALCOHOLIC BEVERAGES AND DRUGS EXCEPT WHEN PRESCRIBED BY HIS/HER TREATING PHYSICIAN; SHALL NOT CONSUME FOOD OR SUBSTANCES CONTAINING POPPYSEEDS; MUST SUBMIT TO WITNESSED RANDOM BIOLOGICAL FLUID COLLECTION; MUST KEEP A LOG OF ANY AND ALL MEDICATIONS PRESCRIBED FOR HIM/HER; SHALL SUBMIT TO ANY EXAMINATIONS OR THERAPY ORDERED BY BOARD; SHALL APPEAR BEFORE BOARD FOR INTERVIEWS UPON REQUEST; SHALL INFORM BOARD OF CHANGE OF ADDRESS OR IF AWAY FOR MORE THAN FIVE DAYS. ARIZONA, IN COMPLIANCE WITH THE AMERICANS WITH DISABILITIES ACT, PROCLAIMS THIS IS NOT A DISCIPLINARY ACTION BUT MERELY A MONITORING PROCEDURE WHICH HE VOLUNTARILY ENTERED INTO.

SHELTON, THOMAS O III MD, LICENSE NUMBER 5608, HAD ACTION TAKEN BY ARIZONA ON JULY 26, 1997

NOTES: STATED ON HIS RENEWAL APPLICATION THAT HE HAD PREVIOUSLY BEEN TREATED FOR SUBSTANCE ABUSE. MUST IMMEDIATELY PARTICIPATE IN A BOARD-APPROVED MONITORED AFTERCARE TREATMENT PROGRAM WHOSE THERAPIST MUST SUBMIT QUARTERLY REPORTS; MUST PARTICIPATE IN 90 12-STEP MEETINGS FOR SUBSTANCE ABUSE WITHIN 90 DAYS; MUST THEN PARTICIPATE IN A 12-STEP RECOVERY PROGRAM AS DETERMINED BY HIS TREATING THERAPIST AND ATTEND AT LEAST THREE WEEKLY MEETINGS; SHALL OBTAIN A BOARD-APPROVED TREATING PHYSICIAN; SHALL ABSTAIN COMPLETELY FROM THE CONSUMPTION OF ALCOHOLIC BEVERAGES AND DRUGS EXCEPT WHEN PRESCRIBED BY HIS TREATING PHYSICIAN; SHALL NOT CONSUME FOOD OR SUBSTANCES CONTAINING POPPYSEEDS; MUST SUBMIT TO WITNESSED RANDOM BIOLOGICAL FLUID COLLECTION; MUST KEEP A LOG OF ANY AND ALL MEDICATIONS PRESCRIBED FOR HIM; SHALL SUBMIT TO ANY EXAMINATIONS OR THERAPY ORDERED BY BOARD; SHALL APPEAR BEFORE BOARD FOR INTERVIEWS UPON REQUEST; SHALL INFORM BOARD OF CHANGE OF ADDRESS OR IF AWAY FOR MORE THAN FIVE DAYS. ARIZONA, IN COMPLIANCE WITH THE AMERICANS WITH DISABILITIES ACT, PROCLAIMS THIS IS NOT A DISCIPLINARY ACTION BUT MERELY A MONITORING PROCEDURE WHICH HE VOLUNTARILY ENTERED INTO.

SHOTTON, RODNEY K MD, LICENSE NUMBER 0011139 OF GILBERT, AZ, HAD ACTION TAKEN BY ARIZONA ON JULY 16, 1993

NOTES: MUST IMMEDIATELY PARTICIPATE IN A BOARD-APPROVED MONITORED AFTERCARE TREATMENT PROGRAM WHOSE THERAPIST MUST SUBMIT QUARTERLY REPORTS; MUST PARTICIPATE IN 90 12-STEP MEETINGS FOR SUBSTANCE ABUSE WITHIN 90 DAYS; MUST THEN PARTICIPATE IN A 12-STEP RECOVERY PROGRAM AS DETERMINED BY HIS TREATING THERAPIST AND ATTEND AT LEAST THREE WEEKLY MEETINGS; SHALL OBTAIN A BOARD-APPROVED TREATING PHYSICIAN; SHALL ABSTAIN COMPLETELY FROM THE CONSUMPTION OF ALCOHOLIC BEVERAGES AND DRUGS EXCEPT WHEN PRESCRIBED BY HIS TREATING PHYSICIAN; MUST SUBMIT TO WITNESSED RANDOM BIOLOGICAL FLUID COLLECTION; KEEP A LOG OF ANY AND ALL MEDICATIONS PRESCRIBED FOR HIM; SHALL SUBMIT TO ANY EXAMINATIONS OR THERAPY ORDERED BY THE BOARD; SHALL APPEAR BEFORE BOARD FOR INTERVIEWS UPON REQUEST; SHALL INFORM BOARD OF CHANGE OF ADDRESS OR IF AWAY FOR MORE THAN FIVE DAYS. ARIZONA, IN COMPLIANCE WITH THE AMERICANS WITH DISABILITIES ACT, PROCLAIMS THIS IS NOT A DISCIPLINARY ACTION BUT MERELY A MONITORING PROCEDURE WHICH HE VOLUNTARILY ENTERED INTO. IN 6/98 ORDER TERMINATED. ON 5/15/98 ORDER TERMINATED IN 90 DAYS.

SIDHU, SARDEV SINGH MD, LICENSE NUMBER 10101, HAD ACTION

TAKEN BY ARIZONA ON JANUARY 25, 1997

NOTES: INFORMATION RECEIVED THAT HIS EMPLOYMENT HAD BEEN TERMINATED DUE TO ALLEGATIONS OF INAPPROPRIATE BEHAVIOR TOWARDS PATIENTS AND STAFF INCLUDING INAPPROPRIATE COMMENTS, SUCH AS INQUIRING ABOUT THEIR SEX LIFE TO SIX PATIENTS TWO OF WHICH HE ALSO INAPPROPRIATELY TOUCHED DURING AN EXAM; HE ASKED ONE OF THESE PATIENTS TO LIE ABOUT THE INCIDENT IN ORDER FOR HIM TO GET HIS JOB BACK. PLACED ON PROBATION FOR INDEFINITE TERM; SHALL NOT SEE, TREAT OR PROVIDE CARE TO ANY FEMALE PATIENT; ALSO ISSUED A DECREE OF CENSURE; BOARD ALSO RECEIVED INFORMATION THAT HE WAS IN TREATMENT FOR ALCOHOLISM. ENTERED INTO THE FOLLOWING MONITORING AGREEMENT: MUST IMMEDIATELY PARTICIPATE IN A BOARD-APPROVED MONITORED AFTERCARE TREATMENT PROGRAM WHOSE THERAPIST MUST SUBMIT QUARTERLY REPORTS; MUST PARTICIPATE IN 90 12-STEP MEETINGS FOR SUBSTANCE ABUSE WITHIN 90 DAYS; MUST THEN PARTICIPATE IN A 12-STEP RECOVERY PROGRAM AS DETERMINED BY HIS TREATING THERAPIST AND ATTEND AT LEAST THREE WEEKLY MEETINGS; SHALL OBTAIN A BOARD-APPROVED TREATING PHYSICIAN; SHALL ABSTAIN COMPLETELY FROM THE CONSUMPTION OF ALCOHOLIC BEVERAGES AND DRUGS EXCEPT WHEN PRESCRIBED BY HIS TREATING PHYSICIAN; SHALL NOT CONSUME FOOD OR SUBSTANCES CONTAINING POPPYSEEDS; MUST SUBMIT TO WITNESSED RANDOM BIOLOGICAL FLUID COLLECTION; MUST KEEP A LOG OF ANY AND ALL MEDICATIONS PRESCRIBED FOR HIM; SHALL SUBMIT TO ANY EXAMINATIONS OR THERAPY ORDERED BY BOARD; SHALL APPEAR BEFORE BOARD FOR INTERVIEWS UPON REQUEST; SHALL INFORM BOARD OF CHANGE OF ADDRESS OR IF AWAY FOR MORE THAN FIVE DAYS; SHALL IMMEDIATELY OBTAIN A TREATING PSYCHIATRIST APPROVED BY BOARD STAFF AND SHALL REMAIN IN TREATMENT WITH THE PSYCHIATRIST UNTIL FURTHER ORDER OF THE BOARD WITH QUARTERLY REPORTS. ARIZONA, IN COMPLIANCE WITH THE AMERICANS WITH DISABILITIES ACT, PROCLAIMS THIS IS NOT A DISCIPLINARY ACTION BUT MERELY A MONITORING PROCEDURE WHICH HE VOLUNTARILY ENTERED INTO. ON 11/1/98 REQUIREMENT TO REMAIN IN PSYCHIATRIC TREATMENT TERMINATED. ON 11/14/97 ORDER MODIFIED ALLOWING HIM TO TREAT FEMALE PATIENTS IN THE PRESENCE OF A CHAPERONE; HE SHALL NOT PERFORM PHYSICAL EXAMINATIONS ON FEMALE PATIENTS.

SILVER, HARRIS S MD, LICENSE NUMBER 0023195, HAD ACTION TAKEN BY ARIZONA ON JULY 13, 1995

NOTES: INTERVIEWED BY THE BOARD RELATIVE TO HIS APPLICATION FOR AN ARIZONA LICENSE; HIS PARTICIPATION IN THE PHYSICIANS' HEALTH PROGRAMS IN PENNSYLVANIA; AND HIS PARTICIPATION IN THE BOARD'S MONITORED AFTERCARE PROGRAM. MUST IMMEDIATELY PARTICIPATE IN A BOARD-APPROVED MONITORED AFTERCARE TREATMENT PROGRAM WHOSE THERAPIST MUST SUBMIT QUARTERLY REPORTS; MUST PARTICIPATE IN A 12-STEP RECOVERY PROGRAM AS DETERMINED BY HIS TREATING THERAPIST AND ATTEND AT LEAST THREE WEEKLY MEETINGS; SHALL OBTAIN A BOARD-APPROVED TREATING PHYSICIAN; SHALL ABSTAIN COMPLETELY FROM THE CONSUMPTION OF ALCOHOLIC BEVERAGES AND DRUGS EXCEPT WHEN PRESCRIBED BY HIS TREATING PHYSICIAN; MUST SUBMIT TO WITNESSED RANDOM BIOLOGICAL FLUID COLLECTION; MUST KEEP A LOG OF ANY AND ALL MEDICATIONS PRESCRIBED FOR HIM; SHALL SUBMIT TO ANY EXAMINATIONS OR THERAPY ORDERED BY THE BOARD; SHALL APPEAR BEFORE THE BOARD FOR INTERVIEWS UPON REQUEST; SHALL INFORM BOARD OF CHANGE OF ADDRESS OR IF AWAY FOR MORE THAN FIVE DAYS; MUST CAUSE THE BOARD OR MONITORING PROGRAM FROM ANY STATE IN WHICH HE PRACTICES OR RESIDES TO FURNISH THE BOARD WITH QUARTERLY REPORTS REGARDING HIS RECOVERY PROGRAM AND URINE DRUG SCREENING; SHALL NOTIFY THE BOARD AT LEAST 90 DAYS PRIOR TO PRACTICING OR RESIDING IN ARIZONA. ARIZONA, IN COMPLIANCE WITH THE AMERICANS WITH DISABILITIES ACT, PROCLAIMS THIS IS NOT A DISCIPLINARY ACTION BUT MERELY A MONITORING PROCEDURE WHICH HE VOLUNTARILY ENTERED INTO. ON 10/19/95 ORDER AMENDED AS FOLLOWS: WHILE HE PRACTICES MEDICINE IN NORTH DAKOTA HE SHALL PARTICIPATE IN THE NORTH DAKOTA IMPAIRED PHYSICIAN'S PROGRAM AND PROVIDE WRITTEN QUARTERLY REPORTS TO THE ARIZONA BOARD; SHALL PROVIDE 90 DAYS ADVANCE NOTICE TO THE ARIZONA BOARD PRIOR TO RETURNING TO ARIZONA TO PRACTICE MEDICINE. ON 5/9/97 THIS ORDER TERMINATED AND AMENDMENT ADDED WITH REQUIREMENT THAT HE OBTAIN A TREATING PSYCHIATRIST WHO SHALL RELEASE ALL TREATMENT RECORDS AND SUBMIT QUARTERLY REPORTS.

SILVER, HARRIS S MD, LICENSE NUMBER 23195, HAD ACTION TAKEN BY ARIZONA ON MARCH 15, 1997

NOTES: MUST IMMEDIATELY PARTICIPATE IN A BOARD-APPROVED MONITORED AFTERCARE TREATMENT PROGRAM WHOSE THERAPIST MUST SUBMIT QUARTERLY REPORTS; MUST PARTICIPATE IN 90 12-STEP MEETINGS FOR SUBSTANCE ABUSE WITHIN 90 DAYS; MUST THEN PARTICIPATE IN A 12-STEP RECOVERY PROGRAM AS DETERMINED BY HIS TREATING THERAPIST AND ATTEND AT LEAST THREE WEEKLY MEETINGS; SHALL OBTAIN A BOARD-APPROVED TREATING PHYSICIAN; SHALL ABSTAIN COMPLETELY FROM THE CONSUMPTION OF ALCOHOLIC BEVERAGES AND DRUGS EXCEPT WHEN PRESCRIBED BY HIS TREATING PHYSICIAN; SHALL NOT CONSUME FOOD OR SUBSTANCES CONTAINING POPPYSEEDS; MUST SUBMIT TO WITNESSED RANDOM BIOLOGICAL FLUID COLLECTION; MUST KEEP A LOG OF ANY AND ALL MEDICATIONS PRESCRIBED FOR HIM; SHALL SUBMIT TO ANY EXAMINATIONS OR THERAPY ORDERED BY BOARD; SHALL APPEAR BEFORE BOARD FOR INTERVIEWS UPON REQUEST; SHALL INFORM BOARD OF CHANGE OF ADDRESS OR IF AWAY FOR MORE THAN FIVE DAYS; ARIZONA, IN COMPLIANCE WITH THE AMERICANS WITH DISABILITIES ACT, PROCLAIMS THIS IS NOT A DISCIPLINARY ACTION BUT MERELY A MONITORING PROCEDURE WHICH HE VOLUNTARILY ENTERED INTO; SHALL IMMEDIATELY OBTAIN A TREATING PSYCHIATRIST APPROVED BY THE BOARD AND SHALL REMAIN IN TREATMENT WITH THE PSYCHIATRIST UNTIL FURTHER ORDER OF THE BOARD WITH QUARTERLY REPORTS; ON 3/28/98 ORDER TERMINATED AND HE ENTERED INTO AN ORDER REQUIRING HE OBTAIN A TREATING PSYCHIATRIST AND SUBMIT QUARTERLY REPORTS AND ALSO SUBMIT TO BIOLOGICAL FLUID TESTING. ON 9/21/99 THE ORDER WAS TERMINATED AND HE SIGNED AN AGREEMENT FOR CONTINUED MONITORING.

SINGH, BALDEV D MD, HAD ACTION TAKEN BY ARIZONA ON JULY 18, 1992

NOTES: MUST IMMEDIATELY PARTICIPATE IN A BOARD-APPROVED MONITORED AFTERCARE PROGRAM WHOSE THERAPIST MUST SUBMIT QUARTERLY

REPORTS; MUST PARTICIPATE IN 90 12-STEP MEETINGS FOR SUBSTANCE ABUSE WITHIN 90 DAYS; MUST THEN PARTICIPATE IN A 12-STEP RECOVERY PROGRAM AS DETERMINED BY HIS TREATING THERAPIST AND ATTEND AT LEAST THREE WEEKLY MEETINGS; SHALL OBTAIN A BOARD-APPROVED TREATING PHYSICIAN; SHALL ABSTAIN COMPLETELY FROM THE CONSUMPTION OF ALCOHOLIC BEVERAGES AND DRUGS EXCEPT WHEN PRESCRIBED BY HIS TREATING PHYSICIAN; MUST SUBMIT TO WITNESSED RANDOM BIOLOGICAL FLUID COLLECTION; KEEP A LOG OF ANY AND ALL MEDICATIONS PRESCRIBED FOR HIM; SHALL SUBMIT TO ANY EXAMINATIONS OR THERAPY ORDERED BY BOARD; SHALL APPEAR BEFORE BOARD FOR INTERVIEWS UPON REQUEST; SHALL INFORM BOARD OF CHANGE OF ADDRESS OR IF AWAY FOR MORE THAN 5 DAYS. ARIZONA, IN COMPLIANCE WITH THE AMERICANS WITH DISABILITIES ACT, PROCLAIMS THIS IS NOT A DISCIPLINARY ACTION BUT MERELY A MONITORING PROCEDURE WHICH HE VOLUNTARILY ENTERED INTO. ORDER TERMINATED ON 4/20/96.

SMITH, RODNEY LESTER MD, LICENSE NUMBER 0016325, HAD ACTION TAKEN BY ARIZONA ON FEBRUARY 15, 1996

NOTES: MUST IMMEDIATELY PARTICIPATE IN A BOARD-APPROVED MONITORED AFTERCARE TREATMENT PROGRAM WHOSE THERAPIST MUST SUBMIT QUARTERLY REPORTS; MUST PARTICIPATE IN 90 12-STEP MEETINGS FOR SUBSTANCE ABUSE WITHIN 90 DAYS; MUST THEN PARTICIPATE IN A 12-STEP RECOVERY PROGRAM AS DETERMINED BY HIS TREATING THERAPIST AND ATTEND AT LEAST THREE WEEKLY MEETINGS; SHALL OBTAIN A BOARD-APPROVED TREATING PHYSICIAN; SHALL NOT CONSUME ANY FOOD OR OTHER SUBSTANCES CONTAINING POPPYSEEDS; SHALL ABSTAIN COMPLETELY FROM THE CONSUMPTION OF ALCOHOLIC BEVERAGES AND DRUGS EXCEPT WHEN PRESCRIBED BY HIS TREATING PHYSICIAN; MUST SUBMIT TO WITNESSED RANDOM BIOLOGICAL FLUID COLLECTION; MUST KEEP A LOG OF ANY AND ALL MEDICATIONS PRESCRIBED FOR HIM; SHALL SUBMIT TO ANY EXAMINATIONS OR THERAPY ORDERED BY BOARD; SHALL APPEAR BEFORE BOARD FOR INTERVIEWS UPON REQUEST; SHALL INFORM BOARD OF CHANGE OF ADDRESS OR IF AWAY FOR MORE THAN FIVE DAYS. IF HE DOES RESIDE IN ANOTHER STATE, SHALL PARTICIPATE IN THAT STATE'S PHYSICIAN REHABILITATION PROGRAM WITH REPORTS TO ARIZONA TWICE YEARLY; TIME SPENT OUT OF ARIZONA MAY BE TOLLED FOR THIS ORDER. ARIZONA, IN COMPLIANCE WITH THE AMERICANS WITH DISABILITIES ACT, PROCLAIMS THIS IS NOT A DISCIPLINARY ACTION BUT MERELY A MONITORING PROCEDURE WHICH HE VOLUNTARILY ENTERED INTO.

SNIPES, FRANK H MD, LICENSE NUMBER 0020832, HAD ACTION TAKEN BY ARIZONA ON OCTOBER 19, 1996

NOTES: MUST IMMEDIATELY PARTICIPATE IN A BOARD-APPROVED MONITORED AFTERCARE TREATMENT PROGRAM WHOSE THERAPIST MUST SUBMIT QUARTERLY REPORTS; MUST PARTICIPATE IN 90 12-STEP MEETINGS FOR SUBSTANCE ABUSE WITHIN 90 DAYS; MUST THEN PARTICIPATE IN A 12-STEP RECOVERY PROGRAM AS DETERMINED BY HIS TREATING THERAPIST AND ATTEND AT LEAST THREE WEEKLY MEETINGS; SHALL OBTAIN A BOARD-APPROVED TREATING PHYSICIAN; SHALL ABSTAIN COMPLETELY FROM THE CONSUMPTION OF ALCOHOLIC BEVERAGES AND DRUGS EXCEPT WHEN PRESCRIBED BY HIS TREATING PHYSICIAN; SHALL NOT CONSUME FOODS OR SUBSTANCES CONTAINING POPPYSEEDS; MUST SUBMIT TO WITNESSED RANDOM BIOLOGICAL FLUID COLLECTION; MUST KEEP A LOG OF ANY AND ALL MEDICATIONS PRESCRIBED FOR HIM; SHALL SUBMIT TO ANY EXAMINATIONS OR THERAPY ORDERED BY THE BOARD; SHALL APPEAR BEFORE BOARD FOR INTERVIEWS UPON REQUEST; SHALL INFORM BOARD OF CHANGE OF ADDRESS OR IF AWAY FOR MORE THAN FIVE DAYS. ARIZONA, IN COMPLIANCE WITH THE AMERICANS WITH DISABILITIES ACT, PROCLAIMS THIS IS NOT A DISCIPLINARY ACTION BUT MERELY A MONITORING PROCEDURE WHICH HE ENTERED INTO VOLUNTARILY.

SOOD, RANJIT K MD, LICENSE NUMBER 0010691, HAD ACTION TAKEN BY ARIZONA ON APRIL 6, 1995

NOTES: ALLEGATIONS THAT HE MAY HAVE AN ALCOHOL ABUSE PROBLEM AND MAY BE SUFFERING FROM DEPRESSION; ALSO IN 3/93 MISMANAGED THE TREATMENT OF A PATIENT; FAILED TO PERFORM ENDOSCOPY FOR A PATIENT WHO HAD SWALLOWED A STRAIGHT PIN ON THE EVENING OF THE HOSPITAL ADMISSION WHEN IT WAS KNOWN THE PIN WAS IN THE STOMACH; FAILED TO ORDER XRAY PRIOR TO PROCEDURE AS WAS NECESSARY AND APPROPRIATE; POSTPONED ENDOSCOPY UNTIL THE FOLLOWING EVENING WHEN THE PIN WAS PROBABLY NO LONGER IN THE STOMACH. SUBJECTED THE PATIENT TO THE RISKS OF AN INVASIVE PROCEDURE THAT HAD LITTLE LIKELIHOOD OF SUCCESS DUE TO THE TIME THAT HAD ELAPSED. BILLED THE HISTORY AND PHYSICAL AS BEING PERFORMED ON 3/10/93, ALTHOUGH THEY WERE PERFORMED ON 3/11/93; CHARGED $150 FOR HIS CONSULTATION AND $520 FOR THE 12-MINUTE ENDOSCOPY. CENSURED. SHALL PAY RESTITUTION TO THE PATIENT OF FEES PAID TO HIM. ALSO CONDITIONS OF REHABILITATION STIPULATION. MUST IMMEDIATELY PARTICIPATE IN A BOARD-APPROVED MONITORED AFTERCARE TREATMENT PROGRAM WHOSE THERAPIST MUST SUBMIT QUARTERLY REPORTS; MUST PARTICIPATE IN 90 12-STEP MEETINGS FOR SUBSTANCE ABUSE WITHIN 90 DAYS; MUST THEN PARTICIPATE IN A 12-STEP RECOVERY PROGRAM AS DETERMINED BY HIS TREATING THERAPIST AND ATTEND AT LEAST THREE WEEKLY MEETINGS; SHALL OBTAIN A BOARD-APPROVED TREATING PHYSICIAN; SHALL ABSTAIN COMPLETELY FROM THE CONSUMPTION OF ALCOHOLIC BEVERAGES AND DRUGS EXCEPT WHEN PRESCRIBED BY HIS TREATING PHYSICIAN; MUST SUBMIT TO WITNESSED RANDOM BIOLOGICAL FLUID COLLECTION; SHALL KEEP A LOG OF ANY AND ALL MEDICATIONS PRESCRIBED FOR HIM; SHALL SUBMIT TO ANY EXAMINATIONS OR THERAPY ORDERED BY THE BOARD; SHALL APPEAR BEFORE BOARD FOR INTERVIEWS UPON REQUEST; SHALL INFORM BOARD OF CHANGE OF ADDRESS OR IF AWAY FOR MORE THAN FIVE DAYS. ARIZONA IN COMPLIANCE WITH THE AMERICANS WITH DISABILITIES ACT, PROCLAIMS THIS IS NOT A DISCIPLINARY ACTION BUT MERELY A MONITORING PROCEDURE WHICH HE ENTERED INTO VOLUNTARILY. ON 7/21/95 CONDITIONS OF THIS REHABILITATION STIPULATION DROPPED.

STANDAGE, GREGG P MD, LICENSE NUMBER 0022289, HAD ACTION TAKEN BY ARIZONA ON APRIL 8, 1995

NOTES: MUST IMMEDIATELY PARTICIPATE IN A BOARD-APPROVED MONITORED AFTERCARE TREATMENT PROGRAM WHOSE THERAPIST MUST SUBMIT QUARTERLY REPORTS; MUST PARTICIPATE IN 90 12-STEP MEETINGS FOR SUBSTANCE ABUSE WITHIN 90 DAYS; MUST THEN PARTICIPATE IN A 12-STEP RECOVERY PROGRAM AS DETERMINED BY HIS TREATING THERAPIST AND ATTEND AT LEAST THREE WEEKLY MEETINGS; SHALL OBTAIN A BOARD-APPROVED TREATING PHYSICIAN; SHALL ABSTAIN

COMPLETELY FROM THE CONSUMPTION OF ALCOHOLIC BEVERAGES AND DRUGS EXCEPT WHEN PRESCRIBED BY HIS TREATING PHYSICIAN; MUST SUBMIT TO WITNESSED RANDOM BIOLOGICAL FLUID COLLECTION; MUST KEEP A LOG OF ANY AND ALL MEDICATIONS PRESCRIBED FOR HIM; SHALL SUBMIT TO ANY EXAMINATIONS OR THERAPY ORDERED BY BOARD; SHALL APPEAR BEFORE BOARD FOR INTERVIEWS UPON REQUEST; SHALL INFORM BOARD OF CHANGE OF ADDRESS OR IF AWAY FOR MORE THAN FIVE DAYS. ARIZONA, IN COMPLIANCE WITH THE AMERICANS WITH DISABILITIES ACT, PROCLAIMS THIS IS NOT A DISCIPLINARY ACTION BUT MERELY A MONITORING PROCEDURE WHICH HE ENTERED INTO VOLUNTARILY. ON 3/24/99 ORDER TERMINATED.

SUFFECOOL, STEVEN L MD, LICENSE NUMBER 0011240, HAD ACTION TAKEN BY ARIZONA ON JULY 16, 1994

NOTES: MUST IMMEDIATELY PARTICIPATE IN A BOARD-APPROVED MONITORED AFTERCARE TREATMENT PROGRAM WHOSE THERAPIST MUST SUBMIT QUARTERLY REPORT; MUST PARTICIPATE IN A 12-STEP RECOVERY PROGRAM AS DETERMINED BY HIS TREATING THERAPIST AND ATTEND AT LEAST THREE WEEKLY MEETINGS; SHALL OBTAIN A BOARD-APPROVED TREATING PHYSICIAN; SHALL ABSTAIN COMPLETELY FROM THE CONSUMPTION OF ALCOHOLIC BEVERAGES AND DRUGS EXCEPT WHEN PRESCRIBED BY HIS TREATING PHYSICIAN; MUST SUBMIT TO WITNESSED RANDOM BIOLOGICAL FLUID COLLECTION; KEEP A LOG OF ANY AND ALL MEDICATIONS PRESCRIBED FOR HIM; SHALL SUBMIT TO ANY EXAMINATIONS OR THERAPY ORDERED BY BOARD; SHALL APPEAR BEFORE BOARD FOR INTERVIEWS UPON REQUEST; SHALL INFORM BOARD OF CHANGE OF ADDRESS OR IF AWAY FOR MORE THAN FIVE DAYS. ARIZONA, IN COMPLIANCE WITH THE AMERICANS WITH DISABILITIES ACT, PROCLAIMS THIS IS NOT A DISCIPLINARY ACTION BUT MERELY A MONITORING PROCEDURE WHICH HE VOLUNTARILY ENTERED INTO. ON 1/25/97 ORDER TERMINATED.

SWEENEY, MICHAEL W MD, LICENSE NUMBER 0022866, HAD ACTION TAKEN BY ARIZONA ON JANUARY 19, 1996

NOTES: ORDER OF 10/21/85 TERMINATED. HE MAY PRACTICE WITH CONDITIONS; SHALL BE FOLLOWED IN INDIVIDUAL THERAPY BY A BOARD-APPROVED PSYCHIATRIST WHO SHALL SUBMIT QUARTERLY REPORTS TO THE BOARD; SHALL ABSTAIN COMPLETELY FROM THE CONSUMPTION OF ALCOHOLIC BEVERAGES AND DRUGS EXCEPT WHEN PRESCRIBED BY HIS TREATING PHYSICIAN; SHALL NOT CONSUME ANY FOOD OR SUBSTANCE CONTAINING POPPYSEEDS; MUST SUBMIT TO WITNESSED RANDOM BIOLOGICAL FLUID COLLECTION; SHALL KEEP A LOG OF ANY AND ALL MEDICATIONS PRESCRIBED FOR HIM; SHALL APPEAR BEFORE THE BOARD FOR INTERVIEWS UPON REQUEST; SHALL INFORM BOARD OF CHANGE OF ADDRESS OR IF AWAY FOR MORE THAN FIVE DAYS; IF HE DOES RESIDE IN ANOTHER STATE, SHALL PARTICIPATE IN THAT STATE'S PHYSICIAN REHABILITATION PROGRAM WITH REPORTS TO ARIZONA TWICE YEARLY; TIME SPENT OUT OF ARIZONA MAY BE TOLLED FOR THIS ORDER. THIS ORDER IS NOT A DISCIPLINARY ACTION, BUT A VOLUNTARY MONITORING PROGRAM TO ENSURE HIS ABILITY TO SAFELY PRACTICE MEDICINE. ON 3/24/99 ORDER TERMINATED.

TELEP, GERALD M MD, LICENSE NUMBER 0012749, HAD ACTION TAKEN BY ARIZONA ON OCTOBER 18, 1996

NOTES: MUST IMMEDIATELY PARTICIPATE IN A BOARD-APPROVED MONITORED AFTERCARE TREATMENT PROGRAM WHOSE THERAPIST MUST SUBMIT QUARTERLY REPORTS; MUST PARTICIPATE IN 90 12-STEP MEETINGS FOR SUBSTANCE ABUSE WITHIN 90 DAYS; MUST THEN PARTICIPATE IN A 12-STEP RECOVERY PROGRAM AS DETERMINED BY HIS TREATING THERAPIST AND ATTEND AT LEAST THREE WEEKLY MEETINGS; SHALL OBTAIN A BOARD-APPROVED TREATING PHYSICIAN; SHALL ABSTAIN COMPLETELY FROM THE CONSUMPTION OF ALCOHOLIC BEVERAGES AND DRUGS EXCEPT WHEN PRESCRIBED BY HIS TREATING PHYSICIAN; SHALL NOT CONSUME FOODS OR SUBSTANCES CONTAINING POPPYSEEDS; MUST SUBMIT TO WITNESSED RANDOM BIOLOGICAL FLUID COLLECTION; MUST KEEP A LOG OF ANY AND ALL MEDICATIONS PRESCRIBED FOR HIM; SHALL SUBMIT TO ANY EXAMINATIONS OR THERAPY ORDERED BY THE BOARD; SHALL APPEAR BEFORE BOARD FOR INTERVIEWS UPON REQUEST; SHALL INFORM BOARD OF CHANGE OF ADDRESS OR IF AWAY FOR MORE THAN FIVE DAYS. IF HE DOES RESIDE IN ANOTHER STATE, SHALL PARTICIPATE IN THAT STATE'S PHYSICIAN REHABILITATION PROGRAM WITH REPORTS TO ARIZONA TWICE YEARLY; TIME SPENT OUT OF ARIZONA MAY BE TOLLED FOR THIS ORDER; ARIZONA, IN COMPLIANCE WITH THE AMERICANS WITH DISABILITIES ACT, PROCLAIMS THIS IS NOT A DISCIPLINARY ACTION BUT MERELY A MONITORING PROCEDURE WHICH HE ENTERED INTO VOLUNTARILY.

TREVELLINE, ERIC E MD, LICENSE NUMBER 0021213, HAD ACTION TAKEN BY ARIZONA ON APRIL 8, 1995

NOTES: CURRENTLY IN LONG-TERM TREATMENT. MUST IMMEDIATELY PARTICIPATE IN A BOARD-APPROVED MONITORED AFTERCARE TREATMENT PROGRAM WHOSE THERAPIST MUST SUBMIT QUARTERLY REPORTS; MUST PARTICIPATE IN 90 12-STEP MEETINGS FOR SUBSTANCE ABUSE WITHIN 90 DAYS; MUST THEN PARTICIPATE IN A 12-STEP RECOVERY PROGRAM AS DETERMINED BY HIS TREATING THERAPIST AND ATTEND AT LEAST THREE WEEKLY MEETINGS; SHALL OBTAIN A BOARD-APPROVED TREATING PHYSICIAN; SHALL ABSTAIN COMPLETELY FROM THE CONSUMPTION OF ALCOHOLIC BEVERAGES AND DRUGS EXCEPT WHEN PRESCRIBED BY HIS TREATING PHYSICIAN; MUST SUBMIT TO WITNESSED RANDOM BIOLOGICAL FLUID COLLECTION; MUST KEEP A LOG OF ANY AND ALL MEDICATIONS PRESCRIBED FOR HIM; SHALL SUBMIT TO ANY EXAMINATIONS OR THERAPY ORDERED BY THE BOARD; SHALL APPEAR BEFORE BOARD FOR INTERVIEWS UPON REQUEST; SHALL INFORM BOARD OF CHANGE OF ADDRESS OR IF AWAY FOR MORE THAN FIVE DAYS. ARIZONA, IN COMPLIANCE WITH THE AMERICANS WITH DISABILITIES ACT, PROCLAIMS THIS IS NOT A DISCIPLINARY ACTION BUT MERELY A MONITORING PROCEDURE WHICH HE ENTERED INTO VOLUNTARILY.

VAN DYKE, SUSAN MD, LICENSE NUMBER 0020156, HAD ACTION TAKEN BY ARIZONA ON JULY 18, 1992

NOTES: MUST IMMEDIATELY PARTICIPATE IN A BOARD-APPROVED MONITORED AFTERCARE TREATMENT PROGRAM WHOSE THERAPIST MUST SUBMIT QUARTERLY REPORTS; MUST PARTICIPATE IN 90 12-STEP MEETINGS FOR SUBSTANCE ABUSE WITHIN 90 DAYS; MUST THEN PARTICIPATE IN A 12-STEP RECOVERY PROGRAM AS DETERMINED BY HER TREATING THERAPIST AND ATTEND AT LEAST THREE WEEKLY MEETINGS; SHALL OBTAIN A BOARD-APPROVED TREATING PHYSICIAN; SHALL ABSTAIN

COMPLETELY FROM THE CONSUMPTION OF ALCOHOLIC BEVERAGES AND DRUGS EXCEPT WHEN PRESCRIBED BY HER TREATING PHYSICIAN; MUST SUBMIT TO WITNESSED RANDOM BIOLOGICAL FLUID COLLECTION; KEEP A LOG OF ANY AND ALL MEDICATIONS PRESCRIBED FOR HER; SHALL SUBMIT TO ANY EXAMINATIONS OR THERAPY ORDERED BY BOARD; SHALL APPEAR BEFORE BOARD FOR INTERVIEWS UPON REQUEST; SHALL INFORM BOARD OF CHANGE OF ADDRESS OR IF AWAY FOR MORE THAN 5 DAYS. ARIZONA, IN COMPLIANCE WITH THE AMERICANS WITH DISABILITIES ACT, PROCLAIMS THIS IS NOT A DISCIPLINARY ACTION BUT MERELY A MONITORING PROCEDURE WHICH SHE VOLUNTARILY ENTERED INTO. AS OF 7/22/95 ORDER TO BE TERMINATED IN 90 DAYS.

VANCE, MICHAEL V MD, LICENSE NUMBER 0007616, HAD ACTION TAKEN BY ARIZONA ON JULY 31, 1995

NOTES: ACKNOWLEDGED THAT HE IS SEEKING TREATMENT REGARDING ALCOHOL USE AFTER BEING COUNSELED AT HOSPITAL FOR APPEARING WITH ALCOHOL ON HIS BREATH. MUST IMMEDIATELY PARTICIPATE IN A BOARD-APPROVED MONITORED AFTERCARE TREATMENT PROGRAM WHOSE THERAPIST MUST SUBMIT QUARTERLY REPORTS; MUST PARTICIPATE IN 90 12-STEP MEETINGS FOR SUBSTANCE ABUSE WITHIN 90 DAYS; MUST THEN PARTICIPATE IN A 12-STEP RECOVERY PROGRAM AS DETERMINED BY HIS TREATING THERAPIST AND ATTEND AT LEAST THREE WEEKLY MEETINGS; SHALL OBTAIN A BOARD-APPROVED TREATING PHYSICIAN; SHALL ABSTAIN COMPLETELY FROM THE CONSUMPTION OF ALCOHOLIC BEVERAGES AND DRUGS EXCEPT WHEN PRESCRIBED BY HIS TREATING PHYSICIAN; MUST SUBMIT TO WITNESSED RANDOM BIOLOGICAL FLUID COLLECTION; MUST KEEP A LOG OF ANY AND ALL MEDICATIONS PRESCRIBED FOR HIM; SHALL SUBMIT TO ANY EXAMINATIONS OR THERAPY ORDERED BY THE BOARD; SHALL APPEAR BEFORE BOARD FOR INTERVIEWS UPON REQUEST; SHALL INFORM BOARD OF CHANGE OF ADDRESS OR IF AWAY FOR MORE THAN FIVE DAYS. ARIZONA, IN COMPLIANCE WITH THE AMERICANS WITH DISABILITIES ACT, PROCLAIMS THIS IS NOT A DISCIPLINARY ACTION BUT MERELY A MONITORING PROCEDURE WHICH HE HAS ENTERED INTO VOLUNTARILY. REQUEST TO PLACE LICENSE IN INACTIVE STATUS GRANTED. AGREES NOT TO PRACTICE MEDICINE ANYWHERE OR WRITE PRESCRIPTIONS WHILE LICENSE IS INACTIVE; AGREES TO ENTER RESIDENTIAL/INPATIENT TREATMENT FOR CHEMICAL DEPENDENCY AND ALCOHOLISM AND TO SUCCESSFULLY COMPLETE ALL TREATMENT RECOMMENDED; AGREES NOT TO REQUEST REACTIVATION OF LICENSE UNTIL MEETS WITH THE BOARD; HE SHALL NOT PRACTICE MEDICINE IN ARIZONA UNTIL FURTHER ORDER OF THE BOARD. ON 10/21/95 ORDER REQUIRING HE NOT PRACTICE WITHOUT FURTHER ORDER OF THE BOARD WAS TERMINATED.

VESPE, JOHN R MD, HAD ACTION TAKEN BY ARIZONA ON JANUARY 23, 1998

NOTES: APPLICATION FOR A RESIDENCY TRAINING PERMIT. MUST IMMEDIATELY PARTICIPATE IN A BOARD-APPROVED MONITORED AFTERCARE TREATMENT PROGRAM WHOSE THERAPIST MUST SUBMIT MONTHLY REPORTS; MUST PARTICIPATE IN 90 12-STEP MEETINGS FOR SUBSTANCE ABUSE WITHIN 90 DAYS; MUST THEN PARTICIPATE IN A 12-STEP RECOVERY PROGRAM AS DETERMINED BY HIS TREATING THERAPIST AND ATTEND AT LEAST THREE WEEKLY MEETINGS; SHALL OBTAIN A BOARD-APPROVED TREATING PHYSICIAN; SHALL ABSTAIN COMPLETELY FROM THE CONSUMPTION OF ALCOHOLIC BEVERAGES AND DRUGS EXCEPT WHEN PRESCRIBED BY HIS TREATING PHYSICIAN; SHALL NOT CONSUME FOOD OR SUBSTANCES CONTAINING POPPYSEEDS; MUST SUBMIT TO WITNESSED RANDOM BIOLOGICAL FLUID COLLECTION; MUST KEEP A LOG OF ANY AND ALL MEDICATIONS PRESCRIBED FOR HIM; SHALL SUBMIT TO ANY EXAMINATIONS OR THERAPY ORDERED BY BOARD; SHALL APPEAR BEFORE BOARD FOR INTERVIEWS UPON REQUEST; SHALL INFORM BOARD OF CHANGE OF ADDRESS OR IF AWAY FOR MORE THAN FIVE DAYS. ARIZONA, IN COMPLIANCE WITH THE AMERICANS WITH DISABILITIES ACT, PROCLAIMS THIS IS NOT A DISCIPLINARY ACTION BUT MERELY A MONITORING PROCEDURE WHICH HE VOLUNTARILY ENTERED INTO. ON 9/21/99 THE BOARD ALLOWED HIM 90 DAYS TO PAY HIS CURRENT ACCOUNT BALANCE AND IF HE FAILS, THAT HE BE PLACED ON PROBATION FOR FIVE YEARS AND THE BALANCE TURNED OVER TO THE ATTORNEY GENERAL'S OFFICE FOR COLLECTION; SHALL REMAIN IN THE MONITORED AFTERCARE PROGRAM.

WAGNER, MITCHELL S MD, HAD ACTION TAKEN BY ARIZONA ON JANUARY 1, 1999

NOTES: MUST IMMEDIATELY PARTICIPATE IN A BOARD-APPROVED MONITORED AFTERCARE TREATMENT PROGRAM WHOSE THERAPIST MUST SUBMIT QUARTERLY REPORTS; MUST PARTICIPATE IN 90 12-STEP MEETINGS FOR SUBSTANCE ABUSE WITHIN 90 DAYS; MUST THEN PARTICIPATE IN A 12-STEP RECOVERY PROGRAM AS DETERMINED BY HIS/HER TREATING THERAPIST AND ATTEND AT LEAST THREE WEEKLY MEETINGS; SHALL OBTAIN A BOARD-APPROVED TREATING PHYSICIAN; SHALL ABSTAIN COMPLETELY FROM THE CONSUMPTION OF ALCOHOLIC BEVERAGES AND DRUGS EXCEPT WHEN PRESCRIBED BY HIS/HER TREATING PHYSICIAN; SHALL NOT CONSUME FOOD OR SUBSTANCES CONTAINING POPPYSEEDS; MUST SUBMIT TO WITNESSED RANDOM BIOLOGICAL FLUID COLLECTION; MUST KEEP A LOG OF ANY AND ALL MEDICATIONS PRESCRIBED FOR HIM/HER; SHALL SUBMIT TO ANY EXAMINATIONS OR THERAPY ORDERED BY BOARD; SHALL APPEAR BEFORE BOARD FOR INTERVIEWS UPON REQUEST; SHALL INFORM BOARD OF CHANGE OF ADDRESS OR IF AWAY FOR MORE THAN FIVE DAYS. ARIZONA, IN COMPLIANCE WITH THE AMERICANS WITH DISABILITIES ACT, PROCLAIMS THIS IS NOT A DISCIPLINARY ACTION BUT MERELY A MONITORING PROCEDURE WHICH HE VOLUNTARILY ENTERED INTO.

WALKER, GREGORY T MD, LICENSE NUMBER 0021091, HAD ACTION TAKEN BY ARIZONA ON OCTOBER 19, 1996

NOTES: MUST IMMEDIATELY PARTICIPATE IN A BOARD-APPROVED MONITORED AFTERCARE TREATMENT PROGRAM WHOSE THERAPIST MUST SUBMIT QUARTERLY REPORTS; MUST PARTICIPATE IN 90 12-STEP MEETINGS FOR SUBSTANCE ABUSE WITHIN 90 DAYS; MUST THEN PARTICIPATE IN A 12-STEP RECOVERY PROGRAM AS DETERMINED BY HIS TREATING THERAPIST AND ATTEND AT LEAST THREE WEEKLY MEETINGS; SHALL OBTAIN A BOARD-APPROVED TREATING PHYSICIAN; SHALL ABSTAIN COMPLETELY FROM THE CONSUMPTION OF ALCOHOLIC BEVERAGES AND DRUGS EXCEPT WHEN PRESCRIBED BY HIS TREATING PHYSICIAN; SHALL NOT CONSUME FOODS OR SUBSTANCES CONTAINING POPPYSEEDS; MUST SUBMIT TO WITNESSED RANDOM BIOLOGICAL FLUID COLLECTION; MUST KEEP A LOG OF ANY AND ALL MEDICATIONS PRESCRIBED FOR HIM; SHALL SUBMIT TO ANY EXAMINATIONS OR THERAPY ORDERED BY THE BOARD; SHALL APPEAR BEFORE

BOARD FOR INTERVIEWS UPON REQUEST; SHALL INFORM BOARD OF CHANGE OF ADDRESS OR IF AWAY FOR MORE THAN FIVE DAYS; IF HE DOES RESIDE IN ANOTHER STATE, SHALL PARTICIPATE IN THAT STATE'S PHYSICIAN REHABILITATION PROGRAM WITH REPORTS TO ARIZONA TWICE YEARLY; TIME SPENT OUT OF ARIZONA MAY BE TOLLED FOR THIS ORDER. ARIZONA, IN COMPLIANCE WITH THE AMERICANS WITH DISABILITIES ACT, PROCLAIMS THIS IS NOT A DISCIPLINARY ACTION BUT MERELY A MONITORING PROCEDURE WHICH HE ENTERED INTO VOLUNTARILY.

WALLACE, STEPHEN A MD, LICENSE NUMBER 0013856, HAD ACTION TAKEN BY ARIZONA ON JANUARY 29, 1994

NOTES: RELATIVE TO TREATMENT FOR SUBSTANCE ABUSE. MUST IMMEDIATELY PARTICIPATE IN A BOARD-APPROVED MONITORED AFTERCARE TREATMENT PROGRAM WHOSE THERAPIST MUST SUBMIT QUARTERLY REPORTS; MUST PARTICIPATE IN 90 12-STEP MEETINGS FOR SUBSTANCE ABUSE WITHIN 90 DAYS; MUST THEN PARTICIPATE IN A 12-STEP RECOVERY PROGRAM AS DETERMINED BY HIS TREATING THERAPIST AND ATTEND AT LEAST THREE WEEKLY MEETINGS; SHALL OBTAIN A BOARD-APPROVED TREATING PHYSICIAN; SHALL ABSTAIN COMPLETELY FROM THE CONSUMPTION OF ALCOHOLIC BEVERAGES AND DRUGS EXCEPT WHEN PRESCRIBED BY HIS TREATING PHYSICIAN; MUST SUBMIT TO WITNESSED RANDOM BIOLOGICAL FLUID COLLECTION; KEEP A LOG OF ANY AND ALL MEDICATIONS PRESCRIBED FOR HIM; SHALL SUBMIT TO ANY EXAMINATIONS OR THERAPY ORDERED BY BOARD; SHALL APPEAR BEFORE BOARD FOR INTERVIEWS UPON REQUEST; SHALL INFORM BOARD OF CHANGE OF ADDRESS OR IF AWAY FOR MORE THAN FIVE DAYS. ARIZONA, IN COMPLIANCE WITH THE AMERICANS WITH DISABILITIES ACT, PROCLAIMS THIS IS NOT A DISCIPLINARY ACTION BUT MERELY A MONITORING PROCEDURE WHICH HE VOLUNTARILY ENTERED INTO. ON 3/28/98 ORDER TERMINATED IN 90 DAYS.

WASSERMAN, SCOTT A MD, LICENSE NUMBER 0023328, HAD ACTION TAKEN BY ARIZONA ON JULY 26, 1995

NOTES: MUST IMMEDIATELY PARTICIPATE IN A BOARD-APPROVED MONITORED AFTERCARE TREATMENT PROGRAM WHOSE THERAPIST MUST SUBMIT QUARTERLY REPORTS; MUST PARTICIPATE IN A 12-STEP RECOVERY PROGRAM FOR SUBSTANCE ABUSE AND ATTEND A MINIMUM OF THREE WEEKLY MEETINGS; SHALL OBTAIN A BOARD-APPROVED TREATING PHYSICIAN; SHALL ABSTAIN COMPLETELY FROM THE CONSUMPTION OF ALCOHOLIC BEVERAGES AND DRUGS EXCEPT WHEN PRESCRIBED BY HIS TREATING PHYSICIAN; MUST SUBMIT TO WITNESSED RANDOM BIOLOGICAL FLUID COLLECTION; MUST KEEP A LOG OF ANY AND ALL MEDICATIONS PRESCRIBED FOR HIM; SHALL SUBMIT TO ANY EXAMINATIONS OR THERAPY ORDERED BY BOARD; SHALL APPEAR BEFORE BOARD FOR INTERVIEWS UPON REQUEST; SHALL INFORM THE BOARD OF CHANGE OF ADDRESS OR IF AWAY FOR MORE THAN FIVE DAYS. ARIZONA, IN COMPLIANCE WITH THE AMERICANS WITH DISABILITIES ACT, PROCLAIMS THIS IS NOT A DISCIPLINARY ACTION BUT MERELY A MONITORING PROCEDURE WHICH HE VOLUNTARILY ENTERED INTO. ON 3/15/97 ORDER WAS TERMINATED EFFECTIVE IN 90 DAYS.

WILLIAMS, RICHARD M MD, HAD ACTION TAKEN BY ARIZONA ON JANUARY 23, 1998

NOTES: MUST IMMEDIATELY PARTICIPATE IN A BOARD-APPROVED MONITORED AFTERCARE TREATMENT PROGRAM WHOSE THERAPIST MUST SUBMIT MONTHLY REPORTS; MUST PARTICIPATE IN A 12-STEP RECOVERY PROGRAM AS DETERMINED BY HIS TREATING THERAPIST AND ATTEND AT LEAST THREE WEEKLY MEETINGS; SHALL OBTAIN A BOARD-APPROVED TREATING PHYSICIAN; SHALL ABSTAIN COMPLETELY FROM THE CONSUMPTION OF ALCOHOLIC BEVERAGES AND DRUGS EXCEPT WHEN PRESCRIBED BY HIS TREATING PHYSICIAN; SHALL NOT CONSUME FOOD OR SUBSTANCES CONTAINING POPPYSEEDS; MUST SUBMIT TO WITNESSED RANDOM BIOLOGICAL FLUID COLLECTION; MUST KEEP A LOG OF ANY AND ALL MEDICATIONS PRESCRIBED FOR HIM; SHALL SUBMIT TO ANY EXAMINATIONS OR THERAPY ORDERED BY BOARD; SHALL APPEAR BEFORE BOARD FOR INTERVIEWS UPON REQUEST; SHALL INFORM BOARD OF CHANGE OF ADDRESS OR IF AWAY FOR MORE THAN FIVE DAYS; ARIZONA, IN COMPLIANCE WITH THE AMERICANS WITH DISABILITIES ACT, PROCLAIMS THIS IS NOT A DISCIPLINARY ACTION BUT MERELY A MONITORING PROCEDURE WHICH HE VOLUNTARILY ENTERED INTO; SHALL IMMEDIATELY OBTAIN A TREATING PSYCHIATRIST APPROVED BY THE BOARD AND SHALL REMAIN IN TREATMENT WITH THE PSYCHIATRIST UNTIL FURTHER ORDER OF THE BOARD WITH QUARTERLY REPORTS.

WILLIAMSON, THOMAS LEE MD, LICENSE NUMBER 21101, HAD ACTION TAKEN BY ARIZONA ON JANUARY 25, 1997

NOTES: MUST IMMEDIATELY PARTICIPATE IN A BOARD-APPROVED MONITORED AFTERCARE TREATMENT PROGRAM WHOSE THERAPIST MUST SUBMIT QUARTERLY REPORTS; MUST PARTICIPATE IN 90 12-STEP MEETINGS FOR SUBSTANCE ABUSE WITHIN 90 DAYS; MUST THEN PARTICIPATE IN A 12-STEP RECOVERY PROGRAM AS DETERMINED BY HIS TREATING THERAPIST AND ATTEND AT LEAST THREE WEEKLY MEETINGS; SHALL OBTAIN A BOARD-APPROVED TREATING PHYSICIAN; SHALL ABSTAIN COMPLETELY FROM THE CONSUMPTION OF ALCOHOLIC BEVERAGES AND DRUGS EXCEPT WHEN PRESCRIBED BY HIS TREATING PHYSICIAN; SHALL NOT CONSUME FOOD OR SUBSTANCES CONTAINING POPPYSEEDS; MUST SUBMIT TO WITNESSED RANDOM BIOLOGICAL FLUID COLLECTION; MUST KEEP A LOG OF ANY AND ALL MEDICATIONS PRESCRIBED FOR HIM; SHALL SUBMIT TO ANY EXAMINATIONS OR THERAPY ORDERED BY BOARD; SHALL APPEAR BEFORE BOARD FOR INTERVIEWS UPON REQUEST; SHALL INFORM BOARD OF CHANGE OF ADDRESS OR IF AWAY FOR MORE THAN FIVE DAYS. ARIZONA, IN COMPLIANCE WITH THE AMERICANS WITH DISABILITIES ACT, PROCLAIMS THIS IS NOT A DISCIPLINARY ACTION BUT MERELY A MONITORING PROCEDURE WHICH HE VOLUNTARILY ENTERED INTO.

WOLF, STEPHEN J MD, LICENSE NUMBER 23479, HAD ACTION TAKEN BY ARIZONA ON MARCH 15, 1997

NOTES: INTERVIEWED BY THE BOARD REGARDING HIS TREATMENT FOR SUBSTANCE ABUSE. MUST IMMEDIATELY PARTICIPATE IN A BOARD-APPROVED MONITORED AFTERCARE TREATMENT PROGRAM WHOSE THERAPIST MUST SUBMIT QUARTERLY REPORTS; MUST PARTICIPATE IN 90 12-STEP MEETINGS FOR SUBSTANCE ABUSE WITHIN 90 DAYS; MUST THEN PARTICIPATE IN A 12-STEP RECOVERY PROGRAM AS DETERMINED BY HIS TREATING THERAPIST AND ATTEND AT LEAST THREE WEEKLY MEETINGS; SHALL OBTAIN A BOARD-APPROVED TREATING PHYSICIAN; SHALL ABSTAIN COMPLETELY FROM THE CONSUMPTION OF ALCOHOLIC BEVERAGES AND DRUGS EXCEPT WHEN PRESCRIBED BY HIS TREATING PHYSICIAN; SHALL NOT CONSUME

FOOD OR SUBSTANCES CONTAINING POPPYSEEDS; MUST SUBMIT TO WITNESSED RANDOM BIOLOGICAL FLUID COLLECTION; MUST KEEP A LOG OF ANY AND ALL MEDICATIONS PRESCRIBED FOR HIM; SHALL SUBMIT TO ANY EXAMINATIONS OR THERAPY ORDERED BY BOARD; SHALL APPEAR BEFORE BOARD FOR INTERVIEWS UPON REQUEST; SHALL INFORM BOARD OF CHANGE OF ADDRESS OR IF AWAY FOR MORE THAN FIVE DAYS; SHALL IMMEDIATELY OBTAIN A TREATING PSYCHIATRIST APPROVED BY THE BOARD AND SHALL REMAIN IN TREATMENT WITH THE PSYCHIATRIST UNTIL FURTHER ORDER OF THE BOARD WITH QUARTERLY REPORTS. ARIZONA, IN COMPLIANCE WITH THE AMERICANS WITH DISABILITIES ACT, PROCLAIMS THIS IS NOT A DISCIPLINARY ACTION BUT MERELY A MONITORING PROCEDURE WHICH HE VOLUNTARILY ENTERED INTO.

WOODS, BRENDA KAY MD, HAD ACTION TAKEN BY ARIZONA ON JULY 26, 1997

NOTES: INTERVIEWED BY THE BOARD REGARDING HER TREATMENT FOR SUBSTANCE ABUSE AND PARTICIPATION IN THE INDIANA PHYSICIANS ASSISTANCE PROGRAM. MUST IMMEDIATELY PARTICIPATE IN A BOARD-APPROVED MONITORED AFTERCARE TREATMENT PROGRAM WHOSE THERAPIST MUST SUBMIT MONTHLY REPORTS; MUST PARTICIPATE IN 90 12-STEP MEETINGS FOR SUBSTANCE ABUSE WITHIN 90 DAYS; MUST THEN PARTICIPATE IN A 12-STEP RECOVERY PROGRAM AS DETERMINED BY HIS TREATING THERAPIST AND ATTEND AT LEAST THREE WEEKLY MEETINGS; SHALL OBTAIN A BOARD-APPROVED TREATING PHYSICIAN; SHALL ABSTAIN COMPLETELY FROM THE CONSUMPTION OF ALCOHOLIC BEVERAGES AND DRUGS EXCEPT WHEN PRESCRIBED BY HIS TREATING PHYSICIAN; SHALL NOT CONSUME FOOD OR SUBSTANCES CONTAINING POPPYSEEDS; MUST SUBMIT TO WITNESSED RANDOM BIOLOGICAL FLUID COLLECTION; MUST KEEP A LOG OF ANY AND ALL MEDICATIONS PRESCRIBED FOR HIM; SHALL SUBMIT TO ANY EXAMINATIONS OR THERAPY ORDERED BY BOARD; SHALL APPEAR BEFORE BOARD FOR INTERVIEWS UPON REQUEST; SHALL INFORM BOARD OF CHANGE OF ADDRESS OR IF AWAY FOR MORE THAN FIVE DAYS. ARIZONA, IN COMPLIANCE WITH THE AMERICANS WITH DISABILITIES ACT, PROCLAIMS THIS IS NOT A DISCIPLINARY ACTION BUT MERELY A MONITORING PROCEDURE WHICH SHE VOLUNTARILY ENTERED INTO; SHALL IMMEDIATELY OBTAIN A TREATING PSYCHIATRIST APPROVED BY BOARD STAFF AND SHALL REMAIN IN TREATMENT WITH THE PSYCHIATRIST UNTIL FURTHER ORDER OF THE BOARD WITH QUARTERLY REPORTS. ORDER TERMINATED ON 11/1/98.

WYLIE, ROBERT J MD, LICENSE NUMBER 18644, HAD ACTION TAKEN BY ARIZONA ON NOVEMBER 14, 1997

NOTES: INTERVIEWED BY BOARD REGARDING HIS TREATMENT FOR SUBSTANCE ABUSE. MUST IMMEDIATELY PARTICIPATE IN A BOARD-APPROVED MONITORED AFTERCARE TREATMENT PROGRAM WHOSE THERAPIST MUST SUBMIT MONTHLY REPORTS; MUST ALSO ATTEND INDIVIDUAL THERAPY IN THE WEEKS HE DOES NOT HAVE GROUP THERAPY; MUST PARTICIPATE IN 90 12-STEP MEETINGS FOR SUBSTANCE ABUSE WITHIN 90 DAYS; MUST THEN PARTICIPATE IN A 12-STEP RECOVERY PROGRAM AS DETERMINED BY HIS TREATING THERAPIST AND ATTEND AT LEAST THREE WEEKLY MEETINGS; SHALL OBTAIN A BOARD-APPROVED TREATING PHYSICIAN; SHALL ABSTAIN COMPLETELY FROM THE CONSUMPTION OF ALCOHOLIC BEVERAGES AND DRUGS EXCEPT WHEN PRESCRIBED BY HIS TREATING PHYSICIAN; SHALL NOT CONSUME FOOD OR SUBSTANCES CONTAINING POPPYSEEDS; MUST SUBMIT TO WITNESSED RANDOM BIOLOGICAL FLUID COLLECTION; MUST KEEP A LOG OF ANY AND ALL MEDICATIONS PRESCRIBED FOR HIM; SHALL SUBMIT TO ANY EXAMINATIONS OR THERAPY ORDERED BY BOARD; SHALL APPEAR BEFORE BOARD FOR INTERVIEWS UPON REQUEST; SHALL INFORM BOARD OF CHANGE OF ADDRESS OR IF AWAY FOR MORE THAN FIVE DAYS. ARIZONA, IN COMPLIANCE WITH THE AMERICANS WITH DISABILITIES ACT, PROCLAIMS THIS IS NOT A DISCIPLINARY ACTION BUT MERELY A MONITORING PROCEDURE WHICH HE VOLUNTARILY ENTERED INTO.

COLORADO

1999 serious action rate: 5.24/1000
1999 ranking: 10th

The Colorado State Board of Medical Examiners sent listings and copies of its newsletters that covered disciplinary actions taken from July 1990 through December 1999. These include the physician's name, degree, license number, date of birth, city and state of residence, the date and a brief description of the type of action taken and the reason for the action. The reports contain no information on modifications and terminations of board actions. Colorado sent separate information on these actions. Colorado informed us no court actions had taken place.

The information provided covers disciplinary actions taken against allopathic physicians (MDs) and osteopathic physicians (DOs).

Besides disciplinary actions taken by the State Medical Board, this listing also includes actions taken by the Medicare/Medicaid programs, the FDA, and the DEA against physicians located in this state. Disciplinary actions taken by other states against physicians located in Colorado or that match a physician disciplined by Colorado (see Appendix 2 for an explanation of the matching protocol) are also included.

Although we have made every effort to match physicians' names correctly, some materials we received did not include complete information on middle names, license numbers, birth dates or addresses. Therefore, consumers should remember that non-disciplined physicians and physicians with different disciplinary actions may have similar names to those disciplined physicians listed in this state. Consumers should also remember that if they want the most current information on the status on a physician's license, they should contact the medical board of the state in which the physician practices or had practiced. (See board address below.) Internet address: *http://www.dora.state.co.us/medical.* This state has a web site which we have graded D on a scale of A (best) to X (worst). This is a measure of the completeness of the information on disciplined doctors. Those state licensing boards with web sites make independent choices about the type of information to be included on their site and how often it is updated.

According to the Federation of State Medical Boards, Colorado took 59 serious disciplinary actions against MDs and DOs in 1999. Compared to the 11,253 MDs practicing in the state, Colorado had a serious disciplinary action rate of 5.24 serious actions per 1,000 MDs and ranked 10th on that list (see Table A, Findings, pg. 14).

The tables below summarize the data Public Citizen received from Colorado.

Table 1. Disciplinary Actions Against MDs and DOs July 1990 through December 1999*

Action	Number	Percent**
Revocation	50	5.7%
Surrender	93	10.5%
Suspension	45	5.1%
Probation	192	21.7%
Practice Restriction	52	5.9%
Action Taken Against Controlled Substance License	16	1.8%
Other Actions	436	49.3%
Total Actions	**884**	**100.0%**

* This table lists only the two most serious disciplinary actions taken against a physician.
** Percentages may not total 100% due to rounding.

Table 2. Offenses for which MDs and DOs were Disciplined July 1990 through December 1999*

Offense	Number	Percent
Criminal Conviction	24	5.7%
Sexual Abuse of or Sexual Misconduct with a Patient	20	4.8%
Substandard Care, Incompetence or Negligence	149	35.4%
Misprescribing or Overprescribing Drugs	5	1.2%
Substance Abuse	79	18.8%
Disciplinary Action Taken Against License by Another State or Agency	13	3.1%
Other Offenses	131	31.1%
Total Records With Offense Listed	**421**	**100%**

* Includes only those actions for which an offense was listed and for which we had a corresponding term in our database.

Table 3. Disciplinary Actions Taken for Sexual Abuse of or Sexual Misconduct with a Patient

Action	Number	Percent
Revocation	3	9.1%
Surrender	2	6.1%
Suspension	8	24.2%
Emergency Suspension	2	6.1%
Probation	11	33.3%
Other Actions	7	21.2%
Total Actions	**33**	**100.0%**

Table 4. Disciplinary Actions Taken for Substandard Care, Incompetence or Negligence

Action	Number	Percent
Revocation	20	9.2%
Surrender	16	7.3%
Suspension	3	1.4%
Emergency Suspension	8	3.7%
Probation	59	27.1%
Practice Restriction	20	9.2%
Reprimand	18	8.3%
Other Actions	74	33.9%
Total Actions	**218**	**100.0%**

Table 5. Disciplinary Actions Taken for Criminal Conviction

Action	Number	Percent
Revocation	11	39.3%
Surrender	4	14.3%
Suspension	1	3.6%
Probation	4	14.3%
Other Actions	8	28.6%
Total Actions	**28**	**100.0%**

Table 6. Disciplinary Actions Taken for Substance Abuse

Action	Number	Percent
Revocation	2	1.5%
Surrender	6	4.5%
Revocation, Surrender, or Suspension of Controlled Substance License	1	0.7%
Suspension	4	3.0%
Emergency Suspension	6	4.5%
Probation	56	41.8%
Restriction of Controlled Substance License	2	1.5%
Required to Enter an Impaired Physician Program or Substance Abuse Treatment	6	4.5%
Other Actions	51	38.1%
Total Actions	**134**	**100.0%**

If you feel that your doctor has not given you proper medical care or has mistreated you in any way--whether or not he or she is listed in this report--it is important that you let your state medical board know. Even if they do not immediately act on your complaint, it is important that the information be recorded in their files because it is possible that other people may have filed or will file complaints about the same doctor. Send a brief written description of what occurred to the addresses below or call the phone numbers listed for more information on how to file a complaint.

Address

Colorado State Board of Medical Examiners
Susan Miller, Program Administrator
1560 Broadway, Suite 1300
Denver, CO 80202-5140
(303) 894-7690
E-mail: medical@dora.state.co.us

Listing of Doctors Sanctioned by Offense

Sexual Abuse of or Sexual Misconduct with a Patient

ADAMS, BARTON JOSEPH
ANGELLO, ANTHONY L
BADZINSKI, GARY L
BELL, JON A
BOSTROM, PAUL D
COLLINS, THOMAS J
COPELAN, RUSSELL I
EMERSON, JOHN H
EPPLER, STEPHEN V
GALLAGHER, MICHAEL J
GERMAN, CHARLES
HERMANN, JOSEPH F
JOHNSON, JOHNNY E
MANUELE, MARK A
NICHOLSON, PETER M
PUSHKIN, JOSHUA R
SANTAGUIDA, RIK
SHAPIRO, JED S
SWEENEY, RICHARD

Substandard Care, Incompetence, or Negligence

ALONSO, KENNETH B
AMANATULLAH, FAISAL F
ANNEBERG, SPENCER K
ASHKAR, LOUIS N
BAGLEY, DAVID L
BARTON, MALCOM DENNIS
BAUMGARDNER, JAN F
BEACH, DON E
BECKWITT, HENRY J
BEDFORD, ALFRED
BENNETT, ALFRED J
BENYI, ELIZABETH R
BHATIA, SOHAN L
BICHON, ROBERT N
BLAKELY, CHARLES A
BRETHOUWER, N ROBERT
BROOKS, BANCROFT
BUGLEWICZ, JOHN
CAMPBELL, BERNARD E
CAMPBELL, WILLIAM M
CARMEL, STEPHEN P
CEDARS, CHESTER M
CHAN, ANTHONY W
COHEN, ELLIOT S
COLE, DON H
COLON-CHANLATTE, IRIS
CONNELLY, JOSEPH W
CORTELYOU, MARIE
COULTER, ROBERT L
CUPPS, JERRY LEE
DAHLBERG, WILLIAM W
DAVIS, HERBERT ALLEN
DAVIS, ROGER WOODS
DAVIS, WILLIAM DUNCAN
DE ALVA, WILLIAM E
DENEGRI, ALBERTO
DOELL, WILLIAM EDWARD
DOTSON, DANIEL A
DOWNING, TERRY
DUNKIN, DONALD E
ECKHARDT, LLOYD O
ECKSTEIN, LARRY
ECOFF, ARTHUR
EDWARDS, JAMES E
ELLIBEE, GARY S
FALZONE, JOSEPH A
FELDMAN, ARMIN
FERN, DONALD EDWIN
FERNON, CHRIS J
FILA, ERNEST G
FOGEL, TIMOTHY J
GALE, JOHN H
GARBER, GEORGE
GARCEAU, ROGER
GARTNER, CHARLES H
GASIS, ALBERT J
GATCHELL, HOMER DALE
GELINAS, MICHAEL P
GIERINGER, GARY V
GLASSMAN, MICHAEL H
GREGG, KELLY R
HAGESETH, CHRISTIAN
HAMILTON, ROBERT
HARRISON, MURKE FRANKLIN
HEIBERGER, JAMES T
HERRIOTT, MICHAEL G
HERSCH, LAWRENCE B
HILBERMAN, MARK
HOFFMAN, JAMES F
HOLDER, SCOTT D
HRDLICKA, JAN F
JESSEL, JOHN M
JOHNSON, VAUGHN A

Caution: This list is designed to be used only in conjunction with the rest of this book which includes additional information on each physician such as license number, date of action and more complete descriptions of the offenses.

Substandard Care, Incompetence, or Negligence (cont'd)

KEELING, MARITA J
KHAN, IMRAN U
KUSESKI, RONALD E
LACONTE, FRANK
LAUER, JAMES W
LEE, RICHARD H
LEHMKUHLE, JOSEPH M
LEMLEY, J STEPHEN
LEONARDI, LEO J
LISONBEE, JOHN E
LOPEZ-SAMAYOA, OMAR
MADAN, VEENA
MARTIN, THEODORE E
MARTINEZ, BENJAMIN
MCCAW, WILLIAM W
MCGUIRE, THOMAS J
MCHUGH, J B
MCLAIN, PHIL C
MEASON, THOMAS M
MERRILL, FRANKLIN B
MONTANTE, JOSEPH R
MOTE, PAUL S
MUBARAK, ASAAD A
MUNOZ, DAVID C
MUSSELMAN, RICHARD P
NEMER, ROBERT J
NORTON, JOHN T
O'NEILL, JOHN J
OVERTURF, BRUCE R
PALU, MARGARET
PATEL, GIRISH
PEOPLES, U S
PETERSON, RICHARD I
POWELL, SCOTT EVAN
PUCKETT, WILLIAM N
RADETSKY, PAUL
RAPAPORT, STEVEN M
RAVIN, THOMAS H
ROSS, MICHAEL H
SCARINZI, HUGO J
SCEATS, DONALD J
SCHACHT, FREDERICK W
SCHWARTZ, KENNETH A
SCOTT, JAMES L
SEERVELD, HAROLD L
SHERMAN, JOSEPH M
SHESOL, BARRY F
SILLS, THERON
SIMMONS-MCNITT, SUZANNE
SIMON, JOHN S
SINGER, JONATHAN W
SLATER, GERALD E
STEVENS, WILLIAM CRAIG
STIRMAN, JERRY A
SULLIVAN, KEVIN P
TOSETTI, JAMES R
TUTT, GEORGE O
UBA, MAHITO
VALENCIA, WARREN H
VERBRUGGE, JOSEPH J
WARWICK, MARK
WIKHOLM, LARRY J
WOLF, ELLIOTT M
YOUNG, PHILIP G
ZIMIK, LUITHUK

Criminal Conviction or Plea of Guilty, Nolo Contendere, or No Contest to a Crime

ANCIER, STEPHEN L
ASKANAZI, JEFFREY
BALDWIN, RICHARD E
BOYLE, CORNELIUS D
CAPALDO, GEORGE R
CUSTODIO, JOSEPH M
FONTANA, N JOHN
GOODLOE, ROBERT K
HALPRIN, ARTHUR H
HARMON, DAVID R
KINNARD, MELINDA M
LIES, BERT A
LINSTRUM, THOMAS E
LISECKI, EDWARD J
LISECKI, MARGARET
MARTIN, RICHARD EDWIN
MILLER, JOHN JOSEPH
MILLER, MARY MARGARET
OLIVA, PHILIP B
PANTER, KENT WOODRUFF
RODRIGUEZ, VINCENT JOHN
SLATER, GERALD E
SNYDER, CHARLES E
WARREN, STEVEN E

Misprescribing or Overprescribing Drugs

GADPAILLE, WARREN
PAUNOVICH, ROBERT P
SARGENT, ROBERT A
TEETER, BRIAN H
WEAVER, JOHN A

Caution: This list is designed to be used only in conjunction with the rest of this book which includes additional information on each physician such as license number, date of action and more complete descriptions of the offenses.

Substance Abuse

ABBOTT, RICHARD D
ARNONE, THOMAS J
AVNER, TED G
BERESFORD, KENNETH W
BOLAND, GREGORY H
BOYD, GWENDOLYN L
BRUNKO, MICHAEL W
BURKS, CHESTER L
BURRIS, WILLIAM T
BUTLER, HARRISON G
BYNUM, RANDALL L
CARLSON, STEVEN R
CHADO, HERBERT N
CLISE, RICHARD K
COBB, DAVID K
CURTIS, KENNETH W
DARNELL, DUANE R
ELGIN, JAMES C
FECTEAU, MICHELE A
FINEMAN, BRUCE G
FISHER, THOMAS C
FLORA, MARK S
FRITZ, ROBERT L
GREEN, EDMON L
HALL, SHANNA D
HARRIS, JOHN CHARLES
HARTMAN, DIANE M
HARVEY, RICHARD L
HEINDEL, TERRY J
HILST, WILBUR D
HOFFNER, MARGARET M
HOLMES, KELLY V
HOWARD, WILLIAM L
HOWE, JOHN J
HUFFORD, JOHN H
KNIGHT, PHILLIP J
MARTIN, DAVID A
MATTHEWSPRICE, LAUREL A
MCALLEN, CULLEN A
MEASON, THOMAS M
METZGER, JAMES R
MILZER, GARY S
MOORE, MICHAEL B
MOSBY, JAMES R
MURPHY, JAMES T
NITKA, ALFRED C
NYMAN, DAVID W
O'NEILL, JOHN J
OSSORIO, JULIO M
OWENS-DUNLOP, CYNTHIA J
PLATT, TERESA
PUGH, MARION
PUMPHREY, ROBERT S
RATHER, DANIEL A
REISER, DAVID E
SAATHOFF, MICHAEL C
SCHLEGEL, KARL J
SCHRADER, NANCY L
SCOTT, GEORGE E
SHAW, ANITA
SICKBERT, SCOTT F
SIMPSON, RUSSELL W
SMITH, JOHN IRVING
SMOLLEY, JOHN
SOLOMON, MAURICE C
SPRINGER, GREGG E
TURLEY, LOREN M
VOSS, RICHARD G
WADE, HENRY KING
WESTENBERGER, PETE D
WHITE, MARK S
WILLIAMS, PAUL C
WILSON, RODDY L
WILSON, SHAWN L

Caution: This list is designed to be used only in conjunction with the rest of this book which includes additional information on each physician such as license number, date of action and more complete descriptions of the offenses.

ABBOTT, RICHARD D MD, DATE OF BIRTH DECEMBER 31, 1963, LICENSE NUMBER 34325, WAS DISCIPLINED BY COLORADO ON APRIL 22, 1999
DISCIPLINARY ACTION: 60-MONTH PROBATION; MONITORING OF PHYSICIAN PERFORMANCE
OFFENSE: SUBSTANCE ABUSE

NOTES: HABITUAL INTEMPERANCE OR EXCESSIVE USE OF A CONTROLLED SUBSTANCE. PROBATIONARY TERMS INCLUDE: ABSTINENCE FROM ALCOHOL AND CONTROLLED SUBSTANCES, TREATMENT MONITORING AND ANESTHESIOLOGY MONITORING.

ABBOTT, RICHARD DALE MD OF 4200 E 9TH AVENUE #B113, DENVER, CO, WAS DISCIPLINED BY DEA ON NOVEMBER 16, 1998
DISCIPLINARY ACTION: SURRENDER OF CONTROLLED SUBSTANCE LICENSE

ADAMS, BARTON J DO, LICENSE NUMBER 00G7150 OF KAHULUI, HI, WAS DISCIPLINED BY TEXAS ON OCTOBER 9, 1992
DISCIPLINARY ACTION: SURRENDER OF LICENSE
OFFENSE: DISCIPLINARY ACTION BY ANOTHER STATE OR AGENCY

NOTES: UNPROFESSIONAL OR DISHONORABLE CONDUCT LIKELY TO DECEIVE, DEFRAUD OR INJURE THE PUBLIC; CONVICTION OF A FELONY OR A CRIME OF A LESSER DEGREE THAT INVOLVES MORAL TURPITUDE; SUSPENSION, REVOCATION OR RESTRICTION BY ANOTHER STATE. LICENSE PERMANENTLY RETIRED.

ADAMS, BARTON J DO OF SAN JOSE, CA, WAS DISCIPLINED BY VERMONT ON DECEMBER 3, 1996
DISCIPLINARY ACTION: EMERGENCY SUSPENSION
OFFENSE: DISCIPLINARY ACTION BY ANOTHER STATE OR AGENCY

NOTES: IN 1992 LICENSES REVOKED IN HAWAII AND TEXAS BECAUSE HE ENGAGED IN SEXUAL CONTACT WITH PATIENTS.

ADAMS, BARTON JOSEPH DO, DATE OF BIRTH NOVEMBER 17, 1951, LICENSE NUMBER 0000516, WAS DISCIPLINED BY HAWAII ON FEBRUARY 24, 1992
DISCIPLINARY ACTION: EMERGENCY SUSPENSION
OFFENSE: SEXUAL ABUSE OF OR SEXUAL MISCONDUCT WITH A PATIENT

NOTES: IN 3/90 SEXUALLY ASSAULTED A FEMALE EMPLOYEE WHILE EXAMINING HER; IN 6/91 PERFORMED A BREAST EXAMINATION ON ONE PATIENT WHO REQUESTED TREATMENT FOR FACIAL ACNE; IN 1991, DURING THE EXAMINATION OF ANOTHER PATIENT FOR AN EAR INFECTION, RESTED HIS HAND ON HER BREAST. SUMMARY SUSPENSION EXTENDED 3/13/92.

ADAMS, BARTON JOSEPH DO, DATE OF BIRTH NOVEMBER 17, 1951, LICENSE NUMBER 0000516 OF 261 LALO STREET, KAHULUI, HI, WAS DISCIPLINED BY HAWAII ON JULY 10, 1992
DISCIPLINARY ACTION: 24-MONTH LICENSE REVOCATION
OFFENSE: SEXUAL ABUSE OF OR SEXUAL MISCONDUCT WITH A PATIENT

NOTES: IN 3/90 SEXUALLY ASSAULTED A FEMALE EMPLOYEE WHILE EXAMINING HER; IN 6/91 PERFORMED A BREAST EXAMINATION ON ONE PATIENT WHO REQUESTED TREATMENT FOR FACIAL ACNE; IN 1991 DURING THE EXAMINATION OF ANOTHER PATIENT FOR AN EAR INFECTION, RESTED HIS HAND ON HER BREAST. REVOCATION RETROACTIVE TO 5/15/92.

ADAMS, BARTON JOSEPH DO, DATE OF BIRTH NOVEMBER 17, 1951, LICENSE NUMBER 0000923, WAS DISCIPLINED BY WEST VIRGINIA ON JANUARY 14, 1993
DISCIPLINARY ACTION: LICENSE REVOCATION

ADAMS, BARTON JOSEPH DO, DATE OF BIRTH NOVEMBER 17, 1951, LICENSE NUMBER 0027020 OF 99902 MOANAHIA HIGHWAY, AIEA, HI, WAS DISCIPLINED BY GEORGIA ON NOVEMBER 9, 1993
DISCIPLINARY ACTION: LICENSE REVOCATION
OFFENSE: DISCIPLINARY ACTION BY ANOTHER STATE OR AGENCY

NOTES: BASED ON ACTION BY HAWAII BOARD, SEXUAL ASSAULT OF FEMALE PATIENTS. CONVICTED OF THREE COUNTS OF SEXUAL ASSAULT IN HAWAII. ON 9/9/94 THE INTERMEDIATE COURT OF APPEALS OF HAWAII VACATED THE JUDGMENT OF CONVICTION WHICH SERVED AS ONE OF THE BASES FOR THE HAWAII BOARD ACTION AND REMANDED THE MATTER TO THE LOWER COURT FOR FURTHER PROCEEDINGS CONSISTENT WITH THIS OPINION. ON 10/16/95 THE CIRCUIT COURT OF THE SECOND CIRCUIT GRANTED HIS MOTION TO DISMISS BASED ON VIOLATION OF SPEEDY TRIAL. HE WILL NEVER BE RETRIED FOR THESE CHARGES. BASED ON THIS DECISION, THE HAWAII BOARD REDACTED ITS ORDER AND EXPUNGED THE CONVICTIONS AS ONE OF THE BASES OF THE REVOCATION.

ADAMS, BARTON JOSEPH DO, DATE OF BIRTH NOVEMBER 17, 1951 OF 261 LALO STREET, KAHULUI, HI, WAS DISCIPLINED BY DEA ON JANUARY 28, 1994
DISCIPLINARY ACTION: REVOCATION OF CONTROLLED SUBSTANCE LICENSE
OFFENSE: DISCIPLINARY ACTION BY ANOTHER STATE OR AGENCY

NOTES: ON 3/29/90 HE SEXUALLY ASSAULTED A PATIENT AND ON 1/30/92 WAS CONVICTED OF THREE COUNTS OF SEXUAL ASSAULT IN THE SECOND DEGREE. AS A RESULT OF THE CONVICTION AND OTHER ALLEGATIONS OF SEXUAL ASSAULT, HAWAII REVOKED HIS LICENSE ON 7/10/92. ON 6/30/92 HIS STATE CONTROLLED SUBSTANCE REGISTRATION EXPIRED. DEA CERTIFICATE OF REGISTRATION REVOKED DUE TO HIS LACK OF AUTHORIZATION TO HANDLE CONTROLLED SUBSTANCES IN HAWAII. ON 9/9/94 THE INTERMEDIATE COURT OF APPEALS OF HAWAII VACATED THE JUDGMENT OF CONVICTION WHICH SERVED AS ONE OF THE BASES FOR THE HAWAII BOARD ACTION AND REMANDED THE MATTER TO THE LOWER COURT FOR FURTHER PROCEEDINGS CONSISTENT WITH THIS OPINION. ON 10/16/95 THE CIRCUIT COURT OF THE SECOND CIRCUIT GRANTED HIS MOTION TO DISMISS BASED ON VIOLATION OF SPEEDY TRIAL. HE WILL NEVER BE RETRIED FOR THESE CHARGES. BASED ON THIS DECISION, THE HAWAII BOARD REDACTED ITS ORDER AND EXPUNGED THE CONVICTIONS AS ONE OF THE BASES OF THE REVOCATION.

ADAMS, BARTON JOSEPH DO, DATE OF BIRTH NOVEMBER 17, 1951, LICENSE NUMBER 0026287 OF COLORADO SPRINGS, CO, WAS DISCIPLINED BY COLORADO ON AUGUST 19, 1994
DISCIPLINARY ACTION: LICENSE REVOCATION
OFFENSE: SEXUAL ABUSE OF OR SEXUAL MISCONDUCT WITH A PATIENT

NOTES: FELONY CONVICTION IN HAWAII. SEXUAL ACT WITH A PATIENT. ON 12/9/96 COLORADO BOARD RECEIVED REQUEST FOR RECONSIDERATION AS APPELLATE COURT HAD OVERTURNED THE CONVICTION AND REMANDED IT FOR A NEW TRIAL; CHARGES WERE THEN DISMISSED DUE TO A VIOLATION OF A RIGHT TO A SPEEDY TRIAL. HE WILL NOT BE RETRIED ON THOSE CHARGES. HOWEVER, COLORADO BOARD DETERMINED THAT BASED ON HAVING ENGAGED IN A SEXUAL ACT WITH A PATIENT IN THE COURSE OF

PATIENT CARE, HE HAD ENGAGED IN UNPROFESSIONAL CONDUCT AND ISSUED A FINAL BOARD ORDER AFTER RECONSIDERATION ON 2/14/97 AFFIRMING THE REVOCATION. REVOCATION STANDS AS OF 2/14/97.

ADEN, GARY CARL MD, DATE OF BIRTH NOVEMBER 18, 1935 OF 2403 CORONA CT, LA JOLLA, CA, WAS DISCIPLINED BY MEDICARE ON MAY 23, 1990
DISCIPLINARY ACTION: EXCLUSION FROM THE MEDICARE AND/OR MEDICAID PROGRAM
OFFENSE: DISCIPLINARY ACTION BY ANOTHER STATE OR AGENCY

NOTES: LICENSE REVOCATION OR SUSPENSION.

ADEN, GARY CARL MD, DATE OF BIRTH NOVEMBER 18, 1935, LICENSE NUMBER 0014167 OF LA JOLLA, CA, WAS DISCIPLINED BY COLORADO ON JUNE 7, 1991
DISCIPLINARY ACTION: SURRENDER OF LICENSE
OFFENSE: DISCIPLINARY ACTION BY ANOTHER STATE OR AGENCY

NOTES: GROSSLY NEGLIGENT MEDICAL PRACTICE, ENGAGING IN A SEXUAL ACT WITH A PATIENT DURING THE COURSE OF PATIENT CARE, AND STIPULATED TO REVOCATION OF HIS CALIFORNIA LICENSE EFFECTIVE 10/9/89 ALTHOUGH HE SPECIFICALLY DENIED ALL CHARGES. AGREEMENT WITH COLORADO NEVER TO REQUEST REINSTATEMENT OR APPLY FOR A NEW LICENSE.

ADEN, GARY CARL MD, DATE OF BIRTH NOVEMBER 18, 1935, LICENSE NUMBER 00D2974 OF 2403 CORONA COURT, LA JOLLA, CA, WAS DISCIPLINED BY TEXAS ON OCTOBER 5, 1991
DISCIPLINARY ACTION: LICENSE REVOCATION
OFFENSE: DISCIPLINARY ACTION BY ANOTHER STATE OR AGENCY

NOTES: CALIFORNIA LICENSE WAS REVOKED BECAUSE OF SEXUALLY ABUSIVE AND VIOLENT TREATMENT OF SEVEN PATIENTS UNDER HIS PSYCHIATRIC CARE; ALSO FAILED TO COMPLY WITH CALIFORNIA BOARD ORDER OF 10/9/89 TO UNDERGO A PSYCHIATRIC EVALUATION.

ADLER, KENNETH G MD, DATE OF BIRTH MAY 3, 1940, LICENSE NUMBER 0020393, WAS DISCIPLINED BY COLORADO ON AUGUST 14, 1996
DISCIPLINARY ACTION: PROBATION; MONITORING OF PHYSICIAN PERFORMANCE
OFFENSE: PHYSICAL OR MENTAL ILLNESS INHIBITING THE ABILITY TO PRACTICE WITH SKILL AND SAFETY

NOTES: PHYSICAL OR MENTAL DISABILITY WHICH RENDERS HIM UNABLE TO PRACTICE MEDICINE. TREATMENT AND PRACTICE MONITORING. ON 5/14/97 AGREES TO REMAIN INACTIVE AND ABSTINENT FROM ALCOHOL AND CONTROLLED SUBSTANCES.

ALDERMAN, JOHN A DO, LICENSE NUMBER E3639 OF ODESSA, TX, WAS DISCIPLINED BY TEXAS ON OCTOBER 24, 1998
DISCIPLINARY ACTION: SURRENDER OF LICENSE

NOTES: VOLUNTARY AND PERMANENT SURRENDER IN LIEU OF FURTHER INVESTIGATION.

ALDERMAN, JOHN ALLEN DO, DATE OF BIRTH SEPTEMBER 11, 1940 OF PO BOX 5000, FLORENCE, CO, WAS DISCIPLINED BY MEDICARE ON JUNE 17, 1999
DISCIPLINARY ACTION: EXCLUSION FROM THE MEDICARE AND/OR MEDICAID PROGRAM
OFFENSE: CRIMINAL CONVICTION OR PLEA OF GUILTY, NOLO CONTENDERE, OR NO CONTEST TO A CRIME

NOTES: CONVICTED OF A CRIME INVOLVING THE MEDICARE, MEDICAID, MATERNAL AND CHILD HEALTH SERVICES BLOCK GRANT OR BLOCK GRANTS TO STATES FOR SOCIAL SERVICES PROGRAMS.

ALEXANDER, J ALAN MD, DATE OF BIRTH NOVEMBER 20, 1931, LICENSE NUMBER 0016714, WAS DISCIPLINED BY COLORADO ON JUNE 13, 1996
DISCIPLINARY ACTION: SURRENDER OF LICENSE
OFFENSE: PHYSICAL OR MENTAL ILLNESS INHIBITING THE ABILITY TO PRACTICE WITH SKILL AND SAFETY

NOTES: PHYSICAL DISABILITY WHICH RENDERS HIM UNABLE TO PRACTICE MEDICINE.

ALONSO, KENNETH B MD, DATE OF BIRTH NOVEMBER 26, 1942, LICENSE NUMBER 0016011 OF 203-B MEDICAL WAY, RIVERDALE, GA, WAS DISCIPLINED BY GEORGIA ON JANUARY 6, 1995
DISCIPLINARY ACTION: 6-MONTH LICENSE SUSPENSION; 36-MONTH PROBATION
OFFENSE: SUBSTANDARD CARE, INCOMPETENCE OR NEGLIGENCE

NOTES: FAILURE TO COMPLY WITH THE MINIMAL STANDARDS OF ACCEPTABLE AND PREVAILING MEDICAL PRACTICE

ALONSO, KENNETH B MD, LICENSE NUMBER 0014228 OF ATLANTA, GA, WAS DISCIPLINED BY FLORIDA ON JUNE 27, 1996
DISCIPLINARY ACTION: LICENSE SUSPENSION; FINE
OFFENSE: DISCIPLINARY ACTION BY ANOTHER STATE OR AGENCY

NOTES: CHARGED WITH HAVING LICENSE ACTED UPON BY ANOTHER JURISDICTION AND FAILING TO REPORT THIS WITHIN 30 DAYS. $2,000 FINE; SUSPENSION UNTIL HIS GEORGIA LICENSE IS FREE OF ENCUMBRANCES; UPON REINSTATEMENT, PROBATION FOR UP TO THREE YEARS WITH TERMS DEEMED APPROPRIATE BY THE BOARD.

ALONSO, KENNETH B MD, DATE OF BIRTH NOVEMBER 26, 1942, LICENSE NUMBER 0031328, WAS DISCIPLINED BY COLORADO ON DECEMBER 12, 1996
DISCIPLINARY ACTION: LICENSE REVOCATION
OFFENSE: SUBSTANDARD CARE, INCOMPETENCE OR NEGLIGENCE

NOTES: SUBSTANDARD CARE.

ALONSO, KENNETH B MD, DATE OF BIRTH NOVEMBER 26, 1942, LICENSE NUMBER 31328, WAS DISCIPLINED BY COLORADO ON JANUARY 9, 1997
DISCIPLINARY ACTION: LICENSE REVOCATION
OFFENSE: SUBSTANDARD CARE, INCOMPETENCE OR NEGLIGENCE

NOTES: SUBSTANDARD CARE.

ALONSO, KENNETH B MD OF ATLANTA, GA, WAS DISCIPLINED BY SOUTH CAROLINA ON DECEMBER 11, 1997
DISCIPLINARY ACTION: LICENSE REVOCATION
OFFENSE: SUBSTANDARD CARE, INCOMPETENCE OR NEGLIGENCE

NOTES: PRACTICE FELL BELOW GENERALLY ACCEPTED STANDARDS OF MEDICAL PRACTICE.

ALONSO, KENNETH BRAULIO MD, LICENSE NUMBER 0G73252 OF ATLANTA, GA, WAS DISCIPLINED BY CALIFORNIA ON MARCH 29, 1996
DISCIPLINARY ACTION: LICENSE REVOCATION
OFFENSE: DISCIPLINARY ACTION BY ANOTHER STATE OR AGENCY

NOTES: ACTION IN GEORGIA. IN HIS TREATMENT OF SIX PATIENTS HE FAILED TO COMPORT WITH THE MINIMAL STANDARDS OF ACCEPTABLE AND PREVAILING MEDICAL PRACTICE. DEFAULT ACTION.

ALONSO, KENNETH BRAULIO MD, DATE OF BIRTH NOVEMBER 26, 1942, LICENSE NUMBER 0027418 OF ATLANTA, GA, WAS DISCIPLINED BY NORTH CAROLINA ON FEBRUARY 19, 1997
DISCIPLINARY ACTION: LICENSE SUSPENSION
OFFENSE: DISCIPLINARY ACTION BY ANOTHER STATE OR AGENCY

NOTES: THE GEORGIA BOARD FOUND THAT HIS TREATMENT OF SIX PATIENTS FELL BELOW MINIMAL STANDARDS; GEORGIA SUSPENDED HIS LICENSE FOR SIX MONTHS AND PROHIBITED HIM FROM TREATING CANCER PATIENTS AT ANY TIME IN THE FUTURE UNLESS HE BECAME A BOARD-CERTIFIED ONCOLOGIST AND PLACED HIM ON PROBATION FOR THREE YEARS.

AMANATULLAH, FAISAL F MD, WAS DISCIPLINED BY NEVADA ON APRIL 3, 1995
DISCIPLINARY ACTION: FINE; REPRIMAND
OFFENSE: OVERCHARGING

NOTES: MAKING UNREASONABLE ADDITIONAL CHARGES FOR LAB TESTS; ENGAGED IN CONDUCT INTENDED TO DECEIVE; AND CHARGED FOR SERVICES NOT RENDERED. SHALL NOT CHARGE ANY PATIENT ANY ADDITIONAL CHARGE OVER AND ABOVE WHAT HE IS CHARGED FOR TESTS IN A LABORATORY, RADIOLOGICAL SERVICES OR OTHER SERVICES FOR TESTING WHICH HE ORDERS AND HAS PERFORMED OUTSIDE HIS OWN OFFICE; MAY CHARGE A PATIENT A DRAWING OR COLLECTION FEE FOR THE COLLECTION OF A SPECIMEN WHICH FEE SHALL BE CONSISTENT WITH WHAT OTHER AREA COMMUNITY PHYSICIANS CHARGE. $5,000 FINE AND $5,000 ADMINISTRATIVE COSTS.

AMANATULLAH, FAISAL F MD, DATE OF BIRTH SEPTEMBER 5, 1948, LICENSE NUMBER 25585, WAS DISCIPLINED BY COLORADO ON MAY 21, 1999
DISCIPLINARY ACTION: LICENSE REVOCATION
OFFENSE: SUBSTANDARD CARE, INCOMPETENCE OR NEGLIGENCE

NOTES: SUBSTANDARD CARE; UNNECESSARY TESTS OR TREATMENT.

ANCIER, STEPHEN L MD, DATE OF BIRTH MAY 1, 1949, LICENSE NUMBER 0025753 OF UPPER MONTCLAIR, NJ, WAS DISCIPLINED BY COLORADO ON OCTOBER 13, 1993
DISCIPLINARY ACTION: LICENSE REVOCATION
OFFENSE: CRIMINAL CONVICTION OR PLEA OF GUILTY, NOLO CONTENDERE, OR NO CONTEST TO A CRIME

NOTES: CONVICTION OF AN OFFENSE INVOLVING MORAL TURPITUDE; RESORTING TO FRAUD, MISREPRESENTATION OR DECEPTION IN APPLYING FOR, SECURING AND SEEKING REINSTATEMENT OF A LICENSE TO PRACTICE MEDICINE IN COLORADO. THIS CASE WAS ON APPEAL TO THE COLORADO COURT OF APPEALS AS OF 8/94.

ANCIER, STEPHEN L MD, LICENSE NUMBER 0019001 OF UPPER MONTCLAIR, NJ, WAS DISCIPLINED BY WASHINGTON ON MARCH 8, 1996

NOTES: SUSPENSION, STAYED UNDER SEVERAL CONDITIONS. ON 3/23/99 REQUEST TO TERMINATE ORDER GRANTED; UNRESTRICTED LICENSE.

ANCIER, STEPHEN LEE MD, DATE OF BIRTH JANUARY 5, 1947, LICENSE NUMBER 032139E OF 21 BROOKFIELD ROAD, PO BOX 4351, UPPER MONTCLAIR, NJ, WAS DISCIPLINED BY PENNSYLVANIA ON FEBRUARY 7, 1995
DISCIPLINARY ACTION: LICENSE REVOCATION
OFFENSE: DISCIPLINARY ACTION BY ANOTHER STATE OR AGENCY

NOTES: RECIPROCAL ACTION FROM COLORADO; TWO COUNTS OF FRAUDULENT REPRESENTATIONS; TWO COUNTS OF IMMORAL CONDUCT; MAKING FALSE BIENNIAL REGISTRATION.

ANCIER, STEPHEN LEE MD, LICENSE NUMBER 0163647 OF PO BOX 4351 21 BROOKFIELD RD, UPPER MOUNTCLAIR, NJ, WAS DISCIPLINED BY NEW YORK ON APRIL 17, 1995
DISCIPLINARY ACTION: LICENSE REVOCATION
OFFENSE: DISCIPLINARY ACTION BY ANOTHER STATE OR AGENCY

NOTES: CONVICTED UNDER THE NEW ZEALAND CRIMES ACT OF 1961 FOR FORGING AIRLINE TICKETS, CREDIT CARD FORGERY AND MARIJUANA POSSESSION. DISCIPLINED BY COLORADO AND PENNSYLVANIA FOR FILING FALSE INFORMATION ON LICENSE APPLICATIONS.

ANCIER, STEPHEN LEE MD, DATE OF BIRTH JANUARY 5, 1947 OF 21 BROOKFIELD ROAD, PO BOX 43451, UPPER MONTCLAIR, NJ, WAS DISCIPLINED BY MEDICARE ON SEPTEMBER 9, 1996
DISCIPLINARY ACTION: EXCLUSION FROM THE MEDICARE AND/OR MEDICAID PROGRAM
OFFENSE: DISCIPLINARY ACTION BY ANOTHER STATE OR AGENCY

NOTES: LICENSE REVOKED FOR REASONS BEARING ON PROFESSIONAL PERFORMANCE. REINSTATED ON 9/26/96.

ANDERSON, MARTIN E JR MD, DATE OF BIRTH FEBRUARY 18, 1918, LICENSE NUMBER 0011254 OF DENVER, CO, WAS DISCIPLINED BY COLORADO ON JUNE 18, 1993
DISCIPLINARY ACTION: SURRENDER OF LICENSE

NOTES: NO SPECIFIC FINDINGS OF UNPROFESSIONAL CONDUCT.

ANGELLO, ANTHONY L MD, DATE OF BIRTH OCTOBER 22, 1934, LICENSE NUMBER 0015626 OF 1601 EAST 19TH AVE #4200, DENVER, CO, WAS DISCIPLINED BY COLORADO ON MAY 1, 1994
DISCIPLINARY ACTION: 2-MONTH LICENSE SUSPENSION; 60-MONTH PROBATION
OFFENSE: SEXUAL ABUSE OF OR SEXUAL MISCONDUCT WITH A PATIENT

NOTES: ENGAGED IN SEXUAL RELATIONSHIPS WITH PATIENTS; IN ONE CASE FROM 6/91 THROUGH 12/92 WHERE HE AND THE PATIENT LIVED TOGETHER FOR SEVERAL MONTHS, AND IN ANOTHER CASE WHERE HE HAD A BRIEF SEXUAL RELATIONSHIP IN THE 1970S. LICENSE SUSPENDED 90 DAYS, 45 DAYS STAYED SUBJECT TO PROBATIONARY TERMS: SHALL CONTINUE TO RECEIVE PSYCHOTHERAPY FROM A BOARD-APPROVED THERAPIST AT LEAST ONCE PER WEEK TO ADDRESS AND PREVENT FUTURE VIOLATIONS OF DOCTOR-PATIENT SEXUAL BOUNDARIES; THERAPIST WILL SUBMIT QUARTERLY REPORTS TO THE BOARD; A CHAPERONE SHALL BE PRESENT DURING THE PHYSICAL EXAMINATIONS OF ANY FEMALE PATIENT; SHALL COMPLETE CONTINUING MEDICAL EDUCATION IN MEDICAL ETHICS WITHIN SIX MONTHS.

ANGELLO, ANTHONY LOUIS MD, DATE OF BIRTH OCTOBER 22, 1934, LICENSE NUMBER 027603L OF 4505 SOUTH YOSEMITE STREET, DENVER, CO, WAS DISCIPLINED BY PENNSYLVANIA ON JANUARY 27, 1998
DISCIPLINARY ACTION: LICENSE REVOCATION
OFFENSE: DISCIPLINARY ACTION BY ANOTHER STATE OR AGENCY

NOTES: DISCIPLINARY ACTION TAKEN BY COLORADO. VOLUNTARY REVOCATION OF LICENSE.

ANNEBERG, SPENCER K MD, DATE OF BIRTH JULY 8, 1946, LICENSE NUMBER 0023426, WAS DISCIPLINED BY COLORADO ON NOVEMBER 9, 1995

NOTES: INTERIM CESSATION OF PRACTICE. AGREED TO STOP PRACTICING MEDICINE UNTIL ASSESSMENT IS REVIEWED BY THE BOARD.

ANNEBERG, SPENCER K MD, DATE OF BIRTH JULY 8, 1946, LICENSE NUMBER 0023426, WAS DISCIPLINED BY COLORADO ON DECEMBER 19, 1996
DISCIPLINARY ACTION: LICENSE REVOCATION
OFFENSE: SUBSTANDARD CARE, INCOMPETENCE OR NEGLIGENCE

NOTES: SUBSTANDARD CARE.

ANNEBERG, SPENCER K MD, LICENSE NUMBER 2763A, WAS DISCIPLINED BY WYOMING ON FEBRUARY 25, 1997
DISCIPLINARY ACTION: LICENSE REVOCATION
OFFENSE: NONCOMPLIANCE WITH A PROFESSIONAL RULE

NOTES: FAILED TO RESPOND TO THE NOTICE OF INTENT TO REVOKE LICENSE WITHIN THE TIME PERIOD PERMITTED.

ARABASZ, JOSEPH A MD, DATE OF BIRTH JUNE 18, 1946, LICENSE NUMBER 20705, WAS DISCIPLINED BY COLORADO ON FEBRUARY 12, 1997
DISCIPLINARY ACTION: LICENSE SUSPENSION

ARABASZ, JOSEPH WALTER MD, LICENSE NUMBER G41169 OF DENVER, CO, WAS DISCIPLINED BY CALIFORNIA ON MAY 8, 1998
DISCIPLINARY ACTION: LICENSE REVOCATION
OFFENSE: DISCIPLINARY ACTION BY ANOTHER STATE OR AGENCY

NOTES: DISCIPLINED BY COLORADO FOR FAILING TO COMPLY WITH AN ORDER FOR AN EVALUATION OF ANY PHYSICAL, EMOTIONAL OR PSYCHOLOGICAL PROBLEMS.

ARNOLD, ROBERT S MD OF 2191 BLACKBERRY LANE, CONWAY, AR, WAS DISCIPLINED BY DEA ON SEPTEMBER 21, 1998
DISCIPLINARY ACTION: SURRENDER OF CONTROLLED SUBSTANCE LICENSE

NOTES: IN LIEU OF PUBLIC INTEREST REVOCATION.

ARNOLD, ROBERT SIDNEY MD, LICENSE NUMBER C7051 OF CONWAY, AR, WAS DISCIPLINED BY ARKANSAS ON JUNE 5, 1998
DISCIPLINARY ACTION: EMERGENCY SUSPENSION

ARNOLD, ROBERT SIDNEY MD, LICENSE NUMBER C7051 OF CONWAY, AR, WAS DISCIPLINED BY ARKANSAS ON SEPTEMBER 17, 1998
DISCIPLINARY ACTION: LICENSE SUSPENSION

NOTES: FIVE YEAR REVOCATION STAYED. SUSPENDED UNTIL CONDITIONS MET.

ARNOLD, ROBERT SIDNEY MD, LICENSE NUMBER C7051 OF CONWAY, AR, WAS DISCIPLINED BY ARKANSAS ON DECEMBER 4, 1998
DISCIPLINARY ACTION: PROBATION

ARNOLD, ROBERT SIDNEY MD, LICENSE NUMBER C7051 OF DENVER, CO, WAS DISCIPLINED BY ARKANSAS ON APRIL 9, 1999
DISCIPLINARY ACTION: EMERGENCY SUSPENSION

ARNONE, THOMAS J MD, DATE OF BIRTH MARCH 14, 1960, LICENSE NUMBER 0035807, WAS DISCIPLINED BY COLORADO ON DECEMBER 19, 1996
DISCIPLINARY ACTION: PROBATION; MONITORING OF PHYSICIAN PERFORMANCE
OFFENSE: SUBSTANCE ABUSE

NOTES: HABITUAL INTEMPERANCE OR EXCESSIVE USE OF A CONTROLLED SUBSTANCE. TREATMENT AND PRACTICE MONITORING.

ARONSON, KARON S MD, DATE OF BIRTH SEPTEMBER 14, 1948, LICENSE NUMBER 0019791, WAS DISCIPLINED BY COLORADO ON SEPTEMBER 26, 1995
DISCIPLINARY ACTION: EMERGENCY SUSPENSION

ARONSON, KARON S MD, DATE OF BIRTH SEPTEMBER 14, 1948, LICENSE NUMBER 0019791, WAS DISCIPLINED BY COLORADO ON APRIL 11, 1996
DISCIPLINARY ACTION: LICENSE REVOCATION
OFFENSE: PHYSICAL OR MENTAL ILLNESS INHIBITING THE ABILITY TO PRACTICE WITH SKILL AND SAFETY

NOTES: MENTAL DISABILITY.

ARONSON, KARON S MD, WAS DISCIPLINED BY IDAHO ON JUNE 24, 1996
DISCIPLINARY ACTION: LICENSE REVOCATION

NOTES: SUPPLEMENTAL ORDER FOR RECIPROCAL DISCIPLINE.

ARONSON, KARON S MD, WAS DISCIPLINED BY NEW MEXICO ON JANUARY 1, 1997
DISCIPLINARY ACTION: LICENSE REVOCATION
OFFENSE: NONCOMPLIANCE WITH A PROFESSIONAL RULE

NOTES: FAILURE TO NOTIFY THE BOARD OF LICENSE REVOCATION IN COLORADO.

ARONSON, KARON SZELWACH MD, LICENSE NUMBER 0G73845 OF DENVER, CO, WAS DISCIPLINED BY CALIFORNIA ON NOVEMBER 21, 1996
DISCIPLINARY ACTION: LICENSE REVOCATION
OFFENSE: DISCIPLINARY ACTION BY ANOTHER STATE OR AGENCY

NOTES: DISCIPLINED BY COLORADO FOR MENTAL IMPAIRMENT. DEFAULT ACTION.

ARORA, SATISH K MD, DATE OF BIRTH DECEMBER 15, 1939, LICENSE NUMBER 0020064 OF DENVER, CO, WAS DISCIPLINED BY COLORADO ON AUGUST 15, 1994
DISCIPLINARY ACTION: REPRIMAND

ARTIST, ELMER J MD, DATE OF BIRTH NOVEMBER 11, 1917, LICENSE NUMBER 0012140, WAS DISCIPLINED BY COLORADO ON MAY 17, 1996
DISCIPLINARY ACTION: SURRENDER OF LICENSE; REPRIMAND

NOTES: NO UNPROFESSIONAL CONDUCT IDENTIFIED. RETIREMENT FROM THE PRACTICE OF MEDICINE EFFECTIVE 9/30/96.

ASHKAR, LOUIS N MD, DATE OF BIRTH JULY 23, 1933, LICENSE NUMBER 14991, WAS DISCIPLINED BY COLORADO ON DECEMBER 10, 1998
DISCIPLINARY ACTION: REPRIMAND; REQUIRED TO TAKE ADDITIONAL MEDICAL EDUCATION
OFFENSE: SUBSTANDARD CARE, INCOMPETENCE OR NEGLIGENCE

NOTES: SUBSTANDARD CARE. HE AGREES TO ENGAGE IN REEDUCATION ACTIVITIES.

ASKANAZI, JEFFREY MD, DATE OF BIRTH MARCH 23, 1951, LICENSE NUMBER 1062515 OF 1033 RIVER STREET, PORT HURON, MI, WAS DISCIPLINED BY MICHIGAN ON APRIL 28, 1998
DISCIPLINARY ACTION: EMERGENCY SUSPENSION
OFFENSE: SUBSTANDARD CARE, INCOMPETENCE OR NEGLIGENCE

NOTES: NEGLIGENCE/INCOMPETENCE.

ASKANAZI, JEFFREY MD, DATE OF BIRTH MARCH 23, 1951, LICENSE NUMBER 35868, WAS DISCIPLINED BY COLORADO ON FEBRUARY 26, 1999
DISCIPLINARY ACTION: EMERGENCY SUSPENSION

ASKANAZI, JEFFREY MD, DATE OF BIRTH MARCH 23, 1951, LICENSE NUMBER 50150 OF 2322 OLDE FARM LANE, HUDSON, OH, WAS DISCIPLINED BY NEW JERSEY ON APRIL 14, 1999
DISCIPLINARY ACTION: LICENSE SUSPENSION
OFFENSE: DISCIPLINARY ACTION BY ANOTHER STATE OR AGENCY

NOTES: A PROVISIONAL ORDER OF DISCIPLINE WAS FILED ON 11/12/98 BASED ON EMERGENCY SUSPENSION BY MICHIGAN ON 4/27/98 DUE TO A VIOLATION OF GENERAL DUTY, NEGLIGENCE OR FAILURE TO EXERCISE DUE CARE, NEGLIGENT DELEGATION TO OR SUPERVISION OF EMPLOYEES OR OTHER INDIVIDUALS, INCOMPETENCE, LACK OF GOOD MORAL CHARACTER AND UNPROFESSIONAL CONDUCT CONSISTING OF PROMOTION FOR PERSONAL GAIN OF UNNECESSARY DRUG, DEVICE, TREATMENT, PROCEDURE OR SERVICE. HE SUBMITTED A RESPONSE TO THE ORDER OF SUMMARY SUSPENSION ISSUED IN MICHIGAN, STATING THAT THE MICHIGAN ACTION WAS POLITICALLY BASED AND COMPLETELY UNJUSTIFIED. THE NEW JERSEY BOARD WAS NOT PERSUADED BY HIS ARGUMENT. PRIOR TO RESUMING ACTIVE PRACTICE IN NEW JERSEY, HE SHALL BE REQUIRED TO APPEAR BEFORE THE BOARD TO DEMONSTRATE HIS POSSESSION OF AN UNRESTRICTED LICENSE IN MICHIGAN.

ASKANAZI, JEFFREY MD, DATE OF BIRTH MARCH 23, 1951, LICENSE NUMBER 35868, WAS DISCIPLINED BY COLORADO ON NOVEMBER 17, 1999
DISCIPLINARY ACTION: LICENSE REVOCATION
OFFENSE: CRIMINAL CONVICTION OR PLEA OF GUILTY, NOLO CONTENDERE, OR NO CONTEST TO A CRIME

NOTES: FELONY CONVICTION.

ASUNSOLO, LEOPOLDO G MD, DATE OF BIRTH JULY 4, 1951, LICENSE NUMBER 0027129 OF DENVER, CO, WAS DISCIPLINED BY COLORADO ON APRIL 5, 1995
DISCIPLINARY ACTION: REPRIMAND

ASUNSOLO, LEOPOLDO G MD, DATE OF BIRTH JULY 4, 1951, LICENSE NUMBER 27129, WAS DISCIPLINED BY COLORADO ON MAY 19, 1999
DISCIPLINARY ACTION: REPRIMAND

AVNER, TED G MD OF 3121 L HONEYWOOD LN, ROANOKE, VA, WAS DISCIPLINED BY VIRGINIA ON APRIL 5, 1990
DISCIPLINARY ACTION: DENIAL OF NEW LICENSE

AVNER, TED G MD, LICENSE NUMBER 0030700 OF CHARLOTTESVILLE, VA, WAS DISCIPLINED BY COLORADO ON JANUARY 9, 1991
DISCIPLINARY ACTION: LICENSE REINSTATEMENT; PROBATION
OFFENSE: SUBSTANCE ABUSE

NOTES: SURRENDERED PREVIOUS COLORADO LICENSE IN 1988 DUE TO EXCESSIVE USE OF HABIT FORMING DRUG OR CONTROLLED SUBSTANCES. LICENSE GRANTED SUBJECT TO PROBATIONARY TERMS AND CONDITIONS.

AVNER, TED G MD, LICENSE NUMBER 0014896 OF BLACKSBURG, VA, WAS DISCIPLINED BY FLORIDA ON JANUARY 8, 1992
DISCIPLINARY ACTION: REPRIMAND
OFFENSE: DISCIPLINARY ACTION BY ANOTHER STATE OR AGENCY

NOTES: RESTRICTION TO REQUIRE THAT HE CONTINUE TO MAINTAIN HIS LICENSE IN GOOD STANDING IN BOTH COLORADO AND VIRGINIA AND THAT HE COMPLY WITH HIS CONTRACT IN VIRGINIA FOR ITS ENTIRE TERM; IF HE COMES TO FLORIDA TO PRACTICE MEDICINE, HE MUST ENROLL IN AND COMPLY WITH REQUIREMENTS OF THE PHYSICIAN'S RECOVERY NETWORK.

BADZINSKI, GARY L DO, DATE OF BIRTH JANUARY 21, 1956, LICENSE NUMBER 0031226, WAS DISCIPLINED BY COLORADO ON APRIL 11, 1996
DISCIPLINARY ACTION: 3-MONTH LICENSE SUSPENSION; 60-MONTH PROBATION
OFFENSE: SEXUAL ABUSE OF OR SEXUAL MISCONDUCT WITH A PATIENT

NOTES: SEXUAL CONTACT WITH A PATIENT. 90 DAY PERIOD OF NO MEDICAL PRACTICE. TREATMENT MONITORING AND AN AGREEMENT TO HAVE A CHAPERONE PRESENT FOR ALL FEMALE PATIENTS.

BADZINSKI, GARY L DO, LICENSE NUMBER 0003416, WAS DISCIPLINED BY OKLAHOMA ON SEPTEMBER 19, 1996
DISCIPLINARY ACTION: 60-MONTH PROBATION; RESTRICTION PLACED ON LICENSE

NOTES: LICENSE GRANTED. SHALL SUBMIT TO THE OKLAHOMA BOARD DOCUMENTATION VERIFYING HIS SUCCESSFUL COMPLETION OF A PROGRAM ON BOUNDARY AND MEDICAL ETHICS ISSUES APPROVED BY THE COLORADO PHYSICIAN'S HEALTH PROGRAM (CPHP) AS REQUIRED BY THE COLORADO BOARD. SHALL RECEIVE SUCH MEDICAL TREATMENT, PARTICULARLY PERSONAL PSYCHOTHERAPY, AS IS DETERMINED TO BE APPROPRIATE BY CPHP; ALL TREATMENT RECOMMENDATIONS BY CPHP SHALL CONSTITUTE TERMS OF THIS ORDER; CPHP SHALL SUBMIT QUARTERLY WRITTEN REPORTS TO THE BOARD WHICH SHALL BRIEFLY DESCRIBE HIS TREATMENT AND STATE WHETHER HE IS COMPLIANCE WITH THIS ORDER; A CHAPERONE SHALL BE PRESENT DURING HIS PHYSICAL EXAMINATIONS OF ANY FEMALE PATIENT AND THE NAME SHALL BE RECORDED IN THE PATIENT'S RECORD; SHALL NOTIFY THE BOARD OF ANY CHANGE OF ADDRESS WITHIN 14 DAYS; SHALL APPEAR BEFORE THE BOARD UPON REQUEST AND SHALL RECEIVE UNANNOUNCED VISITS FROM THE BOARD AT ITS DISCRETION; MAY NOT APPLY FOR MODIFICATION OF THIS ORDER FOR THREE YEARS; SHALL COMPLETE A RELEASE PERMITTING CPHP TO DISCLOSE TO THE BOARD ALL PRIVILEGED INFORMATION CONCERNING HIM IN ITS POSSESSION, INCLUDING INFORMATION GENERATED BY OTHER SOURCES; THE EXPIRATION OF THE PROBATIONARY PERIOD WILL BE TOLLED AND THE PROBATIONARY PERIOD WILL BE EXTENDED FOR ANY PERIOD OF RESIDENCE OR PRACTICE OUTSIDE OF OKLAHOMA OR WHEN HE IS NOT PARTICIPATING WITH CPHP. ON 6/18/98 PROBATION TERMINATED.

BADZINSKI, GARY L DO, DATE OF BIRTH JANUARY 21, 1956, LICENSE NUMBER 1009464 OF 1060 ORCHARD AVENUE STE E,

GRAND JUNCTION, CO, WAS DISCIPLINED BY MICHIGAN ON FEBRUARY 6, 1997
DISCIPLINARY ACTION: FINE; RESTRICTION PLACED ON LICENSE
OFFENSE: DISCIPLINARY ACTION BY ANOTHER STATE OR AGENCY

NOTES: FAILURE TO REPORT/COMPLY. $1000 FINE.

BAGLEY, DAVID L MD, DATE OF BIRTH NOVEMBER 12, 1937, LICENSE NUMBER 0015050 OF GREELEY, CO, WAS DISCIPLINED BY COLORADO ON JANUARY 21, 1994
DISCIPLINARY ACTION: SURRENDER OF CONTROLLED SUBSTANCE LICENSE
OFFENSE: SUBSTANDARD CARE, INCOMPETENCE OR NEGLIGENCE

NOTES: ALLEGATIONS OF UNPROFESSIONAL CONDUCT AND OTHER ISSUES INVOLVING PATIENT CARE. AGREES NOT TO APPLY FOR DRUG ENFORCEMENT ADMINISTRATION CERTIFICATE IN THE FUTURE; PROHIBITED FROM PRESCRIBING/DISPENSING CONTROLLED SUBSTANCES OF ANY TYPE AND FOR ANY PURPOSE.

BAGLEY, DAVID L MD, DATE OF BIRTH NOVEMBER 12, 1937 OF 228 7TH STREET, EATON, CO, WAS DISCIPLINED BY DEA ON FEBRUARY 15, 1994
DISCIPLINARY ACTION: SURRENDER OF CONTROLLED SUBSTANCE LICENSE
OFFENSE: DISCIPLINARY ACTION BY ANOTHER STATE OR AGENCY

NOTES: PROBATION INSOFAR AS LICENSE TO PRACTICE MEDICINE 10/14/88 IN COLORADO.

BALDWIN, RICHARD E DO OF DAVIS, OK, WAS DISCIPLINED BY MISSOURI ON JULY 27, 1990
DISCIPLINARY ACTION: 2-MONTH LICENSE SUSPENSION; 22-MONTH PROBATION
OFFENSE: DISCIPLINARY ACTION BY ANOTHER STATE OR AGENCY

NOTES: TWO MONTH SUSPENSION RETROACTIVE TO 6/15/89, TWENTY-TWO MONTH PROBATION RETROACTIVE TO 8/16/89.

BALDWIN, RICHARD E DO, LICENSE NUMBER 00E3192 OF DAVIS, OK, WAS DISCIPLINED BY TEXAS ON AUGUST 18, 1990
OFFENSE: DISCIPLINARY ACTION BY ANOTHER STATE OR AGENCY

NOTES: STIPULATED ORDER. MUST COMPLY WITH OKLAHOMA BOARD ORDER, RECEIVE PERMISSION OF TEXAS BOARD BEFORE RETURNING TO PRACTICE MEDICINE IN TEXAS, AND BE SUBJECT TO ANY TERMS IMPOSED.

BALDWIN, RICHARD E DO, DATE OF BIRTH JULY 19, 1938, LICENSE NUMBER 0018743 OF DAVIS, OK, WAS DISCIPLINED BY COLORADO ON FEBRUARY 21, 1992
DISCIPLINARY ACTION: SURRENDER OF LICENSE
OFFENSE: CRIMINAL CONVICTION OR PLEA OF GUILTY, NOLO CONTENDERE, OR NO CONTEST TO A CRIME

NOTES: FELONY CONVICTION FOR MEDICAID FRAUD.

BANKER, DEBORAH E MD, DATE OF BIRTH APRIL 14, 1952, LICENSE NUMBER 28591, WAS DISCIPLINED BY COLORADO ON JULY 27, 1998
DISCIPLINARY ACTION: EMERGENCY SUSPENSION

NOTES: DELIBERATE AND WILLFUL VIOLATION OF THE MEDICAL PRACTICE ACT.

BANKER, DEBORAH E MD, DATE OF BIRTH APRIL 14, 1952, LICENSE NUMBER 28591, WAS DISCIPLINED BY COLORADO ON DECEMBER 17, 1998

NOTES: NO UNPROFESSIONAL CONDUCT IDENTIFIED. SHE AGREES NEVER TO REINSTATE HER LAPSED LICENSE, NEVER TO APPLY FOR A NEW LICENSE AND NEVER TO PERFORM ANY ACT REQUIRING A LICENSE ISSUED BY THE BOARD.

BAPTIST, ROBERT MD OF 72 EAGLE DRIVE, NORTH CANON CITY, CO, WAS DISCIPLINED BY DEA ON OCTOBER 4, 1999
DISCIPLINARY ACTION: SURRENDER OF CONTROLLED SUBSTANCE LICENSE
OFFENSE: NONCOMPLIANCE WITH A PROFESSIONAL RULE

NOTES: LACK OF RECORD KEEPING.

BARRICKMAN, LES L DO, DATE OF BIRTH NOVEMBER 2, 1953, LICENSE NUMBER 0001988 OF 938 TALWRN COURT, IOWA CITY, IA, WAS DISCIPLINED BY IOWA ON JUNE 3, 1993
DISCIPLINARY ACTION: 48-MONTH PROBATION; FINE
OFFENSE: CRIMINAL CONVICTION OR PLEA OF GUILTY, NOLO CONTENDERE, OR NO CONTEST TO A CRIME

NOTES: ALLEGATIONS OF CRIMINAL CONVICTIONS RELATED TO ILLEGAL POSSESSION OF CONTROLLED DRUGS. $5,000 CIVIL PENALTY.

BARRICKMAN, LES L DO, DATE OF BIRTH NOVEMBER 2, 1953, LICENSE NUMBER 0099794, WAS DISCIPLINED BY NEW MEXICO ON FEBRUARY 12, 1994
DISCIPLINARY ACTION: PROBATION
OFFENSE: DISCIPLINARY ACTION BY ANOTHER STATE OR AGENCY

NOTES: ACTION IN ANOTHER STATE. ON 10/21/95 A PERMANENT LICENSE WITH FULL PRIVILEGES ISSUED.

BARRICKMAN, LES L DO, DATE OF BIRTH NOVEMBER 2, 1953, LICENSE NUMBER 0002676 OF 2316 CAMIO DE LOS ARTESANOS NW, ALBUQUERQUE, NM, WAS DISCIPLINED BY ARIZONA ON MAY 13, 1994
DISCIPLINARY ACTION: MONITORING OF PHYSICIAN PERFORMANCE
OFFENSE: DISCIPLINARY ACTION BY ANOTHER STATE OR AGENCY

NOTES: ACTION IN NEW MEXICO ON 2/12/94 BASED ON TWO GUILTY PLEAS TO POSSESSION OF A CONTROLLED SUBSTANCE ON 1/15/93 IN IOWA; ON 6/3/93 IOWA LICENSE PLACED ON PROBATION BASED ON THESE ACTIONS. AGREEMENT WITH ARIZONA: SHALL COMPLY WITH THE NEW MEXICO BOARD ORDER; SHALL MEET WITH THE BOARD UPON REQUEST; SHALL AUTHORIZE NEW MEXICO TO RELEASE TO THE BOARD UPON REQUEST A RECORD OF COMPLIANCE WITH THE TERMS AND CONDITIONS IN NEW MEXICO; IF HE CHOOSES TO PRACTICE IN ARIZONA BOARD RESERVES THE RIGHT TO REVIEW THE COMPLIANCE WITH THIS ORDER.

BARRICKMAN, LES L DO, DATE OF BIRTH NOVEMBER 2, 1953, LICENSE NUMBER 0025600 OF IOWA CITY, IA, WAS DISCIPLINED BY COLORADO ON MAY 20, 1994
DISCIPLINARY ACTION: SURRENDER OF LICENSE
OFFENSE: DISCIPLINARY ACTION BY ANOTHER STATE OR AGENCY

NOTES: BASED ON IOWA DISCIPLINE. NO UNPROFESSIONAL CONDUCT IDENTIFIED. PERMANENT LICENSE SURRENDER.

BARRICKMAN, LES L DO OF HI, WAS DISCIPLINED BY IOWA ON MAY 22, 1997
DISCIPLINARY ACTION: SURRENDER OF LICENSE
OFFENSE: DISCIPLINARY ACTION BY ANOTHER STATE OR AGENCY

NOTES: CHARGED WITH VIOLATING THE TERMS OF A PREVIOUS AGREEMENT WITH THE BOARD AS WELL AS IN CONNECTION WITH DISCIPLINE TAKEN BY ARIZONA.

BARRICKMAN, LES L DO, LICENSE NUMBER 782 OF 509 UNIVERSITY AVENUE, #104, HONOLULU, HI, WAS DISCIPLINED BY HAWAII ON DECEMBER 11, 1998
DISCIPLINARY ACTION: FINE
OFFENSE: DISCIPLINARY ACTION BY ANOTHER STATE OR AGENCY
NOTES: FAILED TO TIMELY INFORM THE HAWAII BOARD OF DISCIPLINARY ACTIONS AGAINST HIS LICENSE IN ARIZONA AND IOWA; ACTION ALSO TAKEN IN NEW MEXICO. $500 FINE

BARTON, MALCOLM D MD, LICENSE NUMBER 092813 OF 789 SHERMAN STREET #613, DENVER, CO, WAS DISCIPLINED BY NEW YORK ON JUNE 13, 1997
DISCIPLINARY ACTION: SURRENDER OF LICENSE
OFFENSE: DISCIPLINARY ACTION BY ANOTHER STATE OR AGENCY
NOTES: DISCIPLINED BY THE COLORADO BOARD FOR GROSS NEGLIGENCE AND NEGLIGENCE ON MORE THAN ONE OCCASION INVOLVING HIS CARE OF TWO ANESTHESIA PATIENTS.

BARTON, MALCOLM DENNIS MD, DATE OF BIRTH SEPTEMBER 22, 1937, LICENSE NUMBER 16208, WAS DISCIPLINED BY COLORADO ON SEPTEMBER 10, 1998
DISCIPLINARY ACTION: SURRENDER OF LICENSE
OFFENSE: PHYSICAL OR MENTAL ILLNESS INHIBITING THE ABILITY TO PRACTICE WITH SKILL AND SAFETY
NOTES: PHYSICAL OR MENTAL DISABILITY.

BARTON, MALCOM DENNIS MD, DATE OF BIRTH SEPTEMBER 22, 1937, LICENSE NUMBER 0016208, WAS DISCIPLINED BY COLORADO ON APRIL 24, 1996
DISCIPLINARY ACTION: LICENSE SUSPENSION

BARTON, MALCOM DENNIS MD, DATE OF BIRTH SEPTEMBER 22, 1937, LICENSE NUMBER 0016208, WAS DISCIPLINED BY COLORADO ON AUGUST 14, 1996
DISCIPLINARY ACTION: 60-MONTH PROBATION; REQUIRED TO TAKE ADDITIONAL MEDICAL EDUCATION
OFFENSE: SUBSTANDARD CARE, INCOMPETENCE OR NEGLIGENCE
NOTES: SUBSTANDARD CARE. RE-EDUCATION ACTIVITIES AND PRACTICE MONITORING.

BAUMGARDNER, JAN F MD, LICENSE NUMBER 0015815 OF BOULDER, CO, WAS DISCIPLINED BY COLORADO ON JANUARY 9, 1991
DISCIPLINARY ACTION: 36-MONTH PROBATION; REQUIRED TO TAKE ADDITIONAL MEDICAL EDUCATION
OFFENSE: SUBSTANDARD CARE, INCOMPETENCE OR NEGLIGENCE
NOTES: ACTION BASED ON PRESCRIBING PRACTICES. ALSO PRACTICE MONITORING, OTHER CONDITIONS.

BEACH, DON E MD, DATE OF BIRTH OCTOBER 18, 1948, LICENSE NUMBER 0022847 OF DELTA, CO, WAS DISCIPLINED BY COLORADO ON OCTOBER 13, 1993
OFFENSE: SUBSTANDARD CARE, INCOMPETENCE OR NEGLIGENCE
NOTES: SUBSTANDARD PATIENT CARE. MUST DEMONSTRATE CONTINUED PROFESSIONAL COMPETENCE PRIOR TO REINSTATEMENT OF HIS LICENSE. IN THE EVENT THAT HE IS REINSTATED, A FIVE YEAR PROBATIONARY PERIOD WILL BE REQUIRED, INCLUDING PRACTICE MONITORING AND OTHER SUCH TERMS AND CONDITIONS AS DEEMED APPROPRIATE BY BOARD. THIS CASE WAS APPEALED TO THE COLORADO COURT OF APPEALS BUT THE APPEAL WAS DISMISSED ON 03/01/94.

BEATTY, BRIAN J DO, DATE OF BIRTH AUGUST 8, 1958 OF 7222 E DAVIES PLACE, ENGLEWOOD, CO, WAS DISCIPLINED BY MEDICARE ON OCTOBER 21, 1993
DISCIPLINARY ACTION: EXCLUSION FROM THE MEDICARE AND/OR MEDICAID PROGRAM
OFFENSE: NONCOMPLIANCE WITH A PROFESSIONAL RULE
NOTES: DEFAULTED ON PUBLIC HEALTH SERVICE EDUCATION LOAN. REINSTATED ON 1/21/94.

BECKER, DAVID W JR MD, DATE OF BIRTH FEBRUARY 4, 1942, LICENSE NUMBER 37324, WAS DISCIPLINED BY COLORADO ON AUGUST 13, 1998
DISCIPLINARY ACTION: RESTRICTION PLACED ON LICENSE
OFFENSE: PHYSICAL OR MENTAL ILLNESS INHIBITING THE ABILITY TO PRACTICE WITH SKILL AND SAFETY
NOTES: PHYSICAL DISABILITY. SHALL NOT PERFORM ANY SURGICAL PROCEDURES REQUIRING DEXTERITY WITH THE RIGHT HAND.

BECKWITT, HENRY J MD, DATE OF BIRTH JULY 13, 1930, LICENSE NUMBER 0015307 OF ENGLEWOOD, CO, WAS DISCIPLINED BY COLORADO ON DECEMBER 17, 1993
DISCIPLINARY ACTION: 60-MONTH PROBATION; MONITORING OF PHYSICIAN PERFORMANCE
OFFENSE: SUBSTANDARD CARE, INCOMPETENCE OR NEGLIGENCE
NOTES: ALLEGATIONS OF SUBSTANDARD PATIENT CARE. PROBATIONARY PERIOD INCLUDES PRACTICE MONITORING. ON 12/21/95 THIS ORDER WAS TERMINATED AND MEDICAL LICENSE RESTORED TO AN UNENCUMBERED STATUS.

BECKWITT, HENRY J MD, LICENSE NUMBER 0080374 OF 4770 EAST PRINCETON AVENUE, ENGLEWOOD, CO, WAS DISCIPLINED BY NEW YORK ON JULY 29, 1996
DISCIPLINARY ACTION: 24-MONTH PROBATION
OFFENSE: DISCIPLINARY ACTION BY ANOTHER STATE OR AGENCY
NOTES: ACTION IN COLORADO FOR GROSS NEGLIGENCE AND NEGLIGENCE ON MORE THAN ONE OCCASION. TWO YEAR SUSPENSION, STAYED WITH PROBATION COMMENCING WHEN HE PRACTICES IN NEW YORK.

BECKY, JOSEPH R MD, DATE OF BIRTH MARCH 20, 1926, LICENSE NUMBER 0012269, WAS DISCIPLINED BY COLORADO ON JUNE 20, 1996
DISCIPLINARY ACTION: SURRENDER OF LICENSE

BEDFORD, ALFRED MD, DATE OF BIRTH SEPTEMBER 15, 1921, LICENSE NUMBER 0012900 OF DURANGO, CO, WAS DISCIPLINED BY COLORADO ON NOVEMBER 15, 1991
DISCIPLINARY ACTION: LICENSE REVOCATION
OFFENSE: SUBSTANDARD CARE, INCOMPETENCE OR NEGLIGENCE
NOTES: FAILURE TO MEET GENERALLY ACCEPTED STANDARDS OF MEDICAL PRACTICE.

BEDFORD, ALFRED MD, LICENSE NUMBER 0070911 OF 3705 COLORADO ROAD #250, DURANGO, CO, WAS DISCIPLINED BY NEW YORK ON APRIL 30, 1993
DISCIPLINARY ACTION: SURRENDER OF LICENSE
OFFENSE: DISCIPLINARY ACTION BY ANOTHER STATE OR AGENCY
NOTES: FOUND GUILTY OF IMPROPER PROFESSIONAL PRACTICE BY THE COLORADO BOARD.

BELL, JON A MD, DATE OF BIRTH DECEMBER 12, 1950, LICENSE NUMBER 22981, WAS DISCIPLINED BY COLORADO ON SEPTEMBER 10, 1998

DISCIPLINARY ACTION: 60-MONTH PROBATION; REQUIRED TO TAKE ADDITIONAL MEDICAL EDUCATION
OFFENSE: SEXUAL ABUSE OF OR SEXUAL MISCONDUCT WITH A PATIENT

NOTES: SEXUAL CONTACT WITH A PATIENT. PROBATIONARY TERMS INCLUDE A BOUNDARIES COURSE AND TREATMENT MONITORING.

BENNETT, ALFRED J DO, DATE OF BIRTH NOVEMBER 28, 1926, LICENSE NUMBER 13947, WAS DISCIPLINED BY COLORADO ON SEPTEMBER 17, 1998
DISCIPLINARY ACTION: SURRENDER OF LICENSE
OFFENSE: SUBSTANDARD CARE, INCOMPETENCE OR NEGLIGENCE

NOTES: SUBSTANDARD CARE.

BENNETT, ALFRED J DO, LICENSE NUMBER 00680 OF MOUNTAIN HOME, TN, WAS DISCIPLINED BY KENTUCKY ON NOVEMBER 13, 1998
DISCIPLINARY ACTION: RESTRICTION PLACED ON LICENSE; RESTRICTION PLACED ON CONTROLLED SUBSTANCE LICENSE

NOTES: MAY NOT PRESCRIBE, DISPENSE OR OTHERWISE UTILIZE CONTROLLED SUBSTANCES IN KENTUCKY; MUST PROVIDE NOTIFICATION OF ANY WORK DONE IN STATE WITHIN 30 DAYS.

BENNETT, ALFRED J DO, DATE OF BIRTH NOVEMBER 28, 1926, LICENSE NUMBER 013537 OF PO BOX 818, MOUNTAIN HOME, TN, WAS DISCIPLINED BY GEORGIA ON FEBRUARY 8, 1999
DISCIPLINARY ACTION: SURRENDER OF LICENSE

NOTES: VOLUNTARY SURRENDER.

BENNETT, ALFRED J DO, LICENSE NUMBER 09977 OF 454 MATSON ROAD, ROUTE 3, JONESBOROUGH, TN, WAS DISCIPLINED BY MISSOURI ON JULY 20, 1999
DISCIPLINARY ACTION: RESTRICTION PLACED ON CONTROLLED SUBSTANCE LICENSE
OFFENSE: DISCIPLINARY ACTION BY ANOTHER STATE OR AGENCY

NOTES: ON 10/28/96 PRESCRIPTION WRITING PRIVILEGES WERE SUSPENDED AT A VETERANS ADMINISTRATION CENTER PENDING REVIEW OF HIS PRESCRIBING PRACTICES SPECIFICALLY THAT HIS NARCOTICS PRESCRIBING PRACTICES DEMONSTRATED A GROSS DEVIATION FROM THE STANDARD OF CARE; ON 8/10/97 RETIRED FROM EMPLOYMENT AS PER AGREEMENT; KENTUCKY BOARD RESTRICTED HIS LICENSE ON 11/13/98 . MISSOURI LICENSE LIMITED AS FOLLOWS: SHALL NOT PRESCRIBE, DISPENSE, OR OTHERWISE UTILIZE CONTROLLED SUBSTANCES; SHALL NOT PETITION FOR MODIFICATION FOR FIVE YEARS.

BENNETT, YVONNE ELAINE MD, DATE OF BIRTH NOVEMBER 17, 1952 OF 7930B S DEPEW STREET, LITTLETON, CO, WAS DISCIPLINED BY MEDICARE ON DECEMBER 20, 1998
DISCIPLINARY ACTION: EXCLUSION FROM THE MEDICARE AND/OR MEDICAID PROGRAM
OFFENSE: NONCOMPLIANCE WITH A PROFESSIONAL RULE

NOTES: DEFAULTED ON PUBLIC HEALTH SERVICE EDUCATION LOAN. REINSTATED ON 2/1/99.

BENSON, JOHN M MD, WAS DISCIPLINED BY MAINE ON JANUARY 20, 1994
DISCIPLINARY ACTION: PROBATION
OFFENSE: DISCIPLINARY ACTION BY ANOTHER STATE OR AGENCY

NOTES: ACTION TAKEN BY MINNESOTA. PROBATION TERMINATED ON 12/14/94.

BENSON, JOHN M MD, LICENSE NUMBER 0123756 OF PO BOX 141, BLUE HILL, ME, WAS DISCIPLINED BY NEW YORK ON JULY 22, 1994
DISCIPLINARY ACTION: SURRENDER OF LICENSE
OFFENSE: DISCIPLINARY ACTION BY ANOTHER STATE OR AGENCY

NOTES: DISCIPLINARY ACTION TAKEN IN MINNESOTA.

BENSON, JOHN M MD, LICENSE NUMBER 26982 OF YARDLEY, PA, WAS DISCIPLINED BY IOWA ON AUGUST 26, 1999
DISCIPLINARY ACTION: REPRIMAND
OFFENSE: DISCIPLINARY ACTION BY ANOTHER STATE OR AGENCY

NOTES: DISCIPLINED BY MINNESOTA ON 11/14/92 BASED ON CHARGES OF EMBEZZLEMENT.

BENSON, JOHN MICHAEL MD, DATE OF BIRTH OCTOBER 5, 1943, LICENSE NUMBER 0023160 OF 1467 SILO ROAD, YARDLEY, PA, WAS DISCIPLINED BY MINNESOTA ON NOVEMBER 14, 1992
DISCIPLINARY ACTION: FINE; MONITORING OF PHYSICIAN PERFORMANCE
OFFENSE: PROFESSIONAL MISCONDUCT

NOTES: UNPROFESSIONAL CONDUCT; ENGAGING IN ABUSIVE OR FRAUDULENT BILLING PRACTICES. LICENSE CONDITIONED AS FOLLOWS: WITHIN TWO YEARS HE SHALL COMPLETE 1500 HOURS COMMUNITY SERVICE, NOT NECESSARILY IN THE MEDICAL FIELD; MUST MEET WITH A BOARD MEMBER OR STAFF PERSON OF THE BOARD ON A QUARTERLY BASIS, INCLUDING MONITORING; SHALL PAY A CIVIL PENALTY OF $2,000. UNCONDITIONAL LICENSE AS OF 5/14/94.

BENSON, JOHN MICHAEL MD, DATE OF BIRTH OCTOBER 5, 1943, LICENSE NUMBER 0029328 OF YARDLEY, PA, WAS DISCIPLINED BY COLORADO ON JANUARY 21, 1994
DISCIPLINARY ACTION: SURRENDER OF LICENSE
OFFENSE: DISCIPLINARY ACTION BY ANOTHER STATE OR AGENCY

NOTES: BASED ON DISCIPLINARY ACTION TAKEN BY MINNESOTA BOARD IN NOVEMBER 1992. TWO OR MORE ACTS OR OMISSIONS WHICH FAIL TO MEET GENERALLY ACCEPTED STANDARDS OF MEDICAL PRACTICE. "PRIMA FACIE" ADMISSION ONLY.

BENSON, JOHN MICHAEL MD, LICENSE NUMBER 011139E OF BLUE HILL, ME, WAS DISCIPLINED BY PENNSYLVANIA ON APRIL 26, 1994
DISCIPLINARY ACTION: SURRENDER OF LICENSE
OFFENSE: DISCIPLINARY ACTION BY ANOTHER STATE OR AGENCY

NOTES: RECIPROCAL ACTION TAKEN IN MINNESOTA.

BENSON, JOHN MICHAEL MD, DATE OF BIRTH OCTOBER 5, 1943, LICENSE NUMBER 0025826 OF PO BOX 141, BLUE HILL, ME, WAS DISCIPLINED BY NEW JERSEY ON OCTOBER 14, 1994

NOTES: BASED UPON QUESTIONABLE ACTIVITY IN MINNESOTA. AGREES TO REFRAIN FROM ENGAGING IN THE PRACTICE OF MEDICINE IN NEW JERSEY UNTIL HE PERSONALLY APPEARS BEFORE A COMMITTEE OF THE BOARD FOR A STATUS CONFERENCE.

BENSON, LAUREL J MD, DATE OF BIRTH OCTOBER 19, 1951 OF 1601 E 19TH AVENUE, DENVER, CO, WAS DISCIPLINED BY MEDICARE ON FEBRUARY 13, 1994
DISCIPLINARY ACTION: EXCLUSION FROM THE MEDICARE AND/OR MEDICAID PROGRAM
OFFENSE: NONCOMPLIANCE WITH A PROFESSIONAL RULE

NOTES: DEFAULTED ON PUBLIC HEALTH SERVICE EDUCATION LOAN. REINSTATED ON 4/5/94.

BENYI, ELIZABETH R DO, DATE OF BIRTH SEPTEMBER 16, 1955, LICENSE NUMBER 32940, WAS DISCIPLINED BY COLORADO ON

AUGUST 12, 1998
DISCIPLINARY ACTION: REPRIMAND
OFFENSE: SUBSTANDARD CARE, INCOMPETENCE OR NEGLIGENCE

NOTES: SUBSTANDARD CARE. SHE MUST OBTAIN REEDUCATION ACTIVITIES IF SHE SEEKS TO REINSTATE HER LAPSED LICENSE.

BERESFORD, KENNETH W MD, DATE OF BIRTH AUGUST 4, 1945, LICENSE NUMBER 0020101 OF MORRISON, CO, WAS DISCIPLINED BY COLORADO ON FEBRUARY 16, 1995
DISCIPLINARY ACTION: 60-MONTH PROBATION; MONITORING OF PHYSICIAN PERFORMANCE
OFFENSE: SUBSTANCE ABUSE

NOTES: HABITUAL INTEMPERANCE OR EXCESSIVE USE OF A CONTROLLED SUBSTANCE. PROBATIONARY PERIOD INCLUDES TREATMENT AND PRACTICE MONITORING.

BERG, DALRIE H A DO, DATE OF BIRTH JULY 5, 1927, LICENSE NUMBER 0013215, WAS DISCIPLINED BY COLORADO ON NOVEMBER 9, 1995
DISCIPLINARY ACTION: 60-MONTH PROBATION; RESTRICTION PLACED ON LICENSE

NOTES: NO OBSTETRICAL PRACTICE; PRACTICE MONITORING.

BERG, ROBERT N MD, DATE OF BIRTH AUGUST 11, 1940, LICENSE NUMBER 0017335 OF ENGLEWOOD, CO, WAS DISCIPLINED BY COLORADO ON MARCH 2, 1994
DISCIPLINARY ACTION: REPRIMAND
OFFENSE: PROFESSIONAL MISCONDUCT

BERMAN, MICHAEL MD, DATE OF BIRTH JUNE 5, 1940, LICENSE NUMBER 0015188 OF COLORADO SPRINGS, CO, WAS DISCIPLINED BY COLORADO ON AUGUST 10, 1994
DISCIPLINARY ACTION: REPRIMAND

BESS, ROBERT J MD, DATE OF BIRTH NOVEMBER 10, 1946, LICENSE NUMBER 0023167 OF CASTLE PINES, CO, WAS DISCIPLINED BY COLORADO ON MARCH 11, 1994
DISCIPLINARY ACTION: REPRIMAND
OFFENSE: PROFESSIONAL MISCONDUCT

BHATIA, SOHAN L DR, DATE OF BIRTH DECEMBER 29, 1946, LICENSE NUMBER 0025993 OF BRUSH, CO, WAS DISCIPLINED BY COLORADO ON AUGUST 30, 1990
DISCIPLINARY ACTION: EMERGENCY SUSPENSION
OFFENSE: SUBSTANDARD CARE, INCOMPETENCE OR NEGLIGENCE

NOTES: FAILED TO MEET GENERALLY ACCEPTED STANDARDS OF MEDICAL PRACTICE. HEARING SET FOR 2/26/91. ORDER ENTERED 4/8/92 FOR AN INDEFINITE SUSPENSION UNTIL HE ENTERS AN APPROVED RESIDENCY PROGRAM; SHOULD HE PETITION THE BOARD FOR REINSTATEMENT UPON ENTRY INTO AN APPROVED RESIDENCY PROGRAM, HE WILL BE ALLOWED A LIMITED LICENSE FOR THE PURPOSE OF PARTICIPATING IN THE RESIDENCY PROGRAM ONLY. UPON SUCCESSFUL COMPLETION OF THE APPROVED RESIDENCY PROGRAM HE WILL BE ON PROBATION INVOLVING PRACTICE MONITORING, CONTINUING EDUCATION, AND A PROHIBITION AGAINST PERFORMING SURGERY. SHOULD HE FAIL TO COMPLETE THE RESIDENCY PROGRAM, HE WILL SURRENDER HIS MEDICAL LICENSE.

BHATIA, SOHAN L DR, DATE OF BIRTH DECEMBER 29, 1946, LICENSE NUMBER 0025993 OF BRUSH, CO, WAS DISCIPLINED BY COLORADO ON APRIL 8, 1992
DISCIPLINARY ACTION: LICENSE SUSPENSION; REQUIRED TO TAKE ADDITIONAL MEDICAL EDUCATION

NOTES: FAILURE TO MEET GENERALLY ACCEPTED STANDARDS OF PRACTICE. SUSPENSION UNTIL HE ENTERS AN APPROVED RESIDENCY PROGRAM; THEN LIMITED LICENSE FOR THE PURPOSE OF PARTICIPATING IN THE PROGRAM; UPON SUCCESSFUL COMPLETION WILL BE ON PROBATION INCLUDING PRACTICE MONITORING, CONTINUING EDUCATION, AND A PROHIBITION AGAINST PERFORMING SURGERY. IF HE FAILS TO COMPLETE RESIDENCY PROGRAM WILL SURRENDER LICENSE.

BICHON, ROBERT N DO, DATE OF BIRTH FEBRUARY 25, 1942, LICENSE NUMBER 0016425, WAS DISCIPLINED BY COLORADO ON APRIL 18, 1996
DISCIPLINARY ACTION: SURRENDER OF LICENSE
OFFENSE: SUBSTANDARD CARE, INCOMPETENCE OR NEGLIGENCE

NOTES: ADMINISTERED A CONTROLLED SUBSTANCE OTHER THAN IN THE COURSE OF LEGITIMATE PROFESSIONAL PRACTICE; ENGAGED IN SUBSTANDARD CARE; ENGAGED IN SEXUAL CONTACT WITH A PATIENT; FAILED TO MAKE ESSENTIAL ENTRIES IN PATIENT RECORDS. SHALL NOT REAPPLY FOR A NEW LICENSE.

BICHON, ROBERT NEAL DO OF 554 MAIN STREET P.O. BOX 159, NUCLA, CO, WAS DISCIPLINED BY DEA ON JANUARY 31, 1996
DISCIPLINARY ACTION: SURRENDER OF CONTROLLED SUBSTANCE LICENSE
OFFENSE: PROFESSIONAL MISCONDUCT

NOTES: ALLEGED VIOLATION OF CONTROLLED SUBSTANCE ACT.

BISHOP, DAVID W MD, DATE OF BIRTH MARCH 5, 1933, LICENSE NUMBER 15696, WAS DISCIPLINED BY COLORADO ON FEBRUARY 19, 1999
DISCIPLINARY ACTION: REPRIMAND

BLAKELY, CHARLES A MD, DATE OF BIRTH MARCH 31, 1941, LICENSE NUMBER 0022395, WAS DISCIPLINED BY COLORADO ON NOVEMBER 15, 1996
DISCIPLINARY ACTION: 60-MONTH PROBATION; REQUIRED TO TAKE ADDITIONAL MEDICAL EDUCATION
OFFENSE: SUBSTANDARD CARE, INCOMPETENCE OR NEGLIGENCE

NOTES: PHYSICAL OR MENTAL DISABILITY AND SUBSTANDARD CARE. PROBATIONARY TERMS INCLUDE PRACTICE MONITORING AND REEDUCATION ACTIVITIES.

BLAKELY, CHARLES A MD, DATE OF BIRTH MARCH 31, 1941, LICENSE NUMBER 22395, WAS DISCIPLINED BY COLORADO ON APRIL 17, 1997
DISCIPLINARY ACTION: LICENSE SUSPENSION

BLANEY, DAVID D MD, LICENSE NUMBER 0029788 OF FT. COLLINS, CO, WAS DISCIPLINED BY WASHINGTON ON NOVEMBER 4, 1999
DISCIPLINARY ACTION: LICENSE REVOCATION

BLECK, ROBERT G MD, DATE OF BIRTH MAY 30, 1944, LICENSE NUMBER 19765, WAS DISCIPLINED BY COLORADO ON APRIL 10, 1997
DISCIPLINARY ACTION: REPRIMAND

BLUM, JACK MD, DATE OF BIRTH JANUARY 9, 1934, LICENSE NUMBER 0C28144 OF FAIR OAKS, CA, WAS DISCIPLINED BY CALIFORNIA ON JUNE 22, 1990
DISCIPLINARY ACTION: SURRENDER OF LICENSE

NOTES: VOLUNTARY SURRENDER ACCEPTED WHILE CHARGES PENDING.

BLUM, JACK MD, DATE OF BIRTH JANUARY 9, 1934, LICENSE NUMBER 0005293, WAS DISCIPLINED BY ARIZONA ON JANUARY 23, 1992
DISCIPLINARY ACTION: PROBATION
OFFENSE: DISCIPLINARY ACTION BY ANOTHER STATE OR AGENCY

NOTES: CALIFORNIA LICENSE SURRENDERED EFFECTIVE 6/22/90 IN CONJUNCTION WITH DISCIPLINARY PROCEEDINGS PENDING AGAINST HIM IN CALIFORNIA. ADMITTED THAT HE USED OR ADMINISTERED TO HIMSELF CONTROLLED SUBSTANCES AND DANGEROUS DRUGS WHICH CAUSED URINE SAMPLES TO TEST POSITIVE ON SIX TESTS DURING THE PERIOD FROM 4/18/88 THROUGH 6/22/89. DR. BLUM IS GUILTY OF UNPROFESSIONAL CONDUCT FOR USE OF CONTROLLED SUBSTANCES EXCEPT IF PRESCRIBED BY ANOTHER PHYSICIAN FOR USE DURING A PRESCRIBED COURSE OF TREATMENT. SHALL MEET WITH THE ARIZONA BOARD PRIOR TO PRACTICING MEDICINE IN ARIZONA AND SHALL BE SUBJECT TO ANY PSYCHIATRIC, PSYCHOMETRIC AND PHYSICAL EVALUATION OR COMPETENCY TESTS THAT THE BOARD MAY DEEM NECESSARY PRIOR TO PERMITTING HIM TO PRACTICE MEDICINE.

BLUM, JACK MD, DATE OF BIRTH JANUARY 9, 1934, LICENSE NUMBER 0003057 OF DALLAS, TX, WAS DISCIPLINED BY VERMONT ON OCTOBER 15, 1992
OFFENSE: DISCIPLINARY ACTION BY ANOTHER STATE OR AGENCY

NOTES: SURRENDERED LICENSE IN CALIFORNIA ON 3/29/90. DISCIPLINED FOR UNPROFESSIONAL CONDUCT, IN THAT HE ADMITTED HE USED OR ADMINISTERED TO HIMSELF CONTROLLED SUBSTANCES AND DANGEROUS DRUGS WHICH CAUSED URINE SAMPLES TO TEST POSITIVE BETWEEN 1/19/89 AND 6/22/89. IF HE SHOULD REAPPLY FOR LICENSURE IN CALIFORNIA, HIS APPLICATION SHALL BE TREATED AS AN ORIGINAL APPLICATION AND HE SHALL BE REQUIRED TO MEET ALL THE REQUIREMENTS OF A NEW APPLICANT. BEFORE PRACTICING IN VERMONT, WILL APPEAR BEFORE THE BOARD AND BE SUBJECT TO ANY COMPETENCY TESTS THEY DEEM NECESSARY.

BLUM, JACK MD, DATE OF BIRTH JANUARY 9, 1934, LICENSE NUMBER 00D2660 OF 10044 INWOOD ROAD, DALLAS, TX, WAS DISCIPLINED BY TEXAS ON JANUARY 29, 1993
DISCIPLINARY ACTION: 60-MONTH PROBATION; RESTRICTION PLACED ON CONTROLLED SUBSTANCE LICENSE
OFFENSE: DISCIPLINARY ACTION BY ANOTHER STATE OR AGENCY

NOTES: DISCIPLINED BY CALIFORNIA BOARD FOR SELF-ADMINISTRATION OF DANGEROUS OR CONTROLLED SUBSTANCES LEADING TO SURRENDER OF HIS LICENSE; MISSISSIPPI LICENSE ALSO SURRENDERED ALTHOUGH HE HAD NEVER PRACTICED THERE; DISCIPLINED BY ARIZONA BOARD ALTHOUGH HE NEVER PRACTICED THERE; SELF-ADMINISTERED DIAZEPAM, CODEINE, PHENERGAN, AND PROCARDIA; CURRENTLY PRACTICING IN GEORGIA. 5 YEAR SUSPENSION STAYED. CONDITIONS OF PROBATION: SHALL PARTICIPATE IN ACTIVITIES OF A PHYSICIAN HEALTH AND REHABILITATION COMMITTEE AND ATTEND WEEKLY MEETINGS WITH QUARTERLY REPORTS; SHALL PARTICIPATE IN AA'S 12 STEP PROGRAM NOT LESS THAN 2 TIMES A WEEK WITH QUARTERLY REPORTS; SHALL FURNISH THE BOARD WITH WRITTEN REPORTS ON HIS MEDICAL CONDITION AND COMPLIANCE WITH THIS ORDER WHEN REQUESTED; SHALL ABSTAIN FROM THE CONSUMPTION OF ALCOHOL/CONTROLLED SUBSTANCES IN ANY FORM; SHALL SUBMIT HIMSELF FOR APPROPRIATE EXAMS INCLUDING DRUG OR ALCOHOL SCREENS; SHALL NOT TREAT OR OTHERWISE SERVE AS THE PHYSICIAN, PRESCRIBE, DISPENSE OR ADMINISTER DRUGS THAT MAY BE SUBJECT TO ABUSE TO HIMSELF OR ANY MEMBER OF HIS FAMILY; SHALL NOT POSSESS, ADMINISTER, DISPENSE OR PRESCRIBE SCHEDULE II OR IIN CONTROLLED SUBSTANCES OUTSIDE OF A HOSPITAL SETTING; SHALL MAINTAIN A SEPARATE LOG OF ALL PRESCRIPTIONS WRITTEN FOR CONTROLLED SUBSTANCES WHICH SHALL BE AVAILABLE FOR INSPECTION; SHALL OBTAIN THE SERVICES OF A PRIMARY CARE PHYSICIAN WHO SHALL RELEASE INFORMATION TO THE BOARD; BOARD WILL BE INFORMED IF ANY DRUG HAVING ADDICTION-FORMING OR ADDICTION-SUSTAINING LIABILITY IS PRESCRIBED; SHALL OBTAIN NO PRESCRIPTIONS FROM ANY OTHER PHYSICIAN UNLESS IT IS APPROVED IN WRITING WITHIN 24 HOURS; ANY PRESCRIPTIONS WRITTEN CAN BE FILLED ONLY AT BOARD-APPROVED PHARMACIES; SHALL BE EVALUATED BY A BOARD-APPROVED PSYCHIATRIST TO WHOM HE WILL PROVIDE A COPY OF THE ORDER; SHALL COOPERATE WITH THE BOARD IN VERIFYING COMPLIANCE; SHALL INFORM BOARD OF CHANGE OF ADDRESS WITHIN 10 DAYS; TIME SPENT OUT OF TEXAS OR GEORGIA DOES NOT COUNT TOWARD PROBATION; SHALL APPEAR BEFORE THE BOARD ONCE A YEAR; SHALL APPEAR BEFORE THE BOARD PRIOR TO PRACTICING IN TEXAS. SHALL NOT SEEK MODIFICATION UNTIL FEBRUARY 6, 1994.

BLUM, JACK MD, DATE OF BIRTH JANUARY 9, 1934, LICENSE NUMBER 0016004 OF 101 BOWENS MILL ROAD, DOUGLAS, GA, WAS DISCIPLINED BY GEORGIA ON JUNE 28, 1993
DISCIPLINARY ACTION: EMERGENCY SUSPENSION

NOTES: IMPAIRMENT.

BLUM, JACK MD, DATE OF BIRTH JANUARY 9, 1934, LICENSE NUMBER 0016004 OF 10044 INWOOD ROAD, DALLAS, TX, WAS DISCIPLINED BY GEORGIA ON OCTOBER 7, 1993
DISCIPLINARY ACTION: LICENSE SUSPENSION

NOTES: IMPAIRMENT; SHALL NOT ENGAGE IN OR RETURN TO PRACTICE OF MEDICINE IN GEORGIA UNTIL FURTHER ORDER OF THE BOARD.

BLUM, JACK MD, DATE OF BIRTH JANUARY 9, 1934, LICENSE NUMBER 00D2660 OF DALLAS, TX, WAS DISCIPLINED BY TEXAS ON OCTOBER 14, 1993
DISCIPLINARY ACTION: EMERGENCY SUSPENSION
OFFENSE: FAILURE TO COMPLY WITH PREVIOUS BOARD ORDER

NOTES: VIOLATED 1/29/93 ORDER IN THAT HE REFUSED TO SUPPLY A URINE SAMPLE IN 8/93 AND INGESTED CONTROLLED SUBSTANCES IN 9/93.

BLUM, JACK MD, DATE OF BIRTH JANUARY 9, 1934, LICENSE NUMBER 00D2660 OF DALLAS, TX, WAS DISCIPLINED BY TEXAS ON JUNE 22, 1994
DISCIPLINARY ACTION: PROBATION
OFFENSE: FAILURE TO COMPLY WITH PREVIOUS BOARD ORDER

NOTES: VIOLATED 1/29/93 TEXAS ORDER IN THAT HE REFUSED TO SUPPLY A URINE SAMPLE ON 8/26/93, INGESTED CONTROLLED SUBSTANCES THREE TIMES IN 9/93; SURRENDERED HIS DEA CONTROLLED SUBSTANCES REGISTRATION ON 11/22/93. SUSPENSION STAYED. CONDITIONS OF INDEFINITE PROBATION: SHALL NOT PRACTICE MEDICINE UNTIL HE HAS UNDERGONE A 72

HOUR INPATIENT EVALUATION FOR CHEMICAL DEPENDENCY, HAS OBTAINED A COMPLETE NEUROLOGIC EXAM FROM A BOARD APPROVED PSYCHIATRIST, CAN DEMONSTRATE COMPLIANCE WITH THIS PSYCHIATRIST'S RECOMMENDATIONS AND APPEARS BEFORE THE BOARD TO REQUEST PERMISSION TO PRACTICE. UPON AN ADEQUATE SHOWING BEFORE THE BOARD THAT HE IS ABLE TO SAFELY PRACTICE MEDICINE, HE SHALL BE ALLOWED TO RESUME THE PRACTICE OF MEDICINE UNDER VARIOUS TERMS AND CONDITIONS.

BLUM, JACK MD, DATE OF BIRTH JANUARY 9, 1934, LICENSE NUMBER 00D2660, WAS DISCIPLINED BY TEXAS ON JANUARY 5, 1995
DISCIPLINARY ACTION: 120-MONTH PROBATION; RESTRICTION PLACED ON CONTROLLED SUBSTANCE LICENSE
OFFENSE: FAILURE TO COMPLY WITH PREVIOUS BOARD ORDER

NOTES: SUSPENSION STAYED. CONDITIONS OF PROBATION: SHALL ABSTAIN FROM THE CONSUMPTION OR ALCOHOL OR CONTROLLED SUBSTANCES IN ANY FORM UNLESS PRESCRIBED BY ANOTHER PHYSICIAN FOR A LEGITIMATE AND THERAPEUTIC PURPOSE; SHALL SUBMIT HIMSELF FOR APPROPRIATE EXAMS INCLUDING DRUG OR ALCOHOL SCREENS; SHALL NOT TREAT OR OTHERWISE SERVE AS PHYSICIAN FOR HIMSELF OR ANY MEMBER OF HIS FAMILY AND SHALL NOT PRESCRIBE, DISPENSE OR ADMINISTER ANY DRUGS THAT MAY BE SUBJECT TO ABUSE TO HIMSELF OR ANY MEMBER OF HIS FAMILY; SHALL ONLY ORDER AND ADMINISTER CONTROLLED SUBSTANCES FOR PERSONS UNDERGOING INPATIENT PROCEDURES AND/OR TREATMENTS AT A HOSPITAL FOR PURPOSES OF INPATIENT CARE; SHALL SURRENDER ALL UNUSED TRIPLICATE PRESCRIPTION FORMS AND CONTROLLED SUBSTANCES IN HIS POSSESSION INCLUDING SAMPLES; SHALL BE MONITORED BY A BOARD-APPROVED PHYSICIAN WITH QUARTERLY REPORTS TO THE BOARD; SEPARATE FROM PATIENT RECORDS SHALL MAINTAIN A FILE OF EVERY PRESCRIPTION WRITTEN FOR DANGEROUS DRUGS WHICH SHALL BE AVAILABLE FOR REVIEW; SHALL NOT TELEPHONE ANY PRESCRIPTION TO A PHARMACY FOR DANGEROUS DRUGS THAT MAY BE HABIT-FORMING; SHALL PARTICIPATE IN THE ACTIVITIES OF A PHYSICIANS' HEALTH AND REHABILITATION COMMITTEE AND ABIDE BY TERMS OF AN AFTERCARE PROGRAM CONTRACT WITH QUARTERLY REPORTS; SHALL PARTICIPATE IN AA'S PROGRAMS NOT LESS THAN THREE TIMES A WEEK WITH QUARTERLY REPORTS TO THE BOARD; SHALL SUBMIT HIMSELF FOR EVALUATION AND TREATMENT TO A BOARD-APPROVED PSYCHIATRIST WITH QUARTERLY REPORTS; SHALL ATTEND AT LEAST 40 HOURS OF CONTINUING MEDICAL EDUCATION PER YEAR; SHALL APPEAR BEFORE THE BOARD TWICE A YEAR; SHALL GIVE A COPY OF THIS ORDER TO ANY HEALTH CARE ENTITY WHERE HE HAS PRIVILEGES; SHALL COOPERATE WITH THE BOARD IN VERIFYING COMPLIANCE; SHALL INFORM BOARD OF CHANGE OF ADDRESS WITHIN 10 DAYS OR IF HE LEAVES THE STATE; TIME SPENT OUT OF TEXAS DOES NOT COUNT TOWARD PROBATION. SHALL NOT SEEK MODIFICATION FOR ONE YEAR.

BLUM, JACK MD, DATE OF BIRTH JANUARY 9, 1934, LICENSE NUMBER 00D2660, WAS DISCIPLINED BY TEXAS ON JUNE 28, 1995
DISCIPLINARY ACTION: LICENSE REVOCATION
OFFENSE: FAILURE TO COMPLY WITH PREVIOUS BOARD ORDER

NOTES: BETWEEN 10/6/94 AND 1/5/95 DIAGNOSED, TREATED, AND PRESCRIBED TO PATIENTS IN VIOLATION OF ORDER; NONCOMPLIANCE TO 1/05/95 ORDER IN THAT HE FAILED TO CAUSE HIS TREATING PHYSICIAN TO REPORT THE INGESTION OF FIORCET AND DIRECTED A MEDICAL ASSISTANT OF HIS MONITORING PHYSICIAN TO PREPARE PRESCRIPTIONS OF CHLORAL HYDRATE AND DIAZEPAM IN HIS WIFE'S NAME WHICH HE TRIED TO FILL, NEITHER OF WHICH WERE AUTHORIZED OR DIRECTED BY HIS MONITORING PHYSICIAN. ON 1/29/99 PETITION TO REINSTATE LICENSE DENIED.

BLUM, JACK MD, DATE OF BIRTH JANUARY 9, 1934, LICENSE NUMBER 0003057 OF DALLAS, TX, WAS DISCIPLINED BY VERMONT ON NOVEMBER 3, 1995
DISCIPLINARY ACTION: LICENSE REVOCATION
OFFENSE: DISCIPLINARY ACTION BY ANOTHER STATE OR AGENCY

NOTES: TEXAS BOARD TOOK DISCIPLINARY ACTION AGAINST HIS MEDICAL LICENSE; ON HIS 1994-1996 LICENSE RENEWAL APPLICATION HE FALSELY ANSWERED "NO" TO A QUESTION REGARDING DISCIPLINARY ACTION TAKEN BY ANOTHER STATE WHEN HE HAD ACTIONS TAKEN BY SEVERAL STATES BETWEEN 1990 AND 1993; ALSO ANSWERED "NO" TO A QUESTION REGARDING REDUCTION, SUSPENSION OR REVOCATION OF STAFF PRIVILEGES, EMPLOYMENT OR APPOINTMENT IN A HOSPITAL OR OTHER HEALTH CARE INSTITUTION WHEN HE HAD RESIGNED FROM A HOSPITAL IN GEORGIA IN 4/93.

BLUM, JACK MD, DATE OF BIRTH JANUARY 9, 1934, LICENSE NUMBER 0005293, WAS DISCIPLINED BY ARIZONA ON JANUARY 19, 1996
DISCIPLINARY ACTION: LICENSE REVOCATION
OFFENSE: DISCIPLINARY ACTION BY ANOTHER STATE OR AGENCY

NOTES: VIOLATED TERMS OF TEXAS PROBATION OF 1/93 IN THAT HE REFUSED TO SUPPLY A URINE SAMPLE AT THE REQUEST OF A COMPLIANCE OFFICER IN 8/93; IN 9/93, INGESTED CHLORAL HYDRATE, CODEINE, AND XANAX WITHOUT A PRESCRIPTION FROM HIS PRIMARY PHYSICIAN AS REQUIRED BY PROBATION TERMS; SURRENDERED HIS DEA CONTROLLED SUBSTANCES REGISTRATION ON 11/22/93; PLACED ON 10 YEAR PROBATION IN TEXAS IN 1/95 BASED ON NONCOMPLIANCE. IN 1993,1994 AND 1995 APPLICATIONS FOR LICENSE RENEWAL IN ARIZONA, HE DENIED ANY DISCIPLINARY ACTION TAKEN AGAINST HIS LICENSE DURING THE REGISTRATION PERIODS AND DENIED ANY DENIAL, RESTRICTION, SUSPENSION, OR LOSS/REVOCATION OF DEA OR PRESCRIPTION PERMIT, DESPITE ACTIONS BY ARIZONA, TEXAS AND SURRENDER OF HIS DEA REGISTRATION DURING THOSE PERIODS. PERMANENT REVOCATION; FINAL DECISION WITH NO OPPORTUNITY FOR REHEARING OR REVIEW.

BLUM, JACK MD, DATE OF BIRTH JANUARY 9, 1934, LICENSE NUMBER 18306, WAS DISCIPLINED BY COLORADO ON APRIL 10, 1997
DISCIPLINARY ACTION: SURRENDER OF LICENSE

NOTES: NO UNPROFESSIONAL CONDUCT IDENTIFIED.

BOGNER, PHILLIP MD OF 1280 GRAND AVENUE, DEL NORTE, CO, WAS DISCIPLINED BY DEA ON JUNE 28, 1999
DISCIPLINARY ACTION: SURRENDER OF CONTROLLED SUBSTANCE LICENSE
OFFENSE: NONCOMPLIANCE WITH A PROFESSIONAL RULE

NOTES: FAILURE TO KEEP RECORDS.

BOLAND, GREGORY H MD, DATE OF BIRTH JULY 8, 1953, LICENSE

NUMBER 0032049 OF LOVELAND, CO, WAS DISCIPLINED BY COLORADO ON JULY 16, 1992
DISCIPLINARY ACTION: 60-MONTH PROBATION; MONITORING OF PHYSICIAN PERFORMANCE
OFFENSE: SUBSTANCE ABUSE

NOTES: HABITUAL INTEMPERANCE OR EXCESSIVE USE OF ANY HABIT-FORMING DRUG OR CONTROLLED SUBSTANCE (IN ABEYANCE). LICENSE GRANTED WITH PROBATION INCLUDING TREATMENT AND PRACTICE MONITORING. PROBATION DEEMED COMPLETED ON 2/16/95 AND LICENSE RESTORED TO UNENCUMBERED STATUS.

BOLAND, GREGORY H MD, DATE OF BIRTH JULY 8, 1953, LICENSE NUMBER 0032049, WAS DISCIPLINED BY COLORADO ON NOVEMBER 16, 1995
DISCIPLINARY ACTION: RESTRICTION PLACED ON LICENSE

NOTES: WILL PERFORM NO ACT REQUIRING A LICENSE TO PRACTICE MEDICINE IN COLORADO UNTIL FURTHER BOARD NOTICE. INTERIM CESSATION OF PRACTICE APPROVED; ORDER IN EFFECT UNTIL ADDITIONAL INFORMATION IS REVIEWED.

BOLAND, GREGORY H MD, DATE OF BIRTH JULY 8, 1953, LICENSE NUMBER 0032049, WAS DISCIPLINED BY COLORADO ON OCTOBER 17, 1996
DISCIPLINARY ACTION: SURRENDER OF LICENSE
OFFENSE: PHYSICAL OR MENTAL ILLNESS INHIBITING THE ABILITY TO PRACTICE WITH SKILL AND SAFETY

NOTES: MENTAL DISABILITY.

BOLAND, GREGORY H MD OF 4601 CORBETT DRIVE, FORT COLLINS, CO, WAS DISCIPLINED BY DEA ON DECEMBER 6, 1996
DISCIPLINARY ACTION: SURRENDER OF CONTROLLED SUBSTANCE LICENSE

BOLAND, GREGORY HAROLD MD, LICENSE NUMBER H7045 OF PUEBLO, CO, WAS DISCIPLINED BY TEXAS ON AUGUST 9, 1997
DISCIPLINARY ACTION: SURRENDER OF LICENSE
OFFENSE: DISCIPLINARY ACTION BY ANOTHER STATE OR AGENCY

NOTES: A 6/23/92 COLORADO BOARD ORDER INDICATES HIS ADMISSION AND AGREEMENT TO HAVING BEEN TREATED FOR EMOTIONAL PROBLEMS MANIFESTED BY MALADAPTIVE CHARATEROLOGICAL, DEPRESSIVE AND ANXIETY SYMPTOMS COMPLICATED BY POLYSUBSTANCE ABUSE IN 1975 AND 1976, AND HAVING BEEN HOSPITALIZED IN 1984 FOR SUBSTANCE ABUSE; ON 11/16/95 THE COLORADO BOARD SUSPENDED HIS LICENSE BECAUSE HE HAD RESUMED ALCOHOL AND DRUG USE AND HAD BEEN ARRESTED IN 10/95 FOR ASSAULT; ON 10/25/96 HE WAS CONVICTED OF TWO COUNTS: SECOND DEGREE ASSAULT, AND UNLAWFUL USE OF A CONTROLLED SUBSTANCE. VOLUNTARY SURRENDER; SHALL GIVE A COPY OF THIS ORDER TO ANY HEALTH CARE ENTITY WHERE HE HAS PRIVILEGES.

BOLAND, GREGORY HAROLD MD, DATE OF BIRTH JULY 8, 1953 OF PO BOX 300, UNIT A, 91573, CANYON CITY, CO, WAS DISCIPLINED BY MEDICARE ON DECEMBER 20, 1998
DISCIPLINARY ACTION: EXCLUSION FROM THE MEDICARE AND/OR MEDICAID PROGRAM
OFFENSE: DISCIPLINARY ACTION BY ANOTHER STATE OR AGENCY

NOTES: LICENSE REVOKED, SUSPENDED, SURRENDERED OR OTHERWISE LOST FOR REASONS BEARING ON PROFESSIONAL PERFORMANCE, PROFESSIONAL COMPETENCE OR FINANCIAL INTEGRITY.

BOLAND, JAMES EDWARD MD, LICENSE NUMBER G63321 OF LITTLETON, CO, WAS DISCIPLINED BY CALIFORNIA ON SEPTEMBER 14, 1998
DISCIPLINARY ACTION: LICENSE REVOCATION
OFFENSE: DISCIPLINARY ACTION BY ANOTHER STATE OR AGENCY

NOTES: DISCIPLINED BY COLORADO FOR FAILURE TO RESPOND TO TWO INQUIRY LETTERS FROM THE BOARD REGARDING THE TREATMENT OF A PATIENT'S INJURED KNEE IN THE EMERGENCY ROOM AND FOR FAILURE TO ADEQUATELY TREAT THE INJURED KNEE.

BOOKHARDT, JOHN F MD, WAS DISCIPLINED BY NEBRASKA ON DECEMBER 17, 1990
DISCIPLINARY ACTION: LICENSE REVOCATION
OFFENSE: FAILURE TO COMPLY WITH PREVIOUS BOARD ORDER

NOTES: VIOLATED PROBATION.

BOOKHARDT, JOHN F MD, DATE OF BIRTH JULY 4, 1927, LICENSE NUMBER 0013885 OF AURORA, CO, WAS DISCIPLINED BY COLORADO ON NOVEMBER 6, 1992
DISCIPLINARY ACTION: LICENSE REVOCATION
OFFENSE: DISCIPLINARY ACTION BY ANOTHER STATE OR AGENCY

NOTES: HIS NEBRASKA MEDICAL LICENSE WAS REVOKED FOR NONCOMPLIANCE WITH ORDER THAT HE NOT PRESCRIBE CONTROLLED SUBSTANCES WITHOUT PRIOR APPROVAL OF A SUPERVISING PHYSICIAN.

BOSTROM, PAUL D MD, DATE OF BIRTH JULY 20, 1940, LICENSE NUMBER 0017962, WAS DISCIPLINED BY COLORADO ON JUNE 15, 1995
DISCIPLINARY ACTION: 60-MONTH PROBATION

NOTES: TREATMENT MONITORING.

BOSTROM, PAUL D MD, DATE OF BIRTH JULY 20, 1940, LICENSE NUMBER 0017962, WAS DISCIPLINED BY COLORADO ON JANUARY 18, 1996

NOTES: INTERIM CESSATION OF PRACTICE RETROACTIVE TO 11/24/95.

BOSTROM, PAUL D MD, DATE OF BIRTH JULY 20, 1940, LICENSE NUMBER 17962, WAS DISCIPLINED BY COLORADO ON JUNE 19, 1997
DISCIPLINARY ACTION: SURRENDER OF LICENSE
OFFENSE: SEXUAL ABUSE OF OR SEXUAL MISCONDUCT WITH A PATIENT

NOTES: A SEXUAL ACT WITH A PATIENT; PHYSICAL OR MENTAL DISABILITY.

BOSTROM, PAUL DAVID MD OF CORTEZ, CO, WAS DISCIPLINED BY UTAH ON JANUARY 23, 1996
OFFENSE: DISCIPLINARY ACTION BY ANOTHER STATE OR AGENCY

NOTES: CURRENT DISCIPLINARY ACTION AGAINST HIS LICENSE TO PRACTICE MEDICINE IN COLORADO. UTAH SUSPENSION STAYED DURING THE FIVE YEAR COLORADO PROBATIONARY PERIOD SO LONG AS HE REMAINS IN FULL COMPLIANCE WITH THE TERMS AND CONDITIONS OF HIS COLORADO PROBATION.

BOWMAN, WILLIAM J MD, DATE OF BIRTH SEPTEMBER 25, 1948, LICENSE NUMBER 0021343, WAS DISCIPLINED BY COLORADO ON MAY 18, 1995
DISCIPLINARY ACTION: EMERGENCY SUSPENSION
OFFENSE: FAILURE TO COMPLY WITH PREVIOUS BOARD ORDER

NOTES: DUE TO NONCOMPLIANCE WITH VALID STIPULATION AND BOARD ORDER.

BOWMAN, WILLIAM J MD, DATE OF BIRTH SEPTEMBER 25, 1948, LICENSE NUMBER 0021343, WAS DISCIPLINED BY COLORADO ON MAY 31, 1995
DISCIPLINARY ACTION: MONITORING OF PHYSICIAN PERFORMANCE

NOTES: PERMANENT TREATMENT MONITORING AND FIVE YEAR PRACTICE MONITORING.

BOYD, GWENDOLYN L MD, DATE OF BIRTH APRIL 22, 1943, LICENSE NUMBER 0016941, WAS DISCIPLINED BY COLORADO ON JANUARY 11, 1996
DISCIPLINARY ACTION: 60-MONTH PROBATION; MONITORING OF PHYSICIAN PERFORMANCE
OFFENSE: SUBSTANCE ABUSE

NOTES: PHYSICAL OR MENTAL IMPAIRMENT; ALCOHOL ABUSE. PRACTICE AND TREATMENT MONITORING THROUGH THE COLORADO PHYSICIAN HEALTH PROGRAM. SINCE SHE IS PRESENTLY NOT PRACTICING MEDICINE IN COLORADO, THE PROBATIONARY TERMS ARE BEING TOLLED. ON 3/13/97 ORDER VACATED AND SHE AGREES TO PLACE HER LICENSE IN INACTIVE STATUS AND TO ENTER INTO A NEW AGREEMENT IF SHE WERE TO EVER SEEK TO REACTIVATE HER LICENSE.

BOYLE, CORNELIUS D MD, DATE OF BIRTH APRIL 15, 1937, LICENSE NUMBER 0025112 OF GRAVES COUNTY, KY, WAS DISCIPLINED BY KENTUCKY ON NOVEMBER 30, 1990
DISCIPLINARY ACTION: LICENSE SUSPENSION; REQUIRED TO TAKE ADDITIONAL MEDICAL EDUCATION
OFFENSE: PROFESSIONAL MISCONDUCT

NOTES: CRIMINAL CHARGES WERE FILED AGAINST HIM. REINSTATEMENT WILL NOT BE CONSIDERED UNTIL SUCH TIME AS HE SUCCESSFULLY COMPLETES AT LEAST ONE YEAR OF BOARD-APPROVED, ACCREDITED POSTGRADUATE TRAINING IN OPHTHALMOLOGY. IF REINSTATED, HIS LICENSE WILL BE SUBJECT TO A PERIOD OF PROBATION OF FOUR AND ONE-HALF YEARS, WITH TERMS AND CONDITIONS. COURT RULED THAT SUSPENSION COULD NOT BE INDEFINITE AND VACATED THE ORDER REMANDING IT BACK TO THE BOARD ON 8/24/92. ON 11/19/92 THE BOARD AMENDED THIS ORDER TO LIMIT THE TIME OF SUSPENSION NOT TO EXCEED FIVE YEARS.

BOYLE, CORNELIUS D MD, DATE OF BIRTH APRIL 15, 1937, LICENSE NUMBER 0027279 OF MAYFIELD, KY, WAS DISCIPLINED BY COLORADO ON FEBRUARY 2, 1995
DISCIPLINARY ACTION: LICENSE REVOCATION
OFFENSE: CRIMINAL CONVICTION OR PLEA OF GUILTY, NOLO CONTENDERE, OR NO CONTEST TO A CRIME

NOTES: FELONY CONVICTION. CASE IS ON APPEAL TO THE COLORADO COURT OF APPEALS AS OF THE DATE OF THE ORDER.

BRAMSCHREIBER, JEROME L MD, DATE OF BIRTH SEPTEMBER 25, 1933, LICENSE NUMBER 0017963, WAS DISCIPLINED BY COLORADO ON JUNE 8, 1995
DISCIPLINARY ACTION: REPRIMAND

BRANSON, DONALD E MD, DATE OF BIRTH MARCH 4, 1926 OF PO BOX 246, LAVETA, CO, WAS DISCIPLINED BY MEDICARE ON AUGUST 1, 1990
DISCIPLINARY ACTION: EXCLUSION FROM THE MEDICARE AND/OR MEDICAID PROGRAM
OFFENSE: DISCIPLINARY ACTION BY ANOTHER STATE OR AGENCY

NOTES: LICENSE REVOCATION OR SUSPENSION.

BRANSON, DONALD E MD, LICENSE NUMBER 0C19501 OF RANCHO MIRAGE, CA, WAS DISCIPLINED BY CALIFORNIA ON MAY 13, 1992
DISCIPLINARY ACTION: LICENSE REVOCATION
OFFENSE: DISCIPLINARY ACTION BY ANOTHER STATE OR AGENCY

NOTES: COLORADO BOARD DISCIPLINE FOR LONG-TERM ALCOHOL ABUSE.

BRETHOUWER, N ROBERT DO, DATE OF BIRTH NOVEMBER 6, 1932, LICENSE NUMBER 0015237 OF MONTROSE, CO, WAS DISCIPLINED BY COLORADO ON JANUARY 18, 1995
DISCIPLINARY ACTION: 60-MONTH PROBATION; REQUIRED TO TAKE ADDITIONAL MEDICAL EDUCATION
OFFENSE: SUBSTANDARD CARE, INCOMPETENCE OR NEGLIGENCE

NOTES: SUBSTANDARD CARE. PROBATIONARY PERIOD INCLUDES PRACTICE MONITORING AND REEDUCATION ACTIVITIES.

BROHOLM, RUSSELL MD, DATE OF BIRTH AUGUST 18, 1931, LICENSE NUMBER 0015926 OF 1016 BLUE STEM BLVD, PUEBLO, CO, WAS DISCIPLINED BY IOWA ON AUGUST 16, 1991
DISCIPLINARY ACTION: SURRENDER OF LICENSE

NOTES: LICENSE VOLUNTARILY SURRENDERED AS DISPOSITION TO FORMAL DISCIPLINARY ACTION.

BROOKS, BANCROFT MD, LICENSE NUMBER 0027849 OF TACOMA, WA, WAS DISCIPLINED BY COLORADO ON FEBRUARY 8, 1991
DISCIPLINARY ACTION: LICENSE REVOCATION
OFFENSE: SUBSTANDARD CARE, INCOMPETENCE OR NEGLIGENCE

NOTES: ACTION BASED ON DIAGNOSIS AND TREATMENT OF PSYCHIATRIC PATIENTS AT COLORADO STATE HOSPITAL.

BROWN, DONALD BRUCE MD OF 5885 PARK LANE ROAD, LONGMONT, CO, WAS DISCIPLINED BY DEA ON JUNE 21, 1996
DISCIPLINARY ACTION: SURRENDER OF CONTROLLED SUBSTANCE LICENSE

NOTES: IN LIEU OF ORDER TO SHOW CAUSE.

BROWN, DONALD BRUCE MD OF 2525 4TH STREET, BOULDER, CO, WAS DISCIPLINED BY DEA ON JUNE 26, 1997
DISCIPLINARY ACTION: SURRENDER OF CONTROLLED SUBSTANCE LICENSE

BROWN, FREDERICK B MD, DATE OF BIRTH OCTOBER 16, 1945, LICENSE NUMBER 0019598, WAS DISCIPLINED BY COLORADO ON OCTOBER 14, 1996
DISCIPLINARY ACTION: REPRIMAND

BROWN, JAMES T MD, DATE OF BIRTH AUGUST 20, 1915 OF 310 E 5TH STREET, LOVELAND, CO, WAS DISCIPLINED BY MEDICARE ON AUGUST 1, 1990
DISCIPLINARY ACTION: EXCLUSION FROM THE MEDICARE AND/OR MEDICAID PROGRAM
OFFENSE: DISCIPLINARY ACTION BY ANOTHER STATE OR AGENCY

NOTES: LICENSE REVOCATION OR SUSPENSION.

BROWN, MAURICE D MD, DATE OF BIRTH AUGUST 12, 1960, LICENSE NUMBER 34659, WAS DISCIPLINED BY COLORADO ON MAY 19, 1997
DISCIPLINARY ACTION: REPRIMAND

BRUNKO, MICHAEL W MD, DATE OF BIRTH SEPTEMBER 23, 1955, LICENSE NUMBER 0025609 OF WHEAT RIDGE, CO, WAS

DISCIPLINED BY COLORADO ON JULY 14, 1993
DISCIPLINARY ACTION: 60-MONTH PROBATION; MONITORING OF PHYSICIAN PERFORMANCE
OFFENSE: SUBSTANCE ABUSE

NOTES: EXCESSIVE USE OF A CONTROLLED SUBSTANCE; SELF-PRESCRIBING OF A SCHEDULE II CONTROLLED SUBSTANCE. PROBATIONARY TERM INCLUDES PRACTICE AND TREATMENT MONITORING.

BUDENSIEK, RICHARD L DO, DATE OF BIRTH AUGUST 26, 1953, LICENSE NUMBER 0001854 OF 2513 54TH AVENUE, GREELEY, CO, WAS DISCIPLINED BY IOWA ON DECEMBER 12, 1996
DISCIPLINARY ACTION: FINE; REPRIMAND
OFFENSE: SEXUAL ABUSE OF OR SEXUAL MISCONDUCT WITH A PATIENT

NOTES: ENGAGED IN A CONSENSUAL SEXUAL RELATIONSHIP WITH A FEMALE PATIENT FOR ABOUT SIX MONTHS IN MID-1991. $2,000 CIVIL PENALTY.

BUDENSIEK, RICHARD L DO, DATE OF BIRTH AUGUST 26, 1953, LICENSE NUMBER 32150, WAS DISCIPLINED BY COLORADO ON NOVEMBER 12, 1997
DISCIPLINARY ACTION: REPRIMAND

BUGLEWICZ, JOHN MD, DATE OF BIRTH JUNE 12, 1933, LICENSE NUMBER 13992, WAS DISCIPLINED BY COLORADO ON AUGUST 15, 1997
DISCIPLINARY ACTION: REPRIMAND; REQUIRED TO TAKE ADDITIONAL MEDICAL EDUCATION
OFFENSE: SUBSTANDARD CARE, INCOMPETENCE OR NEGLIGENCE

NOTES: SUBSTANDARD CARE. REEDUCATION ACTIVITIES.

BURKE, LEONARD P JR MD OF DENVER, CO, WAS DISCIPLINED BY ILLINOIS ON SEPTEMBER 1, 1990
DISCIPLINARY ACTION: 36-MONTH PROBATION
OFFENSE: DISCIPLINARY ACTION BY ANOTHER STATE OR AGENCY

NOTES: COLORADO LICENSE PLACED ON PROBATION FOR FIVE YEARS.

BURKE, ROBERT W MD, LICENSE NUMBER 0C18151 OF SAN RAFAEL, CA, WAS DISCIPLINED BY CALIFORNIA ON MARCH 8, 1995
DISCIPLINARY ACTION: 36-MONTH PROBATION
OFFENSE: SUBSTANDARD CARE, INCOMPETENCE OR NEGLIGENCE

NOTES: REPEATED NEGLIGENT ACTS IN THE MANAGEMENT OF A 13-YEAR-OLD WITH GENETIC ABNORMAL BEHAVIOR WITH LITHIUM AND AMITRIPTYLINE, WITHOUT ADEQUATE DOCUMENTATION, RATIONALES AND MONITORING. REVOCATION STAYED.

BURKE, ROBERT W MD, DATE OF BIRTH JULY 6, 1947, LICENSE NUMBER 19565, WAS DISCIPLINED BY COLORADO ON JULY 18, 1997
DISCIPLINARY ACTION: REPRIMAND

BURKS, CHESTER L JR DO, DATE OF BIRTH OCTOBER 20, 1950, LICENSE NUMBER 0027067 OF DENVER, CO, WAS DISCIPLINED BY COLORADO ON AUGUST 21, 1992
DISCIPLINARY ACTION: 60-MONTH PROBATION; MONITORING OF PHYSICIAN PERFORMANCE
OFFENSE: SUBSTANCE ABUSE

NOTES: ALCOHOL ABUSE/HABITUAL INTEMPERANCE. PROBATION INCLUDES TREATMENT AND PRACTICE MONITORING.

BURKS, CHESTER L DO, DATE OF BIRTH OCTOBER 20, 1950, LICENSE NUMBER 0027067 OF AURORA, CO, WAS DISCIPLINED BY COLORADO ON SEPTEMBER 7, 1994
DISCIPLINARY ACTION: REPRIMAND

BURRIS, WILLIAM T MD, LICENSE NUMBER 0024901 OF STOCKTON, CA, WAS DISCIPLINED BY COLORADO ON DECEMBER 7, 1990
DISCIPLINARY ACTION: 36-MONTH PROBATION; MONITORING OF PHYSICIAN PERFORMANCE
OFFENSE: SUBSTANCE ABUSE

NOTES: FAILURE TO MEET GENERALLY ACCEPTED STANDARDS OF MEDICAL PRACTICE; HABITUAL INTEMPERANCE. LICENSE ON PROBATION COMMENCING ON DATE HE RETURNS TO COLORADO AND COMMENCES PRACTICE OF MEDICINE. ALSO TREATMENT MONITORING AND PRACTICE SUPERVISION.

BURRIS, WILLIAM T MD, LICENSE NUMBER 0G60044 OF STOCKTON, CA, WAS DISCIPLINED BY CALIFORNIA ON JANUARY 28, 1993
DISCIPLINARY ACTION: SURRENDER OF LICENSE

NOTES: VOLUNTARY SURRENDER OF LICENSE WHILE CHARGES PENDING.

BURY, RICHARD MD OF 850 E. HARVARD STREET #325, DENVER, CO, WAS DISCIPLINED BY DEA ON MAY 21, 1999
DISCIPLINARY ACTION: SURRENDER OF CONTROLLED SUBSTANCE LICENSE

BURY, RICHARD R MD, DATE OF BIRTH SEPTEMBER 5, 1946, LICENSE NUMBER 23175, WAS DISCIPLINED BY COLORADO ON OCTOBER 21, 1999
DISCIPLINARY ACTION: 60-MONTH PROBATION; RESTRICTION PLACED ON CONTROLLED SUBSTANCE LICENSE
OFFENSE: PROFESSIONAL MISCONDUCT

NOTES: ADMINISTERED A CONTROLLED SUBSTANCE OTHER THAN IN THE COURSE OF LEGITIMATE PROFESSIONAL PRACTICE. PROBATIONARY TERMS INCLUDE: NO PRESCRIPTION OF CONTROLLED SUBSTANCES, ABSTINENCE FROM ALCOHOL AND CONTROLLED SUBSTANCES, TREATMENT MONITORING AND PRACTICE MONITORING.

BUSSEY, WILLIAM J MD, DATE OF BIRTH DECEMBER 23, 1962, LICENSE NUMBER 0032929 OF FT. COLLINS, CO, WAS DISCIPLINED BY COLORADO ON JUNE 17, 1994
DISCIPLINARY ACTION: LICENSE REVOCATION
OFFENSE: FAILURE TO COMPLY WITH PREVIOUS BOARD ORDER

NOTES: VIOLATION OF BOARD ORDER.

BUSSEY, WILLIAM J MD, DATE OF BIRTH DECEMBER 23, 1962 OF 1306 ASH DRIVE, FT COLLINS, CO, WAS DISCIPLINED BY MEDICARE ON DECEMBER 5, 1994
DISCIPLINARY ACTION: EXCLUSION FROM THE MEDICARE AND/OR MEDICAID PROGRAM
OFFENSE: DISCIPLINARY ACTION BY ANOTHER STATE OR AGENCY

NOTES: LICENSE REVOKED FOR REASONS BEARING ON PROFESSIONAL COMPETENCE. REINSTATED ON 12/13/94.

BUSSEY, WILLIAM J MD OF 1306 ASH DRIVE, FT COLLINS, CO, WAS DISCIPLINED BY NEW MEXICO ON JANUARY 1, 1997
OFFENSE: SUBSTANCE ABUSE

NOTES: LICENSE ISSUED UNDER UNSPECIFIED CONDITIONS. IN 1997 STIPULATIONS FOR SUBSTANCE ABUSE REDUCED TO ANNUAL VISITS WITH THE BOARD. IN 11/98 REMOVED ALL STIPULATIONS FOR SUBSTANCE ABUSE; UNRESTRICTED LICENSE.

BUSSEY, WILLIAM J MD, DATE OF BIRTH DECEMBER 23, 1962, LICENSE NUMBER 36582, WAS DISCIPLINED BY COLORADO ON OCTOBER 9, 1997
DISCIPLINARY ACTION: 60-MONTH PROBATION; MONITORING OF PHYSICIAN PERFORMANCE

NOTES: NO UNPROFESSIONAL CONDUCT IDENTIFIED. PROBATIONARY TERMS INCLUDE: ABSTINENCE FROM ADDICTIVE SUBSTANCES, TREATMENT MONITORING AND PRACTICE MONITORING.

BUSSEY, WILLIAM J MD, WAS DISCIPLINED BY IOWA ON MARCH 12, 1998
DISCIPLINARY ACTION: REQUIRED TO ENTER AN IMPAIRED PHYSICIAN PROGRAM OR SUBSTANCE ABUSE TREATMENT; MONITORING OF PHYSICIAN PERFORMANCE

NOTES: RECEIVED AN IOWA MEDICAL LICENSE UNDER TERMS AND CONDITIONS: PROHIBITED FROM USING ALCOHOL OR OTHER CONTROLLED SUBSTANCES NOT PRESCRIBED BY A QUALIFIED HEALTH CARE PROVIDER; REQUIRED TO SEEK CONTINUING SUBSTANCE ABUSE TREATMENT, FILE REGULAR REPORTS ON HIS PROGRESS AND PROVIDE BLOOD OR URINE SAMPLES ON DEMAND.

BUTLER, HARRISON G III MD, DATE OF BIRTH JUNE 30, 1943, LICENSE NUMBER 0019371 OF 1810 E. THIRD AVENUE, DURANGO, CO, WAS DISCIPLINED BY COLORADO ON JULY 21, 1994
DISCIPLINARY ACTION: EMERGENCY SUSPENSION
OFFENSE: SUBSTANCE ABUSE

NOTES: HAS BEEN TREATED FOR AND RELAPSED FROM ALCOHOLISM FROM 1973 UNTIL 7/11/94 WHEN HE LEFT THE HOSPITAL AGAINST MEDICAL ADVICE; WAS CITED FOR DRIVING WHILE INTOXICATED ON 7/13/94; ON THREE OCCASIONS BETWEEN 3/93 AND 7/94 HE DID NOT RESPOND TO HOSPITAL CALLS REGARDING HIS PATIENTS OR HAD TO HAVE ANOTHER PHYSICIAN ATTEND THEM AT LEAST TWO OF WHICH BECAUSE OF HIS PROBLEM.

BUTLER, HARRISON G III MD, DATE OF BIRTH JUNE 30, 1943, LICENSE NUMBER 0019371 OF DURANGO, CO, WAS DISCIPLINED BY COLORADO ON MARCH 16, 1995
DISCIPLINARY ACTION: SURRENDER OF LICENSE
OFFENSE: SUBSTANCE ABUSE

NOTES: PHYSICAL OR MENTAL DISABILITY.

BYNUM, RANDALL L MD, DATE OF BIRTH MAY 17, 1959, LICENSE NUMBER 30249, WAS DISCIPLINED BY COLORADO ON MAY 14, 1997
DISCIPLINARY ACTION: 60-MONTH PROBATION; MONITORING OF PHYSICIAN PERFORMANCE
OFFENSE: SUBSTANCE ABUSE

NOTES: HABITUAL INTEMPERANCE OR EXCESSIVE USE OF A CONTROLLED SUBSTANCE. TERMS OF PROBATION INCLUDE: HE AGREES TO REMAIN ABSTINENT FROM ADDICTIVE SUBSTANCES, TREATMENT MONITORING AND PRACTICE MONITORING.

BYNUM, RANDALL L MD, DATE OF BIRTH MAY 17, 1959, LICENSE NUMBER 30249, WAS DISCIPLINED BY COLORADO ON DECEMBER 18, 1997
DISCIPLINARY ACTION: SURRENDER OF LICENSE
OFFENSE: FAILURE TO COMPLY WITH PREVIOUS BOARD ORDER

NOTES: VIOLATION OF A VALID BOARD ORDER.

BYNUM, RANDALL LEE MD, DATE OF BIRTH MAY 17, 1959 OF 19950 EAST BELLEWOOD DRIVE, AURORA, CO, WAS DISCIPLINED BY MEDICARE ON JULY 20, 1998
DISCIPLINARY ACTION: EXCLUSION FROM THE MEDICARE AND/OR MEDICAID PROGRAM
OFFENSE: DISCIPLINARY ACTION BY ANOTHER STATE OR AGENCY

NOTES: LICENSE REVOKED, SUSPENDED, SURRENDERED OR OTHERWISE LOST FOR REASONS BEARING ON PROFESSIONAL PERFORMANCE, PROFESSIONAL COMPETENCE OR FINANCIAL INTEGRITY.

CALLAHAN, SUSAN M MD, DATE OF BIRTH OCTOBER 20, 1958, LICENSE NUMBER 0032417 OF DENVER, CO, WAS DISCIPLINED BY COLORADO ON MARCH 16, 1995
DISCIPLINARY ACTION: LICENSE SUSPENSION

NOTES: FAILURE TO UNDERGO MEDICAL EVALUATION.

CAMPBELL, BERNARD E MD, DATE OF BIRTH JUNE 12, 1916, LICENSE NUMBER 0010931 OF LAKEWOOD, CO, WAS DISCIPLINED BY COLORADO ON APRIL 10, 1992
DISCIPLINARY ACTION: PROBATION; RESTRICTION PLACED ON LICENSE
OFFENSE: SUBSTANDARD CARE, INCOMPETENCE OR NEGLIGENCE

NOTES: FAILURE TO COMPLY WITH GENERALLY ACCEPTED STANDARDS OF MEDICAL PRACTICE. PERMANENT PRACTICE RESTRICTION (NO INTRA-OCULAR SURGERY), AND INDEFINITE PROBATION.

CAMPBELL, DONALD L MD, DATE OF BIRTH MAY 31, 1932, LICENSE NUMBER 15143, WAS DISCIPLINED BY COLORADO ON AUGUST 18, 1999
DISCIPLINARY ACTION: REPRIMAND

CAMPBELL, WILLIAM M DO, DATE OF BIRTH OCTOBER 20, 1940, LICENSE NUMBER 0016123 OF PUEBLO, CO, WAS DISCIPLINED BY COLORADO ON FEBRUARY 15, 1991
DISCIPLINARY ACTION: 36-MONTH PROBATION; REQUIRED TO TAKE ADDITIONAL MEDICAL EDUCATION
OFFENSE: SUBSTANDARD CARE, INCOMPETENCE OR NEGLIGENCE

NOTES: TWO OR MORE ACTS OR OMISSIONS WHICH FAIL TO MEET GENERALLY ACCEPTED STANDARDS OF MEDICAL PRACTICE. CONDITIONS OF PROBATION INCLUDE: OB/GYN PHYSICIAN PRACTICE MONITOR, AND 30 HOURS OF CONTINUING MEDICAL EDUCATION YEARLY. EFFECTIVE 5/20/94 PROBATION DEEMED COMPLETED AND LICENSE RESTORED TO UNRESTRICTED STATUS.

CAPALDO, GEORGE R MD, DATE OF BIRTH FEBRUARY 17, 1956, LICENSE NUMBER 35308, WAS DISCIPLINED BY COLORADO ON AUGUST 18, 1999
DISCIPLINARY ACTION: 3-MONTH LICENSE SUSPENSION; PROBATION
OFFENSE: CRIMINAL CONVICTION OR PLEA OF GUILTY, NOLO CONTENDERE, OR NO CONTEST TO A CRIME

NOTES: FELONY CONVICTION. PROBATION WILL CEASE UPON SUCCESSFUL TERMINATION OF ALL COURT ORDERED PROBATIONARY TERMS RELATED TO THE FELONY.

CAPALDO, GEORGE R MD, LICENSE NUMBER 180881 OF 6020 EAST FIRST AVENUE, DENVER, CO, WAS DISCIPLINED BY NEW YORK ON DECEMBER 27, 1999
DISCIPLINARY ACTION: SURRENDER OF LICENSE
OFFENSE: CRIMINAL CONVICTION OR PLEA OF GUILTY, NOLO CONTENDERE, OR NO CONTEST TO A CRIME

NOTES: CONVICTED IN U.S. DISTRICT COURT IN COLORADO FOR SUBMITTING FALSE CLAIMS TO THE MEDICARE PROGRAM.

CARLSON, STEVE MD OF 1517 CULEBRA PLACE, COLORADO SPRINGS, CO, WAS DISCIPLINED BY DEA ON SEPTEMBER 21, 1998
DISCIPLINARY ACTION: SURRENDER OF CONTROLLED SUBSTANCE LICENSE

CARLSON, STEVEN R MD, DATE OF BIRTH SEPTEMBER 13, 1964, LICENSE NUMBER 33963, WAS DISCIPLINED BY COLORADO ON OCTOBER 15, 1998
DISCIPLINARY ACTION: 60-MONTH PROBATION; MONITORING OF PHYSICIAN PERFORMANCE
OFFENSE: SUBSTANCE ABUSE

NOTES: HABITUAL INTEMPERANCE OR EXCESSIVE USE OF A CONTROLLED SUBSTANCE. PROBATIONARY TERMS INCLUDE: ABSTINENCE FROM ALCOHOL AND CONTROLLED SUBSTANCES, TREATMENT MONITORING AND PRACTICE MONITORING.

CARMEL, STEPHEN P MD, DATE OF BIRTH MAY 18, 1944, LICENSE NUMBER 18095, WAS DISCIPLINED BY COLORADO ON APRIL 17, 1997
DISCIPLINARY ACTION: REPRIMAND; REQUIRED TO TAKE ADDITIONAL MEDICAL EDUCATION
OFFENSE: SUBSTANDARD CARE, INCOMPETENCE OR NEGLIGENCE

NOTES: SUBSTANDARD CARE (PRIMA FACIA TYPE ADMISSION ONLY). MUST ATTEND A PRESCRIBING AND RECORD KEEPING COURSE.

CARR, CLAY B III MD, DATE OF BIRTH APRIL 29, 1961, LICENSE NUMBER 0031843, WAS DISCIPLINED BY COLORADO ON FEBRUARY 16, 1996
DISCIPLINARY ACTION: REPRIMAND

CEDARS, CHESTER M MD, DATE OF BIRTH MARCH 19, 1945, LICENSE NUMBER 16561, WAS DISCIPLINED BY COLORADO ON JUNE 18, 1998
DISCIPLINARY ACTION: 36-MONTH PROBATION; REQUIRED TO TAKE ADDITIONAL MEDICAL EDUCATION
OFFENSE: SUBSTANDARD CARE, INCOMPETENCE OR NEGLIGENCE

NOTES: SUBSTANDARD CARE; FAILURE TO KEEP PROPER RECORDS. PROBATIONARY TERMS INCLUDE: REEDUCATION ACTIVITIES AND PRACTICE MONITORING.

CELIO, ALBERT DO, DATE OF BIRTH MARCH 9, 1952, LICENSE NUMBER 0027758, WAS DISCIPLINED BY COLORADO ON OCTOBER 7, 1996
DISCIPLINARY ACTION: REPRIMAND

CHADO, HERBERT N MD, DATE OF BIRTH JANUARY 1, 1956 OF 30203 TROUTDALE SCENIC DRIVE, EVERGREEN, CO, WAS DISCIPLINED BY DEA ON FEBRUARY 3, 1994
DISCIPLINARY ACTION: RESTRICTION PLACED ON CONTROLLED SUBSTANCE LICENSE
OFFENSE: SUBSTANCE ABUSE

NOTES: ADMIT TO USING CONTROLLED SUBSTANCE FOR NON-MEDICAL PURPOSES DAILY 02/90 TO 02/93.

CHADO, HERBERT N MD, DATE OF BIRTH JANUARY 1, 1956, LICENSE NUMBER 0027381 OF EVERGREEN, CO, WAS DISCIPLINED BY COLORADO ON JUNE 10, 1994
DISCIPLINARY ACTION: 60-MONTH PROBATION; MONITORING OF PHYSICIAN PERFORMANCE
OFFENSE: SUBSTANCE ABUSE

NOTES: HABITUAL INTEMPERANCE OR EXCESSIVE USE OF A CONTROLLED SUBSTANCE. PROBATION UNDER TERMS AND CONDITIONS INCLUDING TREATMENT AND PRACTICE MONITORING.

CHAHAL, KAMLESHWAR S MD, DATE OF BIRTH AUGUST 6, 1950, LICENSE NUMBER 34290, WAS DISCIPLINED BY COLORADO ON OCTOBER 15, 1998
DISCIPLINARY ACTION: 1-MONTH LICENSE SUSPENSION; REPRIMAND

NOTES: DISCIPLINE IN ANOTHER STATE.

CHAMOUN, CHAMOUN D MD, DATE OF BIRTH APRIL 12, 1931, LICENSE NUMBER 16830, WAS DISCIPLINED BY COLORADO ON JUNE 11, 1998
DISCIPLINARY ACTION: REPRIMAND

CHAN, ANTHONY W MD, DATE OF BIRTH OCTOBER 4, 1935, LICENSE NUMBER 0019743 OF WESTMINSTER, CO, WAS DISCIPLINED BY COLORADO ON OCTOBER 16, 1991
DISCIPLINARY ACTION: 24-MONTH PROBATION; REQUIRED TO TAKE ADDITIONAL MEDICAL EDUCATION
OFFENSE: SUBSTANDARD CARE, INCOMPETENCE OR NEGLIGENCE

NOTES: PRACTICE MONITORING, COLORADO PERSONALIZED EDUCATION FOR PHYSICIANS PROGRAM (CPEPP) INVOLVEMENT OR CONTINUING MEDICAL EDUCATION IN LIEU OF CPEPP. EFFECTIVE 2/11/94 PROBATION DEEMED COMPLETED AND LICENSE RESTORED TO UNENCUMBERED STATUS.

CHANG, FRANKLIN M MD, DATE OF BIRTH FEBRUARY 10, 1949, LICENSE NUMBER 0023714, WAS DISCIPLINED BY COLORADO ON OCTOBER 14, 1996
DISCIPLINARY ACTION: REPRIMAND

CHISHOLM, THOMAS N MD, LICENSE NUMBER 0046864 OF AURORA, CO, WAS DISCIPLINED BY FLORIDA ON DECEMBER 13, 1991
DISCIPLINARY ACTION: FINE; REQUIRED TO TAKE ADDITIONAL MEDICAL EDUCATION
OFFENSE: SUBSTANDARD CARE, INCOMPETENCE OR NEGLIGENCE

NOTES: CHARGED WITH FAILURE TO PRACTICE MEDICINE WITH AN ACCEPTABLE LEVEL OF CARE AND SKILL; FAILURE TO KEEP MEDICAL RECORDS JUSTIFYING THE COURSE OF TREATMENT OF A PATIENT. $3,000 FINE; LETTER OF CONCERN; 20 HOURS CONTINUING MEDICAL EDUCATION COURSES WITHIN ONE YEAR IN EMERGENCY TREATMENT OF EYE INJURIES.

CHISHOLM, THOMAS N MD, LICENSE NUMBER 0046864 OF AURORA, CO, WAS DISCIPLINED BY FLORIDA ON FEBRUARY 25, 1993
DISCIPLINARY ACTION: FINE
OFFENSE: FAILURE TO COMPLY WITH PREVIOUS BOARD ORDER

NOTES: FAILING TO PAY FINE. MUST PAY $500 FINE.

CHOW, FRANKLIN S MD, DATE OF BIRTH APRIL 15, 1956, LICENSE NUMBER 25189, WAS DISCIPLINED BY COLORADO ON MAY 15, 1998
DISCIPLINARY ACTION: 60-MONTH PROBATION; REQUIRED TO TAKE ADDITIONAL MEDICAL EDUCATION
OFFENSE: PROFESSIONAL MISCONDUCT

NOTES: UNPROFESSIONAL CONDUCT. PROBATIONARY TERMS INCLUDE: PRACTICE MONITORING AND A COLORADO PERSONALIZED EDUCATION FOR PHYSICIAN'S EVALUATION AND LEARNING PLAN.

CHOW, FRANKLIN SZU-CHEN MD, LICENSE NUMBER 145123 OF PO BOX 5657, VAIL, CO, WAS DISCIPLINED BY NEW YORK ON JUNE 8, 1999
DISCIPLINARY ACTION: 60-MONTH PROBATION

OFFENSE: DISCIPLINARY ACTION BY ANOTHER STATE OR AGENCY

NOTES: DISCIPLINED BY THE COLORADO BOARD FOR FAILING TO MEET THE ACCEPTED STANDARDS OF PRACTICE. PROBATION TO RUN CONCURRENTLY WITH TERMS IMPOSED BY COLORADO.

CIANFLONE, ALEXANDER G MD, DATE OF BIRTH JULY 14, 1953, LICENSE NUMBER 0022675, WAS DISCIPLINED BY COLORADO ON APRIL 11, 1996
DISCIPLINARY ACTION: REPRIMAND

CIBULL, MURIEL R MD, DATE OF BIRTH MAY 3, 1930, LICENSE NUMBER 0012483 OF DENVER, CO, WAS DISCIPLINED BY COLORADO ON JUNE 19, 1994
DISCIPLINARY ACTION: REPRIMAND
OFFENSE: PROFESSIONAL MISCONDUCT

CIEMIEGA, GERALD J DO, DATE OF BIRTH APRIL 7, 1951, LICENSE NUMBER 0023556 OF VALRICO, FL, WAS DISCIPLINED BY COLORADO ON JANUARY 31, 1994
DISCIPLINARY ACTION: REPRIMAND
OFFENSE: PROFESSIONAL MISCONDUCT

CIENKI, JOHN J MD, DATE OF BIRTH SEPTEMBER 24, 1959, LICENSE NUMBER 0012956 OF JACKSON, MS, WAS DISCIPLINED BY MISSISSIPPI ON AUGUST 13, 1991
DISCIPLINARY ACTION: MONITORING OF PHYSICIAN PERFORMANCE
OFFENSE: SUBSTANCE ABUSE

NOTES: HAS ADMITTED A CHEMICAL DEPENDENCY PROBLEM BUT HAS RECEIVED TREATMENT AND HAS MAINTAINED AT LEAST TWO YEARS OF SOBRIETY. LICENSED UNDER THE FOLLOWING CONDITIONS: SHALL SUBMIT TO RANDOM URINE AND BLOOD SCREENS FOR AT LEAST TWO YEARS; SHALL NOT ADMINISTER, DISPENSE OR PRESCRIBE TO HIMSELF ANY DRUGS HAVING ADDICTION-FORMING OR ADDICTION-SUSTAINING PROPERTIES; SHALL OBTAIN THE SERVICES OF A BOARD-APPROVED PRIMARY CARE PHYSICIAN TO TREAT HIMSELF AND HIS FAMILY; CAN PETITION FOR MODIFICATION IN ONE YEAR.

CIENKI, JOHN J MD, DATE OF BIRTH SEPTEMBER 24, 1959, LICENSE NUMBER 0012956 OF 288 CUMBERLAND STREET, APT 301, HARRISBURG, PA, WAS DISCIPLINED BY MISSISSIPPI ON SEPTEMBER 21, 1995
DISCIPLINARY ACTION: SURRENDER OF LICENSE

NOTES: VOLUNTARILY AND UNCONDITIONALLY SURRENDERED HIS LICENSE TO AVOID A DISCIPLINARY HEARING BEFORE THE BOARD.

CIENKI, JOHN J MD, DATE OF BIRTH SEPTEMBER 24, 1959, LICENSE NUMBER 0033340, WAS DISCIPLINED BY COLORADO ON OCTOBER 11, 1995
DISCIPLINARY ACTION: 60-MONTH PROBATION; MONITORING OF PHYSICIAN PERFORMANCE

NOTES: TREATMENT AND PRACTICE MONITORING.

CIENKI, JOHN J MD, DATE OF BIRTH SEPTEMBER 24, 1959, LICENSE NUMBER 041445E OF 1025 SHORE LANE, MIAMI BEACH, FL, WAS DISCIPLINED BY PENNSYLVANIA ON JULY 3, 1997
DISCIPLINARY ACTION: 60-MONTH PROBATION
OFFENSE: DISCIPLINARY ACTION BY ANOTHER STATE OR AGENCY

NOTES: DISCIPLINARY ACTION TAKEN BY COLORADO AND MISSISSIPPI; CONVICTION OF A MISDEMEANOR RELATING TO THE HEALTH PROFESSION AND MAKING FALSE OR DECEPTIVE BIENNIAL RENEWAL APPLICATION. LICENSE TO BE PLACED ON PROBATION UPON HIS RETURN TO PENNSYLVANIA.

CIENKI, JOHN J MD OF CO, WAS DISCIPLINED BY DEA ON OCTOBER 30, 1998
DISCIPLINARY ACTION: RESTRICTION PLACED ON CONTROLLED SUBSTANCE LICENSE; MONITORING OF PHYSICIAN PERFORMANCE
OFFENSE: PROVIDING FALSE INFORMATION TO THE BOARD OR OTHER HEALTH AGENCY

NOTES: IN THE MID-1980S HE BEGAN ABUSING CONTROLLED SUBSTANCES INCLUDING DEMEROL AND TALWIN; BY 1988 HIS DRUG USE ESCALATED TO A POINT WHERE HE SOUGHT AND RECEIVED 28 DAYS OF INPATIENT TREATMENT FOR HIS ADDICTION THEN SIGNED UP WITH A PHYSICIAN'S RECOVERY NETWORK TO MONITOR HIM FOR FIVE YEARS; IN 1991 HE APPLIED FOR LICENSURE IN MISSISSIPPI ADMITTING HIS DRUG ABUSE; AGREED TO A NON-DISCIPLINARY CONSENT ORDER INCLUDING MONITORING; ON 10/1/93 AND 1/12/95 HE SUBMITTED RENEWAL REGISTRATIONS TO DEA AND ANSWERED NO TO THE QUESTION OF WHETHER HIS LICENSE HAD BEEN SANCTIONED BELIEVING HE DID NOT HAVE TO REPORT THE NON-DISCIPLINARY ACTION; DEA FOUND HE SHOULD HAVE KNOWN TO REPORT IT SINCE IT AFFECTED HIS PRESCRIBING OF CONTROLLED SUBSTANCES; FROM 6/94-3/95 HE RELAPSED ON STADOL AND OBTAINED IT FOR HIS OWN USE BY WRITING FALSE PRESCRIPTIONS AND BY FRAUDULENTLY TELEPHONING PRESCRIPTIONS TO LOCAL PHARMACIES; IN 6/95 PLED GUILTY TO THE MISDEMEANOR CHARGE OF FRAUD AND DECEIT TO OBTAIN A PRESCRIPTION DRUG; COLORADO LICENSE WAS PLACED ON PROBATION AND HE ULTIMATELY DID NOT RENEW IT; SURRENDERED HIS MISSISSIPPI LICENSE ON 9/18/95 AND PENNSYLVANIA LICENSE PLACED ON PROBATION ON 8/23/95; ON 5/18/96 ENTERED INTO A CONTRACT WITH FLORIDA PHYSICIAN'S RECOVERY NETWORK AND ON 6/30/97 FLORIDA SUSPENDED HIS LICENSE; ON 9/24/96 HE ANSWERED YES TO WHETHER DISCIPLINARY ACTION HAD BEEN TAKEN ON ANOTHER DEA RENEWAL REQUEST. DEA RENEWAL APPLICATION GRANTED UNDER THE FOLLOWING CONDITIONS FOR THREE YEARS: SHALL NOT PRESCRIBE OR OTHERWISE DISPENSE CONTROLLED SUBSTANCES OR STADOL FOR HIMSELF OR IMMEDIATE FAMILY MEMBERS; SHALL NOT ORDER, ADMINISTER, PRESCRIBE OR OTHERWISE DISPENSE CONTROLLED SUBSTANCES OR STADOL EXCEPT IN THE COURSE OF HIS EMPLOYMENT IN A MEDICAL CLINIC OR HOSPITAL; SHALL MAINTAIN A LOG OF HANDLING OF CONTROLLED SUBSTANCES AND STADOL WHICH SHALL BE AVAILABLE TO BE SENT TO THE DEA QUARTERLY; SHALL INFORM DEA OF ANY STATE ACTIONS AGAINST HIS LICENSE.

CLAPP, HARRY W DO, DATE OF BIRTH AUGUST 21, 1918, LICENSE NUMBER 11280, WAS DISCIPLINED BY COLORADO ON JANUARY 16, 1997
OFFENSE: NONCOMPLIANCE WITH A PROFESSIONAL RULE

NOTES: VIOLATION OF THE MEDICAL PRACTICE ACT. HE AGREES NEVER TO ACTIVATE HIS LAPSED LICENSE.

CLINE, FOSTER W JR MD, DATE OF BIRTH JUNE 1, 1940, LICENSE NUMBER 0017080, WAS DISCIPLINED BY COLORADO ON SEPTEMBER 27, 1995
DISCIPLINARY ACTION: RESTRICTION PLACED ON LICENSE; REPRIMAND

NOTES: RESTRICTED FROM TREATING OR PARTICIPATING IN

THE TREATMENT OF PATIENTS WHICH INCLUDES THERAPY THAT USES AVERSE PHYSICAL STIMULATION OR VERBAL ABUSE.

CLISE, RICHARD K MD, DATE OF BIRTH OCTOBER 6, 1957, LICENSE NUMBER 0034152 OF FT. MORGAN, CO, WAS DISCIPLINED BY COLORADO ON NOVEMBER 18, 1994
DISCIPLINARY ACTION: 12-MONTH PROBATION; MONITORING OF PHYSICIAN PERFORMANCE
OFFENSE: SUBSTANCE ABUSE

NOTES: HABITUAL INTEMPERANCE OR EXCESSIVE USE OF ANY HABIT-FORMING DRUG OR CONTROLLED SUBSTANCE. GRANTED LICENSE. PROBATIONARY PERIOD INCLUDES ONE YEAR OF TREATMENT MONITORING. PROBATION TERMINATED ON 12/14/95 AND LICENSE RESTORED TO AN UNENCUMBERED AND UNRESTRICTED STATUS.

CLISE, RICHARD KEIT MD, LICENSE NUMBER 1406783, WAS DISCIPLINED BY MICHIGAN ON JULY 18, 1990
DISCIPLINARY ACTION: PROBATION

COBB, DAVID K MD, DATE OF BIRTH MAY 28, 1926, LICENSE NUMBER 32544, WAS DISCIPLINED BY COLORADO ON FEBRUARY 17, 1999
DISCIPLINARY ACTION: 60-MONTH PROBATION; MONITORING OF PHYSICIAN PERFORMANCE
OFFENSE: SUBSTANCE ABUSE

NOTES: HABITUAL INTEMPERANCE OR EXCESSIVE USE OF A CONTROLLED SUBSTANCE. PROBATIONARY TERMS INCLUDE: ABSTINENCE FROM ALCOHOL AND CONTROLLED SUBSTANCES, TREATMENT MONITORING AND PRACTICE MONITORING.

COHEN, ELLIOT S MD, DATE OF BIRTH AUGUST 26, 1942, LICENSE NUMBER 22617, WAS DISCIPLINED BY COLORADO ON JUNE 18, 1998
DISCIPLINARY ACTION: REPRIMAND; REQUIRED TO TAKE ADDITIONAL MEDICAL EDUCATION
OFFENSE: SUBSTANDARD CARE, INCOMPETENCE OR NEGLIGENCE

NOTES: SUBSTANDARD CARE; FAILURE TO KEEP PROPER RECORDS. HE AGREES TO REEDUCATION ACTIVITIES.

COLE, DON H MD, DATE OF BIRTH MARCH 27, 1929, LICENSE NUMBER 0012755 OF PUEBLO, CO, WAS DISCIPLINED BY COLORADO ON JANUARY 31, 1992
DISCIPLINARY ACTION: EMERGENCY SUSPENSION
OFFENSE: SUBSTANDARD CARE, INCOMPETENCE OR NEGLIGENCE

NOTES: PRESCRIBING CONTROLLED SUBSTANCES OTHER THAN IN THE COURSE OF LEGITIMATE MEDICAL PRACTICE AND IN VIOLATION OF BOARD'S "STIMULANT RULE"; GROSSLY NEGLIGENT OR SUBSTANDARD MEDICAL PRACTICE; FALSIFICATION AND REPEATED FAILURE TO MAKE ESSENTIAL ENTRIES IN PATIENT RECORDS.

COLE, DON H MD, DATE OF BIRTH MARCH 27, 1929 OF 3715 CARLILE AVE, PUEBLO, CO, WAS DISCIPLINED BY DEA ON AUGUST 7, 1992
DISCIPLINARY ACTION: REVOCATION OF CONTROLLED SUBSTANCE LICENSE
OFFENSE: DISCIPLINARY ACTION BY ANOTHER STATE OR AGENCY

NOTES: ON 01/29/92, COLORADO SUSPENDED HIS MEDICAL LICENSE, THEREBY TERMINATING HIS AUTHORITY TO PRESCRIBE, DISPENSE, ADMINISTER OR OTHERWISE HANDLE CONTROLLED SUBSTANCES.

COLE, DON H MD, DATE OF BIRTH MARCH 27, 1929, LICENSE NUMBER 0012755 OF PUEBLO, CO, WAS DISCIPLINED BY COLORADO ON MARCH 12, 1993
DISCIPLINARY ACTION: LICENSE REVOCATION
OFFENSE: SUBSTANDARD CARE, INCOMPETENCE OR NEGLIGENCE

NOTES: SUBSTANDARD CARE; PRESCRIBING CONTROLLED SUBSTANCES OTHER THAN IN THE COURSE OF LEGITIMATE PROFESSIONAL PRACTICE.

COLESCOTT, PAULA J MD, DATE OF BIRTH NOVEMBER 5, 1949, LICENSE NUMBER 0020693, WAS DISCIPLINED BY COLORADO ON OCTOBER 11, 1995
DISCIPLINARY ACTION: SURRENDER OF LICENSE

NOTES: PERMANENT SURRENDER.

COLLINS, THOMAS J MD, DATE OF BIRTH APRIL 19, 1952, LICENSE NUMBER 0024911, WAS DISCIPLINED BY COLORADO ON APRIL 11, 1996
DISCIPLINARY ACTION: 3-MONTH LICENSE SUSPENSION; 60-MONTH PROBATION
OFFENSE: SEXUAL ABUSE OF OR SEXUAL MISCONDUCT WITH A PATIENT

NOTES: SEXUAL CONTACT WITH A PATIENT. TREATMENT MONITORING AND AN AGREEMENT TO HAVE A CHAPERONE PRESENT FOR ALL FEMALE PATIENTS.

COLON-CHANLATTE, IRIS MD, DATE OF BIRTH SEPTEMBER 23, 1961, LICENSE NUMBER 0030814, WAS DISCIPLINED BY COLORADO ON FEBRUARY 16, 1996
DISCIPLINARY ACTION: REQUIRED TO TAKE ADDITIONAL MEDICAL EDUCATION; MONITORING OF PHYSICIAN PERFORMANCE
OFFENSE: SUBSTANDARD CARE, INCOMPETENCE OR NEGLIGENCE

NOTES: SUBSTANDARD CARE (PRIMA FACIE TYPE ADMISSION ONLY). PRACTICE MONITORING AND RE-EDUCATION UPON HER RETURN TO PRACTICE. ALSO KNOWN AS IRIS MARRERO.

CONNELLY, JOHN MICHAEL MD, DATE OF BIRTH JULY 12, 1928, LICENSE NUMBER 0019316 OF 8348 EAST JAMISON CIRCLE SOUTH, ENGLEWOOD, CO, WAS DISCIPLINED BY NEW JERSEY ON NOVEMBER 22, 1995
DISCIPLINARY ACTION: LICENSE SUSPENSION
OFFENSE: DISCIPLINARY ACTION BY ANOTHER STATE OR AGENCY

NOTES: MAY REAPPLY FOR REINSTATEMENT UPON SUBMISSION OF PROOF THAT HE HAS COMPLIED WITH THE TERMS OF THE COLORADO ORDER AND HIS LICENSE HAS BEEN RESTORED BY COLORADO.

CONNELLY, JOSEPH W DO, DATE OF BIRTH OCTOBER 7, 1919, LICENSE NUMBER 0011482 OF DENVER, CO, WAS DISCIPLINED BY COLORADO ON APRIL 14, 1994
DISCIPLINARY ACTION: REPRIMAND
OFFENSE: SUBSTANDARD CARE, INCOMPETENCE OR NEGLIGENCE

NOTES: FAILED TO MEET STANDARDS OF PRACTICE IN A PATIENT FOR WHOM HIS PRENATAL CARE WAS NOT ADEQUATE, INCLUDING THE LACK OF FETAL MONITORING, AND HIS CHOICE TO UNDERTAKE MID-FORCEPS DELIVERY REPRESENTED BAD JUDGMENT.

CONNOLLY, JOHN M MD, DATE OF BIRTH JULY 12, 1928, LICENSE NUMBER 0021514 OF ENGLEWOOD, CO, WAS DISCIPLINED BY COLORADO ON JUNE 12, 1992
DISCIPLINARY ACTION: LICENSE SUSPENSION
OFFENSE: FAILURE TO COMPLY WITH PREVIOUS BOARD ORDER

NOTES: FAILED TO COMPLY WITH AN ORDER OF THE BOARD TO SUBMIT TO A MEDICAL EVALUATION.

CONNOLLY, JOHN M MD, LICENSE NUMBER 0078168 OF 8348 EAST JAMISON CIRCLE SOUTH, ENGLEWOOD, CO, WAS DISCIPLINED BY NEW YORK ON JULY 21, 1994
DISCIPLINARY ACTION: LICENSE REVOCATION
OFFENSE: DISCIPLINARY ACTION BY ANOTHER STATE OR AGENCY

NOTES: DISCIPLINED BY COLORADO BOARD.

COPELAN, RUSSELL I MD, DATE OF BIRTH DECEMBER 30, 1947, LICENSE NUMBER 24453, WAS DISCIPLINED BY COLORADO ON JUNE 18, 1998
DISCIPLINARY ACTION: 2-MONTH LICENSE SUSPENSION; 58-MONTH PROBATION
OFFENSE: SEXUAL ABUSE OF OR SEXUAL MISCONDUCT WITH A PATIENT

NOTES: SEXUAL CONTACT WITH A PATIENT. TERMS OF ORDER INCLUDE: A BOUNDARIES COURSE, REEDUCATION ACTIVITIES AND PRACTICE MONITORING.

CORMIA, FRANK E JR MD, WAS DISCIPLINED BY ALASKA ON JULY 11, 1997
DISCIPLINARY ACTION: DENIAL OF NEW LICENSE
OFFENSE: DISCIPLINARY ACTION BY ANOTHER STATE OR AGENCY

NOTES: SUSPENSION OF LICENSE IN TEXAS.

CORMIA, FRANK EDWARD JR MD, LICENSE NUMBER 00E3885, WAS DISCIPLINED BY TEXAS ON AUGUST 17, 1996
DISCIPLINARY ACTION: 60-MONTH PROBATION; REQUIRED TO TAKE ADDITIONAL MEDICAL EDUCATION
OFFENSE: SUBSTANDARD CARE, INCOMPETENCE OR NEGLIGENCE

NOTES: IN 4/91 FAILED TO ADEQUATELY TREAT A PATIENT IN REGARD TO THIS PATIENT'S DIABETES MANAGEMENT; AND THE MEDICAL RECORDS FAILED TO ADEQUATELY DOCUMENT THE PATIENT'S CARE, TREATMENT, AND RECOMMENDATIONS. SUSPENSION, STAYED AS PROBATION WITH TERMS AND CONDITIONS; WITHIN SIX MONTHS SHALL TAKE AND PASS THE SPEX EXAMINATION AND THE MEDICAL JURISPRUDENCE EXAMINATION; SHALL OBTAIN AT LEAST 50 HOURS PER YEAR OF CONTINUING MEDICAL EDUCATION INCLUDING AT LEAST ONE COURSE IN RISK MANAGEMENT AND THE REMAINING HOURS IN FAMILY PRACTICE; SHALL MAINTAIN ADEQUATE MEDICAL RECORDS WHICH SHALL BE AVAILABLE FOR REVIEW; HIS MEDICAL PRACTICE, INCLUDING ANY OFFICE AND SURGICAL PRACTICE, SHALL BE MONITORED BY A BOARD APPROVED TEXAS PHYSICIAN WHO SHALL PROVIDE QUARTERLY REPORTS TO THE BOARD; WITHIN ONE YEAR SHALL TAKE AN ADVANCED CARDIAC LIFE SUPPORT COURSE AND AN ADVANCED TRAUMA LIFE SUPPORT COURSE AND OBTAIN CERTIFICATION OF BOTH; SHALL COOPERATE WITH THE BOARD IN VERIFYING COMPLIANCE; SHALL APPEAR BEFORE THE BOARD AT LEAST TWICE A YEAR; SHALL GIVE A COPY OF THIS ORDER TO ANY HEALTH CARE ENTITY WHERE HE HAS PRIVILEGES; SHALL PROVIDE A COPY OF THIS ORDER TO ANYONE REQUESTING IT WITHIN 10 DAYS; TIME PERIOD OUT OF TEXAS DOES NOT COUNT TOWARD PROBATION; SHALL INFORM THE BOARD OF CHANGE OF ADDRESS WITHIN 10 DAYS OF IF HE LEAVES THE STATE; SHALL NOT SEEK MODIFICATION FOR ONE YEAR.

CORMIA, FRANK EDWARD JR MD, LICENSE NUMBER E3885 OF FORT COLLINS, CO, WAS DISCIPLINED BY TEXAS ON MAY 16, 1998
DISCIPLINARY ACTION: 54-MONTH PROBATION; REQUIRED TO TAKE ADDITIONAL MEDICAL EDUCATION

NOTES: FAILED TO TAKE AND PASS SPEX, AND MEDICAL JURISPRUDENCE EXAM BY 2/17/97, IN VIOLATION OF 8/17/96 ORDER; LICENSE WAS SUSPENDED; ON 10/27/97 HE PASSED THE SPEX WITH A SCORE OF 80. SUSPENSION STAYED FOR PROBATION WITH FOLLOWING TERMS AND CONDITIONS: SHALL OBTAIN 50 HOURS PER YEAR OF CONTINUING MEDICAL EDUCATION WITH AT LEAST ONE COURSE IN RISK MANAGEMENT; SHALL MAINTAIN ADEQUATE MEDICAL RECORDS WHICH SHALL BE AVAILABLE FOR REVIEW; HIS MEDICAL PRACTICE SHALL BE MONITORED BY A BOARD APPROVED TEXAS PHYSICIAN WHO SHALL PROVIDE QUARTERLY REPORTS TO THE BOARD; WITHIN ONE YEAR SHALL TAKE AND SUCCESSFULLY COMPLETE AN ADVANCED CARDIAC LIFE SUPPORT COURSE AND AN ADVANCED TRAUMA LIFE SUPPORT COURSE AND OBTAIN CERTIFICATION; SHALL COOPERATE WITH THE BOARD IN VERIFYING COMPLIANCE; SHALL APPEAR BEFORE THE BOARD TWICE A YEAR; SHALL GIVE A COPY OF THIS ORDER TO ANY HEALTH CARE ENTITY WHERE HE HAS PRIVILEGES; SHALL PROVIDE A COPY OF THIS ORDER TO ANYONE REQUESTING IT WITHIN 10 DAYS; TIME SPENT OUT OF TEXAS DOES NOT COUNT TOWARD PROBATION; SHALL INFORM THE BOARD OF CHANGE OF ADDRESS WITHIN 10 DAYS OR IF HE LEAVES THE STATE; SHALL NOT SEEK MODIFICATION FOR ONE YEAR.

CORTELYOU, MARIE MD, DATE OF BIRTH AUGUST 10, 1935, LICENSE NUMBER 0028069, WAS DISCIPLINED BY COLORADO ON MARCH 21, 1996
DISCIPLINARY ACTION: REQUIRED TO TAKE ADDITIONAL MEDICAL EDUCATION; MONITORING OF PHYSICIAN PERFORMANCE
OFFENSE: SUBSTANDARD CARE, INCOMPETENCE OR NEGLIGENCE

NOTES: SUBSTANDARD CARE AND FAILURE TO MAKE ESSENTIAL CHART ENTRIES. RE-EDUCATION ACTIVITIES, SUPERVISION OF EMERGENCY ROOM PRACTICE, AND PRACTICE MONITORING.

CORTELYOU, MARIE MD, LICENSE NUMBER 0087877 OF 5335 CAMBRIA DRIVE, COLORADO SPRINGS, CO, WAS DISCIPLINED BY NEW YORK ON OCTOBER 7, 1996
DISCIPLINARY ACTION: LICENSE REVOCATION
OFFENSE: DISCIPLINARY ACTION BY ANOTHER STATE OR AGENCY

NOTES: DISCIPLINED BY COLORADO BOARD FOR INCOMPETENCE ON MORE THAN ONE OCCASION AND FAILING TO MAINTAIN ACCURATE PATIENT RECORDS.

CORTELYOU, MARIE MD, DATE OF BIRTH AUGUST 10, 1935, LICENSE NUMBER 28069, WAS DISCIPLINED BY COLORADO ON SEPTEMBER 28, 1998
DISCIPLINARY ACTION: LICENSE SUSPENSION
OFFENSE: FAILURE TO COMPLY WITH PREVIOUS BOARD ORDER

NOTES: FAILURE TO COMPLY WITH A LAWFUL ORDER OF THE BOARD.

COSBY, ROBERT L MD, DATE OF BIRTH SEPTEMBER 10, 1954, LICENSE NUMBER 0027190 OF PHOENIX, AZ, WAS DISCIPLINED BY COLORADO ON JUNE 19, 1992
DISCIPLINARY ACTION: SURRENDER OF LICENSE
OFFENSE: PROFESSIONAL MISCONDUCT

NOTES: PATIENT ABANDONMENT.

COTTMAN, GORDON W MD, DATE OF BIRTH JANUARY 17, 1959, LICENSE NUMBER 0028427 OF KITTREDGE, CO, WAS DISCIPLINED BY COLORADO ON MAY 11, 1994
DISCIPLINARY ACTION: REPRIMAND
OFFENSE: PROFESSIONAL MISCONDUCT

COTTON, RALPH L MD, DATE OF BIRTH DECEMBER 6, 1928, LICENSE NUMBER 0012750, WAS DISCIPLINED BY COLORADO ON SEPTEMBER 14, 1995
DISCIPLINARY ACTION: REPRIMAND

COULTER, ROBERT L MD, DATE OF BIRTH APRIL 29, 1924, LICENSE NUMBER 0013899, WAS DISCIPLINED BY COLORADO ON SEPTEMBER 19, 1996
DISCIPLINARY ACTION: RESTRICTION PLACED ON LICENSE; MONITORING OF PHYSICIAN PERFORMANCE
OFFENSE: SUBSTANDARD CARE, INCOMPETENCE OR NEGLIGENCE

NOTES: SUBSTANDARD CARE. RESTRICTED TO THE DIAGNOSTIC CENTER FOR MEN; PRACTICE MONITORING.

CRANDALL, JACK S MD, LICENSE NUMBER 0014410 OF ASPEN, CO, WAS DISCIPLINED BY COLORADO ON MAY 10, 1991
DISCIPLINARY ACTION: RESTRICTION PLACED ON CONTROLLED SUBSTANCE LICENSE

NOTES: MUST NOT ADMINISTER, DISPENSE OR PRESCRIBE ANY HABIT FORMING DRUGS OR CONTROLLED SUBSTANCES WITHOUT RECEIVING APPROVAL OF THE BOARD.

CRAVEN, E RANDY MD, DATE OF BIRTH SEPTEMBER 14, 1956, LICENSE NUMBER 26080, WAS DISCIPLINED BY COLORADO ON NOVEMBER 17, 1999
DISCIPLINARY ACTION: REPRIMAND

CUPPS, JERRY LEE DO, DATE OF BIRTH MARCH 11, 1941, LICENSE NUMBER 0016337 OF COMMERCE CITY, CO, WAS DISCIPLINED BY COLORADO ON SEPTEMBER 11, 1992
DISCIPLINARY ACTION: 36-MONTH PROBATION; REQUIRED TO TAKE ADDITIONAL MEDICAL EDUCATION
OFFENSE: SUBSTANDARD CARE, INCOMPETENCE OR NEGLIGENCE

NOTES: TWO OR MORE ACTS OR OMISSIONS WHICH FAILED TO MEET GENERALLY ACCEPTED STANDARDS OF MEDICAL PRACTICE. PROBATIONARY PERIOD INCLUDES PRACTICE MONITORING AND COMPLETION OF AN INDIVIDUAL EDUCATION PLAN. SECOND STIPULATION/ORDER FOR ADDITIONAL EDUCATION REQUIREMENT COMPLETION WITHIN 3 MONTHS OF ORDER'S EFFECTIVE DATE.

CUPPS, JERRY LEE DO, DATE OF BIRTH MARCH 11, 1941, LICENSE NUMBER 0016337 OF COMMERCE CITY, CO, WAS DISCIPLINED BY COLORADO ON FEBRUARY 18, 1993
DISCIPLINARY ACTION: 4-MONTH LICENSE SUSPENSION
OFFENSE: FAILURE TO COMPLY WITH PREVIOUS BOARD ORDER

NOTES: FAILURE TO COMPLY WITH VALID BOARD ORDER, SPECIFICALLY, AN EARLIER STIPULATION. LICENSE SUSPENDED UNTIL JUNE 11, 1993 WHEN HE COMPLETED RETRAINING ACTIVITIES.

CURTIS, KENNETH W JR MD, DATE OF BIRTH MAY 8, 1934, LICENSE NUMBER 0024455 OF 939 LOCKNESS COURT, FORT COLLINS, CO, WAS DISCIPLINED BY COLORADO ON NOVEMBER 3, 1994
DISCIPLINARY ACTION: 60-MONTH PROBATION; MONITORING OF PHYSICIAN PERFORMANCE
OFFENSE: SUBSTANCE ABUSE

NOTES: ADMITS THAT HE HAS SUFFERED FROM ALCOHOL DEPENDENCE FOR WHICH HE HAS RECEIVED ONGOING SUCCESSFUL TREATMENT; NO COMPLAINT RECEIVED REGARDING THE QUALITY OF PATIENT CARE. CONDITIONS OF PROBATION: SHALL TOTALLY ABSTAIN FROM THE USE OF ALCOHOL OR HABIT FORMING DRUG OR CONTROLLED SUBSTANCE UNLESS PRESCRIBED BY ANOTHER PERSON; SHALL RECEIVE MEDICAL TREATMENT FROM THE COLORADO PHYSICIAN HEALTH PROGRAM INCLUDING RANDOM URINE SCREENING; THEY SHALL PROVIDE QUARTERLY REPORTS TO THE BOARD; PRACTICE SHALL BE MONITORED BY A BOARD APPROVED PHYSICIAN FOR AT LEAST 18 MONTHS WHO SHALL REVIEW CHARTS MONTHLY AND SUBMIT QUARTERLY REPORTS TO THE BOARD.

CURTIS, KENNETH W JR MD, DATE OF BIRTH MAY 8, 1934, LICENSE NUMBER 0024455, WAS DISCIPLINED BY COLORADO ON MAY 4, 1995
DISCIPLINARY ACTION: EMERGENCY SUSPENSION
OFFENSE: FAILURE TO COMPLY WITH PREVIOUS BOARD ORDER

NOTES: DUE TO NONCOMPLIANCE WITH ORDER OF 11/3/94 WHEN HE AGREED NOT TO USE ALCOHOL OR CONTROLLED SUBSTANCES. THREE TESTS DONE ON HIS URINE IN 12/94 WERE POSITIVE FOR ALCOHOL OR MORPHINE WHICH HE SAID CAME FROM THE INGESTION OF POPPY SEEDS, NEAR BEERS AND/OR MOUTHWASH; A TEST ON HIS URINE IN 4/95 WAS POSITIVE FOR ALCOHOL WHICH HE ADMITTED TO CONSUMING; PLACED ON INVOLUNTARY HOLD IN A TREATMENT FACILITY ON 5/3/95.

CURTIS, KENNETH W JR MD, DATE OF BIRTH MAY 8, 1934, LICENSE NUMBER 0024455, WAS DISCIPLINED BY COLORADO ON NOVEMBER 9, 1995
DISCIPLINARY ACTION: 60-MONTH PROBATION; MONITORING OF PHYSICIAN PERFORMANCE

NOTES: CONDITIONS OF PROBATION: SHALL ABSTAIN FROM THE USE OF ALCOHOL OR ANY HABIT FORMING DRUG OR CONTROLLED SUBSTANCE UNLESS PRESCRIBED BY ANOTHER PERSON AND WITH APPROVAL OF HIS TREATMENT MONITOR; SHALL RECEIVE MEDICAL TREATMENT FROM THE COLORADO PHYSICIAN HEALTH PROGRAM INCLUDING RANDOM URINE SCREENING; THEY SHALL SUBMIT QUARTERLY REPORTS TO THE BOARD; PRACTICE SHALL BE MONITORED BY A BOARD APPROVED PHYSICIAN FOR AT LEAST 18 MONTHS WHO SHALL REVIEW CHARTS MONTHLY AND SUBMIT QUARTERLY REPORTS TO THE BOARD; TIME SPENT OUT OF COLORADO DOES NOT COUNT TOWARD PROBATION.

CURTIS, KENNETH W MD, DATE OF BIRTH MAY 8, 1934, LICENSE NUMBER 24455, WAS DISCIPLINED BY COLORADO ON MAY 14, 1997
DISCIPLINARY ACTION: LICENSE REVOCATION
OFFENSE: FAILURE TO COMPLY WITH PREVIOUS BOARD ORDER

NOTES: FAILURE TO ABIDE BY A PROBATIONARY AGREEMENT.

CUSTODIO, JOSEPH M MD, DATE OF BIRTH OCTOBER 16, 1952, LICENSE NUMBER 0029497 OF VERO BEACH, FL, WAS DISCIPLINED BY COLORADO ON DECEMBER 16, 1994
DISCIPLINARY ACTION: LICENSE REVOCATION
OFFENSE: CRIMINAL CONVICTION OR PLEA OF GUILTY, NOLO CONTENDERE, OR NO CONTEST TO A CRIME

NOTES: FELONY CONVICTION AND FALSIFIED OR REPEATEDLY INCORRECT ESSENTIAL ENTRIES ON PATIENT CHARTS. THIS CASE WAS ON APPEAL TO THE COLORADO COURT OF APPEALS AS OF 6/95 NEWSLETTER.

CUSTODIO, JOSEPH M MD, LICENSE NUMBER 0051502 OF VERO BEACH, FL, WAS DISCIPLINED BY FLORIDA ON APRIL 30, 1996
DISCIPLINARY ACTION: LICENSE REVOCATION
OFFENSE: DISCIPLINARY ACTION BY ANOTHER STATE OR AGENCY

NOTES: BEING FOUND GUILTY OF A CRIME DIRECTLY RELATED

TO THE PRACTICE OF MEDICINE.

CUSTODIO, JOSEPH M MD, DATE OF BIRTH OCTOBER 16, 1952 OF 2708 CARDINAL DRIVE, VERO BEACH, FL, WAS DISCIPLINED BY MEDICARE ON AUGUST 20, 1998
DISCIPLINARY ACTION: EXCLUSION FROM THE MEDICARE AND/OR MEDICAID PROGRAM
OFFENSE: DISCIPLINARY ACTION BY ANOTHER STATE OR AGENCY
NOTES: LICENSE REVOKED, SUSPENDED, SURRENDERED OR OTHERWISE LOST FOR REASONS BEARING ON PROFESSIONAL PERFORMANCE, PROFESSIONAL COMPETENCE OR FINANCIAL INTEGRITY.

CUSTODIO, JOSEPH MANUEL MD, DATE OF BIRTH OCTOBER 16, 1952, LICENSE NUMBER 028959 OF 2708 CARDINAL DRIVE, VERO BEACH, FL, WAS DISCIPLINED BY GEORGIA ON AUGUST 7, 1997
DISCIPLINARY ACTION: LICENSE REVOCATION
OFFENSE: DISCIPLINARY ACTION BY ANOTHER STATE OR AGENCY
NOTES: DISCIPLINARY ACTION IN COLORADO.

DAHLBERG, WILLIAM W MD, DATE OF BIRTH JUNE 17, 1939, LICENSE NUMBER 0016572 OF DENVER, CO, WAS DISCIPLINED BY COLORADO ON MAY 14, 1993
DISCIPLINARY ACTION: PROBATION; 60-MONTH MONITORING OF PHYSICIAN PERFORMANCE
OFFENSE: SUBSTANDARD CARE, INCOMPETENCE OR NEGLIGENCE
NOTES: SUBSTANDARD CARE. STIPULATION AND ORDER OF THIS DATE PROVIDING FOR LIFETIME PROBATION AND TREATMENT MONITORING. FIVE YEAR PERIOD OF PRACTICE MONITORING.

DAHLBERG, WILLIAM W MD OF NEW ORLEANS, LA, WAS DISCIPLINED BY LOUISIANA ON JULY 21, 1994
DISCIPLINARY ACTION: LICENSE SUSPENSION
OFFENSE: DISCIPLINARY ACTION BY ANOTHER STATE OR AGENCY
NOTES: DISCIPLINARY ACTION BY COLORADO; DECEIT OR PERJURY IN OBTAINING A LICENSE OR PERMIT. REINSTATEMENT CONDITIONED ON FULL COMPLIANCE WITH TERMS IMPOSED BY ORDER OF COLORADO BOARD; PRIOR NOTICE OF INTENT TO RELOCATE TO LOUISIANA; REINSTATEMENT OF LICENSE ON PROBATION FOR SUCH TERMS; AND ON SUCH CONDITIONS AS THE BOARD MAY DETERMINE TO BE APPROPRIATE.

DARNELL, DUANE R DO, DATE OF BIRTH AUGUST 17, 1942, LICENSE NUMBER 0033685, WAS DISCIPLINED BY COLORADO ON AUGUST 30, 1996
DISCIPLINARY ACTION: EMERGENCY SUSPENSION

DARNELL, DUANE R DO, DATE OF BIRTH AUGUST 17, 1942, LICENSE NUMBER 0033685, WAS DISCIPLINED BY COLORADO ON NOVEMBER 13, 1996
DISCIPLINARY ACTION: SURRENDER OF LICENSE
OFFENSE: PROFESSIONAL MISCONDUCT
NOTES: FRAUD, MISREPRESENTATION, OR DECEPTION TOWARD THE BOARD OR A HOSPITAL.

DARNELL, DUANE R DO, DATE OF BIRTH AUGUST 17, 1942, WAS DISCIPLINED BY COLORADO ON APRIL 17, 1997
DISCIPLINARY ACTION: PROBATION; MONITORING OF PHYSICIAN PERFORMANCE
OFFENSE: SUBSTANCE ABUSE
NOTES: HISTORY OF HABITUAL INTEMPERANCE OR EXCESSIVE USE OF A CONTROLLED SUBSTANCE. PROBATIONARY TERMS INCLUDE ABSTINENCE FROM ADDICTIVE SUBSTANCES, TREATMENT AND PRACTICE MONITORING.

DARNELL, DUANE R DO, LICENSE NUMBER 20A4863 OF SUN CITY, CA, WAS DISCIPLINED BY CALIFORNIA ON DECEMBER 24, 1997
DISCIPLINARY ACTION: 60-MONTH PROBATION
OFFENSE: DISCIPLINARY ACTION BY ANOTHER STATE OR AGENCY
NOTES: ACTION TAKEN BY ANOTHER STATE FOR FALSIFYING APPLICATION. REVOCATION STAYED.

DARNELL, DUANE R DO, DATE OF BIRTH AUGUST 17, 1942, LICENSE NUMBER 1008269 OF 24850 HANCOCK AVE APT K-104, MURRIETA, CA, WAS DISCIPLINED BY MICHIGAN ON OCTOBER 1, 1998
DISCIPLINARY ACTION: 6-MONTH LICENSE SUSPENSION; 12-MONTH PROBATION
OFFENSE: DISCIPLINARY ACTION BY ANOTHER STATE OR AGENCY
NOTES: FAILURE TO REPORT/COMPLY.

DARTON, LISA ANN MD OF 5220 EAST DAKOTA AVENUE, DENVER, CO, WAS DISCIPLINED BY DEA ON FEBRUARY 15, 1994
DISCIPLINARY ACTION: RESTRICTION PLACED ON CONTROLLED SUBSTANCE LICENSE
OFFENSE: DISCIPLINARY ACTION BY ANOTHER STATE OR AGENCY
NOTES: COLORADO MEDICAL LICENSE PLACED ON PROBATION DUE TO HISTORY OF DRUG AND ALCOHOL ABUSE. RESTRICTED APPROVAL APPLICATION; RESTRICTED TO SCHEDULE III THROUGH V.

DAVIS, HERBERT ALLEN MD, DATE OF BIRTH FEBRUARY 7, 1940, LICENSE NUMBER 0021196 OF TYLER, TX, WAS DISCIPLINED BY COLORADO ON SEPTEMBER 17, 1993
DISCIPLINARY ACTION: SURRENDER OF LICENSE
OFFENSE: SUBSTANDARD CARE, INCOMPETENCE OR NEGLIGENCE
NOTES: ALLEGATIONS OF SUBSTANDARD PATIENT CARE.

DAVIS, HERBERT ALLEN MD, DATE OF BIRTH FEBRUARY 7, 1940, LICENSE NUMBER 00D2408 OF TYLER, TX, WAS DISCIPLINED BY TEXAS ON AUGUST 19, 1994
DISCIPLINARY ACTION: REPRIMAND
OFFENSE: DISCIPLINARY ACTION BY ANOTHER STATE OR AGENCY
NOTES: ON 8/4/93 HE VOLUNTARILY SURRENDERED COLORADO LICENSE IN LIEU OF FURTHER PROCEEDINGS. HE TREATED A PATIENT BETWEEN 1985 AND 1988 AND TOWARDS THE END OF TREATMENT A SOCIAL AND LATER SEXUAL RELATIONSHIP DEVELOPED; HE CLAIMED THE SEXUAL RELATIONSHIP OCCURRED AFTER TERMINATION OF TREATMENT; HE UNDERSTANDS THE RELATIONSHIP WAS NON-THERAPEUTIC AND DETRIMENTAL TO THE PATIENT. NO OTHER COMPLAINTS ABOUT HIS PRACTICE IN TEXAS HAVE BEEN RECEIVED. SHALL SUBMIT TO A FULL EXAMINATION FOR SEXUAL DISORDERS/ADDICTION WITHIN 30 DAYS; SHALL GIVE A COPY OF THIS ORDER TO ANY HEALTH CARE ENTITY WHERE HE HAS PRIVILEGES; SHALL COOPERATE WITH THE BOARD IN VERIFYING COMPLIANCE. SHALL NOT SEEK MODIFICATION FOR ONE YEAR. THE BOARD RESERVES THE RIGHT TO SEEK OR IMPOSE ADDITIONAL DISCIPLINARY ACTION SHOULD AN UNFAVORABLE REPORT BE RECEIVED FROM THE AFOREMENTIONED EXAMINATION.

DAVIS, HERBERT ALLEN MD, DATE OF BIRTH FEBRUARY 7, 1940, LICENSE NUMBER 00D2408 OF 2323 W FRONT STREET, TYLER, TX, WAS DISCIPLINED BY TEXAS ON MARCH 4, 1995
DISCIPLINARY ACTION: RESTRICTION PLACED ON LICENSE; REQUIRED TO TAKE ADDITIONAL MEDICAL EDUCATION

NOTES: ON 11/7/94 BOARD RECEIVED REPORT ORDERED BY 8/19/94 AGREEMENT IN WHICH THE EVALUATOR STATED THAT DR. DAVIS WAS NOT IMPAIRED OR POTENTIALLY IMPAIRED IN HIS PRACTICE OF PSYCHIATRY, ALTHOUGH HE REMAINS VULNERABLE TO BOUNDARY VIOLATIONS AND ROLE BLURRING DUE TO LIMITED INSIGHT TO ENGAGE IN AND COMMIT TO THERAPEUTIC PROCESS; HE IS COMMITTED TO THE THERAPEUTIC PROCESS; THE EVALUATOR SUPPORTED CONTINUED EMPLOYMENT IN HIS CURRENT POSITION WITH APPROPRIATE SAFEGUARDS AND CONTINUED MEDICAL EDUCATION. SHALL NOT ENGAGE IN THE PRACTICE OF PSYCHOTHERAPY UNLESS APPROVED IN ADVANCE BY HIS THERAPIST; SHALL LIMIT HIS PRACTICE TO CRISIS INTERVENTION, MEDICATION MANAGEMENT, AND GROUP WORK WITH A CO-FACILITATOR PRESENT; SHALL SEE PATIENTS IN HIS OFFICE ALONE ONLY FOR BRIEF VISITS AND INITIAL EVALUATIONS WITH OFFICE DOOR OPEN AND OTHERS AT HIS WORKPLACE; SHALL USE A NURSE CHAPERONE IN ALL SITUATIONS WHERE A RISK OF MISINTERPRETATION EXISTS AND THIS WILL BE MARKED ON MEDICAL RECORDS; PRACTICE SHALL BE SUPERVISED BY A BOARD APPROVED MONITOR WHO SHALL HAVE RANDOM ACCESS TO HIS RECORDS AND PROVIDE QUARTERLY REPORTS; SHALL HAVE A BOARD APPROVED EXPERT REVIEW HIS THERAPEUTIC PROCESS; SHALL OBTAIN AT LEAST 30 HOURS PER YEAR OF CONTINUING MEDICAL EDUCATION, INCLUDING AT LEAST ONE COURSE IN MEDICAL ETHICS, SEXUAL ABUSE, OR TRANSFERENCE/COUNTERTRANSFERENCE/PROFESSIONAL BOUNDARIES PER YEAR; CONDITIONS SHALL REMAIN IN EFFECT FOR TWO YEARS; HE HAS A RIGHT TO PETITION FOR MODIFICATION YEARLY. ON 5/15/96 BOARD DENIED A REQUEST TO TERMINATE THIS ORDER. EFFECTIVE 3/4/97 THIS ORDER EXPIRED.

DAVIS, JOSEPH V DO, DATE OF BIRTH SEPTEMBER 17, 1949, LICENSE NUMBER 28673, WAS DISCIPLINED BY COLORADO ON MAY 14, 1997
DISCIPLINARY ACTION: REPRIMAND

DAVIS, KAREN A DO, DATE OF BIRTH APRIL 24, 1957, LICENSE NUMBER 0027763 OF PARKER, CO, WAS DISCIPLINED BY COLORADO ON NOVEMBER 18, 1993
DISCIPLINARY ACTION: REPRIMAND

DAVIS, ROGER WOODS MD, DATE OF BIRTH JUNE 16, 1940, LICENSE NUMBER 0025882 OF COLORADO SPRINGS, CO, WAS DISCIPLINED BY COLORADO ON JUNE 27, 1991
DISCIPLINARY ACTION: EMERGENCY SUSPENSION
OFFENSE: SUBSTANDARD CARE, INCOMPETENCE OR NEGLIGENCE

NOTES: EXCESSIVE USE OF A CONTROLLED SUBSTANCE, HABITUAL INTEMPERANCE; PRESCRIBING, DISTRIBUTING OR GIVING TO HIMSELF CONTROLLED SUBSTANCES NOT ON AN EMERGENCY BASIS; MISLEADING, DECEPTIVE OR FALSE ADVERTISING; PRESCRIBING CONTROLLED SUBSTANCES OTHER THAN IN THE COURSE OF LEGITIMATE PROFESSIONAL PRACTICE; VIOLATION OF A BOARD RULE; FAILURE TO MAKE ESSENTIAL ENTRIES ON PATIENT RECORDS; FAILURE TO MEET GENERALLY ACCEPTED STANDARDS OF MEDICAL PRACTICE; GROSSLY NEGLIGENT MEDICAL PRACTICE.

DAVIS, ROGER WOODS MD, DATE OF BIRTH JUNE 16, 1940, LICENSE NUMBER 0025882 OF COLORADO SPRINGS, CO, WAS DISCIPLINED BY COLORADO ON APRIL 16, 1993
DISCIPLINARY ACTION: LICENSE REVOCATION
OFFENSE: SUBSTANDARD CARE, INCOMPETENCE OR NEGLIGENCE

NOTES: EXCESSIVE USE OF A CONTROLLED SUBSTANCE; PRESCRIBING A CONTROLLED SUBSTANCE OTHER THAN IN THE COURSE OF LEGITIMATE PROFESSIONAL PRACTICE; SUBSTANDARD CARE; ADVERTISING WHICH IS DECEPTIVE, MISLEADING OR FALSE. CASE WAS ON APPEAL TO THE COLORADO COURT OF APPEALS AS OF 1/94.

DAVIS, ROGER WOODS MD, DATE OF BIRTH JUNE 16, 1940 OF 5330 LOMITA ROAD, COLORADO SPRINGS, CO, WAS DISCIPLINED BY MEDICARE ON DECEMBER 5, 1994
DISCIPLINARY ACTION: EXCLUSION FROM THE MEDICARE AND/OR MEDICAID PROGRAM
OFFENSE: DISCIPLINARY ACTION BY ANOTHER STATE OR AGENCY

NOTES: LICENSE REVOKED FOR REASONS BEARING ON PROFESSIONAL PERFORMANCE.

DAVIS, WILLIAM DUNCAN III MD, DATE OF BIRTH MARCH 4, 1953, LICENSE NUMBER 0032421, WAS DISCIPLINED BY COLORADO ON SEPTEMBER 14, 1995
DISCIPLINARY ACTION: REPRIMAND

DAVIS, WILLIAM DUNCAN III MD, DATE OF BIRTH MARCH 4, 1953, LICENSE NUMBER 32421, WAS DISCIPLINED BY COLORADO ON JUNE 12, 1997
DISCIPLINARY ACTION: 60-MONTH PROBATION; RESTRICTION PLACED ON LICENSE
OFFENSE: SUBSTANDARD CARE, INCOMPETENCE OR NEGLIGENCE

NOTES: SUBSTANDARD CARE (PRIMA FACIA TYPE ADMISSION ONLY). TERMS OF PROBATION INCLUDE: MUST BE ASSISTED ON SURGICAL PROCEDURES AND PRACTICE MONITORING.

DAVIS, WILLIAM DUNCAN III MD, LICENSE NUMBER 015255R, WAS DISCIPLINED BY LOUISIANA ON OCTOBER 20, 1999
DISCIPLINARY ACTION: PROBATION
OFFENSE: DISCIPLINARY ACTION BY ANOTHER STATE OR AGENCY

NOTES: IN 6/97 COLORADO PLACED LICENSE ON PROBATION. SHALL NOT PRACTICE IN LOUISIANA UNTIL SUCH TIME AS HE HOLDS AN UNRESTRICTED LICENSE IN COLORADO; SHALL PAY COSTS.

DE ALVA, WILLIAM E MD, DATE OF BIRTH APRIL 2, 1925, LICENSE NUMBER 0015060 OF TUCSON, AZ, WAS DISCIPLINED BY COLORADO ON FEBRUARY 19, 1993
DISCIPLINARY ACTION: REPRIMAND
OFFENSE: SUBSTANDARD CARE, INCOMPETENCE OR NEGLIGENCE

NOTES: SUBSTANDARD CARE.

DEJONG, JITZE MD, DATE OF BIRTH MARCH 15, 1922, LICENSE NUMBER 0015901 OF DENVER, CO, WAS DISCIPLINED BY COLORADO ON MARCH 19, 1993
DISCIPLINARY ACTION: SURRENDER OF LICENSE

NOTES: NO SPECIFIC FINDINGS OF UNPROFESSIONAL CONDUCT. STIPULATION AND ORDER EFFECTIVE ON ACTION DATE.

DENEGRI, ALBERTO MD, DATE OF BIRTH JULY 24, 1944, LICENSE NUMBER 0020339 OF DENVER, CO, WAS DISCIPLINED BY COLORADO ON MARCH 2, 1994
DISCIPLINARY ACTION: REPRIMAND
OFFENSE: PROFESSIONAL MISCONDUCT

DENEGRI, ALBERTO MD, DATE OF BIRTH JULY 24, 1944, LICENSE NUMBER 20339, WAS DISCIPLINED BY COLORADO ON AUGUST 12, 1998
OFFENSE: SUBSTANDARD CARE, INCOMPETENCE OR NEGLIGENCE

NOTES: SUBSTANDARD CARE. MUST COMPLETE RESIDENCY TRAINING.

DENTON, SANDRA M MD, DATE OF BIRTH JANUARY 20, 1946, LICENSE NUMBER 0030084 OF ANCHORAGE, AK, WAS DISCIPLINED BY COLORADO ON DECEMBER 13, 1993
DISCIPLINARY ACTION: SURRENDER OF LICENSE

NOTES: NO UNPROFESSIONAL CONDUCT IDENTIFIED.

DICK, ARTHUR L MD, DATE OF BIRTH JANUARY 11, 1937, LICENSE NUMBER 33181, WAS DISCIPLINED BY COLORADO ON MAY 15, 1998

NOTES: NO UNPROFESSIONAL CONDUCT IDENTIFIED. HE AGREES TO PERMANENTLY RELINQUISH HIS LICENSE ON 8/31/98.

DICKEY, LORRAINE A MD, DATE OF BIRTH DECEMBER 17, 1961, LICENSE NUMBER 37535, WAS DISCIPLINED BY COLORADO ON NOVEMBER 12, 1998
DISCIPLINARY ACTION: 36-MONTH PROBATION; MONITORING OF PHYSICIAN PERFORMANCE

NOTES: NO UNPROFESSIONAL CONDUCT IDENTIFIED. PROBATIONARY TERMS INCLUDE TREATMENT MONITORING AND PRACTICE MONITORING.

DILLINGHAM, BRUCE L MD, DATE OF BIRTH JANUARY 27, 1951, LICENSE NUMBER 23199, WAS DISCIPLINED BY COLORADO ON FEBRUARY 13, 1998
DISCIPLINARY ACTION: LICENSE REVOCATION
OFFENSE: DISCIPLINARY ACTION BY ANOTHER STATE OR AGENCY

NOTES: DISCIPLINE IN ANOTHER STATE; FELONY CONVICTION; ADMINISTERING A CONTROLLED SUBSTANCE OTHER THAN IN THE COURSE OF LEGITIMATE PROFESSIONAL PRACTICE; A VIOLATION OF A LAW REGULATING CONTROLLED SUBSTANCES; SUBSTANDARD CARE.

DILLINGHAM, BRUCE LEE MD, DATE OF BIRTH JANUARY 27, 1951, LICENSE NUMBER 0026098 OF 845 DEAN WAY, LAWRENCEVILLE, GA, WAS DISCIPLINED BY GEORGIA ON FEBRUARY 21, 1996
DISCIPLINARY ACTION: SURRENDER OF CONTROLLED SUBSTANCE LICENSE

NOTES: PRESCRIBING. PUBLIC ORDER. MUST SURRENDER DEA REGISTRATION BY 2/26/96.

DILLINGHAM, BRUCE LEE MD, DATE OF BIRTH JANUARY 27, 1951, LICENSE NUMBER 0026098 OF 845 DEAN WAY, LAWRENCEVILLE, GA, WAS DISCIPLINED BY GEORGIA ON APRIL 14, 1996
DISCIPLINARY ACTION: 4-MONTH LICENSE SUSPENSION; 72-MONTH PROBATION

NOTES: PRESCRIBING VIOLATIONS. NO DEA CERTIFICATE.

DOELL, WILLIAM EDWARD DO, DATE OF BIRTH MAY 26, 1933, LICENSE NUMBER 0015643 OF WHEAT RIDGE, CO, WAS DISCIPLINED BY COLORADO ON AUGUST 17, 1990
DISCIPLINARY ACTION: LICENSE REVOCATION
OFFENSE: SUBSTANDARD CARE, INCOMPETENCE OR NEGLIGENCE

NOTES: FAILED TO MEET GENERALLY ACCEPTED STANDARDS OF MEDICAL PRACTICE AND PRESCRIBED OTHER THAN IN THE COURSE OF LEGITIMATE PROFESSIONAL PRACTICE. APPEAL FILED 8/28/90; STAY DENIED BY MEDICAL BOARD AND COURT OF APPEALS. ON 12/12/91, COLORADO COURT OF APPEALS UPHELD FINDINGS OF SUBSTANDARD CARE, PRESCRIBING OTHER THAN IN THE COURSE OF LEGITIMATE PROFESSIONAL PRACTICE, AND REVOCATION OF MEDICAL LICENSE.

DOELL, WILLIAM EDWARD DO, DATE OF BIRTH MAY 26, 1933 OF 13040 WEST 80TH AVE, ARVADA, CO, WAS DISCIPLINED BY MEDICARE ON MAY 10, 1991
DISCIPLINARY ACTION: EXCLUSION FROM THE MEDICARE AND/OR MEDICAID PROGRAM
OFFENSE: DISCIPLINARY ACTION BY ANOTHER STATE OR AGENCY

NOTES: LICENSE REVOCATION OR SUSPENSION.

DOELL, WILLIAM EDWARD DO, DATE OF BIRTH MAY 26, 1933 OF 13040 WEST 80TH AVE, ARVADA, CO, WAS DISCIPLINED BY ALASKA ON JUNE 19, 1991
DISCIPLINARY ACTION: DENIAL OF NEW LICENSE
OFFENSE: DISCIPLINARY ACTION BY ANOTHER STATE OR AGENCY

NOTES: LICENSE DENIED BASED ON REVOCATION OF COLORADO LICENSE.

DOELL, WILLIAM EDWARD DO, WAS DISCIPLINED BY ALASKA ON DECEMBER 5, 1991
DISCIPLINARY ACTION: DENIAL OF NEW LICENSE
OFFENSE: DISCIPLINARY ACTION BY ANOTHER STATE OR AGENCY

NOTES: BASED ON REVOCATION OF COLORADO LICENSE.

DOELL, WILLIAM EDWARD DO, DATE OF BIRTH MAY 26, 1933 OF 7777 W. 38TH AVENUE #124, WHEAT RIDGE, CO, WAS DISCIPLINED BY DEA ON JULY 12, 1993
DISCIPLINARY ACTION: REVOCATION OF CONTROLLED SUBSTANCE LICENSE
OFFENSE: DISCIPLINARY ACTION BY ANOTHER STATE OR AGENCY

NOTES: COLORADO MEDICAL LICENSE REVOKED ON 8/17/90 DUE TO NUMEROUS INSTANCES OF SUBSTANDARD CARE, IN CONNECTION WITH SEVENTEEN PATIENTS, INCLUDING EXCESSIVE PRESCRIBING OF DILAUDID TO A PATIENT.

DORAN, JOHN H DO, DATE OF BIRTH AUGUST 28, 1954, LICENSE NUMBER 26825, WAS DISCIPLINED BY COLORADO ON JULY 17, 1997
DISCIPLINARY ACTION: LICENSE SUSPENSION

DOTSON, DANIEL A MD, LICENSE NUMBER 00D4096 OF GRAHAM, TX, WAS DISCIPLINED BY TEXAS ON DECEMBER 1, 1990
DISCIPLINARY ACTION: LICENSE REVOCATION
OFFENSE: PROFESSIONAL MISCONDUCT

NOTES: UNPROFESSIONAL OR DISHONORABLE CONDUCT LIKELY TO DECEIVE, DEFRAUD OR INJURE PUBLIC, PROFESSIONAL FAILURE TO PRACTICE MEDICINE IN ACCEPTABLE MANNER CONSISTENT WITH PUBLIC HEALTH AND WELFARE. FILED MOTION FOR REHEARING.

DOTSON, DANIEL A MD, DATE OF BIRTH NOVEMBER 14, 1941, LICENSE NUMBER 0025062 OF PUEBLO, CO, WAS DISCIPLINED BY COLORADO ON SEPTEMBER 11, 1992
DISCIPLINARY ACTION: SURRENDER OF CONTROLLED SUBSTANCE LICENSE
OFFENSE: SUBSTANDARD CARE, INCOMPETENCE OR NEGLIGENCE

NOTES: TWO OR MORE ACTS OR OMISSIONS WHICH FAILED TO MEET GENERALLY ACCEPTED STANDARDS OF MEDICAL PRACTICE. PERMANENT SURRENDER OF DRUG ENFORCEMENT ADMINISTRATION CERTIFICATE (ALL SCHEDULES). NOT TO SEEK CERTIFICATE

REINSTATEMENT IN FUTURE.

DOUGLAS, HOWARD T MD, LICENSE NUMBER 12539 OF 4255 S BUCKLEY ROAD #130, AURORA, CO, WAS DISCIPLINED BY OKLAHOMA ON JUNE 26, 1998
DISCIPLINARY ACTION: DENIAL OF NEW LICENSE
OFFENSE: DISCIPLINARY ACTION BY ANOTHER STATE OR AGENCY

NOTES: LICENSE IN TEXAS WAS SUSPENDED ON 5/12/97 FOR UNPROFESSIONAL CONDUCT, INCLUDING HIS PRESCRIBING WITHOUT EXAMINATION OR EVALUATION AND HIS FAILURE TO CONFORM TO MINIMAL STANDARDS OF ACCEPTABLE MEDICAL PRACTICE. THE LICENSE REMAINS UNDER SUSPENSION AS OF THE DATE OF THIS ORDER. REINSTATEMENT DENIED.

DOUGLAS, HOWARD T III MD, DATE OF BIRTH MARCH 31, 1949, LICENSE NUMBER 24197, WAS DISCIPLINED BY COLORADO ON NOVEMBER 13, 1998
DISCIPLINARY ACTION: REPRIMAND; REQUIRED TO TAKE ADDITIONAL MEDICAL EDUCATION

NOTES: DISCIPLINE IN ANOTHER STATE. HE AGREES TO REEDUCATION ACTIVITIES.

DOUGLAS, HOWARD T III MD, DATE OF BIRTH MARCH 31, 1949, LICENSE NUMBER 24197, WAS DISCIPLINED BY COLORADO ON MAY 19, 1999

NOTES: ISSUE OF COMPLIANCE WITH INITIAL ORDER. LICENSE PLACED IN INACTIVE STATUS.

DOUGLAS, HOWARD THOMAS III MD, LICENSE NUMBER F1511, WAS DISCIPLINED BY TEXAS ON MAY 10, 1997
DISCIPLINARY ACTION: LICENSE SUSPENSION; FINE
OFFENSE: OVERPRESCRIBING OR MISPRESCRIBING DRUGS

NOTES: HE HAD A CONTRACT WITH SOUTHWEST MEDICAL ASSOCIATES, INC., INVOLVING HIS AGREEMENT TO PROVIDE CONTINUOUS PHYSICIAN COVERAGE, INCLUDING ER SERVICES, TO A SPECIFIED HOSPITAL IN SONORA, TEXAS BETWEEN 6 PM ON 7/6/94 AND 6 AM ON 7/11/94, INCLUSIVE. ON 7/10/94 HE BECAME ILL WITH A VIRUS, INCLUDING STOMACH CRAMPS, VOMITING, AND DIARRHEA, DROVE TO THE HOSPITAL ADMINISTRATOR'S HOUSE, AND TOLD HIM HE COULD NOT ADEQUATELY TREAT PATIENTS AND ASSUMED IT WAS ALL RIGHT TO LEAVE THE HOSPITAL WHILE IN FACT THE ADMINISTRATOR WAS SURPRISED AND UPSET THAT THE DOCTOR LEFT BEFORE THE REGULAR PHYSICIAN RETURNED OR A REPLACEMENT WAS SECURED. WITHOUT DEFINITELY TELLING THE NURSING STAFF HE WAS LEAVING, HE LEFT AND DID NOT CONTACT THE HOSPITAL AFTER HE LEFT. ON 7/9/94 HE HAD PRESCRIBED A CONTROLLED SUBSTANCE, VICODIN, TO A PATIENT HE NEVER EXAMINED AND WITHOUT CONSULTING ANY MEDICAL RECORDS ON THE BASIS OF HER TESTIMONY THAT SHE HAD A TOOTHACHE AND NEEDED A NEW SUPPLY OF HER PREVIOUS PRESCRIPTION FOR SAID SUBSTANCE. UNDER THE CIRCUMSTANCES THE PHYSICIAN HAD NO WAY OF KNOWING WHETHER THE DRUG WOULD BE THERAPEUTIC FOR THE PATIENT. LICENSE SUSPENDED UNTIL THE PHYSICIAN SATISFIES THE FOLLOWING: SHALL RECERTIFY IN ATLS AND ADVANCED CARDIAC LIFE SUPPORT; SHALL PASS 100 HOURS IN EMERGENCY ROOM MEDICINE AND CONTINUING MEDICAL EDUCATION; SHALL PASS AN APPROVED PHARMACOLOGY COURSE AND AN APPROVED RISK MANAGEMENT COURSE; SHALL PASS THE SPEX AND THE BOARD'S JURISPRUDENCE EXAM; SHALL SEND A BOARD-APPROVED WRITTEN APOLOGY TO THE CONCERNED HOSPITAL AND TO SOUTHWEST MEDICAL ASSOCIATES, INC.; SHALL INFORM ALL HOSPITALS WHERE HE HAS PRIVILEGES AND ALL ER COMPANIES WITH WHICH HE HAS OR HAS HAD CONTRACTS THAT HIS LICENSE IS SUSPENDED; SHALL SEND A COPY OF THIS ORDER TO ALL STATES WHERE HE IS LICENSED; AND SHALL FURNISH ACCEPTABLE PROOF TO THE BOARD THAT HE HAS NOTIFIED THE ABOVE ENTITIES. UPON FULFILLMENT OF THESE CONDITIONS, HE WILL BE SUSPENDED FOR ANOTHER FIVE YEARS; SUSPENSION STAYED AND LICENSE PLACED ON PROBATION WITH TERMS. $10,000 ADMINISTRATIVE FINE. ON 10/24/98 PETITION FOR REINSTATEMENT DENIED; THE FOLLOWING MODIFICATIONS WERE ORDERED HOWEVER: DELETION OF REQUIREMENT TO TAKE AND PASS A BOARD-APPROVED PHARMACOLOGY COURSE; MAY PASS THE AMERICAN BOARD OF EMERGENCY ROOM MEDICINE CERTIFICATION EXAM AS AN ALTERNATIVE TO PASSING THE SPEX EXAM; FINE REDUCED TO $5,000; LICENSE PLACED ON PROBATION AS SOON AS THESE CONDITIONS ARE MET; ALL OTHER PROVISIONS OF ORDER REMAIN IN EFFECT UNTIL SUPERSEDED BY A SUBSEQUENT BOARD ORDER. ON 5/14/99 REQUEST FOR REINSTATEMENT DENIED.

DOUGLAS, HOWARD THOMAS III MD, DATE OF BIRTH MARCH 31, 1949 OF 729 GRAPEVINE HIGHWAY, HURST, TX, WAS DISCIPLINED BY MEDICARE ON SEPTEMBER 20, 1998
DISCIPLINARY ACTION: EXCLUSION FROM THE MEDICARE AND/OR MEDICAID PROGRAM
OFFENSE: DISCIPLINARY ACTION BY ANOTHER STATE OR AGENCY

NOTES: LICENSE REVOKED, SUSPENDED, SURRENDERED OR OTHERWISE LOST FOR REASONS BEARING ON PROFESSIONAL PERFORMANCE, PROFESSIONAL COMPETENCE OR FINANCIAL INTEGRITY. REINSTATED ON 11/5/99.

DOWNING, TERRY MD, DATE OF BIRTH MAY 24, 1944, LICENSE NUMBER 0018110 OF DENVER, CO, WAS DISCIPLINED BY COLORADO ON FEBRUARY 9, 1995
DISCIPLINARY ACTION: 60-MONTH PROBATION; REQUIRED TO TAKE ADDITIONAL MEDICAL EDUCATION
OFFENSE: SUBSTANDARD CARE, INCOMPETENCE OR NEGLIGENCE

NOTES: PROBATION INCLUDES PRACTICE MONITORING AND REEDUCATION ACTIVITIES.

DOWNING, TERRY ALAN MD, LICENSE NUMBER 0G26727 OF DENVER, CO, WAS DISCIPLINED BY CALIFORNIA ON FEBRUARY 13, 1996
DISCIPLINARY ACTION: 60-MONTH PROBATION
OFFENSE: DISCIPLINARY ACTION BY ANOTHER STATE OR AGENCY

NOTES: ACTION IN COLORADO FOR TWO UNSPECIFIED ACTS OR OMISSIONS WHICH FAIL TO MEET GENERALLY ACCEPTED STANDARDS OF MEDICAL PRACTICE. REVOCATION, STAYED.

DRICKEY, ROBERT E MD, DATE OF BIRTH JANUARY 24, 1944, LICENSE NUMBER 0017983, WAS DISCIPLINED BY COLORADO ON APRIL 14, 1994
DISCIPLINARY ACTION: LICENSE REINSTATEMENT; RESTRICTION PLACED ON LICENSE

NOTES: FOUR YEAR ABSENCE FROM CLINICAL PRACTICE. PRACTICE RESTRICTED TO UCHSC ONLY AND CPEP REQUIREMENTS. LICENSE REINSTATED UNDER INDEFINITE STIPULATION. ON 11/3/94 LICENSE RESTORED TO UNRESTRICTED, UNENCUMBERED STATUS.

DUBLEMAN, ALAN MD, DATE OF BIRTH FEBRUARY 22, 1948, LICENSE NUMBER 0021695 OF THORNTON, CO, WAS DISCIPLINED BY COLORADO ON APRIL 14, 1993
DISCIPLINARY ACTION: SURRENDER OF LICENSE
OFFENSE: PHYSICAL OR MENTAL ILLNESS INHIBITING THE ABILITY TO PRACTICE WITH SKILL AND SAFETY

NOTES: MENTAL DISABILITY.

DUBLEMAN, ALAN MD, LICENSE NUMBER 0G32505 OF DENVER, CO, WAS DISCIPLINED BY CALIFORNIA ON JUNE 27, 1994
DISCIPLINARY ACTION: LICENSE REVOCATION
OFFENSE: DISCIPLINARY ACTION BY ANOTHER STATE OR AGENCY

NOTES: DISCIPLINED BY THE COLORADO BOARD. DEFAULT DECISION.

DUNKIN, DONALD E DO, DATE OF BIRTH SEPTEMBER 24, 1932, LICENSE NUMBER 0014789 OF DENVER, CO, WAS DISCIPLINED BY COLORADO ON AUGUST 14, 1992
DISCIPLINARY ACTION: 60-MONTH PROBATION; REQUIRED TO TAKE ADDITIONAL MEDICAL EDUCATION
OFFENSE: SUBSTANDARD CARE, INCOMPETENCE OR NEGLIGENCE

NOTES: TWO OR MORE ACTS OR OMISSIONS WHICH FAILED TO MEET GENERALLY ACCEPTED STANDARDS OF MEDICAL PRACTICE. EDUCATION ASSESSMENT. PROBATIONARY PERIOD INCLUDES PRACTICE MONITORING.

DUNKIN, DONALD E DO, DATE OF BIRTH SEPTEMBER 24, 1932, LICENSE NUMBER 0014789 OF BRIGHTON, CO, WAS DISCIPLINED BY COLORADO ON JULY 13, 1994
DISCIPLINARY ACTION: SURRENDER OF LICENSE; RESTRICTION PLACED ON LICENSE
OFFENSE: SUBSTANDARD CARE, INCOMPETENCE OR NEGLIGENCE

NOTES: PATIENT CARE ISSUES; PHYSICAL/MENTAL DISABILITY ISSUES. SURRENDER AS OF 10/1/94; UNTIL THEN NO INVASIVE SURGICAL PROCEDURES (IN-OFFICE). ORIGINAL STIPULATION OF 08/14/92 TERMS AND CONDITIONS REMAIN IN EFFECT.

DUNKIN, DONALD E DO, DATE OF BIRTH SEPTEMBER 24, 1932 OF 14531 COUNTRY HILLS DRIVE, BRIGHTON, CO, WAS DISCIPLINED BY MEDICARE ON FEBRUARY 22, 1995
DISCIPLINARY ACTION: EXCLUSION FROM THE MEDICARE AND/OR MEDICAID PROGRAM
OFFENSE: DISCIPLINARY ACTION BY ANOTHER STATE OR AGENCY

NOTES: LICENSE SURRENDERED FOR REASONS BEARING ON PROFESSIONAL COMPETENCE.

DUNLOP, CYNTHIA OWENS MD, DATE OF BIRTH MARCH 21, 1949, LICENSE NUMBER 0021323 OF THORNTON, CO, WAS DISCIPLINED BY COLORADO ON MARCH 19, 1993
DISCIPLINARY ACTION: 2-MONTH LICENSE SUSPENSION
OFFENSE: FAILURE TO COMPLY WITH PREVIOUS BOARD ORDER

NOTES: FAILURE TO COMPLY WITH A VALID BOARD ORDER, SPECIFICALLY, A PREVIOUS STIPULATION. LICENSE SUSPENDED UNTIL SHE CAME BACK INTO COMPLIANCE.

DUNN, TERRY S MD, DATE OF BIRTH NOVEMBER 12, 1954, LICENSE NUMBER 0028675 OF DENVER, CO, WAS DISCIPLINED BY COLORADO ON JUNE 14, 1991
DISCIPLINARY ACTION: LICENSE SUSPENSION; REQUIRED TO TAKE ADDITIONAL MEDICAL EDUCATION
OFFENSE: DISCIPLINARY ACTION BY ANOTHER STATE OR AGENCY

NOTES: SUSPENSION OF LICENSE IN ANOTHER STATE, SUBSTANDARD MEDICAL PRACTICE. INDEFINITE SUSPENSION WITH CONDITIONS FOR REINSTATEMENT INCLUDING COMPLETION OF A 1 YEAR RESIDENCY; IF REINSTATED THAN LICENSURE SHALL BE SUBJECT TO THE PROVISIONS OF A 5 YEAR PROBATION WITH PRACTICE MONITORING, CONSULTATIONS, AND CONTINUING EDUCATION.

DUNN, TERRY S MD, DATE OF BIRTH NOVEMBER 12, 1954, LICENSE NUMBER 0028675 OF DENVER, CO, WAS DISCIPLINED BY COLORADO ON MAY 15, 1992
DISCIPLINARY ACTION: 60-MONTH PROBATION; REQUIRED TO TAKE ADDITIONAL MEDICAL EDUCATION

NOTES: FIRST AMENDMENT TO ORDER DATED 6/14/91; REINSTATED UNDER TERMS AND CONDITIONS OF PROBATION; INCLUDING PRACTICE MONITORING AND EDUCATION REQUIREMENTS.

DUVALL, BRUCE C MD, DATE OF BIRTH FEBRUARY 7, 1943, LICENSE NUMBER 0021201 OF DENVER, CO, WAS DISCIPLINED BY COLORADO ON APRIL 14, 1994
DISCIPLINARY ACTION: REPRIMAND
OFFENSE: PROFESSIONAL MISCONDUCT

DYSART, RICHARD A MD, DATE OF BIRTH APRIL 29, 1949, LICENSE NUMBER 24202, WAS DISCIPLINED BY COLORADO ON JUNE 19, 1997
DISCIPLINARY ACTION: REPRIMAND

EASTER, THOMAS G II MD, DATE OF BIRTH FEBRUARY 26, 1952, LICENSE NUMBER 27470, WAS DISCIPLINED BY COLORADO ON AUGUST 18, 1999
DISCIPLINARY ACTION: SURRENDER OF LICENSE
OFFENSE: DISCIPLINARY ACTION BY ANOTHER STATE OR AGENCY

NOTES: DISCIPLINED IN ANOTHER STATE.

EASTER, THOMAS G II MD, LICENSE NUMBER 049380 OF EL PASO, TX, WAS DISCIPLINED BY VIRGINIA ON NOVEMBER 15, 1999
DISCIPLINARY ACTION: PROBATION
OFFENSE: DISCIPLINARY ACTION BY ANOTHER STATE OR AGENCY

NOTES: DISCIPLINARY ACTION BY THE TEXAS BOARD FOR PRESCRIBING MEDICATIONS TO A PATIENT WITHOUT ADEQUATE MEDICAL INDICATION AND WITHOUT ADEQUATELY DOCUMENTING CARE AND TREATMENT.

EASTER, THOMAS GLENN II MD, LICENSE NUMBER G7801 OF EL PASO, TX, WAS DISCIPLINED BY TEXAS ON AUGUST 22, 1998
DISCIPLINARY ACTION: REPRIMAND; REQUIRED TO TAKE ADDITIONAL MEDICAL EDUCATION
OFFENSE: OVERPRESCRIBING OR MISPRESCRIBING DRUGS

NOTES: FOR SEVERAL YEARS AND UNTIL APPROXIMATELY 7/93, HE PRESCRIBED, DISPENSED AND/OR ADMINISTERED INJECTABLE MORPHINE SULFATE AND DEMEROL TO AN ADULT FEMALE PATIENT, WITHOUT ADEQUATE MEDICATION INDICATION AND WITHOUT ADEQUATELY DOCUMENTING HIS CARE AND TREATMENT OF THIS PATIENT INCLUDING DOCUMENTATION OF THE DRUGS PRESCRIBED, DISPENSED OR ADMINISTERED; WHEN THE PATIENT DEVELOPED ABSCESSES, HE FAILED TO STOP PRESCRIBING MORPHINE AND FAILED TO PROVIDE ADEQUATE ALTERNATIVE TREATMENT IN LIEU OF NARCOTIC MEDICATIONS; HE HAS NOT MAINTAINED HIS UPDATED PRACTICE AND MAILING ADDRESSES WITH THE BOARD, AND HAS NOT RESPONDED TO BOARD'S REQUESTS FOR INFORMATION; CURRENTLY AND DURING THE PERIOD OF PRESCRIBING HE WAS COHABITING WITH THE PATIENT. LICENSE LIMITED FOR FIVE YEARS AS FOLLOWS: SHALL NOT TREAT OR

OTHERWISE SERVE AS PHYSICIAN, PRESCRIBE, DISPENSE OR ADMINISTER DRUGS THAT MAY BE SUBJECT TO ABUSE TO HIMSELF OR TO ANY MEMBER OF HIS FAMILY; SEPARATE FROM PATIENT RECORDS, SHALL MAINTAIN A LOGBOOK OF EVERY PRESCRIPTION WRITTEN BY HIM FOR DANGEROUS DRUGS WITH ADDICTIVE POTENTIAL WHICH SHALL BE MADE AVAILABLE FOR REVIEW; SHALL MAINTAIN ADEQUATE MEDICAL RECORDS WHICH SHALL BE AVAILABLE FOR REVIEW; SHALL OBTAIN 50 HOURS PER YEAR OF CONTINUING MEDICAL EDUCATION; SHALL COOPERATE WITH THE BOARD IN VERIFYING COMPLIANCE INCLUDING PROVIDING COPIES OF PEER REVIEW RECORDS UPON REQUEST; SHALL GIVE A COPY OF THIS ORDER TO ANY HEALTH CARE ENTITY WHERE HE HAS PRIVILEGES; SHALL PROVIDE A COPY OF THIS ORDER TO ANYONE REQUESTING IT WITHIN 10 DAYS; SHALL APPEAR BEFORE THE BOARD UPON REQUEST; TIME SPENT OUT OF TEXAS DOES NOT COUNT TOWARD RESTRICTION; SHALL INFORM THE BOARD OF CHANGE OF ADDRESS WITHIN 10 DAYS OR IF HE LEAVES THE STATE; SHALL NOT SEEK MODIFICATION FOR ONE YEAR.

ECKHARDT, LLOYD O MD, DATE OF BIRTH APRIL 23, 1935, LICENSE NUMBER 0017085, WAS DISCIPLINED BY COLORADO ON AUGUST 14, 1996
DISCIPLINARY ACTION: 60-MONTH PROBATION; MONITORING OF PHYSICIAN PERFORMANCE
OFFENSE: SUBSTANDARD CARE, INCOMPETENCE OR NEGLIGENCE

NOTES: SUBSTANDARD CARE.

ECKHARDT, LLOYD O MD, LICENSE NUMBER 093173 OF 2779 EAST FREMONT PLACE, LITTLETON, CO, WAS DISCIPLINED BY NEW YORK ON APRIL 15, 1997
DISCIPLINARY ACTION: SURRENDER OF LICENSE
OFFENSE: DISCIPLINARY ACTION BY ANOTHER STATE OR AGENCY

NOTES: DISCIPLINED BY THE COLORADO BOARD FOR PRESCRIBING EXCESSIVE PAIN MEDICATIONS AND BENZODIAZEPINES FOR TWO PATIENTS.

ECKSTEIN, LARRY MD, DATE OF BIRTH APRIL 15, 1947, LICENSE NUMBER 33042, WAS DISCIPLINED BY COLORADO ON NOVEMBER 17, 1999
DISCIPLINARY ACTION: 60-MONTH PROBATION; REQUIRED TO TAKE ADDITIONAL MEDICAL EDUCATION
OFFENSE: SUBSTANDARD CARE, INCOMPETENCE OR NEGLIGENCE

NOTES: SUBSTANDARD CARE (PRIMA FACIE TYPE ADMISSION ONLY). TERMS OF PROBATION INCLUDE REEDUCATION ACTIVITIES AND PRACTICE MONITORING.

ECOFF, ARTHUR DO, DATE OF BIRTH APRIL 1, 1931, LICENSE NUMBER 0022426 OF 1241 S PARKER SUITE, DENVER, CO, WAS DISCIPLINED BY COLORADO ON MAY 14, 1993
DISCIPLINARY ACTION: EMERGENCY SUSPENSION
OFFENSE: SUBSTANDARD CARE, INCOMPETENCE OR NEGLIGENCE

NOTES: SUBSTANDARD CARE; ALLEGATIONS OF SEXUAL CONTACT WITH THREE PATIENTS BETWEEN 7/88 AND 9/92; MENTAL DISABILITY. ALLEGATIONS ARE DENIED BY PHYSICIAN. LICENSE SUSPENDED PENDING A HEARINGS PANEL REVIEW OF THE INITIAL DECISION OF THE ADMINISTRATIVE LAW JUDGE.

ECOFF, ARTHUR DO, DATE OF BIRTH APRIL 1, 1931, LICENSE NUMBER 0022426 OF 1241 S PARKER SUITE, DENVER, CO, WAS DISCIPLINED BY COLORADO ON FEBRUARY 18, 1994
DISCIPLINARY ACTION: LICENSE REVOCATION
OFFENSE: SUBSTANDARD CARE, INCOMPETENCE OR NEGLIGENCE

NOTES: SUBSTANDARD CARE; A SEXUAL ACT WITH A PATIENT; MENTAL DISABILITY.

ECOFF, ARTHUR MD, DATE OF BIRTH APRIL 1, 1931, LICENSE NUMBER 0A29185 OF DENVER, CO, WAS DISCIPLINED BY CALIFORNIA ON MAY 26, 1994
DISCIPLINARY ACTION: 12-MONTH LICENSE SUSPENSION
OFFENSE: DISCIPLINARY ACTION BY ANOTHER STATE OR AGENCY

NOTES: ON 5/14/93 COLORADO BOARD SUMMARILY SUSPENDED LICENSE BASED ON THREE COUNTS ALLEGING SEXUAL MISCONDUCT WITH PATIENTS. LICENSE SUSPENDED FOR ONE YEAR DEPENDING ON OUTCOME OF PENDING COLORADO CASE.

ECOFF, ARTHUR DO, DATE OF BIRTH APRIL 10, 1931 OF 3781 S QUEBEC STREET, DENVER, CO, WAS DISCIPLINED BY MEDICARE ON OCTOBER 10, 1994
DISCIPLINARY ACTION: EXCLUSION FROM THE MEDICARE AND/OR MEDICAID PROGRAM
OFFENSE: DISCIPLINARY ACTION BY ANOTHER STATE OR AGENCY

NOTES: LICENSE REVOKED FOR REASONS BEARING ON PROFESSIONAL PERFORMANCE.

ECOFF, ARTHUR DO OF DENVER, CO, WAS DISCIPLINED BY MISSOURI ON JUNE 21, 1995
DISCIPLINARY ACTION: LICENSE REVOCATION
OFFENSE: DISCIPLINARY ACTION BY ANOTHER STATE OR AGENCY

NOTES: LICENSE REVOKED IN COLORADO FOR FAILURE TO RESPECT THE BOUNDARIES BETWEEN A MALE PHYSICIAN AND FEMALE PATIENTS AND NOT COOPERATING WITH A BOARD INVESTIGATION. NO REAPPLICATION FOR SEVEN YEARS.

ECOFF, ARTHUR MD, DATE OF BIRTH APRIL 1, 1931, LICENSE NUMBER 0A29185 OF 3781 SOUTH QUEBEC STREET, DENVER, CO, WAS DISCIPLINED BY CALIFORNIA ON JANUARY 29, 1996
DISCIPLINARY ACTION: LICENSE REVOCATION
OFFENSE: DISCIPLINARY ACTION BY ANOTHER STATE OR AGENCY

NOTES: ON 2/18/94 COLORADO REVOKED HIS LICENSE DUE TO NUMEROUS ACTS OF UNPROFESSIONAL CONDUCT, INCLUDING SEVERAL INSTANCES OF SUBSTANDARD PRACTICE AND SEXUAL CONDUCT WITH PATIENTS; ADDITIONALLY HE HAS A MENTAL DISABILITY WHICH RENDERS HIM UNABLE TO PRACTICE MEDICINE WITH REASONABLE SKILL AND SAFETY. DEFAULT ACTION.

ECOFF, ARTHUR DO, LICENSE NUMBER 0001310 OF 1241 S. PARKER ROAD #201-202, DENVER, CO, WAS DISCIPLINED BY FLORIDA ON OCTOBER 14, 1998
DISCIPLINARY ACTION: LICENSE REVOCATION
OFFENSE: DISCIPLINARY ACTION BY ANOTHER STATE OR AGENCY

NOTES: ON OR ABOUT 2/18/94 THE COLORADO BOARD REVOKED HIS LICENSE DUE TO NUMEROUS ACTS OF UNPROFESSIONAL CONDUCT, INCLUDING SEVERAL INSTANCES OF SUBSTANDARD PRACTICE AND SEXUAL CONDUCT WITH PATIENTS; WAS CONSIDERED UNABLE TO PRACTICE WITH REASONABLE SKILL AND SAFETY TO PATIENTS DUE TO A MENTAL DISABILITY; ON OR ABOUT 6/21/95 THE MISSOURI BOARD REVOKED HIS LICENSE BASED ON THE COLORADO ACTION ALONG WITH THE CALIFORNIA BOARD ON 1/29/96; FAILED TO NOTIFY THE FLORIDA BOARD THAT ACTION WAS TAKEN AGAINST HIS LICENSE IN ANOTHER STATE.

EDWARDS, JAMES E MD, DATE OF BIRTH MARCH 24, 1924, LICENSE

NUMBER 0013098 OF COLORADO SPRINGS, CO, WAS DISCIPLINED BY COLORADO ON AUGUST 20, 1993
DISCIPLINARY ACTION: SURRENDER OF CONTROLLED SUBSTANCE LICENSE
OFFENSE: SUBSTANDARD CARE, INCOMPETENCE OR NEGLIGENCE
NOTES: ALLEGATIONS OF SUBSTANDARD PATIENT CARE.

EDWARDS, JAMES E MD, DATE OF BIRTH MARCH 24, 1924 OF 2727 N CHELTON ROAD, COLORADO SPRINGS, CO, WAS DISCIPLINED BY DEA ON FEBRUARY 16, 1994
DISCIPLINARY ACTION: SURRENDER OF CONTROLLED SUBSTANCE LICENSE
OFFENSE: DISCIPLINARY ACTION BY ANOTHER STATE OR AGENCY
NOTES: HE CAN NO LONGER ADMINISTER, DISPENSE OR PRESCRIBE CONTROLLED SUBSTANCES PER ORDER OF COLORADO MEDICAL BOARD.

ELGIN, JAMES C DO, DATE OF BIRTH JANUARY 30, 1951, LICENSE NUMBER 0023915 OF COLORADO SPRINGS, CO, WAS DISCIPLINED BY COLORADO ON APRIL 14, 1994
DISCIPLINARY ACTION: REPRIMAND
OFFENSE: PROFESSIONAL MISCONDUCT

ELGIN, JAMES C DO, DATE OF BIRTH JANUARY 30, 1951, LICENSE NUMBER 0023915, WAS DISCIPLINED BY COLORADO ON JUNE 13, 1996
DISCIPLINARY ACTION: 60-MONTH PROBATION; MONITORING OF PHYSICIAN PERFORMANCE
OFFENSE: SUBSTANCE ABUSE
NOTES: HABITUAL INTEMPERANCE OR EXCESSIVE USE OF A CONTROLLED SUBSTANCE. TREATMENT AND PRACTICE MONITORING.

ELGIN, JAMES C DO, DATE OF BIRTH JANUARY 30, 1951, LICENSE NUMBER 23915, WAS DISCIPLINED BY COLORADO ON MAY 14, 1997
DISCIPLINARY ACTION: REPRIMAND

ELGIN, JAMES CASEY DO, DATE OF BIRTH JANUARY 30, 1951, LICENSE NUMBER 23915, WAS DISCIPLINED BY COLORADO ON AUGUST 18, 1999
DISCIPLINARY ACTION: 60-MONTH PROBATION; MONITORING OF PHYSICIAN PERFORMANCE
NOTES: NO UNPROFESSIONAL CONDUCT IDENTIFIED. AGREES TO RECOMMENCE PERIOD OF PROBATION, WITH THE FOLLOWING TERMS: ABSTINENCE FROM ALCOHOL AND CONTROLLED SUBSTANCES, TREATMENT MONITORING AND PRACTICE MONITORING.

ELKIN, SCOTT RICHARD DO, DATE OF BIRTH APRIL 8, 1950, LICENSE NUMBER 00G1644 OF 5806 MESA DRIVE SUITE 375, AUSTIN, TX, WAS DISCIPLINED BY TEXAS ON DECEMBER 4, 1991
DISCIPLINARY ACTION: 60-MONTH PROBATION; 60-MONTH REQUIRED TO TAKE ADDITIONAL MEDICAL EDUCATION
OFFENSE: PROFESSIONAL MISCONDUCT
NOTES: SEVERAL TIMES BETWEEN 11/6/89 AND 2/14/90 HE SIGNED INSURANCE FORMS FOR A PATIENT REPRESENTING HE HAD PROVIDED PSYCHOTHERAPY, WHEN IN FACT IT HAD BEEN PERFORMED BY AN UNLICENSED PSYCHOTHERAPIST. SUSPENSION STAYED. CONDITIONS OF PROBATION: SHALL COMPLETE FIVE HOURS PER YEAR OF AN ETHICS COURSE; SHALL REFRAIN FROM SIGNING INSURANCE FORMS AND/OR ATTENDING PHYSICIAN STATEMENTS FOR PATIENTS HE HAS NOT PERSONALLY TREATED; SHALL APPEAR BEFORE THE BOARD ONCE A YEAR; SHALL COOPERATE WITH BOARD IN VERIFYING COMPLIANCE; SHALL ADVISE THE BOARD OF CHANGE OF ADDRESS WITHIN 10 DAYS; TIME SPENT OUT OF TEXAS DOES NOT COUNT TOWARD PROBATION; MAY NOT PETITION FOR MODIFICATION FOR AT LEAST ONE YEAR. ON 8/20/93, ORDER TERMINATED AND LICENSE FREE AND CLEAR OF ANY PREVIOUS RESTRICTIONS.

ELKIN, SCOTT RICHARD DO, DATE OF BIRTH APRIL 8, 1950, LICENSE NUMBER 0023916 OF AUSTIN, TX, WAS DISCIPLINED BY COLORADO ON FEBRUARY 11, 1994
DISCIPLINARY ACTION: REPRIMAND
OFFENSE: DISCIPLINARY ACTION BY ANOTHER STATE OR AGENCY
NOTES: DISCIPLINARY ACTION TAKEN BY TEXAS.

ELLIBEE, GARY S MD, DATE OF BIRTH DECEMBER 29, 1933, LICENSE NUMBER 0024353 OF GRAND JUNCTION, CO, WAS DISCIPLINED BY COLORADO ON SEPTEMBER 10, 1993
DISCIPLINARY ACTION: LICENSE SUSPENSION; REQUIRED TO TAKE ADDITIONAL MEDICAL EDUCATION
OFFENSE: SUBSTANDARD CARE, INCOMPETENCE OR NEGLIGENCE
NOTES: SUBSTANDARD PATIENT CARE. LICENSE SUSPENDED UNTIL HE HAS SUCCESSFULLY COMPLETED A MINIMUM OF ONE YEAR FULL-TIME RESIDENCY TRAINING. UPON COMPLETION OF RETRAINING, AT SUCH TIME, HE MAY REQUEST THAT HIS LICENSE BE REINSTATED, AND IF GRANTED, HE SHALL UNDERGO FIVE YEARS OF TREATMENT AND PRACTICE MONITORING.

EMERSON, JOHN H MD, DATE OF BIRTH AUGUST 21, 1952, LICENSE NUMBER 30269, WAS DISCIPLINED BY COLORADO ON MAY 21, 1999
DISCIPLINARY ACTION: 60-MONTH PROBATION; RESTRICTION PLACED ON LICENSE
OFFENSE: SEXUAL ABUSE OF OR SEXUAL MISCONDUCT WITH A PATIENT
NOTES: SEXUAL CONTACT WITH A PATIENT; FAILURE TO KEEP PROPER RECORDS. PROBATIONARY TERMS INCLUDE: REEDUCATION ACTIVITIES, BOUNDARIES COURSE, USE OF A CHAPERONE AND PRACTICE MONITORING.

EPPLER, STEPHEN V MD, DATE OF BIRTH JANUARY 12, 1952, LICENSE NUMBER 23920, WAS DISCIPLINED BY COLORADO ON OCTOBER 21, 1999
DISCIPLINARY ACTION: 60-MONTH PROBATION; RESTRICTION PLACED ON LICENSE
OFFENSE: SEXUAL ABUSE OF OR SEXUAL MISCONDUCT WITH A PATIENT
NOTES: SEXUAL CONTACT WITH A PATIENT. PROBATIONARY TERMS INCLUDE: BOUNDARIES EDUCATION, REQUIREMENT OF A CHAPERONE AND PRACTICE MONITORING.

ERDOES, LUKE S MD, DATE OF BIRTH FEBRUARY 5, 1958, LICENSE NUMBER 0027079 OF TUCSON, AZ, WAS DISCIPLINED BY COLORADO ON NOVEMBER 19, 1993
DISCIPLINARY ACTION: REPRIMAND

EWING, ROBERT K DO, DATE OF BIRTH JUNE 2, 1946, LICENSE NUMBER 0028915 OF LITTLETON, CO, WAS DISCIPLINED BY COLORADO ON OCTOBER 13, 1994
DISCIPLINARY ACTION: REPRIMAND

EZELL, WILLIAM W MD, DATE OF BIRTH AUGUST 1, 1935, LICENSE NUMBER 16049, WAS DISCIPLINED BY COLORADO ON JULY 17, 1997
DISCIPLINARY ACTION: REPRIMAND

FALZONE, JOSEPH A III MD, DATE OF BIRTH OCTOBER 20, 1954, LICENSE NUMBER 0023925, WAS DISCIPLINED BY COLORADO ON JULY 18, 1996
DISCIPLINARY ACTION: EMERGENCY SUSPENSION

FALZONE, JOSEPH A III MD, DATE OF BIRTH OCTOBER 20, 1954, LICENSE NUMBER 23925, WAS DISCIPLINED BY COLORADO ON AUGUST 13, 1997
DISCIPLINARY ACTION: LICENSE REVOCATION
OFFENSE: SUBSTANDARD CARE, INCOMPETENCE OR NEGLIGENCE

NOTES: SUBSTANDARD CARE; FAILURE TO TIMELY RESPOND TO A 30 DAY LETTER.

FARRIN, JOHN C MD, DATE OF BIRTH JULY 24, 1947, LICENSE NUMBER 22431, WAS DISCIPLINED BY COLORADO ON JULY 9, 1998
DISCIPLINARY ACTION: REPRIMAND

FECTEAU, MICHELE A DO, DATE OF BIRTH MAY 2, 1955, LICENSE NUMBER 27080, WAS DISCIPLINED BY COLORADO ON MAY 2, 1997
DISCIPLINARY ACTION: EMERGENCY SUSPENSION
OFFENSE: SUBSTANCE ABUSE

NOTES: HABITUAL INTEMPERANCE; EXCESSIVE USE OF HABIT-FORMING DRUGS OR CONTROLLED SUBSTANCES. ON 12/18/97 THIS ORDER LIFTED AND SHE AGREED TO NOT PRACTICE FOR AN INDEFINITE TIME; IF SHE DOES RETURN TO PRACTICE SHE MUST BEGIN PROBATION WITH TERMS.

FELDMAN, ARMIN MD, DATE OF BIRTH AUGUST 6, 1949, LICENSE NUMBER 20744, WAS DISCIPLINED BY COLORADO ON MARCH 13, 1997
DISCIPLINARY ACTION: MONITORING OF PHYSICIAN PERFORMANCE

NOTES: NO UNPROFESSIONAL CONDUCT IDENTIFIED. HE AGREES TO CEASE PRACTICING, TO REMAIN ABSTINENT AND TO UNDERGO TREATMENT MONITORING. THIS IS AN INTERIM AGREEMENT PENDING FINAL AGENCY ACTION.

FELDMAN, ARMIN MD, DATE OF BIRTH AUGUST 6, 1949, LICENSE NUMBER 20744, WAS DISCIPLINED BY COLORADO ON FEBRUARY 17, 1999
DISCIPLINARY ACTION: PROBATION; RESTRICTION PLACED ON CONTROLLED SUBSTANCE LICENSE
OFFENSE: SUBSTANDARD CARE, INCOMPETENCE OR NEGLIGENCE

NOTES: ADMINISTERING A CONTROLLED SUBSTANCE OTHER THAN IN THE COURSE OF LEGITIMATE PROFESSIONAL PRACTICE; A VIOLATION OF A LAW REGULATING CONTROLLED SUBSTANCES; HABITUAL INTEMPERANCE OR EXCESSIVE USE OF A CONTROLLED SUBSTANCE; SUBSTANDARD CARE; SEXUAL CONTACT WITH A PATIENT; GIVING A SCHEDULE II SUBSTANCE TO SELF OR A FAMILY MEMBER; AND FAILURE TO ACCURATELY ANSWER A RENEWAL FORM. INDEFINITE PERIOD OF PROBATION WHICH TERMS INCLUDE: A RESTRICTION FROM OBTAINING A DRUG ENFORCEMENT ADMINISTRATION CERTIFICATE; ABSTINENCE FROM ALCOHOL AND CONTROLLED SUBSTANCES; A MEDICAL EDUCATION PLAN; TREATMENT MONITORING AND PRACTICE MONITORING.

FELDMAN, ARMIN IRA MD OF 1644 EMERSON STREET, DENVER, CO, WAS DISCIPLINED BY DEA ON AUGUST 11, 1997
DISCIPLINARY ACTION: SURRENDER OF CONTROLLED SUBSTANCE LICENSE

FERN, DONALD EDWIN DO, DATE OF BIRTH JANUARY 6, 1929, LICENSE NUMBER 0000923 OF FORT LUPTON, CO, WAS DISCIPLINED BY IOWA ON DECEMBER 4, 1990
DISCIPLINARY ACTION: LICENSE SUSPENSION
OFFENSE: DISCIPLINARY ACTION BY ANOTHER STATE OR AGENCY

NOTES: INDEFINITE SUSPENSION.

FERN, DONALD EDWIN DO, DATE OF BIRTH JANUARY 6, 1929, LICENSE NUMBER 0012384 OF FT LUPTON, CO, WAS DISCIPLINED BY COLORADO ON FEBRUARY 14, 1992
DISCIPLINARY ACTION: PROBATION; REQUIRED TO TAKE ADDITIONAL MEDICAL EDUCATION
OFFENSE: SUBSTANDARD CARE, INCOMPETENCE OR NEGLIGENCE

NOTES: FAILURE TO MEET GENERALLY ACCEPTED STANDARDS OF MEDICAL PRACTICE. AMENDMENT TO STIPULATION AND ORDER OF 2/16/88. IMPOSES ADDED DISCIPLINE: MUST PARTICIPATE IN COLORADO PERSONALIZED EDUCATION FOR PHYSICIANS PROGRAM AND PROBATION EXTENDED FOR AN INDEFINITE PERIOD.

FERN, DONALD EDWIN DO, DATE OF BIRTH JANUARY 6, 1929, LICENSE NUMBER 0012384, WAS DISCIPLINED BY COLORADO ON JUNE 12, 1992
DISCIPLINARY ACTION: SURRENDER OF LICENSE

NOTES: SECOND AMENDMENT TO STIPULATION AND ORDER DATED 2/16/88 FOR RETIREMENT AND LICENSE SURRENDER AS OF 9/30/92; ORIGINAL STIPULATION REMAINS IN EFFECT (EXCEPT COMPLIANCE WITH ADDITIONAL EDUCATION REQUIREMENTS OF AMENDMENT DATED 2/14/92).

FERNON, CHRIS J DO, LICENSE NUMBER 5355A, WAS DISCIPLINED BY WYOMING ON JANUARY 31, 1998
DISCIPLINARY ACTION: RESTRICTION PLACED ON CONTROLLED SUBSTANCE LICENSE; REQUIRED TO TAKE ADDITIONAL MEDICAL EDUCATION
OFFENSE: OVERPRESCRIBING OR MISPRESCRIBING DRUGS

NOTES: ALLEGATIONS THAT HE PRESCRIBED SCHEDULE II NARCOTICS FOR A 30 DAY PERIOD WITHOUT HAVING FIRST SEEN HER IN PERSON AS A PATIENT, AND WITHOUT HAVING FIRST ESTABLISHED A MEDICAL JUSTIFICATION FOR SUCH PRESCRIBING BY PERSONALLY PERFORMING A PHYSICAL EXAMINATION. SHALL NOT PRESCRIBE ANY MEDICATION TO ANY PATIENT WHICH HE HAS NOT PERSONALLY SEEN; SHALL SUCCESSFULLY COMPLETE AN INTENSIVE BOARD-APPROVED CONTINUING MEDICAL EDUCATION SEMINAR OR WORKSHOP IN THE AREA OF APPROPRIATE PRESCRIBING OF MEDICATIONS WITHIN 12 MONTHS.

FERNON, CHRIS J DO, DATE OF BIRTH JANUARY 11, 1956, LICENSE NUMBER 34279, WAS DISCIPLINED BY COLORADO ON FEBRUARY 19, 1999
DISCIPLINARY ACTION: REPRIMAND; REQUIRED TO TAKE ADDITIONAL MEDICAL EDUCATION
OFFENSE: SUBSTANDARD CARE, INCOMPETENCE OR NEGLIGENCE

NOTES: SUBSTANDARD CARE. MUST UNDERGO REEDUCATION ACTIVITIES.

FERNON, CHRIS J DO, DATE OF BIRTH JANUARY 11, 1956, LICENSE NUMBER 34279, WAS DISCIPLINED BY COLORADO ON AUGUST 20, 1999
DISCIPLINARY ACTION: SURRENDER OF LICENSE

NOTES: NO UNPROFESSIONAL CONDUCT IDENTIFIED.

FERRIS, JOHN MD OF ARVADA, CO, WAS DISCIPLINED BY ILLINOIS ON JANUARY 1, 1993
DISCIPLINARY ACTION: LICENSE SUSPENSION
OFFENSE: DISCIPLINARY ACTION BY ANOTHER STATE OR AGENCY

NOTES: DISCIPLINED BY ARIZONA. INDEFINITE SUSPENSION.

FILA, ERNEST G MD, DATE OF BIRTH FEBRUARY 5, 1932, LICENSE NUMBER 0022946 OF LITTLETON, CO, WAS DISCIPLINED BY COLORADO ON FEBRUARY 18, 1994
DISCIPLINARY ACTION: 60-MONTH PROBATION; MONITORING OF PHYSICIAN PERFORMANCE
OFFENSE: SUBSTANDARD CARE, INCOMPETENCE OR NEGLIGENCE

NOTES: ALLEGATIONS OF ISSUES INVOLVING PATIENT CARE. PROBATION UNDER TERMS AND CONDITIONS INCLUDING PRACTICE MONITORING.

FILA, ERNEST GEORGE MD, LICENSE NUMBER FE40729 OF LITTLETON, CO, WAS DISCIPLINED BY CALIFORNIA ON JUNE 24, 1996
DISCIPLINARY ACTION: 60-MONTH PROBATION
OFFENSE: DISCIPLINARY ACTION BY ANOTHER STATE OR AGENCY

NOTES: ACTION IN COLORADO FOR SUBSTANDARD MEDICAL CARE AND TREATMENT OF TWO PATIENTS WITH CARDIOPULMONARY PROBLEMS. REVOCATION, STAYED. WILL TAKE EFFECT IF AND WHEN HIS LICENSE IS RETURNED TO ACTIVE STATUS.

FILNER, IVAN M DO, DATE OF BIRTH APRIL 25, 1956, LICENSE NUMBER 29577, WAS DISCIPLINED BY COLORADO ON SEPTEMBER 10, 1998
DISCIPLINARY ACTION: REPRIMAND

FINEMAN, BRUCE G MD, DATE OF BIRTH FEBRUARY 6, 1949, LICENSE NUMBER 0020872 OF DENVER, CO, WAS DISCIPLINED BY COLORADO ON DECEMBER 13, 1991
DISCIPLINARY ACTION: 60-MONTH PROBATION; REQUIRED TO ENTER AN IMPAIRED PHYSICIAN PROGRAM OR SUBSTANCE ABUSE TREATMENT
OFFENSE: SUBSTANCE ABUSE

NOTES: SUBSTANCE ABUSE AND DEPENDENCE. DRUG TREATMENT AND MONITORING AND PRACTICE MONITORING.

FISHER, THOMAS C MD OF 1136 EAST STUART #4202, FORT COLLINS, CO, WAS DISCIPLINED BY DEA ON NOVEMBER 30, 1995
DISCIPLINARY ACTION: SURRENDER OF CONTROLLED SUBSTANCE LICENSE
OFFENSE: DISCIPLINARY ACTION BY ANOTHER STATE OR AGENCY

NOTES: IN LIEU OF ORDER TO SHOW CAUSE.

FISHER, THOMAS C MD, DATE OF BIRTH DECEMBER 11, 1953, LICENSE NUMBER 0028126, WAS DISCIPLINED BY COLORADO ON APRIL 11, 1996
DISCIPLINARY ACTION: 60-MONTH PROBATION; MONITORING OF PHYSICIAN PERFORMANCE
OFFENSE: SUBSTANCE ABUSE

NOTES: HABITUAL INTEMPERANCE OR EXCESSIVE USE OF A CONTROLLED SUBSTANCE AND MENTAL DISABILITY. TREATMENT AND PRACTICE MONITORING PROVISIONS.

FLORA, MARK S MD, DATE OF BIRTH SEPTEMBER 23, 1953, LICENSE NUMBER 0025779 OF WESTMINSTER, CO, WAS DISCIPLINED BY COLORADO ON FEBRUARY 9, 1995
DISCIPLINARY ACTION: 60-MONTH PROBATION; MONITORING OF PHYSICIAN PERFORMANCE
OFFENSE: SUBSTANCE ABUSE

NOTES: HABITUAL INTEMPERANCE OR EXCESSIVE USE OF A CONTROLLED SUBSTANCE. PROBATION INCLUDES PRACTICE AND TREATMENT MONITORING.

FLORA, MARK S MD, DATE OF BIRTH SEPTEMBER 23, 1953, LICENSE NUMBER 25779, WAS DISCIPLINED BY COLORADO ON JUNE 12, 1996
DISCIPLINARY ACTION: EMERGENCY SUSPENSION

FLORA, MARK S MD, DATE OF BIRTH SEPTEMBER 23, 1953, LICENSE NUMBER 25779, WAS DISCIPLINED BY COLORADO ON NOVEMBER 12, 1997
DISCIPLINARY ACTION: 60-MONTH PROBATION; MONITORING OF PHYSICIAN PERFORMANCE
OFFENSE: FAILURE TO COMPLY WITH PREVIOUS BOARD ORDER

NOTES: VIOLATION OF A VALID BOARD ORDER; HABITUAL INTEMPERANCE OR EXCESSIVE USE OF A CONTROLLED SUBSTANCE. PROBATIONARY TERMS INCLUDE: AGREES TO REMAIN ABSTINENT FROM ALCOHOL AND CONTROLLED SUBSTANCES, TREATMENT MONITORING AND PRACTICE MONITORING.

FOGEL, TIMOTHY J MD, LICENSE NUMBER 0013269 OF BEULAH, CO, WAS DISCIPLINED BY COLORADO ON NOVEMBER 9, 1990
DISCIPLINARY ACTION: RESTRICTION PLACED ON LICENSE
OFFENSE: SUBSTANDARD CARE, INCOMPETENCE OR NEGLIGENCE

NOTES: PHYSICAL OR MENTAL DISABILITY WHICH RENDERS HIM UNABLE TO PROVIDE MEDICAL SERVICES WITH REASONABLE SKILL AND SAFETY. ORDER RESTRICTS HIS PERFORMANCE OF SURGERY OR SURGICAL PROCEDURES.

FOGEL, TIMOTHY J MD, LICENSE NUMBER 0A15451 OF BEULAH, CO, WAS DISCIPLINED BY CALIFORNIA ON AUGUST 20, 1993
DISCIPLINARY ACTION: LICENSE REVOCATION
OFFENSE: DISCIPLINARY ACTION BY ANOTHER STATE OR AGENCY

NOTES: DISCIPLINED BY COLORADO BOARD. DEFAULT DECISION.

FONTANA, N JOHN II MD, DATE OF BIRTH NOVEMBER 7, 1932, LICENSE NUMBER 0029501 OF VAIL, CO, WAS DISCIPLINED BY COLORADO ON FEBRUARY 21, 1992
DISCIPLINARY ACTION: SURRENDER OF LICENSE
OFFENSE: CRIMINAL CONVICTION OR PLEA OF GUILTY, NOLO CONTENDERE, OR NO CONTEST TO A CRIME

NOTES: FELONY CONVICTION FOR BANK FRAUD AND TRANSPORTATION OF FRAUDULENT SECURITIES (CHECK KITING).

FOSTER, WILLIAM MD, DATE OF BIRTH OCTOBER 28, 1944, LICENSE NUMBER 0019258 OF WELLINGTON, CO, WAS DISCIPLINED BY COLORADO ON MARCH 18, 1994
DISCIPLINARY ACTION: REPRIMAND
OFFENSE: PROFESSIONAL MISCONDUCT

FRANK, BARRY W MD, DATE OF BIRTH SEPTEMBER 28, 1934, LICENSE NUMBER 0013579 OF DENVER, CO, WAS DISCIPLINED BY COLORADO ON NOVEMBER 3, 1994
DISCIPLINARY ACTION: REPRIMAND

FREED, CHARLES R MD, DATE OF BIRTH FEBRUARY 18, 1918, LICENSE NUMBER 11582, WAS DISCIPLINED BY COLORADO ON NOVEMBER 14, 1997

DISCIPLINARY ACTION: SURRENDER OF LICENSE

NOTES: NO UNPROFESSIONAL CONDUCT IDENTIFIED.

FREUDENBURG, JAMES C MD, DATE OF BIRTH AUGUST 1, 1949, LICENSE NUMBER 0020749, WAS DISCIPLINED BY COLORADO ON NOVEMBER 16, 1996
DISCIPLINARY ACTION: 3-MONTH LICENSE SUSPENSION; REQUIRED TO TAKE ADDITIONAL MEDICAL EDUCATION

NOTES: FIVE YEAR PRACTICE MONITORING, AND ENROLLMENT IN A COURSE ON PRESCRIBING PRACTICES AND RECORDKEEPING.

FRITZ, ROBERT L MD, DATE OF BIRTH OCTOBER 28, 1945, LICENSE NUMBER 0031881, WAS DISCIPLINED BY COLORADO ON MAY 17, 1996
DISCIPLINARY ACTION: EMERGENCY SUSPENSION

FRITZ, ROBERT L MD, DATE OF BIRTH OCTOBER 28, 1945, LICENSE NUMBER 0031881, WAS DISCIPLINED BY COLORADO ON SEPTEMBER 19, 1996
DISCIPLINARY ACTION: SURRENDER OF LICENSE
OFFENSE: SUBSTANCE ABUSE

NOTES: HABITUAL INTEMPERANCE OR EXCESSIVE USE OF A CONTROLLED SUBSTANCE; SUBSTANDARD CARE AND ADMINISTERING A CONTROLLED SUBSTANCE OTHER THAN IN THE COURSE OF LEGITIMATE PROFESSIONAL PRACTICE.

FRITZ, ROBERT LESLIE MD OF 209 SOUTH NEVADA AVENUE, COLORADO SPRINGS, CO, WAS DISCIPLINED BY DEA ON MAY 29, 1996
DISCIPLINARY ACTION: SURRENDER OF CONTROLLED SUBSTANCE LICENSE

NOTES: IN LIEU OF ORDER TO SHOW CAUSE.

GADPAILLE, WARREN MD, DATE OF BIRTH MARCH 12, 1924, LICENSE NUMBER 0013420 OF CONIFER, CO, WAS DISCIPLINED BY COLORADO ON JUNE 11, 1993
DISCIPLINARY ACTION: 60-MONTH PROBATION; MONITORING OF PHYSICIAN PERFORMANCE
OFFENSE: OVERPRESCRIBING OR MISPRESCRIBING DRUGS

NOTES: PRESCRIBING CONTROLLED SUBSTANCES OTHER THAN IN THE COURSE OF LEGITIMATE PROFESSIONAL PRACTICE; SELF-PRESCRIBING OF A SCHEDULE II CONTROLLED SUBSTANCE. CONDITIONS OF PROBATION INCLUDE TREATMENT MONITORING.

GALE, JOHN H MD, DATE OF BIRTH AUGUST 9, 1948, LICENSE NUMBER 0021707 OF GOLDEN, CO, WAS DISCIPLINED BY COLORADO ON JUNE 11, 1993
DISCIPLINARY ACTION: REPRIMAND
OFFENSE: SUBSTANDARD CARE, INCOMPETENCE OR NEGLIGENCE

NOTES: SUBSTANDARD CARE.

GALLAGHER, MICHAEL J MD, DATE OF BIRTH JULY 16, 1951, LICENSE NUMBER 0027393 OF 1036 ROCKAFELLOW COURT, CANON CITY, CO, WAS DISCIPLINED BY COLORADO ON JANUARY 15, 1992
DISCIPLINARY ACTION: LICENSE REVOCATION
OFFENSE: SEXUAL ABUSE OF OR SEXUAL MISCONDUCT WITH A PATIENT

NOTES: ON 10/15/87 ENGAGED IN SEXUAL CONTACT WITH A MINOR PATIENT DURING THE COURSE OF ANESTHESIOLOGY TREATMENT DURING SURGERY WHICH CONSTITUTED GROSS NEGLIGENCE; AT THE TIME HE SUFFERED FROM A PSYCHIATRIC ILLNESS WHICH HAD BEEN DIAGNOSED AS LONGSTANDING DEPRESSION OF SIGNIFICANT PROPORTIONS; ALSO SUFFERED A DISSOCIATIVE DISORDER WHICH CAUSED HIM TO BE FUNDAMENTALLY UNAWARE OF WHAT HE WAS DOING; SHORTLY AFTER THIS INCIDENT HE WAS HOSPITALIZED FOR PSYCHIATRIC CARE AND TREATMENT; COLORADO LICENSE WAS SUSPENDED ON 2/12/88 FOR AN INDEFINITE PERIOD OF TIME AND HE WAS COMMITTED TO A STATE HOSPITAL IN 11/88; SINCE 3/91 HE HAS RECEIVED TREATMENT ON AN OUTPATIENT BASIS; ALTHOUGH HE IS NOT NOW PSYCHIATRICALLY DISABLED, HE STILL DOES NOT UNDERSTAND OR RECALL THE EVENTS DISCUSSED ABOVE. NO PSYCHIATRIC DISABILITY. DR. GALLAGHER APPEALED THE FINAL BOARD ORDER TO THE COLORADO COURT OF APPEALS WHICH AFFIRMED THE BOARD ORDER ON 2/11/93.

GALVIN, JAMES MD, LICENSE NUMBER 0042740 OF 1330 GAYLORD ST, DENVER, CO, WAS DISCIPLINED BY NEW YORK ON OCTOBER 21, 1992
DISCIPLINARY ACTION: SURRENDER OF LICENSE
OFFENSE: DISCIPLINARY ACTION BY ANOTHER STATE OR AGENCY

NOTES: DID NOT CONTEST CHARGES RELATING TO ACTION TAKEN AGAINST HIS LICENSE IN COLORADO.

GARBER, GEORGE MD, LICENSE NUMBER 0018794 OF MCALESTER, OK, WAS DISCIPLINED BY COLORADO ON JULY 17, 1990
DISCIPLINARY ACTION: RESTRICTION PLACED ON LICENSE; MONITORING OF PHYSICIAN PERFORMANCE
OFFENSE: SUBSTANDARD CARE, INCOMPETENCE OR NEGLIGENCE

NOTES: INABILITY TO PRACTICE WITH REASONABLE SKILL AND SAFETY TO PATIENTS. CONSENT ORDER MANDATING FAVORABLE PHYSICAL/MENTAL EXAMINATIONS, PRACTICE MONITORING, AND A GENERAL SURGERY PROHIBITION.

GARCEAU, ROGER MD, LICENSE NUMBER 0024465 OF PORTAGE, MI, WAS DISCIPLINED BY COLORADO ON OCTOBER 12, 1990
DISCIPLINARY ACTION: SURRENDER OF LICENSE
OFFENSE: SUBSTANDARD CARE, INCOMPETENCE OR NEGLIGENCE

NOTES: FAILED TO MEET GENERALLY ACCEPTED STANDARDS OF MEDICAL PRACTICE.

GARCIA, ALFRED G MD, DATE OF BIRTH NOVEMBER 1, 1947, LICENSE NUMBER 23218, WAS DISCIPLINED BY COLORADO ON FEBRUARY 12, 1997
DISCIPLINARY ACTION: REPRIMAND

GARCIA, ALFRED G MD, DATE OF BIRTH NOVEMBER 1, 1947, LICENSE NUMBER 23218, WAS DISCIPLINED BY COLORADO ON APRIL 7, 1997
DISCIPLINARY ACTION: REPRIMAND

GARGAN, THOMAS J III MD, DATE OF BIRTH SEPTEMBER 28, 1952, LICENSE NUMBER 25890, WAS DISCIPLINED BY COLORADO ON JANUARY 8, 1998
DISCIPLINARY ACTION: SURRENDER OF LICENSE
OFFENSE: PHYSICAL OR MENTAL ILLNESS INHIBITING THE ABILITY TO PRACTICE WITH SKILL AND SAFETY

NOTES: PHYSICAL OR MENTAL DISABILITY.

GARLAND, JAMES W DO, DATE OF BIRTH NOVEMBER 21, 1950, LICENSE NUMBER 0022442 OF COLORADO SPRINGS, CO, WAS DISCIPLINED BY COLORADO ON OCTOBER 13, 1993
DISCIPLINARY ACTION: REPRIMAND

GARRY, STEPHEN H MD, DATE OF BIRTH OCTOBER 10, 1952, LICENSE NUMBER 0023735 OF INDIANAPOLIS, IN, WAS DISCIPLINED BY COLORADO ON JUNE 14, 1991
OFFENSE: PHYSICAL OR MENTAL ILLNESS INHIBITING THE ABILITY TO PRACTICE WITH SKILL AND SAFETY

NOTES: PHYSICAL AND/OR MENTAL DISABILITY WHICH AFFECTS THE ABILITY TO PRACTICE MEDICINE WITH REASONABLE SKILL AND SAFETY. CONSENT ORDER WHEREBY HE AGREED NOT TO RENEW COLORADO MEDICAL LICENSE BEYOND 5/31/91.

GARTNER, CHARLES H MD, DATE OF BIRTH JUNE 12, 1942, LICENSE NUMBER 0016580 OF DENVER, CO, WAS DISCIPLINED BY COLORADO ON APRIL 14, 1995
DISCIPLINARY ACTION: 60-MONTH PROBATION; RESTRICTION PLACED ON LICENSE
OFFENSE: SUBSTANDARD CARE, INCOMPETENCE OR NEGLIGENCE

NOTES: SUBSTANDARD CARE. PROBATION INCLUDES RESTRICTIONS, PRACTICE MONITORING AND REEDUCATION ACTIVITIES.

GARTNER, CHARLES H MD, LICENSE NUMBER 0017295, WAS DISCIPLINED BY ARIZONA ON SEPTEMBER 19, 1996

NOTES: SHALL NOT PRACTICE MEDICINE IN ARIZONA UNTIL FIRST MEETING WITH THE BOARD AND UNTIL ORDER OF THE BOARD.

GASIS, ALBERT J MD, DATE OF BIRTH FEBRUARY 16, 1931, LICENSE NUMBER 0017944 OF ALBUQUERQUE, NM, WAS DISCIPLINED BY COLORADO ON OCTOBER 15, 1993
DISCIPLINARY ACTION: 60-MONTH PROBATION; RESTRICTION PLACED ON LICENSE
OFFENSE: SUBSTANDARD CARE, INCOMPETENCE OR NEGLIGENCE

NOTES: ALLEGATIONS OF SUBSTANDARD PATIENT CARE. PROBATIONARY PERIOD INCLUDES PRACTICE MONITORING; ORDER PROHIBITS SURGICAL PRACTICE.

GATCHELL, HOMER DALE DO, DATE OF BIRTH MAY 30, 1924, LICENSE NUMBER 0016452 OF COLORADO SPRINGS, CO, WAS DISCIPLINED BY COLORADO ON OCTOBER 7, 1992
DISCIPLINARY ACTION: RESTRICTION PLACED ON LICENSE
OFFENSE: SUBSTANDARD CARE, INCOMPETENCE OR NEGLIGENCE

NOTES: PRIMA FACIE CASE INVOLVING TWO OR MORE ACTS OR OMISSIONS WHICH FAILED TO MEET GENERALLY ACCEPTED STANDARDS OF MEDICAL PRACTICE. HE DENIES HE PROVIDED SUBSTANDARD CARE. PERMANENT LICENSE RESTRICTION: MAY NO LONGER CARE FOR OR TREAT NURSING HOME PATIENTS OR SERVE AS ON-CALL PHYSICIAN FOR NURSING HOME PATIENTS.

GEER, RICHARD MD OF 137 EAST TENTH STREET, DURANGO, CO, WAS DISCIPLINED BY NEW MEXICO ON JULY 28, 1993
OFFENSE: PROFESSIONAL MISCONDUCT

NOTES: LICENSE PLACED UNDER UNSPECIFIED CONDITIONS. PROBATION TERMINATED IN 1995; DONATED 1,000 FREE PATIENT VISITS.

GELINAS, MICHAEL P MD, DATE OF BIRTH MARCH 11, 1962, LICENSE NUMBER 0030450, WAS DISCIPLINED BY COLORADO ON NOVEMBER 20, 1996
DISCIPLINARY ACTION: MONITORING OF PHYSICIAN PERFORMANCE

NOTES: NO UNPROFESSIONAL CONDUCT IDENTIFIED. PREOPERATIVE APPROVAL FOR ANY OPHTHALMOLOGICAL SURGERY AND A SURGICAL PRECEPTOR AND A PRACTICE MONITOR. THIS IS ONLY AN INTERIM AGREEMENT AND DOES NOT CONSTITUTE FINAL AGENCY ACTION.

GELINAS, MICHAEL P MD, DATE OF BIRTH MARCH 11, 1962, LICENSE NUMBER 30450, WAS DISCIPLINED BY COLORADO ON NOVEMBER 14, 1997
DISCIPLINARY ACTION: 60-MONTH PROBATION; MONITORING OF PHYSICIAN PERFORMANCE
OFFENSE: SUBSTANDARD CARE, INCOMPETENCE OR NEGLIGENCE

NOTES: SUBSTANDARD CARE. FAILURE TO KEEP PROPER RECORDS. PROBATIONARY TERMS INCLUDE PRACTICE MONITORING.

GENTRY, ROBERT P MD, DATE OF BIRTH NOVEMBER 3, 1929, LICENSE NUMBER 14318, WAS DISCIPLINED BY COLORADO ON DECEMBER 31, 1997
DISCIPLINARY ACTION: SURRENDER OF LICENSE

NOTES: NO UNPROFESSIONAL CONDUCT IDENTIFIED.

GERMAN, CHARLES MD, DATE OF BIRTH SEPTEMBER 10, 1948, LICENSE NUMBER 0023464 OF PO BOX 3615, ENGLEWOOD, CO, WAS DISCIPLINED BY COLORADO ON OCTOBER 17, 1994
DISCIPLINARY ACTION: EMERGENCY SUSPENSION
OFFENSE: SEXUAL ABUSE OF OR SEXUAL MISCONDUCT WITH A PATIENT

NOTES: ENGAGED IN A SEXUAL ACT WITH A PATIENT. PENDING PROCEEDINGS TO DETERMINE WHETHER HIS LICENSE SHOULD BE FURTHER DISCIPLINED. CHARGED ON 10/12/94 WITH TWO COUNTS OF SEXUAL ASSAULT IN THE SECOND DEGREE AND ONE COUNT OF SEXUAL ASSAULT IN THE THIRD DEGREE IN ARAPAHOE COUNTY COURT. FELONY COMPLAINT/INFORMATION ALLEGES THAT ON OR ABOUT 8/12/94 DR. GERMAN SUBJECTED A FEMALE PATIENT TO SEXUAL CONTACT WHILE ENGAGED IN TREATMENT AND EXAMINATION FOR OTHER THAN BONAFIDE MEDICAL PURPOSES AND IN A MANNER SUBSTANTIALLY INCONSISTENT WITH REASONABLE MEDICAL PRACTICE.

GERMAN, CHARLES MD, DATE OF BIRTH SEPTEMBER 10, 1948, LICENSE NUMBER 0023464 OF PO BOX 3615, ENGLEWOOD, CO, WAS DISCIPLINED BY COLORADO ON NOVEMBER 18, 1994
DISCIPLINARY ACTION: LICENSE REVOCATION
OFFENSE: PHYSICAL OR MENTAL ILLNESS INHIBITING THE ABILITY TO PRACTICE WITH SKILL AND SAFETY

NOTES: MENTAL DISABILITY ISSUES. HE DENIES ALLEGATIONS. AGREES NEVER TO REAPPLY FOR A COLORADO MEDICAL LICENSE.

GERMAN, CHARLES MD, LICENSE NUMBER 0125071 OF 150 EAST 10TH ST, DENVER, CO, WAS DISCIPLINED BY NEW YORK ON NOVEMBER 7, 1995
DISCIPLINARY ACTION: SURRENDER OF LICENSE
OFFENSE: DISCIPLINARY ACTION BY ANOTHER STATE OR AGENCY

NOTES: ACTION IN COLORADO FOR HAVING A MENTAL DISABILITY WHICH RENDERS HIM UNABLE TO PERFORM MEDICAL SERVICES WITH REASONABLE SKILL AND SAFETY.

GIDWANI, ASHOK M MD, LICENSE NUMBER 140760 OF 9528 COLONIAL DRIVE, BOULDER, CO, WAS DISCIPLINED BY NEW YORK ON MARCH 26, 1997
DISCIPLINARY ACTION: SURRENDER OF LICENSE
OFFENSE: DISCIPLINARY ACTION BY ANOTHER STATE OR AGENCY

NOTES: DISCIPLINED BY THE CALIFORNIA BOARD FOR HAVING

BEEN CONVICTED OF SOLICITING ANOTHER TO COMMIT ASSAULT WITH A DEADLY WEAPON.

GIDWANI, ASHOK MOTILAL MD, LICENSE NUMBER 0A36815 OF LITTLETON, CO, WAS DISCIPLINED BY CALIFORNIA ON MAY 22, 1996
DISCIPLINARY ACTION: 60-MONTH PROBATION
OFFENSE: CRIMINAL CONVICTION OR PLEA OF GUILTY, NOLO CONTENDERE, OR NO CONTEST TO A CRIME
NOTES: CONVICTION FOR SOLICITING ANOTHER TO COMMIT AN ASSAULT. REVOCATION, STAYED.

GIERINGER, GARY V MD, DATE OF BIRTH NOVEMBER 21, 1934, LICENSE NUMBER 0015247 OF COLORADO SPRINGS, CO, WAS DISCIPLINED BY COLORADO ON JULY 15, 1994
DISCIPLINARY ACTION: 60-MONTH PROBATION; REQUIRED TO TAKE ADDITIONAL MEDICAL EDUCATION
OFFENSE: PHYSICAL OR MENTAL ILLNESS INHIBITING THE ABILITY TO PRACTICE WITH SKILL AND SAFETY
NOTES: PHYSICAL OR MENTAL DISABILITY ISSUES. PROBATION INCLUDES LIFETIME TREATMENT MONITORING; FIVE YEAR PROBATION INCLUDING PRACTICE MONITORING AND CONTINUING PROFESSIONAL EDUCATION FOR PHYSICIANS REQUIREMENTS.

GIERINGER, GARY V MD, DATE OF BIRTH NOVEMBER 21, 1934, LICENSE NUMBER 0015247, WAS DISCIPLINED BY COLORADO ON MAY 23, 1995
DISCIPLINARY ACTION: EMERGENCY SUSPENSION
OFFENSE: FAILURE TO COMPLY WITH PREVIOUS BOARD ORDER
NOTES: DUE TO NONCOMPLIANCE WITH A PREVIOUS ORDER.

GIERINGER, GARY V MD, DATE OF BIRTH NOVEMBER 21, 1934, LICENSE NUMBER 0015247, WAS DISCIPLINED BY COLORADO ON APRIL 15, 1996
DISCIPLINARY ACTION: LICENSE SUSPENSION

GIERINGER, GARY V MD, DATE OF BIRTH NOVEMBER 21, 1934, LICENSE NUMBER 15247, WAS DISCIPLINED BY COLORADO ON FEBRUARY 14, 1997
DISCIPLINARY ACTION: PROBATION; MONITORING OF PHYSICIAN PERFORMANCE
OFFENSE: SUBSTANDARD CARE, INCOMPETENCE OR NEGLIGENCE
NOTES: SUBSTANDARD CARE; VIOLATION OF THE MEDICAL PRACTICE ACT. PRACTICE AND TREATMENT MONITORING.

GIERINGER, GARY V MD, DATE OF BIRTH NOVEMBER 21, 1934, LICENSE NUMBER 15247, WAS DISCIPLINED BY COLORADO ON JULY 17, 1997
DISCIPLINARY ACTION: EMERGENCY SUSPENSION

GIERINGER, GARY V MD, DATE OF BIRTH NOVEMBER 21, 1934, LICENSE NUMBER 15247, WAS DISCIPLINED BY COLORADO ON AUGUST 18, 1998
DISCIPLINARY ACTION: REPRIMAND

GIPSTEIN, MILTON MD OF 5205 SOUTH HANOVER WAY, ENGLEWOOD, CO, WAS DISCIPLINED BY DEA ON NOVEMBER 15, 1999
DISCIPLINARY ACTION: SURRENDER OF CONTROLLED SUBSTANCE LICENSE

GLASSER, EDWARD J MD, DATE OF BIRTH AUGUST 23, 1939, LICENSE NUMBER 15274, WAS DISCIPLINED BY COLORADO ON JUNE 24, 1999
DISCIPLINARY ACTION: REPRIMAND

GLASSMAN, MICHAEL H MD, DATE OF BIRTH MAY 20, 1961, LICENSE NUMBER 0030091, WAS DISCIPLINED BY COLORADO ON MARCH 14, 1996
DISCIPLINARY ACTION: MONITORING OF PHYSICIAN PERFORMANCE
OFFENSE: SUBSTANDARD CARE, INCOMPETENCE OR NEGLIGENCE
NOTES: SUBSTANDARD CARE. PRACTICE AND TREATMENT MONITORING, AND RECISION OF PREVIOUS ORDER OF SUSPENSION.

GLASSMAN, MICHAEL H MD, DATE OF BIRTH MAY 20, 1961, LICENSE NUMBER 0030091, WAS DISCIPLINED BY COLORADO ON MAY 15, 1996
DISCIPLINARY ACTION: EMERGENCY SUSPENSION

GOLLADAY, DONALD E MD, DATE OF BIRTH FEBRUARY 11, 1938 OF 1505 E BUENA VENTURA, COLORADO SPRINGS, CO, WAS DISCIPLINED BY MEDICARE ON JULY 26, 1990
DISCIPLINARY ACTION: EXCLUSION FROM THE MEDICARE AND/OR MEDICAID PROGRAM
OFFENSE: DISCIPLINARY ACTION BY ANOTHER STATE OR AGENCY
NOTES: LICENSE REVOCATION OR SUSPENSION.

GOODLOE, ROBERT K DO, LICENSE NUMBER 0001338, WAS DISCIPLINED BY OKLAHOMA ON SEPTEMBER 19, 1991
DISCIPLINARY ACTION: 12-MONTH PROBATION; REQUIRED TO TAKE ADDITIONAL MEDICAL EDUCATION
OFFENSE: CRIMINAL CONVICTION OR PLEA OF GUILTY, NOLO CONTENDERE, OR NO CONTEST TO A CRIME
NOTES: CONVICTED OF HAVING IMPROPERLY PRESCRIBED CONTROLLED SUBSTANCES TO HIS FORMER WIFE; SENTENCED TO 18 MONTHS PROBATION. THE OKLAHOMA BUREAU OF NARCOTICS AND DANGEROUS DRUGS CONTROL SUSPENDED HIS REGISTRATION FOR THREE DAYS BEGINNING 10/11/91. CONDITIONS OF PROBATION: SHALL WITHIN SIX MONTHS ENROLL IN AND ATTEND A COURSE ENTITLED "THE PROPER PRESCRIBING OF CONTROLLED DANGEROUS SUBSTANCES"; AND HIS LICENSE IS DEVOID OF ANY RESTRICTIONS. PROBATION TERMINATED ON 9/17/92, THE BOARD APPROVED A LETTER TO THE DRUG ENFORCEMENT ADMINISTRATION RECOMMENDING THAT HIS SCHEDULE II NARCOTIC AUTHORITY BE REINSTATED.

GOODLOE, ROBERT K DO, DATE OF BIRTH OCTOBER 4, 1937, LICENSE NUMBER 0028511 OF MUSTANG, OK, WAS DISCIPLINED BY COLORADO ON JUNE 19, 1992
DISCIPLINARY ACTION: SURRENDER OF LICENSE
OFFENSE: CRIMINAL CONVICTION OR PLEA OF GUILTY, NOLO CONTENDERE, OR NO CONTEST TO A CRIME
NOTES: CONVICTION OF A FELONY WITH RESPECT TO FURNISHING OF FALSE INFORMATION ON A DOCUMENT PERTAINING TO DEMEROL DISTRIBUTION.

GOODLOE, ROBERT K DO OF MUSTANG, OK, WAS DISCIPLINED BY MISSOURI ON APRIL 27, 1993
DISCIPLINARY ACTION: LICENSE REVOCATION
OFFENSE: CRIMINAL CONVICTION OR PLEA OF GUILTY, NOLO CONTENDERE, OR NO CONTEST TO A CRIME
NOTES: FELONY CONVICTION. NO REINSTATEMENT OF LICENSE FOR SEVEN YEARS.

GOODMAN, EDWARD MD, LICENSE NUMBER 0023388 OF BRUSH, CO, WAS DISCIPLINED BY COLORADO ON OCTOBER 10, 1990

DISCIPLINARY ACTION: SURRENDER OF LICENSE
OFFENSE: PHYSICAL OR MENTAL ILLNESS INHIBITING THE ABILITY TO PRACTICE WITH SKILL AND SAFETY

NOTES: SUCH PHYSICAL OR MENTAL DISABILITY AS TO RENDER HIM UNABLE TO PERFORM MEDICAL SERVICES WITH REASONABLE SKILL AND SAFETY.

GOTTESFELD, STUART A MD, DATE OF BIRTH APRIL 10, 1935, LICENSE NUMBER 13585, WAS DISCIPLINED BY COLORADO ON MAY 13, 1998
DISCIPLINARY ACTION: SURRENDER OF LICENSE
OFFENSE: PHYSICAL OR MENTAL ILLNESS INHIBITING THE ABILITY TO PRACTICE WITH SKILL AND SAFETY

NOTES: PHYSICAL DISABILITY.

GREEN, EDMON L MD, DATE OF BIRTH JULY 27, 1939, LICENSE NUMBER 0031114 OF BRISTOL, TN, WAS DISCIPLINED BY COLORADO ON JULY 15, 1991
DISCIPLINARY ACTION: 60-MONTH PROBATION; MONITORING OF PHYSICIAN PERFORMANCE
OFFENSE: SUBSTANCE ABUSE

NOTES: LICENSE APPLICATION, PAST TREATMENT FOR ALCOHOLISM. TREATMENT MONITORING. IN ABEYANCE.

GREEN, EDMON LEE MD OF 2300 PAVILLION DR, KINGSPORT, TN, WAS DISCIPLINED BY DEA ON AUGUST 17, 1992
DISCIPLINARY ACTION: RESTRICTION PLACED ON CONTROLLED SUBSTANCE LICENSE

NOTES: MEDICAL LICENSE PLACED ON FIVE YEARS PROBATION. RESTRICTION PLACED ON REGISTRATION. APPROVAL OF RENEWAL APPLICATION.

GREGG, KELLY R MD, DATE OF BIRTH JULY 10, 1951, LICENSE NUMBER 0027394 OF COLORADO SPRINGS, CO, WAS DISCIPLINED BY COLORADO ON AUGUST 21, 1992
DISCIPLINARY ACTION: 60-MONTH PROBATION; RESTRICTION PLACED ON LICENSE
OFFENSE: SUBSTANDARD CARE, INCOMPETENCE OR NEGLIGENCE

NOTES: TWO OR MORE ACTS OR OMISSIONS WHICH FAILED TO MEET GENERALLY ACCEPTED STANDARDS OF MEDICAL PRACTICE. PERMANENT PRACTICE RESTRICTION: NO OBSTETRICS CARE AND PRACTICE MONITORING.

GRIFFITH, DILLARD B MD, DATE OF BIRTH NOVEMBER 5, 1934, LICENSE NUMBER 0014490 OF COLORADO SPRINGS, CO, WAS DISCIPLINED BY COLORADO ON DECEMBER 11, 1992
DISCIPLINARY ACTION: MONITORING OF PHYSICIAN PERFORMANCE
OFFENSE: PHYSICAL OR MENTAL ILLNESS INHIBITING THE ABILITY TO PRACTICE WITH SKILL AND SAFETY

NOTES: INDEFINITE PERIOD OF TREATMENT AND PRACTICE MONITORING.

GRIFFITH, DILLARD B MD, DATE OF BIRTH NOVEMBER 5, 1934, LICENSE NUMBER 0014490, WAS DISCIPLINED BY COLORADO ON JULY 31, 1995
DISCIPLINARY ACTION: SURRENDER OF LICENSE

NOTES: RETIREMENT AND RELINQUISHMENT OF HIS MEDICAL LICENSE.

GRIFFITH, EUGENE R MD, DATE OF BIRTH JANUARY 20, 1916, LICENSE NUMBER 0011847 OF COLORADO SPRINGS, CO, WAS DISCIPLINED BY COLORADO ON SEPTEMBER 10, 1993
DISCIPLINARY ACTION: REPRIMAND

GRIMSLEY, JO ANNE MD, DATE OF BIRTH MAY 7, 1950, LICENSE NUMBER 0023226, WAS DISCIPLINED BY COLORADO ON MARCH 21, 1996
DISCIPLINARY ACTION: MONITORING OF PHYSICIAN PERFORMANCE
OFFENSE: PROFESSIONAL MISCONDUCT

NOTES: ADMINISTERING CONTROLLED SUBSTANCES OTHER THAN IN THE COURSE OF LEGITIMATE PROFESSIONAL PRACTICE; EXCESSIVE USE OF A CONTROLLED SUBSTANCE; AND MENTAL DISABILITY. AGREES NOT TO PRACTICE IN COLORADO UNTIL SHE RECEIVES A FAVORABLE PSYCHIATRIC EVALUATION, AT WHICH TIME SHE WILL RECEIVE TREATMENT AND PRACTICE MONITORING.

GUESE, MICHAEL J MD, DATE OF BIRTH FEBRUARY 20, 1952, LICENSE NUMBER 0024675 OF DENVER, CO, WAS DISCIPLINED BY COLORADO ON JANUARY 18, 1995
DISCIPLINARY ACTION: REPRIMAND

GULEVICH, STEVEN J MD, DATE OF BIRTH JANUARY 9, 1959, LICENSE NUMBER 32094, WAS DISCIPLINED BY COLORADO ON AUGUST 14, 1998
DISCIPLINARY ACTION: REPRIMAND; REQUIRED TO TAKE ADDITIONAL MEDICAL EDUCATION
OFFENSE: PROFESSIONAL MISCONDUCT

NOTES: ADMINISTERING A CONTROLLED SUBSTANCE OTHER THAN IN THE COURSE OF LEGITIMATE PROFESSIONAL PRACTICE. HE AGREES TO A BOUNDARIES COURSE AND A COURSE IN PROPER PRESCRIBING.

HAGESETH, CHRISTIAN III MD, DATE OF BIRTH FEBRUARY 23, 1941, LICENSE NUMBER 21721, WAS DISCIPLINED BY COLORADO ON NOVEMBER 19, 1999
DISCIPLINARY ACTION: LICENSE REVOCATION
OFFENSE: SUBSTANDARD CARE, INCOMPETENCE OR NEGLIGENCE

NOTES: SUBSTANDARD CARE; SEXUAL CONTACT WITH A PATIENT; PHYSICAL AND MENTAL DISABILITY.

HALL, DEAN M MD, DATE OF BIRTH NOVEMBER 19, 1924, LICENSE NUMBER 0023019, WAS DISCIPLINED BY COLORADO ON JULY 14, 1994
DISCIPLINARY ACTION: LICENSE REINSTATEMENT; 6-MONTH PROBATION

NOTES: HIS ABSENCE FROM CLINICAL PRACTICE SINCE JANUARY 1991. THERE IS NO EVIDENCE THAT HIS MEDICAL PRACTICE HAS EVER BEEN UNPROFESSIONAL OR IMPROPER; PROBATION WITH PRACTICE MONITORING.

HALL, KAREN A MD, DATE OF BIRTH DECEMBER 1, 1947, LICENSE NUMBER 0020171, WAS DISCIPLINED BY COLORADO ON JUNE 20, 1996
DISCIPLINARY ACTION: REPRIMAND

HALL, SHANNA D MD, LICENSE NUMBER 0018449, WAS DISCIPLINED BY ARIZONA ON MARCH 24, 1990
DISCIPLINARY ACTION: RESTRICTION PLACED ON LICENSE; REQUIRED TO TAKE ADDITIONAL MEDICAL EDUCATION

NOTES: SUMMARY SUSPENSION ORDER OF 8/3/89 RESCINDED AND LICENSE TO PRACTICE IS REINSTATED SUBJECT TO FOLLOWING TERMS AND CONDITIONS: MUST OBTAIN CARE AND TREATMENT FOR AFFECTIVE DISORDERS FROM A BOARD-APPROVED THERAPIST WHO MUST SUBMIT QUARTERLY REPORTS TO THE BOARD; MUST SUBMIT TO ANY EXAMS ORDERED BY THE BOARD; MUST TAKE NO DRUGS; MUST APPEAR

BEFORE BOARD FOR INTERVIEWS UPON REQUEST; MUST AUTHORIZE RELEASE OF ALL DOCUMENTS CONCERNING PROFESSIONAL CONDUCT; MUST PRACTICE ONLY WITHIN A MEDICAL CARE GROUP, HOSPITAL OR MEDICAL FACILITY WITH FOLLOWING CONDITIONS: MUST HAVE IMMEDIATE ACCESS TO A LICENSED PEDIATRICIAN FOR CONSULTATION; A FORMAL PEER REVIEW MECHANISM IN PLACE; MUST HAVE QUARTERLY REPORTS SUBMITTED TO THE BOARD. MUST ALSO TAKE 35 HOURS OF CONTINUING MEDICAL EDUCATION IN PEDIATRICS WITHIN 18 MONTHS FROM AT LEAST 3 DIFFERENT PROVIDERS; SHALL PROVIDE COPY OF ORDER TO THERAPIST AND EMPLOYER. ON 7/17/92 BOARD ACCEPTED THE CONTINUING MEDICAL EDUCATION SUBMITTED BY HER AS FULFILLMENT OF THE REQUIREMENTS OF THIS STIPULATION ORDER.

HALL, SHANNA D MD, DATE OF BIRTH JUNE 24, 1951, LICENSE NUMBER 0033893 OF DENVER, CO, WAS DISCIPLINED BY COLORADO ON OCTOBER 9, 1992
DISCIPLINARY ACTION: DENIAL OF NEW LICENSE
OFFENSE: SUBSTANCE ABUSE

NOTES: MENTAL DISABILITY, EXCESSIVE USE OF A CONTROLLED SUBSTANCE. APPLICATION FOR AN UNRESTRICTED LICENSE DENIED. BOARD WILLING TO OFFER LICENSURE UNDER PROBATIONARY TERMS. THE DENIAL OF THE APPLICATION HAS BEEN APPEALED TO THE COLORADO COURT OF APPEALS.

HALL, SHANNA D MD OF COLUMBIA, MO, WAS DISCIPLINED BY MISSOURI ON JUNE 28, 1993
DISCIPLINARY ACTION: DENIAL OF NEW LICENSE
OFFENSE: DISCIPLINARY ACTION BY ANOTHER STATE OR AGENCY

NOTES: DENIAL BASED ON A DENIAL OF LICENSURE BY ANOTHER STATE.

HALL, SHANNA D MD, DATE OF BIRTH JUNE 24, 1951, LICENSE NUMBER 0033893 OF DENVER, CO, WAS DISCIPLINED BY COLORADO ON JULY 14, 1994
DISCIPLINARY ACTION: 36-MONTH PROBATION; RESTRICTION PLACED ON LICENSE
OFFENSE: SUBSTANCE ABUSE

NOTES: SUBSTANCE ABUSE ISSUES AND MENTAL/PHYSICAL DISABILITY. PROBATION PERIOD INCLUDES TREATMENT AND PRACTICE MONITORING. MAY PRACTICE ONLY WITHIN A HOSPITAL OR MEDICAL CARE GROUP SETTING OF THREE OR MORE PHYSICIANS.

HALPRIN, ARTHUR H MD, DATE OF BIRTH JUNE 15, 1947, LICENSE NUMBER 22256, WAS DISCIPLINED BY COLORADO ON AUGUST 14, 1998
DISCIPLINARY ACTION: EMERGENCY SUSPENSION

HALPRIN, ARTHUR H MD, DATE OF BIRTH JUNE 15, 1947, LICENSE NUMBER 22256, WAS DISCIPLINED BY COLORADO ON MARCH 25, 1999
DISCIPLINARY ACTION: SURRENDER OF LICENSE
OFFENSE: CRIMINAL CONVICTION OR PLEA OF GUILTY, NOLO CONTENDERE, OR NO CONTEST TO A CRIME

NOTES: FELONY CONVICTION; SEXUAL CONTACT WITH A PATIENT; MENTAL DISABILITY.

HALPRIN, ARTHUR HENRY MD, DATE OF BIRTH JUNE 15, 1947 OF 3665 LEE STREET, WHEAT RIDGE, CO, WAS DISCIPLINED BY MEDICARE ON OCTOBER 20, 1999
DISCIPLINARY ACTION: EXCLUSION FROM THE MEDICARE AND/OR MEDICAID PROGRAM
OFFENSE: CRIMINAL CONVICTION OR PLEA OF GUILTY, NOLO CONTENDERE, OR NO CONTEST TO A CRIME

NOTES: CONVICTED OF A CRIME RELATED TO PATIENT ABUSE OR NEGLECT.

HAM, GORDON C MD, DATE OF BIRTH JULY 18, 1944, LICENSE NUMBER 18348, WAS DISCIPLINED BY COLORADO ON DECEMBER 10, 1998
DISCIPLINARY ACTION: SURRENDER OF LICENSE

NOTES: NO UNPROFESSIONAL CONDUCT IDENTIFIED.

HAM, GORDON CLYDE MD, LICENSE NUMBER G30040 OF DENVER, CO, WAS DISCIPLINED BY CALIFORNIA ON JANUARY 16, 1997
DISCIPLINARY ACTION: SURRENDER OF LICENSE

NOTES: WHILE CHARGES PENDING.

HAMILTON, ROBERT MD, LICENSE NUMBER 0022257 OF COLORADO SPRINGS, CO, WAS DISCIPLINED BY COLORADO ON APRIL 12, 1991
DISCIPLINARY ACTION: 24-MONTH PROBATION; MONITORING OF PHYSICIAN PERFORMANCE
OFFENSE: SUBSTANDARD CARE, INCOMPETENCE OR NEGLIGENCE

NOTES: FAILURE TO MEET GENERALLY ACCEPTED STANDARDS OF MEDICAL PRACTICE.

HANNA, SALWA H MD, DATE OF BIRTH JULY 3, 1951, LICENSE NUMBER 0023307, WAS DISCIPLINED BY COLORADO ON JANUARY 11, 1991
DISCIPLINARY ACTION: LICENSE SUSPENSION

NOTES: INABILITY TO PRACTICE MEDICINE WITH REASONABLE SKILL AND SAFETY. CONSENT ORDER, LICENSE SUSPENDED INDEFINITELY.

HANNA, SALWA H MD, DATE OF BIRTH JULY 3, 1951 OF 1355 S COLORADO BLVD #504, DENVER, CO, WAS DISCIPLINED BY MEDICARE ON JULY 22, 1991
DISCIPLINARY ACTION: EXCLUSION FROM THE MEDICARE AND/OR MEDICAID PROGRAM
OFFENSE: DISCIPLINARY ACTION BY ANOTHER STATE OR AGENCY

NOTES: LICENSE REVOCATION OR SUSPENSION. REINSTATED ON 8/29/95.

HANNA, SALWA H MD, DATE OF BIRTH JULY 3, 1951, LICENSE NUMBER 0023307 OF ARVADA, CO, WAS DISCIPLINED BY COLORADO ON JANUARY 20, 1995
DISCIPLINARY ACTION: 60-MONTH PROBATION; RESTRICTION PLACED ON LICENSE

NOTES: APPLICATION FOR REINSTATEMENT OF A LICENSE. NO UNPROFESSIONAL CONDUCT INDICATED. LICENSE REINSTATED, PROVIDING FOR A PRACTICE RESTRICTION AND PROBATION PERIOD, INCLUDING PRACTICE AND TREATMENT MONITORING.

HARDY, RONALD G JR MD, DATE OF BIRTH NOVEMBER 9, 1936, LICENSE NUMBER 17497, WAS DISCIPLINED BY COLORADO ON JULY 22, 1999
DISCIPLINARY ACTION: SURRENDER OF LICENSE

NOTES: NO UNPROFESSIONAL CONDUCT IDENTIFIED. AGREES TO PERMANENTLY RELINQUISH HIS LICENSE.

HARLEY, NED R MD, DATE OF BIRTH MARCH 29, 1942, LICENSE NUMBER 0016887, WAS DISCIPLINED BY COLORADO ON AUGUST 17, 1995
DISCIPLINARY ACTION: PROBATION; RESTRICTION PLACED ON LICENSE

NOTES: INDEFINITE PROBATION WITH PRACTICE AND TREATMENT MONITORING; HIS ACTIVE PATIENT LOAD LIMITED TO 20 OR LESS; SHALL NOT PRESCRIBE SCHEDULE II AND III CONTROLLED SUBSTANCES.

HARLEY, NED R MD, DATE OF BIRTH MARCH 29, 1942, LICENSE NUMBER 16887, WAS DISCIPLINED BY COLORADO ON JULY 10, 1997
DISCIPLINARY ACTION: EMERGENCY SUSPENSION

HARMON, DAVID R DO, DATE OF BIRTH DECEMBER 6, 1947, LICENSE NUMBER 0020974, WAS DISCIPLINED BY COLORADO ON JANUARY 12, 1996
DISCIPLINARY ACTION: EMERGENCY SUSPENSION
OFFENSE: PHYSICAL OR MENTAL ILLNESS INHIBITING THE ABILITY TO PRACTICE WITH SKILL AND SAFETY

NOTES: PHYSICAL OR MENTAL DISABILITY WHICH RENDERS HIM UNABLE TO PERFORM MEDICAL SERVICES WITH REASONABLE SKILL AND SAFETY.

HARMON, DAVID R DO OF 595 OBSERVATORY DRIVE, COLORADO SPRINGS, CO, WAS DISCIPLINED BY DEA ON APRIL 9, 1996
DISCIPLINARY ACTION: SURRENDER OF CONTROLLED SUBSTANCE LICENSE

NOTES: IN LIEU OF ORDER TO SHOW CAUSE.

HARMON, DAVID R DO, DATE OF BIRTH DECEMBER 6, 1947, LICENSE NUMBER 0020974, WAS DISCIPLINED BY COLORADO ON AUGUST 14, 1996
DISCIPLINARY ACTION: LICENSE REVOCATION
OFFENSE: CRIMINAL CONVICTION OR PLEA OF GUILTY, NOLO CONTENDERE, OR NO CONTEST TO A CRIME

NOTES: CONVICTION OF A LAW REGULATING CONTROLLED SUBSTANCES, HABITUAL INTEMPERANCE OR EXCESSIVE USE OF HABIT FORMING DRUG; FRAUD, MISREPRESENTATION OR DECEPTION IN APPLYING FOR A LICENSE; PHYSICAL OR MENTAL DISABILITY; FAILURE TO ACCURATELY ANSWER THE QUESTIONNAIRE ACCOMPANYING THE RENEWAL FORM AND FAILURE TO RESPOND IN A TIMELY MANNER TO A COMPLAINT.

HARMON, DAVID R DO, LICENSE NUMBER E9684 OF GRAND JUNCTION, CO, WAS DISCIPLINED BY TEXAS ON AUGUST 9, 1997
DISCIPLINARY ACTION: LICENSE SUSPENSION; REQUIRED TO ENTER AN IMPAIRED PHYSICIAN PROGRAM OR SUBSTANCE ABUSE TREATMENT
OFFENSE: DISCIPLINARY ACTION BY ANOTHER STATE OR AGENCY

NOTES: IN 8/93, HE WAS NONJUDICIALLY PUNISHED BY THE US NAVY CONCERNING ALLEGATIONS THAT HE WAS ALLEGEDLY UNABLE TO PERFORM HIS MEDICAL DUTIES, WHILE SERVING AS A RESIDENT IN THE NAVAL RESIDENCY PROGRAM, DUE TO ALLEGEDLY BEING UNDER THE INFLUENCE OF A MOOD ALTERING CHEMICAL SUBSTANCE ON A SPECIFIC DATE IN 6/93. IN 5/94, HE WAS TERMINATED FROM THE NAVAL RESIDENCY PROGRAM; FROM SEPTEMBER THROUGH DECEMBER 1995 HE WAS EVALUATED BY THE COLORADO PHYSICIAN HEALTH PROGRAM; HE FAILED TO ENGAGE IN THEIR RECOMMENDED TREATMENT PROGRAM. IN 1/96 THE COLORADO BOARD SUMMARILY SUSPENDED HIS LICENSE AND IN 8/96, REVOKED HIS COLORADO LICENSE. HE DID NOT SELF-REPORT HIS INTEMPERANCE. SUSPENSION UNTIL HE REQUESTS TO HAVE THE SUSPENSION STAYED AND APPEARS BEFORE THE BOARD TO PROVIDE SUFFICIENT EVIDENCE THAT HE IS PHYSICALLY, MENTALLY, AND OTHERWISE COMPETENT TO SAFELY PRACTICE. SUCH EVIDENCE SHALL INCLUDE AT A MINIMUM, A CERTIFIED ORDER OF THE COLORADO BOARD REINSTATING HIS COLORADO LICENSE WITHOUT ANY RESTRICTIONS OR SUBSEQUENT DISCIPLINARY ACTION; COMPLETE MEDICAL RECORDS AND REPORTS OF PSYCHOLOGICAL AND NEUROPSYCHIATRIC EVALUATIONS CONDUCTED BY CERTIFIED PSYCHIATRIST(S); ALL PRIOR MEDICAL RECORDS FROM ANY TREATING PHYSICIAN OR FACILITY INCLUDING CHEMICAL DEPENDENCY TREATMENT FACILITIES, SATISFACTORY EVIDENCE THAT HE IS UNDER AN AFTERCARE MONITORING CONTRACT AND PARTICIPATING IN AA WITH A SPONSOR; COMPLETION OF ALL CONTINUING MEDICAL EDUCATION REQUIREMENTS DURING THE PERIOD OF SUSPENSION. UPON SUCH PROOF HE SHALL BE PLACED ON PROBATION WITH TERMS AND CONDITIONS. HE SHALL COOPERATE WITH THE BOARD IN VERIFYING COMPLIANCE INCLUDING PROVIDING COPIES OF MEDICAL RELEASES AND REPORTS SUBMITTED TO COLORADO UPON REQUEST; SHALL GIVE A COPY OF THIS ORDER TO ANY HEALTH CARE ENTITY WHERE HE HAS PRIVILEGES; SHALL PROVIDE A COPY OF THIS ORDER TO ANYONE REQUESTING IT WITHIN 10 DAYS; SHALL INFORM THE BOARD OF CHANGE OF ADDRESS WITHIN 10 DAYS.

HARPER, CHARLES RICHARD MD, DATE OF BIRTH APRIL 19, 1932, LICENSE NUMBER 0014370 OF PO BOX 20787 ATLANTA AIRPORT, ATLANTA, GA, WAS DISCIPLINED BY GEORGIA ON DECEMBER 5, 1994
DISCIPLINARY ACTION: EMERGENCY SUSPENSION

NOTES: IMPAIRMENT.

HARPER, CHARLES RICHARD MD, DATE OF BIRTH APRIL 19, 1932, LICENSE NUMBER 0014370 OF PO BOX 20787, ATLANTA, GA, WAS DISCIPLINED BY GEORGIA ON MAY 5, 1995
DISCIPLINARY ACTION: 60-MONTH PROBATION

NOTES: IMPAIRED.

HARPER, CHARLES RICHARD MD, DATE OF BIRTH APRIL 19, 1932, LICENSE NUMBER 0014923, WAS DISCIPLINED BY COLORADO ON JUNE 15, 1995
DISCIPLINARY ACTION: EMERGENCY SUSPENSION

HARPER, CHARLES RICHARD MD, LICENSE NUMBER 0022046 OF ATLANTA, GA, WAS DISCIPLINED BY OHIO ON DECEMBER 6, 1995
DISCIPLINARY ACTION: LICENSE REVOCATION
OFFENSE: DISCIPLINARY ACTION BY ANOTHER STATE OR AGENCY

NOTES: PRIOR ACTION BY GEORGIA MEDICAL BOARD DUE TO ALCOHOLISM/CHEMICAL DEPENDENCY. PERMANENT REVOCATION.

HARRIS, JOHN CHARLES MD, DATE OF BIRTH AUGUST 1, 1946, LICENSE NUMBER 23021, WAS DISCIPLINED BY COLORADO ON MAY 19, 1999
DISCIPLINARY ACTION: 60-MONTH PROBATION; RESTRICTION PLACED ON CONTROLLED SUBSTANCE LICENSE
OFFENSE: SUBSTANCE ABUSE

NOTES: EXCESSIVE USE OF A CONTROLLED SUBSTANCE; ADMINISTERING A CONTROLLED SUBSTANCE OTHER THAN IN THE COURSE OF LEGITIMATE PROFESSIONAL PRACTICE. PROBATIONARY TERMS INCLUDE: ABSTINENCE FROM ALCOHOL AND CONTROLLED SUBSTANCES, TREATMENT MONITORING, PRACTICE MONITORING AND A PROHIBITION AGAINST THE PRESCRIBING OF CONTROLLED SUBSTANCES.

HARRISON, MURKE FRANKLIN IV DO, LICENSE NUMBER 0004058 OF BUTTE, MT, WAS DISCIPLINED BY OHIO ON APRIL 15, 1993
DISCIPLINARY ACTION: PROBATION; RESTRICTION PLACED ON LICENSE
OFFENSE: DISCIPLINARY ACTION BY ANOTHER STATE OR AGENCY

NOTES: ACTION BY MONTANA BOARD AND TREATMENT FOR CHEMICAL DEPENDENCY.

HARRISON, MURKE FRANKLIN IV DO, DATE OF BIRTH JUNE 24, 1956, LICENSE NUMBER 0027091 OF BUTTE, MT, WAS DISCIPLINED BY COLORADO ON JUNE 11, 1993
OFFENSE: SUBSTANDARD CARE, INCOMPETENCE OR NEGLIGENCE

NOTES: SUBSTANDARD CARE; MENTAL DISABILITY. ORDER REQUIRES COMPLIANCE WITH TERMS OF AN AGREEMENT WITH THE MONTANA MEDICAL BOARD.

HARRISON, MURKE FRANKLIN IV DO, DATE OF BIRTH JUNE 24, 1956, LICENSE NUMBER 0009497 OF PO BOX 3052, BUTTE, MT, WAS DISCIPLINED BY MICHIGAN ON OCTOBER 15, 1993
DISCIPLINARY ACTION: EMERGENCY SUSPENSION
OFFENSE: PHYSICAL OR MENTAL ILLNESS INHIBITING THE ABILITY TO PRACTICE WITH SKILL AND SAFETY

HARRISON, MURKE FRANKLIN IV DO, DATE OF BIRTH JUNE 24, 1956, LICENSE NUMBER 0006511 OF PO BOX 3052, BUTTE, MT, WAS DISCIPLINED BY MONTANA ON NOVEMBER 5, 1993
DISCIPLINARY ACTION: SURRENDER OF LICENSE
OFFENSE: FAILURE TO COMPLY WITH PREVIOUS BOARD ORDER

NOTES: VIOLATION OF CHEMICAL DEPENDENCY MONITORING AGREEMENT IN THAT URINE SAMPLES TAKEN IN 4/93 AND 6/93 TESTED POSITIVE FOR AMPHETAMINES AND COCAINE. INDEFINITE SURRENDER; SHALL NOT PETITION FOR REINSTATEMENT UNTIL THE FOLLOWING CONDITIONS HAVE BEEN MET: SHALL HAVE SPENT NO LESS THAN ONE YEAR IMMEDIATELY PRIOR TO HIS REQUEST FOR REINSTATEMENT IN ONE WORK AND RESIDENCE LOCATION; SHALL PROVIDE DOCUMENTATION OF COMPLIANCE WITH A RECOVERY PROGRAM, INCLUDING NEGATIVE RANDOM URINE MONITORING; REGULAR AA OR NARCOTICS ANONYMOUS 12-STEP GROUP ATTENDANCE; REGULAR CADUCEUS OR OTHER PROFESSIONAL SUPPORT GROUP ATTENDANCE; QUARTERLY REPORTS FROM A SPONSOR; REEVALUATION AND SATISFACTORY MEDICAL DISCHARGE FROM A TREATMENT OR EVALUATION CENTER OF THE BOARD'S CHOICE.

HARRISON, MURKE FRANKLIN IV DO, DATE OF BIRTH JUNE 24, 1956, LICENSE NUMBER 0009497 OF POST OFFICE BOX 3052, BUTTE, MT, WAS DISCIPLINED BY MICHIGAN ON APRIL 7, 1994
DISCIPLINARY ACTION: 6-MONTH LICENSE SUSPENSION
OFFENSE: SUBSTANCE ABUSE

NOTES: MENTAL/PHYSICAL INABILITY TO PRACTICE-DRUG RELATED.

HARRISON, MURKE FRANKLIN IV DO, DATE OF BIRTH JUNE 24, 1956, LICENSE NUMBER 0027091 OF BUTTE, MT, WAS DISCIPLINED BY COLORADO ON MAY 13, 1994
DISCIPLINARY ACTION: SURRENDER OF LICENSE
OFFENSE: FAILURE TO COMPLY WITH PREVIOUS BOARD ORDER

NOTES: VIOLATION OF MONTANA AND COLORADO STIPULATIONS. HABITUAL INTEMPERANCE OR EXCESSIVE USE OF A CONTROLLED SUBSTANCE.

HARRISON, MURKE FRANKLIN IV DO, LICENSE NUMBER 0004058 OF BUTTE, MT, WAS DISCIPLINED BY OHIO ON JUNE 15, 1994
DISCIPLINARY ACTION: LICENSE REVOCATION
OFFENSE: FAILURE TO COMPLY WITH PREVIOUS BOARD ORDER

NOTES: VIOLATION OF CONDITIONS OF LIMITATION IMPOSED BY 4/15/93 CONSENT AGREEMENT DUE TO FAILURE TO COMPLY WITH TERMS OF PROBATION IMPOSED ON MONTANA MEDICAL LICENSE BY MONTANA BOARD; SUBMISSION OF FALSE STATEMENTS TO OHIO BOARD REGARDING PROBATIONARY COMPLIANCE. PERMANENT REVOCATION. NOTICE OF APPEAL FILED BY DOCTOR WITH FRANKLIN COUNTY COURT OF COMMON PLEAS ON 7/5/94. COMMON PLEAS SUSTAINED BOARD'S MOTION TO DISMISS HIS APPEAL. MOTION FOR RECONSIDERATION OF DISMISSAL OF APPEAL ORDER FILED BY HIM ON 5/19/95. DECISION FROM 10TH DISTRICT COURT OF APPEALS DENYING MOTION FOR RECONSIDERATION FILED ON 6/15/95. NOTICE OF APPEAL TO THE OHIO SUPREME COURT FILED BY HIM ON 6/23/95. ON 10/18/95 THE SUPREME COURT DECLINED TO ACCEPT JURISDICTION OF HIS APPEAL.

HARROD, CHARLES S MD, DATE OF BIRTH OCTOBER 24, 1953, LICENSE NUMBER 0023960, WAS DISCIPLINED BY COLORADO ON FEBRUARY 16, 1996
DISCIPLINARY ACTION: REPRIMAND

HARTMAN, DIANE M MD, DATE OF BIRTH MARCH 19, 1963, LICENSE NUMBER 30949, WAS DISCIPLINED BY COLORADO ON JUNE 11, 1998
DISCIPLINARY ACTION: 60-MONTH PROBATION; MONITORING OF PHYSICIAN PERFORMANCE
OFFENSE: SUBSTANCE ABUSE

NOTES: HABITUAL INTEMPERANCE OR EXCESSIVE USE OF A CONTROLLED SUBSTANCE. PROBATIONARY TERMS INCLUDE: ABSTINENCE FROM ALCOHOL AND CONTROLLED SUBSTANCES, TREATMENT MONITORING AND PRACTICE MONITORING.

HARTMAN, DIANE M MD OF 3555 LUTHERAN PKWAY #230, WHEAT RIDGE, CO, WAS DISCIPLINED BY DEA ON JANUARY 13, 1999
DISCIPLINARY ACTION: RESTRICTION PLACED ON CONTROLLED SUBSTANCE LICENSE

NOTES: MEMO OF AGREEMENT IN LIEU OF PUBLIC INTEREST REVOCATION.

HARTWIG, FRANK E MD, DATE OF BIRTH SEPTEMBER 9, 1946, LICENSE NUMBER 21726, WAS DISCIPLINED BY COLORADO ON NOVEMBER 13, 1998
DISCIPLINARY ACTION: SURRENDER OF LICENSE

NOTES: NO UNPROFESSIONAL CONDUCT IDENTIFIED.

HARVEY, RICHARD L MD, DATE OF BIRTH SEPTEMBER 17, 1932, LICENSE NUMBER 0013368, WAS DISCIPLINED BY COLORADO ON JULY 21, 1994
DISCIPLINARY ACTION: EMERGENCY SUSPENSION
OFFENSE: SUBSTANCE ABUSE

NOTES: HABITUAL INTEMPERANCE OR EXCESSIVE USE OF ANY HABIT-FORMING DRUG OR CONTROLLED SUBSTANCE; PRESCRIBING, DISTRIBUTING OR GIVING TO A FAMILY MEMBER OR TO ONESELF A CONTROLLED SUBSTANCE. PENDING PROCEEDINGS TO DETERMINE WHETHER HIS LICENSE SHOULD BE FURTHER DISCIPLINED.

HARVEY, RICHARD L MD, DATE OF BIRTH SEPTEMBER 17, 1932, LICENSE NUMBER 0013368 OF AURORA, CO, WAS DISCIPLINED BY COLORADO ON AUGUST 11, 1994
DISCIPLINARY ACTION: LICENSE SUSPENSION; REQUIRED TO

ENTER AN IMPAIRED PHYSICIAN PROGRAM OR SUBSTANCE ABUSE TREATMENT
OFFENSE: SUBSTANCE ABUSE

NOTES: SUBSTANCE ABUSE AND PHYSICAL/MENTAL DISABILITY ISSUES. SUSPENSION PENDING SUCCESSFUL COMPLETION OF INPATIENT EVALUATION/TREATMENT FOR SUBSTANCE ABUSE. IF LICENSE REINSTATED, THEN PROBATIONARY TERMS INCLUDING FIVE YEAR PRACTICE AND TREATMENT MONITORING.

HARVEY, RICHARD L MD, DATE OF BIRTH SEPTEMBER 17, 1932 OF 2845 SOUTH MACON COURT, AURORA, CO, WAS DISCIPLINED BY MEDICARE ON MARCH 16, 1995
DISCIPLINARY ACTION: EXCLUSION FROM THE MEDICARE AND/OR MEDICAID PROGRAM
OFFENSE: DISCIPLINARY ACTION BY ANOTHER STATE OR AGENCY

NOTES: LICENSE SUSPENDED FOR REASONS BEARING ON PROFESSIONAL PERFORMANCE.

HARVEY, RICHARD L MD, DATE OF BIRTH SEPTEMBER 17, 1932, LICENSE NUMBER 0013368, WAS DISCIPLINED BY COLORADO ON FEBRUARY 14, 1996
DISCIPLINARY ACTION: LICENSE SUSPENSION

NOTES: FAILURE TO COMPLY WITH CONDITIONS IMPOSED BY THE INQUIRY PANEL. SUSPENSION UNTIL HE COMPLIES WITH PROBATIONARY TERMS. SUSPENSION CONTINUED ON 10/17/96.

HAUGEN, HAROLD M MD, DATE OF BIRTH MARCH 2, 1921, LICENSE NUMBER 0012273 OF FRANKTOWN, CO, WAS DISCIPLINED BY COLORADO ON APRIL 12, 1995
DISCIPLINARY ACTION: PROBATION
OFFENSE: FAILURE TO COMPLY WITH PREVIOUS BOARD ORDER

NOTES: SUBSTANDARD CARE AND VIOLATION OF A BOARD ORDER.

HAUGEN, HAROLD M MD, DATE OF BIRTH MARCH 2, 1921, LICENSE NUMBER 0012273 OF FRANKTOWN, CO, WAS DISCIPLINED BY COLORADO ON APRIL 12, 1996
DISCIPLINARY ACTION: SURRENDER OF LICENSE
OFFENSE: FAILURE TO COMPLY WITH PREVIOUS BOARD ORDER

NOTES: SUBSTANDARD CARE; VIOLATION OF A BOARD ORDER.

HAUN, WILLIAM E MD, DATE OF BIRTH AUGUST 10, 1951, LICENSE NUMBER 21727, WAS DISCIPLINED BY COLORADO ON NOVEMBER 19, 1999
DISCIPLINARY ACTION: REPRIMAND; REQUIRED TO TAKE ADDITIONAL MEDICAL EDUCATION
OFFENSE: PROFESSIONAL MISCONDUCT

NOTES: UNPROFESSIONAL CONDUCT (PRIMA FACIE TYPE ADMISSION ONLY). SHALL TAKE A BOUNDARIES COURSE.

HAYES, JUDE R MD, LICENSE NUMBER 0024565 OF PORTERVILLE, CA, WAS DISCIPLINED BY COLORADO ON NOVEMBER 9, 1990
DISCIPLINARY ACTION: SURRENDER OF LICENSE
OFFENSE: DISCIPLINARY ACTION BY ANOTHER STATE OR AGENCY

NOTES: CONVICTION OF VIOLATION OF FEDERAL LAW REGARDING CONTROLLED SUBSTANCES AND REVOCATION IN ANOTHER STATE.

HAYES, JUDE R MD OF PORTERVILLE, CA, WAS DISCIPLINED BY DEA ON AUGUST 15, 1994
DISCIPLINARY ACTION: DENIAL OF NEW LICENSE
OFFENSE: CRIMINAL CONVICTION OR PLEA OF GUILTY, NOLO CONTENDERE, OR NO CONTEST TO A CRIME

NOTES: ON 7/20/84 CONVICTED OF 281 COUNTS OF UNLAWFUL DISTRIBUTION OF CONTROLLED SUBSTANCES; MOTION TO SET ASIDE SENTENCE GRANTED AND HE WAS RELEASED FROM CUSTODY AND PROBATION TERMINATED ON 12/11/91; ON 4/18/90 CALIFORNIA BOARD RESTORED ALL MEDICAL PRIVILEGES AFTER HE COMPLETED FIVE YEARS PROBATION; STILL EXCLUDED FROM THE MEDI-CAL PROGRAM; TREATED MEDI-CAL PATIENTS WITHOUT AUTHORIZATION AND USED OTHER PHYSICIANS' PRE-SIGNED PRESCRIPTION FORMS; HAD COMPLETE LACK OF REMORSE; TOTAL DISREGARD FOR RULES AND REGULATIONS GOVERNING THE HANDLING OF CONTROLLED SUBSTANCES.

HAYNES, ROBERT G MD, DATE OF BIRTH AUGUST 3, 1926, LICENSE NUMBER 0012739, WAS DISCIPLINED BY COLORADO ON JUNE 8, 1995
DISCIPLINARY ACTION: REPRIMAND

HEAVRIN, JOHN S MD, DATE OF BIRTH OCTOBER 11, 1948, LICENSE NUMBER 0024475, WAS DISCIPLINED BY COLORADO ON AUGUST 2, 1995
DISCIPLINARY ACTION: REPRIMAND

HEIBERGER, JAMES T MD, DATE OF BIRTH NOVEMBER 29, 1941, LICENSE NUMBER 0024223 OF COLORADO SPRINGS, CO, WAS DISCIPLINED BY COLORADO ON MARCH 16, 1995
DISCIPLINARY ACTION: 24-MONTH PROBATION; MONITORING OF PHYSICIAN PERFORMANCE
OFFENSE: SUBSTANDARD CARE, INCOMPETENCE OR NEGLIGENCE

NOTES: SUBSTANDARD CARE. PROBATION INCLUDES PRACTICE MONITORING.

HEINDEL, TERRY J MD, DATE OF BIRTH JUNE 2, 1963, LICENSE NUMBER 34601, WAS DISCIPLINED BY COLORADO ON NOVEMBER 13, 1998
DISCIPLINARY ACTION: 60-MONTH PROBATION; MONITORING OF PHYSICIAN PERFORMANCE
OFFENSE: SUBSTANCE ABUSE

NOTES: HABITUAL INTEMPERANCE OR EXCESSIVE USE OF A CONTROLLED SUBSTANCE. PROBATIONARY TERMS INCLUDE: ABSTINENCE FROM ALCOHOL AND CONTROLLED SUBSTANCES, TREATMENT MONITORING AND PRACTICE MONITORING.

HENSEN, JAMES MD, LICENSE NUMBER 0013284 OF PUEBLO, CO, WAS DISCIPLINED BY COLORADO ON SEPTEMBER 28, 1990

NOTES: ISSUE: RETIREMENT. STIPULATION AND ORDER ESTABLISHING THAT HE WILL NOT NOW, OR IN THE FUTURE, PRACTICE MEDICINE IN THE STATE WITHOUT MAKING APPLICATION AND RECEIVING THE BOARD'S APPROVAL.

HERMANN, JOSEPH F MD, DATE OF BIRTH JUNE 19, 1953, LICENSE NUMBER 22592, WAS DISCIPLINED BY COLORADO ON APRIL 15, 1999
DISCIPLINARY ACTION: 2-MONTH LICENSE SUSPENSION; 60-MONTH PROBATION
OFFENSE: SEXUAL ABUSE OF OR SEXUAL MISCONDUCT WITH A PATIENT

NOTES: SEXUAL CONTACT WITH A PATIENT. PROBATIONARY TERMS INCLUDE: USE OF A CHAPERONE, USE OF A CONSENT FORM AND PRACTICE MONITORING.

HERRIOTT, MICHAEL G DO, DATE OF BIRTH APRIL 13, 1953, LICENSE NUMBER 27649, WAS DISCIPLINED BY COLORADO ON JUNE 17, 1999
OFFENSE: SUBSTANDARD CARE, INCOMPETENCE OR NEGLIGENCE

NOTES: PHYSICAL OR MENTAL DISABILITY; SUBSTANDARD CARE (PRIMA FACIE TYPE ADMISSION ONLY). AGREES TO PLACE HIS LICENSE IN INACTIVE STATUS. AT SUCH TIME AS HE RETURNS TO PRACTICE MEDICINE, HE SHALL COMMENCE A FIVE-YEAR PERIOD OF PROBATION WITH TREATMENT AND PRACTICE MONITORING PROVISIONS.

HERSCH, LAWRENCE B MD, DATE OF BIRTH SEPTEMBER 26, 1940, LICENSE NUMBER 0017277, WAS DISCIPLINED BY COLORADO ON MARCH 21, 1996
DISCIPLINARY ACTION: REQUIRED TO TAKE ADDITIONAL MEDICAL EDUCATION; MONITORING OF PHYSICIAN PERFORMANCE
OFFENSE: SUBSTANDARD CARE, INCOMPETENCE OR NEGLIGENCE

NOTES: SUBSTANDARD CARE. RE-EDUCATION ACTIVITIES AND PRACTICE MONITORING.

HILBERMAN, MARK MD, DATE OF BIRTH MARCH 3, 1938, LICENSE NUMBER 0026371 OF CARBONDALE, CO, WAS DISCIPLINED BY COLORADO ON MAY 13, 1994
DISCIPLINARY ACTION: 60-MONTH PROBATION; MONITORING OF PHYSICIAN PERFORMANCE
OFFENSE: SUBSTANDARD CARE, INCOMPETENCE OR NEGLIGENCE

NOTES: SUBSTANDARD CARE. "PRIMA FACIE" TYPE ADMISSION ONLY. IN ABEYANCE PENDING HIS RELOCATION TO COLORADO. PROBATION PERIOD INCLUDES TREATMENT AND PRACTICE MONITORING. ON 6/12/97 ORDER MODIFIED WHEREBY HE AGREES TO A FIVE YEAR PROBATIONARY TERM UPON THE RETURN TO PRACTICE; PROBATIONARY TERMS INCLUDE REEDUCATION ACTIVITIES, TREATMENT AND PRACTICE MONITORING.

HILBERMAN, MARK MD, LICENSE NUMBER 0G16206 OF CARBONDALE, CO, WAS DISCIPLINED BY CALIFORNIA ON SEPTEMBER 15, 1995
DISCIPLINARY ACTION: 48-MONTH PROBATION
OFFENSE: DISCIPLINARY ACTION BY ANOTHER STATE OR AGENCY

NOTES: ACTION IN COLORADO FOR FAILURE TO MEET GENERALLY ACCEPTED MEDICAL STANDARDS IN ANESTHESIOLOGY PRACTICE. REVOCATION, STAYED.

HILBERMAN, MARK MD, DATE OF BIRTH MARCH 3, 1938, LICENSE NUMBER 0040843 OF 95 COTTON HOLLOW LANE, CARBONDALE, CO, WAS DISCIPLINED BY NEW JERSEY ON MAY 9, 1996
DISCIPLINARY ACTION: 60-MONTH PROBATION
OFFENSE: DISCIPLINARY ACTION BY ANOTHER STATE OR AGENCY

NOTES: ACTION IN COLORADO. PROBATION RETROACTIVE TO 5/13/94. SHALL APPEAR BEFORE THE BOARD PRIOR TO COMMENCING ACTIVE PRACTICE IN NEW JERSEY TO DISCUSS LICENSURE STATUS IN ALL OTHER JURISDICTIONS AND PRACTICE PLANS.

HILST, WILBUR MD, LICENSE NUMBER 412627 OF 1821 N CALHOUN AVENUE, LIBERAL, KS, WAS DISCIPLINED BY KANSAS ON JULY 16, 1997
DISCIPLINARY ACTION: LICENSE REVOCATION
OFFENSE: FAILURE TO COMPLY WITH PREVIOUS BOARD ORDER

NOTES: VIOLATED THE TERMS OF 10/22/96 ORDER AND HIS CONTRACT WITH THE KANSAS IMPAIRED PHYSICIANS PROGRAM.

HILST, WILBUR D MD, LICENSE NUMBER 0412627 OF TOPEKA, KS, WAS DISCIPLINED BY KANSAS ON FEBRUARY 10, 1990
DISCIPLINARY ACTION: LICENSE REVOCATION

HILST, WILBUR D MD, LICENSE NUMBER 0412627 OF 3724 SOUTHWEST 29TH, TOPEKA, KS, WAS DISCIPLINED BY KANSAS ON MARCH 14, 1994
DISCIPLINARY ACTION: LICENSE REINSTATEMENT; RESTRICTION PLACED ON LICENSE

NOTES: ALCOHOLISM PROBLEMS WHICH RESULTED IN A PATTERN OF BEHAVIOR CLEARLY DEMONSTRATING AN INCOMPETENCE TO PRACTICE MEDICINE. LED TO 2/10/90 ORDER OF REVOCATION. LICENSE REINSTATED UNDER THE FOLLOWING CONDITIONS: AGREES TO COMPLETELY ABSTAIN FROM THE CONSUMPTION OR USE OF ANY ALCOHOL OR CEREAL MALT BEVERAGE; SHALL NOT ADMINISTER TO HIMSELF OR ALLOW TO BE DISPENSED OR PRESCRIBED TO HIM ANY CONTROLLED SUBSTANCES OR ANY OTHER MOOD ALTERING SUBSTANCE OR POTENTIALLY ADDICTING SUBSTANCE WITHOUT FIRST OBTAINING A WRITTEN PRESCRIPTION BY A DULY-LICENSED PHYSICIAN; AGREES TO COMPLY WITH ALL TERMS AND CONDITIONS OF HIS REVISED CONTRACT WITH THE KANSAS MEDICAL SOCIETY IMPAIRED PHYSICIANS PROGRAM AND TO FOLLOW ALL RECOMMENDATIONS MADE BY SUCH PROGRAM FOR SUBSEQUENT TREATMENT, MONITORING AND SUPPORT; AGREES TO SUBMIT TO RANDOM URINALYSIS; AGREES TO ATTEND ALCOHOLICS ANONYMOUS MEETINGS AT A MINIMUM OF FOUR TIMES PER WEEK; AGREES HIS PRACTICE OF MEDICINE IS LIMITED TO PERFORMING SERVICES WITHIN THE SCOPE OF HIS EMPLOYMENT AT SOUTHWEST MEDICAL CENTER IN LIBERAL AND AT A.H. THIEMANN MEMORIAL CLINIC IN SUBLETTE; HIS PRACTICE IS LIMITED TO EMERGENCY MEDICINE AND FAMILY PRACTICE, AND SHALL NOT PERFORM GENERAL SURGERY, EXCEPT TO THE EXTENT REQUIRED IN THE COURSE OF PERFORMANCE OF EMERGENCY ROOM SERVICES; MAY PERFORM MINOR CUTANEOUS INCISIONS AND THOSE PROCEDURES PERFORMED UNDER LOCAL ANESTHESIA; SHALL NOT ENGAGE IN THE PRACTICE OF OBSTETRICS, PRENATAL, POSTPARTUM OR NEWBORN MEDICAL CARE; AGREES TO SHOW PROOF OF COMPLETION OF A WEEK-LONG REVIEW SESSION IN FAMILY MEDICINE AT LEAST ONCE A YEAR, THE FIRST SESSION TO BE COMPLETED BY 09/01/94; AGREES TO FOCUS CONTINUING MEDICAL EDUCATION IN THE FOLLOWING AREAS: PEDIATRICS, OFFICE GYNECOLOGY, MODERN IMAGING TECHNIQUES, ACUTE ASTHMA, HYPERTENSION, ANTIMICROBIAL THERAPY, DIABETES, PHYSICIAN-PATIENT COMMUNICATIONS AND MEDICAL DOCUMENTATION; MUST HAVE HIS PATIENT CHARTS REVIEWED; IF FAVORABLE REPORTS WITH RESPECT TO CHART REVIEW ARE DEEMED SATISFACTORY, SUCH REVIEW WILL BE REDUCED TO 10 CHARTS PER MONTH AFTER SIX MONTHS; IF FAVORABLE REPORTS ARE DEEMED SATISFACTORY AFTER THE NEXT SIX MONTHS, SUCH CHART REVIEW MAY BE DISCONTINUED; STIPULATION TO BE IN EFFECT FOR AT LEAST FIVE YEARS; HE MAY PETITION FOR MODIFICATION AFTER ONE YEAR. ON 3/14/94 AN ADDITIONAL HOSPITAL WAS ADDED TO WHERE HE COULD PRACTICE WITH THE SAME CONDITIONS OF CHART MONITORING.

HILST, WILBUR D MD, DATE OF BIRTH DECEMBER 7, 1931, LICENSE NUMBER 0014776 OF TOPEKA, KS, WAS DISCIPLINED BY COLORADO ON NOVEMBER 3, 1994
DISCIPLINARY ACTION: SURRENDER OF LICENSE
OFFENSE: SUBSTANCE ABUSE

NOTES: HABITUAL INTEMPERANCE OR EXCESSIVE USE OF ANY HABIT-FORMING DRUG OR CONTROLLED SUBSTANCE.

HILST, WILBUR D MD, LICENSE NUMBER 0412627 OF 1821 N. CALHOUN AVENUE, LIBERAL, KS, WAS DISCIPLINED BY KANSAS ON JULY 13, 1995
DISCIPLINARY ACTION: EMERGENCY SUSPENSION
OFFENSE: FAILURE TO COMPLY WITH PREVIOUS BOARD ORDER

NOTES: ON 6/24/95 THROUGH 6/27/95 CONSUMED AND WAS UNDER THE INFLUENCE OF ALCOHOL ON SEVERAL OCCASIONS WHERE HE TREATED PATIENTS IN VIOLATION OF HIS PREVIOUS STIPULATION AGREEMENT OF 3/14/94; FAILED TO SUBMIT TO A URINALYSIS ON TWO OCCASIONS. ON 8/29/96 THE EMERGENCY SUSPENSION WAS TERMINATED; HE REMAINS SUBJECT TO THE TERMS OF THE 3/14/94 ORDER.

HILST, WILBUR D MD, LICENSE NUMBER 0412627, WAS DISCIPLINED BY KANSAS ON OCTOBER 22, 1996
DISCIPLINARY ACTION: 14-MONTH LICENSE SUSPENSION; RESTRICTION PLACED ON LICENSE
OFFENSE: FAILURE TO COMPLY WITH PREVIOUS BOARD ORDER

NOTES: VIOLATED A PREVIOUS ORDER BY CONSUMING ALCOHOL ON 6/24 AND 6/25/95; FAILING TO SUBMIT TO REQUESTED URINALYSIS ON THREE OCCASIONS BETWEEN 6/30 AND 7/4/95, TESTING POSITIVE FOR BARBITURATES AND BENZODIAZEPINES ON 7/7/95, AND FAILING TO REPORT HIS POSITIVE TESTING. SUSPENSIONS RETROACTIVE TO 7/07/95 UNTIL 9/01/96. FINAL ORDER: SHALL ABSTAIN FROM THE CONSUMPTION OR USE OF ANY ALCOHOL OR CEREAL MALT BEVERAGE; SHALL NOT ADMINISTER TO HIMSELF OR ALLOW TO BE DISPENSED OR PRESCRIBED TO HIM ANY SUBSTANCES IN ANY SCHEDULE OF THE UNIFORM CONTROLLED SUBSTANCES ACT OR ANY OTHER MOOD OR MIND ALTERING SUBSTANCE OR POTENTIALLY ADDICTING SUBSTANCE WITHOUT FIRST OBTAINING A WRITTEN PRESCRIPTION BY A DULY LICENSED PHYSICIAN FOR MEDICAL NEED; SHALL LIMIT HIS PRACTICE TO EMERGENCY MEDICINE AND FAMILY PRACTICE; SHALL NOT HOLD HIMSELF OUT TO THE PUBLIC AS A GENERAL SURGEON, BUT MAY APPLY FOR PRIVILEGES AS A GENERAL SURGEON; SHALL NOT PERFORM GENERAL SURGERY, EXCEPT TO THE EXTENT REQUIRED IN THE COURSE OF PERFORMANCE OF EMERGENCY ROOM SERVICES; MAY PERFORM MINOR CUTANEOUS INCISIONS, THOSE PERFORMED UNDER LOCAL ANESTHESIA, AND MAY ASSIST AT A SURGERY ONLY IN THE PRESENCE OF A GENERAL OR OTHER SURGEON WITH SURGICAL PRIVILEGES; SHALL NOT ENGAGE IN THE PRACTICE OF OBSTETRICS, PRENATAL, POSTPARTUM, OR NEWBORN MEDICAL CARE; SHALL COMPLY WITH THE RECOMMENDATIONS FROM THE COLORADO PERSONALIZED EDUCATION FOR PHYSICIANS, EXCEPT TO THE EXTENT INCONSISTENT WITH THIS ORDER; SHALL COMPLY WITH ANY REASONABLE PEER REVIEW REPORTS AT ANY HEALTH CARE FACILITY WITH WHICH HE IS AFFILIATED; MAY SEEK EMPLOYMENT AND/OR STAFF PRIVILEGES AS HE DEEMS APPROPRIATE AND NOTIFY THE BOARD OF ANY CHANGE; MUST COMPLETE A CURRENT PSYCHIATRIC EVALUATION AND REPORT RESULTS TO THE BOARD; AND SHALL SEEK ON-GOING PSYCHOTHERAPY, AS A TERM AND CONDITION OF HIS KMS-MAP MONITORING CONTRACT. MUST SEEK ONGOING PSYCHOTHERAPY.

HILST, WILBUR D MD, LICENSE NUMBER 6037 OF 1821 NORTH CALHOUN, LIBERAL, KS, WAS DISCIPLINED BY OKLAHOMA ON JULY 7, 1998
DISCIPLINARY ACTION: 60-MONTH PROBATION; RESTRICTION PLACED ON LICENSE
OFFENSE: DISCIPLINARY ACTION BY ANOTHER STATE OR AGENCY

NOTES: HISTORY OF ALCOHOL ABUSE AND PRIOR DISCIPLINARY ACTION IN COLORADO AND KANSAS. HE PLANS TO LIMIT HIS OKLAHOMA PRACTICE TO EMERGENCY MEDICINE AT A HOSPITAL IN GUYMON, OKLAHOMA. GRANTED LICENSURE WITH CONDITIONS OF PROBATION: SHALL PRACTICE IN A CONTROLLED ENVIRONMENT APPROVED BY THE BOARD LIMITED TO EMERGENCY MEDICINE AT THE SPECIFIED HOSPITAL IN GUYMON, OKLAHOMA AND WILL NOT PRACTICE MORE THAN 60 HOURS IN ANY GIVEN WEEK; MUST OBTAIN APPROVAL FROM THE BOARD PRIOR TO MAKING ANY CHANGE IN HIS PRACTICE OR LOCATION; SHALL REQUEST THE SPECIFIED HOSPITAL AND PRACTICE GROUP, AND ANY AND ALL HOSPITALS SUBSEQUENTLY APPROVED BY THE BOARD TO FURNISH TO THE BOARD A WRITTEN QUARTERLY STATEMENT MONITORING HIS PRACTICE; SHALL SUBMIT TO EVERY STATE IN WHICH HE HOLDS LICENSURE AND TO HOSPITALS, CLINICS OR OTHER INSTITUTIONS IN WHICH HE HOLDS OR ANTICIPATES HOLDING ANY FORM OF STAFF PRIVILEGE A COPY OF THIS ORDER; SHALL NOT SUPERVISE ALLIED HEALTH PROFESSIONALS; SHALL SUBMIT BIOLOGICAL FLUID SPECIMENS AND SHALL NOT INGEST ANY SUBSTANCE WHICH WILL CAUSE A SPECIMEN TO TEST POSITIVE FOR PROHIBITED SUBSTANCES; SHALL SUBMIT HIS WRITTEN WORK SCHEDULE TO THE BOARD AS OFTEN AS NECESSARY TO KEEP THE BOARD INFORMED, AT ALL TIMES, OF THE DATES AND TIMES THAT HE WILL BE PROVIDING MEDICAL SERVICES TO OKLAHOMA; SHALL NOT PRESCRIBE, ADMINISTER OR DISPENSE ANY MEDICATIONS FOR HIS PERSONAL USE AND SHALL TAKE NONE UNLESS AUTHORIZED BY ANOTHER PHYSICIAN FOR A LEGITIMATE MEDICAL NEED; SHALL AFFILIATE WITH THE OKLAHOMA PHYSICIANS' RECOVERY PROGRAM AND AA AND WILL ASK THOSE SUPPORT GROUPS TO SUBMIT QUARTERLY REPORTS ON HIS PROGRESS TO THE BOARD; SHALL MEET PERIODICALLY WITH A BOARD APPROVED PSYCHIATRIST AND SHALL AUTHORIZE THEM TO SUBMIT WRITTEN REPORTS TO THE BOARD FOLLOWING SUCH CONSULTATIONS AND SHALL COMPLY WITH ALL TREATMENT RECOMMENDATIONS; SHALL KEEP THE BOARD INFORMED OF HIS ADDRESS AND PAY COSTS; SHALL APPEAR BEFORE THE BOARD UPON REQUEST; SHALL EXECUTE THE RELEASE OF ANY MEDICAL, COUNSELING, AND PSYCHIATRIC RECORDS AS NECESSARY TO DISCUSS HIS CASE WITH TREATING PHYSICIANS AND/OR ANY PHYSICIANS HOLDING RECORDS; SHALL NOTIFY THE BOARD OF ANY ENTRY, OR RE-ENTRY, INTO AN INPATIENT REHABILITATION, ASSESSMENT, OR EVALUATION PROGRAM AND SHALL PROVIDE AUTHORIZATION FOR ANY AND ALL RECORDS ASSOCIATED WITH TREATMENT. ON 10/2/98 HIS REQUEST TO ADD A SECOND PRACTICE LOCATION WHICH WOULD ALLOW HIM TO PRACTICE IN THE ER OF SPECIFIED MUNICIPAL HOSPITAL, STILL AS AN EMPLOYEE OF THE SAME PRACTICE GROUP WAS GRANTED SUBJECT TO ALL OTHER TERMS OF THIS ORDER.

HILST, WILBUR DEAN MD, DATE OF BIRTH DECEMBER 7, 1931 OF 1821 NORTH CALHOUN AVENUE, LIBERAL, KS, WAS DISCIPLINED BY MEDICARE ON JULY 20, 1998
DISCIPLINARY ACTION: EXCLUSION FROM THE MEDICARE AND/OR MEDICAID PROGRAM

OFFENSE: DISCIPLINARY ACTION BY ANOTHER STATE OR AGENCY

NOTES: LICENSE REVOKED, SUSPENDED, SURRENDERED OR OTHERWISE LOST FOR REASONS BEARING ON PROFESSIONAL PERFORMANCE, PROFESSIONAL COMPETENCE OR FINANCIAL INTEGRITY.

HILTY, RAYMOND W JR MD, DATE OF BIRTH NOVEMBER 29, 1937, LICENSE NUMBER 0016006, WAS DISCIPLINED BY COLORADO ON JUNE 15, 1995
DISCIPLINARY ACTION: REPRIMAND

HITE, JAMES H JR MD, DATE OF BIRTH DECEMBER 26, 1921, LICENSE NUMBER 0014122 OF PUEBLO, CO, WAS DISCIPLINED BY COLORADO ON APRIL 13, 1994

NOTES: NO UNPROFESSIONAL CONDUCT IDENTIFIED. MAY NOT PERFORM ANY ACT DEFINED AS THE PRACTICE OF MEDICINE INCLUDING MEDICATION PRESCRIBING OR FUNCTIONING AS A NURSING HOME MEDICAL DIRECTOR WHILE HIS LICENSE IS INACTIVE. AGREES TO PLACE AND MAINTAIN HIS LICENSE IN INACTIVE STATUS AND NOT TO APPLY TO RESUME THE PRACTICE OF MEDICINE IN COLORADO.

HIX, IVAN E JR MD, DATE OF BIRTH NOVEMBER 24, 1920, LICENSE NUMBER 0010808 OF WHEAT RIDGE, CO, WAS DISCIPLINED BY COLORADO ON AUGUST 22, 1994
DISCIPLINARY ACTION: 60-MONTH PROBATION; RESTRICTION PLACED ON LICENSE
OFFENSE: PHYSICAL OR MENTAL ILLNESS INHIBITING THE ABILITY TO PRACTICE WITH SKILL AND SAFETY

NOTES: PHYSICAL DISABILITY ISSUES. NO HOSPITAL-BASED SURGERY EXCEPT AS ASSISTANT SURGEON OR SURGICAL ASSISTANT.

HOFFMAN, JAMES F JR MD, DATE OF BIRTH FEBRUARY 12, 1938, LICENSE NUMBER 0014835 OF FT COLLINS, CO, WAS DISCIPLINED BY COLORADO ON MARCH 10, 1992
DISCIPLINARY ACTION: EMERGENCY SUSPENSION
OFFENSE: SUBSTANDARD CARE, INCOMPETENCE OR NEGLIGENCE

NOTES: AN ACT OR OMISSION CONSTITUTING GROSSLY NEGLIGENT PRACTICE, OR TWO OR MORE ACTS OF SUBSTANDARD CARE, AND FALSIFYING OR REPEATEDLY FAILING TO MAKE ESSENTIAL ENTRIES ON PATIENT RECORDS.

HOFFMAN, JAMES F JR MD, DATE OF BIRTH FEBRUARY 12, 1938, LICENSE NUMBER 0014835 OF FT COLLINS, CO, WAS DISCIPLINED BY COLORADO ON MAY 15, 1992
DISCIPLINARY ACTION: SURRENDER OF LICENSE
OFFENSE: SUBSTANDARD CARE, INCOMPETENCE OR NEGLIGENCE

NOTES: AN ACT OR OMISSION CONSTITUTING GROSSLY NEGLIGENT PRACTICE, OR TWO OR MORE ACTS OF SUBSTANDARD CARE, AND FALSIFYING OR REPEATEDLY FAILING TO MAKE ESSENTIAL ENTRIES ON PATIENT RECORDS. AGREES NEVER TO REAPPLY FOR LICENSURE IN COLORADO.

HOFFMAN, JAMES F JR MD, WAS DISCIPLINED BY NEVADA ON JANUARY 28, 1993
DISCIPLINARY ACTION: SURRENDER OF LICENSE
OFFENSE: NONCOMPLIANCE WITH A PROFESSIONAL RULE

NOTES: ON 12/04/92 COMPLAINT FILED WHERE HE WAS CHARGED WITH FAILURE TO REPORT WITHIN 30 DAYS, AND CONTINUAL FAILURE TO REPORT TO THE BOARD, THE SURRENDER OF HIS COLORADO LICENSE TO PRACTICE MEDICINE.

HOFFMAN, JAMES F JR MD, DATE OF BIRTH FEBRUARY 12, 1938 OF 1845 KEDRON CIRCLE, FORT COLLINS, CO, WAS DISCIPLINED BY MEDICARE ON AUGUST 13, 1996
DISCIPLINARY ACTION: 180-MONTH EXCLUSION FROM THE MEDICARE AND/OR MEDICAID PROGRAM
OFFENSE: CRIMINAL CONVICTION OR PLEA OF GUILTY, NOLO CONTENDERE, OR NO CONTEST TO A CRIME

NOTES: CONVICTED OF A CRIME INVOLVING THE MEDICARE, MEDICAID, MATERNAL AND CHILD HEALTH SERVICES BLOCK GRANT OR BLOCK GRANTS TO STATES FOR SOCIAL SERVICES PROGRAMS.

HOFFNER, MARGARET M M MD, DATE OF BIRTH DECEMBER 12, 1937, LICENSE NUMBER 0014280 OF FORT COLLINS, CO, WAS DISCIPLINED BY COLORADO ON SEPTEMBER 28, 1990
DISCIPLINARY ACTION: LICENSE REVOCATION
OFFENSE: SUBSTANCE ABUSE

NOTES: HABITUAL INTEMPERANCE. APPEAL FILED 11/9/90. COURT OF APPEALS AFFIRMED BOARD'S ORDER IN 3/92 AND DENIED DR. HOFFNER'S PETITION FOR REHEARING ON 5/7/92.

HOFFNER, MARY M M MD, DATE OF BIRTH DECEMBER 21, 1937 OF 1217 E ELIZABETH ST SUITE 5, FT COLLINS, CO, WAS DISCIPLINED BY MEDICARE ON MAY 10, 1991
DISCIPLINARY ACTION: EXCLUSION FROM THE MEDICARE AND/OR MEDICAID PROGRAM
OFFENSE: DISCIPLINARY ACTION BY ANOTHER STATE OR AGENCY

NOTES: LICENSE REVOCATION OR SUSPENSION.

HOGENKAMP, JON MELVIN MD, LICENSE NUMBER 0028252 OF PUEBLO, CO, WAS DISCIPLINED BY OHIO ON SEPTEMBER 13, 1990
DISCIPLINARY ACTION: SURRENDER OF LICENSE

NOTES: PERMANENT SURRENDER.

HOHM, RICHARD A MD, DATE OF BIRTH NOVEMBER 12, 1944, LICENSE NUMBER 0020609 OF FT COLLINS, CO, WAS DISCIPLINED BY COLORADO ON AUGUST 20, 1993
DISCIPLINARY ACTION: REPRIMAND

HOLDER, SCOTT D MD, DATE OF BIRTH OCTOBER 12, 1963, LICENSE NUMBER 33728, WAS DISCIPLINED BY COLORADO ON MAY 19, 1999
OFFENSE: SUBSTANDARD CARE, INCOMPETENCE OR NEGLIGENCE

NOTES: SUBSTANDARD CARE. AGREES TO PLACE LICENSE IN INACTIVE STATUS; IF HE EVER WERE TO PLACE HIS LICENSE IN ACTIVE STATUS HE MUST COMPLY WITH A FIVE YEAR PERIOD OF PROBATION WHICH INCLUDES REEDUCATION ACTIVITIES AND PRACTICE MONITORING.

HOLLISTER, ELBERT E MD, DATE OF BIRTH FEBRUARY 25, 1930, LICENSE NUMBER 14006, WAS DISCIPLINED BY COLORADO ON FEBRUARY 17, 1999
DISCIPLINARY ACTION: REPRIMAND

HOLMES, KELLY V MD, DATE OF BIRTH JUNE 22, 1964, LICENSE NUMBER 0031434, WAS DISCIPLINED BY COLORADO ON AUGUST 24, 1995
DISCIPLINARY ACTION: EMERGENCY SUSPENSION
OFFENSE: SUBSTANCE ABUSE

NOTES: SUBSTANCE ABUSE.

HOLMES, KELLY V MD, DATE OF BIRTH JUNE 22, 1964, LICENSE

NUMBER 31434, WAS DISCIPLINED BY COLORADO ON APRIL 10, 1997
DISCIPLINARY ACTION: LICENSE SUSPENSION
OFFENSE: SUBSTANCE ABUSE

NOTES: HABITUAL INTEMPERANCE OR EXCESSIVE USE OF A CONTROLLED SUBSTANCE. SHE AGREES TO AN INDEFINITE SUSPENSION, ABSTINENCE FROM ADDICTIVE SUBSTANCES AND ADDITIONAL TERMS.

HOLMES, KELLY V MD, DATE OF BIRTH JUNE 22, 1964, LICENSE NUMBER 31434, WAS DISCIPLINED BY COLORADO ON JULY 10, 1997
DISCIPLINARY ACTION: LICENSE REVOCATION
OFFENSE: FAILURE TO COMPLY WITH PREVIOUS BOARD ORDER

NOTES: FAILED TO COMPLY WITH PROBATIONARY TERMS. STAYED REVOCATION LIFTED AND REVOCATION PUT INTO EFFECT.

HOLTGREWE, JEFFREY L MD, DATE OF BIRTH MARCH 16, 1956, LICENSE NUMBER 0028681 OF COLORADO SPRINGS, CO, WAS DISCIPLINED BY COLORADO ON NOVEMBER 18, 1994
DISCIPLINARY ACTION: PROBATION; REQUIRED TO TAKE ADDITIONAL MEDICAL EDUCATION
OFFENSE: PHYSICAL OR MENTAL ILLNESS INHIBITING THE ABILITY TO PRACTICE WITH SKILL AND SAFETY

NOTES: PHYSICAL DISABILITY ISSUES. LICENSE REACTIVATED UNDER STIPULATION FOR LIFETIME PROBATION INCLUDING PRACTICE AND TREATMENT MONITORING AND REEDUCATION ACTIVITIES.

HORWITZ, MICHAEL L MD, LICENSE NUMBER G50945 OF GRAND JUNCTION, CO, WAS DISCIPLINED BY CALIFORNIA ON DECEMBER 31, 1999
DISCIPLINARY ACTION: REPRIMAND

HOWARD, BARRY MD, LICENSE NUMBER 0G42894 OF BOULDER, CO, WAS DISCIPLINED BY CALIFORNIA ON AUGUST 24, 1994
DISCIPLINARY ACTION: LICENSE REVOCATION
OFFENSE: DISCIPLINARY ACTION BY ANOTHER STATE OR AGENCY

NOTES: DISCIPLINED BY COLORADO BOARD FOR WRITING FALSE PRESCRIPTIONS TO OBTAIN PERCODAN AND PERCOCET FOR SELF USE. DEFAULT DECISION.

HOWARD, WILLIAM L MD, DATE OF BIRTH FEBRUARY 1, 1953, LICENSE NUMBER 0025310 OF BRIGHTON, CO, WAS DISCIPLINED BY COLORADO ON JULY 15, 1992
DISCIPLINARY ACTION: SURRENDER OF CONTROLLED SUBSTANCE LICENSE; 60-MONTH PROBATION
OFFENSE: SUBSTANCE ABUSE

NOTES: ADMINISTERING, DISPENSING OR PRESCRIBING ANY HABIT-FORMING DRUG OR CONTROLLED SUBSTANCE OTHER THAN IN THE COURSE OF LEGITIMATE PROFESSIONAL PRACTICE; HABITUAL INTEMPERANCE OR EXCESSIVE USE OF ANY HABIT-FORMING DRUG OR CONTROLLED SUBSTANCE; PHYSICAL OR MENTAL DISABILITY; AND PRESCRIBING, DISTRIBUTING, OR GIVING TO A FAMILY MEMBER OR TO ONESELF EXCEPT ON AN EMERGENCY BASIS ANY CONTROLLED SUBSTANCE. REVOCATION, STAYED FOR 5 YEARS SUBJECT TO TERMS OF STIPULATION INCLUDING A FIVE YEAR PROBATIONARY PERIOD, SURRENDER OF DEA CERTIFICATE WITH BOARD-APPROVED GRADUATED RETURN OF PRESCRIBING PRIVILEGES; PRACTICE AND TREATMENT MONITORING. 8/14/92: SECOND STIPULATION/ORDER. TERMS AND CONDITIONS OF FIRST ORDER REMAIN IN EFFECT EXCEPT FOR PARAGRAPH 14 (WHICH IS RESCINDED AND REPLACED); MAY ADMINISTER, DISPENSE OR PRESCRIBE CONTROLLED SUBSTANCES ONLY THRU PHARMACY AT PLATTE VALLEY HOSPITAL; MUST RECORD SUCH PRESCRIBING IN A LOG BOOK AND USE NUMBERED PRESCRIPTION PADS.

HOWARD, WILLIAM L MD, DATE OF BIRTH FEBRUARY 1, 1953, LICENSE NUMBER 0025310 OF BOULDER, CO, WAS DISCIPLINED BY COLORADO ON DECEMBER 8, 1994
DISCIPLINARY ACTION: LICENSE SUSPENSION
OFFENSE: PHYSICAL OR MENTAL ILLNESS INHIBITING THE ABILITY TO PRACTICE WITH SKILL AND SAFETY

NOTES: PHYSICAL OR MENTAL DISABILITY ISSUES. LICENSE INDEFINITELY SUSPENDED.

HOWARD, WILLIAM L MD, LICENSE NUMBER 0006039, WAS DISCIPLINED BY RHODE ISLAND ON JULY 12, 1995
DISCIPLINARY ACTION: RESTRICTION PLACED ON LICENSE
OFFENSE: DISCIPLINARY ACTION BY ANOTHER STATE OR AGENCY

NOTES: COLORADO PLACED RESTRICTIONS ON HIS LICENSE TO PRACTICE MEDICINE. RHODE ISLAND HAS ADOPTED THESE RESTRICTIONS. ACTIONS WOULD BE UNPROFESSIONAL CONDUCT IN RHODE ISLAND.

HOWE, JOHN J MD, DATE OF BIRTH JULY 17, 1938, LICENSE NUMBER 0014837 OF PUEBLO, CO, WAS DISCIPLINED BY COLORADO ON JUNE 14, 1991
DISCIPLINARY ACTION: 60-MONTH PROBATION; REQUIRED TO ENTER AN IMPAIRED PHYSICIAN PROGRAM OR SUBSTANCE ABUSE TREATMENT
OFFENSE: SUBSTANCE ABUSE

NOTES: HABITUAL (ALCOHOL) INTEMPERANCE; SUCH PHYSICAL OR MENTAL DISABILITY AS TO RENDER PHYSICIAN UNABLE TO PERFORM MEDICAL SERVICES WITH REASONABLE SKILL AND SAFETY. SUBSTANCE ABSTINENCE, ALCOHOL DEPENDENCY TREATMENT, URINALYSIS 3 TIMES PER WEEK, MONITORED ANTABUSE, AFTER CARE, AA, OFFICE AND HOSPITAL PRACTICE MONITORING.

HOWE, JOHN J MD, DATE OF BIRTH JULY 17, 1938, LICENSE NUMBER 0014837 OF PUEBLO, CO, WAS DISCIPLINED BY COLORADO ON FEBRUARY 18, 1994
DISCIPLINARY ACTION: REPRIMAND
OFFENSE: FAILURE TO COMPLY WITH PREVIOUS BOARD ORDER

NOTES: VIOLATION OF ORDER DATED 6/14/91.

HOWE, JOHN J MD, DATE OF BIRTH JULY 17, 1938, LICENSE NUMBER 0014837 OF PUEBLO, CO, WAS DISCIPLINED BY COLORADO ON APRIL 14, 1994
DISCIPLINARY ACTION: SURRENDER OF LICENSE

NOTES: HAD RETIRED FROM PRACTICE AND CEASED URINE MONITORING. NO UNPROFESSIONAL CONDUCT WAS IDENTIFIED REGARDING CEASING URINE MONITORING.

HRDLICKA, JAN F MD, DATE OF BIRTH APRIL 9, 1939, LICENSE NUMBER 0019210 OF ARVADA, CO, WAS DISCIPLINED BY COLORADO ON SEPTEMBER 8, 1994
DISCIPLINARY ACTION: SURRENDER OF LICENSE
OFFENSE: SUBSTANDARD CARE, INCOMPETENCE OR NEGLIGENCE

NOTES: ALLEGATIONS OF AN ACT OR OMISSION CONSTITUTING GROSSLY NEGLIGENT MEDICAL PRACTICE OR TWO OR MORE ACTS OR OMISSIONS WHICH FAIL TO MEET GENERALLY ACCEPTED STANDARDS WHICH DR. HRDLICKA DENIES.

HUFFORD, JOHN H DO, DATE OF BIRTH AUGUST 1, 1940, LICENSE NUMBER 0016598 OF AURORA, CO, WAS DISCIPLINED BY

COLORADO ON JUNE 10, 1994
DISCIPLINARY ACTION: LICENSE SUSPENSION; MONITORING OF PHYSICIAN PERFORMANCE
OFFENSE: SUBSTANCE ABUSE

NOTES: SUBSTANCE ABUSE ISSUES AND MENTAL AND/OR PHYSICAL DISABILITY ISSUES. SUSPENDED UNTIL HE FULFILLS SPECIFIC REQUIREMENTS INCLUDING AN EVALUATION AND ONGOING PRACTICE AND TREATMENT MONITORING. IF APPROVED BY BOARD OF MEDICAL EXAMINERS TO RETURN TO PRACTICE, THEN PROBATION FOR FIVE YEARS.

HUNT, THEODORE C MD, DATE OF BIRTH AUGUST 27, 1931, LICENSE NUMBER 0014930, WAS DISCIPLINED BY COLORADO ON SEPTEMBER 19, 1996
DISCIPLINARY ACTION: RESTRICTION PLACED ON LICENSE

NOTES: ON 5/31/95 HE PLACED HIS COLORADO MEDICAL LICENSE ON INACTIVE STATUS. PERMANENT RESTRICTION AS AN INDEPENDENT MEDICAL EXAMINER.

HUSTON, JEFFREY D MD, DATE OF BIRTH APRIL 4, 1949, LICENSE NUMBER 24485, WAS DISCIPLINED BY COLORADO ON NOVEMBER 13, 1998
DISCIPLINARY ACTION: REPRIMAND

HUTTNER, DONALD J MD, DATE OF BIRTH FEBRUARY 21, 1935, LICENSE NUMBER 0013829, WAS DISCIPLINED BY COLORADO ON MAY 11, 1995
DISCIPLINARY ACTION: SURRENDER OF LICENSE

NOTES: SURRENDERED HIS LICENSE AFTER A SUMMARY SUSPENSION ORDER.

JACKSON, TAYLOR W MD OF 6 ABILENE STE 201, AURORA, CO, WAS DISCIPLINED BY DEA ON FEBRUARY 8, 1990
DISCIPLINARY ACTION: SURRENDER OF CONTROLLED SUBSTANCE LICENSE
OFFENSE: SUBSTANDARD CARE, INCOMPETENCE OR NEGLIGENCE

NOTES: STATE LICENSE REVOKED BECAUSE OF SUBSTANDARD CARE TO PATIENTS.

JACOBS, ROBERT C MD, DATE OF BIRTH DECEMBER 8, 1936, LICENSE NUMBER 14578, WAS DISCIPLINED BY COLORADO ON JULY 9, 1998
DISCIPLINARY ACTION: REPRIMAND
OFFENSE: PROFESSIONAL MISCONDUCT

NOTES: UNNECESSARY TREATMENT.

JAFEK, BRUCE W MD, DATE OF BIRTH MARCH 4, 1941, LICENSE NUMBER 19991, WAS DISCIPLINED BY COLORADO ON MAY 21, 1999
DISCIPLINARY ACTION: REPRIMAND

JAFEK, BRUCE W MD, LICENSE NUMBER A22587 OF DENVER, CO, WAS DISCIPLINED BY CALIFORNIA ON SEPTEMBER 22, 1999
DISCIPLINARY ACTION: REPRIMAND

JENKINS, CHARLES T DO, DATE OF BIRTH JANUARY 25, 1928, LICENSE NUMBER 0031115 OF DANA POINT, CA, WAS DISCIPLINED BY COLORADO ON JULY 15, 1991
DISCIPLINARY ACTION: PROBATION
OFFENSE: PHYSICAL OR MENTAL ILLNESS INHIBITING THE ABILITY TO PRACTICE WITH SKILL AND SAFETY

NOTES: PHYSICAL OR MENTAL DISABILITY AS TO RENDER HIM UNABLE TO PERFORM MEDICAL SERVICES WITH REASONABLE SKILL AND SAFETY. APPLICANT FOR LICENSURE. LIFETIME PROBATION, PHYSICIAN-PSYCHIATRIST THERAPY FROM ONE LICENSED IN COLORADO. IN ABEYANCE.

JENKINS, KEITH E MD, DATE OF BIRTH NOVEMBER 14, 1955, LICENSE NUMBER 31911, WAS DISCIPLINED BY COLORADO ON SEPTEMBER 10, 1998
DISCIPLINARY ACTION: REPRIMAND

JESSEL, JOHN M MD, DATE OF BIRTH MAY 1, 1944, LICENSE NUMBER 0020194 OF COLORADO SPRINGS, CO, WAS DISCIPLINED BY COLORADO ON JUNE 12, 1992
DISCIPLINARY ACTION: SURRENDER OF LICENSE
OFFENSE: SUBSTANDARD CARE, INCOMPETENCE OR NEGLIGENCE

NOTES: AN ACT OR OMISSION CONSTITUTING GROSSLY NEGLIGENT PRACTICE, OR TWO OR MORE ACTS OF SUBSTANDARD CARE.

JOHNSON, BENJAMIN T MD, DATE OF BIRTH MAY 29, 1967, LICENSE NUMBER 34609, WAS DISCIPLINED BY COLORADO ON OCTOBER 15, 1998
DISCIPLINARY ACTION: REPRIMAND

JOHNSON, BENJAMIN TAYLOR MD, LICENSE NUMBER A67193 OF ENGLEWOOD, CO, WAS DISCIPLINED BY CALIFORNIA ON MAY 11, 1999
DISCIPLINARY ACTION: REPRIMAND
OFFENSE: DISCIPLINARY ACTION BY ANOTHER STATE OR AGENCY

NOTES: DISCIPLINED BY COLORADO FOR PRESCRIBING VIAGRA VIA THE INTERNET AND TELEPHONE FOR INDIVIDUALS WITH WHOM HE HAD NOT ESTABLISHED A PHYSICIAN/PATIENT RELATIONSHIP, HAD NOT PHYSICALLY EXAMINED, AND HAD NOT KEPT APPROPRIATE PATIENT RECORDS.

JOHNSON, CHARLES L DO, DATE OF BIRTH JULY 2, 1945, LICENSE NUMBER 0018812 OF COLORADO SPRINGS, CO, WAS DISCIPLINED BY COLORADO ON AUGUST 12, 1992
DISCIPLINARY ACTION: 60-MONTH PROBATION; RESTRICTION PLACED ON LICENSE

NOTES: TWO OR MORE ACTS OR OMISSIONS WHICH FAILED TO MEET GENERALLY ACCEPTED STANDARDS OF MEDICAL PRACTICE. EDUCATION ASSESSMENT AND PERMANENT PRACTICE RESTRICTION. WILL BE PERMANENTLY LIMITED TO FAMILY PRACTICE, AND SUCH PRACTICE WILL NOT INCLUDE SURGERY, ABORTIONS OR OBSTETRICAL CARE; PRACTICE MONITORING; ASSESSMENT FOR, AND COMPLETION OF, AN INDIVIDUAL EDUCATION PLAN.

JOHNSON, CHARLES L MD, LICENSE NUMBER 154576 OF 503 NORTH OAKLAND AVENUE, PASADENA, CA, WAS DISCIPLINED BY NEW YORK ON JUNE 26, 1998
DISCIPLINARY ACTION: LICENSE REVOCATION
OFFENSE: DISCIPLINARY ACTION BY ANOTHER STATE OR AGENCY

NOTES: DISCIPLINED BY THE CALIFORNIA BOARD FOR GROSS NEGLIGENCE, INCOMPETENCE, REPEATED NEGLIGENCE AND EXCESSIVE PRESCRIBING AND TESTING.

JOHNSON, CHARLES LARUE DO OF MONUMENT, IL, WAS DISCIPLINED BY ILLINOIS ON AUGUST 1, 1993
DISCIPLINARY ACTION: 48-MONTH PROBATION
OFFENSE: DISCIPLINARY ACTION BY ANOTHER STATE OR AGENCY

NOTES: DISCIPLINED IN COLORADO.

JOHNSON, CHARLES LYNNWOOD MD, LICENSE NUMBER G69296 OF PASADENA, CA, WAS DISCIPLINED BY CALIFORNIA ON JUNE 30, 1997
DISCIPLINARY ACTION: 84-MONTH PROBATION

NOTES: GROSS NEGLIGENCE, INCOMPETENCE AND REPEATED NEGLIGENT ACTS IN THE CARE AND TREATMENT OF SEVEN PATIENTS. REVOCATION STAYED.

JOHNSON, CHARLES LYNNWOOD MD, LICENSE NUMBER G69296 OF LOS ANGELES, CA, WAS DISCIPLINED BY CALIFORNIA ON DECEMBER 17, 1999
DISCIPLINARY ACTION: LICENSE REVOCATION

JOHNSON, JOHNNY E JR MD, DATE OF BIRTH MARCH 14, 1945, LICENSE NUMBER 22809, WAS DISCIPLINED BY COLORADO ON NOVEMBER 12, 1997
DISCIPLINARY ACTION: REPRIMAND; REQUIRED TO TAKE ADDITIONAL MEDICAL EDUCATION
OFFENSE: SEXUAL ABUSE OF OR SEXUAL MISCONDUCT WITH A PATIENT

NOTES: SEXUAL CONTACT WITH A PATIENT. MUST COMPLETE A BOUNDARIES COURSE WITHIN ONE YEAR.

JOHNSON, PATRICIA L MD, DATE OF BIRTH MARCH 25, 1953 OF 1254 COOK STREET, DENVER, CO, WAS DISCIPLINED BY MEDICARE ON JULY 26, 1990
DISCIPLINARY ACTION: EXCLUSION FROM THE MEDICARE AND/OR MEDICAID PROGRAM
OFFENSE: DISCIPLINARY ACTION BY ANOTHER STATE OR AGENCY

NOTES: LICENSE REVOCATION OR SUSPENSION.

JOHNSON, VAUGHN A MD, DATE OF BIRTH JULY 12, 1939, LICENSE NUMBER 0014849, WAS DISCIPLINED BY COLORADO ON AUGUST 14, 1996
DISCIPLINARY ACTION: 60-MONTH PROBATION; REQUIRED TO TAKE ADDITIONAL MEDICAL EDUCATION
OFFENSE: SUBSTANDARD CARE, INCOMPETENCE OR NEGLIGENCE

NOTES: SUBSTANDARD CARE (PRIMA FACIE TYPE ADMISSION ONLY. RE-EDUCATION ACTIVITIES AND PRACTICE MONITORING.

JOHNSON, VAUGHN A MD OF DURANGO, CO, WAS DISCIPLINED BY UTAH ON JUNE 12, 1997
DISCIPLINARY ACTION: PROBATION
OFFENSE: DISCIPLINARY ACTION BY ANOTHER STATE OR AGENCY

NOTES: DISCIPLINARY ACTION TAKEN AGAINST HIS MEDICAL LICENSE IN COLORADO. CONDITIONS ON LICENSE FOR THE DURATION OF HIS COLORADO PROBATION. AS OF 1/29/98, THE PROBATION WAS TERMINATED AND HIS MEDICAL LICENSE WAS REINSTATED WITH FULL PRIVILEGES.

JOHNSTON, JAMES C MD, LICENSE NUMBER 0022573, WAS DISCIPLINED BY ARIZONA ON OCTOBER 18, 1995

NOTES: SHALL NOT PRACTICE MEDICINE IN ARIZONA PRIOR TO MEETING WITH THE BOARD.

JOHNSTON, JAMES C MD, LICENSE NUMBER 25337 OF SAN ANTONIO, TX, WAS DISCIPLINED BY WASHINGTON ON JANUARY 24, 1997

NOTES: AGREED ORDER TO APPEAR BEFORE THE COMMISSION PRIOR TO PRACTICING MEDICINE IN WASHINGTON. ON 1/21/99 REQUEST TO TERMINATE THE CONDITIONS OF THIS ORDER GRANTED AND LICENSE IS NOW UNRESTRICTED.

JOHNSTON, JAMES C MD, DATE OF BIRTH NOVEMBER 20, 1954, LICENSE NUMBER 33573, WAS DISCIPLINED BY COLORADO ON APRIL 17, 1997
DISCIPLINARY ACTION: SURRENDER OF LICENSE

NOTES: NO UNPROFESSIONAL CONDUCT IDENTIFIED.

JOHNSTON, JAMES CHRISTOPHER MD, DATE OF BIRTH NOVEMBER 20, 1959, LICENSE NUMBER 00G8880 OF NACOGDOCHES, TX, WAS DISCIPLINED BY TEXAS ON JUNE 22, 1994
DISCIPLINARY ACTION: RESTRICTION PLACED ON LICENSE
OFFENSE: SEXUAL ABUSE OF OR SEXUAL MISCONDUCT WITH A PATIENT

NOTES: AS RECENTLY AS 6/8/94 CRIMINAL COMPLAINTS WERE FILED AGAINST HIM ALLEGING HE ENGAGED IN BEHAVIOR CONSTITUTING ATTEMPTED SEXUAL ASSAULT AGAINST INDIVIDUALS WHO WERE PATIENTS; DENIES ALLEGATIONS; BECAUSE HE DESIRES TO FOCUS RESOURCES AND TIME ON DEFENSE OF THE CRIMINAL CASE. AGREES TO THIS ORDER WITH THE BOARD. LICENSE IS RESTRICTED AS FOLLOWS: SHALL NOT EXAMINE OR TREAT PATIENTS AFTER THE ORDER DATE; WITHIN 30 DAYS SHALL SUBMIT HIMSELF FOR ASSESSMENT THROUGH THE BEHAVIOR CARE NETWORK PROGRAM OR OTHER BOARD-APPROVED PROGRAM WHICH WILL FOCUS ON THE DISPARITY BETWEEN THE COMPLAINTS AGAINST HIM AND HIS OWN VERSION OF EVENTS AND ATTEMPT TO DETERMINE THE DEGREE OF RISK TO THE PUBLIC INVOLVED IN HIS CONTINUED PRACTICE; SHOULD THIS EVALUATION INDICATE HIS PRACTICE CONSTITUTES NO THREAT TO THE PUBLIC HEALTH HE SHALL BE PERMITTED TO RESUME PRACTICE PENDING FURTHER ORDER OF THE BOARD PROVIDED HE SEES PATIENTS ONLY WHEN ACCOMPANIED BY A CHAPERONE APPROVED IN ADVANCE WHO WILL SIGN ALL CHARTS TO INDICATE PRESENCE; SHALL COOPERATE WITH THE BOARD IN VERIFYING COMPLIANCE; SHALL INFORM BOARD OF CHANGE OF ADDRESS WITHIN 10 DAYS.

JOHNSTON, JAMES CHRISTOPHER MD, DATE OF BIRTH NOVEMBER 20, 1959, LICENSE NUMBER 00G8880 OF 5601 BANDERA ROAD SUITE 416, SAN ANTONIO, TX, WAS DISCIPLINED BY TEXAS ON SEPTEMBER 30, 1994
DISCIPLINARY ACTION: RESTRICTION PLACED ON LICENSE
OFFENSE: SEXUAL ABUSE OF OR SEXUAL MISCONDUCT WITH A PATIENT

NOTES: CRIMINAL COMPLAINTS HAVE BEEN FILED AGAINST HIM ALLEGING THAT HE HAS ENGAGED IN BEHAVIOR CONSTITUTING ATTEMPTED SEXUAL ASSAULT AGAINST INDIVIDUALS WHO WERE PATIENTS; HE DENIES ALL OF THESE ALLEGATIONS; AS A CONDITION OF 6/22/94 AGREEMENT HAS UNDERGONE AN EXTENSIVE EVALUATION WHICH CONCLUDED THAT THERE WAS NOTHING TO SUGGEST THAT HE WOULD BE UNABLE TO PROVIDE CLINICAL SERVICES UNDER CERTAIN RESTRICTIONS AND SUPERVISION. CONDITIONS OF RESTRICTION WHICH SUPERSEDE PREVIOUS ORDER: SHALL NOT EXAMINE OR TREAT ANY PATIENT WITHOUT BEING ACCOMPANIED BY A BOARD APPROVED CHAPERONE WHO SHALL VERIFY PRESENCE BY SIGNING ALL CHARTS; SHALL OBTAIN AN EXAM TABLE WITH SPECIFICATIONS; SHALL REPOSITION THIS TABLE SO HE MAY WALK BEHIND PATIENTS TO EXAMINE THE SHOULDER AND PROXIMAL AREAS; SHALL NOT PLACE A PAGER OR INSTRUMENTS IN HIS POCKETS DURING EXAMS; PATIENTS SHALL ONLY BE REPOSITIONED BY A NURSE OR TECHNICIAN; SHALL EXPLAIN TO ALL PATIENTS PROCEDURES WHICH INVOLVE CONTACT

AND ASK THEM IN DETAIL REGARDING ANY PROBLEMS OR CONCERNS REGARDING HIS EXAM; WITHIN 60 DAYS SHALL UNDERGO ADDITIONAL PHALLOMETRIC TESTING; SHALL COOPERATE WITH THE BOARD IN VERIFYING COMPLIANCE; SHALL INFORM THE BOARD OF CHANGE OF ADDRESS WITHIN 10 DAYS; SHALL HAVE THE RIGHT TO PETITION FOR AMENDMENT OR TERMINATION UPON DISMISSAL OR ACQUITTAL ON THE CRIMINAL CHARGES; OTHERWISE MAY SEEK MODIFICATIONS ONCE A YEAR. ON 1/29/99 ORDER TERMINATED.

JOHNSTON, JAMES CHRISTOPHER MD, LICENSE NUMBER 00M5411, WAS DISCIPLINED BY IDAHO ON DECEMBER 14, 1994
DISCIPLINARY ACTION: RESTRICTION PLACED ON LICENSE; MONITORING OF PHYSICIAN PERFORMANCE
OFFENSE: DISCIPLINARY ACTION BY ANOTHER STATE OR AGENCY

NOTES: ON 9/30/94 TEXAS RESTRICTED HIS LICENSE BASED ON CRIMINAL ALLEGATIONS THAT HE HAD ENGAGED IN BEHAVIOR CONSTITUTING ATTEMPTED SEXUAL ASSAULT AGAINST PATIENTS. IDAHO BOARD ADOPTS AND INCORPORATES ALL TERMS AND CONDITIONS OF THE TEXAS ORDER WHICH INCLUDE: SHALL NOT EXAMINE OR TREAT ANY PATIENTS WITHOUT BEING ACCOMPANIED AT ALL TIMES BY A PROCTOR OR CHAPERONE APPROVED BY THE BOARD; SHALL OBTAIN AN EXAM TABLE THAT IS SPECIFICALLY DESIGNED FOR THE PERFORMANCE OF ELECTROMYOGRAPHY WITH A STANDARD ARM BOARD AND THE ABILITY TO ELEVATE THE HEAD OF THE PATIENT; SHALL REPOSITION HIS EXAMINATION TABLE SO THAT HE MAY WALK BEHIND PATIENTS TO EXAMINE THE SHOULDER AND PROXIMAL AREAS; SHALL NOT PLACE A PAGER OR INSTRUMENTS IN HIS POCKETS DURING EXAMINATION OF PATIENTS; PATIENTS SHALL BE REPOSITIONED DURING EVALUATIONS ONLY BY A NURSE OR TECHNICIAN; SHALL EXPLAIN TO ALL PATIENTS THOSE PROCEDURES WHICH INVOLVE CONTACT WITH HIM PRIOR TO SUCH CONTACT; SHALL ASK PATIENTS IN DETAIL REGARDING ANY PROBLEMS OR CONCERNS WHICH THEY MIGHT HAVE CONCERNING HIS EXAMINATIONS OR ANY PROCEDURES PERFORMED; SHALL UNDERGO ADDITIONAL PHALLOMETRIC TESTING WITHIN 60 DAYS. ON 1/13/99 ORDER TERMINATED.

JOHNSTON, JAMES CHRISTOPHER MD, LICENSE NUMBER 0A44527 OF NACOGDOCHES, TX, WAS DISCIPLINED BY CALIFORNIA ON DECEMBER 30, 1995
DISCIPLINARY ACTION: SURRENDER OF LICENSE

NOTES: WHILE CHARGES PENDING.

JOHNSTON, JAMES CHRISTOPHER MD, LICENSE NUMBER 0018716 OF SAN ANTONIO, TX, WAS DISCIPLINED BY OREGON ON NOVEMBER 4, 1996
DISCIPLINARY ACTION: SURRENDER OF LICENSE

NOTES: VOLUNTARY SURRENDER.

JORDAN, KENT MD, DATE OF BIRTH JANUARY 3, 1932, LICENSE NUMBER 0015180 OF VISALIA, CA, WAS DISCIPLINED BY COLORADO ON AUGUST 21, 1992
DISCIPLINARY ACTION: SURRENDER OF LICENSE
OFFENSE: PHYSICAL OR MENTAL ILLNESS INHIBITING THE ABILITY TO PRACTICE WITH SKILL AND SAFETY

NOTES: PHYSICAL OR MENTAL DISABILITY. PERMANENT SURRENDER. AGREES TO NEVER REAPPLY FOR LICENSURE IN COLORADO.

JOSEPH, RONALD B MD, LICENSE NUMBER 8699, WAS DISCIPLINED BY ARIZONA ON NOVEMBER 12, 1997
DISCIPLINARY ACTION: 24-MONTH PROBATION; REQUIRED TO TAKE ADDITIONAL MEDICAL EDUCATION
OFFENSE: PROFESSIONAL MISCONDUCT

NOTES: ON ONE OR MORE OCCASIONS DURING THE BOARD'S INVESTIGATION, HE FAILED TO RESPOND TO SUBPOENAS TO PRODUCE DOCUMENTS OR TO TIMELY OBJECT TO THE SUBPOENAS. THE FOLLOWING CASES WERE INVOLVED IN THE INVESTIGATION: ON 6/22/92, HE PERFORMED SURGERY ON A FEMALE PATIENT; ALTHOUGH THE PATIENT HAD SIGNED A CONSENT FORM, THERE WAS NO DOCUMENTATION INDICATING THAT THE PATIENT HAD REQUESTED THE PROCEDURE, THAT HE HAD EXPLAINED THE RISKS ASSOCIATED WITH THE PROCEDURE OR THAT HE HAD REVIEWED X-RAYS; HE ALSO FAILED TO TIMELY DICTATE A MEDICAL RECORD THAT ANOTHER SURGERY, SCHEDULED FOR THE PATIENT ON 7/2/92, HAD BEEN CANCELED. IN A SECOND CASE ON 8/11/93, A HOSPITAL EMERGENCY DEPARTMENT PHYSICIAN ATTEMPTED TO CONTACT DR. JOSEPH REGARDING A MALE PATIENT THAT HE HAD TREATED ON SEVERAL OCCASIONS BETWEEN JULY AND AUGUST 1993 AND PERFORMED AN ARTHROSCOPY; ON 8/6/93; THE EMERGENCY PHYSICIAN WAS ABLE TO REACH THE DOCTOR'S NURSE; ACCORDING TO THE NURSE, DR. JOSEPH WAS OUT OF TOWN, WAS NOT AVAILABLE, AND THAT TO HER KNOWLEDGE, HE HAD NO ONE COVERING FOR HIM. IN A DEPOSITION HE GAVE ON 6/26/95, IN A THIRD CASE DR. JOSEPH PROVIDED TESTIMONY CONTRARY TO HIS OFFICE NOTES REGARDING A PATIENT HE TREATED BETWEEN 6/11/93 AND 2/15/95. CONDITIONS OF PROBATION: WITHIN 30 DAYS, HE SHALL ENGAGE A BOARD APPROVED OFFICE MANAGEMENT AND BILLING CONSULTANT WHO WITHIN 150 DAYS SHALL MAKE A WRITTEN REPORT, INCLUDING RECOMMENDATIONS, OF HIS EVALUATION OF DR. JOSEPH'S OFFICE AND BILLING PRACTICES; SHALL PERFORM 20 MAJOR SURGERIES WHICH SHALL BE CONCURRENTLY SUPERVISED BY AT LEAST FOUR DIFFERENT BOARD APPROVED SUPERVISORS WHO SHALL SUBMIT A WRITTEN REPORT TO THE BOARD WITHIN 60 DAYS AFTER EACH SURGICAL CASE; THE BOARD SHALL CONDUCT A REVIEW OF HIS PATIENT CARE AND BILLING PRACTICES AT THE END OF ONE YEAR; WITHIN ONE YEAR, SHALL TAKE EIGHT HOURS OF CONTINUING MEDICAL EDUCATION IN FORENSIC ETHICS. WITHIN 90 DAYS, HE SHALL PAY RESTITUTION TO A SPECIFIED PATIENT OF ALL FEES PAID TO THE DOCTOR AND HIS MEDICAL PRACTICE, SHALL REIMBURSE THE PATIENT'S INSURANCE CARRIER(S), AND SHALL PROVIDE SATISFACTORY EVIDENCE TO THE BOARD OF PAYMENT IN FULL.

JOSEPH, RONALD B MD, DATE OF BIRTH OCTOBER 9, 1944, LICENSE NUMBER 19422, WAS DISCIPLINED BY COLORADO ON AUGUST 18, 1999
DISCIPLINARY ACTION: REPRIMAND

KANG, BOBBY C DO, DATE OF BIRTH AUGUST 16, 1950, LICENSE NUMBER 0026022 OF COLORADO SPRINGS, CO, WAS DISCIPLINED BY COLORADO ON JANUARY 17, 1992
DISCIPLINARY ACTION: LICENSE REVOCATION

NOTES: FAILURE TO MEET GENERALLY ACCEPTED STANDARDS OF MEDICAL PRACTICE. REVOCATION VACATED BY COURT OF APPEALS ON 8/13/92; CASE REMANDED WITH DIRECTIONS. SECOND FINAL BOARD ORDER ISSUED 12/11/92 REVOKING HIS MEDICAL LICENSE.

KANG, BOBBY CHU DO, LICENSE NUMBER 0002373, WAS DISCIPLINED BY OKLAHOMA ON APRIL 6, 1992
DISCIPLINARY ACTION: LICENSE REINSTATEMENT; 60-MONTH PROBATION

NOTES: PROBATION UNDER THE FOLLOWING TERMS AND CONDITIONS: THE FIRST TWO YEARS OF THIS PERIOD MUST BE SPENT AS A FAMILY PRACTICE RESIDENT UNDER SUPERVISION; HIS LICENSE WILL BE CANCELED IF HE LEAVES THE RESIDENCY PROGRAM PRIOR TO COMPLETION; MUST CONFINE HIS PRACTICE ACTIVITY TO PARTICIPATION IN THE RESIDENCY PROGRAM. SHALL NOTIFY THE BOARD IN WRITING OF ANY CHANGE OF ADDRESS WITHIN 14 DAYS; SHALL APPEAR BEFORE THE BOARD UPON REQUEST; AGREES TO UNANNOUNCED VISITS FROM THE BOARD AT SUCH TIMES AND PLACES AS WILL BE DETERMINED AT BOARD DISCRETION; TERMS OF RESIDENCE OR PRACTICE OUTSIDE OKLAHOMA WILL RESULT IN THE TOLLING OF THE AGREEMENT AND WILL NOT APPLY TO THE REDUCTION OF PROBATION; SHALL NOT SEEK ANY AUTHORITY FROM THE STATE BUREAU OF NARCOTICS AND DANGEROUS DRUGS OR THE DRUG ENFORCEMENT ADMINISTRATION TO PRESCRIBE, DISPENSE, OR ADMINISTER CONTROLLED DANGEROUS SUBSTANCES, NOR SHALL HE ENGAGE IN THE PRESCRIPTION, DISPENSING, OR ADMINISTRATION OF SUCH CONTROLLED DANGEROUS SUBSTANCES; WITHIN 180 DAYS HE MUST FURNISH EVIDENCE THAT HE HAS COMPLETED A COURSE IN MEDICAL ETHICS; SHALL PROVIDE THE BOARD WITH QUARTERLY REPORTS OF HIS PROGRESS THROUGH THE RESIDENCY PROGRAM. ON 3/17/94 PROBATION AND RESTRICTIONS TERMINATED.

KANTOR, JOHN R MD, LICENSE NUMBER 00C4667 OF ANDREWS, TX, WAS DISCIPLINED BY TEXAS ON AUGUST 18, 1995
DISCIPLINARY ACTION: 60-MONTH RESTRICTION PLACED ON LICENSE; 60-MONTH RESTRICTION PLACED ON CONTROLLED SUBSTANCE LICENSE
OFFENSE: OVERPRESCRIBING OR MISPRESCRIBING DRUGS

NOTES: DURING 1992 AND 1993, HE PRESCRIBED DIETHYLPROPION, A CONTROLLED SUBSTANCE, TO FAMILY MEMBERS WITHOUT AN APPROPRIATE EVALUATION, AN ADEQUATE DIAGNOSIS AND ADEQUATE DOCUMENTATION; DURING 1993, PRESCRIBED RITALIN, A CONTROLLED SUBSTANCE, TO FAMILY MEMBERS WITHOUT AN APPROPRIATE EVALUATION, AN ADEQUATE DIAGNOSIS AND ADEQUATE DOCUMENTATION. RESTRICTION FOR FIVE YEARS WITH TERMS: SHALL NOT TREAT OR OTHERWISE SERVE AS PHYSICIAN, PRESCRIBE, DISPENSE OR ADMINISTER DRUGS THAT MAY BE SUBJECT TO ABUSE TO HIMSELF OR TO ANY MEMBER OF HIS FAMILY; SHALL NOT TELEPHONE TO A PHARMACY A PRESCRIPTION OR REFILL FOR THESE DRUGS NOR PERMIT ANYONE HE IS SUPERVISING TO DO SO; SHALL MAINTAIN A FILE WITH COPIES OF EVERY PRESCRIPTION WRITTEN BY HIM FOR CONTROLLED SUBSTANCES OR DRUGS WITH ADDICTIVE POTENTIAL OR POTENTIAL FOR ABUSE AND SHALL MAINTAIN ADEQUATE MEDICAL RECORDS BOTH OF WHICH SHALL BE AVAILABLE FOR REVIEW; SHALL NOT PRACTICE EMERGENCY ROOM MEDICINE UNTIL HE OBTAINS ADVANCED TRAUMA LIFE SUPPORT (ATLS) AND ADVANCED CARDIAC LIFE SUPPORT (ACLS) CERTIFICATIONS; SHALL OBTAIN AT LEAST 50 HOURS PER YEAR OF CONTINUING MEDICAL EDUCATION; SHALL APPEAR BEFORE THE BOARD AT LEAST ONCE A YEAR OR AT BOARD REQUEST; SHALL COOPERATE WITH BOARD IN VERIFYING COMPLIANCE INCLUDING PROVIDING COPIES OF MEDICAL RELEASES AND PEER REVIEW RECORDS UPON REQUEST; SHALL GIVE A COPY OF THIS ORDER TO ANY HEALTH CARE ENTITY WHERE HE HAS PRIVILEGES; SHALL PROVIDE A COPY OF THIS ORDER TO ANYONE REQUESTING IT WITHIN 10 DAYS; TIME PERIOD OUT OF TEXAS DOES NOT COUNT TOWARD PROBATION; SHALL INFORM BOARD OF CHANGE OF ADDRESS WITHIN 10 DAYS OR IF HE LEAVES THE STATE. SHALL NOT SEEK MODIFICATION FOR ONE YEAR. ON 9/20/97 PETITION TO TERMINATE ORDER DENIED; ORDER MODIFIED DELETING FIFTY HOUR CONTINUING MEDICAL EDUCATION REQUIREMENT EACH YEAR. ON 8/22/98 ORDER TERMINATED.

KANTOR, JOHN R MD, DATE OF BIRTH NOVEMBER 12, 1924, LICENSE NUMBER 15719, WAS DISCIPLINED BY COLORADO ON MARCH 20, 1997
DISCIPLINARY ACTION: REPRIMAND

KARRER, JOHN M MD, DATE OF BIRTH AUGUST 28, 1954, LICENSE NUMBER 0025905 OF DENVER, CO, WAS DISCIPLINED BY COLORADO ON MARCH 18, 1994
DISCIPLINARY ACTION: REPRIMAND
OFFENSE: PROFESSIONAL MISCONDUCT

KATZ, JEREMY MD, LICENSE NUMBER 1035249 OF 692 SOUTH HIGH STREET, DENVER, CO, WAS DISCIPLINED BY INDIANA ON AUGUST 22, 1991
DISCIPLINARY ACTION: 60-MONTH PROBATION; MONITORING OF PHYSICIAN PERFORMANCE
OFFENSE: DISCIPLINARY ACTION BY ANOTHER STATE OR AGENCY

NOTES: UPON APPLYING FOR LICENSURE RENEWAL, HE RESPONDED THAT A DISCIPLINARY ACTION HAD BEEN TAKEN AGAINST HIS LICENSE IN COLORADO. LICENSE PLACED ON FIVE YEARS PROBATION BY COLORADO ON 5/8/90. INTERIM AGREEMENT WITH THE PHYSICIAN'S DIVERSION PROGRAM WITH THE MEDICAL BOARD OF CALIFORNIA ON 12/20/90. LICENSE RENEWED ON THE FOLLOWING CONDITIONS OF PROBATION: SHALL MAINTAIN SOBRIETY AT ALL TIMES AND TOTALLY ABSTAIN FROM ALL ALCOHOL AND CONTROLLED SUBSTANCES EXCEPT AS PRESCRIBED FOR HIM BY ANOTHER PERSON LICENSED TO DO SO; MUST OBTAIN A LICENSED PHYSICIAN WHO SHALL MAINTAIN HIS ACTIVITIES AND REPORT QUARTERLY WITH REGARD TO ALL PERFORMANCES, SOBRIETY TESTS, PROBLEMS, AND DISCIPLINES IMPOSED; URINE AND BLOOD SCREENS SHALL BE REQUIRED ON A MONTHLY BASIS; HE MAY PETITION THE BOARD TO LIFT THIS TERM AFTER ONE YEAR; THE MONITOR SHALL REPORT ANY USE OF ALCOHOL OR CONTROLLED SUBSTANCE WHERE HE FEELS DR. KATZ IS NOT CAPABLE OF PRACTICING MEDICINE WITH REASONABLE SKILL AND SAFETY; HE MUST ATTEND THREE ALCOHOLIC ANONYMOUS AND ONE CADUCEUS MEETING PER WEEK AND PROVIDE WRITTEN VERIFICATION. PROBATION TERMINATED ON 6/07/95.

KEELING, MARITA J MD, DATE OF BIRTH AUGUST 11, 1952, LICENSE NUMBER 0024236, WAS DISCIPLINED BY COLORADO ON FEBRUARY 14, 1996
DISCIPLINARY ACTION: MONITORING OF PHYSICIAN PERFORMANCE

NOTES: NO UNPROFESSIONAL CONDUCT IDENTIFIED. THIS IS AN INTERIM AGREEMENT PENDING SOME FINAL OUTCOME. AGREES TO TREATMENT AND PRACTICE MONITORING.

KEELING, MARITA J MD, DATE OF BIRTH AUGUST 11, 1952, LICENSE NUMBER 24236, WAS DISCIPLINED BY COLORADO ON FEBRUARY 14, 1999
DISCIPLINARY ACTION: REPRIMAND; REQUIRED TO TAKE ADDITIONAL MEDICAL EDUCATION
OFFENSE: SUBSTANDARD CARE, INCOMPETENCE OR NEGLIGENCE

NOTES: SUBSTANDARD CARE. SHE AGREES TO TREATMENT MONITORING, PRACTICE MONITORING AND REEDUCATION ACTIVITIES.

KEHMEIER, DEAN F MD, DATE OF BIRTH JANUARY 23, 1947, LICENSE NUMBER 0023989, WAS DISCIPLINED BY COLORADO ON JULY 8, 1996
DISCIPLINARY ACTION: REPRIMAND

KELLY, TERRANCE E MD, DATE OF BIRTH AUGUST 23, 1940, LICENSE NUMBER 0017355, WAS DISCIPLINED BY COLORADO ON AUGUST 17, 1995
DISCIPLINARY ACTION: 60-MONTH PROBATION; MONITORING OF PHYSICIAN PERFORMANCE

NOTES: PRACTICE MONITORING AND EVALUATION AND LEARNING PLAN.

KELLY, TERRANCE E MD, DATE OF BIRTH AUGUST 23, 1940, LICENSE NUMBER 17355, WAS DISCIPLINED BY COLORADO ON JUNE 20, 1997
DISCIPLINARY ACTION: EMERGENCY SUSPENSION
OFFENSE: FAILURE TO COMPLY WITH PREVIOUS BOARD ORDER

NOTES: FAILURE TO SUBMIT PRACTICE MONITORING REPORTS AS REQUIRED BY 8/18/95 ORDER.

KELLY, TERRANCE E MD, DATE OF BIRTH AUGUST 23, 1940, LICENSE NUMBER 17355, WAS DISCIPLINED BY COLORADO ON NOVEMBER 13, 1998
DISCIPLINARY ACTION: REPRIMAND

KELLY, TERRANCE E MD, DATE OF BIRTH AUGUST 23, 1940, LICENSE NUMBER 17355, WAS DISCIPLINED BY COLORADO ON NOVEMBER 17, 1999
DISCIPLINARY ACTION: EMERGENCY SUSPENSION

KENNEDY, TIMOTHY C MD, DATE OF BIRTH NOVEMBER 8, 1942, LICENSE NUMBER 0018011 OF DENVER, CO, WAS DISCIPLINED BY COLORADO ON JULY 15, 1994
DISCIPLINARY ACTION: REPRIMAND
OFFENSE: PROFESSIONAL MISCONDUCT

KHAN, IMRAN U MD, DATE OF BIRTH NOVEMBER 2, 1956, LICENSE NUMBER 0029305, WAS DISCIPLINED BY COLORADO ON OCTOBER 17, 1996
DISCIPLINARY ACTION: EMERGENCY SUSPENSION

KHAN, IMRAN U MD, DATE OF BIRTH NOVEMBER 2, 1956, LICENSE NUMBER 29305, WAS DISCIPLINED BY COLORADO ON MARCH 12, 1998
DISCIPLINARY ACTION: LICENSE REVOCATION
OFFENSE: SUBSTANDARD CARE, INCOMPETENCE OR NEGLIGENCE

NOTES: SUBSTANDARD CARE; UNNECESSARY TESTS OR TREATMENT; FAILURE TO KEEP PROPER RECORDS.

KHAN, IMRAN U MD, LICENSE NUMBER D38932 OF 14 COUNTRY CLUB VILLAGE, PUEBLO, CO, WAS DISCIPLINED BY MARYLAND ON SEPTEMBER 29, 1999
DISCIPLINARY ACTION: DENIAL OF NEW LICENSE
OFFENSE: DISCIPLINARY ACTION BY ANOTHER STATE OR AGENCY

NOTES: DISCIPLINED BY THE COLORADO BOARD (REVOCATION OF LICENSE) FOR VIOLATION OF STANDARDS OF CARE, OVERUTILIZATION OF TESTS, STUDIES AND TREATMENT, AND FAILING TO MAKE ESSENTIAL ENTRIES ON PATIENT RECORDS.

KIM, YOUNGHOO MD, LICENSE NUMBER 00H7442 OF LOVELAND, CO, WAS DISCIPLINED BY TEXAS ON JUNE 17, 1992
DISCIPLINARY ACTION: SURRENDER OF LICENSE

KINNARD, MELINDA M MD, DATE OF BIRTH JUNE 9, 1955, LICENSE NUMBER 0024951 OF GOLDEN, CO, WAS DISCIPLINED BY COLORADO ON OCTOBER 14, 1994
DISCIPLINARY ACTION: SURRENDER OF CONTROLLED SUBSTANCE LICENSE; 60-MONTH PROBATION
OFFENSE: CRIMINAL CONVICTION OR PLEA OF GUILTY, NOLO CONTENDERE, OR NO CONTEST TO A CRIME

NOTES: FELONY CONVICTION; ADMINISTERING, DISPENSING OR PRESCRIBING ANY HABIT-FORMING DRUG OR ANY CONTROLLED SUBSTANCES OTHER THAN IN THE COURSE OF LEGITIMATE PROFESSIONAL PRACTICE OR TO A FAMILY MEMBER; HABITUAL INTEMPERANCE OR EXCESSIVE USE OF A CONTROLLED SUBSTANCE; SELF-ADMINISTRATION OF A CLASS II CONTROLLED SUBSTANCE. REVOCATION STAYED FIVE YEARS UNDER TERMS AND CONDITIONS: SHALL COMPLETE AN INPATIENT TREATMENT PROGRAM; SHALL SURRENDER HER DEA CERTIFICATE; AND PRACTICE AND TREATMENT MONITORING.

KINNARD, MELINDA M MD OF 1353 BROOKCRESS DRIVE, GOLDEN, CO, WAS DISCIPLINED BY DEA ON NOVEMBER 22, 1994
DISCIPLINARY ACTION: SURRENDER OF CONTROLLED SUBSTANCE LICENSE

NOTES: IN LIEU OF ORDER TO SHOW CAUSE.

KIRBENS, DREW J MD, LICENSE NUMBER 4421A, WAS DISCIPLINED BY WYOMING ON APRIL 9, 1998
DISCIPLINARY ACTION: LICENSE REVOCATION; FINE
OFFENSE: LOSS OR RESTRICTION OF HOSPITAL PRIVILEGES

NOTES: IN TREATING THREE PATIENTS, THE ENDOSCOPIC SURGERY TREATMENT HE RENDERED WHEN THE PRE OPERATIVE CT SCAN DISCLOSED NO ACTIVE SINUS DISEASE, WAS NEGLIGENT, INAPPROPRIATE AND UNNECESSARY; HOSPITAL SUSPENDED HIS PRIVILEGES FOR AN INDEFINITE PERIOD EFFECTIVE 1/14/97; AGREED NOT TO SCHEDULE ANY SURGERIES AT ANOTHER HOSPITAL EFFECTIVE 6/12/97. SHALL PAY A $5,000 FINE AND COSTS.

KIRBENS, DREW JOSEPH MD, DATE OF BIRTH MAY 19, 1949 OF 13691 E MARINA DRIVE #207, AURORA, CO, WAS DISCIPLINED BY MEDICARE ON SEPTEMBER 20, 1998
DISCIPLINARY ACTION: EXCLUSION FROM THE MEDICARE AND/OR MEDICAID PROGRAM
OFFENSE: DISCIPLINARY ACTION BY ANOTHER STATE OR AGENCY

NOTES: LICENSE REVOKED, SUSPENDED, SURRENDERED OR OTHERWISE LOST FOR REASONS BEARING ON PROFESSIONAL PERFORMANCE, PROFESSIONAL COMPETENCE OR FINANCIAL INTEGRITY.

KIRBENS, DREW JOSEPH MD, LICENSE NUMBER G33256 OF LARAMIE, WY, WAS DISCIPLINED BY CALIFORNIA ON DECEMBER 24, 1998
DISCIPLINARY ACTION: LICENSE REVOCATION
OFFENSE: DISCIPLINARY ACTION BY ANOTHER STATE OR AGENCY

NOTES: DISCIPLINED BY WYOMING FOR PERFORMING

ENDOSCOPIC SINUS SURGERIES ON THREE PATIENTS WHICH WERE INAPPROPRIATE AND UNNECESSARY.

KIRK, HARRY L III MD, DATE OF BIRTH APRIL 10, 1945, LICENSE NUMBER 0021745, WAS DISCIPLINED BY COLORADO ON JANUARY 11, 1996
DISCIPLINARY ACTION: 60-MONTH PROBATION; MONITORING OF PHYSICIAN PERFORMANCE

NOTES: HIS COLORADO MEDICAL LICENSE WAS REINSTATED HE WAS PLACED ON PROBATION WITH MONITORING BY HIS RESIDENCY DIRECTOR, SUBSEQUENT PRACTICE MONITORING, AND TREATMENT MONITORING THROUGH THE COLORADO PHYSICIANS HEALTH PROGRAM.

KLEIN, JORDAN R MD, DATE OF BIRTH AUGUST 13, 1948, LICENSE NUMBER 20776, WAS DISCIPLINED BY COLORADO ON JUNE 13, 1996
DISCIPLINARY ACTION: REPRIMAND

KLUCK, JOHN JAMES MD, DATE OF BIRTH NOVEMBER 3, 1944, LICENSE NUMBER 0021549 OF LOUISVILLE, CO, WAS DISCIPLINED BY COLORADO ON NOVEMBER 19, 1993
DISCIPLINARY ACTION: REPRIMAND

KLUCK, JOHN JAMES MD, DATE OF BIRTH NOVEMBER 3, 1944, LICENSE NUMBER 0021549 OF LOUISVILLE, CO, WAS DISCIPLINED BY COLORADO ON JANUARY 21, 1994
DISCIPLINARY ACTION: REPRIMAND
OFFENSE: PROFESSIONAL MISCONDUCT

KNIGHT, PHILLIP J MD, DATE OF BIRTH JULY 3, 1950, LICENSE NUMBER 0022197 OF PONCA CITY, OK, WAS DISCIPLINED BY COLORADO ON JULY 12, 1991
DISCIPLINARY ACTION: 60-MONTH PROBATION; REQUIRED TO ENTER AN IMPAIRED PHYSICIAN PROGRAM OR SUBSTANCE ABUSE TREATMENT
OFFENSE: SUBSTANCE ABUSE

NOTES: HABITUAL INTEMPERANCE OR EXCESSIVE USE OF CONTROLLED SUBSTANCES. ALCOHOL AND SUBSTANCE ABUSE TREATMENT, AND PRACTICE AND TREATMENT MONITORS. IN ABEYANCE. ORDER BECOMES EFFECTIVE UPON HIS RETURN TO COLORADO.

KNIGHT, PHILLIP JOSEPH MD, LICENSE NUMBER 0012150, WAS DISCIPLINED BY OKLAHOMA ON SEPTEMBER 27, 1990
DISCIPLINARY ACTION: LICENSE SUSPENSION; REQUIRED TO ENTER AN IMPAIRED PHYSICIAN PROGRAM OR SUBSTANCE ABUSE TREATMENT
OFFENSE: SUBSTANCE ABUSE

NOTES: ON 2/26/90 LEFT INPATIENT TREATMENT FOR SUBSTANCE ABUSE BEFORE TREATMENT WAS COMPLETED AGAINST MEDICAL ADVICE. SUSPENSION UNTIL HE CAN PROVIDE TO THE BOARD EVIDENCE OF SUCCESSFUL COMPLETION OF IN-PATIENT TREATMENT AND RELATED RESIDENTIAL OUT-PATIENT TREATMENT FROM THE PHYSICIAN RECOVERY CENTER IN JACKSON, MISSISSIPPI, OR AN EQUIVALENT BOARD APPROVED PROGRAM. ON 11/1/90 SUSPENSION WAS RETAINED.

KNIGHT, PHILLIP JOSEPH MD, LICENSE NUMBER 0012150, WAS DISCIPLINED BY OKLAHOMA ON MARCH 6, 1991
DISCIPLINARY ACTION: 60-MONTH PROBATION; RESTRICTION PLACED ON CONTROLLED SUBSTANCE LICENSE
OFFENSE: SUBSTANCE ABUSE

NOTES: IN 1990 WAS PLACED ON SUSPENSION WHILE SUCCESSFULLY COMPLETING IN-PATIENT TREATMENT FOR SUBSTANCE ABUSE. CONDITIONS OF PROBATION: SHALL NOT PRESCRIBE, ADMINISTER OR DISPENSE ANY MEDICATIONS FOR HIS PERSONAL USE AND SHALL TAKE NONE UNLESS AUTHORIZED BY ANOTHER PHYSICIAN FOR LEGITIMATE MEDICAL NEED; SHALL NOT PRESCRIBE, ADMINISTER OR DISPENSE ANY CONTROLLED DANGEROUS SUBSTANCES OR NARCOTIC DRUGS TO ANY PATIENT FOR ANY CONDITION; SHALL ABSTAIN FROM CONSUMING ALCOHOL OR ANY SUBSTANCE WHICH WOULD ADVERSELY AFFECT HIS ABILITY TO PRACTICE; SHALL SUBMIT BIOLOGICAL FLUID SPECIMENS; SHALL CONTINUE REGULAR PARTICIPATION IN PHYSICIAN RECOVERY COMMITTEE AND AA OR NARCOTICS ANONYMOUS; SHALL FURNISH TO BOARD ADDRESS AND/OR CHANGE OF ADDRESS; SHALL APPEAR BEFORE BOARD UPON REQUEST; SHALL NOTIFY ANY HOSPITAL WHERE HE HOLDS STAFF PRIVILEGES OR CLINIC OR GROUP, OF THE TERMS AND CONDITIONS.

KNIGHT, PHILLIP JOSEPH MD, LICENSE NUMBER 0012150 OF 400 FAIRVIEW AVE, PONCA CITY, OK, WAS DISCIPLINED BY OKLAHOMA ON NOVEMBER 8, 1991
DISCIPLINARY ACTION: 6-MONTH PROBATION; REPRIMAND
OFFENSE: FAILURE TO COMPLY WITH PREVIOUS BOARD ORDER

NOTES: FAILED TO APPEAR BEFORE BOARD; FAILED TO PAY COSTS WITHIN 30 DAYS. REPRIMAND FOR NON-PAYMENT OF COSTS; PROBATION OF 3/6/91 EXTENDED AN ADDITIONAL SIX MONTHS. ON 10/22/92 ORDER MODIFIED TO ALLOW HIM TO PRESCRIBE, ADMINISTER OR DISPENSE SCHEDULE III, IV OR V DRUGS TO HOSPITAL IN-PATIENTS, HOSPITAL EMERGENCY ROOM PATIENTS, AND NURSING HOME PATIENTS, AND TO REDUCE HIS LEVEL OF PROBATION FROM LEVEL I TO LEVEL II AND TO APPLY FOR STATE AND FEDERAL REGISTRATION FOR CONTROLLED DANGEROUS SUBSTANCES. ON 7/23/94, THE PROBATION IF FURTHER MODIFIED TO ALLOW HIM TO PRESCRIBE SCHEDULE III, IV AND V CONTROLLED DANGEROUS SUBSTANCES ON AN OUTPATIENT BASIS USING SEQUENTIALLY NUMBERED, DUPLICATE PRESCRIPTION FORMS, COPIES OF WHICH SHALL BE SUBMITTED MONTHLY TO THE BOARD. OTHER TERMS AND CONDITIONS REMAIN IN EFFECT. ON 12/7/95 PROBATION MODIFIED ALLOWING HIM TO PRESCRIBE, ADMINISTER OR DISPENSE SCHEDULE II SUBSTANCES TO INPATIENTS IN AN INSTITUTIONAL SETTING BY WAY OF A SPECIFIC WRITTEN ORDER UNTIL 9/6/96 UNDER THE REMAINING CONDITIONS.

KNIGHT, ROBERT A MD OF 8580 RALSTON ROAD, ARVADA, CO, WAS DISCIPLINED BY DEA ON OCTOBER 7, 1997
DISCIPLINARY ACTION: SURRENDER OF CONTROLLED SUBSTANCE LICENSE

KNIGHT, ROBERT A MD, DATE OF BIRTH AUGUST 31, 1954, LICENSE NUMBER 23997, WAS DISCIPLINED BY COLORADO ON OCTOBER 22, 1997
DISCIPLINARY ACTION: CEASE AND DESIST ORDER
OFFENSE: PROFESSIONAL MISCONDUCT

NOTES: ILLEGALLY DISPENSING CONTROLLED SUBSTANCES. HE AGREES TO PERFORM NO ACT REQUIRING A COLORADO MEDICAL LICENSE. INTERIM ORDER.

KNIGHT, ROBERT A MD, DATE OF BIRTH AUGUST 31, 1954, LICENSE NUMBER 23997, WAS DISCIPLINED BY COLORADO ON NOVEMBER 13, 1998

DISCIPLINARY ACTION: SURRENDER OF LICENSE

NOTES: NO UNPROFESSIONAL CONDUCT IDENTIFIED.

KOMPUS, LARRY L MD OF 4166 STODDARD ROAD, ORCHARD LAKE, MI, WAS DISCIPLINED BY DEA ON AUGUST 6, 1990
DISCIPLINARY ACTION: RESTRICTION PLACED ON CONTROLLED SUBSTANCE LICENSE
OFFENSE: PROFESSIONAL MISCONDUCT

NOTES: SUSPENSION OF MEDICAL LICENSE DUE TO ADMINISTRATIVE COMPLAINT INVOLVING SEXUAL MISCONDUCT 04/18/90. ARRESTED 04/19/90 FOR MEDICAID FRAUD AND CONTRIBUTING TO THE DELINQUENCY OF A MINOR.

KOMPUS, LARRY L MD, DATE OF BIRTH MARCH 25, 1938 OF 4166 STODDARD ROAD, ORCHARD LAKE, MI, WAS DISCIPLINED BY MEDICARE ON MARCH 5, 1991
DISCIPLINARY ACTION: 60-MONTH EXCLUSION FROM THE MEDICARE AND/OR MEDICAID PROGRAM
OFFENSE: CRIMINAL CONVICTION OR PLEA OF GUILTY, NOLO CONTENDERE, OR NO CONTEST TO A CRIME

NOTES: PROGRAM-RELATED CONVICTION.

KOMPUS, LARRY L MD, DATE OF BIRTH MARCH 25, 1938, LICENSE NUMBER 0413281 OF 4166 STODDARD RD, ORCHARD LAKE, MI, WAS DISCIPLINED BY KANSAS ON NOVEMBER 18, 1992
DISCIPLINARY ACTION: SURRENDER OF LICENSE
OFFENSE: DISCIPLINARY ACTION BY ANOTHER STATE OR AGENCY

NOTES: ON 4/18/90, MICHIGAN FILED A SUMMARY SUSPENSION AGAINST HIS LICENSE BECAUSE OF ALLEGATIONS THAT HE TRADED DRUGS, ALCOHOL AND OTHER GIFTS FOR SEXUAL FAVORS WITH A MINOR MALE PATIENT; WAS CHARGED WITH MEDICAID FRAUD FOR WHICH HE WAS FOUND GUILTY AND CONVICTED IN MICHIGAN IN 10/90. NO ADMISSION OF VIOLATION OR LIABILITY OR FINDINGS RELATED TO THE ALLEGATIONS. VOLUNTARILY AGREES TO THE SURRENDER OF HIS LICENSE AND SHALL NOT APPLY FOR REINSTATEMENT OF LICENSURE IN KANSAS.

KOMPUS, LARRY L MD, DATE OF BIRTH MARCH 25, 1938, LICENSE NUMBER 0016611 OF MEDICAL DENTAL PLAZA, BLOOMFIELD HILLS, MI, WAS DISCIPLINED BY COLORADO ON MAY 21, 1993
DISCIPLINARY ACTION: SURRENDER OF LICENSE
OFFENSE: DISCIPLINARY ACTION BY ANOTHER STATE OR AGENCY

NOTES: SEXUAL CONTACT WITH A PATIENT (HE NEITHER ADMITTED NOR DENIED THIS CONDUCT); FELONY CONVICTION ON 10/25/90 OF 12 COUNTS OF FALSE MEDICAID CLAIM FILING; PERMANENTLY SURRENDERED LICENSE IN MICHIGAN ON 10/11/90.

KRAGOR, HUGH F DO, DATE OF BIRTH JANUARY 25, 1933 OF 8090 OAK STREET, ARVADA, CO, WAS DISCIPLINED BY MEDICARE ON MARCH 19, 1990
DISCIPLINARY ACTION: EXCLUSION FROM THE MEDICARE AND/OR MEDICAID PROGRAM
OFFENSE: DISCIPLINARY ACTION BY ANOTHER STATE OR AGENCY

NOTES: LICENSE REVOCATION OR SUSPENSION.

KRAMISH, DAVID MD, DATE OF BIRTH NOVEMBER 4, 1919, LICENSE NUMBER 10612, WAS DISCIPLINED BY COLORADO ON JUNE 19, 1997
DISCIPLINARY ACTION: RESTRICTION PLACED ON LICENSE
OFFENSE: PHYSICAL OR MENTAL ILLNESS INHIBITING THE ABILITY TO PRACTICE WITH SKILL AND SAFETY

NOTES: HAS HAD A HEALTH CONDITION THAT HAD PREVIOUSLY REQUIRED HIM TO PLACE HIS LICENSE IN INACTIVE STATUS. HE IS TO REACTIVATE AN INACTIVE MEDICAL LICENSE. NO ISSUES OF UNPROFESSIONAL CONDUCT HAVE BEEN IDENTIFIED. HE MAY NOT PERFORM SURGERY OR DIRECT PATIENT CARE AND MAY PERFORM ADMINISTRATIVE WORK.

KUBOWICZ, SCOTT MD, DATE OF BIRTH JULY 13, 1958, LICENSE NUMBER 0029263 OF LITTLETON, CO, WAS DISCIPLINED BY COLORADO ON NOVEMBER 11, 1994
DISCIPLINARY ACTION: REPRIMAND

KUHN, KENNETH L MD, DATE OF BIRTH JANUARY 26, 1941, LICENSE NUMBER 0015383 OF ANDOVER, MN, WAS DISCIPLINED BY KENTUCKY ON SEPTEMBER 7, 1993
DISCIPLINARY ACTION: PROBATION
OFFENSE: DISCIPLINARY ACTION BY ANOTHER STATE OR AGENCY

NOTES: ACTION TAKEN BY COLORADO BOARD. WILL BE PLACED ON PROBATION UPON RELOCATION TO KENTUCKY.

KUHN, KENNETH LEE MD, DATE OF BIRTH JANUARY 26, 1941, LICENSE NUMBER 0017665 OF MINNEAPOLIS, MN, WAS DISCIPLINED BY COLORADO ON AUGUST 16, 1991
DISCIPLINARY ACTION: SURRENDER OF LICENSE

NOTES: SURRENDER OF DR. KUHN'S COLORADO MEDICAL LICENSE IN EXCHANGE FOR TERMINATION OF HIS SUSPENSION.

KUHN, KENNETH LEE MD, LICENSE NUMBER 0035175, WAS DISCIPLINED BY MINNESOTA ON JANUARY 11, 1992
DISCIPLINARY ACTION: RESTRICTION PLACED ON LICENSE

NOTES: UNCONDITIONAL LICENSE GRANTED ON 3/12/94.

KUNA, GUPTA B MD, DATE OF BIRTH MAY 4, 1942, LICENSE NUMBER 0021004 OF PUEBLO, CO, WAS DISCIPLINED BY COLORADO ON APRIL 14, 1995
DISCIPLINARY ACTION: REPRIMAND

KUNA, GUPTA B MD, DATE OF BIRTH MAY 4, 1942, LICENSE NUMBER 21004, WAS DISCIPLINED BY COLORADO ON MARCH 25, 1999

NOTES: NO UNPROFESSIONAL CONDUCT IDENTIFIED. HE AGREES HIS LICENSE WILL BECOME PERMANENTLY INACTIVE EFFECTIVE 6/15/00.

KUSESKI, RONALD E MD, DATE OF BIRTH OCTOBER 21, 1946, LICENSE NUMBER 0018602 OF BOULDER, CO, WAS DISCIPLINED BY COLORADO ON JANUARY 20, 1995
DISCIPLINARY ACTION: REPRIMAND; REQUIRED TO TAKE ADDITIONAL MEDICAL EDUCATION
OFFENSE: SUBSTANDARD CARE, INCOMPETENCE OR NEGLIGENCE

NOTES: SUBSTANDARD CARE. SHALL SUCCESSFULLY COMPLETE A CPR/ACLS COURSE.

KUSKA, HARRY D MD, DATE OF BIRTH APRIL 14, 1932, LICENSE NUMBER 0017360, WAS DISCIPLINED BY COLORADO ON FEBRUARY 14, 1996
DISCIPLINARY ACTION: RESTRICTION PLACED ON LICENSE; REQUIRED TO TAKE ADDITIONAL MEDICAL EDUCATION
OFFENSE: PROFESSIONAL MISCONDUCT

NOTES: VIOLATION OF A PROVISION OF THE MEDICAL PRACTICE ACT (SUPERVISION OF PHYSICIAN EXTENDERS). AGREES NOT TO TREAT PATIENTS FOR PSYCHIATRIC OR PSYCHOLOGICAL CONDITIONS OR TO USE HYPNOTHERAPY; AGREES NOT TO

REACTIVATE HIS LICENSE WITHOUT FIRST UNDERGOING RE-EDUCATION ACTIVITIES AND UNDERGOING PRACTICE MONITORING.

LACEY, RONALD L MD, LICENSE NUMBER 0424503 OF 1010 NORTH KANSAS, WICHITA, KS, WAS DISCIPLINED BY KANSAS ON JANUARY 6, 1993
DISCIPLINARY ACTION: PROBATION; MONITORING OF PHYSICIAN PERFORMANCE
OFFENSE: DISCIPLINARY ACTION BY ANOTHER STATE OR AGENCY
NOTES: DISCIPLINARY ACTIONS HAVE BEEN TAKEN BY IOWA, HAWAII, AND COLORADO. HE AGREES TO ENTER INTO A MONITORING CONTRACT WITH THE KANSAS MEDICAL SOCIETY IMPAIRED PHYSICIAN PROGRAM WITHIN 30 DAYS; AGREES TO COMPLY WITH TERMS OF MONITORING CONTRACT AND THAT PROGRAM MAY DISCUSS OR OTHERWISE COMMUNICATE WITH BOARD DETAILS OF HIS CASE NECESSARY TO PLAN AND COORDINATE HIS INDIVIDUAL PROGRAM FOR POST-TREATMENT MONITORING; SHALL CONTINUE PSYCHOTHERAPY FOR THREE YEARS AND SHALL BE RESPONSIBLE TO HAVE HIS THERAPIST SUBMIT QUARTERLY REPORTS TO THE BOARD; SHALL ALSO HAVE PROGRAM DIRECTOR SUBMIT QUARTERLY REPORTS; SHALL MAKE A PERSONAL APPEARANCE BEFORE THE BOARD UPON COMPLETION OF HIS RESIDENCY AT WHICH TIME BOARD WILL CONSIDER MODIFICATIONS TO RESTRICTIONS ON HIS LICENSE. ON 08/18/94, THIS STIPULATION AND AGREEMENT AND ENFORCEMENT ORDER WERE TERMINATED AND ANY AND ALL RESTRICTIONS AND LIMITATIONS WHICH WERE IMPOSED ARE REMOVED.

LACEY, RONALD LEE MD, DATE OF BIRTH APRIL 20, 1952, LICENSE NUMBER 0028058 OF ENGLEWOOD, CO, WAS DISCIPLINED BY IOWA ON AUGUST 3, 1990
NOTES: LICENSE AUTHORIZED FOR REINSTATEMENT UPON COMPLETION OF 100 HOURS OF CONTINUING MEDICAL EDUCATION CREDIT AND PAYMENT OF FEES. WHEN REINSTATED, LICENSE WILL BE PLACED ON INDEFINITE PROBATION WITH TERMS AND CONDITIONS: SHALL ONLY PARTICIPATE IN AN ACGME APPROVED PSYCHIATRIC RESIDENCY PROGRAM INVOLVING CLOSE SUPERVISION WHICH SHALL MAKE QUARTERLY REPORTS TO THE BOARD; SHALL CONTINUE PSYCHOTHERAPY FOR A MINIMUM OF THREE YEARS; SHALL APPEAR BEFORE THE BOARD UPON COMPLETION OF RESIDENCY.

LACEY, RONALD LEE MD, DATE OF BIRTH APRIL 20, 1952, LICENSE NUMBER 0028058 OF 8214 INDIANAPOLIS, WICHITA, KS, WAS DISCIPLINED BY IOWA ON APRIL 30, 1991
DISCIPLINARY ACTION: LICENSE REINSTATEMENT; PROBATION
NOTES: LICENSE ISSUED ON IMMEDIATE INDEFINITE PROBATION. EFFECTIVE 12/10/94 INDEFINITE PROBATION TERMINATED; MEDICAL LICENSE RESTRICTED TO ALLOW HEALTH CARE SERVICES TO MALE PATIENTS ONLY. ON 8/8/96 PROBATION TERMINATED AND LICENSE RETURNED TO ITS FULL PRIVILEGES FREE AND CLEAR OF ALL RESTRICTIONS.

LACONTE, FRANK JR DO, DATE OF BIRTH DECEMBER 3, 1931, LICENSE NUMBER 0015568 OF DENVER, CO, WAS DISCIPLINED BY COLORADO ON APRIL 12, 1995
DISCIPLINARY ACTION: 36-MONTH PROBATION; REQUIRED TO TAKE ADDITIONAL MEDICAL EDUCATION
OFFENSE: SUBSTANDARD CARE, INCOMPETENCE OR NEGLIGENCE
NOTES: SUBSTANDARD CARE. PROBATIONARY PERIOD INCLUDES PRACTICE MONITORING AND REEDUCATION ACTIVITIES.

LACONTE, FRANK JR DO OF DENVER, CO, WAS DISCIPLINED BY MISSOURI ON APRIL 12, 1995
DISCIPLINARY ACTION: 36-MONTH PROBATION; REPRIMAND
OFFENSE: DISCIPLINARY ACTION BY ANOTHER STATE OR AGENCY
NOTES: ACTION IN ANOTHER STATE FOR ALLEGATIONS OF FAILURE TO MAKE ESSENTIAL ENTRIES ON PATIENT RECORDS AND ENTERING INCORRECT ESSENTIAL ENTRIES. PROBATION RETROACTIVE TO 4/12/95.

LACONTE, FRANK JR DO OF DENVER, CO, WAS DISCIPLINED BY MISSOURI ON OCTOBER 3, 1996
DISCIPLINARY ACTION: 36-MONTH PROBATION; REPRIMAND
OFFENSE: DISCIPLINARY ACTION BY ANOTHER STATE OR AGENCY
NOTES: BASED UPON DISCIPLINE IN ANOTHER STATE FOR ALLEGATIONS OF FAILURE TO MAKE ESSENTIAL ENTRIES ON PATIENT RECORDS AND ENTERING INCORRECT ESSENTIAL ENTRIES. PROBATION RETROACTIVE TO 4/12/95.

LAMKIN, KENNETH R MD, DATE OF BIRTH APRIL 6, 1946, LICENSE NUMBER 19665, WAS DISCIPLINED BY COLORADO ON FEBRUARY 12, 1997
DISCIPLINARY ACTION: REPRIMAND

LANDRETH, KNUTE JR MD, WAS DISCIPLINED BY WYOMING ON JUNE 20, 1990
NOTES: LETTER OF CENSURE.

LANDRETH, KNUTE JR MD, DATE OF BIRTH AUGUST 15, 1945, LICENSE NUMBER 0022198 OF SHERIDAN, WY, WAS DISCIPLINED BY COLORADO ON APRIL 14, 1993
DISCIPLINARY ACTION: LICENSE SUSPENSION
OFFENSE: FAILURE TO COMPLY WITH PREVIOUS BOARD ORDER
NOTES: FAILURE TO SUBMIT TO MENTAL OR PHYSICAL EXAMINATION. LICENSE SUSPENDED UNTIL HE SUBMITS TO EXAMINATION.

LARKIN, JAMES M MD, DATE OF BIRTH MAY 18, 1943, LICENSE NUMBER 0024710, WAS DISCIPLINED BY COLORADO ON OCTOBER 11, 1995
DISCIPLINARY ACTION: 60-MONTH PROBATION; RESTRICTION PLACED ON LICENSE
NOTES: PRACTICE MONITORING AND COMPLETION OF A LEARNING PLAN; PERMANENT RESTRICTION TO A SINGLE HOSPITAL OR HOSPITAL SYSTEM; PROHIBITED FROM PERFORMING VASCULAR SURGERY OR TAKING TRAUMA CALL EXCEPT FOR EMERGENCY ROOM CALL; PROHIBITED FROM PERFORMING SURGICAL PROCEDURES ON A PERSON LESS THAN TWO YEARS OLD.

LARKIN, JAMES M MD, DATE OF BIRTH MAY 18, 1943, LICENSE NUMBER 0024710, WAS DISCIPLINED BY COLORADO ON NOVEMBER 15, 1996
DISCIPLINARY ACTION: RESTRICTION PLACED ON LICENSE; REQUIRED TO TAKE ADDITIONAL MEDICAL EDUCATION
OFFENSE: FAILURE TO COMPLY WITH PREVIOUS BOARD ORDER
NOTES: VIOLATION OF A VALID BOARD ORDER AND SUBSTANDARD CARE. MAY ACT AS AN ASSISTANT SURGEON ONLY UNTIL SUCH TIME AS HE COMPLETES A SURGERY RESIDENCY; AND MAY CONTINUE TO HAVE AN OFFICE PRACTICE BUT HIS OFFICE SURGICAL PRACTICE WILL BE LIMITED TO CERTAIN LISTED PROCEDURES.

LAUER, JAMES W MD, DATE OF BIRTH MAY 30, 1935, LICENSE NUMBER 16264, WAS DISCIPLINED BY COLORADO ON JULY 18, 1996
DISCIPLINARY ACTION: REPRIMAND

LAUER, JAMES W MD, DATE OF BIRTH MAY 30, 1935, LICENSE NUMBER 16264, WAS DISCIPLINED BY COLORADO ON JUNE 24, 1999
DISCIPLINARY ACTION: 36-MONTH PROBATION; MONITORING OF PHYSICIAN PERFORMANCE
OFFENSE: SUBSTANDARD CARE, INCOMPETENCE OR NEGLIGENCE

NOTES: SUBSTANDARD CARE. PRACTICE MONITORING. HE AGREES NOT TO PRACTICE MEDICINE AFTER 5/1/02.

LAUER, JAMES WARD MD, LICENSE NUMBER G20834 OF GRAND JUNCTION, CO, WAS DISCIPLINED BY CALIFORNIA ON FEBRUARY 3, 1997
DISCIPLINARY ACTION: REPRIMAND
OFFENSE: DISCIPLINARY ACTION BY ANOTHER STATE OR AGENCY

NOTES: DISCIPLINED BY COLORADO FOR DEFICIENCY IN HIS RECORDKEEPING.

LAWTON, WILLIS H MD, DATE OF BIRTH APRIL 5, 1934, LICENSE NUMBER 35687, WAS DISCIPLINED BY COLORADO ON JULY 15, 1999
DISCIPLINARY ACTION: CEASE AND DESIST ORDER
OFFENSE: NONCOMPLIANCE WITH A PROFESSIONAL RULE

NOTES: FAILURE TO KEEP PROPER RECORDS. AGREES TO CEASE PRACTICING AND NOT TO RENEW HIS LICENSE WHEN IT NEXT EXPIRES ON 5/31/01.

LEE, RICHARD H MD, DATE OF BIRTH JUNE 17, 1925, LICENSE NUMBER 0019009 OF HICKORY HILLS, IL, WAS DISCIPLINED BY COLORADO ON JANUARY 22, 1993
DISCIPLINARY ACTION: SURRENDER OF LICENSE
OFFENSE: SUBSTANDARD CARE, INCOMPETENCE OR NEGLIGENCE

NOTES: SUBSTANDARD CARE; PHYSICAL OR MENTAL DISABILITY.

LEETE, RICHARD C MD, DATE OF BIRTH JULY 12, 1939 OF 1245 S BELLAIRE #609, DENVER, CO, WAS DISCIPLINED BY MEDICARE ON FEBRUARY 24, 1994
DISCIPLINARY ACTION: 60-MONTH EXCLUSION FROM THE MEDICARE AND/OR MEDICAID PROGRAM

NOTES: EXCLUDED AS A RESULT OF A SETTLEMENT AGREEMENT.

LEETE, RICHARD C MD, LICENSE NUMBER 0013619 OF DENVER, CO, WAS DISCIPLINED BY CONNECTICUT ON MAY 21, 1996

NOTES: AGREEMENT NOT TO SEEK REINSTATEMENT OR REAPPLICATION OF LICENSURE.

LEETE, RICHARD C MD, DATE OF BIRTH JULY 12, 1939, LICENSE NUMBER 0016908, WAS DISCIPLINED BY COLORADO ON JULY 11, 1996
DISCIPLINARY ACTION: REPRIMAND

LEHMKUHLE, JOSEPH M DO, DATE OF BIRTH APRIL 28, 1932, LICENSE NUMBER 0014521 OF GRAND JUNCTION, CO, WAS DISCIPLINED BY COLORADO ON JUNE 17, 1994
DISCIPLINARY ACTION: LICENSE REVOCATION
OFFENSE: SUBSTANDARD CARE, INCOMPETENCE OR NEGLIGENCE

NOTES: PATIENT CARE ISSUES.

LEHMKUHLE, JOSEPH M DO, DATE OF BIRTH APRIL 28, 1932 OF 1060 ORCHARD AVENUE, GRAND JUNCTION, CO, WAS DISCIPLINED BY MEDICARE ON DECEMBER 5, 1994
DISCIPLINARY ACTION: EXCLUSION FROM THE MEDICARE AND/OR MEDICAID PROGRAM
OFFENSE: DISCIPLINARY ACTION BY ANOTHER STATE OR AGENCY

NOTES: LICENSE REVOKED FOR REASONS BEARING ON PROFESSIONAL PERFORMANCE.

LEMLEY, J STEPHEN MD, DATE OF BIRTH MARCH 24, 1947, LICENSE NUMBER 27587, WAS DISCIPLINED BY COLORADO ON JUNE 19, 1997
DISCIPLINARY ACTION: REPRIMAND
OFFENSE: SUBSTANDARD CARE, INCOMPETENCE OR NEGLIGENCE

NOTES: SUBSTANDARD CARE.

LEONARDI, LEO J MD, DATE OF BIRTH JANUARY 11, 1924, LICENSE NUMBER 0011372 OF SALIDA, CO, WAS DISCIPLINED BY COLORADO ON SEPTEMBER 13, 1991
DISCIPLINARY ACTION: 60-MONTH PROBATION; REQUIRED TO TAKE ADDITIONAL MEDICAL EDUCATION
OFFENSE: SUBSTANDARD CARE, INCOMPETENCE OR NEGLIGENCE

NOTES: FAILURE TO MEET GENERALLY ACCEPTED STANDARDS OF MEDICAL PRACTICE. MUST PARTICIPATE IN THE COLORADO PERSONALIZED EDUCATION FOR PHYSICIANS PROGRAM, AS WELL AS A PRACTICE MONITOR THROUGHOUT PROBATIONARY PERIOD.

LEVALLEY, STEVE A MD, LICENSE NUMBER 0008158 OF 185 S ELM STREET, DENVER, CO, WAS DISCIPLINED BY OKLAHOMA ON FEBRUARY 8, 1990
DISCIPLINARY ACTION: 7-MONTH PROBATION; MONITORING OF PHYSICIAN PERFORMANCE
OFFENSE: DISCIPLINARY ACTION BY ANOTHER STATE OR AGENCY

NOTES: CURRENTLY PRACTICING MEDICINE AND SURGERY IN COLORADO. THE COLORADO BOARD FOUND THAT FROM 3/84 TO 2/01/88 HE DID NOT PRACTICE MEDICINE AND SURGERY. WAS DETERMINED TO HAVE A DISABILITY WHICH RENDERED HIM UNABLE TO PERFORM MEDICAL SERVICES WITH REASONABLE SKILL AND SAFETY TO THE PATIENTS. ON 8/12/88 THE COLORADO BOARD FOUND THAT HE HAD NO DIAGNOSIS OR PSYCHOPATHOLOGY THAT PREVENTED HIM FROM PRACTICING WITH REASONABLE SKILL AND SAFETY TO PATIENTS, BUT FOUND A CASE OF UNPROFESSIONAL CONDUCT AND PLACED HIM ON TWO YEAR PROBATION. OKLAHOMA PLACES HIM ON PROBATION BEGINNING 2/2/90 UNDER THE FOLLOWING TERMS AND CONDITIONS: HIS MEDICAL PRACTICE IN COLORADO SHALL BE MONITORED BY A BOARD APPROVED LICENSED COLORADO PHYSICIAN WHO SHALL BE RESPONSIBLE FOR OVERSIGHT OF THE HIS ENTIRE MEDICAL PRACTICE WHICH INCLUDES, BUT IS NOT LIMITED TO ANY HOSPITAL WHERE HE PRACTICES; SHALL REVIEW A RANDOM SAMPLING OF ANY RECORDS MAINTAINED, TO DETERMINE WHETHER HE HAS PRACTICED IN ACCORDANCE WITH THE GENERALLY ACCEPTED STANDARD OF MEDICAL CARE; THE MONITOR SHALL REPORT QUARTERLY TO THE BOARD; SHALL OBTAIN PSYCHIATRIC TREATMENT ON A REGULAR, CONTINUING BASIS, NO LESS THAN ONCE EVERY 30 DAYS, BY A BOARD APPROVED PHYSICIAN WHO SHALL SUBMIT TO THE BOARD IN WRITING, ON A REGULAR BASIS, A REPORT CONCERNING HIS MENTAL STABILITY; SHALL UNDERGO AN EVALUATION FOR SUBSTANCE ABUSE AT ANY TIME THAT THE PRACTICE MONITOR OR TREATMENT MONITOR BELIEVES IT TO BE APPROPRIATE; SHALL NOTIFY THE BOARD OF HIS CHANGE IN ADDRESS SHOULD HE RELOCATE TO ANOTHER STATE; IF HE RETURNS TO THE ACTIVE PRACTICE OF MEDICINE AND SURGERY IN

OKLAHOMA, HE SHALL REAPPEAR BEFORE THE BOARD AND SHALL PROVIDE THE BOARD WITH A COPY OF THE FINAL REPORT FROM HIS PSYCHIATRIST THAT WAS SUBMITTED TO THE COLORADO BOARD IN 8/90.

LEVY, ALAN B MD, DATE OF BIRTH FEBRUARY 17, 1938, LICENSE NUMBER 0017285 OF DENVER, CO, WAS DISCIPLINED BY COLORADO ON AUGUST 10, 1994
DISCIPLINARY ACTION: REPRIMAND

LIES, BERT A MD, LICENSE NUMBER 0029966 OF SANTA FE, NM, WAS DISCIPLINED BY WASHINGTON ON NOVEMBER 15, 1996
DISCIPLINARY ACTION: PROBATION

NOTES: PROBATION UNDER TERMS AND CONDITIONS.

LIES, BERT A MD, DATE OF BIRTH APRIL 22, 1939, LICENSE NUMBER 30316, WAS DISCIPLINED BY COLORADO ON AUGUST 13, 1997
DISCIPLINARY ACTION: LICENSE REVOCATION
OFFENSE: CRIMINAL CONVICTION OR PLEA OF GUILTY, NOLO CONTENDERE, OR NO CONTEST TO A CRIME

NOTES: FELONY CONVICTION.

LIM, DANIEL MD, LICENSE NUMBER FE41398 OF HIGHLANDS RANCH, CO, WAS DISCIPLINED BY CALIFORNIA ON JULY 22, 1995
DISCIPLINARY ACTION: REPRIMAND
OFFENSE: LOSS OR RESTRICTION OF HOSPITAL PRIVILEGES

NOTES: RESTRICTION OF PRIVILEGES OF MILITARY DOCTOR BY THE U.S. ARMY RELATED TO A LAPAROSCOPIC INCIDENT.

LIM, DANIEL MD, LICENSE NUMBER 157077 OF 29 SUTHERLAND COURT, HIGHLANDS RANCH, CO, WAS DISCIPLINED BY NEW YORK ON MARCH 3, 1999
DISCIPLINARY ACTION: SURRENDER OF LICENSE; FINE
OFFENSE: DISCIPLINARY ACTION BY ANOTHER STATE OR AGENCY

NOTES: COLORADO BOARD DENIED HIS APPLICATION FOR A MEDICAL LICENSE. $1000 FINE.

LINDSAY, A L DO OF 1060 ORCHARD AVENUE SUITE L, GRAND JUNCTION, CO, WAS DISCIPLINED BY DEA ON JULY 27, 1995
DISCIPLINARY ACTION: SURRENDER OF CONTROLLED SUBSTANCE LICENSE

NOTES: IN LIEU OF ORDER TO SHOW CAUSE.

LINDSAY, ALBERT L DO, DATE OF BIRTH MARCH 29, 1924, LICENSE NUMBER 0013422, WAS DISCIPLINED BY COLORADO ON JUNE 8, 1995
DISCIPLINARY ACTION: 60-MONTH PROBATION; MONITORING OF PHYSICIAN PERFORMANCE

NOTES: PRACTICE MONITORING AND ASSESSMENT.

LINDSAY, ALBERT L DO, DATE OF BIRTH MARCH 29, 1924, LICENSE NUMBER 0013422, WAS DISCIPLINED BY COLORADO ON OCTOBER 11, 1995
DISCIPLINARY ACTION: SURRENDER OF LICENSE

LINGLE, JEFFREY W DO, DATE OF BIRTH AUGUST 17, 1949, LICENSE NUMBER 0022199, WAS DISCIPLINED BY COLORADO ON DECEMBER 19, 1996

NOTES: NO UNPROFESSIONAL CONDUCT IDENTIFIED. AGREES NEVER TO ACTIVATE HIS LAPSED LICENSE.

LINSTRUM, THOMAS E MD, DATE OF BIRTH MARCH 23, 1925, LICENSE NUMBER 0031390 OF MCKINNEY, TX, WAS DISCIPLINED BY COLORADO ON FEBRUARY 9, 1995
DISCIPLINARY ACTION: LICENSE REVOCATION
OFFENSE: CRIMINAL CONVICTION OR PLEA OF GUILTY, NOLO CONTENDERE, OR NO CONTEST TO A CRIME

NOTES: FELONY CONVICTION.

LISECKI, EDWARD J MD, DATE OF BIRTH JANUARY 7, 1952, LICENSE NUMBER 24873, WAS DISCIPLINED BY COLORADO ON OCTOBER 8, 1998
DISCIPLINARY ACTION: REPRIMAND
OFFENSE: CRIMINAL CONVICTION OR PLEA OF GUILTY, NOLO CONTENDERE, OR NO CONTEST TO A CRIME

NOTES: FELONY CONVICTION.

LISECKI, MARGARET MD, DATE OF BIRTH FEBRUARY 8, 1953, LICENSE NUMBER 35164, WAS DISCIPLINED BY COLORADO ON APRIL 10, 1998
DISCIPLINARY ACTION: LICENSE REVOCATION
OFFENSE: CRIMINAL CONVICTION OR PLEA OF GUILTY, NOLO CONTENDERE, OR NO CONTEST TO A CRIME

NOTES: UNPROFESSIONAL CONDUCT BASED ON TWO FELONY CONVICTIONS.

LISONBEE, JOHN E DO, DATE OF BIRTH NOVEMBER 10, 1947, LICENSE NUMBER 0027111 OF AGUILAR, CO, WAS DISCIPLINED BY COLORADO ON AUGUST 11, 1994
DISCIPLINARY ACTION: RESTRICTION PLACED ON LICENSE; REQUIRED TO TAKE ADDITIONAL MEDICAL EDUCATION
OFFENSE: SUBSTANDARD CARE, INCOMPETENCE OR NEGLIGENCE

NOTES: SUBSTANDARD CARE; FALSIFYING ESSENTIAL ENTRIES IN PATIENT RECORDS. MUST IMMEDIATELY CEASE HIS PRACTICE OF OBSTETRICS; SPECIFIC EDUCATION AND CERTIFICATION REQUIREMENTS TO BE MET PRIOR TO ANY RESUMPTION OF OBSTETRICAL PRACTICE.

LLOYD, JUDSON F MD, DATE OF BIRTH DECEMBER 22, 1934, LICENSE NUMBER 0022206 OF DENVER, CO, WAS DISCIPLINED BY COLORADO ON JANUARY 15, 1992

NOTES: AMENDMENT TO STIPULATION AND ORDER DATED 12/1/89. RE: PRACTICE MONITORING ARRANGEMENT. ON 2/24/92 HE APPEALED THE BOARD'S DENIAL OF HIS REQUEST FOR UNRESTRICTED LICENSE. ON 4/23/92 THE COURT OF APPEALS DISMISSED THE APPEAL WITHOUT PREJUDICE FOR LACK OF A FINAL APPEALABLE ORDER. AMENDMENT ISSUED ON 12/3/92 PERMITTING HIM TO HAVE SEPARATE PRACTICE MONITORS AT EACH OF HIS PRACTICE LOCATIONS.

LOEFFLER, ANNA MD, DATE OF BIRTH AUGUST 9, 1921, LICENSE NUMBER 0012730 OF ENGLEWOOD, CO, WAS DISCIPLINED BY COLORADO ON MAY 21, 1993
DISCIPLINARY ACTION: SURRENDER OF LICENSE

NOTES: NO SPECIFIC FINDINGS OF UNPROFESSIONAL CONDUCT. IS ALLOWED TO MAINTAIN AN INACTIVE LICENSE; SURRENDERED HER ACTIVE MEDICAL LICENSE.

LOPEZ-SAMAYOA, OMAR MD, DATE OF BIRTH NOVEMBER 21, 1948, LICENSE NUMBER 0026263 OF JULESBURG, CO, WAS DISCIPLINED BY COLORADO ON MAY 8, 1992
DISCIPLINARY ACTION: 60-MONTH PROBATION; REQUIRED TO TAKE ADDITIONAL MEDICAL EDUCATION
OFFENSE: SUBSTANDARD CARE, INCOMPETENCE OR NEGLIGENCE

NOTES:

TWO OR MORE ACTS OR OMISSIONS OF SUBSTANDARD PATIENT CARE AND FAILURE TO COMPLY WITH ORDERS OF THE BOARD. PRACTICE MONITORING, MANDATORY EDUCATION AND TRAINING REQUIREMENTS. HE APPEALED FINAL BOARD ORDER AND THE SUBSEQUENT SUPPLEMENTAL FINAL BOARD ORDER TO THE COLORADO COURT OF APPEALS. DECISION PENDING.

LOPEZ-SAMAYOA, OMAR MD, DATE OF BIRTH NOVEMBER 21, 1948, LICENSE NUMBER 0026263 OF JULESBURG, CO, WAS DISCIPLINED BY COLORADO ON JUNE 17, 1992
DISCIPLINARY ACTION: LICENSE SUSPENSION
OFFENSE: FAILURE TO COMPLY WITH PREVIOUS BOARD ORDER

NOTES: FAILED TO COMPLY WITH PROVISIONS OF THE FINAL BOARD ORDER WITH RESPECT TO PRACTICE MONITORING (ORDER DATED 5/8/92). SUPPLEMENTAL FINAL BOARD ORDER OF 10/7/92 REQUIRES COMPLETION OF RESIDENCY PROGRAM AND OTHER ADDITIONAL EDUCATION REQUIREMENTS; NO PRACTICE OUTSIDE OF RESIDENCY; MUST ACHIEVE CERTIFICATION BY SPECIAL BOARD. HE APPEALED FINAL BOARD ORDER AND SUPPLEMENTAL FINAL BOARD ORDER TO THE COLORADO COURT OF APPEALS. DECISION PENDING AS OF MARCH 1993.

LOPEZ-SAMAYOA, OMAR MD, DATE OF BIRTH NOVEMBER 21, 1948, LICENSE NUMBER 0023139 OF CLAY COUNTY, KY, WAS DISCIPLINED BY KENTUCKY ON OCTOBER 29, 1993
DISCIPLINARY ACTION: 60-MONTH PROBATION; FINE
OFFENSE: DISCIPLINARY ACTION BY ANOTHER STATE OR AGENCY

NOTES: ACTION TAKEN BY COLORADO BOARD AND ALSO FALSIFIED ANNUAL RENEWAL APPLICATION. MUST PROVIDE NOTIFICATION OF OUTCOME REGARDING STATUS OF HIS COLORADO LICENSE. ON 5/20/98 ORDER TERMINATED.

LOPEZ-SAMAYOA, OMAR MD, DATE OF BIRTH NOVEMBER 21, 1948, LICENSE NUMBER 0026263, WAS DISCIPLINED BY COLORADO ON AUGUST 17, 1995
DISCIPLINARY ACTION: 60-MONTH PROBATION; MONITORING OF PHYSICIAN PERFORMANCE

NOTES: PRACTICE MONITORING AND COMPLETION OF A LEARNING PLAN.

LUNDGREN, JOHN C MD, DATE OF BIRTH OCTOBER 1, 1911, LICENSE NUMBER 0009998 OF JULESBURG, CO, WAS DISCIPLINED BY COLORADO ON NOVEMBER 6, 1992

NOTES: AGREES TO MAINTAIN HIS LICENSE IN INACTIVE STATUS AND FURTHER AGREES NOT TO APPLY FOR AN ACTIVE MEDICAL LICENSE. RESTRICTIONS OF STIPULATION DATED 11/3/83 ARE REMOVED.

MACON, PHILIP F MD, DATE OF BIRTH SEPTEMBER 11, 1940, LICENSE NUMBER 20224, WAS DISCIPLINED BY COLORADO ON APRIL 17, 1997
DISCIPLINARY ACTION: REPRIMAND

MACON, PHILIP FREDERICK MD, LICENSE NUMBER C30168 OF CORTEZ, CO, WAS DISCIPLINED BY CALIFORNIA ON MARCH 26, 1999
DISCIPLINARY ACTION: LICENSE REVOCATION
OFFENSE: DISCIPLINARY ACTION BY ANOTHER STATE OR AGENCY

NOTES: DISCIPLINED BY COLORADO FOR MISCOMMUNICATION IN CONJUNCTION WITH HIS REFERRAL OF A PATIENT TO AN ORTHOPEDIC SURGEON.

MADAN, VEENA MD, DATE OF BIRTH NOVEMBER 11, 1944, LICENSE NUMBER 0022595 OF DENVER, CO, WAS DISCIPLINED BY COLORADO ON FEBRUARY 21, 1993
DISCIPLINARY ACTION: 60-MONTH PROBATION; MONITORING OF PHYSICIAN PERFORMANCE
OFFENSE: SUBSTANDARD CARE, INCOMPETENCE OR NEGLIGENCE

NOTES: SUBSTANDARD CARE. PROBATION INCLUDES RESIDENCY TRAINING AND PRACTICE MONITORING.

MADAN, VEENA MD, DATE OF BIRTH NOVEMBER 11, 1944, LICENSE NUMBER 00F1768 OF PLANO, TX, WAS DISCIPLINED BY TEXAS ON AUGUST 19, 1994
DISCIPLINARY ACTION: RESTRICTION PLACED ON LICENSE; REQUIRED TO TAKE ADDITIONAL MEDICAL EDUCATION
OFFENSE: DISCIPLINARY ACTION BY ANOTHER STATE OR AGENCY

NOTES: ON 2/12/93 ENTERED INTO A STIPULATION AND ORDER WITH THE COLORADO BOARD RESTRICTED COLORADO LICENSE. CONDITIONS ON TEXAS LICENSE: SHALL NOT INDEPENDENTLY TREAT ANY PATIENT UNTIL SHE COMPLETES A BOARD-APPROVED THREE MONTH REFRESHER MINI-RESIDENCY IN ANESTHESIOLOGY AND PERSONALLY APPEARS BEFORE THE BOARD AND PROVIDES SUFFICIENT INFORMATION WHICH SHOWS THAT SHE IS ABLE TO SAFELY PRACTICE. ON 5/13/95 BOARD GRANTED HER PETITION REQUESTING TERMINATION OF ORDER SINCE SHE HAD SATISFIED ALL CONDITIONS.

MAGOUN, HAROLD I JR DO, DATE OF BIRTH JUNE 11, 1927, LICENSE NUMBER 11808, WAS DISCIPLINED BY COLORADO ON AUGUST 20, 1999
DISCIPLINARY ACTION: REPRIMAND; REQUIRED TO TAKE ADDITIONAL MEDICAL EDUCATION

NOTES: NO UNPROFESSIONAL CONDUCT IDENTIFIED. HE MUST OBTAIN EDUCATION IN BOUNDARY ISSUES AND MUST NOT EMPLOY A PARTICULAR PATIENT WHILE HE IS TREATING THAT PATIENT.

MAHAFFEY, GENE F DO OF 2465 S DOWNING #103, DENVER, CO, WAS DISCIPLINED BY DEA ON MARCH 12, 1990
DISCIPLINARY ACTION: SURRENDER OF CONTROLLED SUBSTANCE LICENSE
OFFENSE: DISCIPLINARY ACTION BY ANOTHER STATE OR AGENCY

NOTES: REVOCATION OF STATE LICENSE DUE TO CONTINUING TO PRESCRIBE AMPHETAMINES AND DIURETICS WITHOUT MEDICAL INDICATION AND PRACTICING MEDICINE WHILE STATE LICENSE SUSPENDED.

MAHAFFEY, GENE F DO, DATE OF BIRTH OCTOBER 13, 1927 OF 3537 SOUTH HILLCREST DR, DENVER, CO, WAS DISCIPLINED BY MEDICARE ON JULY 26, 1990
DISCIPLINARY ACTION: EXCLUSION FROM THE MEDICARE AND/OR MEDICAID PROGRAM
OFFENSE: DISCIPLINARY ACTION BY ANOTHER STATE OR AGENCY

NOTES: LICENSE REVOCATION OR SUSPENSION.

MAHAFFEY, GENE F DO OF DENVER, CO, WAS DISCIPLINED BY MISSOURI ON JANUARY 25, 1991
DISCIPLINARY ACTION: LICENSE REVOCATION
OFFENSE: DISCIPLINARY ACTION BY ANOTHER STATE OR AGENCY

NOTES: REVOCATION OF COLORADO LICENSE BASED ON VIOLATION OF COLORADO BOARD STIPULATION/ORDER BY PRESCRIBING DRUGS RESTRICTED BY THE BOARD'S ORDER AND FAILING TO MEET WITH PATIENTS; FAILING TO KEEP CHARTS AND ADEQUATELY SUPERVISE STAFF IN THE TREATMENT OF ONE PATIENT; PRACTICING MEDICINE WHILE UNDER ORDER OF SUMMARY SUSPENSION.

MAHAFFEY, GENE FRANCIS DO, LICENSE NUMBER 00C3141 OF DENVER, CO, WAS DISCIPLINED BY TEXAS ON JULY 1, 1990
DISCIPLINARY ACTION: SURRENDER OF LICENSE

NOTES: LICENSE CANCELED WITH PROVISIONS; EARLIER BOARD ORDER (LICENSE REVOCATION, STAY OF REVOCATION, THREE YEAR PROBATION) TO BE REINSTATED SHOULD PHYSICIAN APPLY FOR LICENSE REINSTATEMENT. IF HE APPLIES FOR REINSTATEMENT FIVE YEARS FROM 1/27/90, HE MUST ALSO PASS A SPECIAL PURPOSE EXAMINATION.

MALASHOCK, MARK HOWARD MD, LICENSE NUMBER G045858 OF BOULDER, CO, WAS DISCIPLINED BY CALIFORNIA ON MARCH 11, 1991
DISCIPLINARY ACTION: SURRENDER OF LICENSE

NOTES: VOLUNTARY SURRENDER WHILE CHARGES PENDING.

MANUELE, MARK A DO, DATE OF BIRTH APRIL 8, 1958, LICENSE NUMBER 28942, WAS DISCIPLINED BY COLORADO ON AUGUST 14, 1996
DISCIPLINARY ACTION: SURRENDER OF LICENSE
OFFENSE: PROFESSIONAL MISCONDUCT

NOTES: UNPROFESSIONAL CONDUCT.

MANUELE, MARK A DO, DATE OF BIRTH APRIL 8, 1958, LICENSE NUMBER 28942, WAS DISCIPLINED BY COLORADO ON NOVEMBER 13, 1996
DISCIPLINARY ACTION: SURRENDER OF LICENSE
OFFENSE: SEXUAL ABUSE OF OR SEXUAL MISCONDUCT WITH A PATIENT

NOTES: SEXUAL ACTS WITH PATIENTS.

MANUELE, MARK A DO OF CAMERON, MO, WAS DISCIPLINED BY MISSOURI ON MAY 28, 1998
DISCIPLINARY ACTION: REPRIMAND
OFFENSE: DISCIPLINARY ACTION BY ANOTHER STATE OR AGENCY

NOTES: SURRENDERED COLORADO LICENSE.

MANUELE, MARK ALLEN DO, LICENSE NUMBER 20A5681 OF CAMERON, MO, WAS DISCIPLINED BY CALIFORNIA ON JULY 15, 1998
DISCIPLINARY ACTION: REPRIMAND
OFFENSE: DISCIPLINARY ACTION BY ANOTHER STATE OR AGENCY

NOTES: ACTION TAKEN BY ANOTHER STATE.

MARQUIS, KATHY A, WAS DISCIPLINED BY COLORADO ON OCTOBER 9, 1996

NOTES: ORDER ISSUED BY THE GUNNISON COUNTY DISTRICT COURT ENJOINING HER FROM THE UNLICENSED PRACTICE OF MEDICINE.

MARTIN, DAVID A MD, DATE OF BIRTH OCTOBER 28, 1941, LICENSE NUMBER 0016271 OF EVERGREEN, CO, WAS DISCIPLINED BY COLORADO ON JUNE 22, 1990
DISCIPLINARY ACTION: EMERGENCY SUSPENSION
OFFENSE: FAILURE TO COMPLY WITH PREVIOUS BOARD ORDER

NOTES: ACTION BASED ON FAILURE TO SUBMIT TO BOARD ORDERED PHYSICAL AND PSYCHIATRIC EXAMINATIONS. SUSPENSION AFFIRMED BY ORDER OF 4/10/91, PENDING COMPLIANCE.

MARTIN, DAVID A MD, DATE OF BIRTH OCTOBER 28, 1941 OF 701C LINWOOD DRIVE, HARRISONVILLE, MO, WAS DISCIPLINED BY MEDICARE ON JULY 23, 1991
DISCIPLINARY ACTION: EXCLUSION FROM THE MEDICARE AND/OR MEDICAID PROGRAM
OFFENSE: DISCIPLINARY ACTION BY ANOTHER STATE OR AGENCY

NOTES: LICENSE REVOCATION OR SUSPENSION.

MARTIN, DAVID A MD, DATE OF BIRTH OCTOBER 28, 1941, LICENSE NUMBER 0016271 OF EVERGREEN, CO, WAS DISCIPLINED BY COLORADO ON JANUARY 28, 1992
DISCIPLINARY ACTION: EMERGENCY SUSPENSION
OFFENSE: SUBSTANCE ABUSE

NOTES: HABITUAL INTEMPERANCE AND EXCESSIVE USE OF A CONTROLLED SUBSTANCE.

MARTIN, DAVID A MD, DATE OF BIRTH OCTOBER 28, 1941, LICENSE NUMBER 0016271 OF EVERGREEN, CO, WAS DISCIPLINED BY COLORADO ON JULY 15, 1992
DISCIPLINARY ACTION: LICENSE REVOCATION
OFFENSE: SUBSTANCE ABUSE

NOTES: DISPENSED ANABOLIC STEROIDS FOR ATHLETIC PURPOSES AND WITHOUT MEDICAL JUSTIFICATION; HABITUAL INTEMPERANCE AND EXCESSIVE USE OF A CONTROLLED SUBSTANCE.

MARTIN, RICHARD EDWIN MD, DATE OF BIRTH NOVEMBER 20, 1953, LICENSE NUMBER 26303, WAS DISCIPLINED BY COLORADO ON OCTOBER 8, 1998
DISCIPLINARY ACTION: 42-MONTH PROBATION; MONITORING OF PHYSICIAN PERFORMANCE
OFFENSE: CRIMINAL CONVICTION OR PLEA OF GUILTY, NOLO CONTENDERE, OR NO CONTEST TO A CRIME

NOTES: FELONY CONVICTION. PROBATIONARY TERMS INCLUDE TREATMENT MONITORING AND ABSTINENCE FROM ALCOHOL AND CONTROLLED SUBSTANCES.

MARTIN, RICHARD EDWIN MD, LICENSE NUMBER 51323 OF DENVER, CO, WAS DISCIPLINED BY OHIO ON MAY 13, 1999
DISCIPLINARY ACTION: EMERGENCY SUSPENSION
OFFENSE: CRIMINAL CONVICTION OR PLEA OF GUILTY, NOLO CONTENDERE, OR NO CONTEST TO A CRIME

NOTES: MEDICAL LICENSE AUTOMATICALLY SUSPENDED RETROACTIVE TO 4/4/97 BASED ON HIS PLEA OF GUILTY TO ONE FELONY COUNT OF SEXUAL ASSAULT ON A CHILD.

MARTIN, RICHARD EDWIN MD, LICENSE NUMBER 51323 OF ENGLEWOOD, CO, WAS DISCIPLINED BY OHIO ON OCTOBER 14, 1999
DISCIPLINARY ACTION: LICENSE REVOCATION
OFFENSE: DISCIPLINARY ACTION BY ANOTHER STATE OR AGENCY

NOTES: PLEA OF GUILTY TO ONE FELONY COUNT OF SEXUAL ASSAULT ON A CHILD; AND PRIOR ACTION AGAINST HIS COLORADO LICENSE BASED ON THAT GUILTY PLEA. PERMANENT REVOCATION.

MARTIN, THEODORE E MD, DATE OF BIRTH MAY 28, 1929, LICENSE NUMBER 0014039 OF ROCKY FORD, CO, WAS DISCIPLINED BY COLORADO ON APRIL 12, 1995
DISCIPLINARY ACTION: 60-MONTH PROBATION; RESTRICTION PLACED ON CONTROLLED SUBSTANCE LICENSE
OFFENSE: SUBSTANDARD CARE, INCOMPETENCE OR NEGLIGENCE

NOTES: PRESCRIBING A CONTROLLED SUBSTANCE OTHER THAN IN THE COURSE OF LEGITIMATE PROFESSIONAL PRACTICE. SUBSTANDARD CARE. FALSIFYING OR REPEATEDLY MAKING INCORRECT ESSENTIAL ENTRIES ON PATIENT RECORDS. PERMANENT PRACTICE RESTRICTION PROHIBITING HIM FROM

PRESCRIBING OR PROVIDING CONTROLLED SUBSTANCES TO PATIENTS. PROBATION INCLUDES PRACTICE MONITORING.

MARTIN, THEODORE E MD, DATE OF BIRTH MAY 28, 1929, LICENSE NUMBER 0014039, WAS DISCIPLINED BY COLORADO ON JULY 13, 1995
DISCIPLINARY ACTION: EMERGENCY SUSPENSION

MARTIN, THEODORE E MD OF 903 SOUTH 12TH STREET, ROCKY FORD, CO, WAS DISCIPLINED BY DEA ON FEBRUARY 27, 1996
DISCIPLINARY ACTION: SURRENDER OF CONTROLLED SUBSTANCE LICENSE

NOTES: IN LIEU OF ORDER TO SHOW CAUSE.

MARTIN, THEODORE E MD, DATE OF BIRTH MAY 28, 1929, LICENSE NUMBER 0014039, WAS DISCIPLINED BY COLORADO ON NOVEMBER 13, 1996
DISCIPLINARY ACTION: SURRENDER OF LICENSE
OFFENSE: PHYSICAL OR MENTAL ILLNESS INHIBITING THE ABILITY TO PRACTICE WITH SKILL AND SAFETY

NOTES: PHYSICAL OR MENTAL DISABILITY.

MARTINEZ, BENJAMIN MD, DATE OF BIRTH APRIL 23, 1945, LICENSE NUMBER 0023493 OF PUEBLO, CO, WAS DISCIPLINED BY COLORADO ON SEPTEMBER 11, 1992
DISCIPLINARY ACTION: 36-MONTH PROBATION; RESTRICTION PLACED ON LICENSE
OFFENSE: SUBSTANDARD CARE, INCOMPETENCE OR NEGLIGENCE

NOTES: ALLEGED SUBSTANDARD CARE. ADDITIONAL EDUCATION EVALUATION AND LICENSE RESTRICTIONS, RE: NO OBSTETRICS PRACTICE EXCEPT AS REQUIRED TO DIAGNOSE PREGNANCY; NOT TO SUPERVISE PHYSICIAN'S ASSISTANTS, ETC, UNLESS SUCH POSITION IS ROUTINELY EMPLOYED IN OFFICE; PRACTICE MONITORING AND PARTICIPATION IN AN INDIVIDUALIZED EDUCATIONAL PLAN.

MARTINEZ, JOHN G MD, DATE OF BIRTH AUGUST 15, 1950, LICENSE NUMBER 0026394, WAS DISCIPLINED BY COLORADO ON MARCH 14, 1996
DISCIPLINARY ACTION: REPRIMAND

MASFERRER, MAURICIO MD, LICENSE NUMBER 0418009 OF 1215 DAHLIA STREET, DENVER, CO, WAS DISCIPLINED BY KANSAS ON JUNE 18, 1996
DISCIPLINARY ACTION: RESTRICTION PLACED ON LICENSE; REQUIRED TO TAKE ADDITIONAL MEDICAL EDUCATION
OFFENSE: CRIMINAL CONVICTION OR PLEA OF GUILTY, NOLO CONTENDERE, OR NO CONTEST TO A CRIME

NOTES: ON 7/25/94 PLED GUILTY TO TWO VIOLATIONS OF THE UNIFORM CODE OF MILITARY JUSTICE FOR CONDUCT UNBECOMING AN OFFICER AND GENTLEMAN WHICH WOULD CONSTITUTE A FELONY COUNT IN KANSAS; IN CONJUNCTION WITH THESE TWO VIOLATIONS HE PLED GUILTY TO COMMITTING ACTS OF SEXUAL ABUSE, MISCONDUCT OR EXPLOITATION RELATED TO PROFESSIONAL PRACTICE. FOLLOWING RESTRICTIONS AND REQUIREMENTS PLACED ON HIS LICENSE FOR A PERIOD OF AT LEAST THREE YEARS: SHALL MAINTAIN CONTRACT WITH KANSAS MEDICAL SOCIETY-MEDICAL ADVOCACY PROGRAM; CLINICAL WORK SHALL BE CLOSELY SUPERVISED BY A BOARD-APPROVED MONITOR WHO SHALL PROVIDE MONTHLY REPORTS TO THE KANSAS MEDICAL SOCIETY-MEDICAL ADVOCACY PROGRAM; SHALL UNDERGO PERSONAL PSYCHOTHERAPY WITH A BOARD-APPROVED THERAPIST WHO SHALL SUBMIT MONTHLY REPORTS; SHALL TAKE FIVE CONTINUING MEDICAL EDUCATION HOURS PER YEAR ON PROFESSIONAL BOUNDARY ISSUES; WILL IMMEDIATELY TAKE ALL NECESSARY STEPS TO REMOVE HIS LICENSE FROM "MILITARY" STATUS TO "ACTIVE" STATUS. ON 6/22/98 ORDER TERMINATED.

MATTHEWSPRICE, LAUREL A MD, DATE OF BIRTH APRIL 11, 1956, LICENSE NUMBER 0028520 OF CLEVELAND, OH, WAS DISCIPLINED BY COLORADO ON JUNE 7, 1991
OFFENSE: SUBSTANCE ABUSE

NOTES: HABITUAL INTEMPERANCE OR EXCESSIVE USE OF ANY HABIT FORMING DRUG OR CONTROLLED SUBSTANCE, PHYSICAL OR MENTAL DISABILITY RENDERING THE LICENSEE UNABLE TO PERFORM MEDICAL SERVICES WITH REASONABLE SKILL AND SAFETY TO THE PATIENT. STIPULATION AND ORDER RELINQUISHING LICENSE.

MAXWELL, MARY S MD, DATE OF BIRTH JULY 14, 1957, LICENSE NUMBER 0026903, WAS DISCIPLINED BY COLORADO ON FEBRUARY 16, 1996
DISCIPLINARY ACTION: REPRIMAND

MAXWELL, MARY SUSAN MD, LICENSE NUMBER 0G56377 OF BOULDER, CO, WAS DISCIPLINED BY CALIFORNIA ON SEPTEMBER 30, 1996
DISCIPLINARY ACTION: REPRIMAND

MCALLEN, CULLEN A MD, DATE OF BIRTH NOVEMBER 15, 1960, LICENSE NUMBER 0030764 OF DECATUR, GA, WAS DISCIPLINED BY COLORADO ON OCTOBER 12, 1994
DISCIPLINARY ACTION: 60-MONTH PROBATION; MONITORING OF PHYSICIAN PERFORMANCE
OFFENSE: SUBSTANCE ABUSE

NOTES: HABITUAL INTEMPERANCE OR EXCESSIVE USE OF ANY HABIT-FORMING DRUG OR CONTROLLED SUBSTANCE. FIVE YEAR PROBATION INCLUDING PRACTICE AND TREATMENT MONITORING IN ABEYANCE PENDING HIS RELOCATION TO COLORADO TO PRACTICE MEDICINE.

MCALLEN, CULLEN A MD, LICENSE NUMBER 00H3827 OF ATLANTA, GA, WAS DISCIPLINED BY TEXAS ON MAY 11, 1995
DISCIPLINARY ACTION: 60-MONTH PROBATION; RESTRICTION PLACED ON LICENSE
OFFENSE: DISCIPLINARY ACTION BY ANOTHER STATE OR AGENCY

NOTES: ON 10/12/94, COLORADO LICENSE PLACED ON PROBATION WITH RESTRICTIONS DUE TO THE ABUSE OF HALOTHANE AND ALCOHOL; REPORTS A SOBRIETY DATE OF 11/21/93; REPORTS ATTENDING AN AVERAGE OF THREE AA MEETINGS PER WEEK; RECEIVED INPATIENT SUBSTANCE ABUSE TREATMENT AT A COLORADO HOSPITAL FROM 11/20/93 TO 12/6/93; RECEIVED OUTPATIENT TREATMENT FROM THE HOSPITAL BETWEEN 12/7/93 AND 3/9/94. SUSPENSION STAYED. PROBATION WITH TERMS: SHALL NOT PRACTICE MEDICINE IN TEXAS INVOLVING DIRECT PATIENT CARE UNTIL HE HAS TAKEN AND PASSED THE SPECIAL PURPOSE EXAMINATION; SHALL NOT PRACTICE ANESTHESIA UNTIL HE PERSONALLY APPEARS BEFORE THE BOARD AND ASKS PERMISSION; SHALL ABSTAIN FROM THE CONSUMPTION OF ALCOHOL/DRUGS IN ANY FORM UNLESS PRESCRIBED BY ANOTHER PHYSICIAN FOR A LEGITIMATE AND THERAPEUTIC PURPOSE; SHALL SUBMIT HIMSELF FOR APPROPRIATE EXAMS

INCLUDING DRUG OR ALCOHOL SCREENS; SHALL SUBMIT HIMSELF FOR EVALUATION AND TREATMENT BY A BOARD-APPROVED PSYCHIATRIST AT LEAST MONTHLY WHO SHALL SUBMIT REPORTS; SHALL PARTICIPATE IN AA'S PROGRAM NOT LESS THAN THREE TIMES A WEEK WITH QUARTERLY REPORTS TO THE BOARD; SHALL PARTICIPATE IN ACTIVITIES OF AN IMPAIRED PHYSICIAN'S GROUP AND ATTEND WEEKLY MEETINGS WITH QUARTERLY REPORTS; SHALL NOT POSSESS ALCOHOL OR CONTROLLED SUBSTANCES EXCEPT AS PROVIDED FOR BY TERMS OF THIS ORDER; SHALL SURRENDER CONTROLLED SUBSTANCES AND, ANY DRUG SAMPLES IN HIS POSSESSION; SHALL NOT TREAT OR OTHERWISE SERVE AS A PHYSICIAN, PRESCRIBE, DISPENSE OR ADMINISTER DRUGS WITH POTENTIAL FOR ABUSE TO HIMSELF OR ANY MEMBER OF HIS FAMILY; SHALL NOT TELEPHONE TO A PHARMACY A PRESCRIPTION OR REFILL FOR CONTROLLED SUBSTANCES OR ALLOW ANY INDIVIDUAL UNDER HIS SUPERVISION TO DO SO; SHALL KEEP A SEPARATE LOG OF ALL PRESCRIPTIONS WHICH SHALL BE SUBJECT TO REVIEW; SHALL MAINTAIN ADEQUATE MEDICAL RECORDS WHICH SHALL BE AVAILABLE FOR REVIEW; SHALL OBTAIN AT LEAST 50 HOURS PER YEAR OF CONTINUING MEDICAL EDUCATION; SHALL COMPLY WITH TERMS OF THE COLORADO ORDER; SHALL APPEAR BEFORE BOARD AT LEAST ONCE A YEAR OR AT BOARD REQUEST; SHALL COOPERATE WITH BOARD IN VERIFYING COMPLIANCE INCLUDING PROVIDING COPIES OF MEDICAL RELEASES UPON REQUEST; SHALL PROVIDE A COPY OF THIS ORDER TO ANYONE REQUESTING IT WITHIN 10 DAYS; SHALL GIVE A COPY OF THIS ORDER TO ANY HEALTH CARE ENTITY WHERE HE HAS PRIVILEGES; TIME PERIOD OUT OF TEXAS DOES NOT COUNT TOWARD PROBATION; SHALL INFORM BOARD OF ANY CHANGE OF ADDRESS WITHIN 10 DAYS OR IF HE LEAVES THE STATE. SHALL NOT SEEK MODIFICATION FOR ONE YEAR. ON 2/7/98 PETITION TO MODIFY ORDER GRANTED; SHALL BE ALLOWED TO PRACTICE ANESTHESIA PROVIDED THAT THERE IS A BOARD-APPROVED MONITOR ON-SITE; HIS PSYCHIATRIST SHALL DETERMINE THE TREATMENT SCHEDULE; CONTINUING MEDICAL EDUCATION HOURS IN EXCESS OF FIFTY HOURS PER YEAR SHALL BE CARRIED FORWARD FOR TWELVE MONTHS. 1/29/99 ORDER TERMINATED.

MCCANN, JAMES R, WAS DISCIPLINED BY COLORADO ON FEBRUARY 13, 1998
OFFENSE: PRACTICING WITHOUT A VALID LICENSE

NOTES: STIPULATION ENJOINS HIM FROM THE UNLICENSED PRACTICE OF MEDICINE.

MCCAW, WILLIAM W MD, DATE OF BIRTH MARCH 15, 1925, LICENSE NUMBER 0012075, WAS DISCIPLINED BY COLORADO ON NOVEMBER 13, 1996
DISCIPLINARY ACTION: 60-MONTH PROBATION; RESTRICTION PLACED ON CONTROLLED SUBSTANCE LICENSE
OFFENSE: SUBSTANDARD CARE, INCOMPETENCE OR NEGLIGENCE

NOTES: SUBSTANDARD CARE. PROBATIONARY TERMS INCLUDE REEDUCATION ACTIVITIES, A REQUIREMENT FOR TRIPLICATE PRESCRIPTIONS, AND PRACTICE MONITORING.

MCCREEDY, PHILIP A MD, DATE OF BIRTH APRIL 9, 1936, LICENSE NUMBER 34350 OF 430 ASPEN PLACE, GOLDEN, CO, WAS DISCIPLINED BY WISCONSIN ON MAY 21, 1998
DISCIPLINARY ACTION: SURRENDER OF LICENSE
OFFENSE: LOSS OR RESTRICTION OF HOSPITAL PRIVILEGES

NOTES: FOR PERSONAL REASONS, HE DID NOT RENEW HIS REGISTRATION WHEN IT EXPIRED ON 11/1/97; BETWEEN 2/5/94 AND 2/28/94 HE WAS EMPLOYED BY THE BELOIT CLINIC TO PROVIDE COVERAGE IN THE DEPARTMENT OF OBSTETRICS/GYNECOLOGY; MEDICAL ASSISTANTS REPORTED THE FOLLOWING: RATHER THAN DRAPING HIS PATIENTS' BREAST, STOMACH AND ABDOMINAL AREAS WITH THEIR GOWNS AND/OR SHEETS WHILE PERFORMING BREAST AND PELVIC EXAMS, HE REPEATEDLY PULLED UP HIS PATIENT'S GOWNS AND SHEETS SO THAT THEIR BODIES WERE COMPLETELY EXPOSED FROM THE NECK DOWN THROUGHOUT ENTIRE EXAMINATION; WHILE IN THE PROCESS OF PERFORMING PELVIC EXAMS ON PATIENTS HE REPEATEDLY SANG THE SONG "OH WHERE, OH WHERE HAS MY WINNIE GONE?"; PELVIC EXAMS TOOK LONGER THAN PERFORMED BY OTHER PHYSICIANS AND THAT IT APPEARED THAT RATHER THAN PROPERLY FEELING PATIENTS' REPRODUCTIVE ORGANS, HE WOULD MOVE HIS FINGER(S) IN AND OUT OF PATIENT'S VAGINA; ON AT LEAST ONE OCCASION WHILE PERFORMING A PELVIC EXAM, HE PUT ONE HAND ON A PATIENT'S BREAST WHILE HE HAD THE FINGERS OF HIS OTHER HAND IN HER VAGINA; THERE WAS NO MEDICAL PURPOSE FOR DOING SO; ON 2/13/94 HE HUGGED AND KISSED A PATIENT AFTER DELIVERING HER BABY; THE PATIENT WAS CAUGHT BY SURPRISE AND WAS UNCOMFORTABLE SINCE HE WAS HER TEMPORARY DOCTOR AND SHE DID NOT REALLY KNOW HIM; ON 2/18/94 NEVER HAVING MET ONE PATIENT ADMITTED FOR DELIVERY, HE STOOD UP AFTER DELIVERY, REMOVED HIS MASK AND KISSED HER; WHILE HE KISSED HER, HIS HAND MADE CONTACT WITH HER BREAST; HE CONTENDS THAT SUCH CONTACT WAS UNINTENTIONAL; THE PATIENT CONTENDS THAT THE NATURE OF THE CONTACT WAS SUCH THAT IT HAD TO BE INTENTIONAL. ON 2/19/94 HE WAS DISMISSED FROM THE HOSPITAL IMMEDIATELY WITH HIS PRIVILEGES REVOKED. MAY APPLY FOR REINSTATEMENT OF LICENSE UNDER STATED CONDITIONS IN TWO YEARS.

MCCREEDY, PHILIP A MD, DATE OF BIRTH APRIL 9, 1936, LICENSE NUMBER 14284, WAS DISCIPLINED BY COLORADO ON JULY 16, 1998
DISCIPLINARY ACTION: SURRENDER OF LICENSE

NOTES: DISCIPLINE IN ANOTHER STATE.

MCCREEDY, PHILIP A MD, LICENSE NUMBER 5607A, WAS DISCIPLINED BY WYOMING ON NOVEMBER 17, 1998
DISCIPLINARY ACTION: SURRENDER OF LICENSE
OFFENSE: DISCIPLINARY ACTION BY ANOTHER STATE OR AGENCY

NOTES: IN 7/94 AND 3/98, LIED ON HIS LICENSE APPLICATION AND RENEWAL REGARDING A 2/19/94 REVOCATION OF HIS HOSPITAL PRIVILEGES IN WISCONSIN, AND A 5/21/98 ORDER AGAINST HIS WISCONSIN LICENSE; ALSO ALLEGATIONS OF SEXUAL ABUSE OF A PATIENT. AGREES TO RELINQUISH HIS LICENSE AND SHALL NOT REAPPLY FOR LICENSURE AT ANY TIME IN THE FUTURE.

MCCREEDY, PHILIP A MD, LICENSE NUMBER 73845 OF 13950 WEST 30TH PLACE, GOLDEN, CO, WAS DISCIPLINED BY MASSACHUSETTS ON APRIL 28, 1999
DISCIPLINARY ACTION: SURRENDER OF LICENSE
OFFENSE: DISCIPLINARY ACTION BY ANOTHER STATE OR AGENCY

NOTES: ALLEGATIONS THAT HE WAS DISCIPLINED BY THE WISCONSIN BOARD FOR SEXUAL MISCONDUCT; AND DISCIPLINED BY THE WYOMING BOARD BASED UPON THE WISCONSIN ACTION. RESIGNATION

PERMANENT(MASSACHUSETTS ONLY).

MCCREEDY, PHILIP A MD, LICENSE NUMBER 28963 OF GOLDEN, CO, WAS DISCIPLINED BY IOWA ON JUNE 23, 1999
DISCIPLINARY ACTION: SURRENDER OF LICENSE

NOTES: HE VOLUNTARILY RELINQUISHED HIS WISCONSIN AND WYOMING LICENSES AS RESOLUTION OF PENDING DISCIPLINARY MATTERS. VOLUNTARY SURRENDER AS RESOLUTION OF A PENDING DISCIPLINARY MATTER.

MCCREEDY, PHILIP A MD, LICENSE NUMBER 29610 OF GOLDEN, CO, WAS DISCIPLINED BY WASHINGTON ON JULY 9, 1999
DISCIPLINARY ACTION: SURRENDER OF LICENSE

NOTES: AGREED TO SURRENDER HIS LICENSE.

MCCREEDY, PHILLIP ALLEN MD, DATE OF BIRTH APRIL 9, 1936, LICENSE NUMBER 39852 OF GOLDEN, CO, WAS DISCIPLINED BY NORTH CAROLINA ON MAY 7, 1999
DISCIPLINARY ACTION: SURRENDER OF LICENSE
OFFENSE: DISCIPLINARY ACTION BY ANOTHER STATE OR AGENCY

NOTES: ON 5/21/98, THE WISCONSIN BOARD ACCEPTED THE SURRENDER OF HIS LICENSE BASED ON ALLEGATIONS OF VARIOUS BOUNDARY VIOLATIONS; IN 11/98, HE RELINQUISHED HIS WYOMING LICENSE BASED ON FALSE ANSWERS HE SUBMITTED ON HIS 1994 LICENSE APPLICATION, HIS 1995 LICENSING INTERVIEW, AND HIS 1998 APPLICATION FOR LICENSE RENEWAL.

MCCREERY, RICHARD A DO, DATE OF BIRTH APRIL 6, 1945, LICENSE NUMBER 0019454, WAS DISCIPLINED BY COLORADO ON OCTOBER 10, 1996
DISCIPLINARY ACTION: RESTRICTION PLACED ON LICENSE
OFFENSE: PHYSICAL OR MENTAL ILLNESS INHIBITING THE ABILITY TO PRACTICE WITH SKILL AND SAFETY

NOTES: PHYSICAL DISABILITY. LIMITED TO 14 HOURS OF PRACTICE PER WEEK.

MCCROSKEY, BRIAN L MD, DATE OF BIRTH SEPTEMBER 28, 1954, LICENSE NUMBER 0027420 OF OVERLAND PARK, KS, WAS DISCIPLINED BY COLORADO ON JULY 15, 1992
DISCIPLINARY ACTION: REPRIMAND

NOTES: TWO OR MORE ACTS OR OMISSIONS WHICH FAILED TO MEET GENERALLY ACCEPTED STANDARDS OF MEDICAL PRACTICE. HE HAS APPEALED TO THE COLORADO COURT OF APPEALS. DECISION PENDING AS OF MARCH 1993 NEWSLETTER.

MCDIVITT, ROBERT B MD, DATE OF BIRTH JULY 13, 1921, LICENSE NUMBER 0011911, WAS DISCIPLINED BY COLORADO ON MARCH 14, 1996
DISCIPLINARY ACTION: RESTRICTION PLACED ON LICENSE; REPRIMAND

NOTES: NO UNPROFESSIONAL CONDUCT IDENTIFIED. WILL ONLY TREAT FAMILY MEMBERS.

MCFARLAND, BRUCE D DO, DATE OF BIRTH AUGUST 11, 1961, LICENSE NUMBER 0034896, WAS DISCIPLINED BY COLORADO ON NOVEMBER 9, 1995
DISCIPLINARY ACTION: 60-MONTH PROBATION; MONITORING OF PHYSICIAN PERFORMANCE

NOTES: PRACTICE AND TREATMENT MONITORING.

MCFARLAND, BRUCE D DO, DATE OF BIRTH AUGUST 11, 1961, LICENSE NUMBER 1011550 OF 2370 FOLSOM UNIT B, BOULDER, CO, WAS DISCIPLINED BY MICHIGAN ON JUNE 6, 1996
DISCIPLINARY ACTION: PROBATION
OFFENSE: DISCIPLINARY ACTION BY ANOTHER STATE OR AGENCY

NOTES: FAILURE TO REPORT/COMPLY.

MCFARLAND, DOUGLAS M MD, DATE OF BIRTH NOVEMBER 9, 1941, LICENSE NUMBER 0022493 OF TRINIDAD, CO, WAS DISCIPLINED BY COLORADO ON NOVEMBER 19, 1993
DISCIPLINARY ACTION: REPRIMAND

MCFARLAND, JOHN Z IV MD, DATE OF BIRTH MARCH 1, 1939, LICENSE NUMBER 18379, WAS DISCIPLINED BY COLORADO ON OCTOBER 21, 1999
DISCIPLINARY ACTION: SURRENDER OF LICENSE

NOTES: NO UNPROFESSIONAL CONDUCT IDENTIFIED.

MCFARLAND, ROBERT MD OF BOULDER, CO, WAS DISCIPLINED BY MISSOURI ON NOVEMBER 24, 1997
DISCIPLINARY ACTION: LICENSE REVOCATION
OFFENSE: DISCIPLINARY ACTION BY ANOTHER STATE OR AGENCY

NOTES: ACTION BASED ON REVOCATION OF HIS COLORADO LICENSE, WHICH WAS BASED UPON FOUR COUNTS OF UNPROFESSIONAL CONDUCT BY COMMITTING ACTS OR OMISSIONS WHICH FAIL TO MEET GENERALLY ACCEPTED STANDARDS OF MEDICINE AND ENGAGING IN UNPROFESSIONAL CONDUCT BY PRESCRIBING A SCHEDULE II CONTROLLED SUBSTANCE IN VIOLATION OF A COLORADO BOARD ORDER DATED 10/11/89. NO REAPPLICATION FOR SEVEN YEARS.

MCFARLAND, ROBERT B MD, DATE OF BIRTH SEPTEMBER 18, 1929, LICENSE NUMBER 0013876 OF BOULDER, CO, WAS DISCIPLINED BY COLORADO ON OCTOBER 13, 1993
DISCIPLINARY ACTION: LICENSE REVOCATION
OFFENSE: FAILURE TO COMPLY WITH PREVIOUS BOARD ORDER

NOTES: VIOLATION OF A VALID BOARD ORDER; SUBSTANDARD PATIENT CARE AND GROSSLY NEGLIGENT MEDICAL PRACTICE.

MCFARLAND, ROBERT B MD, LICENSE NUMBER 0025254 OF 2300 KALMIA AVE, BOULDER, CO, WAS DISCIPLINED BY MASSACHUSETTS ON MARCH 8, 1995
DISCIPLINARY ACTION: NONRENEWAL OF LICENSE
OFFENSE: DISCIPLINARY ACTION BY ANOTHER STATE OR AGENCY

NOTES: DISCIPLINARY ACTION IN COLORADO; FAILURE TO RESPOND TO BOARD. REVOCATION OF INCHOATE RIGHT TO RENEW LICENSE.

MCFARLAND, ROBERT B MD, DATE OF BIRTH SEPTEMBER 18, 1929 OF 2300 KALMIA AVENUE, BOULDER, CO, WAS DISCIPLINED BY MEDICARE ON MAY 4, 1995
DISCIPLINARY ACTION: EXCLUSION FROM THE MEDICARE AND/OR MEDICAID PROGRAM
OFFENSE: DISCIPLINARY ACTION BY ANOTHER STATE OR AGENCY

NOTES: LICENSE REVOKED FOR REASONS BEARING ON PROFESSIONAL PERFORMANCE.

MCFARLAND, ROBERT BRUCE MD OF 2660 13TH STREET, BOULDER, CO, WAS DISCIPLINED BY DEA ON APRIL 13, 1994
DISCIPLINARY ACTION: SURRENDER OF CONTROLLED SUBSTANCE LICENSE
OFFENSE: DISCIPLINARY ACTION BY ANOTHER STATE OR AGENCY

NOTES: STATE BOARD.

MCGRATH, RICHARD W DO, DATE OF BIRTH NOVEMBER 17, 1943, LICENSE NUMBER 0017557, WAS DISCIPLINED BY COLORADO ON MARCH 14, 1996
DISCIPLINARY ACTION: REPRIMAND

MCGUIRE, THOMAS J MD, DATE OF BIRTH JULY 15, 1955, LICENSE NUMBER 31790, WAS DISCIPLINED BY COLORADO ON JANUARY 14, 1999
DISCIPLINARY ACTION: 60-MONTH PROBATION; REQUIRED TO TAKE ADDITIONAL MEDICAL EDUCATION
OFFENSE: SUBSTANDARD CARE, INCOMPETENCE OR NEGLIGENCE

NOTES: SUBSTANDARD CARE (PRIMA FACIE TYPE ADMISSION ONLY). TERMS OF PROBATION INCLUDE: RE-EDUCATION ACTIVITIES AND PRACTICE MONITORING.

MCHUGH, J B DUKE MD, DATE OF BIRTH NOVEMBER 13, 1951, LICENSE NUMBER 0027804 OF WEST MONROE, LA, WAS DISCIPLINED BY COLORADO ON DECEMBER 16, 1994
DISCIPLINARY ACTION: PROBATION
OFFENSE: SUBSTANDARD CARE, INCOMPETENCE OR NEGLIGENCE

NOTES: DENIES HE PROVIDED SUBSTANDARD MEDICAL CARE. PROBATIONARY TERMS TO BE DETERMINED IF/WHEN HE RESUMES HIS COLORADO PRACTICE. THE PROBATION IS IN ABEYANCE, PENDING HIS RELOCATION TO COLORADO TO PRACTICE MEDICINE.

MCINTOSH, GERALD C MD, DATE OF BIRTH JUNE 6, 1946, LICENSE NUMBER 0022494, WAS DISCIPLINED BY COLORADO ON OCTOBER 14, 1996
DISCIPLINARY ACTION: REPRIMAND

MCINTYRE, ROBERT F MD, DATE OF BIRTH MARCH 28, 1951, LICENSE NUMBER 0033349 OF GARLAND, TX, WAS DISCIPLINED BY COLORADO ON JANUARY 20, 1994
DISCIPLINARY ACTION: 12-MONTH PROBATION; RESTRICTION PLACED ON LICENSE
OFFENSE: PHYSICAL OR MENTAL ILLNESS INHIBITING THE ABILITY TO PRACTICE WITH SKILL AND SAFETY

NOTES: PHYSICAL OR MENTAL DISABILITY ISSUES. APPLICATION FOR LICENSURE. PROBATION FOR AT LEAST ONE YEAR INCLUDING PRACTICE MONITORING; AND STIPULATION FOR PERMANENT PRACTICE RESTRICTION (LIMITED TO DISABILITY EVALUATIONS AND NONCLINICAL RISK MANAGEMENT ACTIVITIES). PROBATION IN ABEYANCE PENDING HIS RELOCATION TO COLORADO MEDICAL PRACTICE.

MCLAIN, PHIL C III MD, DATE OF BIRTH MARCH 30, 1952, LICENSE NUMBER 0024726 OF ESTES PARK, CO, WAS DISCIPLINED BY COLORADO ON MARCH 16, 1995
DISCIPLINARY ACTION: RESTRICTION PLACED ON LICENSE
OFFENSE: SUBSTANDARD CARE, INCOMPETENCE OR NEGLIGENCE

NOTES: SUBSTANDARD CARE. SHALL REFRAIN FROM THE PRACTICE OF EMERGENCY MEDICINE.

MCLAIN, PHIL C III MD, DATE OF BIRTH MARCH 30, 1952, LICENSE NUMBER 0024726, WAS DISCIPLINED BY COLORADO ON APRIL 18, 1996
DISCIPLINARY ACTION: REPRIMAND

MEACHAM, STEPHEN R MD, DATE OF BIRTH APRIL 16, 1942, LICENSE NUMBER 15950, WAS DISCIPLINED BY COLORADO ON MARCH 19, 1998
DISCIPLINARY ACTION: REPRIMAND

MEASON, THOMAS M MD, DATE OF BIRTH SEPTEMBER 11, 1951, LICENSE NUMBER 0022499, WAS DISCIPLINED BY COLORADO ON OCTOBER 10, 1996
DISCIPLINARY ACTION: REPRIMAND
OFFENSE: SUBSTANDARD CARE, INCOMPETENCE OR NEGLIGENCE

MEASON, THOMAS M MD, DATE OF BIRTH SEPTEMBER 11, 1951, LICENSE NUMBER 22499, WAS DISCIPLINED BY COLORADO ON DECEMBER 18, 1997
DISCIPLINARY ACTION: 60-MONTH PROBATION; MONITORING OF PHYSICIAN PERFORMANCE
OFFENSE: SUBSTANCE ABUSE

NOTES: HABITUAL INTEMPERANCE OR EXCESSIVE USE OF A CONTROLLED SUBSTANCE. PROBATIONARY TERMS INCLUDE: ABSTINENCE FROM ALCOHOL AND CONTROLLED SUBSTANCES; TREATMENT MONITORING AND PRACTICE MONITORING.

MERRILL, FRANKLIN MD OF 425 SOUTH CHERRY STREET #140, DENVER, CO, WAS DISCIPLINED BY DEA ON AUGUST 12, 1999
DISCIPLINARY ACTION: RESTRICTION PLACED ON CONTROLLED SUBSTANCE LICENSE

NOTES: IN LIEU OF ORDER TO SHOW CAUSE.

MERRILL, FRANKLIN B MD, DATE OF BIRTH JUNE 14, 1927, LICENSE NUMBER 0012377, WAS DISCIPLINED BY COLORADO ON NOVEMBER 13, 1996
DISCIPLINARY ACTION: 60-MONTH PROBATION; RESTRICTION PLACED ON CONTROLLED SUBSTANCE LICENSE
OFFENSE: SUBSTANDARD CARE, INCOMPETENCE OR NEGLIGENCE

NOTES: SUBSTANDARD CARE. REVOCATION STAYED. PROBATION UNDER TERMS AND CONDITIONS: REEDUCATION ACTIVITIES; A RESTRICTION AGAINST PRESCRIBING SCHEDULE II AND III CONTROLLED SUBSTANCES; PRACTICE AND TREATMENT MONITORING.

MERRITT, EDWARD G MD, DATE OF BIRTH OCTOBER 13, 1921, LICENSE NUMBER 0011315 OF DELORES, CO, WAS DISCIPLINED BY COLORADO ON SEPTEMBER 17, 1993
DISCIPLINARY ACTION: SURRENDER OF LICENSE

NOTES: NO UNPROFESSIONAL CONDUCT IDENTIFIED. ACCORDING TO ORDER, AGREES TO PERMANENTLY RETIRE FROM THE PRACTICE OF MEDICINE EFFECTIVE 03/31/94.

MERRITT, EDWARD GEORGE MD OF CORTEZ, CO, WAS DISCIPLINED BY UTAH ON MARCH 10, 1994
DISCIPLINARY ACTION: SURRENDER OF LICENSE
OFFENSE: DISCIPLINARY ACTION BY ANOTHER STATE OR AGENCY

NOTES: SURRENDER OF LICENSE ON OFFER TO RETIRE PENDING INQUIRY INTO BASIS FOR CAUSE FOR DISCIPLINARY ACTION IN COLORADO. AGREED TO PERMANENTLY RETIRE FROM PRACTICE OF MEDICINE IN UTAH EFFECTIVE 03/31/94 AND AGREES HE WILL NOT REAPPLY FOR LICENSURE TO PRACTICE MEDICINE IN UTAH.

METZGER, JAMES MD OF 3535 S. LAFAYETTE #105, ENGLEWOOD, CO, WAS DISCIPLINED BY DEA ON MAY 3, 1999
DISCIPLINARY ACTION: SURRENDER OF CONTROLLED SUBSTANCE LICENSE
OFFENSE: PROFESSIONAL MISCONDUCT

NOTES: OBTAINING CONTROLLED SUBSTANCES BY FRAUD.

METZGER, JAMES R MD, DATE OF BIRTH MAY 5, 1961, LICENSE NUMBER 29735, WAS DISCIPLINED BY COLORADO ON DECEMBER

9, 1999
DISCIPLINARY ACTION: 60-MONTH PROBATION; RESTRICTION PLACED ON CONTROLLED SUBSTANCE LICENSE
OFFENSE: SUBSTANCE ABUSE

NOTES: HABITUAL INTEMPERANCE OR EXCESSIVE USE OF A CONTROLLED SUBSTANCE; ADMINISTERING A CONTROLLED SUBSTANCE OTHER THAN IN THE COURSE OF LEGITIMATE PROFESSIONAL PRACTICE. PROBATIONARY TERMS INCLUDE: A RESTRICTION AGAINST PRESCRIBING CONTROLLED SUBSTANCES; ABSTINENCE FROM ALCOHOL AND CONTROLLED SUBSTANCES; AND, TREATMENT MONITORING AND PRACTICE MONITORING.

MEZA-DEZA, FELIX MD, DATE OF BIRTH FEBRUARY 21, 1937, LICENSE NUMBER 19916, WAS DISCIPLINED BY COLORADO ON MAY 13, 1998

NOTES: NO UNPROFESSIONAL CONDUCT IDENTIFIED. HE AGREES TO RETIRE AS OF 9/30/98.

MICHELSON, ABRAHAM K MD, DATE OF BIRTH APRIL 4, 1942, LICENSE NUMBER 18286, WAS DISCIPLINED BY COLORADO ON MAY 14, 1997
DISCIPLINARY ACTION: SURRENDER OF LICENSE

NOTES: NO UNPROFESSIONAL CONDUCT IDENTIFIED.

MICKISH, ALAN B MD, LICENSE NUMBER 00E1059 OF FORT WORTH, TX, WAS DISCIPLINED BY TEXAS ON OCTOBER 9, 1992
DISCIPLINARY ACTION: 36-MONTH PROBATION
OFFENSE: PROFESSIONAL MISCONDUCT

NOTES: COMMITTED SEVERAL VIOLATIONS OF THE MEDICAL PRACTICE ACT, INCLUDING AIDING AND ABETTING, DIRECTLY OR INDIRECTLY, THE PRACTICE OF MEDICINE BY ANY PERSON, PARTNERSHIP, ASSOCIATION, OR CORPORATION NOT DULY LICENSED TO PRACTICE MEDICINE BY THE BOARD. SUSPENSION STAYED. PROBATION ON TERMS AND CONDITIONS.

MICKISH, ALAN B MD, DATE OF BIRTH JANUARY 2, 1947, LICENSE NUMBER 0021568 OF IRVING, TX, WAS DISCIPLINED BY COLORADO ON AUGUST 20, 1993
DISCIPLINARY ACTION: REPRIMAND

MILANO, WILLIAM J MD, DATE OF BIRTH DECEMBER 25, 1952, LICENSE NUMBER 0023497 OF LOVELAND, CO, WAS DISCIPLINED BY COLORADO ON MARCH 9, 1995
DISCIPLINARY ACTION: EMERGENCY SUSPENSION

MILANO, WILLIAM J MD, DATE OF BIRTH DECEMBER 25, 1952, LICENSE NUMBER 0023497, WAS DISCIPLINED BY COLORADO ON JULY 12, 1995
DISCIPLINARY ACTION: 60-MONTH PROBATION; RESTRICTION PLACED ON LICENSE

NOTES: REVOCATION, STAYED AS PROBATION WITH TREATMENT AND PRACTICE MONITORING. CHAPERONE REQUIRED FOR EXAM OR TREATMENT OF ANY FEMALE PATIENT OR JUVENILE PATIENT AND WHEN ANY JUVENILE'S FEMALE PARENT OR GUARDIAN IS PRESENT.

MILBURN, WILLIAM HAMPTON MD, DATE OF BIRTH MAY 17, 1936 OF BOX 727, LYONS, CO, WAS DISCIPLINED BY MEDICARE ON AUGUST 2, 1990
DISCIPLINARY ACTION: EXCLUSION FROM THE MEDICARE AND/OR MEDICAID PROGRAM

OFFENSE: DISCIPLINARY ACTION BY ANOTHER STATE OR AGENCY

NOTES: LICENSE REVOCATION OR SUSPENSION.

MILLER, JOHN J MD, WAS DISCIPLINED BY NEVADA ON OCTOBER 17, 1995
DISCIPLINARY ACTION: LICENSE REVOCATION
OFFENSE: DISCIPLINARY ACTION BY ANOTHER STATE OR AGENCY

NOTES: CONVICTION OF A FELONY; CHARGED WITH BEING FOUND GUILTY OF TWO FELONIES IN MONTANA; DISCIPLINARY ACTION AGAINST HIS LICENSE IN MONTANA; SUSPENSION OF LICENSE BY ANY OTHER JURISDICTION; FAILURE TO REPORT, WITHIN 30 DAYS, THE SUSPENSION OF HIS LICENSE TO PRACTICE MEDICINE IN ANOTHER JURISDICTION.

MILLER, JOHN J MD OF JACKSONVILLE, FL, WAS DISCIPLINED BY UTAH ON OCTOBER 28, 1995
DISCIPLINARY ACTION: LICENSE REVOCATION; REVOCATION OF CONTROLLED SUBSTANCE LICENSE
OFFENSE: PHYSICAL OR MENTAL ILLNESS INHIBITING THE ABILITY TO PRACTICE WITH SKILL AND SAFETY

NOTES: ADMISSION OF INABILITY TO SAFELY ENGAGE IN THE PRACTICE OF MEDICINE BECAUSE OF A MENTAL OR PHYSICAL CONDITION.

MILLER, JOHN J MD, LICENSE NUMBER 0D27191 OF HIDDEN LAKE DRIVE, JACKSONVILLE, FL, WAS DISCIPLINED BY MARYLAND ON NOVEMBER 7, 1995
DISCIPLINARY ACTION: PROBATION
OFFENSE: DISCIPLINARY ACTION BY ANOTHER STATE OR AGENCY

NOTES: ACTION BY MONTANA. REVOCATION STAYED.

MILLER, JOHN J MD, LICENSE NUMBER 0039841 OF DEER LODGE, MT, WAS DISCIPLINED BY FLORIDA ON MARCH 6, 1996
DISCIPLINARY ACTION: LICENSE REVOCATION
OFFENSE: DISCIPLINARY ACTION BY ANOTHER STATE OR AGENCY

NOTES: CONVICTED OF A CRIME DIRECTLY RELATING TO THE PRACTICE OF MEDICINE.

MILLER, JOHN JOSEPH MD, DATE OF BIRTH FEBRUARY 14, 1942, LICENSE NUMBER 0003980 OF 310 SUNNYVIEW LANE, KALISPELL, MT, WAS DISCIPLINED BY MONTANA ON AUGUST 23, 1994
DISCIPLINARY ACTION: EMERGENCY SUSPENSION
OFFENSE: SUBSTANCE ABUSE

NOTES: UNTREATED CHEMICAL DEPENDENCY. STIPULATION NOT TO SEEK REINSTATEMENT OF LICENSE UNTIL AFTER COMPLETION OF EVALUATION AND TREATMENT FOR ILLNESSES ON 8/31/94.

MILLER, JOHN JOSEPH MD, DATE OF BIRTH FEBRUARY 14, 1942, LICENSE NUMBER 00M5606, WAS DISCIPLINED BY IDAHO ON NOVEMBER 18, 1994
DISCIPLINARY ACTION: LICENSE SUSPENSION
OFFENSE: DISCIPLINARY ACTION BY ANOTHER STATE OR AGENCY

NOTES: ON 8/24/94 MONTANA ORDERED THAT LICENSE BE PLACED ON EMERGENCY SUSPENSION; ALSO REQUIRED HIM TO HAVE A COMPLETE MENTAL AND PHYSICAL EXAMINATION. THE IDAHO BOARD FOR THE PURPOSE OF THIS RECIPROCAL DISCIPLINE INCORPORATES THE TERMS AND CONDITIONS OF THIS ORDER AND ORDERS HIM TO FULLY COMPLY WITH THEM.

MILLER, JOHN JOSEPH MD, DATE OF BIRTH FEBRUARY 14, 1942, LICENSE NUMBER 0021472 OF JACKSONVILLE, FL, WAS DISCIPLINED BY TENNESSEE ON FEBRUARY 23, 1995

DISCIPLINARY ACTION: LICENSE REVOCATION
OFFENSE: DISCIPLINARY ACTION BY ANOTHER STATE OR AGENCY

NOTES: DISCIPLINARY ACTION TAKEN BY MONTANA BOARD. SUBSTANCE ABUSE. MUST APPEAR BEFORE BOARD IF REINSTATEMENT SOUGHT.

MILLER, JOHN JOSEPH MD, DATE OF BIRTH FEBRUARY 14, 1942, LICENSE NUMBER 00M5606, WAS DISCIPLINED BY IDAHO ON MAY 1, 1995
DISCIPLINARY ACTION: LICENSE REVOCATION
OFFENSE: DISCIPLINARY ACTION BY ANOTHER STATE OR AGENCY

NOTES: IN 8/94 ENGAGED IN THE EXCESSIVE USE OF ALCOHOL OR OTHER SUBSTANCES TO THE EXTENT THAT THE USE IMPAIRED HIM PHYSICALLY OR MENTALLY; AS A RESULT HE WAS IN AN AUTO ACCIDENT WHICH CAUSED THE DEATH OF TWO PERSONS; LICENSE IN TENNESSEE WAS REVOKED ON 2/23/95. THE IDAHO BOARD ADOPTS THE FINDING OF THE TENNESSEE ORDER AND INCORPORATES ALL OF THE TERMS AND CONDITIONS OF THE TENNESSEE ORDER.

MILLER, JOHN JOSEPH MD, DATE OF BIRTH FEBRUARY 14, 1942 OF 215 SUNNYVIEW LANE #7, KALISPELL, MT, WAS DISCIPLINED BY MEDICARE ON MAY 4, 1995
DISCIPLINARY ACTION: EXCLUSION FROM THE MEDICARE AND/OR MEDICAID PROGRAM
OFFENSE: DISCIPLINARY ACTION BY ANOTHER STATE OR AGENCY

NOTES: LICENSE SUSPENDED FOR REASONS BEARING ON PROFESSIONAL PERFORMANCE.

MILLER, JOHN JOSEPH MD, DATE OF BIRTH FEBRUARY 14, 1942, LICENSE NUMBER 0003980 OF 3459 HIDDEN LAKE DRIVE WEST, JACKSONVILLE, FL, WAS DISCIPLINED BY MONTANA ON MAY 19, 1995
DISCIPLINARY ACTION: PROBATION
OFFENSE: CRIMINAL CONVICTION OR PLEA OF GUILTY, NOLO CONTENDERE, OR NO CONTEST TO A CRIME

NOTES: CONVICTION OF FELONY; CHEMICAL DEPENDENCY. REVOCATION STAYED.

MILLER, JOHN JOSEPH MD, LICENSE NUMBER 0049431 OF JACKSONVILLE, FL, WAS DISCIPLINED BY VIRGINIA ON JUNE 13, 1995
DISCIPLINARY ACTION: LICENSE SUSPENSION
OFFENSE: DISCIPLINARY ACTION BY ANOTHER STATE OR AGENCY

NOTES: REVOCATION BY TENNESSEE AND SUSPENSION BY MONTANA AFTER HE ENGAGED IN THE EXCESSIVE USE OF ALCOHOL OR OTHER SUBSTANCES.

MILLER, JOHN JOSEPH MD, DATE OF BIRTH FEBRUARY 14, 1942, LICENSE NUMBER 0031991 OF 3459 HIDDEN LAKE DR W, JACKSONVILLE, FL, WAS DISCIPLINED BY GEORGIA ON AUGUST 3, 1995
DISCIPLINARY ACTION: LICENSE SUSPENSION
OFFENSE: CRIMINAL CONVICTION OR PLEA OF GUILTY, NOLO CONTENDERE, OR NO CONTEST TO A CRIME

NOTES: CONVICTION OF A CRIME. SUSPENDED INDEFINITELY.

MILLER, JOHN JOSEPH MD, DATE OF BIRTH FEBRUARY 14, 1942, LICENSE NUMBER 0009752 OF 3459 HIDDEN LAKE DRIVE WEST, JACKSONVILLE, FL, WAS DISCIPLINED BY WEST VIRGINIA ON NOVEMBER 20, 1995
DISCIPLINARY ACTION: LICENSE REVOCATION
OFFENSE: DISCIPLINARY ACTION BY ANOTHER STATE OR AGENCY

NOTES: FOUND GUILTY OF TWO FELONY COUNTS OF NEGLIGENT HOMICIDE IN 2/95 IN MONTANA; HIS EXCESSIVE USE OF ALCOHOL CAUSED HIM TO BE IMPAIRED AND TO CAUSE THE DEATHS OF TWO PERSONS IN A MOTOR VEHICLE ACCIDENT. IN 2/95 THE TENNESSEE BOARD REVOKED HIS LICENSE. IN 11/94 THE IDAHO BOARD SUSPENDED HIS LICENSE AND IN 5/95 REVOKED HIS LICENSE. IN 8/94 MONTANA SUSPENDED HIS LICENSE AND IN 4/95 REVOKED HIS LICENSE AND THEN STAYED THE REVOCATION AS PROBATION UNDER SEVERAL TERMS AND CONDITIONS.

MILLER, JOHN JOSEPH MD, DATE OF BIRTH FEBRUARY 14, 1942, LICENSE NUMBER 0030589, WAS DISCIPLINED BY COLORADO ON JANUARY 11, 1996
OFFENSE: CRIMINAL CONVICTION OR PLEA OF GUILTY, NOLO CONTENDERE, OR NO CONTEST TO A CRIME

NOTES: PLED GUILTY TO TWO FELONY CHARGES (NEGLIGENT HOMICIDE AS A RESULT OF A MOTOR VEHICLE ACCIDENT). ORDERED TO PERMANENTLY RELINQUISH HIS LICENSE TO PRACTICE MEDICINE IN COLORADO.

MILLER, JOHN JOSEPH MD, LICENSE NUMBER 0060453 OF DEER LODGE, MT, WAS DISCIPLINED BY OHIO ON FEBRUARY 14, 1996
DISCIPLINARY ACTION: LICENSE REVOCATION
OFFENSE: DISCIPLINARY ACTION BY ANOTHER STATE OR AGENCY

NOTES: PRIOR ACTION BY MONTANA MEDICAL BOARD WHICH WAS BASED ON HIS ADMISSIONS THAT HE HAD ENGAGED IN EXCESSIVE USE OF ALCOHOL SO THAT HE WAS MENTALLY AND PHYSICALLY IMPAIRED AND THAT WHILE HE WAS IMPAIRED, HE WAS INVOLVED IN A MOTOR VEHICLE ACCIDENT THAT CAUSED THE DEATH OF TWO PEOPLE. CONVICTION OF TWO FELONY COUNTS OF NEGLIGENT HOMICIDE. PERMANENT REVOCATION.

MILLER, MARY MARGARET MD, DATE OF BIRTH DECEMBER 21, 1937, LICENSE NUMBER 0021635 OF FORT COLLINS, CO, WAS DISCIPLINED BY KENTUCKY ON DECEMBER 1, 1992
DISCIPLINARY ACTION: NONRENEWAL OF LICENSE
OFFENSE: DISCIPLINARY ACTION BY ANOTHER STATE OR AGENCY

NOTES: ACTION BASED ON HEARING OFFICER'S FINDINGS, ACTION TAKEN BY COLORADO, AND PREVIOUS SUBSTANCE ABUSE PROBLEM.

MILLER, MARY MARGARET MD, DATE OF BIRTH DECEMBER 21, 1937, LICENSE NUMBER 00IP113 OF JEFFERSON COUNTY, KY, WAS DISCIPLINED BY KENTUCKY ON APRIL 1, 1994
DISCIPLINARY ACTION: SURRENDER OF LICENSE; MONITORING OF PHYSICIAN PERFORMANCE

NOTES: INSTITUTIONAL PRACTICE LIMITED LICENSE ISSUED TO UNIVERSITY OF LOUISVILLE FOR 1 YEAR SUBJECT TO FOLLOWING TERMS AND CONDITIONS: MUST MAINTAIN RELATIONSHIP WITH COMMITTEE ON IMPAIRED PHYSICIANS WITH REGULAR REPORTS; BIOLOGICAL FLUID TESTING.

MILLER, MARY MARGARET MD, DATE OF BIRTH DECEMBER 21, 1937, LICENSE NUMBER 0035089, WAS DISCIPLINED BY COLORADO ON FEBRUARY 15, 1996
DISCIPLINARY ACTION: RESTRICTION PLACED ON LICENSE
OFFENSE: CRIMINAL CONVICTION OR PLEA OF GUILTY, NOLO CONTENDERE, OR NO CONTEST TO A CRIME

NOTES: FELONY CONVICTION; CONVICTION OF A LAW REGARDING CONTROLLED SUBSTANCES; PRESCRIBING OTHER THAN IN THE COURSE OF LEGITIMATE PROFESSIONAL PRACTICE; HABITUAL INTEMPERANCE; PHYSICAL OR MENTAL DISABILITY.

GRANTED A LICENSE TO PRACTICE MEDICINE, BUT IS PROHIBITED FROM PRACTICING UNDER THE AUTHORITY OF THE LICENSE.

MILLER, MARY MARGARET MD OF LOUISVILLE, KY, WAS DISCIPLINED BY DEA ON JANUARY 21, 1999
DISCIPLINARY ACTION: RESTRICTION PLACED ON CONTROLLED SUBSTANCE LICENSE; MONITORING OF PHYSICIAN PERFORMANCE
OFFENSE: DISCIPLINARY ACTION BY ANOTHER STATE OR AGENCY

NOTES: IN 1983 DEA INITIATED AN INVESTIGATION WHEN HER NAME CAME UP AS A LARGE PRESCRIBER OF SCHEDULE II SUBSTANCES AND AN UNDERCOVER AGENT WENT TO HER OFFICE ON FIVE OCCASIONS TO ATTEMPT TO OBTAIN CONTROLLED SUBSTANCE PRESCRIPTIONS FOR NO LEGITIMATE MEDICAL PURPOSES; THE AGENT WAS ABLE TO OBTAIN PRESCRIPTIONS FOR BIPHETAMINE, SECONAL AND VALIUM WITHOUT GIVING A MEDICAL REASON; SHE TOLD THE "PATIENT" TO FILL THE PRESCRIPTIONS AT DIFFERENT PHARMACIES; CONVICTED ON 10/22/84 IN THE U.S. DISTRICT COURT OF COLORADO OF 15 COUNTS OF DISTRIBUTION OF CONTROLLED SUBSTANCES AND PRESCRIPTIONS NOT ISSUED FOR A LEGITIMATE MEDICAL PURPOSE; IN 10/84 THE COLORADO BOARD SUSPENDED HER LICENSE WHICH WAS REINSTATED IN 1986; SHE ABUSED ALCOHOL BETWEEN 1986 AND 1989 BUT HAS CONSUMED NONE SINCE 1/29/90; COLORADO BOARD REVOKED HER LICENSE ON 9/28/90; KENTUCKY BOARD DENIED HER A LICENSE IN 11/92; HAS PARTICIPATED IN TREATMENT AND PHYSICIAN'S HEALTH PROGRAMS; IN 3/95 KENTUCKY GRANTED HER A FULL LICENSE WITH MONITORING CONDITIONS; ON 5/1/95 APPLIED FOR DEA REGISTRATION IN SCHEDULES III, IV AND V, FULLY DISCLOSING CONVICTION AND REHABILITATION; ON 9/22/97 KENTUCKY DROPPED MORE STRINGENT CONDITIONS AND REQUIRED HER TO KEEP A LOG OF CONTROLLED SUBSTANCES PRESCRIPTIONS; ON 2/15/96 COLORADO REINSTATED HER LICENSE SOLELY FOR HER TO BE RECERTIFIED WITH THE CONDITION SHE NOT PRACTICE IN COLORADO; TAKES FULL RESPONSIBILITY FOR HER ACTIONS. DEA REGISTRATION GRANTED FOR SCHEDULES III THROUGH V WITH THE FOLLOWING RESTRICTIONS FOR THREE YEARS: SHALL PROVIDE THE DEA WITH A LOG QUARTERLY OF ALL CONTROLLED SUBSTANCES PRESCRIPTIONS WRITTEN; MUST MAINTAIN CONTRACT WITH IMPAIRED PHYSICIANS PROGRAM; SHALL INFORM DEA OF ANY ACTION TAKEN AGAINST LICENSE WITHIN 30 DAYS; SHALL CONSENT TO DEA INSPECTIONS.

MILZER, GARY S MD, DATE OF BIRTH APRIL 9, 1949, LICENSE NUMBER 0022288 OF AURORA, CO, WAS DISCIPLINED BY COLORADO ON JUNE 12, 1992
DISCIPLINARY ACTION: 60-MONTH PROBATION
OFFENSE: SUBSTANCE ABUSE

NOTES: SUBSTANCE ABUSE AND DEPENDENCE; SELF TREATMENT OF MIGRAINE HEADACHES WITH FIORINAL.

MILZER, GARY S MD, DATE OF BIRTH APRIL 9, 1949, LICENSE NUMBER 0022288, WAS DISCIPLINED BY COLORADO ON SEPTEMBER 12, 1996
DISCIPLINARY ACTION: 60-MONTH PROBATION; MONITORING OF PHYSICIAN PERFORMANCE
OFFENSE: FAILURE TO COMPLY WITH PREVIOUS BOARD ORDER

NOTES: VIOLATION OF A VALID BOARD ORDER. TREATMENT AND MONITORING PROVISIONS.

MILZER, GARY S MD, DATE OF BIRTH APRIL 9, 1949, LICENSE NUMBER 0022288, WAS DISCIPLINED BY COLORADO ON SEPTEMBER 23, 1996
DISCIPLINARY ACTION: EMERGENCY SUSPENSION

MILZER, GARY S MD, DATE OF BIRTH APRIL 9, 1949, LICENSE NUMBER 0022288, WAS DISCIPLINED BY COLORADO ON NOVEMBER 13, 1996
DISCIPLINARY ACTION: SURRENDER OF LICENSE
OFFENSE: PHYSICAL OR MENTAL ILLNESS INHIBITING THE ABILITY TO PRACTICE WITH SKILL AND SAFETY

NOTES: PHYSICAL OR MENTAL DISABILITY.

MILZER, GARY STEVEN MD OF 1421 S POTOMAC SUITE 300, AURORA, CO, WAS DISCIPLINED BY DEA ON MARCH 8, 1994
DISCIPLINARY ACTION: RESTRICTION PLACED ON CONTROLLED SUBSTANCE LICENSE
OFFENSE: SUBSTANCE ABUSE

NOTES: PLACED ON PROBATION FOR EXCESSIVE USE OF FIORINAL AND WRITING FRAUDULENT PRESCRIPTIONS. RESTRICTED TO SCHEDULES II, IV AND V ONLY.

MIRCHANDANI, RAJAN K MD, DATE OF BIRTH NOVEMBER 2, 1956, LICENSE NUMBER 0033934, WAS DISCIPLINED BY COLORADO ON NOVEMBER 21, 1996
DISCIPLINARY ACTION: EMERGENCY SUSPENSION

MIRCHANDANI, RAJAN K MD, DATE OF BIRTH NOVEMBER 2, 1956, LICENSE NUMBER 33934, WAS DISCIPLINED BY COLORADO ON MAY 16, 1997
DISCIPLINARY ACTION: SURRENDER OF LICENSE
OFFENSE: PROVIDING FALSE INFORMATION TO THE BOARD OR OTHER HEALTH AGENCY

NOTES: FRAUD, MISREPRESENTATION OR DECEPTION IN OBTAINING LICENSURE; HABITUAL INTEMPERANCE OR EXCESSIVE USE OF A CONTROLLED SUBSTANCE.

MITCHELL, LAUREN E DO, DATE OF BIRTH DECEMBER 12, 1915 OF P O BOX 322, RIMROCK, AZ, WAS DISCIPLINED BY MEDICARE ON FEBRUARY 12, 1990
DISCIPLINARY ACTION: EXCLUSION FROM THE MEDICARE AND/OR MEDICAID PROGRAM
OFFENSE: DISCIPLINARY ACTION BY ANOTHER STATE OR AGENCY

NOTES: LICENSE REVOCATION OR SUSPENSION.

MITCHELL, LAUREN E DO, DATE OF BIRTH DECEMBER 12, 1915, LICENSE NUMBER 0010261 OF LONGMONT, CO, WAS DISCIPLINED BY COLORADO ON JULY 6, 1994
DISCIPLINARY ACTION: REPRIMAND
OFFENSE: PROFESSIONAL MISCONDUCT

MITCHELL, ORDERIA F MD, DATE OF BIRTH NOVEMBER 14, 1949, LICENSE NUMBER 25103, WAS DISCIPLINED BY COLORADO ON JUNE 19, 1997
DISCIPLINARY ACTION: REPRIMAND

MIXTER, BRUCE R MD, DATE OF BIRTH MARCH 13, 1954, LICENSE NUMBER 0031939, WAS DISCIPLINED BY COLORADO ON JUNE 15, 1995
DISCIPLINARY ACTION: REPRIMAND

MIXTER, BRUCE ROBERT MD, LICENSE NUMBER 0G49879 OF FAYETTEVILLE, NC, WAS DISCIPLINED BY CALIFORNIA ON JULY 12, 1996

DISCIPLINARY ACTION: LICENSE REVOCATION
OFFENSE: DISCIPLINARY ACTION BY ANOTHER STATE OR AGENCY

NOTES: DISCIPLINARY ACTION IN COLORADO AS HIS CARE OF A PATIENT FELL BELOW THE ACCEPTED STANDARD OF MEDICAL PRACTICE; FAILED TO APPROPRIATELY MANAGE THE PATIENT'S POSITIVE RH STATUS; AND FAILED TO TRANSFER IMPORTANT INFORMATION TO THE PATIENT'S PRENATAL FLOW SHEET. DEFAULT ACTION.

MOHLER, NELSON E DO, DATE OF BIRTH JUNE 30, 1937 OF 7233 LOWELL BLVD, WESTMINSTER, CO, WAS DISCIPLINED BY MEDICARE ON OCTOBER 20, 1994
DISCIPLINARY ACTION: EXCLUSION FROM THE MEDICARE AND/OR MEDICAID PROGRAM; FINE

NOTES: IMPOSITION OF A CIVIL MONEY PENALTY OR ASSESSMENT.

MONAGIN, JOHN A MD, DATE OF BIRTH MARCH 27, 1946, LICENSE NUMBER 28244, WAS DISCIPLINED BY COLORADO ON FEBRUARY 17, 1999
DISCIPLINARY ACTION: 60-MONTH PROBATION; REQUIRED TO TAKE ADDITIONAL MEDICAL EDUCATION
OFFENSE: NONCOMPLIANCE WITH A PROFESSIONAL RULE

NOTES: VIOLATION OF THE MEDICAL PRACTICE ACT. PROBATIONARY TERMS INCLUDE: TREATMENT AND PRACTICE MONITORING AND REEDUCATION ACTIVITIES.

MONSOUR, JAMES W MD, LICENSE NUMBER 0011773 OF PRATT, KS, WAS DISCIPLINED BY FLORIDA ON MAY 7, 1991
DISCIPLINARY ACTION: FINE; RESTRICTION PLACED ON LICENSE
OFFENSE: DISCIPLINARY ACTION BY ANOTHER STATE OR AGENCY

NOTES: $1,000 FINE; REPRIMAND; RESTRICTED FROM TREATING OBESE PATIENTS WITH AMPHETAMINES OR SYMPATHOMIMETIC AMINES IN FLORIDA UNTIL HE PETITIONS BOARD AND APPEARS BEFORE THE BOARD FOR LIFTING OF THE RESTRICTION. SUCH PETITION TO INCLUDE PROOF OF COMPLETION OF CATEGORY I CONTINUING MEDICAL EDUCATION IN TREATMENT OF OBESITY AND AN AFFIDAVIT WHICH DEMONSTRATES HIS FAMILIARITY WITH FLORIDA LAW REGARDING RESTRICTIONS ON USE OF AMPHETAMINES AND SYMPATHOMIMETIC AMINES AND RESPONSIBLE SUPERVISION OF ALLIED HEALTH PERSONNEL.

MONSOUR, JAMES W MD, LICENSE NUMBER 0C28031 OF DENVER, CO, WAS DISCIPLINED BY CALIFORNIA ON OCTOBER 24, 1993
DISCIPLINARY ACTION: LICENSE REVOCATION
OFFENSE: DISCIPLINARY ACTION BY ANOTHER STATE OR AGENCY

NOTES: DISCIPLINED BY COLORADO BOARD FOR SUBSTANDARD PRACTICE IN DISPENSING AMPHETAMINES FOR OBESITY. DEFAULT DECISION.

MONTAGUE, JOHN F MD, DATE OF BIRTH NOVEMBER 6, 1924, LICENSE NUMBER 0013052 OF LITTLETON, CO, WAS DISCIPLINED BY COLORADO ON SEPTEMBER 11, 1992
OFFENSE: PHYSICAL OR MENTAL ILLNESS INHIBITING THE ABILITY TO PRACTICE WITH SKILL AND SAFETY

NOTES: PHYSICAL OR MENTAL DISABILITY. CONDITIONS TO BE MET FOR LICENSE RENEWAL. IF RENEWED, THEN INDEFINITE PROBATION. AGREES NOT TO PRACTICE MEDICINE IN COLORADO WITHOUT PRIOR BOARD APPROVAL, AND COMPLIANCE WITH BOARD REQUIREMENTS AS MAY BE NECESSARY TO PROTECT PUBLIC SAFETY.

MONTAGUE, JOHN FRANCIS MD, LICENSE NUMBER 0AA2603, WAS DISCIPLINED BY ALASKA ON MARCH 18, 1991
DISCIPLINARY ACTION: EMERGENCY SUSPENSION

NOTES: QUESTION ABOUT ABILITY TO SAFELY PRACTICE MEDICINE.

MONTAGUE, JOHN FRANCIS MD, LICENSE NUMBER 0002603, WAS DISCIPLINED BY ALASKA ON JANUARY 7, 1993
DISCIPLINARY ACTION: RESTRICTION PLACED ON LICENSE; MONITORING OF PHYSICIAN PERFORMANCE

NOTES: SUBMIT RENEWAL WITH ALL FEES AND CONTINUING MEDICAL EDUCATION; EXAM BY PSYCHIATRIST; BE UNDER ONGOING CARE FOR BIPOLAR DISORDER; MAY NOT PRACTICE ALONE AND WILL BE SUPERVISED BY ANOTHER PHYSICIAN; RANDOM REVIEW OF CHARTS.

MONTANTE, JOSEPH R MD, DATE OF BIRTH JULY 23, 1948, LICENSE NUMBER 0022290 OF BOULDER, CO, WAS DISCIPLINED BY COLORADO ON AUGUST 21, 1992
DISCIPLINARY ACTION: 60-MONTH PROBATION; MONITORING OF PHYSICIAN PERFORMANCE
OFFENSE: SUBSTANDARD CARE, INCOMPETENCE OR NEGLIGENCE

NOTES: TWO OR MORE ACTS OR OMISSIONS WHICH FAILED TO MEET GENERALLY ACCEPTED STANDARDS OF MEDICAL PRACTICE. PROBATIONARY PERIOD INCLUDES PRACTICE MONITORING. ON 8/21/95 ORDER AMENDED TO CLARIFY THE PRACTICE MONITOR'S RESPONSIBILITIES.

MOONEY, HERBERT S MD, LICENSE NUMBER 0A19982 OF LONGMONT, CO, WAS DISCIPLINED BY CALIFORNIA ON AUGUST 17, 1994
DISCIPLINARY ACTION: 60-MONTH PROBATION
OFFENSE: DISCIPLINARY ACTION BY ANOTHER STATE OR AGENCY

NOTES: DISCIPLINE BY COLORADO BOARD FOR ENGAGING IN 2 OR MORE ACTS WHICH FAILED TO MEET GENERALLY ACCEPTED STANDARDS OF MEDICAL PRACTICE WHILE TREATING 3 EMERGENCY ROOM PATIENTS. REVOCATION STAYED.

MOONEY, WILLIAM M DO, DATE OF BIRTH FEBRUARY 8, 1948 OF PO BOX 1894, SILVERTHORNE, CO, WAS DISCIPLINED BY MEDICARE ON APRIL 10, 1996
DISCIPLINARY ACTION: EXCLUSION FROM THE MEDICARE AND/OR MEDICAID PROGRAM
OFFENSE: DISCIPLINARY ACTION BY ANOTHER STATE OR AGENCY

NOTES: LICENSE REVOKED FOR REASONS BEARING ON PROFESSIONAL PERFORMANCE.

MOONEY, WILLIAM PATRICK DO, LICENSE NUMBER 0002379 OF SILVERTHORNE, CO, WAS DISCIPLINED BY OHIO ON APRIL 21, 1995
DISCIPLINARY ACTION: LICENSE REVOCATION
OFFENSE: SUBSTANDARD CARE, INCOMPETENCE OR NEGLIGENCE

NOTES: FAILURE TO CONFORM TO MINIMAL STANDARDS OF CARE WITH RESPECT TO TREATMENT AND SUPERVISION OF SEVEN OBSTETRICAL PATIENTS WHICH RESULTED IN INFANT INJURIES AND/OR DEATH. PERMANENT REVOCATION.

MOORE, JOHN B MD, DATE OF BIRTH APRIL 8, 1949, LICENSE NUMBER 0020487, WAS DISCIPLINED BY COLORADO ON JULY 15, 1996
DISCIPLINARY ACTION: REPRIMAND

MOORE, MICHAEL B MD, DATE OF BIRTH MARCH 2, 1963, LICENSE

NUMBER 0031513 OF DENVER, CO, WAS DISCIPLINED BY COLORADO ON JANUARY 16, 1992
DISCIPLINARY ACTION: 36-MONTH PROBATION; MONITORING OF PHYSICIAN PERFORMANCE
OFFENSE: SUBSTANCE ABUSE

NOTES: ALCOHOL ABUSE. LICENSED UNDER STIPULATION FOR PROBATION WITH TREATMENT MONITORING.

MOORE, MICHAEL B MD, DATE OF BIRTH MARCH 2, 1963, LICENSE NUMBER 0031513 OF DENVER, CO, WAS DISCIPLINED BY COLORADO ON JUNE 19, 1992
DISCIPLINARY ACTION: 60-MONTH PROBATION; MONITORING OF PHYSICIAN PERFORMANCE
OFFENSE: FAILURE TO COMPLY WITH PREVIOUS BOARD ORDER

NOTES: SUBSTANCE ABUSE AND VIOLATION OF FIRST ORDER. REVOCATION, STAYED FOR 5 YEARS CONDITIONED UPON FIVE YEARS PROBATION WITH TREATMENT MONITORING.

MOORE, MICHAEL B MD, DATE OF BIRTH MARCH 2, 1963, LICENSE NUMBER 0031513 OF DENVER, CO, WAS DISCIPLINED BY COLORADO ON NOVEMBER 18, 1992
DISCIPLINARY ACTION: LICENSE REVOCATION
OFFENSE: FAILURE TO COMPLY WITH PREVIOUS BOARD ORDER

NOTES: VIOLATED SECOND STIPULATION/ORDER DATED 6/19/92. STAY OF REVOCATION VACATED BASED ON CONTINUED DRUG ABUSE.

MORAN, LAURA B DO, DATE OF BIRTH MARCH 5, 1955, LICENSE NUMBER 0030243, WAS DISCIPLINED BY COLORADO ON FEBRUARY 14, 1996
DISCIPLINARY ACTION: REPRIMAND

MORITZ, TERRELL C MD, DATE OF BIRTH AUGUST 5, 1937, LICENSE NUMBER 16162, WAS DISCIPLINED BY COLORADO ON JULY 10, 1997
DISCIPLINARY ACTION: SURRENDER OF LICENSE

NOTES: NO UNPROFESSIONAL CONDUCT IDENTIFIED.

MORITZ, TERRELL CONWAY MD, LICENSE NUMBER 0020323, WAS DISCIPLINED BY ARIZONA ON OCTOBER 10, 1991
DISCIPLINARY ACTION: 60-MONTH PROBATION; FINE
OFFENSE: PROVIDING FALSE INFORMATION TO THE BOARD OR OTHER HEALTH AGENCY

NOTES: KNOWINGLY MAKING A FALSE OR MISLEADING STATEMENT TO THE BOARD IN THAT IN HIS 2/14/91 APPLICATION FOR HIS ARIZONA LICENSE, HE DENIED HAVING EVER BEEN TREATED FOR THE USE OF OR MISUSE OF ANY CHEMICAL SUBSTANCES, DESPITE THE FACT THAT HE HAD BEEN AN INPATIENT AT A TREATMENT CENTER IN COLORADO IN 8/90 FOR 28 DAYS AND AN INPATIENT AT A RECOVERY CENTER IN GEORGIA FOR THREE MONTHS IN THE FALL OF 1990 BOTH FOR THE TREATMENT OF ALCOHOLISM; ALSO PRIVILEGES AT A MEDICAL CENTER IN COLORADO WERE TEMPORARILY SUSPENDED IN 12/89 DUE TO HIS MISREADING AN EKG AND HE WAS REQUIRED TO GET ADDITIONAL TRAINING; PRIVILEGES WERE RESTORED IN 4/90. PROBATION WITH CONDITIONS: MUST IMMEDIATELY PARTICIPATE IN A BOARD-APPROVED MONITORED AFTERCARE TREATMENT PROGRAM WHOSE THERAPIST MUST SUBMIT QUARTERLY REPORTS; SHALL ATTEND A MINIMUM OF THREE WEEKLY MEETINGS OF AA AND SHALL OBTAIN A SPONSOR IN AA WITH WHOM HE SHALL HAVE CONTACT AT LEAST ONCE A WEEK; SHALL OBTAIN A BOARD-APPROVED TREATING PHYSICIAN; SHALL ABSTAIN COMPLETELY FROM THE CONSUMPTION OF ALCOHOL AND DRUGS EXCEPT WHEN PRESCRIBED BY HIS TREATING PHYSICIAN; MUST SUBMIT TO WITNESSED RANDOM BIOLOGICAL FLUID COLLECTION; SHALL KEEP A LOG OF ANY AND ALL MEDICATIONS PRESCRIBED FOR HIM; SHALL SUBMIT TO ANY EXAMINATIONS OR THERAPY ORDERED BY THE BOARD; SHALL APPEAR BEFORE BOARD FOR INTERVIEWS UPON REQUEST; SHALL INFORM BOARD OF CHANGE OF ADDRESS OR IF AWAY FOR MORE THAN FIVE DAYS; SHALL PAY $2,500 ADMINISTRATIVE PENALTY WITHIN ONE YEAR.

MORITZ, TERRELL CONWAY MD, LICENSE NUMBER 0020323, WAS DISCIPLINED BY ARIZONA ON JANUARY 25, 1992
DISCIPLINARY ACTION: EMERGENCY SUSPENSION
OFFENSE: SUBSTANCE ABUSE

NOTES: IS CURRENTLY IN TREATMENT FOR ALCOHOL ABUSE.

MORITZ, TERRELL CONWAY MD, LICENSE NUMBER 0020323, WAS DISCIPLINED BY ARIZONA ON SEPTEMBER 11, 1992
DISCIPLINARY ACTION: 120-MONTH PROBATION; REQUIRED TO ENTER AN IMPAIRED PHYSICIAN PROGRAM OR SUBSTANCE ABUSE TREATMENT
OFFENSE: FAILURE TO COMPLY WITH PREVIOUS BOARD ORDER

NOTES: VIOLATED A PREVIOUS BOARD ORDER OF 10/10/91 IN THAT HE DID NOT MAINTAIN MEDICATION LOG AS REQUIRED, STATED HE WAS TAKING ONLY ASPIRIN, MULTIVITAMINS AND MINERALS, BUT TESTED POSITIVE ON 11/8/91 FOR PSEUDOEPHEDRINE AND DEXTROMETHORPHAN, ON 12/2/91 FOR TERPIN HYDRATE, ACETAMINOPHEN, DOXYLAMINE, DEXTROMETHORPHAN, AND PSEUDOEPHEDRINE, ON 12/12/91 FOR DOXYLAMINE, PSEUDOEPHEDRINE, DEXTROMETHORPHAN, AND ACETAMINOPHEN. FROM 1/9/92 TO AT LEAST 1/14/92, DRANK ALCOHOL EVERY DAY RESULTING IN SUBSTANTIAL INTOXICATION. BOARD SUMMARILY SUSPENDED LICENSE ON 1/25/92. ADMITTED HIMSELF FOR ALCOHOL ABUSE TREATMENT TO REHABILITATION CENTER IN ARIZONA. FROM 3/16/92 TO 5/8/92, PARTICIPATED IN TREATMENT AT AN OUTPATIENT CENTER FOR ALCOHOLISM AND DEPRESSION. ORDERED TO PAY COSTS OF $500. MUST IMMEDIATELY PARTICIPATE IN A BOARD-APPROVED MONITORED AFTERCARE TREATMENT PROGRAM WHOSE THERAPIST MUST SUBMIT QUARTERLY REPORTS; MUST PARTICIPATE IN 90 12-STEP MEETINGS FOR SUBSTANCE ABUSE WITHIN 90 DAYS; MUST THEN PARTICIPATE IN A 12-STEP RECOVERY PROGRAM AS DETERMINED BY HIS TREATING THERAPIST AND ATTEND AT LEAST 3 WEEKLY MEETINGS; SHALL OBTAIN A BOARD-APPROVED TREATING PHYSICIAN; SHALL ABSTAIN COMPLETELY FROM THE CONSUMPTION OF ALCOHOLIC BEVERAGES AND DRUGS EXCEPT WHEN PRESCRIBED BY HIS TREATING PHYSICIAN; MUST SUBMIT TO WITNESSED RANDOM BIOLOGICAL FLUID COLLECTION; IF BOARD RECEIVES NOTIFICATION OF A POSITIVE SCREEN, LICENSE SHALL BE CANCELED WITH CAUSE WITHIN 15 DAYS. KEEP A LOG OF ANY AND ALL MEDICATIONS PRESCRIBED FOR HIM; SHALL SUBMIT TO ANY EXAMINATIONS OR THERAPY ORDERED BY BOARD; SHALL APPEAR BEFORE BOARD FOR INTERVIEWS UPON REQUEST; SHALL HAVE EMPLOYER SUBMIT QUARTERLY REPORTS TO THE BOARD; SHALL INFORM BOARD OF CHANGE OF ADDRESS OR EMPLOYMENT OR IF AWAY FOR MORE THAN 5 DAYS. ON 2/15/96 PROBATION TERMINATED.

MORRIS, ROBERT S MD, DATE OF BIRTH MARCH 5, 1951, LICENSE NUMBER 25106, WAS DISCIPLINED BY COLORADO ON MARCH 25, 1999
DISCIPLINARY ACTION: REPRIMAND; REQUIRED TO TAKE

ADDITIONAL MEDICAL EDUCATION
OFFENSE: DISCIPLINARY ACTION BY ANOTHER STATE OR AGENCY

NOTES: DISCIPLINE IN ANOTHER STATE. WHEN HE RETURNS TO COLORADO TO PRACTICE, HE WILL BE REQUIRED TO TAKE REEDUCATION ACTIVITIES.

MOSBY, JAMES R MD, DATE OF BIRTH JUNE 9, 1947, LICENSE NUMBER 0018845 OF EVERGREEN, CO, WAS DISCIPLINED BY COLORADO ON SEPTEMBER 17, 1993
DISCIPLINARY ACTION: 60-MONTH PROBATION; REPRIMAND
OFFENSE: SUBSTANCE ABUSE

NOTES: HABITUAL INTEMPERANCE. PROBATIONARY PERIOD INCLUDES PRACTICE AND TREATMENT MONITORING. ALSO, A SEPARATE LETTER OF ADMONITION ISSUED 10/15/93.

MOTE, PAUL S MD, DATE OF BIRTH AUGUST 28, 1947, LICENSE NUMBER 0029142, WAS DISCIPLINED BY COLORADO ON APRIL 18, 1996
DISCIPLINARY ACTION: 60-MONTH PROBATION; REQUIRED TO TAKE ADDITIONAL MEDICAL EDUCATION
OFFENSE: SUBSTANDARD CARE, INCOMPETENCE OR NEGLIGENCE

NOTES: SUBSTANDARD CARE. FIVE YEAR PROBATION WITH RE-EDUCATION ACTIVITIES AND PRACTICE MONITORING.

MOTE, PAUL S MD, DATE OF BIRTH AUGUST 28, 1947, LICENSE NUMBER 0029142, WAS DISCIPLINED BY COLORADO ON JUNE 20, 1996
DISCIPLINARY ACTION: SURRENDER OF LICENSE

NOTES: NO UNPROFESSIONAL CONDUCT IDENTIFIED.

MOTE, PAUL S MD, WAS DISCIPLINED BY NEW MEXICO ON JANUARY 1, 1997
DISCIPLINARY ACTION: SURRENDER OF LICENSE
OFFENSE: PROVIDING FALSE INFORMATION TO THE BOARD OR OTHER HEALTH AGENCY

NOTES: PROVIDED FALSE INFORMATION TO THE BOARD ON A LICENSE RENEWAL AND FAILURE TO NOTIFY THE BOARD; VOLUNTARY SURRENDER OF NEW MEXICO LICENSE WITH THE CONDITION THAT HE MAY NEVER REAPPLY.

MOYER, JOHN P MD, DATE OF BIRTH JANUARY 15, 1941, LICENSE NUMBER 0017760, WAS DISCIPLINED BY COLORADO ON MARCH 14, 1996
DISCIPLINARY ACTION: REPRIMAND

MROZEK, JOHN R MD, DATE OF BIRTH OCTOBER 10, 1959, LICENSE NUMBER 26911, WAS DISCIPLINED BY COLORADO ON AUGUST 14, 1998
DISCIPLINARY ACTION: SURRENDER OF LICENSE
OFFENSE: PHYSICAL OR MENTAL ILLNESS INHIBITING THE ABILITY TO PRACTICE WITH SKILL AND SAFETY

NOTES: PHYSICAL OR MENTAL DISABILITY.

MUBARAK, ASAAD A MD, DATE OF BIRTH APRIL 5, 1933, LICENSE NUMBER 0015118 OF WHEAT RIDGE, CO, WAS DISCIPLINED BY COLORADO ON SEPTEMBER 10, 1993
DISCIPLINARY ACTION: 60-MONTH PROBATION; RESTRICTION PLACED ON LICENSE
OFFENSE: SUBSTANDARD CARE, INCOMPETENCE OR NEGLIGENCE

NOTES: ALLEGATIONS OF SUBSTANDARD PATIENT CARE. PROHIBITION AGAINST PERFORMING ANY MAJOR ARTERIAL RECONSTRUCTIVE SURGERY.

MUBARAK, ASAAD A MD, DATE OF BIRTH APRIL 5, 1933, LICENSE NUMBER 0015118, WAS DISCIPLINED BY COLORADO ON NOVEMBER 9, 1995
DISCIPLINARY ACTION: RESTRICTION PLACED ON LICENSE

NOTES: VOLUNTARY RELINQUISHMENT OF SURGICAL PRACTICE.

MUNOZ, DAVID C MD, DATE OF BIRTH JULY 19, 1951, LICENSE NUMBER 0033332, WAS DISCIPLINED BY COLORADO ON JUNE 13, 1996
DISCIPLINARY ACTION: 60-MONTH PROBATION; REQUIRED TO TAKE ADDITIONAL MEDICAL EDUCATION
OFFENSE: SUBSTANDARD CARE, INCOMPETENCE OR NEGLIGENCE

NOTES: SUBSTANDARD CARE. REQUIRED TO COMPLETE RESIDENCY PROGRAM IN FAMILY PRACTICE.

MURPHY, JAMES T MD, DATE OF BIRTH AUGUST 30, 1944, LICENSE NUMBER 0019868 OF BOULDER, CO, WAS DISCIPLINED BY COLORADO ON OCTOBER 9, 1992
DISCIPLINARY ACTION: 60-MONTH PROBATION; MONITORING OF PHYSICIAN PERFORMANCE
OFFENSE: SUBSTANCE ABUSE

NOTES: EXCESSIVE USE OF A HABIT-FORMING DRUG OR CONTROLLED SUBSTANCE. PROBATIONARY PERIOD INCLUDES TREATMENT AND PRACTICE MONITORING.

MURRAY, KEVIN K MD, DATE OF BIRTH SEPTEMBER 30, 1960, LICENSE NUMBER 31745, WAS DISCIPLINED BY COLORADO ON MARCH 13, 1998
DISCIPLINARY ACTION: REPRIMAND

MUSSELMAN, RICHARD P DO, DATE OF BIRTH APRIL 3, 1948, LICENSE NUMBER 0001544 OF PO BOX 372, ATTICA, KS, WAS DISCIPLINED BY IOWA ON NOVEMBER 14, 1991
DISCIPLINARY ACTION: SURRENDER OF LICENSE

NOTES: LICENSE SURRENDERED DURING INVESTIGATION.

MUSSELMAN, RICHARD P DO, DATE OF BIRTH APRIL 3, 1948, LICENSE NUMBER 0018730 OF ATTICA, KS, WAS DISCIPLINED BY COLORADO ON JANUARY 22, 1993
DISCIPLINARY ACTION: SURRENDER OF LICENSE
OFFENSE: SUBSTANDARD CARE, INCOMPETENCE OR NEGLIGENCE

NOTES: ALLEGATIONS OF SUBSTANDARD CARE.

NAGASHIMA, RAYMOND J MD, DATE OF BIRTH NOVEMBER 11, 1957, LICENSE NUMBER 0029271, WAS DISCIPLINED BY COLORADO ON AUGUST 17, 1995
DISCIPLINARY ACTION: REPRIMAND

NAGEL, JOHN K JR MD, DATE OF BIRTH FEBRUARY 14, 1944, LICENSE NUMBER 18209, WAS DISCIPLINED BY COLORADO ON SEPTEMBER 18, 1997
DISCIPLINARY ACTION: REPRIMAND

NARAMORE, LLOYD S MD, WAS DISCIPLINED BY ALASKA ON DECEMBER 9, 1994
DISCIPLINARY ACTION: DENIAL OF NEW LICENSE
OFFENSE: DISCIPLINARY ACTION BY ANOTHER STATE OR AGENCY

NOTES: ACTION IN ANOTHER STATE.

NARAMORE, LLOYD S DO, DATE OF BIRTH MARCH 2, 1945, LICENSE NUMBER 1006969 OF 225 N COURT AVE, COLBY, KS, WAS DISCIPLINED BY MICHIGAN ON DECEMBER 1, 1995

DISCIPLINARY ACTION: LICENSE REVOCATION
OFFENSE: DISCIPLINARY ACTION BY ANOTHER STATE OR AGENCY

NOTES: FAILURE TO REPORT/COMPLY.

NARAMORE, LLOYD S DO, DATE OF BIRTH MARCH 2, 1945, LICENSE NUMBER 0002235 OF COLBY, KS, WAS DISCIPLINED BY KENTUCKY ON MAY 28, 1996
DISCIPLINARY ACTION: LICENSE REVOCATION
OFFENSE: DISCIPLINARY ACTION BY ANOTHER STATE OR AGENCY

NOTES: DISCIPLINARY ACTION TAKEN BY OTHER STATE BOARDS.

NARAMORE, LLOYD STAN DO, WAS DISCIPLINED BY WYOMING ON FEBRUARY 18, 1995
DISCIPLINARY ACTION: SURRENDER OF LICENSE

NOTES: VOLUNTARY SURRENDER.

NARAMORE, LLOYD STAN DO, LICENSE NUMBER 0524020, WAS DISCIPLINED BY KANSAS ON MAY 2, 1995
DISCIPLINARY ACTION: SURRENDER OF LICENSE
OFFENSE: SUBSTANDARD CARE, INCOMPETENCE OR NEGLIGENCE

NOTES: IN 8/92 COMMITTED ONE OR MORE INSTANCES INVOLVING GROSS NEGLIGENCE IN WHICH HE HAD ADMINISTERED DRUGS TO TWO PATIENTS; HAD AN ADVERSE EFFECT ON ONE AND THE OTHER ULTIMATELY DIED. CONDITION OF SURRENDER, IF HE APPLIES FOR REINSTATEMENT, HE MUST TAKE AND PASS THE SPEX TEST WITHIN THE PRECEDING SIX MONTHS PRIOR TO BOARD CONSIDERATION.

NARAMORE, LLOYD STAN DO, LICENSE NUMBER 2001095, WAS DISCIPLINED BY INDIANA ON DECEMBER 7, 1995
DISCIPLINARY ACTION: SURRENDER OF LICENSE
OFFENSE: DISCIPLINARY ACTION BY ANOTHER STATE OR AGENCY

NOTES: SURRENDER IN LIEU OF FURTHER DISCIPLINARY PROCEEDINGS. PENDING MURDER AND ATTEMPTED MURDER CHARGES, ON 5/2/95 KANSAS REVOKED HIS LICENSE. ON 2/18/95 VOLUNTARILY RELINQUISHED LICENSE TO WISCONSIN FOR NOT ANSWERING TRUTHFULLY THAT HE WAS UNDER INVESTIGATION BY ANOTHER LICENSING BOARD. SHALL PAY COSTS OF $318.52.

NARAMORE, LLOYD STANLEY DO, DATE OF BIRTH MARCH 2, 1945, LICENSE NUMBER 0030724, WAS DISCIPLINED BY COLORADO ON JUNE 15, 1995
DISCIPLINARY ACTION: SURRENDER OF LICENSE

NAVRKAL, HARVEY J MD, DATE OF BIRTH JANUARY 8, 1963, LICENSE NUMBER 0033552 OF FT. COLLINS, CO, WAS DISCIPLINED BY COLORADO ON APRIL 14, 1994
DISCIPLINARY ACTION: 60-MONTH PROBATION
OFFENSE: FAILURE TO COMPLY WITH PREVIOUS BOARD ORDER

NOTES: HABITUAL INTEMPERANCE OR EXCESSIVE USE OF A CONTROLLED SUBSTANCE; PHYSICAL OR MENTAL DISABILITY; VIOLATION OF A BOARD ORDER. GRANTED A LICENSE WITH PROBATION.

NAVRKAL, HARVEY J MD, DATE OF BIRTH JANUARY 8, 1963, LICENSE NUMBER 0033552 OF FT. COLLINS, CO, WAS DISCIPLINED BY COLORADO ON JUNE 22, 1994
DISCIPLINARY ACTION: LICENSE SUSPENSION
OFFENSE: FAILURE TO COMPLY WITH PREVIOUS BOARD ORDER

NOTES: VIOLATION OF STIPULATION.

NAVRKAL, HARVEY J MD, DATE OF BIRTH JANUARY 8, 1963 OF 1613 EAST PITKIN, FT COLLINS, CO, WAS DISCIPLINED BY MEDICARE ON DECEMBER 5, 1994
DISCIPLINARY ACTION: EXCLUSION FROM THE MEDICARE AND/OR MEDICAID PROGRAM
OFFENSE: DISCIPLINARY ACTION BY ANOTHER STATE OR AGENCY

NOTES: LICENSE SUSPENDED FOR REASONS BEARING ON PROFESSIONAL COMPETENCE. REINSTATED ON 5/1/96.

NAVRKAL, HARVEY JOSEPH MD, WAS DISCIPLINED BY NEBRASKA ON APRIL 4, 1996
DISCIPLINARY ACTION: 60-MONTH PROBATION

NAVRKAL, HARVEY JOSEPH MD, WAS DISCIPLINED BY NEBRASKA ON OCTOBER 17, 1997
DISCIPLINARY ACTION: LICENSE REVOCATION
OFFENSE: FAILURE TO COMPLY WITH PREVIOUS BOARD ORDER

NOTES: PROBATION VIOLATION; DISHONORABLE CONDUCT; UNPROFESSIONAL CONDUCT.

NELSON, JERRY A MD, DATE OF BIRTH SEPTEMBER 8, 1950, LICENSE NUMBER 0021042, WAS DISCIPLINED BY COLORADO ON SEPTEMBER 14, 1995
DISCIPLINARY ACTION: 60-MONTH PROBATION; RESTRICTION PLACED ON LICENSE

NOTES: TREATMENT AND PRACTICE MONITORING; RESTRICTED ANESTHESIA PRACTICE.

NELSON, JERRY ALAN MD, LICENSE NUMBER 24196 OF DENVER, CO, WAS DISCIPLINED BY WASHINGTON ON MARCH 5, 1998
DISCIPLINARY ACTION: PROBATION
OFFENSE: DISCIPLINARY ACTION BY ANOTHER STATE OR AGENCY

NOTES: ALLEGATIONS OF DISCIPLINARY ACTION IN ANOTHER STATE. ON 12/31/98, REQUEST TO TERMINATE THE CONDITIONS OF THIS ORDER GRANTED AND LICENSE IS UNRESTRICTED.

NEMER, ROBERT J DO, DATE OF BIRTH MAY 11, 1934, LICENSE NUMBER 0024384 OF OSAGE BEACH, MO, WAS DISCIPLINED BY COLORADO ON MAY 14, 1993
DISCIPLINARY ACTION: 60-MONTH PROBATION; MONITORING OF PHYSICIAN PERFORMANCE
OFFENSE: SUBSTANDARD CARE, INCOMPETENCE OR NEGLIGENCE

NOTES: SUBSTANDARD CARE. PROBATION INCLUDES PRACTICE MONITORING.

NEUMEIER, JOHN A MD, DATE OF BIRTH MARCH 1, 1941, LICENSE NUMBER 0033350 OF DENVER, CO, WAS DISCIPLINED BY COLORADO ON JANUARY 20, 1994
DISCIPLINARY ACTION: RESTRICTION PLACED ON LICENSE
OFFENSE: PHYSICAL OR MENTAL ILLNESS INHIBITING THE ABILITY TO PRACTICE WITH SKILL AND SAFETY

NOTES: PHYSICAL OR MENTAL DISABILITY ISSUES. GRANTED A MEDICAL LICENSE. LIMITED TO DUTIES OF PATHOLOGIST ASSISTANT ONLY.

NICHOLSON, PETER M MD, DATE OF BIRTH AUGUST 16, 1961, LICENSE NUMBER 0032584, WAS DISCIPLINED BY COLORADO ON APRIL 11, 1996
DISCIPLINARY ACTION: 2-MONTH LICENSE SUSPENSION; 60-MONTH PROBATION
OFFENSE: SEXUAL ABUSE OF OR SEXUAL MISCONDUCT WITH A PATIENT

NOTES: SEXUAL CONTACT WITH A PATIENT. CHAPERONING, PRACTICE, AND TREATMENT MONITORING.

NICHOLSON, PETER M MD, DATE OF BIRTH AUGUST 16, 1961, LICENSE NUMBER 32584, WAS DISCIPLINED BY COLORADO ON APRIL 15, 1999
DISCIPLINARY ACTION: REPRIMAND

NITKA, ALFRED C MD, DATE OF BIRTH NOVEMBER 11, 1952, LICENSE NUMBER 0025578, WAS DISCIPLINED BY COLORADO ON AUGUST 22, 1996
DISCIPLINARY ACTION: EMERGENCY SUSPENSION
OFFENSE: NONCOMPLIANCE WITH A PROFESSIONAL RULE

NOTES: VIOLATION OF THE MEDICAL PRACTICE ACT.

NITKA, ALFRED C MD OF 711 LYRA DRIVE, COLORADO SPRINGS, CO, WAS DISCIPLINED BY DEA ON OCTOBER 31, 1996
DISCIPLINARY ACTION: SURRENDER OF CONTROLLED SUBSTANCE LICENSE

NOTES: IN LIEU OF PUBLIC INTEREST REVOCATION.

NITKA, ALFRED C MD, DATE OF BIRTH NOVEMBER 11, 1952, LICENSE NUMBER 0025578, WAS DISCIPLINED BY COLORADO ON NOVEMBER 15, 1996
DISCIPLINARY ACTION: LICENSE SUSPENSION; REQUIRED TO ENTER AN IMPAIRED PHYSICIAN PROGRAM OR SUBSTANCE ABUSE TREATMENT
OFFENSE: SUBSTANCE ABUSE

NOTES: HABITUAL INTEMPERANCE OR EXCESSIVE USE OF A CONTROLLED SUBSTANCE; AND GIVING A SCHEDULE II SUBSTANCE TO SELF OR A FAMILY MEMBER. SUSPENDED UNTIL HE COMPLETES AN IN-PATIENT TREATMENT AND A RECOMMENDATION FOR A RETURN TO PRACTICE BY THE TREATMENT MONITOR. AFTER TERMINATION OF THE SUSPENSION, HIS LICENSE SHALL BE PLACED ON FIVE YEAR PROBATION INCLUDING TREATMENT AND PRACTICE MONITORING PROVISIONS.

NITKA, ALFRED C MD, LICENSE NUMBER 70752 OF 711 LYRA DRIVE, COLORADO SPRINGS, CO, WAS DISCIPLINED BY MASSACHUSETTS ON JANUARY 21, 1998
DISCIPLINARY ACTION: PROBATION
OFFENSE: DISCIPLINARY ACTION BY ANOTHER STATE OR AGENCY

NOTES: DISCIPLINE--COLORADO; PRACTICING WHILE IMPAIRED. SUSPENSION STAYED.

NORTON, JOHN T MD, LICENSE NUMBER 0012526 OF DENVER, CO, WAS DISCIPLINED BY COLORADO ON DECEMBER 14, 1990
DISCIPLINARY ACTION: LICENSE REVOCATION
OFFENSE: SUBSTANDARD CARE, INCOMPETENCE OR NEGLIGENCE

NOTES: FAILURE TO MEET GENERALLY ACCEPTED STANDARDS OF MEDICAL PRACTICE. REVOCATION STAYED BY COURT OF APPEALS ON 1/7/91 PENDING JUDICIAL REVIEW. COURT OF APPEALS AFFIRMED THE BOARD'S ORDER ON 9/12/91, DISSOLVED STAY OF BOARD'S ORDER ON 10/11/91. THE COLORADO SUPREME COURT STAYED BOARD'S ORDER PENDING FURTHER JUDICIAL REVIEW ON 12/11/91. COLORADO SUPREME COURT DENIED HIS PETITION FOR WRIT OF CERTIORI ON 1/13/92; THE BOARD'S REVOCATION ORDER OF 12/14/90 IS FULLY IN EFFECT.

NORTON, JOHN T MD, DATE OF BIRTH OCTOBER 12, 1926 OF 5459 S KEARNEY, ENGLEWOOD, CO, WAS DISCIPLINED BY MEDICARE ON OCTOBER 29, 1992
DISCIPLINARY ACTION: EXCLUSION FROM THE MEDICARE AND/OR MEDICAID PROGRAM
OFFENSE: DISCIPLINARY ACTION BY ANOTHER STATE OR AGENCY

NOTES: LICENSE REVOCATION OR SUSPENSION.

NYMAN, DAVID W DO, DATE OF BIRTH NOVEMBER 9, 1950, LICENSE NUMBER 0026920 OF COLORADO SPRINGS, CO, WAS DISCIPLINED BY COLORADO ON MARCH 24, 1994
DISCIPLINARY ACTION: EMERGENCY SUSPENSION
OFFENSE: SUBSTANCE ABUSE

NOTES: SUBSTANCE ABUSE ISSUES. SUSPENSION PENDING PROCEEDINGS TO DETERMINE WHETHER HIS LICENSE SHOULD BE DISCIPLINED.

NYMAN, DAVID W DO OF 5780 NORTH CAREFREE, COLORADO SPRINGS, CO, WAS DISCIPLINED BY DEA ON SEPTEMBER 15, 1994
DISCIPLINARY ACTION: SURRENDER OF CONTROLLED SUBSTANCE LICENSE
OFFENSE: DISCIPLINARY ACTION BY ANOTHER STATE OR AGENCY

NOTES: STATE BOARD.

NYMAN, DAVID W DO, DATE OF BIRTH NOVEMBER 9, 1950 OF 5780 N CAREFREE CIRCLE #B, COLORADO SPRINGS, CO, WAS DISCIPLINED BY MEDICARE ON FEBRUARY 15, 1995
DISCIPLINARY ACTION: EXCLUSION FROM THE MEDICARE AND/OR MEDICAID PROGRAM
OFFENSE: DISCIPLINARY ACTION BY ANOTHER STATE OR AGENCY

NOTES: LICENSE REVOCATION OR SUSPENSION.

NYMAN, DAVID W DO, DATE OF BIRTH NOVEMBER 9, 1950, LICENSE NUMBER 0026920, WAS DISCIPLINED BY COLORADO ON NOVEMBER 9, 1995
DISCIPLINARY ACTION: LICENSE SUSPENSION; MONITORING OF PHYSICIAN PERFORMANCE

NOTES: SUSPENSION PENDING ACCEPTANCE INTO A RESIDENCY PROGRAM. PERMANENT PRACTICE AND TREATMENT MONITORING.

NYMAN, DAVID WILLIAM DO OF COLORADO SPRINGS, CO, WAS DISCIPLINED BY DEA ON MARCH 10, 1997
DISCIPLINARY ACTION: DENIAL OF LICENSE REINSTATEMENT
OFFENSE: DISCIPLINARY ACTION BY ANOTHER STATE OR AGENCY

NOTES: ON 3/23/94 THE COLORADO BOARD SUMMARILY SUSPENDED HIS LICENSE BASED ON FINDINGS THAT IN 7/86 HE COLLAPSED AND AN EMERGENCY TOXICOLOGY REPORT REVEALED DARVON AND COCAINE; RELAPSED IN 1/94 AND 2//94 INCLUDING USING BUPRENEX; IN 3/94 HE CALLED A PHARMACY REPEATEDLY IN AN ATTEMPT TO OBTAIN A PERSONAL ORDER FOR VALIUM AND BUPRENEX; SURRENDERED PREVIOUS DEA CERTIFICATE; ON 11/9/95 COLORADO BOARD SUSPENDED LICENSE UNTIL HE ENTERS INTO A RESIDENCY PROGRAM WHICH HE HAD NOT DONE AS OF THE DATE OF THIS ORDER.

NYMAN, DAVID WILLIAM DO, DATE OF BIRTH NOVEMBER 9, 1950, LICENSE NUMBER 046629 OF 1301 LINCOLN COURT AVENUE, NE, ATLANTA, GA, WAS DISCIPLINED BY GEORGIA ON DECEMBER 2, 1998
DISCIPLINARY ACTION: PROBATION

NOTES: IMPAIRMENT.

O'DONNELL, RICHARD S MD, DATE OF BIRTH FEBRUARY 4, 1943, LICENSE NUMBER 0021799, WAS DISCIPLINED BY COLORADO ON AUGUST 14, 1996
DISCIPLINARY ACTION: REPRIMAND; REQUIRED TO TAKE ADDITIONAL MEDICAL EDUCATION

NOTES: NO UNPROFESSIONAL CONDUCT IDENTIFIED. RE-EDUCATION ACTIVITIES.

O'LEARY, MICHAEL PATRICK MD, DATE OF BIRTH AUGUST 7, 1954, LICENSE NUMBER 29406, WAS DISCIPLINED BY COLORADO ON SEPTEMBER 12, 1996
DISCIPLINARY ACTION: REPRIMAND

O'NEILL, JOHN J MD, DATE OF BIRTH JANUARY 23, 1939, LICENSE NUMBER 0017570 OF FT COLLINS, CO, WAS DISCIPLINED BY COLORADO ON OCTOBER 15, 1993
DISCIPLINARY ACTION: 60-MONTH PROBATION; MONITORING OF PHYSICIAN PERFORMANCE
OFFENSE: SUBSTANCE ABUSE

NOTES: EXCESSIVE USE OF A CONTROLLED SUBSTANCE. PROBATIONARY PERIOD INCLUDES PRACTICE AND TREATMENT MONITORING.

O'NEILL, JOHN J MD OF FORT COLLINS, CO, WAS DISCIPLINED BY MISSOURI ON DECEMBER 20, 1996
DISCIPLINARY ACTION: 60-MONTH PROBATION
OFFENSE: DISCIPLINARY ACTION BY ANOTHER STATE OR AGENCY

NOTES: BASED ON DISCIPLINE BY THE COLORADO BOARD AND THE RESTRICTION OF HIS DEA REGISTRATION ON OR ABOUT 11/16/93.

O'NEILL, JOHN J MD, DATE OF BIRTH JANUARY 23, 1939, LICENSE NUMBER 17570, WAS DISCIPLINED BY COLORADO ON AUGUST 20, 1999
DISCIPLINARY ACTION: REPRIMAND; REQUIRED TO TAKE ADDITIONAL MEDICAL EDUCATION
OFFENSE: SUBSTANDARD CARE, INCOMPETENCE OR NEGLIGENCE

NOTES: SUBSTANDARD CARE (PRIMA FACIE TYPE ADMISSION ONLY). HE MUST UNDERGO REEDUCATION ACTIVITIES

OBA, DAVID M MD, DATE OF BIRTH JANUARY 12, 1955, LICENSE NUMBER 0030326, WAS DISCIPLINED BY COLORADO ON MARCH 14, 1996
DISCIPLINARY ACTION: REPRIMAND

OGIN, GARY A MD, DATE OF BIRTH JUNE 23, 1947, LICENSE NUMBER 0026922, WAS DISCIPLINED BY COLORADO ON JULY 15, 1996
DISCIPLINARY ACTION: REPRIMAND

OLIVA, PHILIP B MD, DATE OF BIRTH FEBRUARY 23, 1939, LICENSE NUMBER 0017234, WAS DISCIPLINED BY COLORADO ON MARCH 18, 1994
DISCIPLINARY ACTION: EMERGENCY SUSPENSION
OFFENSE: PROFESSIONAL MISCONDUCT

NOTES: FELONIOUS OBTAINING SCHEDULED DRUGS BY FRAUD/DECEIT AND FAILURE TO APPEAR. SUSPENSION PENDING PROCEEDINGS TO DETERMINE WHETHER HIS LICENSE SHOULD BE DISCIPLINED.

OLIVA, PHILIP B MD, DATE OF BIRTH FEBRUARY 23, 1939, LICENSE NUMBER 0017234 OF DENVER, CO, WAS DISCIPLINED BY COLORADO ON MARCH 16, 1995
DISCIPLINARY ACTION: LICENSE REVOCATION
OFFENSE: CRIMINAL CONVICTION OR PLEA OF GUILTY, NOLO CONTENDERE, OR NO CONTEST TO A CRIME

NOTES: RESORTING TO FRAUD, MISREPRESENTATION, OR DECEPTION IN RENEWING A LICENSE. PRESCRIBING A CONTROLLED SUBSTANCE OTHER THAN IN THE COURSE OF LEGITIMATE PROFESSIONAL PRACTICE. FELONY CONVICTION. CONVICTION OF A LAW REGULATING CONTROLLED SUBSTANCES. HABITUAL INTEMPERANCE OR EXCESSIVE USE OF A CONTROLLED SUBSTANCE. SUBSTANDARD CARE. SELF ADMINISTRATION OF A SCHEDULE II CONTROLLED SUBSTANCE.

OLIVA, PHILLIP B MD, DATE OF BIRTH FEBRUARY 23, 1939 OF 1065 MAPLETON AVE, BOULDER, CO, WAS DISCIPLINED BY MEDICARE ON FEBRUARY 15, 1995
DISCIPLINARY ACTION: EXCLUSION FROM THE MEDICARE AND/OR MEDICAID PROGRAM
OFFENSE: CRIMINAL CONVICTION OR PLEA OF GUILTY, NOLO CONTENDERE, OR NO CONTEST TO A CRIME

NOTES: CONVICTION RELATING TO CONTROLLED SUBSTANCES.

OLSON, DAVID MARK MD, DATE OF BIRTH MARCH 31, 1958, LICENSE NUMBER 34559, WAS DISCIPLINED BY COLORADO ON NOVEMBER 13, 1998
DISCIPLINARY ACTION: 60-MONTH PROBATION; MONITORING OF PHYSICIAN PERFORMANCE
OFFENSE: PHYSICAL OR MENTAL ILLNESS INHIBITING THE ABILITY TO PRACTICE WITH SKILL AND SAFETY

NOTES: PHYSICAL OR MENTAL DISABILITY. MUST HAVE TREATMENT MONITORING.

ONISCHUK, ROBERT T DO, LICENSE NUMBER 0026261 OF NUCLA, CO, WAS DISCIPLINED BY COLORADO ON NOVEMBER 9, 1990
DISCIPLINARY ACTION: LICENSE SUSPENSION
OFFENSE: FAILURE TO COMPLY WITH PREVIOUS BOARD ORDER

NOTES: ACTION BASED ON FAILURE TO SUBMIT TO ORDERED PSYCHIATRIC AND PHYSICAL EXAMINATIONS. LICENSE TO REMAIN SUSPENDED UNTIL HE SUBMITS TO SUCH EXAMINATIONS.

ONISCHUK, ROBERT T DO, DATE OF BIRTH JUNE 11, 1941 OF PO BOX 578, NUCLA, CO, WAS DISCIPLINED BY MEDICARE ON JULY 22, 1991
DISCIPLINARY ACTION: EXCLUSION FROM THE MEDICARE AND/OR MEDICAID PROGRAM
OFFENSE: DISCIPLINARY ACTION BY ANOTHER STATE OR AGENCY

NOTES: LICENSE REVOCATION OR SUSPENSION.

ONISCHUK, ROBERT T DO, LICENSE NUMBER 003585L OF P.O. BOX 203, NUCLA, CO, WAS DISCIPLINED BY PENNSYLVANIA ON OCTOBER 4, 1994
DISCIPLINARY ACTION: LICENSE REVOCATION
OFFENSE: DISCIPLINARY ACTION BY ANOTHER STATE OR AGENCY

NOTES: ON 11/04/90 HIS COLORADO LICENSE WAS REVOKED WHEN HE DID NOT COMPLY WITH REQUIRED EXAMINATIONS. ON HIS PENNSYLVANIA APPLICATION ON 11/22/92 HE ANSWERED "NO" TO THE QUESTION, "SINCE YOUR LAST RENEWAL, HAS ANY DISCIPLINARY ACTION BEEN TAKEN AGAINST YOUR LICENSE IN ANOTHER STATE, TERRITORY, OR COUNTRY?"

OSSORIO, JULIO M MD, DATE OF BIRTH JULY 9, 1948, LICENSE NUMBER 0032219 OF CANON CITY, CO, WAS DISCIPLINED BY COLORADO ON DECEMBER 1, 1992
DISCIPLINARY ACTION: EMERGENCY SUSPENSION
OFFENSE: PROVIDING FALSE INFORMATION TO THE BOARD OR OTHER HEALTH AGENCY

NOTES: RESORTING TO FRAUD, MISREPRESENTATION, OR DECEPTION IN APPLYING FOR AND SECURING A MEDICAL LICENSE; HABITUAL INTEMPERANCE; PHYSICAL OR MENTAL DISABILITY WHICH RENDERS HIM UNABLE TO PRACTICE WITH SKILL AND SAFETY; FAILURE TO MEET GENERALLY ACCEPTED STANDARDS OF MEDICAL PRACTICE.

OSSORIO, JULIO M MD, DATE OF BIRTH JULY 9, 1948, LICENSE NUMBER 0032219 OF CANON CITY, CO, WAS DISCIPLINED BY COLORADO ON MARCH 19, 1993
DISCIPLINARY ACTION: SURRENDER OF LICENSE
OFFENSE: SUBSTANCE ABUSE

NOTES: HABITUAL INTEMPERANCE.

OSSORIO, JULIO M MD OF 3695 HOT SPRINGS BLVD, LAS VEGAS, NM, WAS DISCIPLINED BY NEW MEXICO ON AUGUST 26, 1993
OFFENSE: SUBSTANCE ABUSE

NOTES: LICENSE PLACED UNDER UNSPECIFIED CONDITIONS. IN 11/98 REMOVED ALL STIPULATIONS FOR SUBSTANCE ABUSE, GIVING HIM AN UNRESTRICTED LICENSE.

OSSORIO, JULIO M MD, LICENSE NUMBER 0117727 OF 1001 RUPPEL STREET APT 521, PUEBLO, CO, WAS DISCIPLINED BY NEW YORK ON NOVEMBER 15, 1993
DISCIPLINARY ACTION: LICENSE REVOCATION
OFFENSE: DISCIPLINARY ACTION BY ANOTHER STATE OR AGENCY

NOTES: SURRENDERED HIS LICENSE IN COLORADO.

OVERETT, THOMAS K MD, DATE OF BIRTH OCTOBER 2, 1946, LICENSE NUMBER 25260, WAS DISCIPLINED BY COLORADO ON DECEMBER 10, 1998
DISCIPLINARY ACTION: REPRIMAND

OVERTURF, BRUCE R MD, DATE OF BIRTH MAY 1, 1937, LICENSE NUMBER 0014811 OF FT MORGAN, CO, WAS DISCIPLINED BY COLORADO ON JULY 14, 1993
DISCIPLINARY ACTION: 60-MONTH PROBATION; MONITORING OF PHYSICIAN PERFORMANCE
OFFENSE: SUBSTANDARD CARE, INCOMPETENCE OR NEGLIGENCE

NOTES: ALLEGATIONS OF SUBSTANDARD PATIENT CARE. PROBATIONARY PERIOD INCLUDES PRACTICE AND TREATMENT MONITORING.

OWENS, CYNTHIA J MD, DATE OF BIRTH MARCH 21, 1949, LICENSE NUMBER 0021323, WAS DISCIPLINED BY COLORADO ON JANUARY 11, 1996
DISCIPLINARY ACTION: 60-MONTH PROBATION; MONITORING OF PHYSICIAN PERFORMANCE
OFFENSE: FAILURE TO COMPLY WITH PREVIOUS BOARD ORDER

NOTES: VIOLATION OF A PREVIOUS ORDER AND SUBSTANCE ABUSE. PRACTICE AND TREATMENT MONITORING THROUGH THE COLORADO PHYSICIANS HEALTH PROGRAM.

OWENS, CYNTHIA J MD, DATE OF BIRTH MARCH 21, 1949, LICENSE NUMBER 0021323, WAS DISCIPLINED BY COLORADO ON JULY 1, 1996
DISCIPLINARY ACTION: EMERGENCY SUSPENSION

OWENS, CYNTHIA J MD, DATE OF BIRTH MARCH 21, 1949, LICENSE NUMBER 0021323, WAS DISCIPLINED BY COLORADO ON DECEMBER 12, 1996
DISCIPLINARY ACTION: LICENSE REVOCATION
OFFENSE: FAILURE TO COMPLY WITH PREVIOUS BOARD ORDER

NOTES: VIOLATION OF A VALID BOARD ORDER.

OWENS-DUNLOP, CYNTHIA J MD, DATE OF BIRTH MARCH 21, 1949, LICENSE NUMBER 0021323 OF DENVER, CO, WAS DISCIPLINED BY COLORADO ON NOVEMBER 13, 1992
DISCIPLINARY ACTION: 60-MONTH PROBATION; MONITORING OF PHYSICIAN PERFORMANCE
OFFENSE: SUBSTANCE ABUSE

NOTES: EXCESSIVE USE OF A HABIT-FORMING DRUG OR CONTROLLED SUBSTANCE. TERM INCLUDES PRACTICE AND TREATMENT MONITORING.

PALMER, MARVIN M MD OF 4516 S 4TH ST TRAFFICWAY, LEAVENWORTH, KS, WAS DISCIPLINED BY DEA ON MAY 8, 1990
DISCIPLINARY ACTION: SURRENDER OF CONTROLLED SUBSTANCE LICENSE
OFFENSE: OVERPRESCRIBING OR MISPRESCRIBING DRUGS

NOTES: WRITING FRAUDULENT PRESCRIPTIONS FOR PERSONAL USE AND FOR OTHERS.

PALMER, MARVIN MILES MD, LICENSE NUMBER 0017889 OF LEAVENWORTH, KS, WAS DISCIPLINED BY COLORADO ON JULY 13, 1990
DISCIPLINARY ACTION: 60-MONTH LICENSE SUSPENSION; 36-MONTH PROBATION
OFFENSE: FAILURE TO COMPLY WITH PREVIOUS BOARD ORDER

NOTES: RELAPSED IN RECOVERY FROM DRUG USE AND ADDICTION DURING A PERIOD WHEN HIS LICENSE WAS SUBJECT TO A BOARD STIPULATION AND ORDER. SUSPENSION WITH CONDITIONS FOR REINSTATEMENT INCLUDING, BUT NOT LIMITED TO, DRUG-FREE URINE SCREENS. THEREAFTER, HIS LICENSE WOULD BE PLACED ON PROBATION STARTING FROM THE DAY HE ESTABLISHES A MEDICAL PRACTICE IN COLORADO. TERMS OF PROBATION INCLUDE DRUG TREATMENT AND MONITORING AND PRACTICE SUPERVISION.

PALMER, MARVIN MILES MD OF LEAVENWORTH, KS, WAS DISCIPLINED BY KANSAS ON OCTOBER 18, 1990

NOTES: STIPULATION AND ENFORCEMENT ORDER.

PALMER, MARVIN MILES MD, LICENSE NUMBER 0417054 OF 4512 S 4TH STREET TRAFFICWAY - A, LEAVENWORTH, KS, WAS DISCIPLINED BY KANSAS ON FEBRUARY 2, 1994
DISCIPLINARY ACTION: LICENSE SUSPENSION; 36-MONTH REQUIRED TO ENTER AN IMPAIRED PHYSICIAN PROGRAM OR SUBSTANCE ABUSE TREATMENT
OFFENSE: SUBSTANCE ABUSE

NOTES: INFORMATION PRESENTED TO BOARD ON 7/21/93 WHICH HE LATER ADMITTED, THAT HE WAS SELF-ADMINISTERING DALGAN WHICH HAD BEEN PRESCRIBED AFTER HE SUSTAINED TRAUMATIC INJURIES; BECAME DEPENDENT ON THIS MEDICATION AND EXPERIENCED A RELAPSE; SOUGHT AND OBTAINED TREATMENT AND DISCONTINUED THE ACTIVE PRACTICE OF MEDICINE; HAD ENTERED PREVIOUS STIPULATIONS WITH KANSAS ON 10/10/87 AND 10/18/90 AND WITH COLORADO ON 7/13/90. SUSPENSION FOR A MINIMUM OF SIX MONTHS RETROACTIVE FROM 07/21/93 AND A MAXIMUM OF THREE YEARS; HE HAS NOT PRACTICED MEDICINE FROM THAT DATE; WILL CONTINUE IN TREATMENT FOR HIS SUBSTANCE ABUSE AND DEPENDENCY PROBLEMS DURING THE ENTIRE PERIOD OF SUSPENSION; AT THE END OF THE SIX MONTH PERIOD WILL HAVE THE RIGHT TO APPLY FOR LIFTING OF THE SUSPENSION; UPON LIFTING OF SUSPENSION WILL BE PLACED UPON PROBATION FOR THREE YEARS, REQUIRED TO STAY UNDER THE CONSTANT CARE OF A PHYSICIAN OF THE BOARD'S CHOOSING WITH EXPERTISE IN SUBSTANCE ABUSE; WILL BE SUBJECT TO RANDOM URINE OR BLOOD ANALYSIS FOR THE DETECTION OF SUBSTANCE ABUSE; MUST KEEP THE BOARD APPRISED OF LOCATION OF HIS PRACTICE;

WILL BE AVAILABLE FOR PHYSICAL OR MENTAL EXAMS; WILL MAKE ANY CHARTS AVAILABLE FOR REVIEW.

PALU, MARGARET MD, LICENSE NUMBER 0022513 OF FT MORGAN, CO, WAS DISCIPLINED BY COLORADO ON AUGUST 1, 1990
DISCIPLINARY ACTION: REQUIRED TO TAKE ADDITIONAL MEDICAL EDUCATION; MONITORING OF PHYSICIAN PERFORMANCE
OFFENSE: SUBSTANDARD CARE, INCOMPETENCE OR NEGLIGENCE

NOTES: FAILED TO MEET GENERALLY ACCEPTED STANDARDS OF MEDICAL PRACTICE. CONSENT ORDER PROVIDED FOR A PRACTICE MONITOR, REVIEW OR REPORTS, SECOND OPINIONS/CONSULTATIONS, AND CONTINUING EDUCATION.

PANIAN, STEVE P MD, DATE OF BIRTH SEPTEMBER 21, 1958, LICENSE NUMBER 28253, WAS DISCIPLINED BY COLORADO ON JANUARY 8, 1998
DISCIPLINARY ACTION: REPRIMAND

PANTER, EDWARD MD, DATE OF BIRTH JULY 21, 1918, LICENSE NUMBER 0011851 OF DENVER, CO, WAS DISCIPLINED BY COLORADO ON APRIL 14, 1993
DISCIPLINARY ACTION: 3-MONTH LICENSE SUSPENSION
OFFENSE: PHYSICAL OR MENTAL ILLNESS INHIBITING THE ABILITY TO PRACTICE WITH SKILL AND SAFETY

NOTES: MENTAL DISABILITY.

PANTER, EDWARD MD, DATE OF BIRTH JULY 21, 1918, LICENSE NUMBER 0011851 OF DENVER, CO, WAS DISCIPLINED BY COLORADO ON JULY 14, 1993
DISCIPLINARY ACTION: 24-MONTH PROBATION; MONITORING OF PHYSICIAN PERFORMANCE

PANTER, KENT MD OF 1245 EAST COLFAX #100, DENVER, CO, WAS DISCIPLINED BY DEA ON NOVEMBER 13, 1997
DISCIPLINARY ACTION: SURRENDER OF CONTROLLED SUBSTANCE LICENSE

PANTER, KENT WOODRUFF MD, DATE OF BIRTH JULY 18, 1951, LICENSE NUMBER 0027925, WAS DISCIPLINED BY COLORADO ON JUNE 14, 1991
DISCIPLINARY ACTION: 36-MONTH PROBATION

NOTES: LICENSE REINSTATED UNDER STIPULATION AND ORDER DATED 05/23/90. EFFECTIVE 6/17/94 PROBATION DEEMED COMPLETED AND LICENSE RESTORED TO UNENCUMBERED STATUS.

PANTER, KENT WOODRUFF MD, DATE OF BIRTH JULY 18, 1951, LICENSE NUMBER 0029062 OF 1245 E COLFAX AVENUE, DENVER, CO, WAS DISCIPLINED BY GEORGIA ON NOVEMBER 7, 1991
DISCIPLINARY ACTION: 12-MONTH LICENSE SUSPENSION; PROBATION
OFFENSE: CRIMINAL CONVICTION OR PLEA OF GUILTY, NOLO CONTENDERE, OR NO CONTEST TO A CRIME

NOTES: CONVICTION OF FELONY IN COLORADO. SUSPENSION DEEMED TO HAVE RUN CONCURRENTLY WITH SUSPENSION IMPOSED BY COLORADO. PLACED ON PROBATION ON 11/7/91, TO RUN CONCURRENTLY WITH PROBATION IMPOSED BY COLORADO ORDER, AND $1,000 FINE. EFFECTIVE 10/7/94 ORDER TERMINATED AND HE HOLDS AN UNRESTRICTED LICENSE.

PANTER, KENT WOODRUFF MD, DATE OF BIRTH JULY 18, 1951, LICENSE NUMBER 27925, WAS DISCIPLINED BY COLORADO ON JULY 17, 1997

NOTES: INTERIM CESSATION OF PRACTICE. AGREEMENT PROVIDES THAT THE BOARD WILL NOT SUSPEND HIM WITHOUT GIVING 30 DAYS NOTICE. HE AGREES NOT TO PRACTICE AND NOT TO RETURN TO PRACTICE WITHOUT PROVIDING 30 DAYS NOTICE. THIS IS NOT A FINAL AGENCY ORDER.

PANTER, KENT WOODRUFF MD, DATE OF BIRTH JULY 18, 1951, LICENSE NUMBER 27925, WAS DISCIPLINED BY COLORADO ON NOVEMBER 13, 1998
DISCIPLINARY ACTION: EMERGENCY SUSPENSION

PANTER, KENT WOODRUFF MD, DATE OF BIRTH JULY 18, 1951, LICENSE NUMBER 27925, WAS DISCIPLINED BY COLORADO ON NOVEMBER 17, 1999
DISCIPLINARY ACTION: LICENSE REVOCATION
OFFENSE: CRIMINAL CONVICTION OR PLEA OF GUILTY, NOLO CONTENDERE, OR NO CONTEST TO A CRIME

NOTES: FELONY CONVICTION.

PARDOS, GEORGE J MD, DATE OF BIRTH JANUARY 24, 1949, LICENSE NUMBER 0024332 OF GOLDEN, CO, WAS DISCIPLINED BY COLORADO ON MAY 16, 1994
DISCIPLINARY ACTION: REPRIMAND
OFFENSE: PROFESSIONAL MISCONDUCT

PARKER, ROBERT K MD, DATE OF BIRTH MARCH 4, 1958, LICENSE NUMBER 35915, WAS DISCIPLINED BY COLORADO ON APRIL 17, 1997
DISCIPLINARY ACTION: RESTRICTION PLACED ON LICENSE

NOTES: NO UNPROFESSIONAL CONDUCT IDENTIFIED. LICENSE ISSUED WITH THE CONDITION THAT HE SHALL NOT TREAT PATIENTS.

PATEL, GIRISH MD, LICENSE NUMBER 0027162 OF AKRON, CO, WAS DISCIPLINED BY COLORADO ON AUGUST 17, 1990
DISCIPLINARY ACTION: EMERGENCY SUSPENSION
OFFENSE: SUBSTANDARD CARE, INCOMPETENCE OR NEGLIGENCE

NOTES: FAILURE TO MEET GENERALLY ACCEPTED STANDARDS OF MEDICAL PRACTICE.

PATTERSON, WILLIAM R MD, DATE OF BIRTH JANUARY 4, 1935, LICENSE NUMBER 0015581, WAS DISCIPLINED BY COLORADO ON AUGUST 24, 1995
DISCIPLINARY ACTION: REPRIMAND

PAUNOVICH, ROBERT P DO, DATE OF BIRTH DECEMBER 3, 1941, LICENSE NUMBER 0016392 OF WESTMINSTER, CO, WAS DISCIPLINED BY COLORADO ON JUNE 12, 1992
DISCIPLINARY ACTION: PROBATION; REQUIRED TO TAKE ADDITIONAL MEDICAL EDUCATION
OFFENSE: OVERPRESCRIBING OR MISPRESCRIBING DRUGS

NOTES: IMPROPER PRESCRIBING PRACTICES. AMENDMENT TO ORDER DATED 6/3/88; ADDITIONAL DISCIPLINE; INDEFINITE PROBATION; PRACTICE MONITORING AND PARTICIPATION IN AN EDUCATION PLAN.

PAUNOVICH, ROBERT P DO, LICENSE NUMBER 0005397 OF PALM HARBOR, FL, WAS DISCIPLINED BY FLORIDA ON SEPTEMBER 1, 1995
DISCIPLINARY ACTION: 24-MONTH PROBATION; FINE
OFFENSE: DISCIPLINARY ACTION BY ANOTHER STATE OR AGENCY

NOTES: CHARGED WITH HAVING DISCIPLINARY ACTION TAKEN AGAINST LICENSE BY ANOTHER JURISDICTION. $1,000

FINE; PROBATION WITH INDIRECT SUPERVISION AND RESTRICTION ON PRESCRIBING; SHALL COMPLETE THE COURSE "CLINICAL, LEGAL AND ETHICAL ISSUES IN PRESCRIBING ABUSABLE DRUGS."

PAUNOVICH, ROBERT PETER DO, LICENSE NUMBER 0003094 OF WESTMINSTER, CO, WAS DISCIPLINED BY OHIO ON FEBRUARY 8, 1994
DISCIPLINARY ACTION: DENIAL OF LICENSE REINSTATEMENT
OFFENSE: DISCIPLINARY ACTION BY ANOTHER STATE OR AGENCY

NOTES: PRIOR DISCIPLINARY ACTION BY COLORADO BOARD FOR FAILURE TO PROPERLY AND ADEQUATELY SUPERVISE NON-PHYSICIAN PERSONNEL AT WEIGHT CONTROL CLINICS, IMPROPERLY PRESCRIBING AMPHETAMINES FOR TREATMENT OF OBESITY, AND IMPROPERLY PRESCRIBING AND/OR ADMINISTERING LINCOCIN (SIC), TESTOSTERONE, AND HUMAN CHORIONIC GONADOTROPIN TO PATIENTS.

PENSACK, ROBERT J MD, DATE OF BIRTH MAY 4, 1950, LICENSE NUMBER 0024744, WAS DISCIPLINED BY COLORADO ON SEPTEMBER 19, 1996
DISCIPLINARY ACTION: RESTRICTION PLACED ON LICENSE

NOTES: ON 6/01/93 HE PLACED HIS COLORADO MEDICAL LICENSE ON INACTIVE STATUS. PERMANENT EMPLOYMENT RESTRICTION AS THE MEDICAL DIRECTOR FOR HOSPICE SERVICES OF NORTHWEST COLORADO.

PEOPLES, U S GRANT III MD, DATE OF BIRTH MARCH 27, 1950, LICENSE NUMBER 0021047 OF ENGLEWOOD, CO, WAS DISCIPLINED BY COLORADO ON JULY 15, 1994
DISCIPLINARY ACTION: RESTRICTION PLACED ON CONTROLLED SUBSTANCE LICENSE
OFFENSE: SUBSTANDARD CARE, INCOMPETENCE OR NEGLIGENCE

NOTES: ALLEGATIONS OF AN ACT OR OMISSION CONSTITUTING GROSSLY NEGLIGENT MEDICAL PRACTICE OR TWO OR MORE ACTS OR OMISSIONS WHICH FAIL TO MEET GENERALLY ACCEPTED STANDARDS. HE DENIES ALLEGATIONS OF SUBSTANDARD CARE BUT CONSENTS TO AGREEMENT/PRACTICE RESTRICTION. PERMANENT PRACTICE RESTRICTION REQUIRING HIM TO PRESCRIBE CONTROLLED SUBSTANCES ONLY IN ACCORDANCE WITH USUAL PUBLISHED MANUFACTURERS' RECOMMENDATIONS FOR ANXIOLITIC OR ANALGESIC USES. ON 10/17/96 THIS RESTRICTION LIFTED AND REPLACED BY A LETTER OF ADMONITION.

PETERS, MARK L MD, DATE OF BIRTH JUNE 2, 1956, LICENSE NUMBER 30870, WAS DISCIPLINED BY COLORADO ON JULY 16, 1998
DISCIPLINARY ACTION: REPRIMAND

PETERSON, RICHARD I MD, DATE OF BIRTH SEPTEMBER 2, 1947, LICENSE NUMBER 0022904 OF COLORADO SPRINGS, CO, WAS DISCIPLINED BY COLORADO ON AUGUST 13, 1990
DISCIPLINARY ACTION: EMERGENCY SUSPENSION
OFFENSE: SUBSTANDARD CARE, INCOMPETENCE OR NEGLIGENCE

NOTES: SELF-ADMINISTERING A HABIT-FORMING DRUG OR CONTROLLED SUBSTANCE NOT IN THE COURSE OF LEGITIMATE MEDICAL PRACTICE; EXCESSIVE USE OF A HABIT-FORMING DRUG OR CONTROLLED SUBSTANCE; PHYSICAL OR MENTAL DISABILITY WHICH RENDERS HIM UNABLE TO PERFORM MEDICAL SERVICES WITH REASONABLE SKILL AND SAFETY TO PATIENTS; ACTS OR OMISSIONS WHICH CONSTITUTE GROSSLY NEGLIGENT MEDICAL PRACTICE OR WHICH FAIL TO MEET GENERALLY ACCEPTED STANDARDS OF MEDICAL PRACTICE; SELF-ADMINISTERING A CONTROLLED SUBSTANCE NOT ON AN EMERGENCY BASIS. LICENSE SUMMARILY SUSPENDED PENDING COMPLETION OF FORMAL DISCIPLINARY PROCEEDINGS, BASED UPON FINDINGS THAT HE WAS GUILTY OF DELIBERATE AND WILLFUL VIOLATION AND THAT THE PUBLIC HEALTH, SAFETY AND WELFARE IMPERATIVELY REQUIRED EMERGENCY ACTION. FORMAL DISCIPLINARY HEARING CONCLUDED 11/9/90; FINAL DECISION PENDING.

PETERSON, RICHARD I MD, DATE OF BIRTH SEPTEMBER 2, 1947, LICENSE NUMBER 0022904 OF SCOTTSDALE, AZ, WAS DISCIPLINED BY COLORADO ON MAY 10, 1991
DISCIPLINARY ACTION: 12-MONTH LICENSE SUSPENSION; 12-MONTH PROBATION
OFFENSE: SUBSTANDARD CARE, INCOMPETENCE OR NEGLIGENCE

NOTES: SELF-ADMINISTERING A CONTROLLED SUBSTANCE NOT IN THE COURSE OF LEGITIMATE MEDICAL PRACTICE; EXCESSIVE USE OF A CONTROLLED SUBSTANCE; PHYSICAL OR MENTAL DISABILITY WHICH RENDERS HIM UNABLE TO PERFORM MEDICAL SERVICES WITH REASONABLE SKILL AND SAFETY; ACTS OR OMISSIONS WHICH CONSTITUTE GROSSLY NEGLIGENT MEDICAL PRACTICE. SUSPENSION RETROACTIVE TO 8/15/90. ON 08/16/91 STIPULATION: HE ADMITS FELONY CONVICTION RE: PERSONAL USE OF CONTROLLED SUBSTANCES AND AGREES NOT TO CHALLENGE PREVIOUS ORDER SUSPENDING LICENSE. BOARD AGREES NOT TO IMPOSE FURTHER DISCIPLINE.

PETTY, WENDELL M MD, DATE OF BIRTH DECEMBER 4, 1931, LICENSE NUMBER 0017299 OF 849 25 ROAD, GRAND JUNCTION, CO, WAS DISCIPLINED BY IOWA ON AUGUST 26, 1993
DISCIPLINARY ACTION: SURRENDER OF LICENSE

PETTY, WENDELL M MD, DATE OF BIRTH DECEMBER 4, 1931, LICENSE NUMBER 0015505 OF GRAND JUNCTION, CO, WAS DISCIPLINED BY COLORADO ON SEPTEMBER 16, 1994
DISCIPLINARY ACTION: LICENSE SUSPENSION
OFFENSE: NONCOMPLIANCE WITH A PROFESSIONAL RULE

NOTES: FAILURE TO UNDERGO PHYSICAL/MENTAL EXAMINATIONS ORDERED BY THE BOARD.

PETTY, WENDELL MEARL DR, LICENSE NUMBER 0015367, WAS DISCIPLINED BY ARIZONA ON JULY 15, 1994
DISCIPLINARY ACTION: LICENSE SUSPENSION
OFFENSE: NONCOMPLIANCE WITH A PROFESSIONAL RULE

NOTES: FAILURE TO PAY RENEWAL FEE DURING PENDING INVESTIGATION.

PETTY, WENDELL MEARL MD, LICENSE NUMBER 15367, WAS DISCIPLINED BY ARIZONA ON JANUARY 23, 1998
DISCIPLINARY ACTION: LICENSE REVOCATION
OFFENSE: DISCIPLINARY ACTION BY ANOTHER STATE OR AGENCY

NOTES: IN A PATIENT HE SAW IN 1990 FAILED TO FOLLOW THROUGH ON HIS TREATMENT FOR DEPRESSION AND BLURRING THE BOUNDARIES OF A THERAPEUTIC ALLIANCE BY ENTERING INTO A BUSINESS TRANSACTION WITH HIM; THE DOCTOR MADE A LOAN TO THE PATIENT WHOM HE HAD SIGN A NOTE; WHEN THE LOAN WAS NOT PAID, DR. PETTY RETAINED AN ATTORNEY TO COLLECT THE MONEY; DR. PETTY WAS APPROVED FOR DISABILITY BENEFITS ON 11/7/91 BASED ON HIS SUFFERING "ONGOING ANXIETY, DEPRESSION AND STRESS DISORDER;" VOLUNTARILY

SURRENDERED IOWA LICENSE ON 8/3/93.

PHILIP, WILLIAM W MD, DATE OF BIRTH MARCH 2, 1946, LICENSE NUMBER 0019536, WAS DISCIPLINED BY COLORADO ON MAY 18, 1995
DISCIPLINARY ACTION: REPRIMAND

PLATT, FREDERIC W MD, DATE OF BIRTH MAY 14, 1938, LICENSE NUMBER 15781, WAS DISCIPLINED BY COLORADO ON SEPTEMBER 18, 1997
DISCIPLINARY ACTION: REPRIMAND

PLATT, TERESA MD, DATE OF BIRTH DECEMBER 4, 1953, LICENSE NUMBER 26172, WAS DISCIPLINED BY COLORADO ON OCTOBER 8, 1998
DISCIPLINARY ACTION: 60-MONTH PROBATION; MONITORING OF PHYSICIAN PERFORMANCE
OFFENSE: SUBSTANCE ABUSE

NOTES: HABITUAL INTEMPERANCE OR EXCESSIVE USE OF A CONTROLLED SUBSTANCE. PROBATIONARY TERMS INCLUDE: ABSTINENCE FROM ALCOHOL AND CONTROLLED SUBSTANCES, TREATMENT MONITORING AND PRACTICE MONITORING.

POLLACK, NATHAN M MD OF 620 HARRISON STREET, DENVER, CO, WAS DISCIPLINED BY DEA ON APRIL 7, 1995
DISCIPLINARY ACTION: RESTRICTION PLACED ON CONTROLLED SUBSTANCE LICENSE
OFFENSE: PROFESSIONAL MISCONDUCT

NOTES: PRIOR ALLEGED CONTROLLED SUBSTANCE VIOLATIONS.

POLO, KATHLEEN BROOKE MD, DATE OF BIRTH JUNE 18, 1930, LICENSE NUMBER 1053790 OF 515 BEWICK PT., COLORADO SPRINGS, CO, WAS DISCIPLINED BY MICHIGAN ON AUGUST 18, 1999
DISCIPLINARY ACTION: PROBATION
OFFENSE: DISCIPLINARY ACTION BY ANOTHER STATE OR AGENCY

NOTES: SISTER STATE DISCIPLINARY ACTION; FAILURE TO REPORT/COMPLY.

POST, GARY L MD, DATE OF BIRTH JULY 4, 1948, LICENSE NUMBER 20261, WAS DISCIPLINED BY COLORADO ON JULY 15, 1999
DISCIPLINARY ACTION: REPRIMAND

POUSMA, DOUGLAS J MD, DATE OF BIRTH JANUARY 24, 1961 OF DENVER, CO, WAS DISCIPLINED BY COLORADO ON JULY 25, 1991
DISCIPLINARY ACTION: EMERGENCY SUSPENSION
OFFENSE: PROVIDING FALSE INFORMATION TO THE BOARD OR OTHER HEALTH AGENCY

NOTES: MENTAL OR PHYSICAL DISABILITY AS TO RENDER HIM UNABLE TO PERFORM MEDICAL SERVICES WITH SAFETY TO THE PATIENT; AND RESORTING TO FRAUD, MISREPRESENTATION, OR DECEPTION IN APPLYING FOR A LICENSE.

POUSMA, DOUGLAS J MD, DATE OF BIRTH JANUARY 24, 1961, LICENSE NUMBER 0035198 OF DENVER, CO, WAS DISCIPLINED BY COLORADO ON JUNE 19, 1992
DISCIPLINARY ACTION: LICENSE REVOCATION
OFFENSE: PROVIDING FALSE INFORMATION TO THE BOARD OR OTHER HEALTH AGENCY

NOTES: MENTAL DISABILITY AND RESORTING TO FRAUD, MISREPRESENTATION OR DECEPTION IN APPLYING FOR A LICENSE.

POUSMA, DOUGLAS J MD, DATE OF BIRTH JANUARY 27, 1961 OF 1660 WYNKOOP ST, STE 900, DENVER, CO, WAS DISCIPLINED BY MEDICARE ON NOVEMBER 20, 1992
DISCIPLINARY ACTION: EXCLUSION FROM THE MEDICARE AND/OR MEDICAID PROGRAM
OFFENSE: DISCIPLINARY ACTION BY ANOTHER STATE OR AGENCY

NOTES: LICENSE REVOCATION OR SUSPENSION.

POUSMA, DOUGLAS J MD, DATE OF BIRTH JANUARY 24, 1961, LICENSE NUMBER 0035198, WAS DISCIPLINED BY COLORADO ON APRIL 11, 1996
DISCIPLINARY ACTION: 36-MONTH RESTRICTION PLACED ON LICENSE
OFFENSE: PHYSICAL OR MENTAL ILLNESS INHIBITING THE ABILITY TO PRACTICE WITH SKILL AND SAFETY

NOTES: THIS IS A NEW APPLICATION. HIS LICENSE HAD BEEN REVOKED IN 6/92 FOR FRAUD AND MENTAL DISABILITY. HE IS ISSUED A NEW LICENSE, BUT NOT PERMITTED TO ENGAGE IN PATIENT CARE. THE PROBATIONARY LICENSE MAY BE REVIEWED IN THREE YEARS.

POWELL, SCOTT EVAN MD, DATE OF BIRTH AUGUST 13, 1948, LICENSE NUMBER 0033894 OF LOS ANGELES, CA, WAS DISCIPLINED BY COLORADO ON JULY 14, 1994
DISCIPLINARY ACTION: 60-MONTH PROBATION; MONITORING OF PHYSICIAN PERFORMANCE
OFFENSE: SUBSTANDARD CARE, INCOMPETENCE OR NEGLIGENCE

NOTES: ALLEGATIONS OF SUBSTANDARD CARE WHICH, IF UNREBUTTED, WOULD CONSTITUTE TWO OR MORE ACTS OF SUBSTANDARD CARE. APPLICATION FOR LICENSURE. PROBATION UNDER TERMS AND CONDITIONS INCLUDING PRACTICE MONITORING. IN ABEYANCE PENDING HIS LOCATION TO COLORADO.

POWELL, SCOTT EVAN MD, LICENSE NUMBER 0G73757 OF LOS ANGELES, CA, WAS DISCIPLINED BY CALIFORNIA ON APRIL 8, 1996
DISCIPLINARY ACTION: REPRIMAND
OFFENSE: DISCIPLINARY ACTION BY ANOTHER STATE OR AGENCY

NOTES: ACTION IN COLORADO RELATED TO DEFICIENCIES IN RECORD KEEPING AND DOCUMENTATION ON DIAGNOSIS, TESTING, PRESCRIBING, AND TREATMENT AS REVEALED IN AN AUDIT OF 25 PATIENT CHARTS BY NEW YORK SOCIAL SERVICES.

POWELL, VANNA M DO, DATE OF BIRTH MAY 24, 1947, LICENSE NUMBER 0021813, WAS DISCIPLINED BY COLORADO ON NOVEMBER 15, 1996
DISCIPLINARY ACTION: REPRIMAND

PUCKETT, WILLIAM N MD, DATE OF BIRTH MAY 21, 1928, LICENSE NUMBER 0013253 OF DENVER, CO, WAS DISCIPLINED BY COLORADO ON JANUARY 22, 1993
DISCIPLINARY ACTION: SURRENDER OF LICENSE
OFFENSE: SUBSTANDARD CARE, INCOMPETENCE OR NEGLIGENCE

NOTES: SUBSTANDARD CARE; PHYSICAL OR MENTAL DISABILITY.

PUGH, MARION MD, LICENSE NUMBER 0021586 OF DALLAS, TX, WAS DISCIPLINED BY COLORADO ON OCTOBER 10, 1990
DISCIPLINARY ACTION: SURRENDER OF LICENSE
OFFENSE: SUBSTANCE ABUSE

NOTES: HABITUAL INTEMPERANCE AND EXCESSIVE USE OF ALCOHOLIC BEVERAGES.

PUMPHREY, ROBERT S MD, DATE OF BIRTH DECEMBER 7, 1948,

LICENSE NUMBER 0020507 OF COLORADO SPRINGS, CO, WAS DISCIPLINED BY COLORADO ON JUNE 12, 1992
DISCIPLINARY ACTION: 60-MONTH PROBATION; MONITORING OF PHYSICIAN PERFORMANCE
OFFENSE: SUBSTANCE ABUSE

NOTES: SUBSTANCE ABUSE AND DEPENDENCE. PROBATION INCLUDES TREATMENT AND PRACTICE MONITORING.

PUSHKIN, JOSHUA R MD, DATE OF BIRTH OCTOBER 8, 1952, LICENSE NUMBER 0022653, WAS DISCIPLINED BY COLORADO ON JUNE 15, 1995
DISCIPLINARY ACTION: RESTRICTION PLACED ON LICENSE; MONITORING OF PHYSICIAN PERFORMANCE
OFFENSE: SEXUAL ABUSE OF OR SEXUAL MISCONDUCT WITH A PATIENT

NOTES: HAD A SEXUAL RELATIONSHIP WITH A PATIENT HE SAW FROM APPROXIMATELY 5/92 THROUGH 10/93, DISCUSSED HIS PERSONAL PROBLEMS WITH HER AND HIRED HER TO PERFORM PERSONAL DUTIES SUCH AS SECRETARIAL AND CHAUFFEUR; IN 8/93 HE ARRANGED FOR HER TO SEE ANOTHER PSYCHIATRIST BUT DID NOT INFORM THAT PSYCHIATRIST OF THIS RELATIONSHIP; PATIENT ATTEMPTED SUICIDE IN 9/93. A BOARD REQUESTED EVALUATION ADVISED HE HAD A SERIOUS AND DEGENERATIVE ILLNESS, MULTIPLE SCLEROSIS, THAT WAS BEGINNING TO EFFECT HIS COGNITIVE FUNCTIONING. AGREES TO SURRENDER HIS MEDICAL LICENSE ON 6/15/97 AND DURING THE INTERIM AGREES TO PRACTICE AND TREATMENT MONITORING, TO DECLINE NEW PATIENTS, AND NEVER EMPLOY OR REQUEST A PATIENT PERFORM A SERVICE IN LIEU OF PAYMENT; SHALL RECEIVE MEDICAL TREATMENT FROM THE COLORADO PHYSICIAN HEALTH PROGRAM AND MEET WITH THEM AT LEAST QUARTERLY; THEY SHALL PROVIDE QUARTERLY REPORTS TO THE BOARD; PRACTICE SHALL BE MONITORED BY A BOARD-APPROVED PHYSICIAN WHO SHALL REVIEW ALL CHARTS WEEKLY AND SUBMIT QUARTERLY REPORTS TO THE BOARD. ON 11/14/97 ORDER MODIFIED WHEREBY HIS EARLIER SURRENDER WAS RESCINDED AND LICENSE PLACED ON INACTIVE STATUS.

RABINOWITZ, JAY S MD, DATE OF BIRTH MAY 15, 1951, LICENSE NUMBER 23508, WAS DISCIPLINED BY COLORADO ON MARCH 20, 1997
DISCIPLINARY ACTION: REPRIMAND

RADETSKY, PAUL MD, LICENSE NUMBER 0013336 OF ARVADA, CO, WAS DISCIPLINED BY COLORADO ON SEPTEMBER 7, 1990
DISCIPLINARY ACTION: 36-MONTH PROBATION; REQUIRED TO TAKE ADDITIONAL MEDICAL EDUCATION
OFFENSE: SUBSTANDARD CARE, INCOMPETENCE OR NEGLIGENCE

NOTES: STIPULATION AND ORDER REQUIRING PROBATION, PRACTICE MONITORING AND CONTINUING MEDICAL EDUCATION.

RAFAL, KENNETH M MD, DATE OF BIRTH DECEMBER 10, 1954, LICENSE NUMBER 24529, WAS DISCIPLINED BY COLORADO ON MARCH 25, 1999
DISCIPLINARY ACTION: REPRIMAND

RAO, YARLAGADDA N MD, DATE OF BIRTH JUNE 1, 1944, LICENSE NUMBER 24128, WAS DISCIPLINED BY COLORADO ON AUGUST 15, 1997
DISCIPLINARY ACTION: REPRIMAND

RAPAPORT, STEVEN M MD, DATE OF BIRTH JULY 22, 1956, LICENSE NUMBER 0028576 OF REDONDO BEACH, CA, WAS DISCIPLINED BY COLORADO ON JUNE 19, 1992
DISCIPLINARY ACTION: SURRENDER OF LICENSE
OFFENSE: SUBSTANDARD CARE, INCOMPETENCE OR NEGLIGENCE

NOTES: AN ACT OR OMISSION CONSTITUTING GROSSLY NEGLIGENT PRACTICE, OR TWO OR MORE ACTS OF SUBSTANDARD CARE. PERMANENT SURRENDER.

RASKIN, DOUGLAS J MD, DATE OF BIRTH SEPTEMBER 27, 1950, LICENSE NUMBER 0025809 OF COLORADO SPRINGS, CO, WAS DISCIPLINED BY COLORADO ON SEPTEMBER 8, 1994
DISCIPLINARY ACTION: REPRIMAND

RATHER, DANIEL A MD, DATE OF BIRTH APRIL 22, 1934, LICENSE NUMBER 0014885 OF PEORIA, AZ, WAS DISCIPLINED BY COLORADO ON OCTOBER 16, 1991
OFFENSE: SUBSTANCE ABUSE

NOTES: HABITUAL INTEMPERANCE, AND ALCOHOL DEPENDENCE AND ABUSE. STIPULATION AND ORDER IMPOSING CONDITIONS FOR RETURN TO THE PRACTICE OF MEDICINE IN COLORADO.

RAVIN, THOMAS H MD, DATE OF BIRTH MARCH 21, 1941, LICENSE NUMBER 0016838 OF DENVER, CO, WAS DISCIPLINED BY COLORADO ON APRIL 16, 1993
DISCIPLINARY ACTION: 36-MONTH PROBATION; REQUIRED TO TAKE ADDITIONAL MEDICAL EDUCATION
OFFENSE: SUBSTANDARD CARE, INCOMPETENCE OR NEGLIGENCE

NOTES: ALLEGATIONS OF SUBSTANDARD CARE. PROBATIONARY TERM INCLUDES PRACTICE MONITORING.

RAVIN, THOMAS H MD, DATE OF BIRTH MARCH 21, 1941, LICENSE NUMBER 0016838, WAS DISCIPLINED BY COLORADO ON AUGUST 24, 1995
DISCIPLINARY ACTION: REPRIMAND

NOTES: LETTER OF ADMONITION.

REDAL, LEIF A MD, DATE OF BIRTH MAY 26, 1956, LICENSE NUMBER 30471, WAS DISCIPLINED BY COLORADO ON FEBRUARY 17, 1999
DISCIPLINARY ACTION: REPRIMAND

REDELS, SIDNEY L DO, DATE OF BIRTH JUNE 13, 1951, LICENSE NUMBER 35399, WAS DISCIPLINED BY COLORADO ON AUGUST 18, 1999
DISCIPLINARY ACTION: REPRIMAND

REED, DAVID J MD, DATE OF BIRTH JANUARY 31, 1938, LICENSE NUMBER 0022024 OF DENVER, CO, WAS DISCIPLINED BY COLORADO ON APRIL 5, 1995
DISCIPLINARY ACTION: REPRIMAND

REINER, MICHAEL DAVID MD, LICENSE NUMBER 0026184 OF HOUSTON, TX, WAS DISCIPLINED BY COLORADO ON OCTOBER 10, 1990
DISCIPLINARY ACTION: PROBATION

NOTES: REINSTATEMENT SOUGHT FROM SUSPENSION ORDER ENTERED ON 12/5/88. REINSTATEMENT SUBJECT TO PROBATIONARY TERMS AND CONDITIONS.

REISER, DAVID E MD, DATE OF BIRTH APRIL 6, 1946, LICENSE NUMBER 0018237 OF GOLDEN, CO, WAS DISCIPLINED BY COLORADO ON OCTOBER 18, 1991

DISCIPLINARY ACTION: 60-MONTH PROBATION; MONITORING OF PHYSICIAN PERFORMANCE
OFFENSE: SUBSTANCE ABUSE

NOTES: ALCOHOL ABUSE; SUCH PHYSICAL OR MENTAL DISABILITY AS TO RENDER HIM UNABLE TO PRACTICE MEDICINE WITH REASONABLE SKILL AND SAFETY. TERMS OF PROBATION INCLUDE TREATMENT AND MONITORING FOR ALCOHOL AND SUBSTANCE ABUSE AND DEPENDENCE AND PRACTICE MONITORING.

REISER, DAVID E MD, DATE OF BIRTH APRIL 6, 1946, LICENSE NUMBER 0018237, WAS DISCIPLINED BY COLORADO ON DECEMBER 21, 1995
DISCIPLINARY ACTION: 120-MONTH PROBATION; MONITORING OF PHYSICIAN PERFORMANCE

NOTES: PRACTICE AND TREATMENT MONITORING.

REISER, DAVID E MD, LICENSE NUMBER 0151164 OF 3300 EAST FIRST STREET, DENVER, CO, WAS DISCIPLINED BY NEW YORK ON SEPTEMBER 27, 1996
DISCIPLINARY ACTION: SURRENDER OF LICENSE
OFFENSE: DISCIPLINARY ACTION BY ANOTHER STATE OR AGENCY

NOTES: DISCIPLINED BY THE COLORADO BOARD FOR FAILING TO COMPLY WITH A PREVIOUS ORDER REQUIRING HIM TO MAINTAIN SOBRIETY AND TOTALLY ABSTAIN FROM THE USE OF ALCOHOL.

REISER, DAVID E MD, DATE OF BIRTH APRIL 6, 1946, LICENSE NUMBER 0018237, WAS DISCIPLINED BY COLORADO ON NOVEMBER 15, 1996
DISCIPLINARY ACTION: SURRENDER OF LICENSE
OFFENSE: FAILURE TO COMPLY WITH PREVIOUS BOARD ORDER

NOTES: VIOLATION OF A VALID BOARD ORDER.

RIBER, JOSHUA I MD, DATE OF BIRTH FEBRUARY 21, 1943, LICENSE NUMBER 0022814, WAS DISCIPLINED BY COLORADO ON MARCH 14, 1996
DISCIPLINARY ACTION: REPRIMAND

RITCHEY, ELIZABETH E MD, DATE OF BIRTH SEPTEMBER 28, 1946, LICENSE NUMBER 29083, WAS DISCIPLINED BY COLORADO ON AUGUST 14, 1998
DISCIPLINARY ACTION: REQUIRED TO TAKE ADDITIONAL MEDICAL EDUCATION; MONITORING OF PHYSICIAN PERFORMANCE
OFFENSE: NONCOMPLIANCE WITH A PROFESSIONAL RULE

NOTES: FAILURE TO KEEP PROPER MEDICAL RECORDS. SHE AGREES TO REEDUCATION ACTIVITIES AND EKG OVERREADS.

ROBERTS, CHARLES C MD, DATE OF BIRTH FEBRUARY 6, 1946 OF 1551 GAYLORD STREET #1, DENVER, CO, WAS DISCIPLINED BY MEDICARE ON JANUARY 12, 1997
DISCIPLINARY ACTION: EXCLUSION FROM THE MEDICARE AND/OR MEDICAID PROGRAM
OFFENSE: NONCOMPLIANCE WITH A PROFESSIONAL RULE

NOTES: DEFAULTED ON PUBLIC HEALTH SERVICE EDUCATION LOAN.

ROBERTS, EMIL DO OF 1111 BONFORTE BLVD #1010, PUEBLO, CO, WAS DISCIPLINED BY DEA ON NOVEMBER 17, 1999
DISCIPLINARY ACTION: SURRENDER OF CONTROLLED SUBSTANCE LICENSE

ROBERTS, JERRY R MD, DATE OF BIRTH AUGUST 19, 1933, LICENSE NUMBER 0015023 OF COLORADO SPRINGS, CO, WAS DISCIPLINED BY COLORADO ON MAY 11, 1994
DISCIPLINARY ACTION: REPRIMAND
OFFENSE: PROFESSIONAL MISCONDUCT

ROBERTSON, LAWRENCE M JR MD, DATE OF BIRTH FEBRUARY 4, 1932, LICENSE NUMBER 0013177 OF DENVER, CO, WAS DISCIPLINED BY COLORADO ON DECEMBER 10, 1993
DISCIPLINARY ACTION: REPRIMAND

RODRIGUEZ, VINCENT J MD, DATE OF BIRTH AUGUST 23, 1959 OF PO BOX 1, HUNT, TX, WAS DISCIPLINED BY MEDICARE ON DECEMBER 20, 1991
DISCIPLINARY ACTION: EXCLUSION FROM THE MEDICARE AND/OR MEDICAID PROGRAM
OFFENSE: DISCIPLINARY ACTION BY ANOTHER STATE OR AGENCY

NOTES: LICENSE REVOCATION OR SUSPENSION.

RODRIGUEZ, VINCENT J MD OF 704 NORTH THIRD STREET, PLAINVIEW, NE, WAS DISCIPLINED BY DEA ON MAY 8, 1995
DISCIPLINARY ACTION: SURRENDER OF CONTROLLED SUBSTANCE LICENSE

NOTES: IN LIEU OF ORDER TO SHOW CAUSE.

RODRIGUEZ, VINCENT JOHN MD, LICENSE NUMBER 0053547 OF TALLAHASSEE, FL, WAS DISCIPLINED BY FLORIDA ON FEBRUARY 6, 1990
DISCIPLINARY ACTION: EMERGENCY SUSPENSION
OFFENSE: OVERPRESCRIBING OR MISPRESCRIBING DRUGS

NOTES: INABILITY TO PRACTICE WITH REASONABLE SKILL BY REASON OF THE USE OF DRUGS OR AS A RESULT OF A MENTAL OR PHYSICAL CONDITION; PRESCRIBING TO HIMSELF.

RODRIGUEZ, VINCENT JOHN MD, LICENSE NUMBER 0028371 OF HUNT, TX, WAS DISCIPLINED BY COLORADO ON APRIL 10, 1991
DISCIPLINARY ACTION: LICENSE REVOCATION
OFFENSE: CRIMINAL CONVICTION OR PLEA OF GUILTY, NOLO CONTENDERE, OR NO CONTEST TO A CRIME

NOTES: ACTION BASED ON HABITUAL OR EXCESSIVE USE OF CONTROLLED SUBSTANCES AND FELONY CONVICTION FOR CARRYING A CONCEALED WEAPON.

RODRIGUEZ, VINCENT JOHN MD, LICENSE NUMBER 0053547 OF HUNT, TX, WAS DISCIPLINED BY FLORIDA ON MAY 6, 1991
DISCIPLINARY ACTION: LICENSE SUSPENSION; 60-MONTH

NOTES: CHARGED WITH BEING UNABLE TO PRACTICE BY REASON OF THE USE OF DRUGS OR AS A RESULT OF ANY MENTAL OR PHYSICAL CONDITION. IN LIEU OF FURTHER PROSECUTION, STIPULATED TO SUSPENSION UNTIL HE CAN PROVE HE IS ABLE TO PRACTICE WITH REASONABLE SKILL AND SAFETY, WHICH SHALL INCLUDE SATISFACTORY PSYCHIATRIC AND PHYSICAL EVALUATIONS; ACTIVE PHYSICIANS RECOVERY NETWORK CONTRACT; BOARD APPROVED PLAN FOR REENTRY TO PRACTICE. UPON REINSTATEMENT, PROBATION WITH TERMS AND CONDITIONS TO BE SET, WHICH SHALL INCLUDE CONTINUATION OF ACTIVE PHYSICIAN'S RECOVERY NETWORK CONTRACT.

RODRIGUEZ, VINCENT JOHN MD OF 9950 W 80TH AVENUE #16, ARVADA, CO, WAS DISCIPLINED BY DEA ON AUGUST 1, 1991
DISCIPLINARY ACTION: REVOCATION OF CONTROLLED SUBSTANCE LICENSE
OFFENSE: DISCIPLINARY ACTION BY ANOTHER STATE OR AGENCY

NOTES: ON 4/10/91 COLORADO REVOKED HIS LICENSE. IN HIS

STATEMENT HE CONTENDS COLORADO ACTION WAS BASED ON FLORIDA'S EMERGENCY SUSPENSION OF HIS LICENSE ON 2/6/90 AND THAT HE HAD ENTERED INTO AN AGREEMENT WITH FLORIDA PERMITTING HIM TO SEEK REINSTATEMENT ON 5/6/91. DEA FOUND THESE FACTS IRRELEVANT TO THE FACT THAT HE DID NOT HAVE PRESCRIBING AUTHORITY IN COLORADO.

RODRIGUEZ, VINCENT JOHN MD, LICENSE NUMBER 0053547 OF PLAINVIEW, NE, WAS DISCIPLINED BY FLORIDA ON DECEMBER 29, 1995
DISCIPLINARY ACTION: LICENSE REVOCATION
OFFENSE: DISCIPLINARY ACTION BY ANOTHER STATE OR AGENCY

NOTES: VIOLATING BOARD RULE IN THAT HE FAILED TO NOTIFY THE BOARD OF THE ADDRESS OF HIS NEW PRIMARY PLACE OF PRACTICE; VIOLATING PREVIOUS BOARD ORDER IN THAT HE FAILED TO COMPLY WITH THE PHYSICIAN'S RECOVERY NETWORK CONTRACT AS REQUIRED; NEBRASKA BOARD ACCEPTED THE VOLUNTARY SURRENDER OF HIS LICENSE AND CONTROLLED SUBSTANCE REGISTRATION AFTER FILING A PETITION FOR DISCIPLINARY ACTION.

ROLAND, RALPH D MD, DATE OF BIRTH NOVEMBER 10, 1943, LICENSE NUMBER 0018866, WAS DISCIPLINED BY COLORADO ON JUNE 8, 1995
DISCIPLINARY ACTION: REPRIMAND

ROMERO, ERNEST F DO, DATE OF BIRTH JUNE 14, 1919 OF PO BOX 116, SALIDA, CO, WAS DISCIPLINED BY MEDICARE ON JANUARY 15, 1992
DISCIPLINARY ACTION: 60-MONTH EXCLUSION FROM THE MEDICARE AND/OR MEDICAID PROGRAM
OFFENSE: CRIMINAL CONVICTION OR PLEA OF GUILTY, NOLO CONTENDERE, OR NO CONTEST TO A CRIME

NOTES: PROGRAM-RELATED CONVICTION. REINSTATED ON 6/2/97.

ROSS, MICHAEL H MD, DATE OF BIRTH NOVEMBER 11, 1939, LICENSE NUMBER 0017592 OF GOLDEN, CO, WAS DISCIPLINED BY COLORADO ON JANUARY 20, 1995
DISCIPLINARY ACTION: PROBATION
OFFENSE: SUBSTANDARD CARE, INCOMPETENCE OR NEGLIGENCE

NOTES: SUBSTANDARD CARE. PROBATIONARY PERIOD UPON RETURN TO PRACTICE IN COLORADO.

ROSS, MICHAEL H MD, DATE OF BIRTH NOVEMBER 11, 1939, LICENSE NUMBER 1026987 OF 9950 W 80TH AVE, ARVADA, CO, WAS DISCIPLINED BY MICHIGAN ON DECEMBER 15, 1995
DISCIPLINARY ACTION: RESTRICTION PLACED ON LICENSE
OFFENSE: DISCIPLINARY ACTION BY ANOTHER STATE OR AGENCY

NOTES: FAILURE TO REPORT/COMPLY.

ROWAN, ALOYSIUS I JR MD, DATE OF BIRTH SEPTEMBER 4, 1923, LICENSE NUMBER 0012134 OF AURORA, CO, WAS DISCIPLINED BY COLORADO ON MAY 11, 1994
DISCIPLINARY ACTION: REPRIMAND
OFFENSE: PROFESSIONAL MISCONDUCT

ROWAN, ALOYSIUS I JR MD, DATE OF BIRTH SEPTEMBER 4, 1923, LICENSE NUMBER 12134, WAS DISCIPLINED BY COLORADO ON NOVEMBER 12, 1997

NOTES: NO UNPROFESSIONAL CONDUCT IDENTIFIED. HE AGREES TO RELINQUISH HIS LICENSE.

ROWAN, ALOYSIUS IGNATIUS MD, DATE OF BIRTH SEPTEMBER 4, 1923 OF 1279 QUARI STREET, AURORA, CO, WAS DISCIPLINED BY MEDICARE ON JULY 20, 1998
DISCIPLINARY ACTION: EXCLUSION FROM THE MEDICARE AND/OR MEDICAID PROGRAM
OFFENSE: DISCIPLINARY ACTION BY ANOTHER STATE OR AGENCY

NOTES: LICENSE REVOKED, SUSPENDED, SURRENDERED OR OTHERWISE LOST FOR REASONS BEARING ON PROFESSIONAL PERFORMANCE, PROFESSIONAL COMPETENCE OR FINANCIAL INTEGRITY.

RUFF, ALAN C MD, LICENSE NUMBER 0G51561 OF BRIGHTON, CO, WAS DISCIPLINED BY CALIFORNIA ON FEBRUARY 2, 1993
DISCIPLINARY ACTION: SURRENDER OF LICENSE

NOTES: VOLUNTARY SURRENDER OF LICENSE WHILE CHARGES PENDING.

RZEPPA, BRENDA L DO, DATE OF BIRTH NOVEMBER 20, 1957, LICENSE NUMBER 0031297 OF GRAND JUNCTION, CO, WAS DISCIPLINED BY COLORADO ON JANUARY 18, 1995
DISCIPLINARY ACTION: REPRIMAND

SAATHOFF, MICHAEL C MD, DATE OF BIRTH NOVEMBER 15, 1964, LICENSE NUMBER 36371, WAS DISCIPLINED BY COLORADO ON DECEMBER 10, 1998
DISCIPLINARY ACTION: 60-MONTH PROBATION; MONITORING OF PHYSICIAN PERFORMANCE
OFFENSE: SUBSTANCE ABUSE

NOTES: HABITUAL INTEMPERANCE OR EXCESSIVE USE OF A CONTROLLED SUBSTANCE. PROBATIONARY TERMS INCLUDE: ABSTINENCE FROM ADDICTIVE SUBSTANCES, TREATMENT MONITORING AND PRACTICE MONITORING.

SAATHOFF, MICHAEL C MD, DATE OF BIRTH NOVEMBER 15, 1964, LICENSE NUMBER 36371, WAS DISCIPLINED BY COLORADO ON MARCH 18, 1999
DISCIPLINARY ACTION: REPRIMAND

SAKAMOTO, ARTHUR DR OF LAKEWOOD, CO, WAS DISCIPLINED BY ILLINOIS ON JULY 1, 1995
DISCIPLINARY ACTION: LICENSE SUSPENSION
OFFENSE: DISCIPLINARY ACTION BY ANOTHER STATE OR AGENCY

NOTES: DISCIPLINED IN CALIFORNIA. INDEFINITE SUSPENSION.

SANTAGUIDA, RIK MD, DATE OF BIRTH OCTOBER 25, 1949, LICENSE NUMBER 0022538 OF PO BOX 1930, IDAHO SPRINGS, CO, WAS DISCIPLINED BY COLORADO ON APRIL 1, 1993
DISCIPLINARY ACTION: 2-MONTH LICENSE SUSPENSION; 60-MONTH PROBATION
OFFENSE: SEXUAL ABUSE OF OR SEXUAL MISCONDUCT WITH A PATIENT

NOTES: IN 7/91 HE BECAME INVOLVED IN A FOUR WEEK SEXUAL AFFAIR WITH A FEMALE PATIENT; AT THE TIME OF THE AFFAIR HAD NOT FORMALLY TERMINATED THE DOCTOR-PATIENT RELATIONSHIP. ALSO, FOLLOWING AN INJURY AND SUBSEQUENT SURGERY HE BEGAN SELF-ADMINISTERING DEMEROL TO THE POINT OF ADDICTION; IN 4/90 HE SELF-REFERRED TO THE COLORADO PHYSICIAN HEALTH PROGRAM FOR HELP AFTER BEING HOSPITALIZED FOR SIDE EFFECTS OF HIS DRUG ABUSE; AFTER A RELAPSE IN 6/90 UNDERWENT A 30-DAY INPATIENT TREATMENT PROGRAM; HAS HAD NO INDICATION OF RELAPSE SINCE 8/90. SUSPENSION FOR 90 DAYS, 45 DAYS STAYED. FOLLOWING SUSPENSION, TERMS OF PROBATION INCLUDE: SHALL RECEIVE TREATMENT

MONITORING BY COLORADO PHYSICIANS HEALTH PROGRAM WHO SHALL PERFORM RANDOM URINE SCREENS AND SUBMIT QUARTERLY REPORTS TO THE BOARD; SHALL HAVE A BOARD APPROVED PRACTICE MONITOR WHO SHALL VISIT HIS OFFICE AT LEAST ONCE PER MONTH AND REVIEW AT LEAST FIVE PATIENT CHARTS AND SHALL SUBMIT QUARTERLY REPORTS TO THE BOARD; WITHIN SIX MONTHS SHALL COMPLETE A BOARD APPROVED CONTINUING MEDICAL EDUCATION COURSE ON THE ETHICAL PROHIBITIONS OF SEXUAL RELATIONSHIPS BETWEEN PHYSICIANS AND PATIENTS; SHALL TOTALLY ABSTAIN FROM THE USE OF DEMEROL OR ANY OTHER HABIT-FORMING OR CONTROLLED SUBSTANCE UNLESS ADMINISTERED, DISPENSED OR PRESCRIBED BY AN AUTHORIZED PERSON OTHER THAN HIMSELF; SHALL REPORT TO THE BOARD WHEN HE GAINS HOSPITAL PRIVILEGES.

SARGENT, ROBERT A MD OF 7720 S BROADWAY #200, LITTLETON, CO, WAS DISCIPLINED BY DEA ON NOVEMBER 9, 1993
DISCIPLINARY ACTION: RESTRICTION PLACED ON CONTROLLED SUBSTANCE LICENSE
OFFENSE: SUBSTANCE ABUSE

NOTES: VOLUNTARY SURRENDER OF SCHEDULE II AND IIN PRIVILEGES FOR ABUSE OF SECONAL.

SARGENT, ROBERT A MD, DATE OF BIRTH MAY 30, 1940, LICENSE NUMBER 0017605 OF LITTLETON, CO, WAS DISCIPLINED BY COLORADO ON NOVEMBER 19, 1993
DISCIPLINARY ACTION: 60-MONTH PROBATION; RESTRICTION PLACED ON CONTROLLED SUBSTANCE LICENSE
OFFENSE: OVERPRESCRIBING OR MISPRESCRIBING DRUGS

NOTES: ADMINISTERING, DISPENSING OR PRESCRIBING A CONTROLLED SUBSTANCE OTHER THAN IN THE COURSE OF LEGITIMATE PROFESSIONAL PRACTICE. CONDITIONS OF PROBATION: COMPLIANCE WITH DRUG ENFORCEMENT ADMINISTRATION RESTRICTIONS AND TREATMENT MONITORING.

SARGENT, ROBERT A MD, LICENSE NUMBER 0G19908 OF LITTLETON, CO, WAS DISCIPLINED BY CALIFORNIA ON JUNE 5, 1995
DISCIPLINARY ACTION: 60-MONTH PROBATION
OFFENSE: DISCIPLINARY ACTION BY ANOTHER STATE OR AGENCY

NOTES: DISCIPLINE BY COLORADO BOARD FOR BARBITURATE ABUSE (SECONAL). REVOCATION STAYED.

SAVONEN, STEVEN J MD, DATE OF BIRTH OCTOBER 27, 1940, LICENSE NUMBER 0035711, WAS DISCIPLINED BY COLORADO ON OCTOBER 25, 1996
DISCIPLINARY ACTION: 60-MONTH PROBATION; MONITORING OF PHYSICIAN PERFORMANCE
OFFENSE: PHYSICAL OR MENTAL ILLNESS INHIBITING THE ABILITY TO PRACTICE WITH SKILL AND SAFETY

NOTES: PHYSICAL OR MENTAL INCAPACITY. EVALUATION BY THE COLORADO PHYSICIAN HEALTH PROGRAM. TREATMENT MONITORING.

SAYRE, MICHAEL C MD, LICENSE NUMBER 0029156 OF WALLA WALLA, WA, WAS DISCIPLINED BY WASHINGTON ON MARCH 19, 1993
DISCIPLINARY ACTION: REQUIRED TO TAKE ADDITIONAL MEDICAL EDUCATION; FINE
OFFENSE: SUBSTANDARD CARE, INCOMPETENCE OR NEGLIGENCE

NOTES: PRIOR TO SURGERY IN WHICH HE WAS THE ATTENDING ANESTHESIOLOGIST FAILED TO ENSURE THAT THE VENTILATOR WAS ON THEREBY DEPRIVING THE PATIENT OF OXYGEN DURING SURGERY; FAILED TO RECOGNIZE AND/OR REACT TO THIS CAUSING THE PATIENT TO SUFFER ANOXIC ENCEPHALOPATHY AND DIE 20 DAYS LATER. SHALL COMPLETE 25 HOURS OF CONTINUING MEDICAL EDUCATION IN THE AREA OF ANESTHESIOLOGY BY 6/1/94; SHALL SUCCESSFULLY COMPLETE A SPECIFIED PROCTORING PLAN; SHALL PAY A $500 FINE. ON 9/2/93 ORDER TERMINATED.

SAYRE, MICHAEL C MD, DATE OF BIRTH NOVEMBER 29, 1946, LICENSE NUMBER 0D39621, WAS DISCIPLINED BY MARYLAND ON APRIL 5, 1994
OFFENSE: DISCIPLINARY ACTION BY ANOTHER STATE OR AGENCY

NOTES: ON 3/16/93 HE ENTERED INTO AN AGREED ORDER WITH THE WASHINGTON BOARD IN WHICH HE ADMITS THAT, PRIOR TO A SURGERY IN WHICH HE WAS THE ATTENDING ANESTHESIOLOGIST, HE FAILED TO ENSURE THAT THE VENTILATOR WAS ON THEREBY DEPRIVING THE PATIENT OF OXYGEN DURING SURGERY AND FAILED TO RECOGNIZE AND/OR REACT TO THE FALLING OXYGEN SATURATION RATE; AS A RESULT THE PATIENT SUFFERED ANOXIC ENCEPHALOPATHY, WAS PLACED ON LIFE SUPPORT AND DIED 20 DAYS LATER AFTER THE FAMILY DECIDED TO REMOVE HIM FROM LIFE SUPPORT; CONDITIONS OF WASHINGTON ORDER INCLUDED CONTINUING MEDICAL EDUCATION AND A FINE; ON 9/2/93 WASHINGTON ORDER WAS TERMINATED. CONDITION OF MARYLAND ORDER: SHALL NOT PRACTICE IN THE STATE UNTIL HE APPEARS BEFORE AND OBTAINS APPROVAL OF THE BOARD.

SAYRE, MICHAEL C MD, DATE OF BIRTH NOVEMBER 29, 1946, LICENSE NUMBER 0030053, WAS DISCIPLINED BY COLORADO ON JULY 8, 1996
DISCIPLINARY ACTION: REPRIMAND

SAYRE, MICHAEL C MD, LICENSE NUMBER 0006962 OF 330 LILLIAN LANE, WATERLOO, IA, WAS DISCIPLINED BY HAWAII ON DECEMBER 20, 1996
DISCIPLINARY ACTION: FINE
OFFENSE: DISCIPLINARY ACTION BY ANOTHER STATE OR AGENCY

NOTES: ACTION IN VERMONT AND DOCUMENTS RECEIVED FROM WASHINGTON, CONNECTICUT, AND IOWA BOARDS. FAILED TO REPORT DISCIPLINARY DECISION IN ANOTHER JURISDICTION. $500 ADMINISTRATIVE FINE. LICENSE EXPIRED ON 1/31/96.

SCARINZI, HUGO DO OF FLAGLER, CO, WAS DISCIPLINED BY MISSOURI ON AUGUST 18, 1995
DISCIPLINARY ACTION: RESTRICTION PLACED ON LICENSE
OFFENSE: DISCIPLINARY ACTION BY ANOTHER STATE OR AGENCY

NOTES: COLORADO RESTRICTED HIS LICENSE.

SCARINZI, HUGO J DO, DATE OF BIRTH JULY 25, 1932, LICENSE NUMBER 0013868 OF HUGO, CO, WAS DISCIPLINED BY COLORADO ON MARCH 18, 1994
DISCIPLINARY ACTION: PROBATION; RESTRICTION PLACED ON LICENSE
OFFENSE: SUBSTANDARD CARE, INCOMPETENCE OR NEGLIGENCE

NOTES: ISSUES INVOLVING PATIENT CARE. ORDER FOR PERMANENT PRACTICE RESTRICTION BY PROHIBITING HOSPITAL ADMISSIONS AND OBSTETRICAL CARE AND INDEFINITE PROBATION INCLUDING MONITORING.

SCEATS, DONALD J MD, LICENSE NUMBER 0013031 OF PUEBLO, CO, WAS DISCIPLINED BY COLORADO ON FEBRUARY 15, 1991
OFFENSE: SUBSTANDARD CARE, INCOMPETENCE OR NEGLIGENCE

NOTES: MAY NOT NOW OR IN THE FUTURE PRACTICE MEDICINE IN COLORADO WITHOUT MAKING APPLICATION AND RECEIVING BOARD'S APPROVAL.

SCEATS, DONALD J MD, DATE OF BIRTH MARCH 16, 1922, LICENSE NUMBER 0004683 OF PUEBLO, CO, WAS DISCIPLINED BY WASHINGTON ON MAY 18, 1991
DISCIPLINARY ACTION: SURRENDER OF LICENSE
OFFENSE: DISCIPLINARY ACTION BY ANOTHER STATE OR AGENCY

NOTES: ON 8/14/87 COLORADO RESTRICTED HIS LICENSE BY PROHIBITING CARE OF LEVEL II OR III INFANTS AND FURTHER RESTRICTED HIS NEONATAL PRACTICE; ON 2/27/88, WHILE APPLYING FOR RENEWAL OF MONTANA LICENSE, STATED HE HAD NOT HAD ANY DISCIPLINARY ACTIONS TAKEN AGAINST HIM; MONTANA ENTERED INTO ORDER ON 5/17/89 REQUIRING HIM TO REPORT ANY DISCIPLINARY PROCEEDINGS OR VOLUNTARY LICENSE SURRENDERS WITHIN 30 DAYS; ACCEPTED THE SURRENDER OF HIS LICENSE ON 11/27/89 IN LIEU OF PROCEEDING TO HEARING ON CHARGES THAT HE HAD FAILED TO REPORT SURRENDERING HIS CALIFORNIA LICENSE WITHIN 30 DAYS; HE SURRENDERED CALIFORNIA LICENSE ON 6/7/89. AGREES NOT TO APPLY FOR REINSTATEMENT FOR AT LEAST ONE YEAR; MUST CONCLUDE ALL MEDICAL BUSINESS AND FORMALLY CLOSE PRACTICE WITHIN 90 DAYS.

SCHACHT, FREDERICK W JR MD, DATE OF BIRTH APRIL 30, 1934, LICENSE NUMBER 15735, WAS DISCIPLINED BY COLORADO ON JULY 17, 1997
DISCIPLINARY ACTION: 60-MONTH PROBATION; REQUIRED TO TAKE ADDITIONAL MEDICAL EDUCATION
OFFENSE: SUBSTANDARD CARE, INCOMPETENCE OR NEGLIGENCE

NOTES: SUBSTANDARD CARE (PRIMA FACIE TYPE ADMISSION ONLY). TERMS OF PROBATION INCLUDE REEDUCATION ACTIVITIES AND PRACTICE MONITORING.

SCHACHT, FREDERICK W JR MD, DATE OF BIRTH APRIL 30, 1934, LICENSE NUMBER 15735, WAS DISCIPLINED BY COLORADO ON SEPTEMBER 18, 1997
DISCIPLINARY ACTION: EMERGENCY SUSPENSION
OFFENSE: FAILURE TO COMPLY WITH PREVIOUS BOARD ORDER

NOTES: FAILURE TO COMPLY WITH A LAWFUL ORDER OF THE BOARD. ON 9/23/97 SUSPENSION LIFTED.

SCHACHT, FREDERICK W JR MD, DATE OF BIRTH APRIL 30, 1934, LICENSE NUMBER 15735, WAS DISCIPLINED BY COLORADO ON MARCH 19, 1998
DISCIPLINARY ACTION: RESTRICTION PLACED ON LICENSE; CEASE AND DESIST ORDER
OFFENSE: SUBSTANDARD CARE, INCOMPETENCE OR NEGLIGENCE

NOTES: SUBSTANDARD CARE (PRIMA FACIE TYPE ADMISSION ONLY). MAY NOT PERFORM OBSTETRICS OR SURGERY EXCEPT FOR SPECIFICALLY IDENTIFIED CURRENT OBSTETRICAL PATIENTS. HE AGREES TO CEASE THE PRACTICE OF MEDICINE BY 2/28/99.

SCHACHT, FREDERICK WILLIAM JR MD, LICENSE NUMBER 8473 OF 1907 N. BOISE AVENUE, LOVELAND, CO, WAS DISCIPLINED BY OKLAHOMA ON SEPTEMBER 24, 1998
DISCIPLINARY ACTION: 60-MONTH PROBATION; RESTRICTION PLACED ON LICENSE
OFFENSE: DISCIPLINARY ACTION BY ANOTHER STATE OR AGENCY

NOTES: ON 7/17/97 THE COLORADO BOARD PLACED HIS LICENSE ON PROBATION FOR FIVE YEARS AFTER REVIEWING A MALPRACTICE SETTLEMENT HE ENTERED INTO. HE WAS ALSO ORDERED TO HAVE HIS PRACTICE, AND PARTICULARLY HIS GYNECOLOGICAL CARE AND SURGERY PRACTICE, EVALUATED. HE HAD FAILED TO MEET THE GENERALLY ACCEPTED STANDARDS OF MEDICAL PRACTICE IN THE TREATMENT OF ONE PATIENT BY FAILING TO OBTAIN AN APPROPRIATE CONSULTATION AND MEDICAL CLEARANCE PRIOR TO PERFORMING SURGERY ON A PATIENT WHO HAD SEVERE ALCOHOLIC LIVER DISEASE, WHICH REMAINED UNDIAGNOSED AT THE TIME OF SURGERY, AND FAILED TO DOCUMENT THE PATIENT'S HEAVY ALCOHOL USE IN EITHER HIS OFFICE CHART OR PREOPERATIVE HISTORY AND PHYSICAL. ON 3/19/98 THE COLORADO BOARD TOOK FURTHER ACTION AGAINST HIM AFTER LEARNING THAT HIS PRIVILEGES HAD BEEN LIMITED BY A MEDICAL CENTER IN LOVELAND, COLORADO. THE 3/19/98 ORDER PROHIBITS HIM FROM PERFORMING SURGERY OR OBSTETRICS IN THE FUTURE. EFFECTIVE 2/28/99, THE COLORADO BOARD ENTIRELY BARS HIM FROM PRACTICING. CONDITIONS OF OKLAHOMA PROBATION: HE WILL COMPLY WITH ALL TERMS, INCLUDING THOSE WITHOUT LIMITATION, THOSE OF EDUCATION AND MONITORING, DESCRIBED IN COLORADO ORDERS UP TO HIS RETIREMENT ON 2/28/99, HE MAY CONTINUE THE PRACTICE OF MEDICINE EXCEPT THAT HE MAY NOT PERFORM SURGERY OR OBSTETRICS UNLESS AS PART OF CONTINUING CARE FOR CURRENT PATIENTS. AFTER 2/28/99, HE SHALL PERFORM NO ACT REQUIRING A LICENSE ISSUED BY THE BOARD. UPON SUCCESSFUL COMPLETION OF THE CPEP LEARNING PLAN, HE MAY PETITION THE COLORADO BOARD TO RETURN TO PRACTICE IN A LIMITED CAPACITY SUCH AS AT A CLINIC OR OFFICE SETTING. SHALL SUBMIT TO EVERY STATE IN WHICH HE HOLDS LICENSURE AND TO HOSPITALS, CLINICS OR OTHER INSTITUTIONS IN WHICH HE HOLDS OR ANTICIPATES HOLDING ANY FORM OF STAFF PRIVILEGE A COPY OF THIS ORDER; SHALL NOT SUPERVISE ALLIED HEALTH PROFESSIONALS; SHALL KEEP THE BOARD INFORMED OF HIS ADDRESS AND PAY COSTS; SHALL APPEAR BEFORE THE BOARD UPON REQUEST. THE PROBATION IS TOLLED UNTIL HE BEGINS PRACTICING IN OKLAHOMA OR IN ANY FEDERAL OR NATIVE AMERICAN FACILITY LOCATED WITHIN ITS BOUNDARIES. SHOULD HE DESIRE TO ESTABLISH ACTIVE PRACTICE OR CONSULTATION PRIVILEGES IN OKLAHOMA, HE SHALL FIRST NOTIFY THE BOARD IN WRITING OF HIS INTENTIONS AND PERSONALLY APPEAR FOR A REVIEW OF THESE MATTERS AND HIS PRESENT STATE OF MEDICAL TRAINING AND COMPETENCE.

SCHAEFER, MARTIN W MD, DATE OF BIRTH JANUARY 11, 1939, LICENSE NUMBER 0017038, WAS DISCIPLINED BY COLORADO ON JUNE 8, 1995
DISCIPLINARY ACTION: MONITORING OF PHYSICIAN PERFORMANCE

NOTES: TREATMENT AND PRACTICE MONITORING. REVOCATION STAYED.

SCHAEFER, MARTIN W MD, DATE OF BIRTH JANUARY 11, 1939, LICENSE NUMBER 0017038, WAS DISCIPLINED BY COLORADO ON MARCH 20, 1996
DISCIPLINARY ACTION: LICENSE REVOCATION
OFFENSE: FAILURE TO COMPLY WITH PREVIOUS BOARD ORDER

NOTES: VIOLATION OF AN AGREEMENT NOT TO DRINK ALCOHOL OR CONSUME A CONTROLLED SUBSTANCE. STAY OF PREVIOUS REVOCATION LIFTED.

SCHAFER, LARRY A MD OF WHEAT RIDGE, CO, WAS DISCIPLINED BY MISSOURI ON SEPTEMBER 4, 1990
DISCIPLINARY ACTION: 84-MONTH PROBATION
OFFENSE: DISCIPLINARY ACTION BY ANOTHER STATE OR AGENCY

NOTES: DISCIPLINARY ACTION TAKEN IN COLORADO BASED ON PERSONAL IMPAIRMENT. PROBATION RETROACTIVE TO 11/03/89.

SCHLECHTER, WILLIAM G MD, LICENSE NUMBER 21342 OF SPOKANE, WA, WAS DISCIPLINED BY WASHINGTON ON JANUARY 23, 1998
DISCIPLINARY ACTION: FINE; RESTRICTION PLACED ON CONTROLLED SUBSTANCE LICENSE

NOTES: $1000 FINE; SHALL REFRAIN FROM PRESCRIBING CONTROLLED SUBSTANCES TO FAMILY MEMBERS AND NON-PATIENTS AND COMPLETE CONTINUING MEDICAL EDUCATION COURSE HOURS IN PAIN MANAGEMENT AND PRESCRIBING. ON 10/6/99 ORDER TERMINATED; LICENSE UNRESTRICTED.

SCHLECHTER, WILLIAM G MD, DATE OF BIRTH DECEMBER 7, 1949, LICENSE NUMBER 22762, WAS DISCIPLINED BY COLORADO ON JULY 15, 1999
DISCIPLINARY ACTION: REPRIMAND

SCHLEGEL, KARL J DO, DATE OF BIRTH AUGUST 29, 1954, LICENSE NUMBER 0027741 OF BOULDER, CO, WAS DISCIPLINED BY COLORADO ON NOVEMBER 19, 1993
DISCIPLINARY ACTION: 60-MONTH PROBATION; MONITORING OF PHYSICIAN PERFORMANCE
OFFENSE: SUBSTANCE ABUSE

NOTES: ALLEGATIONS OF HABITUAL INTEMPERANCE. PROBATIONARY PERIOD INCLUDES PRACTICE AND TREATMENT MONITORING.

SCHLEGEL, KARL J DO, DATE OF BIRTH AUGUST 29, 1954, LICENSE NUMBER 27741, WAS DISCIPLINED BY COLORADO ON DECEMBER 18, 1997
DISCIPLINARY ACTION: REPRIMAND

SCHLOM, LOUIS MD, LICENSE NUMBER 0A28614 OF COLORADO SPRINGS, CO, WAS DISCIPLINED BY CALIFORNIA ON MAY 2, 1992
DISCIPLINARY ACTION: SURRENDER OF LICENSE

NOTES: VOLUNTARY SURRENDER WHILE CHARGES PENDING.

SCHMUCKER, MARION LEE MD, DATE OF BIRTH JUNE 29, 1951, LICENSE NUMBER 0022033 OF LA JUNTA, CO, WAS DISCIPLINED BY COLORADO ON JANUARY 31, 1994
DISCIPLINARY ACTION: REPRIMAND
OFFENSE: PROFESSIONAL MISCONDUCT

SCHRADER, NANCY L MD, LICENSE NUMBER 0197671 OF 4301 WEST MARKHAM SLOT 584, LITTLE ROCK, AR, WAS DISCIPLINED BY NEW YORK ON NOVEMBER 26, 1996
DISCIPLINARY ACTION: SURRENDER OF LICENSE
OFFENSE: DISCIPLINARY ACTION BY ANOTHER STATE OR AGENCY

NOTES: ACTION IN ARKANSAS FOR WRITING FRAUDULENT PRESCRIPTIONS FOR CONTROLLED SUBSTANCES FOR HER OWN USE AND FOR BEING A HABITUAL USER OF DRUGS.

SCHRADER, NANCY L MD, DATE OF BIRTH FEBRUARY 3, 1955, LICENSE NUMBER 30826, WAS DISCIPLINED BY COLORADO ON AUGUST 13, 1997
DISCIPLINARY ACTION: 60-MONTH PROBATION; MONITORING OF PHYSICIAN PERFORMANCE
OFFENSE: SUBSTANCE ABUSE

NOTES: HABITUAL INTEMPERANCE OR EXCESSIVE USE OF A CONTROLLED SUBSTANCE. TERMS OF PROBATION INCLUDE: TREATMENT AND PRACTICE MONITORING; MUST REMAIN ABSTINENT FROM ADDICTIVE SUBSTANCES.

SCHRADER, NANCY LYNN MD, LICENSE NUMBER 00N7571 OF LITTLE ROCK, AR, WAS DISCIPLINED BY ARKANSAS ON JULY 11, 1996
DISCIPLINARY ACTION: 24-MONTH EMERGENCY SUSPENSION

NOTES: TERMINATED ON 9/12/96.

SCHRADER, NANCY LYNN MD OF 4301 W. MARKHAM #584, LITTLE ROCK, AR, WAS DISCIPLINED BY DEA ON AUGUST 19, 1996
DISCIPLINARY ACTION: SURRENDER OF CONTROLLED SUBSTANCE LICENSE

SCHRADER, NANCY LYNN MD, LICENSE NUMBER 00N7571 OF LITTLE ROCK, AR, WAS DISCIPLINED BY ARKANSAS ON SEPTEMBER 27, 1996
DISCIPLINARY ACTION: 60-MONTH PROBATION; FINE

NOTES: $1,000 FINE.

SCHRADER, NANCY LYNN MD, LICENSE NUMBER 0004470 OF 7249 GERMAN CREEK PARK, MEMPHIS, TN, WAS DISCIPLINED BY DELAWARE ON FEBRUARY 25, 1997
DISCIPLINARY ACTION: SURRENDER OF LICENSE

NOTES: DISCIPLINARY ACTION TAKEN IN ANOTHER STATE. VOLUNTARY SURRENDER OF CERTIFICATE WHILE UNDER INVESTIGATION.

SCHRADER, NANCY LYNN MD, DATE OF BIRTH FEBRUARY 3, 1955, LICENSE NUMBER 36087 OF 7249 GERMAN CREEK PARK, MEMPHIS, TN, WAS DISCIPLINED BY WISCONSIN ON OCTOBER 22, 1997
DISCIPLINARY ACTION: LICENSE SUSPENSION
OFFENSE: DISCIPLINARY ACTION BY ANOTHER STATE OR AGENCY

NOTES: ON 9/27/96, DISCIPLINED BY THE ARKANSAS BOARD FOR ALLEGATIONS OF IMPROPER SELF-PRESCRIPTION OF CONTROLLED SUBSTANCES. MAY PETITION THE BOARD FOR PERMISSION TO PRACTICE AT ANY TIME WHICH SHALL REQUIRE DOCUMENTATION OF FULL COMPLIANCE WITH THE ARKANSAS ORDER.

SCHRANDT, DONALD L MD, DATE OF BIRTH SEPTEMBER 23, 1935, LICENSE NUMBER 0015355 OF DENVER, CO, WAS DISCIPLINED BY COLORADO ON DECEMBER 4, 1992
DISCIPLINARY ACTION: 60-MONTH PROBATION; MONITORING OF PHYSICIAN PERFORMANCE

NOTES: TWO OR MORE ACTS OR OMISSIONS WHICH FAILED TO MEET GENERALLY ACCEPTED STANDARDS OF MEDICAL PRACTICE. PROBATIONARY PERIOD INCLUDES PRACTICE MONITORING.

SCHREIBER, DAVID P MD, DATE OF BIRTH FEBRUARY 29, 1956, LICENSE NUMBER 26553, WAS DISCIPLINED BY COLORADO ON JUNE 12, 1997
DISCIPLINARY ACTION: REPRIMAND

SCHROEDER, WILLIAM R DO, DATE OF BIRTH SEPTEMBER 15, 1956, LICENSE NUMBER 32902, WAS DISCIPLINED BY COLORADO ON OCTOBER 8, 1998
DISCIPLINARY ACTION: REPRIMAND

SCHWARTZ, KENNETH A MD, DATE OF BIRTH AUGUST 18, 1954, LICENSE NUMBER 0024397 OF RIFLE, CO, WAS DISCIPLINED BY COLORADO ON SEPTEMBER 13, 1991
DISCIPLINARY ACTION: 24-MONTH PROBATION; MONITORING OF PHYSICIAN PERFORMANCE
OFFENSE: SUBSTANDARD CARE, INCOMPETENCE OR NEGLIGENCE

NOTES: FAILURE TO MEET GENERALLY ACCEPTED STANDARDS OF MEDICAL PRACTICE IN FAILING TO PROPERLY DIAGNOSE A PATIENT'S DIABETES. SHALL SUBMIT TO PRACTICE MONITORING AND UNDERGO EVALUATION BY THE COLORADO PERSONALIZED EDUCATION PROGRAM FOR PHYSICIANS.

SCOTT, GEORGE E MD, DATE OF BIRTH NOVEMBER 9, 1924, LICENSE NUMBER 0011390 OF LA JUNTA, CO, WAS DISCIPLINED BY COLORADO ON SEPTEMBER 13, 1991
DISCIPLINARY ACTION: PROBATION; MONITORING OF PHYSICIAN PERFORMANCE
OFFENSE: SUBSTANCE ABUSE

NOTES: EXCESSIVE USE OF CONTROLLED SUBSTANCES AND HABITUAL INTEMPERANCE. INDEFINITE PROBATION. TREATMENT AND PRACTICE MONITORING.

SCOTT, JAMES L MD, LICENSE NUMBER 0030031 OF DENVER, CO, WAS DISCIPLINED BY COLORADO ON MARCH 15, 1991
DISCIPLINARY ACTION: SURRENDER OF LICENSE
OFFENSE: SUBSTANDARD CARE, INCOMPETENCE OR NEGLIGENCE

SCOTT, JAMES L JR MD, LICENSE NUMBER 0C21706 OF DENVER, CO, WAS DISCIPLINED BY CALIFORNIA ON FEBRUARY 25, 1993
DISCIPLINARY ACTION: LICENSE REVOCATION

SEERVELD, HAROLD L MD, DATE OF BIRTH JUNE 17, 1933, LICENSE NUMBER 0015221 OF WHEAT RIDGE, CO, WAS DISCIPLINED BY COLORADO ON MARCH 18, 1994
DISCIPLINARY ACTION: RESTRICTION PLACED ON LICENSE
OFFENSE: SUBSTANDARD CARE, INCOMPETENCE OR NEGLIGENCE

NOTES: ALLEGATIONS OF ISSUES INVOLVING PATIENT CARE. DOCTOR DENIES SUBSTANDARD PRACTICE. NO OB CARE.

SENFT, OTTO E MD, DATE OF BIRTH JUNE 15, 1922, LICENSE NUMBER 0015430 OF LONGMONT, CO, WAS DISCIPLINED BY IOWA ON FEBRUARY 19, 1990
DISCIPLINARY ACTION: 2-MONTH LICENSE SUSPENSION; FINE

NOTES: FINE $1000.

SENFT, OTTO E MD, DATE OF BIRTH JUNE 15, 1922, LICENSE NUMBER 0029202 OF LONGMONT, CO, WAS DISCIPLINED BY COLORADO ON OCTOBER 13, 1993
DISCIPLINARY ACTION: REPRIMAND

SENFT, OTTO ERNST MD, LICENSE NUMBER 0028887 OF 706 AZALEA DRIVE, LA FAYETTE, GA, WAS DISCIPLINED BY GEORGIA ON MAY 22, 1990
DISCIPLINARY ACTION: NONRENEWAL OF LICENSE
OFFENSE: DISCIPLINARY ACTION BY ANOTHER STATE OR AGENCY

NOTES: LICENSE PLACED ON INACTIVE STATUS BASED ON DISCIPLINARY ACTION BY IOWA. CONVICTION IN IOWA FOR MEDICARE FRAUD. REVOKED BY PROCESS OF LAW FOR NONRENEWAL.

SHAPIRO, JED S MD, DATE OF BIRTH OCTOBER 6, 1946, LICENSE NUMBER 19891, WAS DISCIPLINED BY COLORADO ON AUGUST 13, 1997
DISCIPLINARY ACTION: 2-MONTH LICENSE SUSPENSION; 58-MONTH PROBATION
OFFENSE: SEXUAL ABUSE OF OR SEXUAL MISCONDUCT WITH A PATIENT

NOTES: SEXUAL ACT WITH A PATIENT. TERMS OF PROBATION INCLUDE A BOUNDARIES COURSE AND PRACTICE MONITORING.

SHAPLEIGH, MARGARET L MD, DATE OF BIRTH OCTOBER 8, 1951, LICENSE NUMBER 0026556 OF COLORADO SPRINGS, CO, WAS DISCIPLINED BY COLORADO ON NOVEMBER 12, 1993
DISCIPLINARY ACTION: REPRIMAND

SHAW, ANITA DR, DATE OF BIRTH NOVEMBER 11, 1953, LICENSE NUMBER 0026963 OF AURORA, CO, WAS DISCIPLINED BY COLORADO ON APRIL 14, 1993
DISCIPLINARY ACTION: 60-MONTH PROBATION; MONITORING OF PHYSICIAN PERFORMANCE
OFFENSE: SUBSTANCE ABUSE

NOTES: EXCESSIVE USE OF A CONTROLLED SUBSTANCE. PROBATIONARY TERMS INCLUDE PRACTICE AND TREATMENT MONITORING.

SHEINER, SETH A MD, DATE OF BIRTH MAY 3, 1958, LICENSE NUMBER 31987, WAS DISCIPLINED BY COLORADO ON MAY 5, 1997
DISCIPLINARY ACTION: EMERGENCY SUSPENSION
OFFENSE: PROFESSIONAL MISCONDUCT

NOTES: ADMINISTERING, DISPENSING OR PRESCRIBING A CONTROLLED SUBSTANCE OTHER THAN IN THE COURSE OF LEGITIMATE PROFESSIONAL PRACTICE.

SHERMAN, JOSEPH M MD, DATE OF BIRTH JANUARY 9, 1946, LICENSE NUMBER 0019940 OF LITTLETON, CO, WAS DISCIPLINED BY COLORADO ON APRIL 13, 1994
DISCIPLINARY ACTION: RESTRICTION PLACED ON LICENSE
OFFENSE: SUBSTANDARD CARE, INCOMPETENCE OR NEGLIGENCE

NOTES: ALLEGATIONS OF SUBSTANDARD CARE. HE DENIES THAT HIS OB PRACTICE WAS SUBSTANDARD. IF UNREBUTTED, WOULD CONSTITUTE TWO OR MORE ACTS OF SUBSTANDARD CARE. NO OB PRACTICE; HE AGREES NOT TO APPLY FOR OR OBTAIN HOSPITAL PRIVILEGES TO PRACTICE OB. PRACTICE OF GYNECOLOGY IS NOT RESTRICTED BY THIS ORDER.

SHERMAN, JOSEPH MARTIN MD, LICENSE NUMBER 0184687 OF 2855 VALMONT, BOULDER, CO, WAS DISCIPLINED BY NEW YORK ON SEPTEMBER 13, 1995
DISCIPLINARY ACTION: 12-MONTH PROBATION; RESTRICTION PLACED ON LICENSE
OFFENSE: DISCIPLINARY ACTION BY ANOTHER STATE OR AGENCY

NOTES: ACTION IN COLORADO FOR NEGLIGENCE AND INCOMPETENCE INCLUDING THE INAPPROPRIATE MANAGEMENT OF THIRD STAGE LABOR, ABNORMAL OR NONPROGRESSIVE LABOR AND THE INAPPROPRIATE USE OF BLOOD AND BLOOD PRODUCTS. LICENSE LIMITED TO PROHIBIT THE PRACTICE OF OBSTETRICS.

SHESOL, BARRY F MD, DATE OF BIRTH OCTOBER 2, 1944, LICENSE NUMBER 0023106 OF PO BOX 460728, AURORA, CO, WAS DISCIPLINED BY COLORADO ON APRIL 16, 1993
DISCIPLINARY ACTION: SURRENDER OF LICENSE
OFFENSE: SUBSTANDARD CARE, INCOMPETENCE OR NEGLIGENCE

NOTES: SUBSTANDARD CARE OF TWO PATIENTS; HAS DIFFICULTY IN RECOGNIZING AND RESPECTING APPROPRIATE DOCTOR-PATIENT BOUNDARIES WHICH

HAS LED TO UNPROVEN ALLEGATIONS OF SEXUAL CONTACT WITH A PATIENT. SEXUAL CONTACT ISSUE IS SET OUT SPECIFICALLY AS AN UNRESOLVED ALLEGATION. HAS SOUGHT PSYCHOTHERAPY TO RESOLVE BOUNDARY ISSUES.

SHESOL, BARRY F MD, DATE OF BIRTH OCTOBER 2, 1944 OF 750 POTOMAC ST SUITE 201, AURORA, CO, WAS DISCIPLINED BY DEA ON SEPTEMBER 23, 1993
DISCIPLINARY ACTION: SURRENDER OF CONTROLLED SUBSTANCE LICENSE
NOTES: VOLUNTARY SURRENDER OF REGISTRATION IN LIEU OF IMPOSING DISCIPLINARY ACTIONS - BY COLORADO STATE BOARD.

SHROYER, JOSEPH M MD, DATE OF BIRTH AUGUST 4, 1932, LICENSE NUMBER 0015964, WAS DISCIPLINED BY COLORADO ON AUGUST 23, 1995
DISCIPLINARY ACTION: EMERGENCY SUSPENSION

SHROYER, JOSEPH M MD, DATE OF BIRTH AUGUST 4, 1932, LICENSE NUMBER 0015964, WAS DISCIPLINED BY COLORADO ON NOVEMBER 9, 1995
DISCIPLINARY ACTION: SURRENDER OF LICENSE
NOTES: RELINQUISHMENT OF LICENSE AND RETIREMENT.

SHROYER, JOSEPH M MD, LICENSE NUMBER 0084520 OF 1302 LONGWOOD AVENUE, PUEBLO, CO, WAS DISCIPLINED BY NEW YORK ON MAY 16, 1996
DISCIPLINARY ACTION: SURRENDER OF LICENSE
OFFENSE: DISCIPLINARY ACTION BY ANOTHER STATE OR AGENCY
NOTES: DISCIPLINED BY THE COLORADO BOARD FOR BEING IMPAIRED.

SHUKERT, SAMUEL A MD, DATE OF BIRTH AUGUST 2, 1938, LICENSE NUMBER 15357, WAS DISCIPLINED BY COLORADO ON FEBRUARY 17, 1999
DISCIPLINARY ACTION: RESTRICTION PLACED ON LICENSE; RESTRICTION PLACED ON CONTROLLED SUBSTANCE LICENSE
NOTES: NO UNPROFESSIONAL CONDUCT IDENTIFIED. RESTRICTIONS INCLUDE: NO OBSTETRICS, SURGERY OR THE PRESCRIPTION OF CONTROLLED SUBSTANCES; SHALL NOT ACCEPT COMPENSATION FROM MEDICAID, MEDICARE OR ANY INSURANCE COMPANY.

SICKBERT, SCOTT MD OF COLORADO SPRINGS, CO, WAS DISCIPLINED BY ILLINOIS ON MARCH 1, 1994
DISCIPLINARY ACTION: LICENSE SUSPENSION
OFFENSE: DISCIPLINARY ACTION BY ANOTHER STATE OR AGENCY
NOTES: DISCIPLINED IN COLORADO. SUSPENSION FOR A MINIMUM OF 5 YEARS.

SICKBERT, SCOTT F MD, DATE OF BIRTH AUGUST 31, 1954, LICENSE NUMBER 0025001 OF COLORADO SPRINGS, CO, WAS DISCIPLINED BY COLORADO ON AUGUST 21, 1992
DISCIPLINARY ACTION: 60-MONTH PROBATION; MONITORING OF PHYSICIAN PERFORMANCE
OFFENSE: SUBSTANCE ABUSE
NOTES: ALCOHOL/SUBSTANCE ABUSE/HABITUAL INTEMPERANCE. PROBATIONARY PERIOD INCLUDES TREATMENT AND PRACTICE MONITORING.

SILLS, THERON MD, DATE OF BIRTH APRIL 9, 1936, LICENSE NUMBER 0015418, WAS DISCIPLINED BY COLORADO ON FEBRUARY 16, 1996
DISCIPLINARY ACTION: RESTRICTION PLACED ON LICENSE
OFFENSE: SUBSTANDARD CARE, INCOMPETENCE OR NEGLIGENCE
NOTES: SUBSTANDARD CARE. AGREES NOT TO SUPERVISE MENTAL HEALTH CARE WORKERS OTHER THAN AT THE WELD COUNTY MENTAL HEALTH CENTER.

SIMERVILLE, JAMES J MD, DATE OF BIRTH SEPTEMBER 15, 1939, LICENSE NUMBER 0022165, WAS DISCIPLINED BY COLORADO ON OCTOBER 14, 1996
DISCIPLINARY ACTION: REPRIMAND

SIMMONS-MCNITT, SUZANNE MD, DATE OF BIRTH JUNE 29, 1954, LICENSE NUMBER 29156, WAS DISCIPLINED BY COLORADO ON JULY 9, 1998
DISCIPLINARY ACTION: REPRIMAND
OFFENSE: SUBSTANDARD CARE, INCOMPETENCE OR NEGLIGENCE
NOTES: SUBSTANDARD CARE.

SIMON, JOHN S MD, DATE OF BIRTH APRIL 18, 1941, LICENSE NUMBER 0019180 OF DENVER, CO, WAS DISCIPLINED BY COLORADO ON NOVEMBER 13, 1992
DISCIPLINARY ACTION: REPRIMAND
OFFENSE: SUBSTANDARD CARE, INCOMPETENCE OR NEGLIGENCE
NOTES: TWO OR MORE ACTS OR OMISSIONS WHICH FAILED TO MEET GENERALLY ACCEPTED STANDARDS OF MEDICAL PRACTICE.

SIMONS, JACK M JR MD, DATE OF BIRTH AUGUST 17, 1914, LICENSE NUMBER 0010277, WAS DISCIPLINED BY COLORADO ON MAY 11, 1995
DISCIPLINARY ACTION: REPRIMAND

SIMPSON, RUSSELL W MD, DATE OF BIRTH JUNE 7, 1944, LICENSE NUMBER 0021847 OF DENVER, CO, WAS DISCIPLINED BY COLORADO ON MARCH 15, 1995
DISCIPLINARY ACTION: 60-MONTH PROBATION; MONITORING OF PHYSICIAN PERFORMANCE
OFFENSE: SUBSTANCE ABUSE
NOTES: HABITUAL INTEMPERANCE OR EXCESSIVE USE OF A CONTROLLED SUBSTANCE. PROBATION INCLUDES PRACTICE AND TREATMENT MONITORING.

SIMPSON, RUSSELL W MD, DATE OF BIRTH JUNE 7, 1944, LICENSE NUMBER 21847, WAS DISCIPLINED BY COLORADO ON MARCH 19, 1998
DISCIPLINARY ACTION: 60-MONTH PROBATION; MONITORING OF PHYSICIAN PERFORMANCE
OFFENSE: FAILURE TO COMPLY WITH PREVIOUS BOARD ORDER
NOTES: VIOLATION OF A VALID BOARD ORDER. PROBATIONARY TERMS INCLUDE: ABSTINENCE FROM ALCOHOL AND CONTROLLED SUBSTANCES, TREATMENT MONITORING AND PRACTICE MONITORING.

SINGER, JONATHAN W DO, LICENSE NUMBER 0003723 OF CHEYENNE, WY, WAS DISCIPLINED BY OHIO ON MARCH 19, 1990
DISCIPLINARY ACTION: LICENSE SUSPENSION; 60-MONTH PROBATION
OFFENSE: PROVIDING FALSE INFORMATION TO THE BOARD OR OTHER HEALTH AGENCY
NOTES: COMMISSION OF FRAUD, MISREPRESENTATION OR DECEPTION IN APPLYING FOR RENEWAL OF OHIO LICENSE, DISCIPLINARY ACTION AGAINST CLINICAL PRIVILEGES BY THE DEPARTMENT OF THE AIR FORCE. REVOCATION STAYED, INDEFINITE

SUSPENSION, MINIMUM ONE YEAR, CONDITIONS FOR REINSTATEMENT. SUSPENSION AFFIRMED BY COURT OF APPEALS. ON 2/26/92 THE OHIO SUPREME COURT REFUSED JURISDICTION OF THE APPEAL OF THIS DECISION. LICENSE REINSTATED ON 1/12/94 SUBJECT TO PROBATIONARY TERMS AND CONDITIONS OF THIS ORDER.

SINGER, JONATHAN W DO, DATE OF BIRTH FEBRUARY 26, 1954, LICENSE NUMBER 29309, WAS DISCIPLINED BY COLORADO ON APRIL 22, 1999
DISCIPLINARY ACTION: 1-MONTH LICENSE SUSPENSION; 60-MONTH PROBATION
OFFENSE: SUBSTANDARD CARE, INCOMPETENCE OR NEGLIGENCE

NOTES: SUBSTANDARD CARE. PROBATIONARY TERMS INCLUDE: A RESTRICTION AGAINST PROVIDING ANY TYPE OF HORMONE THERAPY, PRACTICE MONITORING AND REEDUCATION ACTIVITIES.

SISK, JERALD LEE MD, LICENSE NUMBER 0169696 OF 15797 FORTUNE COURT, BRIGHTON, CO, WAS DISCIPLINED BY NEW YORK ON JUNE 21, 1993
DISCIPLINARY ACTION: 24-MONTH PROBATION
OFFENSE: DISCIPLINARY ACTION BY ANOTHER STATE OR AGENCY

NOTES: DISCIPLINED BY COLORADO BOARD. 2 YEAR SUSPENSION STAYED.

SLATER, GERALD E MD, DATE OF BIRTH JUNE 1, 1944, LICENSE NUMBER 0018882, WAS DISCIPLINED BY COLORADO ON MAY 17, 1996
DISCIPLINARY ACTION: 60-MONTH PROBATION; REQUIRED TO TAKE ADDITIONAL MEDICAL EDUCATION
OFFENSE: SUBSTANDARD CARE, INCOMPETENCE OR NEGLIGENCE

NOTES: SUBSTANDARD CARE AND FALSE, FRAUDULENT, MISLEADING, OR DECEPTIVE STATEMENT OR CLAIM. RE-EDUCATION ACTIVITIES AND PRACTICE MONITORING. REQUIRED TO CEASE AND DESIST FROM REPRESENTING THAT HE HOLDS ANY BOARD CERTIFICATION WHICH IN FACT HE DOES NOT HAVE.

SLATER, GERALD E MD, DATE OF BIRTH JUNE 1, 1944, LICENSE NUMBER 18882, WAS DISCIPLINED BY COLORADO ON AUGUST 15, 1997
DISCIPLINARY ACTION: REPRIMAND
OFFENSE: CRIMINAL CONVICTION OR PLEA OF GUILTY, NOLO CONTENDERE, OR NO CONTEST TO A CRIME

NOTES: FELONY CONVICTION.

SMALLWOOD, THOMAS E MD, DATE OF BIRTH AUGUST 21, 1965, LICENSE NUMBER 0032431, WAS DISCIPLINED BY COLORADO ON FEBRUARY 14, 1996
DISCIPLINARY ACTION: REPRIMAND

SMERNOFF, DEAN G MD, DATE OF BIRTH APRIL 29, 1928, LICENSE NUMBER 13317, WAS DISCIPLINED BY COLORADO ON DECEMBER 17, 1998
DISCIPLINARY ACTION: REPRIMAND

SMITH, CATHY DIANE MD, DATE OF BIRTH JULY 13, 1952, LICENSE NUMBER 26256, WAS DISCIPLINED BY COLORADO ON JANUARY 21, 1999
DISCIPLINARY ACTION: REPRIMAND

SMITH, ERIC H DO, DATE OF BIRTH APRIL 3, 1952, LICENSE NUMBER 0022553 OF WESTMINSTER, CO, WAS DISCIPLINED BY COLORADO ON FEBRUARY 15, 1994
DISCIPLINARY ACTION: EMERGENCY SUSPENSION

NOTES: PENDING PROCEEDINGS TO DETERMINE WHETHER HIS LICENSE SHOULD BE DISCIPLINED.

SMITH, ERIC H DO, DATE OF BIRTH APRIL 3, 1952 OF 3633 WEST 90TH AVENUE, WESTMINSTER, CO, WAS DISCIPLINED BY MEDICARE ON SEPTEMBER 1, 1994
DISCIPLINARY ACTION: EXCLUSION FROM THE MEDICARE AND/OR MEDICAID PROGRAM
OFFENSE: DISCIPLINARY ACTION BY ANOTHER STATE OR AGENCY

NOTES: LICENSE SUSPENDED FOR REASONS BEARING ON PROFESSIONAL COMPETENCE. REINSTATED ON 11/12/98.

SMITH, ERIC H DO, DATE OF BIRTH APRIL 3, 1952, LICENSE NUMBER 0022553, WAS DISCIPLINED BY COLORADO ON SEPTEMBER 14, 1995
DISCIPLINARY ACTION: 60-MONTH PROBATION; MONITORING OF PHYSICIAN PERFORMANCE

NOTES: TREATMENT AND PRACTICE MONITORING.

SMITH, ERIC H DO OF 1022 DEPOT HILL ROAD, BROOMFIELD, CO, WAS DISCIPLINED BY DEA ON FEBRUARY 23, 1996
DISCIPLINARY ACTION: RESTRICTION PLACED ON CONTROLLED SUBSTANCE LICENSE

NOTES: MEMO OF UNDERSTANDING.

SMITH, JOHN I MD, DATE OF BIRTH NOVEMBER 14, 1931, LICENSE NUMBER 0014232 OF AURORA, CO, WAS DISCIPLINED BY COLORADO ON SEPTEMBER 10, 1993
DISCIPLINARY ACTION: SURRENDER OF LICENSE
OFFENSE: FAILURE TO COMPLY WITH PREVIOUS BOARD ORDER

NOTES: VIOLATION OF BOARD ORDER ISSUED 8/14/92.

SMITH, JOHN I MD, DATE OF BIRTH NOVEMBER 14, 1931 OF PO BOX 2368, DILLON, CO, WAS DISCIPLINED BY MEDICARE ON MAY 4, 1995
DISCIPLINARY ACTION: EXCLUSION FROM THE MEDICARE AND/OR MEDICAID PROGRAM
OFFENSE: DISCIPLINARY ACTION BY ANOTHER STATE OR AGENCY

NOTES: LICENSE SURRENDERED FOR REASONS BEARING ON PROFESSIONAL COMPETENCE. REINSTATED ON 9/21/95.

SMITH, JOHN IRVING MD, DATE OF BIRTH NOVEMBER 14, 1931, LICENSE NUMBER 0014232 OF AURORA, CO, WAS DISCIPLINED BY COLORADO ON AUGUST 14, 1992
DISCIPLINARY ACTION: 60-MONTH PROBATION; MONITORING OF PHYSICIAN PERFORMANCE
OFFENSE: SUBSTANCE ABUSE

NOTES: ALCOHOL ABUSE/HABITUAL INTEMPERANCE; PHYSICAL OR MENTAL DISABILITY WHICH RENDERS HIM UNABLE TO PRACTICE WITH SKILL AND SAFETY. PROBATIONARY PERIOD INCLUDES TREATMENT AND PRACTICE MONITORING.

SMITH, JOHN IRVING MD, DATE OF BIRTH NOVEMBER 14, 1931, LICENSE NUMBER 0014232, WAS DISCIPLINED BY COLORADO ON NOVEMBER 6, 1992
DISCIPLINARY ACTION: LICENSE SUSPENSION
OFFENSE: FAILURE TO COMPLY WITH PREVIOUS BOARD ORDER

NOTES: VIOLATION OF STIPULATION/ORDER DATED 8/14/92.

SMITH, JOHN M MD, DATE OF BIRTH AUGUST 23, 1942, LICENSE NUMBER 0016403 OF COLORADO SPRINGS, CO, WAS DISCIPLINED BY COLORADO ON SEPTEMBER 30, 1994

DISCIPLINARY ACTION: REPRIMAND

SMITH, URBY DUANE MD, LICENSE NUMBER 0420504 OF P.O. BOX 366, ELLSWORTH, KS, WAS DISCIPLINED BY KANSAS ON DECEMBER 30, 1993
DISCIPLINARY ACTION: 2-MONTH LICENSE SUSPENSION; RESTRICTION PLACED ON LICENSE
OFFENSE: SUBSTANDARD CARE, INCOMPETENCE OR NEGLIGENCE

NOTES: COMMITTED REPEATED INSTANCES INVOLVING FAILURE TO ADHERE TO THE APPLICABLE STANDARD OF CARE TO A DEGREE CONSTITUTING ORDINARY NEGLIGENCE. PROVIDED FALSE INFORMATION IN APPLICATIONS FOR PRIVILEGES TO ONE HOSPITAL AND PRISON HEALTH SERVICES. DECISION WAS AFFIRMED BY DISTRICT COURT ON 5/13/94. PUBLIC CENSURE. MAY NOT PERFORM COLONOSCOPIES AND BONE MARROW ASPIRATIONS FOR A PERIOD OF AT LEAST ONE YEAR, AT WHICH TIME HE MAY PETITION FOR TERMINATION OF THIS LIMITATION; THE BURDEN OF PROOF SHALL BE UPON HIM TO SHOW COMPETENCY AND PROFICIENCY IN THE PERFORMANCE OF THESE PROCEDURES AND FAILING SUCH A SHOWING, THE ABOVE-MENTIONED LIMITATION SHALL REMAIN IN EFFECT.

SMITH, URBY DUANE MD, DATE OF BIRTH JUNE 10, 1942, LICENSE NUMBER 0018049 OF ELLSWORTH, KS, WAS DISCIPLINED BY COLORADO ON APRIL 12, 1995
DISCIPLINARY ACTION: 24-MONTH PROBATION; MONITORING OF PHYSICIAN PERFORMANCE
OFFENSE: DISCIPLINARY ACTION BY ANOTHER STATE OR AGENCY

NOTES: NO UNPROFESSIONAL CONDUCT IDENTIFIED. COMPLIANCE WITH A KANSAS STIPULATION.

SMITH-RUDNICK, ANN KATHLEEN MD, LICENSE NUMBER 170459 OF 8966 W BOWLES AVENUE, LITTLETON, CO, WAS DISCIPLINED BY NEW YORK ON OCTOBER 7, 1999
DISCIPLINARY ACTION: 60-MONTH PROBATION
OFFENSE: DISCIPLINARY ACTION BY ANOTHER STATE OR AGENCY

NOTES: DISCIPLINED BY THE COLORADO BOARD FOR FAILING TO MAINTAIN PERTINENT INFORMATION REGARDING CONTROLLED SUBSTANCES PRESCRIPTIONS. PROBATION RETROACTIVE TO 8/18/98.

SMITH-RUDNIK, ANN K MD, DATE OF BIRTH JULY 29, 1958, LICENSE NUMBER 30352, WAS DISCIPLINED BY COLORADO ON AUGUST 14, 1998
DISCIPLINARY ACTION: 60-MONTH PROBATION; MONITORING OF PHYSICIAN PERFORMANCE
OFFENSE: NONCOMPLIANCE WITH A PROFESSIONAL RULE

NOTES: FAILURE TO KEEP PROPER RECORDS. PROBATIONARY TERMS INCLUDE PRACTICE MONITORING AND TREATMENT MONITORING.

SMOLLEY, JOHN JR MD, DATE OF BIRTH JUNE 7, 1956, LICENSE NUMBER 36742, WAS DISCIPLINED BY COLORADO ON JANUARY 8, 1998
DISCIPLINARY ACTION: 120-MONTH PROBATION; MONITORING OF PHYSICIAN PERFORMANCE
OFFENSE: SUBSTANCE ABUSE

NOTES: HISTORY OF HABITUAL INTEMPERANCE OR EXCESSIVE USE OF A CONTROLLED SUBSTANCE. PROBATIONARY TERMS INCLUDE ABSTINENCE FROM ALCOHOL AND CONTROLLED SUBSTANCES, TREATMENT MONITORING AND PRACTICE MONITORING.

SNIVELY, STEVEN L MD, DATE OF BIRTH AUGUST 15, 1950, LICENSE NUMBER 0027144 OF ENGLEWOOD, CO, WAS DISCIPLINED BY COLORADO ON JULY 16, 1993
DISCIPLINARY ACTION: REPRIMAND

SNOOK, RANDALL MD OF 7780 S. BROADWAY #100, LITTLETON, CO, WAS DISCIPLINED BY DEA ON AUGUST 27, 1999
DISCIPLINARY ACTION: SURRENDER OF CONTROLLED SUBSTANCE LICENSE

SNYDER, CHARLES E MD, DATE OF BIRTH SEPTEMBER 13, 1944, LICENSE NUMBER 20838, WAS DISCIPLINED BY COLORADO ON JULY 9, 1998
DISCIPLINARY ACTION: PROBATION; MONITORING OF PHYSICIAN PERFORMANCE
OFFENSE: CRIMINAL CONVICTION OR PLEA OF GUILTY, NOLO CONTENDERE, OR NO CONTEST TO A CRIME

NOTES: FRAUD, MISREPRESENTATION OR DECEPTION IN OBTAINING OR RENEWING A LICENSE; FELONY CONVICTION; HABITUAL INTEMPERANCE OR EXCESSIVE USE OF A CONTROLLED SUBSTANCE AND PHYSICAL OR MENTAL DISABILITY. HE AGREES TO AN INDEFINITE PERIOD OF PROBATION WITH TERMS THAT INCLUDE: ABSTINENCE FROM ALCOHOL AND CONTROLLED SUBSTANCES, TREATMENT MONITORING AND PRACTICE MONITORING.

SNYDER, CHARLES E MD, DATE OF BIRTH SEPTEMBER 13, 1944, LICENSE NUMBER 20838, WAS DISCIPLINED BY COLORADO ON FEBRUARY 17, 1999
DISCIPLINARY ACTION: EMERGENCY SUSPENSION

SOLOMON, MAURICE C MD, DATE OF BIRTH AUGUST 23, 1939, LICENSE NUMBER 0017622 OF COLORADO SPRINGS, CO, WAS DISCIPLINED BY COLORADO ON SEPTEMBER 17, 1993
DISCIPLINARY ACTION: 60-MONTH PROBATION; MONITORING OF PHYSICIAN PERFORMANCE
OFFENSE: SUBSTANCE ABUSE

NOTES: EXCESSIVE USE OF A CONTROLLED SUBSTANCE; SELF PRESCRIBING A SCHEDULE II CONTROLLED SUBSTANCE; ADMINISTERING, DISPENSING, OR PRESCRIBING A CONTROLLED SUBSTANCE OTHER THAN IN THE COURSE OF LEGITIMATE PROFESSIONAL PRACTICE. PROBATIONARY PERIOD INCLUDES PRACTICE AND TREATMENT MONITORING.

SOLOMON, MAURICE C MD, LICENSE NUMBER 0G23212 OF COLORADO SPRINGS, CO, WAS DISCIPLINED BY CALIFORNIA ON JANUARY 30, 1995
DISCIPLINARY ACTION: 60-MONTH PROBATION
OFFENSE: DISCIPLINARY ACTION BY ANOTHER STATE OR AGENCY

NOTES: DISCIPLINED BY COLORADO BOARD FOR SUBSTANCE ABUSE. REVOCATION STAYED.

SOLOMON, MAURICE COCHRAN MD OF 1622 RAINIER DRIVE, COLORADO SPRINGS, CO, WAS DISCIPLINED BY DEA ON MAY 31, 1995
DISCIPLINARY ACTION: SURRENDER OF CONTROLLED SUBSTANCE LICENSE
OFFENSE: DISCIPLINARY ACTION BY ANOTHER STATE OR AGENCY

NOTES: STATE BOARD.

SPAULDING, LYMAN B MD, DATE OF BIRTH FEBRUARY 16, 1943, LICENSE NUMBER 0030034, WAS DISCIPLINED BY COLORADO ON NOVEMBER 16, 1995
DISCIPLINARY ACTION: REPRIMAND

SPAULDING, LYMAN BLAINE MD, LICENSE NUMBER 0G39247 OF FORT MORGAN, CO, WAS DISCIPLINED BY CALIFORNIA ON DECEMBER 5, 1996
DISCIPLINARY ACTION: REPRIMAND
OFFENSE: DISCIPLINARY ACTION BY ANOTHER STATE OR AGENCY

NOTES: DISCIPLINED BY COLORADO FOR MISTAKENLY REMOVING A PATIENT'S OVARIES DURING A HYSTERECTOMY AND FOR PERFORMING A CIRCUMCISION WITHOUT THE APPROPRIATE PARENTAL CONSENT FORM.

SPIEGELMAN, WILLARD G MD, DATE OF BIRTH OCTOBER 28, 1942, LICENSE NUMBER 0028879 OF VAIL, CO, WAS DISCIPLINED BY COLORADO ON MARCH 15, 1991
DISCIPLINARY ACTION: PROBATION
OFFENSE: FAILURE TO COMPLY WITH PREVIOUS BOARD ORDER

NOTES: PROBATION IS EXTENDED SIX MONTHS FOR FAILURE TO COMPLY WITH PROBATIONARY CONDITIONS. PROBATION DEEMED CONCLUDED EFFECTIVE 6/14/91.

SPRINGER, GREGG E MD, DATE OF BIRTH MARCH 7, 1945, LICENSE NUMBER 0017915 OF COLORADO SPRINGS, CO, WAS DISCIPLINED BY COLORADO ON DECEMBER 10, 1993
DISCIPLINARY ACTION: 60-MONTH PROBATION; MONITORING OF PHYSICIAN PERFORMANCE
OFFENSE: SUBSTANCE ABUSE

NOTES: ALLEGATIONS OF EXCESSIVE USE OF A CONTROLLED SUBSTANCE. PROBATIONARY PERIOD INCLUDES TREATMENT AND PRACTICE MONITORING.

SPRINGER, GREGG E MD, DATE OF BIRTH MARCH 7, 1945, LICENSE NUMBER 0017915, WAS DISCIPLINED BY COLORADO ON OCTOBER 10, 1996
DISCIPLINARY ACTION: EMERGENCY SUSPENSION

SPRINGER, GREGG E MD, DATE OF BIRTH MARCH 7, 1945, LICENSE NUMBER 17915, WAS DISCIPLINED BY COLORADO ON JANUARY 9, 1997
DISCIPLINARY ACTION: MONITORING OF PHYSICIAN PERFORMANCE
OFFENSE: FAILURE TO COMPLY WITH PREVIOUS BOARD ORDER

NOTES: VIOLATION OF A VALID BOARD ORDER AND GIVING A SCHEDULE II SUBSTANCE TO SELF OR A FAMILY MEMBER. REVOCATION STAYED FOR AN INDEFINITE PERIOD. HE MAY NOT PRACTICE UNTIL TREATERS STATE THAT HE IS SAFE TO RESUME PRACTICE; SHALL BE SUBJECT TO TREATMENT AND PRACTICE MONITORING PROVISIONS.

SPRINGER, GREGG E MD, DATE OF BIRTH MARCH 7, 1945, LICENSE NUMBER 1048010 OF 509 BEAR PAW LANE, COLORADO SPRINGS, CO, WAS DISCIPLINED BY MICHIGAN ON AUGUST 15, 1997
DISCIPLINARY ACTION: PROBATION; FINE
OFFENSE: DISCIPLINARY ACTION BY ANOTHER STATE OR AGENCY

NOTES: FAILURE TO REPORT/COMPLY. $2000 FINE.

SPRINGER, GREGG EDWARD MD, LICENSE NUMBER 0017379, WAS DISCIPLINED BY ARIZONA ON MAY 4, 1995

NOTES: 90 DAYS PRIOR TO PRACTICING MEDICINE IN ARIZONA, SHALL NOTIFY THE ARIZONA BOARD OF HIS INTENT TO DO SO.

STEINBERG, MARTIN MD OF 300 S JACKSON STREET #203, DENVER, CO, WAS DISCIPLINED BY DEA ON SEPTEMBER 9, 1991
DISCIPLINARY ACTION: DENIAL OF NEW LICENSE
OFFENSE: PRACTICING WITHOUT A VALID CONTROLLED SUBSTANCE LICENSE

NOTES: IN LATE 1989 AN INDIVIDUAL AND HIS WIFE GAVE STATEMENTS TO DENVER POLICE ALLEGING THAT HE KNOWINGLY MAINTAINED THE INDIVIDUAL'S DRUG ADDICTION BY PRESCRIBING HIM VARIOUS CONTROLLED SUBSTANCES ON A REGULAR BASIS OVER A 2 YEAR PERIOD. THE PATIENT HAD SUSTAINED BONE FRACTURES TO HIS RIGHT ARM IN 1986 AND WAS GIVEN CONTROLLED SUBSTANCES WHILE HOSPITALIZED. UPON HIS RELEASE THE INDIVIDUAL BELIEVED HE WAS ADDICTED TO DRUGS. IN THE FALL OF 1987, HE WENT TO DR. STEINBERG FOR COUNSELING AND ASKED FOR PERCODAN. DR. STEINBERG PRESCRIBED HIM PERCODAN, DEXEDRINE AND RITALIN. PATIENT CLAIMED THE DOCTOR NEVER FILLED OUT A PATIENT/MEDICAL HISTORY NOR WAS HE EVER EXAMINED. DR. STEINBERG DID NOT MAINTAIN A PATIENT CHART FOR THIS PERSON; HE ALSO HAD NOT BEEN REGISTERED WITH DEA SINCE 1972. DEA OFFICIALS MET WITH HIM 1/26/90 INFORMING HIM HE WAS NOT AUTHORIZED TO PRESCRIBE CONTROLLED SUBSTANCES. HE WROTE 12 PRESCRIPTIONS AFTER THIS MEETING.

STEINBERG, MARTIN C MD, DATE OF BIRTH FEBRUARY 6, 1928, LICENSE NUMBER 0012793 OF DENVER, CO, WAS DISCIPLINED BY COLORADO ON APRIL 13, 1994
OFFENSE: PHYSICAL OR MENTAL ILLNESS INHIBITING THE ABILITY TO PRACTICE WITH SKILL AND SAFETY

NOTES: NO UNPROFESSIONAL CONDUCT IDENTIFIED. PHYSICAL CONDITION HAS AFFECTED HIS ABILITY TO PRACTICE MEDICINE WITH REASONABLE SKILL AND SAFETY TO PATIENTS. HE AGREES TO CEASE THE PRACTICE OF MEDICINE IN COLORADO AND TO PERMANENTLY MAINTAIN HIS COLORADO MEDICAL LICENSE IN INACTIVE STATUS.

STEVENS, WILLIAM CRAIG DO, DATE OF BIRTH AUGUST 23, 1938, LICENSE NUMBER 0021085, WAS DISCIPLINED BY COLORADO ON APRIL 10, 1991
DISCIPLINARY ACTION: 60-MONTH PROBATION; REQUIRED TO TAKE ADDITIONAL MEDICAL EDUCATION
OFFENSE: SUBSTANDARD CARE, INCOMPETENCE OR NEGLIGENCE

NOTES: TWO OR MORE ACTS OR OMISSIONS WHICH FAIL TO MEET GENERALLY ACCEPTED STANDARDS OF MEDICAL PRACTICE. ORDER INCLUDES PHYSICIAN PRACTICE MONITORING, 50 HOURS OF CONTINUING MEDICAL EDUCATION YEARLY, AND NO SUPERVISION OF PHYSICIAN ASSISTANTS OR PHYSICIAN EXTENDERS.

STEVENS, WILLIAM CRAIG DO, DATE OF BIRTH AUGUST 23, 1938, LICENSE NUMBER 0021085, WAS DISCIPLINED BY COLORADO ON FEBRUARY 17, 1992
DISCIPLINARY ACTION: EMERGENCY SUSPENSION
OFFENSE: SUBSTANDARD CARE, INCOMPETENCE OR NEGLIGENCE

NOTES: TWO OR MORE ACTS OF SUBSTANDARD PATIENT CARE.

STEVENS, WILLIAM CRAIG DO, DATE OF BIRTH AUGUST 23, 1938, LICENSE NUMBER 0021085, WAS DISCIPLINED BY COLORADO ON SEPTEMBER 18, 1992
DISCIPLINARY ACTION: LICENSE REVOCATION
OFFENSE: SUBSTANDARD CARE, INCOMPETENCE OR NEGLIGENCE

NOTES: ACTS OR OMISSIONS OF GROSSLY NEGLIGENT MEDICAL PRACTICE AND/OR SUBSTANDARD MEDICAL PRACTICE. HAS APPEALED TO THE COLORADO COURT OF APPEALS. COURT REVERSED ORDER AND CASE REMANDED WITH DIRECTIONS ON 10/28/93.

STEVENS, WILLIAM CRAIG DO, DATE OF BIRTH AUGUST 23, 1938, LICENSE NUMBER 0021085 OF MOORESTOWN, CO, WAS DISCIPLINED BY COLORADO ON MARCH 16, 1995
DISCIPLINARY ACTION: LICENSE REVOCATION
OFFENSE: SUBSTANDARD CARE, INCOMPETENCE OR NEGLIGENCE

NOTES: SUBSTANDARD CARE. CASE ON APPEAL WITH COLORADO COURT OF APPEALS AS OF 4/30/95.

STEVENS, WILLIAM CRAIG DO, DATE OF BIRTH AUGUST 23, 1938, LICENSE NUMBER 0002464 OF DULUTH, GA, WAS DISCIPLINED BY KENTUCKY ON APRIL 13, 1996
DISCIPLINARY ACTION: 24-MONTH PROBATION; MONITORING OF PHYSICIAN PERFORMANCE

NOTES: GRANTED LICENSURE WITH PROBATIONARY PERIOD; MUST CONSULT WITH IMPAIRED PHYSICIANS PROGRAM; SUBJECT TO PATIENT CHART REVIEWS.

STINSON, MICHAEL MD, LICENSE NUMBER 000T327 OF AURORA, CO, WAS DISCIPLINED BY SOUTH CAROLINA ON FEBRUARY 27, 1991

NOTES: TEMPORARY LICENSE ISSUED WITH CONDITIONS.

STIRMAN, JERRY A MD, DATE OF BIRTH OCTOBER 13, 1924, LICENSE NUMBER 0013957 OF 653 CANYON ROAD #6, SANTA FE, NM, WAS DISCIPLINED BY COLORADO ON JANUARY 24, 1994
OFFENSE: SUBSTANDARD CARE, INCOMPETENCE OR NEGLIGENCE

NOTES: ACTION BASED ON ALLEGATIONS OF SUBSTANDARD CARE--TWO OR MORE ACTS OR OMISSIONS WHICH FAIL TO MEET GENERALLY ACCEPTED STANDARDS OF MEDICAL PRACTICE IN PRACTICE HE PROVIDED TO PATIENTS IN THE EMERGENCY ROOM IN 4/91. HE DENIES SUBSTANDARD CARE. AGREES TO NO FURTHER MEDICAL PRACTICE IN COLORADO, TO ALLOW HIS LICENSE TO PERMANENTLY LAPSE.

STIRMAN, JERRY A MD, DATE OF BIRTH OCTOBER 13, 1924 OF 653 CANYON ROAD #6, SANTA FE, NM, WAS DISCIPLINED BY MEDICARE ON NOVEMBER 9, 1994
DISCIPLINARY ACTION: EXCLUSION FROM THE MEDICARE AND/OR MEDICAID PROGRAM
OFFENSE: DISCIPLINARY ACTION BY ANOTHER STATE OR AGENCY

NOTES: LICENSE REVOKED FOR REASONS BEARING ON PROFESSIONAL PERFORMANCE.

STIRMAN, JERRY A MD OF 653 CANYON ROAD, SANTA FE, NM, WAS DISCIPLINED BY NEW MEXICO ON DECEMBER 1, 1994
DISCIPLINARY ACTION: SURRENDER OF LICENSE

NOTES: IN LIEU OF ACTION.

STUART, WALLACE E MD, DATE OF BIRTH MAY 13, 1934, LICENSE NUMBER 20666, WAS DISCIPLINED BY COLORADO ON JUNE 12, 1997
DISCIPLINARY ACTION: SURRENDER OF LICENSE

NOTES: NO UNPROFESSIONAL CONDUCT IDENTIFIED.

SULLIVAN, KEVIN P MD, DATE OF BIRTH OCTOBER 21, 1951, LICENSE NUMBER 0023423, WAS DISCIPLINED BY COLORADO ON AUGUST 17, 1995
DISCIPLINARY ACTION: 60-MONTH PROBATION; MONITORING OF PHYSICIAN PERFORMANCE

NOTES: PRACTICE MONITORING.

SULLIVAN, KEVIN P MD, DATE OF BIRTH OCTOBER 21, 1951, LICENSE NUMBER 23423, WAS DISCIPLINED BY COLORADO ON OCTOBER 16, 1997
DISCIPLINARY ACTION: LICENSE REVOCATION
OFFENSE: SUBSTANDARD CARE, INCOMPETENCE OR NEGLIGENCE

NOTES: SUBSTANDARD CARE.

SULLIVAN, KEVIN P MD, LICENSE NUMBER 7632 OF PUYALLUP, WA, WAS DISCIPLINED BY NEW HAMPSHIRE ON SEPTEMBER 8, 1998
DISCIPLINARY ACTION: LICENSE REVOCATION
OFFENSE: DISCIPLINARY ACTION BY ANOTHER STATE OR AGENCY

NOTES: ACTION TAKEN IN COLORADO FOR GROSS NEGLIGENCE.

SULLIVAN, KEVIN P MD, LICENSE NUMBER 31847 OF PUYALLUP, WA, WAS DISCIPLINED BY WASHINGTON ON NOVEMBER 20, 1998
DISCIPLINARY ACTION: LICENSE REVOCATION
OFFENSE: DISCIPLINARY ACTION BY ANOTHER STATE OR AGENCY

NOTES: ENGAGED IN ACTS OF MORAL TURPITUDE; MISREPRESENTATION IN OBTAINING A LICENSE OR REINSTATEMENT OF A LICENSE; DISCIPLINE IN ANOTHER STATE; AND WILLFULLY MISREPRESENTING FACTS DURING A DISCIPLINARY PROCEEDING.

SULLIVAN, KEVIN P MD, LICENSE NUMBER 57163 OF 5922 100TH STREET SW SUITE 26, TACOMA, WA, WAS DISCIPLINED BY MASSACHUSETTS ON DECEMBER 16, 1998
DISCIPLINARY ACTION: LICENSE REVOCATION
OFFENSE: DISCIPLINARY ACTION BY ANOTHER STATE OR AGENCY

NOTES: IN 7/95 AND 10/97 DISCIPLINED BY THE COLORADO BOARD FIRST FOR FAILING TO DOCUMENT INFORMATION ON THE RECORDS OF TWO PATIENTS, AND SECOND FOR COMMITTING GROSS NEGLIGENCE IN THE TREATMENT OF ONE PATIENT; ALSO, FRAUDULENTLY PROCURED HIS MASSACHUSETTS LICENSE RENEWAL BY FAILING TO DISCLOSE THE COLORADO DISCIPLINE.

SULLIVAN, KEVIN PAUL MD, LICENSE NUMBER 0G35765 OF CHICAGO, IL, WAS DISCIPLINED BY CALIFORNIA ON JULY 31, 1996
DISCIPLINARY ACTION: REPRIMAND
OFFENSE: DISCIPLINARY ACTION BY ANOTHER STATE OR AGENCY

NOTES: DISCIPLINARY ACTION IN COLORADO FOR FAILING TO DOCUMENT PATIENT FILES.

SULLIVAN, KEVIN PAUL MD, LICENSE NUMBER G35765 OF CHICAGO, IL, WAS DISCIPLINED BY CALIFORNIA ON NOVEMBER 2, 1998
DISCIPLINARY ACTION: 12-MONTH LICENSE SUSPENSION
OFFENSE: DISCIPLINARY ACTION BY ANOTHER STATE OR AGENCY

NOTES: DISCIPLINED BY COLORADO FOR GROSS NEGLIGENCE RESULTING FROM HIS FAILURE TO PROPERLY TREAT A LEG INJURY RESULTING IN THE PATIENT'S DEATH. IF WITHIN THE 12 MONTH SUSPENSION, THE ORDER OF THE COLORADO BOARD IS OVERTURNED, THIS ORDER WILL BE VACATED; IF THE COLORADO ORDER IS NOT OVERTURNED WITHIN 12 MONTHS HE SHALL IMMEDIATELY SURRENDER HIS CALIFORNIA LICENSE.

SULLIVAN, KEVIN PAUL MD, DATE OF BIRTH OCTOBER 21, 1951, LICENSE NUMBER 32178 OF PUYALLUP, WA, WAS DISCIPLINED BY NORTH CAROLINA ON MARCH 10, 1999
DISCIPLINARY ACTION: LICENSE REVOCATION
OFFENSE: DISCIPLINARY ACTION BY ANOTHER STATE OR AGENCY

NOTES: ON 10/18/97, COLORADO REVOKED HIS MEDICAL LICENSE UPON FINDINGS THAT INCLUDED GROSSLY NEGLIGENT MEDICAL PRACTICE.

SULLIVAN, KEVIN PAUL MD, DATE OF BIRTH OCTOBER 21, 1951 OF

4441 S MENDION, PUYALLUP, WA, WAS DISCIPLINED BY MEDICARE ON APRIL 20, 1999
DISCIPLINARY ACTION: EXCLUSION FROM THE MEDICARE AND/OR MEDICAID PROGRAM
OFFENSE: DISCIPLINARY ACTION BY ANOTHER STATE OR AGENCY

NOTES: LICENSE REVOKED, SUSPENDED, SURRENDERED OR OTHERWISE LOST FOR REASONS BEARING ON PROFESSIONAL PERFORMANCE, PROFESSIONAL COMPETENCE OR FINANCIAL INTEGRITY.

SULLIVAN, KEVIN PAUL MD, LICENSE NUMBER G35765 OF CHICAGO, IL, WAS DISCIPLINED BY CALIFORNIA ON DECEMBER 2, 1999
DISCIPLINARY ACTION: LICENSE REVOCATION

SUTHERLAND, JESSE O JR MD, DATE OF BIRTH SEPTEMBER 4, 1945, LICENSE NUMBER 0022563 OF DENVER, CO, WAS DISCIPLINED BY COLORADO ON APRIL 14, 1994
DISCIPLINARY ACTION: REPRIMAND
OFFENSE: PROFESSIONAL MISCONDUCT

SWARTZ, JOE M MD, DATE OF BIRTH OCTOBER 7, 1947, LICENSE NUMBER 0025956 OF BOULDER, CO, WAS DISCIPLINED BY COLORADO ON NOVEMBER 10, 1994
DISCIPLINARY ACTION: REPRIMAND

SWARTZ, JOE M MD, DATE OF BIRTH OCTOBER 7, 1947, LICENSE NUMBER 0025956, WAS DISCIPLINED BY COLORADO ON JUNE 8, 1995
DISCIPLINARY ACTION: REPRIMAND

SWARTZ, JOE M MD, LICENSE NUMBER 0C36167 OF BOULDER, CO, WAS DISCIPLINED BY CALIFORNIA ON FEBRUARY 13, 1996
DISCIPLINARY ACTION: REPRIMAND
OFFENSE: DISCIPLINARY ACTION BY ANOTHER STATE OR AGENCY

NOTES: ACTION IN COLORADO FOR UNJUSTIFIED USE OF NARCOTICS FOR MANAGEMENT OF PATIENT'S ABUSIVE MEMORY AND POST-TRAUMATIC STRESS DISORDER.

SWARTZ, JOE MATTHEW MD, LICENSE NUMBER 00E1145 OF BOULDER, CO, WAS DISCIPLINED BY TEXAS ON AUGUST 18, 1995
DISCIPLINARY ACTION: REPRIMAND
OFFENSE: DISCIPLINARY ACTION BY ANOTHER STATE OR AGENCY

NOTES: IN 10/91, COLORADO BOARD ISSUED HIM A LETTER OF ADMONITION BASED ON HIS PRESCRIBING CONTROLLED SUBSTANCES INCLUDING, BUT NOT LIMITED TO, HYDROCODONE, PERCOCET AND VICODIN TO A PATIENT WITHOUT ADEQUATE INDICATIONS OF A LEGITIMATE MEDICAL PURPOSE; MAINTAINS PRESCRIBING WAS MEDICALLY APPROPRIATE; IN APPROXIMATELY 1/95, HE ENTERED A PLEA OF GUILTY AND WAS CONVICTED FOR A FEDERAL CRIMINAL OFFENSE FOR MAKING A FALSE STATEMENT ON AN APPLICATION FOR MEDICARE PAYMENT. LICENSE RESTRICTED WITH TERMS: SHALL NOT PRACTICE MEDICINE IN TEXAS UNTIL HE APPEARS BEFORE BOARD WITH SUFFICIENT EVIDENCE WHICH INDICATES THAT HE IS PHYSICALLY, MENTALLY AND OTHERWISE COMPETENT TO SAFELY PRACTICE MEDICINE, HAS COMPLIED WITH ALL TERMS OF PROBATION AS SET FORTH IN COURT'S JUDGMENT AND HAS FULLY COMPLIED WITH AND SATISFIED ALL TERMS OF ANY ACTION TAKEN BY ANOTHER STATE; SHALL COOPERATE WITH BOARD IN VERIFYING COMPLIANCE; SHALL GIVE A COPY OF THIS ORDER TO ANY HEALTH CARE ENTITY WHERE HE HAS PRIVILEGES; TIME PERIOD OUT OF TEXAS DOES NOT COUNT TOWARD RESTRICTION; SHALL INFORM BOARD OF CHANGE OF ADDRESS WITHIN 10 DAYS OR IF HE LEAVES THE STATE. SHALL NOT SEEK MODIFICATION FOR ONE YEAR.

SWARTZ, JOSEPH MATTHEW MD, DATE OF BIRTH OCTOBER 7, 1947 OF 3061 4TH STREET, BOULDER, CO, WAS DISCIPLINED BY MEDICARE ON APRIL 11, 1995
DISCIPLINARY ACTION: 60-MONTH EXCLUSION FROM THE MEDICARE AND/OR MEDICAID PROGRAM
OFFENSE: CRIMINAL CONVICTION OR PLEA OF GUILTY, NOLO CONTENDERE, OR NO CONTEST TO A CRIME

NOTES: CONVICTED OF A CRIME INVOLVING THE MEDICARE, MEDICAID, MATERNAL AND CHILD HEALTH SERVICES BLOCK GRANT OR BLOCK GRANTS TO STATES FOR SOCIAL SERVICES PROGRAMS.

SWEENEY, RICHARD MD, DATE OF BIRTH JANUARY 14, 1956, LICENSE NUMBER 0026441 OF 7720 SOUTH BROADWAY #580, LITTLETON, CO, WAS DISCIPLINED BY COLORADO ON AUGUST 19, 1992
DISCIPLINARY ACTION: EMERGENCY SUSPENSION
OFFENSE: SEXUAL ABUSE OF OR SEXUAL MISCONDUCT WITH A PATIENT

NOTES: ENGAGING IN SEXUAL ACTS WITH FOUR PATIENTS. THIS CONDUCT CONSTITUTES UNPROFESSIONAL CONDUCT; SUFFERS FROM A MENTAL CONDITION THAT MANIFESTS ITSELF IN SEXUALLY EXPLOITATIVE BEHAVIOR OF WOMEN.

SWEENEY, RICHARD MD, DATE OF BIRTH JANUARY 14, 1956, LICENSE NUMBER 0026441 OF 7720 SOUTH BROADWAY #580, LITTLETON, CO, WAS DISCIPLINED BY COLORADO ON JUNE 11, 1993
DISCIPLINARY ACTION: LICENSE REVOCATION
OFFENSE: SEXUAL ABUSE OF OR SEXUAL MISCONDUCT WITH A PATIENT

NOTES: SUBSTANDARD CARE IN THAT HE HAD A SEXUAL AFFAIR WITH A FEMALE EMPLOYEE STARTING IN 9/88 WHILE CONCURRENTLY PROVIDING INFERTILITY COUNSELING AND CARE TO HER AND HER HUSBAND; PERFORMED AN ABORTION UPON A FETUS WHEN HE COULD HAVE BEEN THE FATHER, THEREBY CLEARLY NOT BEING ABLE TO PROVIDE OBJECTIVE COUNSELING; FAILED TO CREATE A RECORD OF THE PROCEDURE; NO EVIDENCE THAT THE ABORTION PERFORMED WAS TECHNICALLY DEFICIENT; BETWEEN 10/90 AND 4/92 HAD SEXUAL RELATIONSHIPS WITH TWO ADDITIONAL PATIENTS, WHO WERE ALSO EMPLOYEES, ONE WHO WAS A PATIENT FROM 8/91 THROUGH 4/92 AND ANOTHER WHOM HE SAW ONLY OCCASIONALLY; ALL THREE OF THESE RELATIONSHIPS WERE MUTUALLY CONSENSUAL, NEVER OCCURRED DURING ACTUAL MEDICAL TREATMENT AND IN TWO CASES OFTEN OCCURRED OUTSIDE THE OFFICE SETTING; IN 7/92 HE SOUGHT PSYCHIATRIC TREATMENT IN CONNECTION WITH HIS SEXUAL BEHAVIOR AND WAS EVALUATED UPON REQUEST OF THE BOARD; HAS A MENTAL CONDITION AND DISABILITY WHICH MANIFESTS ITSELF IN SEXUALLY EXPLOITATIVE BEHAVIOR TOWARD WOMEN AND WHICH RENDERS HIM UNABLE TO PERFORM MEDICAL SERVICES WITH REASONABLE SKILL AND SAFETY; THERE IS NO EVIDENCE HE HAS EVER PREVIOUSLY ENGAGED IN SEXUAL RELATIONS WITH A PATIENT WHO IS NOT ALSO HIS EMPLOYEE; RECEIVING TREATMENT FOR THIS DISABILITY.

TAYLOR, JAMES K MD, DATE OF BIRTH MARCH 3, 1939, LICENSE NUMBER 0026717 OF DENVER, CO, WAS DISCIPLINED BY

COLORADO ON SEPTEMBER 11, 1992
DISCIPLINARY ACTION: 12-MONTH PROBATION; 12-MONTH RESTRICTION PLACED ON LICENSE

NOTES: APPLICATION FOR LICENSURE REINSTATEMENT. LICENSE HAD LAPSED FOR NON-RENEWAL ON 3/31/85 AND HE HAD NOT PRACTICED IN HIS SPECIALTY SINCE THAT TIME. LICENSE REINSTATED UNDER PROBATIONARY CONDITIONS: LIMITS PRACTICE TO TRAINING PROGRAM AT DENVER GENERAL HOSPITAL. A FINDING OF UNPROFESSIONAL CONDUCT WAS SPECIFICALLY NOT MADE.

TEETER, BRIAN H MD, DATE OF BIRTH JUNE 17, 1950, LICENSE NUMBER 0027329 OF JOPLIN, MO, WAS DISCIPLINED BY COLORADO ON MAY 20, 1994
DISCIPLINARY ACTION: SURRENDER OF LICENSE
OFFENSE: OVERPRESCRIBING OR MISPRESCRIBING DRUGS

NOTES: NO UNPROFESSIONAL CONDUCT IDENTIFIED. CONTROLLED SUBSTANCE PRESCRIBING TO FAMILY MEMBER IN MISSOURI. PERMANENT SURRENDER.

TELLO, ROBERT J MD, DATE OF BIRTH MARCH 3, 1947, LICENSE NUMBER 0022781, WAS DISCIPLINED BY COLORADO ON JULY 11, 1996
DISCIPLINARY ACTION: REPRIMAND

THAYER, DAVID O MD, DATE OF BIRTH FEBRUARY 11, 1949, LICENSE NUMBER 0027055, WAS DISCIPLINED BY COLORADO ON MAY 17, 1996
DISCIPLINARY ACTION: 60-MONTH PROBATION; REQUIRED TO TAKE ADDITIONAL MEDICAL EDUCATION
OFFENSE: PROFESSIONAL MISCONDUCT

NOTES: UNPROFESSIONAL CONDUCT, NO SPECIFIC TYPE. RE-EDUCATION ACTIVITIES AND PRACTICE MONITORING.

THAYER, DAVID ORR MD, LICENSE NUMBER 139229 OF 2100 RIVERSIDE LANE, BOULDER, CO, WAS DISCIPLINED BY NEW YORK ON JUNE 17, 1997
DISCIPLINARY ACTION: 60-MONTH PROBATION
OFFENSE: DISCIPLINARY ACTION BY ANOTHER STATE OR AGENCY

NOTES: DISCIPLINED BY THE COLORADO BOARD FOR GROSS NEGLIGENCE INVOLVING HIS CARE AND TREATMENT OF A SURGICAL PATIENT. PROBATION COMMENCING UPON PRACTICING IN NEW YORK AND RENEWAL OF NEW YORK LICENSE. ON 10/27/97 LICENSE SURRENDERED.

THERMOS, ALEXANDER W DO, DATE OF BIRTH AUGUST 23, 1959, LICENSE NUMBER 38279, WAS DISCIPLINED BY COLORADO
DISCIPLINARY ACTION: PROBATION; MONITORING OF PHYSICIAN PERFORMANCE
OFFENSE: PHYSICAL OR MENTAL ILLNESS INHIBITING THE ABILITY TO PRACTICE WITH SKILL AND SAFETY

NOTES: HE HAS A MENTAL DISABILITY. PROBATIONARY TERMS INCLUDE TREATMENT MONITORING.

THERMOS, ALEXANDER W DO, WAS DISCIPLINED BY NEBRASKA ON NOVEMBER 14, 1997
DISCIPLINARY ACTION: FINE
OFFENSE: PROFESSIONAL MISCONDUCT

NOTES: UNPROFESSIONAL CONDUCT; VIOLATION OF UNIFORMED CONTROLLED SUBSTANCE ACT.

THOMAS, IVAL R IV MD, DATE OF BIRTH JANUARY 4, 1944, LICENSE NUMBER 0017311, WAS DISCIPLINED BY COLORADO ON MARCH 14, 1996
DISCIPLINARY ACTION: REPRIMAND

THOMAS, IVAL R IV MD, DATE OF BIRTH JANUARY 4, 1944, LICENSE NUMBER 0017311, WAS DISCIPLINED BY COLORADO ON JUNE 10, 1996
DISCIPLINARY ACTION: REPRIMAND

THOMAS, JOSEPH D MD, DATE OF BIRTH SEPTEMBER 8, 1946, LICENSE NUMBER 0021094, WAS DISCIPLINED BY COLORADO ON JULY 14, 1995

NOTES: RELINQUISHMENT OF HIS MEDICAL LICENSE AND PERMANENT RETIREMENT.

THOMPSON, LLOYD G MD, LICENSE NUMBER 00C9161 OF DALLAS, TX, WAS DISCIPLINED BY TEXAS ON JUNE 17, 1992
DISCIPLINARY ACTION: REPRIMAND
OFFENSE: NONCOMPLIANCE WITH A PROFESSIONAL RULE

NOTES: SEVERAL VIOLATIONS OF THE MEDICAL PRACTICE ACT, INCLUDING MISLEADING ADVERTISEMENT.

THOMPSON, LLOYD G MD, DATE OF BIRTH OCTOBER 15, 1934, LICENSE NUMBER 0016951, WAS DISCIPLINED BY COLORADO ON JULY 14, 1995
DISCIPLINARY ACTION: 24-MONTH LICENSE SUSPENSION

THOMPSON, LLOYD GILBERT MD, LICENSE NUMBER C9161 OF DALLAS, TX, WAS DISCIPLINED BY TEXAS ON AUGUST 28, 1999
DISCIPLINARY ACTION: 60-MONTH PROBATION; FINE
OFFENSE: CRIMINAL CONVICTION OR PLEA OF GUILTY, NOLO CONTENDERE, OR NO CONTEST TO A CRIME

NOTES: ON 8/7/96 HE PLED GUILTY TO ONE COUNT OF WIRE FRAUD IN THE U.S. DISTRICT COURT MIDDLE DISTRICT OF LOUISIANA; THE BOARD DETERMINED THAT HE FAILED TO MAINTAIN ADEQUATE MEDICAL RECORDS, USED NON-STANDARD ABBREVIATIONS AND FAILED TO RECORD VITAL SIGNS ON SOME OFFICE VISITS. SUSPENSION STAYED FOR PROBATION WITH FOLLOWING TERMS AND CONDITIONS: $5,000 FINE; SHALL OBTAIN 50 HOURS PER YEAR OF CONTINUING MEDICAL EDUCATION WITH 20 HOURS IN RISK MANAGEMENT AND/OR MEDICAL RECORD KEEPING; WITHIN 6 MONTHS SHALL SUCCESSFULLY COMPLETE A BOARD-APPROVED COURSE IN MEDICAL RECORD KEEPING; WITHIN 6 MONTHS SHALL IMPLEMENT A NEW MEDICAL RECORD FORMAT; SHALL APPEAR BEFORE THE BOARD AT LEAST TWICE A YEAR; TIME SPENT OUT OF TEXAS DOES NOT COUNT TOWARD PROBATION; SHALL INFORM THE BOARD OF CHANGE OF ADDRESS WITHIN 10 DAYS OR IF HE LEAVES THE STATE; SHALL NOT SEEK MODIFICATION FOR ONE YEAR.

THOMPSON, RICHARD G MD, LICENSE NUMBER G049719 OF COLORADO SPRINGS, CO, WAS DISCIPLINED BY CALIFORNIA ON FEBRUARY 7, 1991
DISCIPLINARY ACTION: LICENSE REVOCATION
OFFENSE: DISCIPLINARY ACTION BY ANOTHER STATE OR AGENCY

NOTES: DISCIPLINED BY COLORADO BOARD FOR SURGICAL DEFICIENCIES. DEFAULT DECISION.

TOSETTI, JAMES R MD, DATE OF BIRTH JULY 24, 1934, LICENSE NUMBER 0014356 OF COLORADO SPRINGS, CO, WAS DISCIPLINED BY COLORADO ON OCTOBER 16, 1991
DISCIPLINARY ACTION: RESTRICTION PLACED ON LICENSE; REQUIRED TO TAKE ADDITIONAL MEDICAL EDUCATION
OFFENSE: SUBSTANDARD CARE, INCOMPETENCE OR NEGLIGENCE

NOTES: GROSSLY NEGLIGENT OR SUBSTANDARD MEDICAL PRACTICE. AMENDED STIPULATION AND ORDER ADDING TERMS TO ALREADY EFFECTIVE INDEFINITE PERIOD OF PROBATION IMPOSED 3/2/90. ADDITIONAL TERMS INCLUDE EDUCATION AND TRAINING REQUIREMENTS AND PROHIBITION OF THE PERFORMANCE OF IN-OFFICE SURGICAL PROCEDURES.

TROUP, ROGER C MD, DATE OF BIRTH DECEMBER 15, 1921, LICENSE NUMBER 0014380 OF JOHNSON, KS, WAS DISCIPLINED BY COLORADO ON FEBRUARY 12, 1993
DISCIPLINARY ACTION: SURRENDER OF LICENSE

NOTES: NO UNPROFESSIONAL CONDUCT SET OUT.

TULLIUS, DANIEL L MD, DATE OF BIRTH SEPTEMBER 23, 1948, LICENSE NUMBER 0021099, WAS DISCIPLINED BY COLORADO ON FEBRUARY 14, 1996
OFFENSE: PROFESSIONAL MISCONDUCT

NOTES: SELF-PRESCRIBING OF A CONTROLLED SUBSTANCE. WILL CEASE PRACTICING 05/01/96 AND SHALL NOT RESUME PRACTICING IN COLORADO UNLESS INVOLVED IN RESIDENCY TRAINING OR OTHER RE-EDUCATION ACTIVITIES.

TULLIUS, DANIEL L MD, DATE OF BIRTH SEPTEMBER 23, 1948, LICENSE NUMBER 0021099, WAS DISCIPLINED BY COLORADO ON AUGUST 22, 1996
DISCIPLINARY ACTION: EMERGENCY SUSPENSION
OFFENSE: NONCOMPLIANCE WITH A PROFESSIONAL RULE

NOTES: VIOLATION OF THE MEDICAL PRACTICE ACT.

TULLIUS, DANIEL L MD, DATE OF BIRTH SEPTEMBER 23, 1948, LICENSE NUMBER 0021099, WAS DISCIPLINED BY COLORADO ON NOVEMBER 13, 1996
DISCIPLINARY ACTION: LICENSE SUSPENSION; PROBATION
OFFENSE: FAILURE TO COMPLY WITH PREVIOUS BOARD ORDER

NOTES: VIOLATION OF A VALID BOARD ORDER. SUSPENDED UNTIL HE ENTERS A RESIDENCY WHEREUPON A PROBATIONARY PERIOD WILL BEGIN: REQUIRED TO COMPLETE THE RESIDENCY AND REMAIN ABSTINENT. IF HE IS PRACTICING IN COLORADO DURING THE PROBATIONARY PERIOD, HE IS REQUIRED TO ENGAGE IN TREATMENT AND PRACTICE MONITORING.

TULLIUS, DANIEL L MD, WAS DISCIPLINED BY ALASKA ON APRIL 4, 1997
DISCIPLINARY ACTION: DENIAL OF NEW LICENSE
OFFENSE: DISCIPLINARY ACTION BY ANOTHER STATE OR AGENCY

NOTES: LICENSE SUSPENDED IN COLORADO AT TIME OF APPLICATION FOR ALASKA LICENSURE.

TURLEY, LOREN M DO, LICENSE NUMBER 0002638, WAS DISCIPLINED BY ARIZONA ON SEPTEMBER 14, 1992
DISCIPLINARY ACTION: LICENSE SUSPENSION; MONITORING OF PHYSICIAN PERFORMANCE
OFFENSE: PROFESSIONAL MISCONDUCT

NOTES: ON 9/10/92 ADMITTED TO THE BOARD THAT HE HAD SELF-MEDICATED WITH CONTROLLED AND/OR PRESCRIPTION ONLY MEDICATIONS (FLEXERIL) ON ONE OR MORE OCCASIONS PRIOR TO THAT DATE WHILE NOT UNDER THE CARE AND TREATMENT OF A PHYSICIAN AND NOT PRESCRIBED AS PART OF A RECOGNIZED COURSE OF TREATMENT. SHALL UNDERGO AN IN-PATIENT EVALUATION PROGRAM FOR SUSPECTED ALCOHOL AND SUBSTANCE ABUSE AND CHEMICAL DEPENDENCE FOR NOT LESS THAN FIVE DAYS; SHALL AUTHORIZE TREATING PERSONNEL AT THE IN-PATIENT EVALUATION PROGRAM TO RELEASE TO THE BOARD FINDINGS OF HIS EVALUATION AND ANY NECESSARY RECOMMENDATIONS FOR TREATMENT; SHALL MEET WITH THE BOARD FOLLOWING THE COMPLETION OF THE EVALUATION PROGRAM TO DETERMINE WHETHER OR NOT ANY ADDITIONAL ACTIONS ARE REQUIRED; SHALL USE NO CONTROLLED SUBSTANCES OR PRESCRIPTION-ONLY MEDICATIONS UNLESS PRESCRIBED BY HIS ATTENDING PHYSICIAN; SHALL REFRAIN FROM THE USE OF ALCOHOL.

TURLEY, LOREN M DO, LICENSE NUMBER 0002638, WAS DISCIPLINED BY ARIZONA ON SEPTEMBER 19, 1992
DISCIPLINARY ACTION: PROBATION; RESTRICTION PLACED ON LICENSE
OFFENSE: PROFESSIONAL MISCONDUCT

NOTES: SUBMITTED DOCUMENTATION OF COMPLIANCE WITH TERMS OF 9/14/92 ORDER. REINSTATED WITH MINIMUM THREE YEAR PROBATION UNDER TERMS AND CONDITIONS: SHALL COMPLETE AN INTENSIVE OUTPATIENT CHEMICAL DEPENDENCE PROGRAM; SHALL SECURE AND MAINTAIN A SPONSOR FOR 12 STEP RECOVERY PROGRAM; SHALL ATTEND AT LEAST FOUR 12 STEP MEETINGS PER WEEK FOR THE FIRST 12 MONTHS; SHALL MEET REGULARLY WITH HIS ATTENDING PHYSICIAN; SHALL ATTEND NO LESS THAN THREE GROUP THERAPY MEETINGS PER MONTH WITH A BOARD APPROVED COUNSELOR; SHALL SUBMIT TO RANDOM BODY FLUID TESTING UPON BOARD REQUEST; SHALL MEET WITH THE BOARD REGULARLY UPON REQUEST; SHALL USE NO CONTROLLED SUBSTANCE OR PRESCRIPTION-ONLY MEDICATION UNLESS PRESCRIBED BY HIS ATTENDING PHYSICIAN; SHALL REFRAIN FROM THE USE OF ALCOHOL; SHALL WORK NO MORE THAN 14 EMERGENCY DEPARTMENT SHIFTS PER MONTH UNLESS AUTHORIZED BY THE BOARD; SHALL AUTHORIZE ALL TREATING PERSONNEL INVOLVED IN HIS CARE TO RELEASE INFORMATION ON HIS PROGRESS AND PROGNOSIS TO THE BOARD UPON REQUEST. ORDER AMENDED ON 1/14/94 ALLOWING HIM TO WORK 17 RATHER THAN 14 EMERGENCY DEPARTMENT SHIFTS PER MONTH. OTHER PROVISIONS REMAIN IN FULL FORCE AND EFFECT.

TURLEY, LOREN M DO, LICENSE NUMBER 0002331 OF 19155 NORTH 94TH PLACE, SCOTTSDALE, AZ, WAS DISCIPLINED BY OKLAHOMA ON MARCH 12, 1993
DISCIPLINARY ACTION: 60-MONTH PROBATION
OFFENSE: DISCIPLINARY ACTION BY ANOTHER STATE OR AGENCY

NOTES: LICENSE SUSPENSION IN ARIZONA ON 9/14/92 WHICH WAS REINSTATED SUBJECT TO TERMS AND CONDITIONS. CONDITIONS OF PROBATION: SHALL REMAIN IN STRICT COMPLIANCE WITH THE ARIZONA ORDER; SHALL APPEAR BEFORE THE BOARD UPON REQUEST AND BEFORE HE REENTERS PRACTICE IN OKLAHOMA.

TURLEY, LOREN M MD, DATE OF BIRTH MARCH 7, 1945, LICENSE NUMBER 0028104 OF SCOTTSDALE, AZ, WAS DISCIPLINED BY COLORADO ON NOVEMBER 19, 1993
DISCIPLINARY ACTION: 60-MONTH PROBATION; MONITORING OF PHYSICIAN PERFORMANCE
OFFENSE: SUBSTANCE ABUSE

NOTES: EXCESSIVE USE OF A CONTROLLED SUBSTANCE AND HABITUAL INTEMPERANCE. PROBATIONARY PERIOD INCLUDES TREATMENT AND PRACTICE MONITORING.

TURNER, DONN M MD, DATE OF BIRTH SEPTEMBER 19, 1952, LICENSE NUMBER 0023363, WAS DISCIPLINED BY COLORADO ON APRIL 18, 1996
DISCIPLINARY ACTION: REPRIMAND

TUTT, GEORGE O JR MD, DATE OF BIRTH NOVEMBER 21, 1948, LICENSE NUMBER 23364, WAS DISCIPLINED BY COLORADO ON FEBRUARY 13, 1998
DISCIPLINARY ACTION: REPRIMAND
OFFENSE: SUBSTANDARD CARE, INCOMPETENCE OR NEGLIGENCE

NOTES: SUBSTANDARD CARE.

TUTT, GEORGE OLIVER JR MD, LICENSE NUMBER G30230 OF FORT COLLINS, CO, WAS DISCIPLINED BY CALIFORNIA ON AUGUST 25, 1998
DISCIPLINARY ACTION: REPRIMAND
OFFENSE: DISCIPLINARY ACTION BY ANOTHER STATE OR AGENCY

NOTES: DISCIPLINED BY COLORADO FOR FAILING TO ADEQUATELY DOCUMENT OPTIONS, RISKS, RATIONALE AND ADVICE, AND FAILING TO INCLUDE ANY REFERENCE TO NEEDLE BIOPSY FOR A PATIENT WHO HAD SUSPECTED BREAST CANCER.

TYLER, JOHN M JR MD, DATE OF BIRTH MAY 2, 1959, LICENSE NUMBER 30232, WAS DISCIPLINED BY COLORADO ON MARCH 20, 1997
DISCIPLINARY ACTION: 60-MONTH PROBATION; MONITORING OF PHYSICIAN PERFORMANCE
OFFENSE: PHYSICAL OR MENTAL ILLNESS INHIBITING THE ABILITY TO PRACTICE WITH SKILL AND SAFETY

NOTES: MENTAL DISABILITY. TERMS OF PROBATION INCLUDE: MUST AGREE TO REMAIN ABSTINENT FROM ADDICTIVE SUBSTANCES, TREATMENT MONITORING AND PRACTICE MONITORING.

TYLER, JOHN M JR MD, LICENSE NUMBER H2853 OF COLORADO SPRINGS, CO, WAS DISCIPLINED BY TEXAS ON MAY 16, 1998
DISCIPLINARY ACTION: MONITORING OF PHYSICIAN PERFORMANCE
OFFENSE: DISCIPLINARY ACTION BY ANOTHER STATE OR AGENCY

NOTES: ON OR ABOUT 3/20/97 HE ENTERED INTO AN AGREED ORDER WITH THE COLORADO BOARD, WHICH STIPULATED THAT FROM APPROXIMATELY 5/96- 8/96 HE CONSUMED 1-2 ALCOHOLIC DRINKS OVER LUNCH ONCE OR TWICE WEEKLY; HE WAS DIAGNOSED WITH ALCOHOL ABUSE IN EARLY REMISSION; THE COLORADO BOARD PLACED HIM ON PROBATIONARY STATUS FOR 5 YEARS. SHALL NOT PRACTICE IN TEXAS UNTIL HE APPEARS BEFORE THE BOARD WITH SUFFICIENT EVIDENCE THAT HE IS PHYSICALLY, MENTALLY AND OTHERWISE COMPETENT TO SAFELY PRACTICE INCLUDING AT A MINIMUM: SHALL ABSTAIN FROM THE CONSUMPTION OF ALCOHOL/DRUGS IN ANY FORM UNLESS PRESCRIBED BY ANOTHER PHYSICIAN FOR A LEGITIMATE AND THERAPEUTIC PURPOSE; SHALL PROVIDE EVIDENCE THAT HE HAS COMPLETED THE TERMS OF HIS COLORADO BOARD ORDER; SHALL COOPERATE WITH THE BOARD IN VERIFYING COMPLIANCE INCLUDING PROVIDING COPIES OF REPORTS SENT TO COLORADO; SHALL INFORM THE BOARD OF CHANGE OF ADDRESS WITHIN 10 DAYS OR IF HE LEAVES THE STATE; SHALL NOT SEEK MODIFICATION FOR ONE YEAR.

UBA, MAHITO DO, DATE OF BIRTH APRIL 8, 1919, LICENSE NUMBER 0010876 OF DENVER, CO, WAS DISCIPLINED BY COLORADO ON NOVEMBER 6, 1992
DISCIPLINARY ACTION: SURRENDER OF LICENSE
OFFENSE: SUBSTANDARD CARE, INCOMPETENCE OR NEGLIGENCE

NOTES: TWO OR MORE ACTS OR OMISSIONS WHICH FAILED TO MEET GENERALLY ACCEPTED STANDARDS OF MEDICAL PRACTICE.

URE, JOHN D JR DO, LICENSE NUMBER 0520207 OF 4046 PONDEROSA DRIVE, EVERGREEN, CO, WAS DISCIPLINED BY KANSAS ON MAY 1, 1996
DISCIPLINARY ACTION: FINE; REPRIMAND
OFFENSE: NONCOMPLIANCE WITH A PROFESSIONAL RULE

NOTES: FAILED TO MAINTAIN PROPER PROFESSIONAL LIABILITY INSURANCE AND PAY HIS ANNUAL PREMIUM SURCHARGE TO THE HEALTHCARE STABILIZATION FUND. SHALL PAY A FINE OF $1,300.

URIOSTE, DEBBIE D MD, DATE OF BIRTH FEBRUARY 14, 1961, LICENSE NUMBER 0033351 OF WALSENBURG, CO, WAS DISCIPLINED BY COLORADO ON JANUARY 20, 1994
DISCIPLINARY ACTION: MONITORING OF PHYSICIAN PERFORMANCE
OFFENSE: PHYSICAL OR MENTAL ILLNESS INHIBITING THE ABILITY TO PRACTICE WITH SKILL AND SAFETY

NOTES: PHYSICAL OR MENTAL DISABILITY ISSUES. MUST REMAIN IN APPROPRIATE MEDICAL TREATMENT; LIFETIME TREATMENT MONITORING. ON 5/14/97 ORDER MODIFIED; AGREES TO RECEIVE TREATMENT MONITORING FROM THE BOARD'S PEER ASSISTANCE PROGRAM.

VALENCIA, WARREN H MD, DATE OF BIRTH AUGUST 2, 1947, LICENSE NUMBER 0020313 OF LONGMONT, CO, WAS DISCIPLINED BY COLORADO ON DECEMBER 17, 1993
DISCIPLINARY ACTION: REPRIMAND
OFFENSE: SUBSTANDARD CARE, INCOMPETENCE OR NEGLIGENCE

NOTES: SUBSTANDARD PATIENT CARE.

VERBRUGGE, JOSEPH J JR MD, DATE OF BIRTH JANUARY 18, 1940, LICENSE NUMBER 0018269 OF ENGLEWOOD, CO, WAS DISCIPLINED BY COLORADO ON DECEMBER 16, 1994
DISCIPLINARY ACTION: LICENSE REVOCATION
OFFENSE: SUBSTANDARD CARE, INCOMPETENCE OR NEGLIGENCE

NOTES: GROSSLY NEGLIGENT MEDICAL PRACTICE AND TWO OR MORE ACTS OR OMISSIONS WHICH FAILED TO MEET GENERALLY ACCEPTED STANDARDS OF CARE AND FALSIFYING AND REPEATEDLY MAKING INCORRECT ESSENTIAL ENTRIES OR REPEATEDLY FAILING TO MAKE ESSENTIAL ENTRIES ON PATIENT RECORDS.

VERBRUGGE, JOSEPH J JR MD, DATE OF BIRTH JANUARY 18, 1940 OF 6390 SOUTH LOCUST WAY, ENGLEWOOD, CO, WAS DISCIPLINED BY MEDICARE ON APRIL 20, 1998
DISCIPLINARY ACTION: 60-MONTH EXCLUSION FROM THE MEDICARE AND/OR MEDICAID PROGRAM
OFFENSE: CRIMINAL CONVICTION OR PLEA OF GUILTY, NOLO CONTENDERE, OR NO CONTEST TO A CRIME

NOTES: CONVICTED OF A CRIME RELATED TO PATIENT ABUSE OR NEGLECT.

VERBRUGGE, JOSEPH JAMES MD, LICENSE NUMBER 0C34826 OF ENGLEWOOD, CO, WAS DISCIPLINED BY CALIFORNIA ON JULY 25, 1994
DISCIPLINARY ACTION: 60-MONTH PROBATION
OFFENSE: DISCIPLINARY ACTION BY ANOTHER STATE OR AGENCY

NOTES: DISCIPLINED BY COLORADO FOR GROSS NEGLIGENCE IN ANESTHESIOLOGY PRACTICE; FALSIFIED MEDICAL RECORDS AND FAILED TO INCLUDE ESSENTIAL ENTRIES IN PATIENT RECORDS. REVOCATION STAYED.

VERBRUGGE, JOSEPH JAMES MD, LICENSE NUMBER C34826 OF ENGLEWOOD, CO, WAS DISCIPLINED BY CALIFORNIA ON APRIL 27, 1998
DISCIPLINARY ACTION: LICENSE REVOCATION
OFFENSE: DISCIPLINARY ACTION BY ANOTHER STATE OR AGENCY

NOTES: DISCIPLINED BY COLORADO BASED ON HIS CRIMINAL CONVICTION FOR CRIMINAL MEDICAL NEGLIGENCE.

VIALPANDO, ARTHUR B MD OF 807 WEST CEDAR ST, WALSENBURG, CO, WAS DISCIPLINED BY DEA ON MAY 15, 1990
DISCIPLINARY ACTION: RESTRICTION PLACED ON CONTROLLED SUBSTANCE LICENSE
OFFENSE: PROFESSIONAL MISCONDUCT

NOTES: EXCESSIVE PURCHASE. REGISTRATION RESTRICTED TO SCHEDULES III THROUGH V.

VOSS, RICHARD G MD, DATE OF BIRTH MARCH 7, 1929, LICENSE NUMBER 0014987 OF FT. COLLINS, CO, WAS DISCIPLINED BY COLORADO ON AUGUST 11, 1994
DISCIPLINARY ACTION: SURRENDER OF LICENSE
OFFENSE: SUBSTANCE ABUSE

NOTES: ALCOHOL DEPENDENCE ISSUES.

VOSS, RICHARD G MD, DATE OF BIRTH MARCH 7, 1929 OF 1217 E ELIZABETH STREET, FORT COLLINS, CO, WAS DISCIPLINED BY MEDICARE ON APRIL 11, 1995
DISCIPLINARY ACTION: EXCLUSION FROM THE MEDICARE AND/OR MEDICAID PROGRAM
OFFENSE: DISCIPLINARY ACTION BY ANOTHER STATE OR AGENCY

NOTES: LICENSE REVOKED FOR REASONS BEARING ON PROFESSIONAL PERFORMANCE.

VOSTINAK, WILLIAM J MD, DATE OF BIRTH JUNE 4, 1951, LICENSE NUMBER 0027707 OF WHEAT RIDGE, CO, WAS DISCIPLINED BY COLORADO ON FEBRUARY 18, 1994
DISCIPLINARY ACTION: REPRIMAND
OFFENSE: PROFESSIONAL MISCONDUCT

VOSTINAK, WILLIAM JEROME MD, DATE OF BIRTH JUNE 4, 1951, LICENSE NUMBER 067381E OF 832 WILLOBE WAY, GOLDEN, CO, WAS DISCIPLINED BY PENNSYLVANIA ON JULY 27, 1999
DISCIPLINARY ACTION: 12-MONTH PROBATION
OFFENSE: DISCIPLINARY ACTION BY ANOTHER STATE OR AGENCY

NOTES: DISCIPLINARY ACTION TAKEN BY CALIFORNIA AND COLORADO.

VOSTINAL, WILLIAM ALAN MD, LICENSE NUMBER 0G44481 OF WESTMINSTER, CO, WAS DISCIPLINED BY CALIFORNIA ON FEBRUARY 5, 1996
DISCIPLINARY ACTION: LICENSE REVOCATION
OFFENSE: DISCIPLINARY ACTION BY ANOTHER STATE OR AGENCY

NOTES: ACTION IN COLORADO FOR COMMENCEMENT OF SURGERY UPON THE WRONG LEG. DEFAULT ACTION.

WADE, HENRY KING III MD, DATE OF BIRTH FEBRUARY 23, 1943, LICENSE NUMBER 0017328 OF DENVER, CO, WAS DISCIPLINED BY COLORADO ON FEBRUARY 19, 1993
DISCIPLINARY ACTION: 60-MONTH PROBATION; MONITORING OF PHYSICIAN PERFORMANCE
OFFENSE: SUBSTANCE ABUSE

NOTES: HABITUAL INTEMPERANCE. PROBATIONARY TERMS INCLUDE TREATMENT AND PRACTICE MONITORING. PROBATION TERMINATED ON 12/21/95 AND LICENSE RESTORED TO AN UNENCUMBERED AND UNRESTRICTED STATUS.

WALLIS, GLENN P MD, DATE OF BIRTH MARCH 14, 1950, LICENSE NUMBER 21105, WAS DISCIPLINED BY COLORADO ON JUNE 19, 1997
DISCIPLINARY ACTION: REPRIMAND

WALSH, JAMES A MD, DATE OF BIRTH JULY 23, 1935, LICENSE NUMBER 0015796, WAS DISCIPLINED BY COLORADO ON NOVEMBER 9, 1995
DISCIPLINARY ACTION: 60-MONTH PROBATION; MONITORING OF PHYSICIAN PERFORMANCE

NOTES: LEARNING PLAN AND PRACTICE MONITORING.

WALSH, JAMES A MD, DATE OF BIRTH JULY 23, 1935, LICENSE NUMBER 028286L OF 21 TUPELO ROAD SEA PINES, HILTON HEAD ISLAND, SC, WAS DISCIPLINED BY PENNSYLVANIA ON NOVEMBER 18, 1997
DISCIPLINARY ACTION: FINE; REPRIMAND
OFFENSE: DISCIPLINARY ACTION BY ANOTHER STATE OR AGENCY

NOTES: DISCIPLINARY ACTION TAKEN BY OHIO.

WALSH, JAMES ALOYSIUS MD, DATE OF BIRTH JULY 23, 1935, LICENSE NUMBER 0036285 OF HILTON HEAD, SC, WAS DISCIPLINED BY NORTH CAROLINA ON AUGUST 14, 1998
DISCIPLINARY ACTION: 60-MONTH RESTRICTION PLACED ON LICENSE; REQUIRED TO TAKE ADDITIONAL MEDICAL EDUCATION
OFFENSE: DISCIPLINARY ACTION BY ANOTHER STATE OR AGENCY

NOTES: IN COLORADO, HIS ABILITY TO EVALUATE MAMMOGRAMS WAS QUESTIONED; THE COLORADO BOARD ON 10/26/95 PLACED HIS LICENSE ON PROBATION FOR FIVE YEARS. HE APPEARS TO BE IN COMPLIANCE WITH THE COLORADO ORDER; HE HAS DOCUMENTED TO THE NORTH CAROLINA BOARD THAT HE HAS OBTAINED 89 HOURS OF CONTINUING MEDICAL EDUCATION IN MAMMOGRAPHY IN THE LAST DECADE AND HAS READ AT LEAST 120 MEDICAL JOURNAL ARTICLES ON MAMMOGRAPHY IN ABOUT THAT TIME; HE STATES HIS INTENTION TO OBTAIN FURTHER CONTINUING MEDICAL EDUCATION ON MAMMOGRAPHY. FOR THE NEXT FIVE YEARS WHEN PRACTICING ON A PATIENT IN NORTH CAROLINA, SHALL HAVE A LICENSED BOARD-APPROVED NORTH CAROLINA PHYSICIAN MONITOR HIS PRACTICE ACTIVITIES IN THE OFFICE AND HOSPITAL; DURING ANY MONTH IN WHICH HE PRACTICES ON A PATIENT OR PATIENTS IN NORTH CAROLINA, HE SHALL HAVE THE MONITOR REVIEW AT LEAST FIVE RANDOM CASES, THREE OF WHICH SHALL BE MAMMOGRAMS AND TWO OF WHICH SHALL BE OTHER THAN MAMMOGRAMS; IF HE HAS FEWER THAN FIVE PATIENTS IN A MONTH, THE MONITOR SHALL REVIEW ALL THE CASES, IF HE DOES NOT PRACTICE ON ANY NORTH CAROLINA PATIENTS, HE SHALL SUBMIT QUARTERLY REPORTS TO THE BOARD SO STATING; IF HE HAS PRACTICED ON A PATIENT IN NORTH CAROLINA DURING ANY QUARTER, THE MONITOR SHALL SUBMIT QUARTERLY REPORTS; SHALL NOT INTERPRET MORE THAN 20 MAMMOGRAMS A DAY; HE SHALL OBTAIN AND DOCUMENT 50 HOURS OF CONTINUING MEDICAL EDUCATION RELEVANT TO HIS PRACTICE EACH YEAR; MUST COMPLY WITH OTHER CONDITIONS.

WARREN, STEVEN E MD OF MONTICELLO, UT, WAS DISCIPLINED BY UTAH ON MAY 5, 1993
DISCIPLINARY ACTION: 60-MONTH PROBATION
OFFENSE: PROFESSIONAL MISCONDUCT

NOTES: UNLAWFULLY USING AND OBTAINING CONTROLLED

SUBSTANCES; CONTAMINATION OF MULTI-DOSE CONTROLLED SUBSTANCE; FAILURE TO MAINTAIN ADEQUATE CONTROLLED SUBSTANCE RECORDS; FALSIFYING PRESCRIPTIONS FOR CONTROLLED SUBSTANCES. DEA REGISTRATION REVOKED. LICENSE REVOKED WITH A STAY OF ENFORCEMENT ON HIS REVOCATION. LICENSE TO PRESCRIBE AND ADMINISTER CONTROLLED SUBSTANCES HAD BEEN VOLUNTARILY SURRENDERED IN 10/92. SHALL NOT APPLY FOR REINSTATEMENT OF THAT LICENSE FOR AT LEAST TWO YEARS. ON 6/5/95 HIS LICENSE TO PRESCRIBE AND ADMINISTER CONTROLLED SUBSTANCES SCHEDULES II-V WAS REINSTATED AND ISSUED WITH FULL PRIVILEGES. ON 8/28/95 LICENSE TO PRESCRIBE AND ADMINISTER CONTROLLED SUBSTANCES CHANGED TO SCHEDULES III-V ONLY TO COMPLY WITH FEDERAL RULES AND THE ASSESSMENT MADE BY DEA. ON 6/19/97 ORDER AMENDED ADDING SCHEDULE II TO HIS LICENSE TO PRESCRIBE AND ADMINISTER CONTROLLED SUBSTANCES.

WARREN, STEVEN E MD, DATE OF BIRTH APRIL 7, 1952, LICENSE NUMBER 0026991 OF MONTICELLO, UT, WAS DISCIPLINED BY COLORADO ON DECEMBER 17, 1993
DISCIPLINARY ACTION: 36-MONTH RESTRICTION PLACED ON LICENSE; MONITORING OF PHYSICIAN PERFORMANCE
OFFENSE: CRIMINAL CONVICTION OR PLEA OF GUILTY, NOLO CONTENDERE, OR NO CONTEST TO A CRIME

NOTES: CONVICTION OF A FELONY; CONVICTION OF A VIOLATION OF FEDERAL LAW REGULATING THE POSSESSION, DISTRIBUTION, OR USE OF ANY CONTROLLED SUBSTANCE; ADMINISTERING, DISPENSING OR PRESCRIBING OR A CONTROLLED SUBSTANCE OTHER THAN IN THE COURSE OF LEGITIMATE PROFESSIONAL PRACTICE; EXCESSIVE USE OF A CONTROLLED SUBSTANCE; SELF-PRESCRIBING OF A CONTROLLED SUBSTANCE. REVOCATION STAYED FOR FIVE YEARS, PENDING COMPLIANCE WITH ALL TERMS OF THE STIPULATION, INCLUDING A PROHIBITION OF ANY MEDICAL PRACTICE IN COLORADO FOR THREE YEARS AND PRACTICE AND TREATMENT MONITORING UPON RESUMPTION OF ANY PRACTICE IN THIS STATE.

WARREN, STEVEN E MD OF 2075 NORTH 1200 WEST, LAYTON, UT, WAS DISCIPLINED BY DEA ON MAY 23, 1996
DISCIPLINARY ACTION: RESTRICTION PLACED ON CONTROLLED SUBSTANCE LICENSE
OFFENSE: CRIMINAL CONVICTION OR PLEA OF GUILTY, NOLO CONTENDERE, OR NO CONTEST TO A CRIME

NOTES: CONTROLLED SUBSTANCES.

WARREN, STEVEN E MD OF OGDEN, UT, WAS DISCIPLINED BY UTAH ON MARCH 11, 1999
DISCIPLINARY ACTION: 12-MONTH PROBATION; 12-MONTH CONTROLLED SUBSTANCE LICENSE PLACED ON PROBATION
OFFENSE: PROFESSIONAL MISCONDUCT

NOTES: HE PRESCRIBED THE MEDICATION STADOL TO FAMILY MEMBERS AND HE FAILED TO MAINTAIN PATIENT RECORDS. PROBATION WITH CONDITIONS AND RESTRICTIONS.

WARWICK, MARK MD, LICENSE NUMBER 0024113 OF BURLINGTON, CO, WAS DISCIPLINED BY COLORADO ON FEBRUARY 15, 1991
DISCIPLINARY ACTION: PROBATION; MONITORING OF PHYSICIAN PERFORMANCE
OFFENSE: SUBSTANDARD CARE, INCOMPETENCE OR NEGLIGENCE

NOTES: INDEFINITE PROBATION, ALSO REQUIRED TO PASS COMPONENT II OF THE FLEX EXAMINATION.

WEAVER, JOHN A JR MD, DATE OF BIRTH MARCH 10, 1903, LICENSE NUMBER 0009152 OF GREELEY, CO, WAS DISCIPLINED BY COLORADO ON OCTOBER 12, 1994
DISCIPLINARY ACTION: SURRENDER OF LICENSE
OFFENSE: OVERPRESCRIBING OR MISPRESCRIBING DRUGS

NOTES: ALLEGATIONS OF PRESCRIBING, DISTRIBUTING OR GIVING TO A FAMILY MEMBER OR TO ONESELF A CONTROLLED SUBSTANCE. HE DENIES ALLEGATIONS.

WEBB, WILLIAM M MD OF 1736 S VAN DYKE WAY, LAKEWOOD, CO, WAS DISCIPLINED BY DEA ON MAY 6, 1998
DISCIPLINARY ACTION: SURRENDER OF CONTROLLED SUBSTANCE LICENSE

WELLER, WILLIAM J MD, DATE OF BIRTH JUNE 28, 1939, LICENSE NUMBER 0017059, WAS DISCIPLINED BY COLORADO ON DECEMBER 19, 1996
DISCIPLINARY ACTION: REPRIMAND

WELLER, WILLIAM J MD, LICENSE NUMBER G13938 OF COLORADO SPRINGS, CO, WAS DISCIPLINED BY CALIFORNIA ON APRIL 9, 1998
DISCIPLINARY ACTION: REPRIMAND
OFFENSE: NONCOMPLIANCE WITH A PROFESSIONAL RULE

NOTES: DISCIPLINED BY COLORADO FOR FAILING TO NOTE IN A PATIENT'S CHART A DIAGNOSIS OF AN INFILTRATE IN HER UPPER LEFT LUNG.

WERMERS, JOSEPH J MD, DATE OF BIRTH MAY 3, 1946, LICENSE NUMBER 0019512, WAS DISCIPLINED BY COLORADO ON NOVEMBER 9, 1995
DISCIPLINARY ACTION: 60-MONTH PROBATION; MONITORING OF PHYSICIAN PERFORMANCE

NOTES: PRACTICE MONITORING.

WESTENBERGER, PETE D MD, DATE OF BIRTH JUNE 30, 1951, LICENSE NUMBER 0025542 OF LITTLETON, CO, WAS DISCIPLINED BY COLORADO ON JANUARY 15, 1992
DISCIPLINARY ACTION: 60-MONTH PROBATION; MONITORING OF PHYSICIAN PERFORMANCE
OFFENSE: SUBSTANCE ABUSE

NOTES: ALCOHOL/SUBSTANCE ABUSE; MENTAL DISABILITY WHICH RENDERS HIM UNABLE TO PRACTICE WITH SKILL AND SAFETY WITHOUT APPROPRIATE TREATMENT. PROBATIONARY PERIOD WITH TREATMENT AND PRACTICE MONITORING.

WESTENBERGER, PETE D MD, DATE OF BIRTH JUNE 30, 1951, LICENSE NUMBER 0025542 OF LITTLETON, CO, WAS DISCIPLINED BY COLORADO ON MAY 11, 1994
DISCIPLINARY ACTION: REPRIMAND
OFFENSE: PROFESSIONAL MISCONDUCT

WETZIG, RICHARD P MD, DATE OF BIRTH AUGUST 23, 1953, LICENSE NUMBER 0028283 OF COLORADO SPRINGS, CO, WAS DISCIPLINED BY COLORADO ON SEPTEMBER 13, 1991
DISCIPLINARY ACTION: PROBATION; MONITORING OF PHYSICIAN PERFORMANCE
OFFENSE: PHYSICAL OR MENTAL ILLNESS INHIBITING THE ABILITY TO PRACTICE WITH SKILL AND SAFETY

NOTES: SUCH MENTAL OR PHYSICAL DISABILITY AS TO RENDER HIM UNABLE TO PERFORM MEDICAL SERVICES WITH REASONABLE SKILL AND SAFETY TO THE PATIENT. LICENSE ON PROBATIONARY STATUS

FOR AS LONG AS HE HOLDS A LICENSE TO PRACTICE MEDICINE IN COLORADO AND REQUIRING HIM TO UNDERGO SPECIFIED MEDICAL TREATMENT WITH APPROPRIATE TREATMENT MONITORING.

WHITE, MARK S DO, DATE OF BIRTH OCTOBER 11, 1953, LICENSE NUMBER 0023863, WAS DISCIPLINED BY COLORADO ON MARCH 14, 1996
DISCIPLINARY ACTION: MONITORING OF PHYSICIAN PERFORMANCE
OFFENSE: SUBSTANCE ABUSE

NOTES: HABITUAL INTEMPERANCE OR EXCESSIVE USE OF A CONTROLLED SUBSTANCE. TREATMENT AND PRACTICE MONITORING UPON RESUMPTION OF PRACTICE IN COLORADO.

WHITELOCK, PAUL MD, LICENSE NUMBER D7364 OF DURANGO, CO, WAS DISCIPLINED BY TEXAS ON AUGUST 9, 1997
DISCIPLINARY ACTION: FINE; REPRIMAND
OFFENSE: NONCOMPLIANCE WITH A PROFESSIONAL RULE

NOTES: VIOLATION OF BOARD RULES RELATING TO MANDATORY COMPLETION AND REPORTING OF CONTINUING MEDICAL EDUCATION. $100 FINE.

WIKHOLM, LARRY J MD, DATE OF BIRTH DECEMBER 30, 1942, LICENSE NUMBER 0020058 OF GREELEY, CO, WAS DISCIPLINED BY COLORADO ON DECEMBER 16, 1994
DISCIPLINARY ACTION: REPRIMAND

WIKHOLM, LARRY J MD, DATE OF BIRTH DECEMBER 30, 1942, LICENSE NUMBER 0020058, WAS DISCIPLINED BY COLORADO ON SEPTEMBER 19, 1996
DISCIPLINARY ACTION: 60-MONTH PROBATION; REQUIRED TO TAKE ADDITIONAL MEDICAL EDUCATION
OFFENSE: SUBSTANDARD CARE, INCOMPETENCE OR NEGLIGENCE

NOTES: SUBSTANDARD CARE (PRIMA FACIE TYPE ADMISSION ONLY). RE-EDUCATION ACTIVITIES AND PRACTICE MONITORING. ON 11/14/97 ORDER MODIFIED WHEREBY HE AGREES TO A RESTRICTION ON HIS LICENSE: ACTING ONLY AS AN ASSISTANT SURGEON.

WIKHOLM, LARRY J MD, DATE OF BIRTH DECEMBER 30, 1942, LICENSE NUMBER 20058, WAS DISCIPLINED BY COLORADO ON FEBRUARY 19, 1999
DISCIPLINARY ACTION: SURRENDER OF LICENSE

NOTES: NO UNPROFESSIONAL CONDUCT IDENTIFIED.

WILKINS, ROLLAND W MD, DATE OF BIRTH OCTOBER 11, 1924, LICENSE NUMBER 0011822, WAS DISCIPLINED BY COLORADO ON JULY 14, 1995
DISCIPLINARY ACTION: SURRENDER OF LICENSE

WILLIAMS, C REX MD, DATE OF BIRTH SEPTEMBER 13, 1932, LICENSE NUMBER 0015035, WAS DISCIPLINED BY COLORADO ON OCTOBER 11, 1995

NOTES: SHALL PERMANENTLY RELINQUISH HIS LICENSE TO PRACTICE.

WILLIAMS, CONRAD R MD, WAS DISCIPLINED BY NEBRASKA ON AUGUST 13, 1999
DISCIPLINARY ACTION: 6-MONTH LICENSE SUSPENSION; RESTRICTION PLACED ON LICENSE
OFFENSE: PROFESSIONAL MISCONDUCT

NOTES: DISHONORABLE, UNPROFESSIONAL CONDUCT.

WILLIAMS, CONRAD REX MD, LICENSE NUMBER 00C7512 OF COLORADO SPRINGS, CO, WAS DISCIPLINED BY TEXAS ON MARCH 31, 1990
DISCIPLINARY ACTION: SURRENDER OF LICENSE

NOTES: STIPULATED ORDER.

WILLIAMS, CONRAD ROBERT MD, DATE OF BIRTH JANUARY 28, 1949, LICENSE NUMBER 0038690 OF 1115 RIVINGTON STREET, ROSELLE, NJ, WAS DISCIPLINED BY NEW JERSEY ON MARCH 8, 1990
DISCIPLINARY ACTION: SURRENDER OF LICENSE
OFFENSE: OVERPRESCRIBING OR MISPRESCRIBING DRUGS

NOTES: ACTION BASED ON QUESTIONABLE CONTROLLED DANGEROUS SUBSTANCE PRESCRIBING. SHALL NOT REAPPLY.

WILLIAMS, CONRAD ROBERT MD OF 44 ROOSEVELT AVE PO BOX 398, CARTERET, NJ, WAS DISCIPLINED BY DEA ON MAY 14, 1990
DISCIPLINARY ACTION: SURRENDER OF CONTROLLED SUBSTANCE LICENSE
OFFENSE: DISCIPLINARY ACTION BY ANOTHER STATE OR AGENCY

NOTES: LICENSE TO PRACTICE MEDICINE AND SURGERY IN NEW JERSEY PERMANENTLY SURRENDERED.

WILLIAMS, PAUL C MD, LICENSE NUMBER 0014868, WAS DISCIPLINED BY ARIZONA ON JANUARY 19, 1990
DISCIPLINARY ACTION: 60-MONTH PROBATION; REQUIRED TO ENTER AN IMPAIRED PHYSICIAN PROGRAM OR SUBSTANCE ABUSE TREATMENT
OFFENSE: FAILURE TO COMPLY WITH PREVIOUS BOARD ORDER

NOTES: VIOLATED 5/24/89 ORDER IN THE FOLLOWING WAYS: IN 10/89 A BLOOD SAMPLE TESTED POSITIVE FOR ALCOHOL; ALSO FAILED TO OBTAIN A BOARD-APPROVED TREATING PHYSICIAN AND MAINTAIN A LOG OF ALL MEDICATIONS TAKEN. CONDITIONS OF PROBATION: MUST IMMEDIATELY ENROLL IN THE LEVEL III AFTERCARE PROGRAM OF NAVAL HOSPITAL AND ATTEND 4 12-STEP AA WEEKLY MEETINGS; WEEKLY MEETINGS WITH AFTERCARE PROGRAM MANAGER; MANDATORY URINALYSIS TWICE WEEKLY; MANDATORY USE OF ANTABUSE. MUST CONTINUE TO PARTICIPATE IN A SUBSTANCE ABUSE TREATMENT PROGRAM EVEN WHEN FORMAL REGIMEN ENDS ON 12/11/90. QUARTERLY REPORTS MUST BE SUBMITTED TO BOARD BY PROGRAM OR THERAPIST; WILL ALSO ABIDE BY TERMS OF 5/24/89 ORDER.

WILLIAMS, PAUL C MD, DATE OF BIRTH DECEMBER 4, 1942, LICENSE NUMBER 0017317 OF LAKE OSWEGO, OR, WAS DISCIPLINED BY COLORADO ON JULY 12, 1991
DISCIPLINARY ACTION: 60-MONTH PROBATION; REQUIRED TO ENTER AN IMPAIRED PHYSICIAN PROGRAM OR SUBSTANCE ABUSE TREATMENT
OFFENSE: SUBSTANCE ABUSE

NOTES: HABITUAL INTEMPERANCE, ALCOHOL ABUSE AND ALCOHOL DEPENDENCE. ALCOHOL TREATMENT AND MONITORING AND PRACTICE MONITORING. IN ABEYANCE.

WILLIAMS, PAUL CARROLL MD, LICENSE NUMBER 0017419 OF PORTLAND, OR, WAS DISCIPLINED BY OREGON ON AUGUST 15, 1991
DISCIPLINARY ACTION: 120-MONTH PROBATION
OFFENSE: SUBSTANCE ABUSE

NOTES: ALLEGED PERSONAL SUBSTANCE ABUSE. REVOCATION STAYED. AS OF 2/22/95 NO LONGER LISTED AS ON PROBATION.

WILLIAMS, PAUL CARROLL MD, LICENSE NUMBER 0C34650 OF LAKE OSWEGO, OR, WAS DISCIPLINED BY CALIFORNIA ON JUNE 18, 1992
DISCIPLINARY ACTION: 60-MONTH PROBATION
OFFENSE: DISCIPLINARY ACTION BY ANOTHER STATE OR AGENCY

NOTES: DISCIPLINED BY ARIZONA BOARD RELATED TO ALCOHOL ABUSE. REVOCATION, STAYED. PROBATION WITH TERMS AND CONDITIONS.

WILSON, JAMES P MD, DATE OF BIRTH MARCH 28, 1944, LICENSE NUMBER 0018578 OF AURORA, CO, WAS DISCIPLINED BY COLORADO ON MARCH 2, 1994
DISCIPLINARY ACTION: REPRIMAND
OFFENSE: PROFESSIONAL MISCONDUCT

WILSON, JAMES P MD, DATE OF BIRTH MARCH 28, 1944, LICENSE NUMBER 1030102 OF 18556 E LONG AVE, AURORA, CO, WAS DISCIPLINED BY MICHIGAN ON OCTOBER 18, 1995
DISCIPLINARY ACTION: REPRIMAND
OFFENSE: SUBSTANDARD CARE, INCOMPETENCE OR NEGLIGENCE

NOTES: NEGLIGENCE.

WILSON, ROBERT S DO, DATE OF BIRTH AUGUST 20, 1949, LICENSE NUMBER 0027467, WAS DISCIPLINED BY COLORADO ON NOVEMBER 16, 1995
DISCIPLINARY ACTION: 60-MONTH PROBATION; MONITORING OF PHYSICIAN PERFORMANCE

NOTES: PRACTICE AND TREATMENT MONITORING.

WILSON, ROBERT STOREY DO, LICENSE NUMBER 00E4770 OF GRANBURY, TX, WAS DISCIPLINED BY TEXAS ON MAY 11, 1995
DISCIPLINARY ACTION: RESTRICTION PLACED ON CONTROLLED SUBSTANCE LICENSE; REQUIRED TO TAKE ADDITIONAL MEDICAL EDUCATION
OFFENSE: SUBSTANCE ABUSE

NOTES: IN 8/93 HE BEGAN SELF-ADMINISTERING DILAUDID WITHOUT A LEGITIMATE MEDICAL PURPOSE AND AS A RESULT OF EMOTIONAL HARDSHIP AND DEPRESSION HE EXPERIENCED DUE TO HIS WIFE'S MEDICAL CONDITION; WROTE FALSE AND FICTITIOUS PRESCRIPTIONS IN ORDER TO OBTAIN DILAUDID; IN 7/94, HE ENTERED AN INTERIM CONTRACT WITH THE TEXAS OSTEOPATHIC MEDICAL ASSOCIATION TO REFRAIN FROM THE PRACTICE OF MEDICINE UNTIL HE SUCCESSFULLY COMPLETED TREATMENT FOR SUBSTANCE ADDICTION; ENTERED A 24-MONTH AFTERCARE RECOVERY CONTRACT; VOLUNTARILY ENTERED A TREATMENT FACILITY IN 7/94 AND SUBSEQUENTLY VOLUNTARILY TRANSFERRED TO INPATIENT TREATMENT WHICH LASTED 97 DAYS; REPORTS SOBRIETY DATE OF 7/17/94; HAS BEEN IN COMPLIANCE WITH HIS AFTERCARE CONTRACT; REPORTS ATTENDING APPROXIMATELY FIVE AA OR NARCOTICS ANONYMOUS MEETINGS PER WEEK. LICENSE RESTRICTED FOR FIVE YEARS UNDER TERMS: SHALL ABSTAIN FROM THE CONSUMPTION OF ALCOHOL/DRUGS IN ANY FORM UNLESS PRESCRIBED BY ANOTHER PHYSICIAN FOR A LEGITIMATE AND THERAPEUTIC PURPOSE; SHALL SUBMIT HIMSELF FOR APPROPRIATE EXAMS INCLUDING DRUG OR ALCOHOL SCREENS; SHALL SUBMIT HIMSELF FOR EVALUATION AND TREATMENT BY A BOARD-APPROVED PSYCHIATRIST AT LEAST ONCE A MONTH WHO WILL SUBMIT REPORTS TO THE BOARD; SHALL CONTINUE TO PARTICIPATE IN AA OR NARCOTICS ANONYMOUS PROGRAM NOT LESS THAN THREE TIMES A WEEK WITH QUARTERLY REPORTS TO THE BOARD; SHALL CONTINUE TO PARTICIPATE IN THE ACTIVITIES OF AN IMPAIRED PHYSICIAN'S GROUP AND ABIDE BY TERMS OF ANY AFTERCARE PROGRAM REQUIRED WITH QUARTERLY REPORTS; SHALL COMPLY WITH TERMS OF ANY CONTRACT ENTERED INTO FOR HOSPITAL PRIVILEGES AND SHALL INFORM BOARD OF ANY DISCIPLINE; EXCEPT AS OTHERWISE PROVIDED FOR BY THIS ORDER, SHALL NOT POSSESS ALCOHOL, CONTROLLED SUBSTANCES OR DRUGS WITH ADDICTIVE POTENTIAL; SHALL SURRENDER SAMPLES OF ANY SUCH DRUGS IN HIS POSSESSION; SHALL NOT OTHERWISE SERVE AS PHYSICIAN, PRESCRIBE, DISPENSE OR ADMINISTER DRUGS THAT MAY BE SUBJECT TO ABUSE TO HIMSELF OR TO ANY MEMBER OF HIS FAMILY; SHALL NOT TELEPHONE TO A PHARMACY A PRESCRIPTION FOR CONTROLLED SUBSTANCES NOR PERMIT ANYONE HE SUPERVISES TO TELEPHONE; MAY NOT POSSESS, ADMINISTER, DISPENSE, ORDER OR PRESCRIBE CONTROLLED SUBSTANCES EXCEPT ORDER FOR HOSPITAL INPATIENTS OR NURSING HOME PATIENTS; MAY PRESCRIBE RITALIN TO PEDIATRIC PATIENTS DIAGNOSED WITH ATTENTION DEFICIT ORDER; SHALL KEEP A SEPARATE LOG OF ALL PRESCRIPTIONS FOR CONTROLLED SUBSTANCES WHICH SHALL BE AVAILABLE FOR REVIEW; SHALL MAINTAIN ADEQUATE MEDICAL RECORDS WHICH SHALL BE AVAILABLE FOR REVIEW; SHALL OBTAIN AT LEAST 50 HOURS PER YEAR OF CONTINUING MEDICAL EDUCATION; SHALL APPEAR BEFORE BOARD AT LEAST ONCE A YEAR; SHALL COOPERATE WITH THE BOARD IN VERIFYING COMPLIANCE INCLUDING PROVIDING COPIES OF MEDICAL RELEASES OR PEER REVIEW RECORDS UPON REQUEST; SHALL GIVE A COPY OF THIS ORDER TO ANY HEALTH CARE ENTITY WHERE HE HAS PRIVILEGES; SHALL PROVIDE A COPY OF THE ORDER TO ANYONE REQUESTING IT WITHIN 10 DAYS; TIME PERIOD OUT OF TEXAS DOES NOT COUNT TOWARD PROBATION; SHALL INFORM BOARD OF CHANGE OF ADDRESS WITHIN 10 DAYS OR IF HE LEAVES THE STATE. SHALL NOT SEEK MODIFICATION FOR ONE YEAR. ON 5/10/97 PETITION TO TERMINATE ORDER DENIED. ON 8/10/97 PETITION TO TERMINATE ORDER DENIED. ON 8/22/98 ORDER TERMINATED.

WILSON, RODDY L DO, DATE OF BIRTH MARCH 20, 1951, LICENSE NUMBER 21882, WAS DISCIPLINED BY COLORADO ON JULY 9, 1998
OFFENSE: SUBSTANCE ABUSE

NOTES: HABITUAL INTEMPERANCE AND DEPRESSION. COLORADO MEDICAL LICENSE INACTIVATED. WHEN HIS LICENSE IS RETURNED TO ACTIVE STATUS HE SHALL BEGIN A FIVE YEAR PROBATIONARY PERIOD WITH PRACTICE AND TREATMENT MONITORING.

WILSON, RODDY L DO, DATE OF BIRTH MARCH 20, 1951, LICENSE NUMBER 21882, WAS DISCIPLINED BY COLORADO ON MARCH 18, 1999
DISCIPLINARY ACTION: SURRENDER OF LICENSE
OFFENSE: FAILURE TO COMPLY WITH PREVIOUS BOARD ORDER

NOTES: VIOLATION OF A VALID BOARD ORDER.

WILSON, RODDY LYNN MD, WAS DISCIPLINED BY NEBRASKA ON JULY 17, 1998
DISCIPLINARY ACTION: LICENSE REVOCATION
OFFENSE: SUBSTANCE ABUSE

NOTES: ALCOHOL ADDICTION.

WILSON, SHAWN L MD, DATE OF BIRTH JANUARY 5, 1960, LICENSE NUMBER 36177, WAS DISCIPLINED BY COLORADO ON JUNE 19, 1997
DISCIPLINARY ACTION: PROBATION; MONITORING OF PHYSICIAN PERFORMANCE
OFFENSE: SUBSTANCE ABUSE

NOTES: HISTORY OF HABITUAL INTEMPERANCE OR EXCESSIVE USE OF A CONTROLLED SUBSTANCE. PROBATIONARY TERMS INCLUDE ABSTINENCE FROM ADDICTIVE SUBSTANCES, TREATMENT AND PRACTICE MONITORING.

WOLF, ELLIOTT M MD, DATE OF BIRTH JANUARY 26, 1943, LICENSE NUMBER 0017253 OF OKEMOS, MI, WAS DISCIPLINED BY COLORADO ON FEBRUARY 14, 1992
DISCIPLINARY ACTION: SURRENDER OF LICENSE
OFFENSE: SUBSTANDARD CARE, INCOMPETENCE OR NEGLIGENCE

NOTES: PATIENT CARE ISSUES; FAILURE TO MEET GENERALLY ACCEPTED STANDARDS OF MEDICAL PRACTICE.

WOLFE, ALVIN E DO, LICENSE NUMBER 00D7715 OF WICHITA, KS, WAS DISCIPLINED BY TEXAS ON APRIL 21, 1990

NOTES: STIPULATED ORDER. MUST REQUEST PERSONAL INTERVIEW BEFORE BOARD TO DISCUSS PRESENT STATUS, LOCATION AND TYPE OF PRACTICE DESIRED TO ENTER INTO, AND RECEIVE APPROVAL PRIOR TO PRACTICING IN TEXAS.

WOLFE, ALVIN E DO, DATE OF BIRTH AUGUST 15, 1932, LICENSE NUMBER 0015428 OF WICHITA, KS, WAS DISCIPLINED BY COLORADO ON OCTOBER 18, 1991
DISCIPLINARY ACTION: SURRENDER OF LICENSE
OFFENSE: DISCIPLINARY ACTION BY ANOTHER STATE OR AGENCY

NOTES: ADMINISTERING, DISPENSING OR PRESCRIBING A HABIT FORMING DRUG NOT IN THE COURSE OF LEGITIMATE MEDICAL PRACTICE. PERMANENT SURRENDER OF COLORADO MEDICAL LICENSE. ACTION TAKEN BY KANSAS BOARD.

WOLFF, QUENTIN A MD, DATE OF BIRTH OCTOBER 11, 1949, LICENSE NUMBER 0020333, WAS DISCIPLINED BY COLORADO ON OCTOBER 18, 1996
DISCIPLINARY ACTION: EMERGENCY SUSPENSION

WOLFF, QUENTIN A MD, DATE OF BIRTH OCTOBER 11, 1949, LICENSE NUMBER 20333, WAS DISCIPLINED BY COLORADO ON APRIL 17, 1997
DISCIPLINARY ACTION: LICENSE REVOCATION
OFFENSE: PHYSICAL OR MENTAL ILLNESS INHIBITING THE ABILITY TO PRACTICE WITH SKILL AND SAFETY

NOTES: PHYSICAL OR MENTAL DISABILITY.

WOOD, DAVID L MD, LICENSE NUMBER 0074992 OF 504 BARRE ROAD, OAKHAM, MA, WAS DISCIPLINED BY MASSACHUSETTS ON AUGUST 10, 1992
DISCIPLINARY ACTION: EMERGENCY SUSPENSION

WOOD, DAVID L MD, LICENSE NUMBER 0074992 OF 504 BARRE ROAD, OAKHAM, MA, WAS DISCIPLINED BY MASSACHUSETTS ON AUGUST 25, 1993
DISCIPLINARY ACTION: LICENSE REVOCATION
OFFENSE: CRIMINAL CONVICTION OR PLEA OF GUILTY, NOLO CONTENDERE, OR NO CONTEST TO A CRIME

NOTES: CRIMINAL CONVICTION; SEXUAL MISCONDUCT: MINOR.

WOOD, DAVID L MD, DATE OF BIRTH NOVEMBER 16, 1949 OF 504 BARRE ROAD, OAKHAM, MA, WAS DISCIPLINED BY MEDICARE ON DECEMBER 8, 1993
DISCIPLINARY ACTION: 60-MONTH EXCLUSION FROM THE MEDICARE AND/OR MEDICAID PROGRAM
OFFENSE: CRIMINAL CONVICTION OR PLEA OF GUILTY, NOLO CONTENDERE, OR NO CONTEST TO A CRIME

NOTES: CONVICTED OF PATIENT ABUSE.

WOOD, DAVID LLOYD DO OF 200 W COUNTY LINE ROAD, HIGHLANDS RANCH, CO, WAS DISCIPLINED BY DEA ON JANUARY 27, 1994
DISCIPLINARY ACTION: RESTRICTION PLACED ON CONTROLLED SUBSTANCE LICENSE
OFFENSE: OVERPRESCRIBING OR MISPRESCRIBING DRUGS

NOTES: REGISTRATION ON PROBATION FOR IMPROPER PRESCRIPTION INVOLVING PERCOCET, FIORINAL, CLORAZEPATE, HYCOTUSS AND TUSSEND. RENEWAL APPLICATION FOR REGISTRATION 06/06/92. ENTERED INTO MEMORANDUM OF UNDERSTANDING 03/10/93.

WOOD, DAVID LLOYD DO OF 200 WEST COUNTY LINE ROAD, HIGHLANDS RANCH, CO, WAS DISCIPLINED BY DEA ON AUGUST 21, 1995
DISCIPLINARY ACTION: RESTRICTION PLACED ON CONTROLLED SUBSTANCE LICENSE

NOTES: MEMO OF UNDERSTANDING.

YOUNG, KENNETH S MD, DATE OF BIRTH MARCH 23, 1947, LICENSE NUMBER 30729, WAS DISCIPLINED BY COLORADO ON MAY 15, 1998
DISCIPLINARY ACTION: LICENSE SUSPENSION
OFFENSE: FAILURE TO COMPLY WITH PREVIOUS BOARD ORDER

NOTES: FAILURE TO COMPLY WITH A PREVIOUS BOARD ORDER FOR A MEDICAL EXAM.

YOUNG, LUCIEN DAVID DO, DATE OF BIRTH FEBRUARY 3, 1942, LICENSE NUMBER 0017816 OF ORANGE PARK, FL, WAS DISCIPLINED BY COLORADO ON OCTOBER 14, 1994
DISCIPLINARY ACTION: 60-MONTH PROBATION; MONITORING OF PHYSICIAN PERFORMANCE
OFFENSE: PHYSICAL OR MENTAL ILLNESS INHIBITING THE ABILITY TO PRACTICE WITH SKILL AND SAFETY

NOTES: PROBATION PERIOD INCLUDES PRACTICE/TREATMENT MONITORING FOR FIVE YEARS AND LIFETIME MENTAL STATUS MONITORING. IN ABEYANCE PENDING HIS RELOCATION TO COLORADO TO PRACTICE MEDICINE.

YOUNG, PHILIP G MD, DATE OF BIRTH FEBRUARY 3, 1938, LICENSE NUMBER 16963, WAS DISCIPLINED BY COLORADO ON APRIL 15, 1996
DISCIPLINARY ACTION: LICENSE REVOCATION
OFFENSE: SUBSTANDARD CARE, INCOMPETENCE OR NEGLIGENCE

NOTES: SUBSTANDARD CARE.

YOUNG, PHILIP G MD, DATE OF BIRTH FEBRUARY 3, 1938, LICENSE NUMBER 16963, WAS DISCIPLINED BY COLORADO ON JANUARY 29, 1998
DISCIPLINARY ACTION: EMERGENCY SUSPENSION

ZAJAC, JOHN J MD, DATE OF BIRTH DECEMBER 16, 1944, LICENSE NUMBER 0022332 OF WOODLAND PARK, CO, WAS DISCIPLINED BY COLORADO ON NOVEMBER 6, 1992
DISCIPLINARY ACTION: SURRENDER OF LICENSE
OFFENSE: FAILURE TO COMPLY WITH PREVIOUS BOARD ORDER

NOTES: PHYSICAL AND MENTAL DISABILITIES WHICH RENDER HIM UNABLE TO PRACTICE WITH SKILL AND SAFETY; EXCESSIVE USE OF A CONTROLLED SUBSTANCE; NON EMERGENCY SELF-MEDICATION WITH SCHEDULE II CONTROLLED SUBSTANCE; FAILURE TO MEET GENERALLY ACCEPTED STANDARDS OF MEDICAL PRACTICE; REPEATEDLY FAILING TO MAKE ESSENTIAL

ENTRIES ON PATIENT RECORDS; FAILURE TO COMPLY WITH A BOARD ORDER.

ZIMIK, LUITHUK MD, DATE OF BIRTH APRIL 2, 1939, LICENSE NUMBER 0021490 OF BRIGHTON, CO, WAS DISCIPLINED BY COLORADO ON OCTOBER 14, 1994
DISCIPLINARY ACTION: 60-MONTH PROBATION; REQUIRED TO TAKE ADDITIONAL MEDICAL EDUCATION
OFFENSE: SUBSTANDARD CARE, INCOMPETENCE OR NEGLIGENCE

NOTES: ALLEGATIONS OF AN ACT OR OMISSION CONSTITUTING GROSSLY NEGLIGENT MEDICAL PRACTICE OR TWO OR MORE ACTS OR OMISSIONS WHICH FAIL TO MEET GENERALLY ACCEPTED STANDARDS. PROBATION PERIOD INCLUDES PRACTICE MONITORING AND CONTINUING MEDICAL EDUCATION REQUIREMENTS.

ZIMIK, LUITHUK MD, DATE OF BIRTH APRIL 2, 1939, LICENSE NUMBER 21490, WAS DISCIPLINED BY COLORADO ON JANUARY 16, 1997
DISCIPLINARY ACTION: REPRIMAND

ZIOLKOWSKI, THOMAS J MD, DATE OF BIRTH JULY 15, 1957, LICENSE NUMBER 0027236, WAS DISCIPLINED BY COLORADO ON MARCH 14, 1996
DISCIPLINARY ACTION: REPRIMAND

ZIOLKOWSKI, THOMAS J MD, DATE OF BIRTH JULY 25, 1927, LICENSE NUMBER 27236, WAS DISCIPLINED BY COLORADO ON JUNE 18, 1998

NOTES: NO UNPROFESSIONAL CONDUCT IDENTIFIED. HE AGREES TO PERMANENTLY PLACE HIS LICENSE IN INACTIVE STATUS.

ZUCKERMAN, JAMES E MD, DATE OF BIRTH JANUARY 14, 1937, LICENSE NUMBER 36813, WAS DISCIPLINED BY COLORADO ON FEBRUARY 11, 1998
DISCIPLINARY ACTION: REPRIMAND

NOTES: OUT-OF-STATE DISCIPLINE.

NEVADA

1999 serious action rate: 3.26/1000
1999 ranking: 25th

The Nevada State Board of Medical Examiners sent copies of newsletters containing all disciplinary actions from 1990 through 1999. The listings include the physician's name, degree, the type of action taken and the reason for the action. In early newsletters, the actual action date was not provided. The date of the newsletter was entered as a proxy. The newsletters contain some information on modifications and terminations of board actions and no information on court decisions affecting board actions. Nevada sent separate information on these actions.

The information provided covers disciplinary actions taken against allopathic physicians (MDs) only. Nevada's separate osteopathic board has taken no actions since 1996.

Besides disciplinary actions taken by the State Medical Board, this listing also includes actions taken by the Medicare/Medicaid programs, the FDA, and the DEA against physicians located in this state. Disciplinary actions taken by other states against physicians located in Nevada or that match a physician disciplined by Nevada (see Appendix 2 for an explanation of the matching protocol) are also included.

Although we have made every effort to match physicians' names correctly, some materials we received did not include complete information on middle names, license numbers, birth dates or addresses. Therefore, consumers should remember that non-disciplined physicians and physicians with different disciplinary actions may have similar names to those disciplined physicians listed in this state. Consumers should also remember that if they want the most current information on the status on a physician's license, they should contact the medical board of the state in which the physician practices or had practiced. (See board address below.) Internet address: *http://www.state.nv.us/medical.* This state has a web site which we have graded B on a scale of A (best) to X (worst). This is a measure of the completeness of the information on disciplined doctors. Those state licensing boards with web sites make independent choices about the type of information to be included on their site and how often it is updated.

According to the Federation of State Medical Boards, Nevada took 11 serious disciplinary actions against MDs in 1999. Compared to the 3,373 MDs practicing in the state, Nevada had a serious disciplinary action rate of 3.26 serious actions per 1,000 MDs and a ranking of 25th on that list (see Table A, Findings, pg. 14).

The tables below summarize the data Public Citizen received from Nevada.

Table 1. Disciplinary Actions Against MDs 1990 through 1999*

Action	Number	Percent**
Revocation	25	16.6%
Surrender	11	7.3%
Suspension	2	1.3%
Probation	22	14.6%
Practice Restriction	10	6.6%
Action Taken Against Controlled Substance License	5	3.3%
Other Actions	76	50.3%
Total Actions	**151**	**100.0%**

* This table lists only the two most serious disciplinary actions taken against a physician.
** Percentages may not total 100% due to rounding.

Table 2. Offenses for which MDs were Disciplined 1990 through 1999*		
Offense	**Number**	**Percent**
Criminal Conviction	10	9.5%
Sexual Abuse of or Sexual Misconduct with a Patient	0	0.0%
Substandard Care, Incompetence or Negligence	13	12.4%
Misprescribing or Overprescribing Drugs	8	7.6%
Substance Abuse	3	2.9%
Disciplinary Action Taken Against License by Another State or Agency	31	29.5%
Other Offenses	40	38.1%
Total Records With Offense Listed	**105**	**100.0%**

* Includes only those actions for which an offense was listed and for which we had a corresponding term in our database.

Table 3. Disciplinary Actions Taken for Substandard Care, Incompetence or Negligence		
Action	**Number**	**Percent**
Revocation	5	31.3%
Emergency Suspension	3	18.8%
Probation	2	12.5%
Practice Restriction	2	12.5%
Fine	1	6.3%
Reprimand	2	12.5%
Other Actions	1	6.3%
Total Actions	**16**	**100.0%**

Table 4. Disciplinary Actions Taken for Criminal Conviction		
Action	**Number**	**Percent**
Revocation	3	21.4%
Probation	2	14.3%
Fine	2	14.3%
Other Actions	7	50.0%
Total Actions	**14**	**100.0%**

Table 5. Disciplinary Actions Taken for Misprescribing or Overprescribing Drugs		
Action	**Number**	**Percent**
Surrender	1	7.1%
Emergency Suspension	1	7.1%
Probation	4	28.6%
Restriction of Controlled Substance License	4	28.6%
Fine	1	7.1%
Education	1	7.1%
Other Actions	2	14.3%
Total Actions	**14**	**100.0%**

Addresses

Nevada State Board of Medical Examiners
Larry D. Lessly, JD, Executive Director
P.O. Box 7238
Reno, NV 89510
(775) 688-2559
Fax: (775) 688-2321
E-mail: nsbme@govmail.state.nv.us

Nevada State Board of Osteopathic Medicine
Larry J. Tarno, DO, Executive Director
2950 East Flamingo Road, Suite E-3
Las Vegas, NV 89121-5208
(702) 732-2147

Listing of Doctors Sanctioned by Offense

Substandard Care, Incompetence, or Negligence

BASS, HARRISTON LEE
CAPPIELLO, RAFAEL M
CAVANAGH, JAMES G
CHANCELLOR, ROBERT S
CHOMIAK, BRYANT D
DE LEE, SOL T
EVANGELISTA, LUISITO A
MARTELL, ALGIS
MEISENHEIMER, KARL W
MINTON, GREGORY A
MOLDE, DONALD A
WYCKOFF, STUART M

Criminal Conviction or Plea of Guilty, Nolo Contendere, or No Contest to a Crime

CSERNA, GEZA JED
EMERY, CLYDE K
GHARAVI, NAJM M
GLADSTONE, SCOTT B
KELLY, RONALD K
MARLON, ANTHONY
MCCORMICK, THOMAS M
MCNAIR, KIMBLE
RIDENOUR, GARY C
WILCOURT, ROBIN J

Misprescribing or Overprescribing Drugs

EMETERIO, LOUIS C
GILBERT, WARREN S
MARTELL, ALGIS
ONG, TENG C
RUECA, CARLOS N
STOERMER, DIETRICH A
THORP, THEODORE M

Substance Abuse

CHOMIAK, BRYANT D
FRANCO, ALLEN I

Caution: This list is designed to be used only in conjunction with the rest of this book which includes additional information on each physician such as license number, date of action and more complete descriptions of the offenses.

ADAMSON, KIM A MD, WAS DISCIPLINED BY NEVADA ON NOVEMBER 9, 1994
DISCIPLINARY ACTION: 120-MONTH PROBATION; FINE
OFFENSE: FAILURE TO COMPLY WITH PREVIOUS BOARD ORDER

NOTES: ON 08/10/94 CHARGED WITH NONCOMPLIANCE OF PROBATION IMPOSED 6/10/88. STAY OF REVOCATION CONTINUED. CONDITIONS OF PROBATION: $2,500 FINE AND COST OF HEARING; RANDOM URINE DRUG TESTING; PROHIBITED FROM PRESCRIBING SCHEDULES II AND III AND STADOL AND NUBAIN; PRACTICE LIMITED TO A BOARD APPROVED STRUCTURE; MUST ABIDE BY ALL CONDITIONS OF AGREEMENT WITH PHYSICIANS ASSISTANCE COMMITTEE.

ADAMSON, KIM A MD, WAS DISCIPLINED BY NEVADA ON MAY 5, 1995
DISCIPLINARY ACTION: 6-MONTH EMERGENCY SUSPENSION
OFFENSE: FAILURE TO COMPLY WITH PREVIOUS BOARD ORDER

NOTES: VIOLATION OF TERMS OF PROBATION IMPOSED BY ORDER EFFECTIVE 11/9/94. PETITION FOR LIFT OF STAY OF LICENSE REVOCATION FILED 5/5/95. SUSPENSION ORDERED TO REMAIN IN EFFECT UNTIL 11/5/95 AT 6/09/95 HEARING.

ADAMSON, KIM A MD, WAS DISCIPLINED BY NEVADA ON DECEMBER 29, 1995
DISCIPLINARY ACTION: 120-MONTH PROBATION; RESTRICTION PLACED ON LICENSE
OFFENSE: FAILURE TO COMPLY WITH PREVIOUS BOARD ORDER

NOTES: VIOLATED A PROVISION OF 11/1/94 PROBATION, SPECIFICALLY, WORKING IN OTHER THAN A CLOSELY SUPERVISED, STRUCTURED WORK ENVIRONMENT IN AN URBAN AREA; HE ENTERED INTO A CHANGE OF EMPLOYMENT TO PERFORM MEDICAL CARE AT A COUNTY JAIL WITHOUT PRIOR APPROVAL OF THE BOARD AND CONTINUED TO PERFORM MEDICAL CARE AT THE COUNTY JAIL AFTER BEING DENIED APPROVAL BY THE BOARD. REVOCATION STAYED; PROBATION RETROACTIVE TO 11/9/94 WITH CONDITIONS AS FOLLOWS: SHALL BE ALLOWED TO OPEN AND ENGAGE IN A PRIVATE PRACTICE AND WORK IN THE EMERGENCY ROOM OF A SPECIFIED HOSPITAL; SHALL ABIDE BY ALL TERMS OF PREVIOUS PROBATION AND WITH HIS AGREEMENT WITH NEVADA DIVERSION PROGRAM.

ADAMSON, KIM A MD, WAS DISCIPLINED BY NEVADA ON JANUARY 27, 1997
DISCIPLINARY ACTION: LICENSE REVOCATION
OFFENSE: FAILURE TO COMPLY WITH PREVIOUS BOARD ORDER

NOTES: VIOLATED 1/5/96 ORDER BY NOT COMPLYING WITH TERMS OF AGREEMENT WITH NEVADA DIVERSION PROGRAM FOR PHYSICIANS AND PHYSICIAN ASSISTANTS.

ADAMSON, KIM A MD, DATE OF BIRTH MAY 11, 1956 OF 430 PINTAIL DRIVE, FALLON, NV, WAS DISCIPLINED BY MEDICARE ON OCTOBER 20, 1998
DISCIPLINARY ACTION: EXCLUSION FROM THE MEDICARE AND/OR MEDICAID PROGRAM
OFFENSE: DISCIPLINARY ACTION BY ANOTHER STATE OR AGENCY

NOTES: LICENSE REVOKED, SUSPENDED, SURRENDERED OR OTHERWISE LOST FOR REASONS BEARING ON PROFESSIONAL PERFORMANCE, PROFESSIONAL COMPETENCE OR FINANCIAL INTEGRITY.

ADAMSON, KIM ALAN MD, LICENSE NUMBER G054258 OF FALLON, NV, WAS DISCIPLINED BY CALIFORNIA ON NOVEMBER 16, 1990
DISCIPLINARY ACTION: 120-MONTH PROBATION
OFFENSE: DISCIPLINARY ACTION BY ANOTHER STATE OR AGENCY

NOTES: DISCIPLINED BY NEVADA BOARD FOR SELF USE OF DRUGS. REVOCATION STAYED.

AGRONIN, IRINA Z MD, LICENSE NUMBER 00LL602, WAS DISCIPLINED BY NEVADA ON JUNE 7, 1991
DISCIPLINARY ACTION: LICENSE REVOCATION
OFFENSE: PROVIDING FALSE INFORMATION TO THE BOARD OR OTHER HEALTH AGENCY

NOTES: INTENTIONALLY MADE A FALSE, MISLEADING, INACCURATE AND INCOMPLETE STATEMENT ON HER APPLICATION FOR LICENSURE AS A RESIDENT PHYSICIAN IN NEVADA. REVOCATION OF RESIDENCE LICENSE. NOT LICENSED AS OF 9/9/92.

AHMED, TARIQ MD, WAS DISCIPLINED BY NEVADA ON MARCH 20, 1992
DISCIPLINARY ACTION: DENIAL OF NEW LICENSE
OFFENSE: PROVIDING FALSE INFORMATION TO THE BOARD OR OTHER HEALTH AGENCY

NOTES: ENGAGED IN CONDUCT INTENDED TO DECEIVE THE BOARD BY INTENTIONALLY MAKING A FALSE, MISLEADING, INACCURATE AND INCOMPLETE STATEMENT ON HIS APPLICATION FOR LICENSURE AS A RESIDENT PHYSICIAN IN NEVADA. LIMITED LICENSE DENIED.

AMANATULLAH, FAISAL F MD, WAS DISCIPLINED BY NEVADA ON APRIL 3, 1995
DISCIPLINARY ACTION: FINE; REPRIMAND
OFFENSE: OVERCHARGING

NOTES: MAKING UNREASONABLE ADDITIONAL CHARGES FOR LAB TESTS; ENGAGED IN CONDUCT INTENDED TO DECEIVE; AND CHARGED FOR SERVICES NOT RENDERED. SHALL NOT CHARGE ANY PATIENT ANY ADDITIONAL CHARGE OVER AND ABOVE WHAT HE IS CHARGED FOR TESTS IN A LABORATORY, RADIOLOGICAL SERVICES OR OTHER SERVICES FOR TESTING WHICH HE ORDERS AND HAS PERFORMED OUTSIDE HIS OWN OFFICE; MAY CHARGE A PATIENT A DRAWING OR COLLECTION FEE FOR THE COLLECTION OF A SPECIMEN WHICH FEE SHALL BE CONSISTENT WITH WHAT OTHER AREA COMMUNITY PHYSICIANS CHARGE. $5,000 FINE AND $5,000 ADMINISTRATIVE COSTS.

AMANATULLAH, FAISAL F MD, DATE OF BIRTH SEPTEMBER 5, 1948, LICENSE NUMBER 25585, WAS DISCIPLINED BY COLORADO ON MAY 21, 1999
DISCIPLINARY ACTION: LICENSE REVOCATION
OFFENSE: SUBSTANDARD CARE, INCOMPETENCE OR NEGLIGENCE

NOTES: SUBSTANDARD CARE; UNNECESSARY TESTS OR TREATMENT.

ARANAS, ROMEO S DR OF PEKIN, IL, WAS DISCIPLINED BY ILLINOIS ON APRIL 1, 1991
DISCIPLINARY ACTION: 24-MONTH PROBATION; 36-MONTH CONTROLLED SUBSTANCE LICENSE PLACED ON PROBATION
OFFENSE: NONCOMPLIANCE WITH A PROFESSIONAL RULE

NOTES: VIOLATED NUMEROUS PROVISIONS OF THE MEDICAL PRACTICE ACT OF 1987 AND THE CONTROLLED SUBSTANCES ACT.

ARANAS, ROMEO S MD, LICENSE NUMBER 0119926 OF 610 PARK AVENUE, PEKIN, IL, WAS DISCIPLINED BY NEW YORK ON AUGUST 23, 1994

DISCIPLINARY ACTION: REPRIMAND
OFFENSE: DISCIPLINARY ACTION BY ANOTHER STATE OR AGENCY

NOTES: DID NOT CONTEST THAT HE WAS DISCIPLINED BY THE ILLINOIS BOARD.

ARANAS, ROMEO S MD, WAS DISCIPLINED BY NEVADA ON MARCH 27, 1995
DISCIPLINARY ACTION: REPRIMAND
OFFENSE: DISCIPLINARY ACTION BY ANOTHER STATE OR AGENCY

NOTES: IN 4/91, ILLINOIS PLACED LICENSE ON PROBATION AS A RESULT OF A FAILURE TO KEEP PROPER DISPENSING RECORDS, FAILURE TO PROVIDE EFFECTIVE CONTROLS TO GUARD AGAINST THE DIVERSION OF CONTROLLED SUBSTANCES AND PRESCRIBING ANOREXIC MEDICATIONS; IN 8/94 NEW YORK BOARD REPRIMANDED HIM BASED ON THE ILLINOIS ACTION. $300 ADMINISTRATIVE COSTS.

AZLEIN, KIT GEOFFREY MD MD, LICENSE NUMBER G35286 OF RENO, NV, WAS DISCIPLINED BY CALIFORNIA ON MAY 29, 1997
DISCIPLINARY ACTION: SURRENDER OF LICENSE

NOTES: WHILE CHARGES PENDING.

AZLEIN, KIT GEOFFREY MD, DATE OF BIRTH APRIL 18, 1950 OF 1949 VILLA WAY SOUTH, RENO, NV, WAS DISCIPLINED BY MEDICARE ON AUGUST 20, 1998
DISCIPLINARY ACTION: EXCLUSION FROM THE MEDICARE AND/OR MEDICAID PROGRAM
OFFENSE: DISCIPLINARY ACTION BY ANOTHER STATE OR AGENCY

NOTES: LICENSE REVOKED, SUSPENDED, SURRENDERED OR OTHERWISE LOST FOR REASONS BEARING ON PROFESSIONAL PERFORMANCE, PROFESSIONAL COMPETENCE OR FINANCIAL INTEGRITY.

BAIG, KHALIQ R MD, WAS DISCIPLINED BY NEVADA ON JUNE 6, 1998
DISCIPLINARY ACTION: 36-MONTH PROBATION; RESTRICTION PLACED ON LICENSE
OFFENSE: PROFESSIONAL MISCONDUCT

NOTES: AIDING, ASSISTING, EMPLOYING OR ADVISING ANY UNLICENSED PERSON TO ENGAGE IN THE PRACTICE OF MEDICINE; SIGNING A BLANK PRESCRIPTION FORM. REVOCATION STAYED. CONDITIONS OF PROBATION AS FOLLOWS: SHALL BE PRECLUDED FROM BEING A SPONSORING PHYSICIAN FOR ANY PHYSICIAN SEEKING THE RIGHTS TO PRACTICE MEDICINE IN NEVADA UNDER ANY DEPARTMENT OF JUSTICE, IMMIGRATION AND NATURALIZATION SERVICE OR OTHER FEDERAL GOVERNMENT PROGRAM; SHALL BE PRECLUDED FROM BEING A SUPERVISING PHYSICIAN FOR A PHYSICIAN ASSISTANT OR A COLLABORATING PHYSICIAN FOR AN ADVANCED PRACTITIONER OF NURSING WITHOUT BOARD APPROVAL; MUST COMPLETE 10 HOURS OF CONTINUING MEDICAL EDUCATION IN ETHICS IN ADDITION; MUST PAY INVESTIGATORY COSTS OF $15,000; REPRIMAND.

BASS, HARRISTON LEE JR MD, WAS DISCIPLINED BY NEVADA ON DECEMBER 2, 1993
DISCIPLINARY ACTION: 36-MONTH PROBATION; RESTRICTION PLACED ON LICENSE
OFFENSE: SUBSTANDARD CARE, INCOMPETENCE OR NEGLIGENCE

NOTES: ON 06/05/92, HE WAS CHARGED WITH GROSS MALPRACTICE AND FAILURE TO PROVIDE MEDICAL CARE TO THE POINT OF ENTIRE DISREGARD FOR AND INDIFFERENCE TO THE SAFETY AND WELFARE OF A PATIENT. ON 11/19/92, TWO ADDITIONAL COUNTS CHARGED: MALPRACTICE AND CONTINUAL FAILURE TO EXERCISE SKILL OR DILIGENCE IN THE SPECIALTY OF GENERAL SURGERY IN 2 CASES. LICENSE REVOKED, REVOCATION STAYED. TERMS AND CONDITIONS OF PROBATION ARE AS FOLLOWS: MUST CEASE PERFORMING LAPAROSCOPIC SURGERIES; ALL SURGERIES PERFORMED, OTHER THAN MINOR OFFICE PROCEDURES WHICH CAN BE SAFELY PERFORMED IN THAT SETTING, WILL BE PERFORMED IN A JCAHO-APPROVED HEALTH CARE FACILITY ASSISTED BY AN AMERICAN BOARD OF SURGERY CERTIFIED SURGEON; WILL FILE WITH THE BOARD A TIMELY REPORT CONCERNING ANY SURGERY PERFORMED, INCLUDING A COPY OF THE HISTORY AND PHYSICAL, ANY LABORATORY TESTS AND X-RAYS PERFORMED, THE OPERATIVE NOTES, AND WILL IMMEDIATELY REPORT ANY ADVERSE SURGICAL OUTCOMES; MUST COMPLETE, IN ADDITION TO OTHER CONTINUING EDUCATION REQUIREMENTS IMPOSED BY LAW, 120 HOURS OF MEDICAL EDUCATION IN THE AREA OF SURGERY BEFORE THE EXPIRATION OF THE PROBATION INCLUDING TAKING AND SUCCESSFULLY PASSING THE 1994 AMERICAN COLLEGE OF SURGEONS SURGICAL EDUCATION AND SELF ASSESSMENT PROGRAM.

BOUCHER, ALAN A DO, DATE OF BIRTH MARCH 18, 1943 OF 308 SIMON BOLIVAR, HENDERSON, NV, WAS DISCIPLINED BY MEDICARE ON MARCH 1, 1990
DISCIPLINARY ACTION: 60-MONTH EXCLUSION FROM THE MEDICARE AND/OR MEDICAID PROGRAM
OFFENSE: CRIMINAL CONVICTION OR PLEA OF GUILTY, NOLO CONTENDERE, OR NO CONTEST TO A CRIME

NOTES: PROGRAM-RELATED CONVICTION.

BRADLEY, BRUCE S MD, DATE OF BIRTH MARCH 12, 1954 OF 298 LYRA LANE, LAS VEGAS, NV, WAS DISCIPLINED BY MEDICARE ON FEBRUARY 16, 1995
DISCIPLINARY ACTION: EXCLUSION FROM THE MEDICARE AND/OR MEDICAID PROGRAM
OFFENSE: NONCOMPLIANCE WITH A PROFESSIONAL RULE

NOTES: DEFAULT ON HEALTH EDUCATION LOAN OR SCHOLARSHIP OBLIGATIONS.

BRALY, JIMMY L MD, WAS DISCIPLINED BY NEVADA ON OCTOBER 26, 1990
OFFENSE: NONCOMPLIANCE WITH A PROFESSIONAL RULE

NOTES: FAILED TO NOTIFY BOARD OF CALIFORNIA DISCIPLINARY ACTION. NEVADA LICENSE STATUS TO REMAIN INACTIVE UNTIL FULL COMPLIANCE WITH CALIFORNIA MEDICAL BOARD ORDER.

BRIGHAM, STEVEN CHASE MD, LICENSE NUMBER 0172457 OF 1 ALPHA AVENUE APT 27, VOORHEES, NJ, WAS DISCIPLINED BY NEW YORK ON JANUARY 1, 1994
DISCIPLINARY ACTION: EMERGENCY SUSPENSION

NOTES: LICENSE SUSPENDED PENDING RESOLUTION OF CHARGES ON APPEAL; CONTINUED PRACTICE OF MEDICINE POSES AN IMMINENT DANGER TO PUBLIC HEALTH.

BRIGHAM, STEVEN CHASE MD, LICENSE NUMBER 0172457 OF 1 ALPHA AVENUE, VOORHEES, NJ, WAS DISCIPLINED BY NEW YORK ON NOVEMBER 30, 1994
DISCIPLINARY ACTION: LICENSE REVOCATION
OFFENSE: SUBSTANDARD CARE, INCOMPETENCE OR NEGLIGENCE

NOTES: GROSS NEGLIGENCE AND NEGLIGENCE ON MORE THAN ONE OCCASION.

BRIGHAM, STEVEN CHASE MD, DATE OF BIRTH AUGUST 29, 1956, LICENSE NUMBER 0051068 OF 143 PINEHURST AVENUE, NEW YORK, NY, WAS DISCIPLINED BY NEW JERSEY ON DECEMBER 14, 1994
OFFENSE: DISCIPLINARY ACTION BY ANOTHER STATE OR AGENCY

NOTES: ALLEGED THAT LICENSE WAS REVOKED IN NEW YORK FOR GROSS NEGLIGENCE IN THE CASE OF ONE PATIENT AND GROSS AND REPEATED NEGLIGENCE IN ANOTHER. DOCTOR CLAIMS THAT NEW YORK DECISION WAS NOT FINAL BUT OFFERED TO REFRAIN FROM THE PRACTICE OF MEDICINE AND SURGERY UNTIL THE STATE BOARD ISSUES A FINAL DECISION ON THE COMPLAINTS FILED BY THE ATTORNEY GENERAL.

BRIGHAM, STEVEN CHASE MD, LICENSE NUMBER 0052183 OF VOORHEES, NV, WAS DISCIPLINED BY FLORIDA ON FEBRUARY 2, 1995
DISCIPLINARY ACTION: EMERGENCY SUSPENSION
OFFENSE: DISCIPLINARY ACTION BY ANOTHER STATE OR AGENCY

NOTES: VIOLATED A BOARD RULE OR ORDER OR FAILED TO COMPLY WITH A SUBPOENA OF THE DEPARTMENT; FAILED TO REPORT TO THE BOARD WITHIN 30 DAYS THAT ACTION HAD BEEN TAKEN BY ANOTHER JURISDICTION.

BRIGHAM, STEVEN CHASE MD, DATE OF BIRTH AUGUST 29, 1956 OF 1 ALPHA AVENUE, VOORHEES, NJ, WAS DISCIPLINED BY MEDICARE ON OCTOBER 10, 1995
DISCIPLINARY ACTION: EXCLUSION FROM THE MEDICARE AND/OR MEDICAID PROGRAM
OFFENSE: DISCIPLINARY ACTION BY ANOTHER STATE OR AGENCY

NOTES: LICENSE REVOKED FOR REASONS BEARING ON PROFESSIONAL COMPETENCE. REINSTATED ON 10/15/96.

BRIGHAM, STEVEN CHASE MD, DATE OF BIRTH AUGUST 29, 1956, LICENSE NUMBER 0051068 OF 1 ALPHA AVENUE SUITE 27, VOORHEES, NJ, WAS DISCIPLINED BY NEW JERSEY ON APRIL 29, 1996
DISCIPLINARY ACTION: RESTRICTION PLACED ON LICENSE

NOTES: LICENSE TO PRACTICE FULLY REINSTATED ON 8/14/96 WHEN ALL CHARGES WERE DISMISSED EXCEPT TWO COMPLAINTS REGARDING MISLEADING ADVERTISEMENTS. SHALL CEASE AND DESIST FROM ANY ADVERTISING THAT MISLEADS OR HAS THE CAPACITY TO MISLEAD AND SHALL CEASE FROM USING THE TERMS "SAFE" AND "PAINLESS" IN ANY ADVERTISING.

BRIGHAM, STEVEN CHASE MD, LICENSE NUMBER 0052183 OF VOORHEES, NY, WAS DISCIPLINED BY FLORIDA ON JULY 5, 1996
DISCIPLINARY ACTION: LICENSE REVOCATION
OFFENSE: DISCIPLINARY ACTION BY ANOTHER STATE OR AGENCY

NOTES: HAD LICENSE OR THE AUTHORITY TO PRACTICE MEDICINE REVOKED, SUSPENDED OR DENIED BY LICENSING AUTHORITY OF ANY JURISDICTION. FAILED TO REPORT DISCIPLINARY ACTION BY ANOTHER JURISDICTION OR STATE; AND VIOLATED A RULE OR ORDER OF THE BOARD OR FAILING TO COMPLY WITH A LAWFUL SUBPOENA. APPEAL PENDING.

BRIGHAM, STEVEN CHASE MD, LICENSE NUMBER G62438 OF VOORHEES, NJ, WAS DISCIPLINED BY CALIFORNIA ON APRIL 24, 1997
DISCIPLINARY ACTION: 36-MONTH PROBATION
OFFENSE: DISCIPLINARY ACTION BY ANOTHER STATE OR AGENCY

NOTES: DISCIPLINED BY NEW JERSEY AND NEW YORK FOR COMMITTING ACTS OF NEGLIGENCE AND INCOMPETENCE IN PERFORMING SECOND TRIMESTER ABORTIONS AND FOR INCOMPETENCE IN HIS TREATMENT OF OBSTETRICAL/GYNECOLOGICAL PATIENTS. ONE YEAR SUSPENSION STAYED.

BRUCE, ROBERT L MD, WAS DISCIPLINED BY NEVADA ON OCTOBER 26, 1990
DISCIPLINARY ACTION: LICENSE REVOCATION

BRUMFIELD, THOMAS J MD, WAS DISCIPLINED BY NEVADA ON MARCH 15, 1991
DISCIPLINARY ACTION: RESTRICTION PLACED ON CONTROLLED SUBSTANCE LICENSE

NOTES: SHALL NOT PRESCRIBE, DISPENSE OR ADMINISTER CONTROLLED SUBSTANCES WITHOUT ORDER OF THE BOARD; LICENSE TO RETIRE NO LATER THAN 7/8/91 SUBJECT TO CONDITIONS FOR REINSTATEMENT TO ACTIVE STATUS.

BRUMFIELD, THOMAS J MD, LICENSE NUMBER 0C35869 OF LAS VEGAS, NV, WAS DISCIPLINED BY CALIFORNIA ON MARCH 18, 1993
DISCIPLINARY ACTION: SURRENDER OF LICENSE

NOTES: VOLUNTARY SURRENDER OF LICENSE WHILE CHARGES PENDING.

BURTON, ROBERT C MD, WAS DISCIPLINED BY NEVADA ON JANUARY 9, 1995
DISCIPLINARY ACTION: FINE; REPRIMAND
OFFENSE: DISCIPLINARY ACTION BY ANOTHER STATE OR AGENCY

NOTES: IN 2/92 IDAHO LICENSE SUSPENDED FOR 30 DAYS AND HE PAID A FINE AS A RESULT OF PATIENT COMPLAINTS OF FAILURE TO COMMUNICATE. THIS ACTION RESULTED IN 8/94 REVOCATION OF HIS LICENSE IN CALIFORNIA AND HE FAILED TO REPORT THIS REVOCATION WITHIN 30 DAYS TO NEVADA. $1,000 FINE.

BURTON, ROBERT CALVIN MD, LICENSE NUMBER 0A29533 OF BOISE, ID, WAS DISCIPLINED BY CALIFORNIA ON MARCH 7, 1994
DISCIPLINARY ACTION: LICENSE REVOCATION
OFFENSE: DISCIPLINARY ACTION BY ANOTHER STATE OR AGENCY

NOTES: BASED UPON DISCIPLINE BY IDAHO BOARD OF MEDICINE. DEFAULT DECISION.

CAPPIELLO, RAFAEL M MD, WAS DISCIPLINED BY NEVADA ON FEBRUARY 4, 1998
DISCIPLINARY ACTION: EMERGENCY SUSPENSION
OFFENSE: SUBSTANDARD CARE, INCOMPETENCE OR NEGLIGENCE

NOTES: MALPRACTICE; REPEATED MALPRACTICE.

CAPPIELLO, RAFAEL M MD, WAS DISCIPLINED BY NEVADA ON JUNE 6, 1998
DISCIPLINARY ACTION: LICENSE REVOCATION
OFFENSE: PROFESSIONAL MISCONDUCT

NOTES: MALPRACTICE; REPEATED MALPRACTICE.

CAPPIELLO, RAFAEL M MD, DATE OF BIRTH JULY 20, 1930 OF 2704 BRIENZA WAY, LAS VEGAS, NV, WAS DISCIPLINED BY MEDICARE ON OCTOBER 20, 1998
DISCIPLINARY ACTION: EXCLUSION FROM THE MEDICARE AND/OR MEDICAID PROGRAM
OFFENSE: DISCIPLINARY ACTION BY ANOTHER STATE OR AGENCY

NOTES: LICENSE REVOKED, SUSPENDED, SURRENDERED OR OTHERWISE LOST FOR REASONS BEARING ON

PROFESSIONAL PERFORMANCE, PROFESSIONAL COMPETENCE OR FINANCIAL INTEGRITY.

CAPPIELLO, RAFAEL M MD, LICENSE NUMBER 110175 OF 2704 BRIENZA WAY, LAS VEGAS, NV, WAS DISCIPLINED BY NEW YORK ON MARCH 5, 1999
DISCIPLINARY ACTION: EMERGENCY SUSPENSION
OFFENSE: DISCIPLINARY ACTION BY ANOTHER STATE OR AGENCY
NOTES: DISCIPLINED BY THE NEVADA BOARD FOR MALPRACTICE.

CAPPIELLO, RAFAEL M MD, LICENSE NUMBER 110175 OF 2704 BRIENZA WAY, LAS VEGAS, NV, WAS DISCIPLINED BY NEW YORK ON JUNE 2, 1999
DISCIPLINARY ACTION: LICENSE REVOCATION
OFFENSE: DISCIPLINARY ACTION BY ANOTHER STATE OR AGENCY
NOTES: DISCIPLINED BY THE NEVADA BOARD FOR MALPRACTICE.

CAPPIELLO, RAFAEL M MD OF LAS VEGAS, NV, WAS DISCIPLINED BY DEA ON SEPTEMBER 7, 1999
DISCIPLINARY ACTION: REVOCATION OF CONTROLLED SUBSTANCE LICENSE
OFFENSE: DISCIPLINARY ACTION BY ANOTHER STATE OR AGENCY
NOTES: ON 6/6/98 THE NEVADA BOARD REVOKED HIS LICENSE.

CARTER-PONZOO, CATHERINE MD, DATE OF BIRTH FEBRUARY 14, 1959 OF 3964 ACAPULCO AVENUE, LAS VEGAS, NV, WAS DISCIPLINED BY MEDICARE ON APRIL 2, 1997
DISCIPLINARY ACTION: EXCLUSION FROM THE MEDICARE AND/OR MEDICAID PROGRAM
OFFENSE: NONCOMPLIANCE WITH A PROFESSIONAL RULE
NOTES: DEFAULTED ON PUBLIC HEALTH SERVICE EDUCATION LOAN.

CAVANAGH, JAMES G MD, WAS DISCIPLINED BY NEVADA ON MARCH 15, 1999
DISCIPLINARY ACTION: LICENSE REVOCATION
OFFENSE: SUBSTANDARD CARE, INCOMPETENCE OR NEGLIGENCE
NOTES: ENGAGING IN THE PRACTICE OF WRITING PRESCRIPTIONS FOR CONTROLLED SUBSTANCES IN EXCESSIVE AMOUNTS; CONTINUAL FAILURE TO EXERCISE APPROPRIATE SKILL AND DILIGENCE IN THE PRACTICE OF MEDICINE.

CAVANAGH, JAMES G MD, DATE OF BIRTH APRIL 25, 1930 OF PO BOX 639, HAWTHORNE, NV, WAS DISCIPLINED BY MEDICARE ON AUGUST 19, 1999
DISCIPLINARY ACTION: EXCLUSION FROM THE MEDICARE AND/OR MEDICAID PROGRAM
OFFENSE: DISCIPLINARY ACTION BY ANOTHER STATE OR AGENCY
NOTES: LICENSE REVOKED, SUSPENDED, SURRENDERED OR OTHERWISE LOST FOR REASONS BEARING ON PROFESSIONAL PERFORMANCE, PROFESSIONAL COMPETENCE OR FINANCIAL INTEGRITY.

CHAKMAKIAN, VACHE MD, DATE OF BIRTH MARCH 21, 1957 OF 17820 ORNA DRIVE, GRANADA HILLS, CA, WAS DISCIPLINED BY NEVADA ON DECEMBER 7, 1996
DISCIPLINARY ACTION: DENIAL OF NEW LICENSE
OFFENSE: DISCIPLINARY ACTION BY ANOTHER STATE OR AGENCY
NOTES: ACTION PENDING IN CALIFORNIA.

CHAMBERS, CHARLES H MD, LICENSE NUMBER 0G40189 OF RENO, NV, WAS DISCIPLINED BY CALIFORNIA ON JULY 27, 1991
DISCIPLINARY ACTION: LICENSE REVOCATION
OFFENSE: FAILURE TO COMPLY WITH PREVIOUS BOARD ORDER
NOTES: VIOLATED TERMS OF PROBATION UNDER PRIOR DISCIPLINE. DEFAULT DECISION.

CHANCELLOR, ROBERT S MD, WAS DISCIPLINED BY NEVADA ON JUNE 6, 1998
DISCIPLINARY ACTION: LICENSE REVOCATION
OFFENSE: SUBSTANDARD CARE, INCOMPETENCE OR NEGLIGENCE
NOTES: MALPRACTICE; REPEATED MALPRACTICE.

CHANCELLOR, ROBERT S MD, DATE OF BIRTH JUNE 30, 1945 OF 2200 S RANCHO #222, LAS VEGAS, NV, WAS DISCIPLINED BY MEDICARE ON NOVEMBER 19, 1998
DISCIPLINARY ACTION: EXCLUSION FROM THE MEDICARE AND/OR MEDICAID PROGRAM
OFFENSE: DISCIPLINARY ACTION BY ANOTHER STATE OR AGENCY
NOTES: LICENSE REVOKED, SUSPENDED, SURRENDERED OR OTHERWISE LOST FOR REASONS BEARING ON PROFESSIONAL PERFORMANCE, PROFESSIONAL COMPETENCE OR FINANCIAL INTEGRITY.

CHANCELLOR, ROBERT S MD OF LAS VEGAS, NV, WAS DISCIPLINED BY NEVADA ON MARCH 15, 1999
DISCIPLINARY ACTION: LICENSE REVOCATION
NOTES: INABILITY TO PRACTICE MEDICINE WITH REASONABLE SKILL AND SAFETY BECAUSE OF ILLNESS, A MENTAL OR PHYSICAL CONDITION OR THE USE OF ALCOHOL, DRUGS, NARCOTICS OR ANY OTHER SUBSTANCE; RENDERING PROFESSIONAL SERVICES TO A PATIENT WHILE UNDER THE INFLUENCE OF ALCOHOL OR ANY CONTROLLED SUBSTANCE OR DUE TO ANY IMPAIRED MENTAL OR PHYSICAL CONDITION.

CHANCELLOR, ROBERT S MD OF LAS VEGAS, NV, WAS DISCIPLINED BY DEA ON SEPTEMBER 7, 1999
DISCIPLINARY ACTION: REVOCATION OF CONTROLLED SUBSTANCE LICENSE
OFFENSE: DISCIPLINARY ACTION BY ANOTHER STATE OR AGENCY
NOTES: ON 6/6/98 THE NEVADA BOARD REVOKED HIS LICENSE.

CHINGROS, WILLIAM N MD, LICENSE NUMBER 0165349 OF 843 FRANKLIN STREET, OGDEN, UT, WAS DISCIPLINED BY NEW YORK ON JULY 21, 1993
DISCIPLINARY ACTION: FINE; REPRIMAND
OFFENSE: CRIMINAL CONVICTION OR PLEA OF GUILTY, NOLO CONTENDERE, OR NO CONTEST TO A CRIME
NOTES: HAD BEEN FOUND GUILTY OF STUDENT LOAN FRAUD. $1,000 FINE.

CHINGROS, WILLIAM N MD, WAS DISCIPLINED BY NEVADA ON DECEMBER 3, 1993
DISCIPLINARY ACTION: REPRIMAND
OFFENSE: DISCIPLINARY ACTION BY ANOTHER STATE OR AGENCY
NOTES: ON 11/15/93, STATE BOARD IN NEW YORK IMPOSED A CENSURE AND REPRIMAND AND A $1,000 FINE UPON HIS LICENSE TO PRACTICE MEDICINE IN NEW YORK.

CHOMIAK, BRYANT D MD, WAS DISCIPLINED BY NEVADA ON OCTOBER 25, 1993
DISCIPLINARY ACTION: EMERGENCY SUSPENSION
OFFENSE: SUBSTANCE ABUSE
NOTES: ON 10/25/93 COMPLAINT FILED WHERE HE WAS CHARGED WITH WILLFUL FAILURE TO COMPLY WITH AN ORDER OF THE INVESTIGATIVE COMMITTEE OF

THE BOARD FOR PHYSICAL EXAMINATION, CONSISTING OF AN ANALYSIS OF BODILY FLUIDS, HABITUAL DEPENDENCY UPON ALCOHOL OR CONTROLLED SUBSTANCES, INABILITY TO PRACTICE MEDICINE WITH REASONABLE SKILL OR SAFETY BECAUSE OF THE USE OF ALCOHOL, DRUGS, NARCOTICS OR OTHER SUBSTANCES AND RENDERING PROFESSIONAL SERVICES TO PATIENTS WHILE UNDER THE INFLUENCE OF ALCOHOL OR CONTROLLED SUBSTANCES.

CHOMIAK, BRYANT D MD, WAS DISCIPLINED BY NEVADA ON JANUARY 22, 1994
DISCIPLINARY ACTION: REPRIMAND; MONITORING OF PHYSICIAN PERFORMANCE
OFFENSE: SUBSTANCE ABUSE

NOTES: EMERGENCY SUSPENSION LIFTED; HE DID COMPLY WITH ORDER. MUST CONTINUE THERAPY FOR SIX MONTHS WITH MONTHLY REPORTS; SHALL SUBMIT TO RANDOM TESTS OF BODILY FLUIDS FOR SIX MONTHS.

CHOMIAK, BRYANT D MD, WAS DISCIPLINED BY NEVADA ON APRIL 24, 1997
DISCIPLINARY ACTION: EMERGENCY SUSPENSION
OFFENSE: SUBSTANDARD CARE, INCOMPETENCE OR NEGLIGENCE

NOTES: ENGAGING IN CONDUCT WHICH THE BOARD HAS DETERMINED IS A VIOLATION OF THE STANDARDS OF PRACTICE ESTABLISHED BY THE BOARD; RENDERING PROFESSIONAL SERVICES TO A PATIENT WHILE UNDER THE INFLUENCE OF ALCOHOL OR ANY CONTROLLED SUBSTANCE.

CHOMIAK, BRYANT D MD, WAS DISCIPLINED BY NEVADA ON JULY 16, 1997
DISCIPLINARY ACTION: LICENSE REVOCATION
OFFENSE: SUBSTANDARD CARE, INCOMPETENCE OR NEGLIGENCE

NOTES: ENGAGING IN CONDUCT WHICH THE BOARD HAS DETERMINED IS A VIOLATION OF THE STANDARDS OF PRACTICE ESTABLISHED BY THE BOARD; RENDERING PROFESSIONAL SERVICES TO A PATIENT WHILE UNDER THE INFLUENCE OF ALCOHOL OR ANY CONTROLLED SUBSTANCE.

CHOMIAK, BRYANT D MD, DATE OF BIRTH OCTOBER 10, 1953 OF 1229 PARK CIRCLE, LAS VEGAS, NV, WAS DISCIPLINED BY MEDICARE ON OCTOBER 20, 1998
DISCIPLINARY ACTION: EXCLUSION FROM THE MEDICARE AND/OR MEDICAID PROGRAM
OFFENSE: DISCIPLINARY ACTION BY ANOTHER STATE OR AGENCY

NOTES: LICENSE REVOKED, SUSPENDED, SURRENDERED OR OTHERWISE LOST FOR REASONS BEARING ON PROFESSIONAL PERFORMANCE, PROFESSIONAL COMPETENCE OR FINANCIAL INTEGRITY.

CHOMIAK, BRYANT D MD OF LAS VEGAS, NV, WAS DISCIPLINED BY DEA ON SEPTEMBER 7, 1999
DISCIPLINARY ACTION: REVOCATION OF CONTROLLED SUBSTANCE LICENSE
OFFENSE: DISCIPLINARY ACTION BY ANOTHER STATE OR AGENCY

NOTES: ON 4/24/97 THE NEVADA BOARD SUMMARILY SUSPENDED HIS LICENSE AND ON 7/15/97 REVOKED IT.

CHOMIAK, BRYANT DOUGLAS MD, LICENSE NUMBER 0G60553 OF LAS VEGAS, NV, WAS DISCIPLINED BY CALIFORNIA ON JUNE 24, 1996
DISCIPLINARY ACTION: 60-MONTH PROBATION
OFFENSE: DISCIPLINARY ACTION BY ANOTHER STATE OR AGENCY

NOTES: ACTION IN NEVADA FOR FAILING TO COMPLY WITH AN ORDER FOR A PHYSICAL EXAM. REVOCATION, STAYED.

CHOMIAK, BRYANT DOUGLAS MD, LICENSE NUMBER G60553 OF LAS VEGAS, NV, WAS DISCIPLINED BY CALIFORNIA ON AUGUST 5, 1998
DISCIPLINARY ACTION: LICENSE REVOCATION
OFFENSE: DISCIPLINARY ACTION BY ANOTHER STATE OR AGENCY

NOTES: DISCIPLINED BY NEVADA FOR PRACTICING WHILE UNDER THE INFLUENCE OF CONTROLLED SUBSTANCES; FAILED TO COMPLY WITH THE TERMS AND CONDITIONS OF PROBATION IMPOSED BY CALIFORNIA BOARD.

CLARK, CORYDON G MD, LICENSE NUMBER 0G20348 OF MARYSVILLE, CA, WAS DISCIPLINED BY CALIFORNIA ON SEPTEMBER 13, 1995
DISCIPLINARY ACTION: 72-MONTH PROBATION
OFFENSE: SUBSTANDARD CARE, INCOMPETENCE OR NEGLIGENCE

NOTES: UNPROFESSIONAL CONDUCT, GROSS NEGLIGENCE, AND REPEATED NEGLIGENT ACTS IN PSYCHIATRIC PRACTICE IN USING INAPPROPRIATE THERAPEUTIC TECHNIQUES IN TREATING ADOLESCENT PATIENTS DIAGNOSED WITH ADHD OR ATTENTION DEFICIT DISORDER. REVOCATION, STAYED.

CLARK, CORYDON G MD, WAS DISCIPLINED BY NEVADA ON FEBRUARY 12, 1996
DISCIPLINARY ACTION: 72-MONTH PROBATION; RESTRICTION PLACED ON LICENSE
OFFENSE: DISCIPLINARY ACTION BY ANOTHER STATE OR AGENCY

NOTES: CHARGED WITH HAVING LICENSE SUBJECT TO SUSPENSION, MODIFICATION, SURRENDER OR LIMITATION BY ANY LICENSING AUTHORITY, A MEDICAL FACILITY, A BRANCH OF THE ARMED SERVICES OF THE UNITED STATES, AN INSURANCE COMPANY, AN AGENCY OF THE FEDERAL GOVERNMENT OR AN EMPLOYER. REVOCATION STAYED. CONDITIONS OF PROBATION ARE AS FOLLOWS: PROBATION SHALL RUN CONCURRENT WITH HIS PROBATIONARY TIME IN CALIFORNIA; WITHIN 30 DAYS OF RECEIPT OF WRITTEN PSYCHIATRIC EVALUATION AND ON A PERIODIC BASIS THEREAFTER HE SHALL PROVIDE THE NEVADA BOARD WITH COMPLETE WRITTEN PSYCHIATRIC EVALUATION(S); IF HE IS REQUIRED TO UNDERGO PSYCHIATRIC TREATMENT BY THE CALIFORNIA BOARD HE SHALL WITHIN 30 DAYS SUBMIT THE NAME OF THE TREATING PSYCHIATRIST TO THE NEVADA BOARD AND HAVE THE TREATING PSYCHIATRIST SUBMIT QUARTERLY STATUS REPORTS; SHALL HAVE A THIRD PARTY PRESENT WHILE EXAMINING OR TREATING PATIENTS UNDER THE AGE OF 18 AND HAVE NO PHYSICAL CONTACT WITH THESE PATIENTS EXCEPT WHEN IT IS MEDICALLY NECESSARY IN ORDER TO CONDUCT AN APPROPRIATE PHYSICAL EXAMINATION; SHALL NOT ENGAGE IN WATER THERAPY WITH THESE PATIENTS; WITHIN 90 DAYS OF THIS ORDER HE SHALL SUBMIT, FOR BOARD APPROVAL, EDUCATIONAL PROGRAMS OR COURSES WHICH SHALL NOT BE LESS THAN 20 HOURS PER YEAR FOR THE FIRST THREE YEARS OF PROBATION; $1,000 COSTS; SHALL COMPLY WITH BOARD PROBATION SURVEILLANCE PROGRAM; SHALL BE PROHIBITED FROM SUPERVISING PHYSICIAN ASSISTANTS DURING THE PERIOD OF PROBATION; SHALL APPEAR BEFORE THE BOARD FOR INTERVIEWS UPON REQUEST; THE PERIOD OF PROBATION SHALL NOT RUN DURING TIME HE IS PRACTICING OR RESIDING OUTSIDE THE JURISDICTION OF CALIFORNIA

OR NEVADA; MAY PETITION THE BOARD FOR A FULL RESTORATION OF HIS LICENSE UPON SUCCESSFUL COMPLETION OF THE PROBATION.

COHEN, DAVID B MD, WAS DISCIPLINED BY NEVADA ON DECEMBER 5, 1998
DISCIPLINARY ACTION: FINE; REPRIMAND
OFFENSE: PRACTICING WITHOUT A VALID LICENSE

NOTES: PRACTICING MEDICINE AFTER HIS LICENSE HAD BEEN SUSPENDED FOR NON-PAYMENT OF FEES; PRACTICING WITHOUT A LICENSE. MUST PAY THE SUM OF $5,876.77 FOR COSTS AND FINES TOTALING $1000.

CONNELLY, CHRISTOPHER F DO, LICENSE NUMBER 0075983, WAS DISCIPLINED BY NEW MEXICO ON APRIL 8, 1991
DISCIPLINARY ACTION: SURRENDER OF LICENSE
OFFENSE: NONCOMPLIANCE WITH A PROFESSIONAL RULE

NOTES: FAILED TO APPEAR BEFORE THE BOARD. VOLUNTARY SURRENDER.

CONNELLY, CHRISTOPHER FOUST DO, DATE OF BIRTH MARCH 6, 1955 OF 3675 LAKEVIEW ROAD, CARSON CITY, NV, WAS DISCIPLINED BY MEDICARE ON FEBRUARY 19, 1998
DISCIPLINARY ACTION: EXCLUSION FROM THE MEDICARE AND/OR MEDICAID PROGRAM
OFFENSE: NONCOMPLIANCE WITH A PROFESSIONAL RULE

NOTES: DEFAULTED ON PUBLIC HEALTH SERVICE EDUCATION LOAN.

CONTE, MAURICE S MD, DATE OF BIRTH SEPTEMBER 4, 1937, LICENSE NUMBER 00E7036 OF HOUSTON, TX, WAS DISCIPLINED BY TEXAS ON MAY 24, 1990
DISCIPLINARY ACTION: REQUIRED TO TAKE ADDITIONAL MEDICAL EDUCATION; MONITORING OF PHYSICIAN PERFORMANCE

NOTES: STIPULATED ORDER. SHALL ATTEND CONTINUING MEDICAL EDUCATION COURSES, UTILIZE PATIENT RECORD-KEEPING SYSTEM TO ACCURATELY REFLECT CERTAIN INFORMATION, AND MAKE ANNUAL APPEARANCES BEFORE BOARD OR BOARD COMMITTEE.

CONTE, MAURICE S MD, DATE OF BIRTH SEPTEMBER 4, 1937, LICENSE NUMBER 00E7036 OF HOUSTON, TX, WAS DISCIPLINED BY TEXAS ON MARCH 6, 1992
DISCIPLINARY ACTION: RESTRICTION PLACED ON LICENSE

NOTES: PROFESSIONAL FAILURE TO PRACTICE MEDICINE IN AN ACCEPTABLE MANNER CONSISTENT WITH PUBLIC HEALTH AND WELFARE.

CONTE, MAURICE S MD, DATE OF BIRTH SEPTEMBER 4, 1937, LICENSE NUMBER 00E7036 OF HENDERSON, NV, WAS DISCIPLINED BY TEXAS ON FEBRUARY 8, 1993
DISCIPLINARY ACTION: LICENSE SUSPENSION
OFFENSE: FAILURE TO COMPLY WITH PREVIOUS BOARD ORDER

NOTES: HE WAS REQUIRED BY AN ORDER OF 3/6/92 TO TAKE AND PASS THE SPEX EXAM; HE HAS TAKEN THE EXAM TWICE IN 9/92 AND 12/92 AND FAILED BOTH TIMES. LICENSE SUSPENDED UNTIL HE PASSES THE SPEX EXAM. ON 3/3/95 SUSPENSION TERMINATED.

CONTE, MAURICE S MD, DATE OF BIRTH SEPTEMBER 4, 1937, LICENSE NUMBER 0021080 OF 1313 SPYGLASS, AUSTIN, TX, WAS DISCIPLINED BY NEW JERSEY ON JUNE 27, 1994
DISCIPLINARY ACTION: LICENSE SUSPENSION

NOTES: MUST APPEAR BEFORE A COMMITTEE OF THIS BOARD FOR A STATUS CONFERENCE PRIOR TO RESUMING NEW JERSEY PRACTICE. LICENSE IS SUSPENDED UNTIL SUCH TIME THAT HE DEMONSTRATES TO THE BOARD THAT HIS LICENSE TO PRACTICE MEDICINE IN TEXAS IS REINSTATED.

CSERNA, GEZA J MD OF RENO, NV, WAS DISCIPLINED BY MISSOURI ON AUGUST 17, 1998
DISCIPLINARY ACTION: LICENSE REVOCATION
OFFENSE: DISCIPLINARY ACTION BY ANOTHER STATE OR AGENCY

NOTES: NEVADA LICENSE REVOKED. MAY NOT APPLY FOR REINSTATEMENT OF LICENSE FOR SEVEN YEARS.

CSERNA, GEZA JED MD, DATE OF BIRTH APRIL 18, 1952, LICENSE NUMBER 0007221 OF 802 AVENUE E, ELY, NV, WAS DISCIPLINED BY NEVADA ON DECEMBER 10, 1996
DISCIPLINARY ACTION: LICENSE REVOCATION; REPRIMAND
OFFENSE: CRIMINAL CONVICTION OR PLEA OF GUILTY, NOLO CONTENDERE, OR NO CONTEST TO A CRIME

NOTES: CONVICTED OF TWO COUNTS OF A FELONY: UNLAWFUL POSSESSION OF A MACHINE GUN AND UNLAWFUL POSSESSION OF A SHORT-BARRELED RIFLE. SENTENCED TO 33 MONTHS AND $10,000 FINE.

CSERNA, GEZA JED MD, DATE OF BIRTH APRIL 18, 1952, LICENSE NUMBER 030606E OF 802 AVENUE E, ELY, NV, WAS DISCIPLINED BY PENNSYLVANIA ON NOVEMBER 27, 1997
DISCIPLINARY ACTION: LICENSE REVOCATION
OFFENSE: DISCIPLINARY ACTION BY ANOTHER STATE OR AGENCY

NOTES: DISCIPLINARY ACTION TAKEN IN NEVADA AND FELONY WEAPONS CONVICTION.

CSERNA, GEZA JED MD, LICENSE NUMBER A41419 OF ELY, NV, WAS DISCIPLINED BY CALIFORNIA ON MAY 15, 1998
DISCIPLINARY ACTION: LICENSE REVOCATION
OFFENSE: DISCIPLINARY ACTION BY ANOTHER STATE OR AGENCY

NOTES: DISCIPLINED BY NEVADA BASED ON A FELONY CONVICTION FOR UNLAWFUL POSSESSION OF A MACHINE GUN AND SHORT-BARRELED RIFLE.

DAVIES, JOSEPH ALAN MD, LICENSE NUMBER G64976 OF SAN DIEGO, CA, WAS DISCIPLINED BY CALIFORNIA ON JULY 8, 1998
DISCIPLINARY ACTION: LICENSE REVOCATION
OFFENSE: DISCIPLINARY ACTION BY ANOTHER STATE OR AGENCY

NOTES: REPRIMANDED BY THE U.S. NAVY FOR USE OF CONTROLLED SUBSTANCES, AMPHETAMINE/METHAMPHETAMINE, WHILE ON ACTIVE DUTY.

DAVIES, JOSEPH ALAN MD, DATE OF BIRTH NOVEMBER 25, 1958 OF 2204 MICHAEL DRIVE, CARSON CITY, NV, WAS DISCIPLINED BY MEDICARE ON JANUARY 20, 1999
DISCIPLINARY ACTION: EXCLUSION FROM THE MEDICARE AND/OR MEDICAID PROGRAM
OFFENSE: DISCIPLINARY ACTION BY ANOTHER STATE OR AGENCY

NOTES: LICENSE REVOKED, SUSPENDED, SURRENDERED OR OTHERWISE LOST FOR REASONS BEARING ON PROFESSIONAL PERFORMANCE, PROFESSIONAL COMPETENCE OR FINANCIAL INTEGRITY.

DE FONSEKA, MAHENDRA MD, DATE OF BIRTH JANUARY 2, 1945, LICENSE NUMBER 0003983 OF 700 SHADOW LANE #165A, LAS VEGAS, NV, WAS DISCIPLINED BY NEVADA ON OCTOBER 23, 1996
OFFENSE: PROFESSIONAL MISCONDUCT

NOTES: PLACED YELLOW PAGE ADVERTISING STATING THAT HE WAS BOARD CERTIFIED IN GASTROENTEROLOGY

WHEN IN FACT HE WAS NOT. $5,000 AS DISGORGEMENT OF PAYMENTS WHICH MAY HAVE BEEN RECEIVED AS A RESULT OF THE AD.

DE LEE, SOL T MD, WAS DISCIPLINED BY NEVADA ON JUNE 5, 1992
DISCIPLINARY ACTION: EMERGENCY SUSPENSION
OFFENSE: SUBSTANDARD CARE, INCOMPETENCE OR NEGLIGENCE

NOTES: CHARGED WITH FAILURE TO BE FOUND COMPETENT TO PRACTICE MEDICINE AS A RESULT OF AN EXAMINATION TO DETERMINE MEDICAL COMPETENCY.

DE LEE, SOL T MD, WAS DISCIPLINED BY NEVADA ON JANUARY 16, 1993
DISCIPLINARY ACTION: SURRENDER OF LICENSE

NOTES: WHILE UNDER INVESTIGATION.

DEFRIEZ, CURTIS B MD OF SALT LAKE CITY, UT, WAS DISCIPLINED BY UTAH ON SEPTEMBER 27, 1994
DISCIPLINARY ACTION: SURRENDER OF CONTROLLED SUBSTANCE LICENSE

NOTES: VOLUNTARY SURRENDER WITHOUT ADMITTING OR DENYING ALLEGATIONS UNTIL SUCH TIME AS THE DIVISION'S DISCIPLINARY ACTION IS RESOLVED COMPLETELY.

DEFRIEZ, CURTIS B MD OF LOVELOCK, NV, WAS DISCIPLINED BY UTAH ON AUGUST 10, 1995
DISCIPLINARY ACTION: REVOCATION OF CONTROLLED SUBSTANCE LICENSE; LICENSE SUSPENSION
OFFENSE: OVERPRESCRIBING OR MISPRESCRIBING DRUGS

NOTES: POSSESSED AND USED CONTROLLED SUBSTANCES NOT OBTAINED UNDER A VALID PRESCRIPTION; ISSUED CONTROLLED SUBSTANCE PRESCRIPTIONS FOR OTHER THAN LEGITIMATE MEDICAL PURPOSES; PRESCRIBED CONTROLLED SUBSTANCES IN QUANTITIES IN EXCESS OF THAT MEDICALLY NECESSARY; MADE FALSE PRESCRIPTIONS AND GAVE FALSE INFORMATION TO OBTAIN PRESCRIPTIONS FOR CONTROLLED SUBSTANCES. MEDICAL LICENSE INDEFINITELY SUSPENDED WITH CONDITIONS TO BE MET DURING PERIOD OF SUSPENSION.

DEFRIEZ, CURTIS B MD, LICENSE NUMBER 0G59725 OF SALT LAKE CITY, UT, WAS DISCIPLINED BY CALIFORNIA ON OCTOBER 7, 1996
DISCIPLINARY ACTION: LICENSE REVOCATION

DESAI, DIPAK KANTILAL MD, DATE OF BIRTH NOVEMBER 30, 1949, LICENSE NUMBER 0004050 OF 700 SHADOW LANE #165A, LAS VEGAS, NV, WAS DISCIPLINED BY NEVADA ON OCTOBER 23, 1996
OFFENSE: PROFESSIONAL MISCONDUCT

NOTES: YELLOW PAGE ADVERTISING STATING THAT CERTAIN MEMBERS OF HIS GROUP WERE BOARD CERTIFIED IN GASTROENTEROLOGY, WHEN IN FACT THEY WERE NOT. $2,500 AS DISGORGEMENT OF PAYMENTS WHICH MAY HAVE BEEN RECEIVED AS A RESULT OF THE AD.

DESMARAIS, GILLES M K MD, LICENSE NUMBER 0030536 OF 2975 S RAINBOW, LAS VEGAS, NV, WAS DISCIPLINED BY MASSACHUSETTS ON DECEMBER 28, 1994
DISCIPLINARY ACTION: NONRENEWAL OF LICENSE
OFFENSE: PROFESSIONAL MISCONDUCT

NOTES: SEXUAL RELATIONS. REVOCATION OF INCHOATE RIGHT TO RENEW LICENSE.

DESMARAIS, GILLES MARK KILDA MD, LICENSE NUMBER 0017915, WAS DISCIPLINED BY ARIZONA ON APRIL 16, 1996
OFFENSE: DISCIPLINARY ACTION BY ANOTHER STATE OR AGENCY

NOTES: DISCIPLINARY ACTION BY MASSACHUSETTS. SHALL NOT PRACTICE MEDICINE IN ARIZONA.

DEVINE, JAMES S MD, LICENSE NUMBER 00G3938 OF LAS VEGAS, NV, WAS DISCIPLINED BY CALIFORNIA ON MARCH 10, 1995
DISCIPLINARY ACTION: LICENSE SUSPENSION; 60-MONTH PROBATION
OFFENSE: OVERPRESCRIBING OR MISPRESCRIBING DRUGS

NOTES: REPEATED ACTS OF CLEARLY EXCESSIVE PRESCRIBING OF CONTROLLED DRUGS. PRIOR DISCIPLINE. REVOCATION STAYED. SUSPENSION UNTIL HE PASSES AN ORAL CLINICAL EXAMINATION.

DEVINE, JAMES S MD, LICENSE NUMBER G3938 OF LAS VEGAS, NV, WAS DISCIPLINED BY CALIFORNIA ON JUNE 29, 1998
DISCIPLINARY ACTION: LICENSE REVOCATION
OFFENSE: FAILURE TO COMPLY WITH PREVIOUS BOARD ORDER

NOTES: VIOLATED TERMS AND CONDITIONS OF BOARD PROBATION, PRACTICED MEDICINE WHILE SUSPENDED, FAILED TO MAINTAIN ADEQUATE MEDICAL RECORDS, AND FAILED TO NOTIFY BOARD OF A CHANGE OF ADDRESS.

DEVINE, JAMES S MD, DATE OF BIRTH DECEMBER 12, 1922 OF 6029 LINDA WAY, CULVER CITY, CA, WAS DISCIPLINED BY MEDICARE ON JUNE 17, 1999
DISCIPLINARY ACTION: EXCLUSION FROM THE MEDICARE AND/OR MEDICAID PROGRAM
OFFENSE: DISCIPLINARY ACTION BY ANOTHER STATE OR AGENCY

NOTES: LICENSE REVOKED, SUSPENDED, SURRENDERED OR OTHERWISE LOST FOR REASONS BEARING ON PROFESSIONAL PERFORMANCE, PROFESSIONAL COMPETENCE OR FINANCIAL INTEGRITY.

DIGREGORIO, MICHAEL MD, WAS DISCIPLINED BY NEVADA ON JUNE 18, 1990
DISCIPLINARY ACTION: RESTRICTION PLACED ON LICENSE
OFFENSE: DISCIPLINARY ACTION BY ANOTHER STATE OR AGENCY

NOTES: ON CALIFORNIA PROBATION. ON ACTIVE STATUS WITH RESTRICTIONS IN NEVADA. AS OF 7/28/94 HE WAS GRANTED AN UNRESTRICTED LICENSE.

DIGREGORIO, MICHAEL DAVID MD OF 3233 W CHARLESTON BLVD, LAS VEGAS, NV, WAS DISCIPLINED BY DEA ON JANUARY 6, 1993
DISCIPLINARY ACTION: RESTRICTION PLACED ON CONTROLLED SUBSTANCE LICENSE
OFFENSE: CRIMINAL CONVICTION OR PLEA OF GUILTY, NOLO CONTENDERE, OR NO CONTEST TO A CRIME

NOTES: PLED GUILTY 02/19/85 TO UNLAWFULLY PRESCRIBING PRELUDIN. SENTENCED 03/22/85 TO THREE YEARS PROBATION AND 200 HOURS COMMUNITY SERVICE. MODIFICATION OF REGISTRATION. REPORTEDLY WROTE A PRESCRIPTION FOR PHENMETRAZINE FOR A NON-LEGITIMATE PURPOSE. PLACED ON FIVE YEARS PROBATION 06/27/87. ALIAS: MICHAEL DAVID DEGREGORIO.

DUBIN, STEPHEN MD OF 625 WEST WILLIAMS AVENUE, FALLON, NV, WAS DISCIPLINED BY DEA ON JUNE 11, 1999
DISCIPLINARY ACTION: SURRENDER OF CONTROLLED SUBSTANCE LICENSE
OFFENSE: DISCIPLINARY ACTION BY ANOTHER STATE OR AGENCY

NOTES: STATE BOARD.

DUBIN, STEPHEN P MD, WAS DISCIPLINED BY NEVADA ON JULY 15, 1997
DISCIPLINARY ACTION: LICENSE REVOCATION
OFFENSE: PROFESSIONAL MISCONDUCT

NOTES: HE OBTAINED A LICENSE BY FRAUD OR MISREPRESENTATION, OR BY A FALSE, MISLEADING, INACCURATE OR INCOMPLETE STATEMENT; HE ENGAGED IN CONDUCT INTENDED TO DECEIVE.

DUBIN, STEPHEN PAUL MD, WAS DISCIPLINED BY HAWAII ON JULY 10, 1998
DISCIPLINARY ACTION: LICENSE REVOCATION
OFFENSE: DISCIPLINARY ACTION BY ANOTHER STATE OR AGENCY

NOTES: ON 7/15/97 NEVADA REVOKED HIS LICENSE DUE TO HIS FAILURE TO REPORT THE INDICTMENT AGAINST HIM IN HAWAII OF FIVE COUNTS OF VIOLATIONS OF THE LAWS OF THE U.S.

DUBIN, STEPHEN PAUL MD, LICENSE NUMBER 4950, WAS DISCIPLINED BY HAWAII ON DECEMBER 11, 1998
DISCIPLINARY ACTION: LICENSE REVOCATION
OFFENSE: SEXUAL ABUSE OF OR SEXUAL MISCONDUCT WITH A PATIENT

NOTES: DURING THE LATE 1980S AND EARLY 1990S REVEALED A PATTERN OF CONDUCT BY ATTEMPTING TO BECOME SEXUALLY OR SOCIALLY INVOLVED WITH YOUNG FEMALE PATIENTS. ON ONE COUNT, SEXUALLY ASSAULTED PATIENT WHEN SHE WAS COMING OUT OF ANESTHESIA FROM SURGERY, HE WAS TOUCHING HER BREASTS INAPPROPRIATELY; IN A TAPED CONVERSATION, SAID HE WOULD MAKE IT UP TO HER BY TAKING HER OUT FOR DINNER; ON ANOTHER COUNT, CAME-ON TO HIS PATIENT IN A SEXUAL WAY IN THE EXAMINING ROOM; HAD ORAL SEX WITH THE PATIENT IN HIS OFFICE AND HAD SEXUAL INTERCOURSE; FAILURE TO TERMINATE THE PHYSICIAN-PATIENT RELATIONSHIP BEFORE INITIATING A SEXUAL RELATIONSHIP WITH HER; ON THIRD COUNT, ATTEMPTED TO INITIATE A SOCIAL RELATIONSHIP WITH A PATIENT.

DURANTE, JOSEPH R MD, LICENSE NUMBER 00G3711 OF PALM DESERT, CA, WAS DISCIPLINED BY CALIFORNIA ON SEPTEMBER 3, 1996
DISCIPLINARY ACTION: 60-MONTH PROBATION

NOTES: REVOCATION, STAYED.

DURANTE, JOSEPH R MD, LICENSE NUMBER G3711 OF BOULDER CITY, NV, WAS DISCIPLINED BY CALIFORNIA ON NOVEMBER 19, 1999
DISCIPLINARY ACTION: 2-MONTH LICENSE SUSPENSION; 58-MONTH PROBATION

NOTES: REVOCATION STAYED.

EMERY, CLYDE K JR MD, WAS DISCIPLINED BY NEVADA ON MARCH 15, 1991
DISCIPLINARY ACTION: REPRIMAND
OFFENSE: CRIMINAL CONVICTION OR PLEA OF GUILTY, NOLO CONTENDERE, OR NO CONTEST TO A CRIME

NOTES: CONVICTED OF PERJURY, A FELONY, IN THE SECOND JUDICIAL DISTRICT COURT OF NEVADA, IN THE COUNTY OF WASHOE. LICENSE TO REMAIN INACTIVE FOR 3 YEARS AND $1,000 REIMBURSEMENT FOR EXPENSES INCURRED BY BOARD.

EMETERIO, LOUIS C MD, WAS DISCIPLINED BY NEVADA ON JUNE 19, 1998
DISCIPLINARY ACTION: 24-MONTH PROBATION; RESTRICTION PLACED ON CONTROLLED SUBSTANCE LICENSE
OFFENSE: OVERPRESCRIBING OR MISPRESCRIBING DRUGS

NOTES: HE ENGAGED IN THE PRACTICE OF WRITING PRESCRIPTIONS FOR CONTROLLED SUBSTANCES IN EXCESSIVE AMOUNTS; MALPRACTICE; HE WROTE A PRESCRIPTION FOR CONTROLLED SUBSTANCES WITHOUT AN APPROPRIATE EXAMINATION TO CONFIRM THE MEDICAL NECESSITY FOR THE CONTROLLED SUBSTANCES; FAILURE TO EXERCISE APPROPRIATE SKILL; REPEATED MALPRACTICE. REVOCATION STAYED. PROBATIONARY CONDITIONS INCLUDE: HE SHALL COMPLETE 80 HOURS OF CONTINUING MEDICAL EDUCATION IN NARCOTICS PRESCRIBING, PAIN MANAGEMENT AND RECORD KEEPING; MUST PAY $10, 465 FOR ADMINISTRATIVE COSTS; MAY NOT PRESCRIBE SCHEDULE II AND SCHEDULE III CONTROLLED SUBSTANCES DURING THE FIRST 6 MONTHS OF PROBATION. ON 8/28/99 BOARD DENIED RECONSIDERATION OF ORDER.

EMETERIO, LOUIS CLINTON MD, DATE OF BIRTH OCTOBER 24, 1932, LICENSE NUMBER 026645L OF 3196 MARYLAND PARKWAY, LAS VEGAS, NV, WAS DISCIPLINED BY PENNSYLVANIA ON DECEMBER 23, 1999
DISCIPLINARY ACTION: LICENSE SUSPENSION
OFFENSE: DISCIPLINARY ACTION BY ANOTHER STATE OR AGENCY

NOTES: DISCIPLINED BY NEVADA BOARD. LICENSE CANNOT BE REINSTATED UNTIL NEVADA LICENSE IS REINSTATED TO UNRESTRICTED STATUS.

EVANGELISTA, LUISITO A MD, WAS DISCIPLINED BY NEVADA ON SEPTEMBER 20, 1997
DISCIPLINARY ACTION: LICENSE REVOCATION
OFFENSE: SUBSTANDARD CARE, INCOMPETENCE OR NEGLIGENCE

NOTES: FAILURE TO MAKE MEDICAL RECORDS OF A PATIENT AVAILABLE FOR INSPECTION AND COPYING; ENGAGING IN CONDUCT INTENDED TO DECEIVE; WILLFUL FAILURE TO COMPLY WITH A SUBPOENA OF THE BOARD; ENGAGING IN CONDUCT WHICH THE BOARD HAS DETERMINED IS A VIOLATION OF THE STANDARDS OF PRACTICE ESTABLISHED BY THE BOARD; WRITING PRESCRIPTIONS FOR CONTROLLED SUBSTANCES IN EXCESSIVE AMOUNTS; FAILURE TO TREAT A PATIENT, USING REASONABLE CARE, SKILL OR KNOWLEDGE; GROSS OR REPEATED MALPRACTICE; FAILURE TO OBTAIN A MEDICAL HISTORY AND PERFORM A PHYSICAL EXAMINATION OF THE PATIENT AND CONDUCT APPROPRIATE STUDIES TO DETERMINE IF THERE ARE ANY CONTRAINDICATIONS TO THE USE OF APPETITE SUPPRESSANTS.

EVANGELISTA, LUISITO A MD, DATE OF BIRTH OCTOBER 31, 1929 OF 4332 EAST HACIENDA, LAS VEGAS, NV, WAS DISCIPLINED BY MEDICARE ON OCTOBER 20, 1998
DISCIPLINARY ACTION: EXCLUSION FROM THE MEDICARE AND/OR MEDICAID PROGRAM
OFFENSE: DISCIPLINARY ACTION BY ANOTHER STATE OR AGENCY

NOTES: LICENSE REVOKED, SUSPENDED, SURRENDERED OR OTHERWISE LOST FOR REASONS BEARING ON PROFESSIONAL PERFORMANCE, PROFESSIONAL COMPETENCE OR FINANCIAL INTEGRITY.

EVANGELISTA, LUISITO A DR OF LAS VEGAS, NV, WAS DISCIPLINED BY ILLINOIS ON FEBRUARY 1, 1999
DISCIPLINARY ACTION: EMERGENCY SUSPENSION
OFFENSE: PROFESSIONAL MISCONDUCT

NOTES: PURCHASED NARCOTIC PRESCRIPTION DRUGS WHICH HE TOOK TO NEVADA TO SELL.

FAJARDO, DEMETRIO MD, LICENSE NUMBER 152673 OF NIAGARA FALLS CLINIC 775 3RD ST, NIAGARA FALLS, NY, WAS DISCIPLINED BY NEW YORK ON OCTOBER 14, 1997
DISCIPLINARY ACTION: 60-MONTH PROBATION; RESTRICTION PLACED ON LICENSE
OFFENSE: SUBSTANDARD CARE, INCOMPETENCE OR NEGLIGENCE

NOTES: GROSS NEGLIGENCE AND INCOMPETENCE; NEGLIGENCE AND INCOMPETENCE ON MORE THAN ONE OCCASION; FAILING TO MAINTAIN ACCURATE PATIENT RECORDS.

FAJARDO, DEMETRIO MD, LICENSE NUMBER 152673 OF 60 SUMMERSHADE COURT, EAST AMHERST, NY, WAS DISCIPLINED BY NEW YORK ON OCTOBER 14, 1998
DISCIPLINARY ACTION: 12-MONTH LICENSE SUSPENSION; 60-MONTH PROBATION
OFFENSE: FAILURE TO COMPLY WITH PREVIOUS BOARD ORDER

NOTES: VIOLATED THE TERMS OF PROBATION AND/OR LICENSE LIMITATION PREVIOUSLY IMPOSED. REMAINDER OF FIVE YEAR SUSPENSION STAYED; PERMANENT LICENSE LIMITATION RESTRICTING HIS PRACTICE TO A SUPERVISED SETTING; $10,000 FINE.

FAJARDO, DEMETRIO MD, LICENSE NUMBER 152673 OF 5832 SPRING RANCH PARKWAY, LAS VEGAS, NV, WAS DISCIPLINED BY NEW YORK ON MAY 26, 1999
DISCIPLINARY ACTION: SURRENDER OF LICENSE
OFFENSE: FAILURE TO COMPLY WITH PREVIOUS BOARD ORDER

NOTES: VIOLATED TERMS OF PROBATION PREVIOUSLY IMPOSED.

FARBER, LESLIE MD, LICENSE NUMBER A38649 OF LAS VEGAS, NV, WAS DISCIPLINED BY CALIFORNIA ON AUGUST 6, 1999
DISCIPLINARY ACTION: REPRIMAND

FORSYTHE, JAMES W MD, WAS DISCIPLINED BY NEVADA ON NOVEMBER 3, 1995
DISCIPLINARY ACTION: FINE
OFFENSE: PROFESSIONAL MISCONDUCT

NOTES: PLED NOLO CONTENDERE TO ONE COUNT OF MAKING AN UNREASONABLE ADDITIONAL CHARGE FOR TESTS IN A LABORATORY, RADIOLOGICAL SERVICES OR OTHER SERVICES FOR TESTING WHICH ARE ORDERED BY THE PHYSICIAN AND PERFORMED OUTSIDE HIS OWN OFFICE. $1,000 FINE AND SHALL PAY $44,000 AS DISGORGEMENT OF PAYMENTS WHICH MAY HAVE BEEN RECEIVED BY HIM IN CONNECTION WITH MEDICAL LABORATORY TESTS PERFORMED IN THE PAST WHICH HAVE BEEN IMPROPERLY BILLED TO PATIENTS AND CANNOT PRACTICALLY BE RETURNED TO THOSE PATIENTS FROM WHOM IT MAY HAVE BEEN RECEIVED.

FRANCO, ALLEN I MD, WAS DISCIPLINED BY NEVADA ON MARCH 15, 1999
DISCIPLINARY ACTION: SURRENDER OF LICENSE
OFFENSE: SUBSTANCE ABUSE

NOTES: CHARGED WITH INABILITY TO PRACTICE MEDICINE WITH SKILL AND SAFETY BECAUSE OF ILLNESS, A MENTAL OR PHYSICAL CONDITION OR THE USE OF ALCOHOL, DRUGS, NARCOTICS OR ANY OTHER SUBSTANCE; WRITING A PRESCRIPTION FOR CONTROLLED SUBSTANCES FOR ANY PERSON WITHOUT AN APPROPRIATE EXAMINATION WHICH CONFIRMS THE MEDICAL NECESSITY FOR THE CONTROLLED SUBSTANCES; ACQUIRING ANY CONTROLLED SUBSTANCES FROM ANY PHARMACY OR OTHER SOURCE BY MISREPRESENTATION, FRAUD, DECEPTION OR SUBTERFUGE; ENGAGING IN CONDUCT WHICH IS INTENDED TO DECEIVE; HABITUAL INTOXICATION FROM ALCOHOL OR DEPENDENCY ON CONTROLLED SUBSTANCES. VOLUNTARY SURRENDER WHILE UNDER INVESTIGATION. MUST PAY $5,688.95 FOR ADMINISTRATIVE EXPENSES.

FRANCO, ALLEN I MD, DATE OF BIRTH MAY 24, 1960 OF 801 RANCHO DRIVE #D-18, LAS VEGAS, NV, WAS DISCIPLINED BY MEDICARE ON SEPTEMBER 20, 1999
DISCIPLINARY ACTION: EXCLUSION FROM THE MEDICARE AND/OR MEDICAID PROGRAM
OFFENSE: DISCIPLINARY ACTION BY ANOTHER STATE OR AGENCY

NOTES: LICENSE REVOKED, SUSPENDED, SURRENDERED OR OTHERWISE LOST FOR REASONS BEARING ON PROFESSIONAL PERFORMANCE, PROFESSIONAL COMPETENCE OR FINANCIAL INTEGRITY.

FRANK, KENNETH A MD, LICENSE NUMBER G038038 OF BAKERSFIELD, CA, WAS DISCIPLINED BY CALIFORNIA ON APRIL 5, 1991
DISCIPLINARY ACTION: LICENSE REVOCATION
OFFENSE: SUBSTANDARD CARE, INCOMPETENCE OR NEGLIGENCE

NOTES: ACTION BASED ON NEGLIGENCE AND INCOMPETENCE IN THE CASE OF AN ASTHMA PATIENT IN DISTRESS WHO DIED. DEFAULT DECISION.

FRANK, KENNETH A MD, DATE OF BIRTH MARCH 7, 1950 OF 3001 CATALINA DR, BAKERSFIELD, CA, WAS DISCIPLINED BY MEDICARE ON JUNE 9, 1992
DISCIPLINARY ACTION: EXCLUSION FROM THE MEDICARE AND/OR MEDICAID PROGRAM
OFFENSE: DISCIPLINARY ACTION BY ANOTHER STATE OR AGENCY

NOTES: LICENSE REVOCATION OR SUSPENSION.

FRANK, KENNETH AARON MD OF WHITE LANE MEDICAL 5401 WHITE LN, BAKERSFIELD, CA, WAS DISCIPLINED BY DEA ON MAY 30, 1990
DISCIPLINARY ACTION: SURRENDER OF CONTROLLED SUBSTANCE LICENSE
OFFENSE: CRIMINAL CONVICTION OR PLEA OF GUILTY, NOLO CONTENDERE, OR NO CONTEST TO A CRIME

NOTES: CONVICTED OF RAPE. DEA REGISTRATION REINSTATED ON OR ABOUT 8/26/91.

FRANK, KENNETH ARON MD, LICENSE NUMBER 00N5509 OF LAS VEGAS, NV, WAS DISCIPLINED BY ARKANSAS ON MAY 12, 1993
DISCIPLINARY ACTION: LICENSE REVOCATION
OFFENSE: SUBSTANDARD CARE, INCOMPETENCE OR NEGLIGENCE

NOTES: GROSSLY NEGLIGENT OR IGNORANT MALPRACTICE.

GALVEZ, TIMOTEO L MD, LICENSE NUMBER 0C40709 OF MADISON, WI, WAS DISCIPLINED BY CALIFORNIA ON NOVEMBER 7, 1994
DISCIPLINARY ACTION: SURRENDER OF LICENSE

NOTES: VOLUNTARY SURRENDER WHILE CHARGES PENDING.

GALVEZ, TIMOTEO L MD, WAS DISCIPLINED BY NEVADA ON MAY 5, 1995
DISCIPLINARY ACTION: REPRIMAND
OFFENSE: DISCIPLINARY ACTION BY ANOTHER STATE OR AGENCY

NOTES: IN 12/92 WISCONSIN ORDER REQUIRED HIM TO CEASE

THE USE OF SPECIFIC DIAGNOSIS SYSTEMS; IN 10/94 CALIFORNIA ACCEPTED SURRENDER OF LICENSE WHILE ALLEGATIONS WERE PENDING; IN 4/93 NEVADA LICENSE APPLICATION SAID NO CHARGES WERE FILED BY STATE BOARDS AND DID NOT INFORM NEVADA OF THE WISCONSIN AND CALIFORNIA ACTIONS. $300 ADMINISTRATIVE COSTS.

GHARAVI, NAJM M MD OF 1700 SOUTH EASTERN, LAS VEGAS, NV, WAS DISCIPLINED BY MEDICARE ON AUGUST 10, 1994
DISCIPLINARY ACTION: 60-MONTH EXCLUSION FROM THE MEDICARE AND/OR MEDICAID PROGRAM
OFFENSE: CRIMINAL CONVICTION OR PLEA OF GUILTY, NOLO CONTENDERE, OR NO CONTEST TO A CRIME

NOTES: CONVICTED OF A CRIME INVOLVING THE MEDICARE, MEDICAID, MATERNAL AND CHILD HEALTH SERVICES BLOCK GRANT OR BLOCK GRANTS TO STATES FOR SOCIAL SERVICES PROGRAMS.

GHARAVI, NAJM M MD, WAS DISCIPLINED BY NEVADA ON DECEMBER 7, 1994
DISCIPLINARY ACTION: REPRIMAND; COMMUNITY SERVICE
OFFENSE: CRIMINAL CONVICTION OR PLEA OF GUILTY, NOLO CONTENDERE, OR NO CONTEST TO A CRIME

NOTES: CONVICTED IN THE JUSTICE COURT OF LAS VEGAS FOR MEDICAID FRAUD. MUST COMPLETE 20 HOURS OF UNCOMPENSATED PUBLIC SERVICE WITHIN 6 MONTHS.

GHARAVI, NAJM M MD, LICENSE NUMBER 0008065, WAS DISCIPLINED BY ARIZONA ON JANUARY 18, 1996
DISCIPLINARY ACTION: LICENSE REVOCATION
OFFENSE: DISCIPLINARY ACTION BY ANOTHER STATE OR AGENCY

NOTES: IN 6/94, EXCLUDED BY THE NEVADA DEPARTMENT OF HUMAN RESOURCES, WELFARE DIVISION-NEVADA MEDICAID FROM THE MEDICAID PROGRAM FOR THREE YEARS DUE TO A GUILTY PLEA TO MEDICAID FRAUD; IN 8/94, EXCLUDED FOR FIVE YEARS FROM PARTICIPATION IN THE MEDICARE, MEDICAID, MATERNAL AND CHILD HEALTH SERVICES BLOCK GRANT AND BLOCK GRANTS TO STATES FOR SOCIAL SERVICES PROGRAMS; EXCLUSION BASED ON CONVICTION IN NEVADA OF A CRIMINAL OFFENSE RELATED TO THE DELIVERY OF AN ITEM OR SERVICE UNDER THE MEDICAID PROGRAM; IN 5/95, RECEIVED NOTIFICATION THAT A COMPLAINT AGAINST HIM HAD BEEN FILED WITH THE BOARD; WITH NOTIFICATION RECEIVED A COPY OF THE DHHS CORRESPONDENCE; ON FOUR OCCASIONS BETWEEN 5/95 AND 10/95, HE WAS REQUESTED TO FILE A NARRATIVE STATEMENT CONCERNING THE MATTER WITH SUPPORTING DOCUMENTATION REGARDING THE COMPLAINT, BUT FAILED TO PROVIDE THIS INFORMATION AS HE WAS LEGALLY REQUESTED; IN 9/95, INTERVIEWED BY THE BOARD, BUT FAILED TO PROVIDE MEANINGFUL INFORMATION OR DOCUMENTATION; ATTEMPTS BY THE BOARD TO COMMUNICATE WITH HIM HAVE BEEN UNSUCCESSFUL, WITH ALL CORRESPONDENCE TO HIS HOME OR OFFICE RETURNED UNCLAIMED; HAS FAILED TO KEEP THE BOARD INFORMED OF HIS CURRENT OFFICE AND/OR RESIDENCE ADDRESS AS REQUIRED; IN 1/96, BOARD RECEIVED INFORMATION THAT IN 12/94, HE WAS REPRIMANDED BY THE NEVADA BOARD AND REQUIRED TO COMPLETE 20 HOURS OF PUBLIC SERVICE.

GHARAVI, NAJM MOOSAVI MD, LICENSE NUMBER C41322 OF LAS VEGAS, NV, WAS DISCIPLINED BY CALIFORNIA ON JANUARY 6, 1997
DISCIPLINARY ACTION: LICENSE REVOCATION
OFFENSE: DISCIPLINARY ACTION BY ANOTHER STATE OR AGENCY

NOTES: DISCIPLINED BY NEVADA FOR MEDICAID FRAUD.

GIBSON, L DEAN MD, WAS DISCIPLINED BY NEVADA ON MARCH 15, 1999
DISCIPLINARY ACTION: SURRENDER OF LICENSE
OFFENSE: PROFESSIONAL MISCONDUCT

NOTES: CHARGED WITH TWO COUNTS OF MALPRACTICE AND ONE COUNT OF REPEATED MALPRACTICE. VOLUNTARY SURRENDER WHILE UNDER INVESTIGATION.

GIBSON, LEONARD DEAN MD, DATE OF BIRTH NOVEMBER 3, 1923 OF 130 E HASKELL STREET #A, WINNEMUCCA, NV, WAS DISCIPLINED BY MEDICARE ON SEPTEMBER 20, 1999
DISCIPLINARY ACTION: EXCLUSION FROM THE MEDICARE AND/OR MEDICAID PROGRAM
OFFENSE: DISCIPLINARY ACTION BY ANOTHER STATE OR AGENCY

NOTES: LICENSE REVOKED, SUSPENDED, SURRENDERED OR OTHERWISE LOST FOR REASONS BEARING ON PROFESSIONAL PERFORMANCE, PROFESSIONAL COMPETENCE OR FINANCIAL INTEGRITY.

GILBERT, WARREN S MD, WAS DISCIPLINED BY NEVADA ON JANUARY 16, 1993
DISCIPLINARY ACTION: 24-MONTH PROBATION; FINE
OFFENSE: OVERPRESCRIBING OR MISPRESCRIBING DRUGS

NOTES: ON 10/19/92 COMPLAINT FILED WHERE HE WAS CHARGED WITH 33 COUNTS INVOLVING 32 PATIENTS AND INCLUDING VIOLATIONS CONSTITUTING ILLEGAL PRESCRIBING (PRESCRIBING SYNTHROID FOR WEIGHT CONTROL), OVER-PRESCRIBING AND INAPPROPRIATE PRESCRIBING OF CONTROLLED SUBSTANCES AND REPEATED MALPRACTICE. MUST PAY A $5,000 FINE, TAKE CONTINUING MEDICAL EDUCATION COURSES ON THE PRESCRIBING OF CONTROLLED SUBSTANCES, AND RECEIVE A PUBLIC REPRIMAND.

GILBERT, WARREN S MD, WAS DISCIPLINED BY NEVADA ON JANUARY 17, 1996
DISCIPLINARY ACTION: 48-MONTH PROBATION
OFFENSE: PROFESSIONAL MISCONDUCT

NOTES: AIDING, ASSISTING, EMPLOYING OR ADVISING ANY UNLICENSED PERSON TO ENGAGE IN THE PRACTICE OF MEDICINE; DELEGATING RESPONSIBILITY FOR THE CARE OF A PATIENT TO A PERSON WHEN HE KNOWS OR HAS REASON TO KNOW THAT THIS PERSON IS NOT QUALIFIED TO UNDERTAKE THAT RESPONSIBILITY. REVOCATION STAYED. CONDITIONS OF PROBATION: DOCUMENT PERSONAL DIRECTION REGARDING THE DISPENSATION OF CARE TO THOSE INMATES ON THE SICK CALL ROSTER AND DISPENSATION OF CARE BY THE TRIAGE NURSES; SHALL ENSURE THAT ALL PHYSICAL EXAMINATIONS WILL BE DONE BY APPROPRIATELY TRAINED AND LICENSED PERSONNEL; WHILE WORKING AT WASHOE COUNTY JAIL SHALL PROVIDE A QUARTERLY REPORT REGARDING DEFICIENCIES AND SUGGESTIONS FOR CORRECTIVE ACTION; SHALL REIMBURSE BOARD FOR COSTS.

GLADSTONE, SCOTT B MD, WAS DISCIPLINED BY NEVADA ON DECEMBER 7, 1994
DISCIPLINARY ACTION: REPRIMAND
OFFENSE: CRIMINAL CONVICTION OR PLEA OF GUILTY, NOLO CONTENDERE, OR NO CONTEST TO A CRIME

NOTES: CONVICTED IN THE LAS VEGAS JUSTICE COURT FOR MEDICAID FRAUD.

GLADSTONE, SCOTT B MD, LICENSE NUMBER 0007841 OF 77-6365 KENIKA PLACE, KAILUA-KONA, HI, WAS DISCIPLINED BY HAWAII ON JUNE 21, 1995
DISCIPLINARY ACTION: FINE; MONITORING OF PHYSICIAN PERFORMANCE
OFFENSE: DISCIPLINARY ACTION BY ANOTHER STATE OR AGENCY

NOTES: VIOLATED STATUTES INVOLVING ACTION TAKEN BY ANOTHER AGENCY AND FAILURE TO REPORT THIS TO THE BOARD WITHIN 30 DAYS; CONVICTION OR GUILTY PLEA TO A CRIME RELATED TO THE PRACTICE OF MEDICINE. HAS AGREED TO PAY A FINE OF $5,000; WILL HAVE A BOARD-APPROVED LICENSED PSYCHIATRIST OR PHYSICIAN WHO IS FAMILIAR WITH HIS PRACTICE MONITOR HIS PRACTICE AND BILLING PROCEDURES AND ISSUE WRITTEN REPORTS ON A QUARTERLY BASIS FOR A ONE YEAR PERIOD; SHALL ABIDE BY ALL TERMS OF CRIMINAL SENTENCE.

GLADSTONE, SCOTT BRUCE MD, LICENSE NUMBER 0G60406 OF LAS VEGAS, NV, WAS DISCIPLINED BY CALIFORNIA ON AUGUST 12, 1996
DISCIPLINARY ACTION: 60-MONTH PROBATION

NOTES: REVOCATION, STAYED.

GLADSTONE, SCOTT V MD, DATE OF BIRTH NOVEMBER 22, 1959 OF PO BOX 97017, LAS VEGAS, NV, WAS DISCIPLINED BY MEDICARE ON APRIL 12, 1993
DISCIPLINARY ACTION: 120-MONTH EXCLUSION FROM THE MEDICARE AND/OR MEDICAID PROGRAM
OFFENSE: CRIMINAL CONVICTION OR PLEA OF GUILTY, NOLO CONTENDERE, OR NO CONTEST TO A CRIME

NOTES: CONVICTED OF OBTAINING MEDICAID MONEY UNDER FALSE PRETENSES.

GOODMAN, BRYAN J MD, WAS DISCIPLINED BY NEVADA ON DECEMBER 5, 1998
DISCIPLINARY ACTION: SURRENDER OF LICENSE

NOTES: VOLUNTARY SURRENDER WHILE UNDER INVESTIGATION.

GOODMAN, HERBERT D MD, LICENSE NUMBER 0007607, WAS DISCIPLINED BY ARIZONA ON JANUARY 21, 1992
OFFENSE: SUBSTANDARD CARE, INCOMPETENCE OR NEGLIGENCE

NOTES: INADEQUATE AND INCOMPLETE MANAGEMENT OF A PATIENT, SPECIFICALLY, FAILURE TO EVALUATE PERSISTENT ANEMIA AND PAINFUL PROTRUDING HEMORRHOIDS, LEADING TO AN ADVANCED CARCINOMA OF THE RECTUM WHICH HAD TO BE TREATED BY AN ABDOMINAL PERINEAL RESECTION. AFTER A MEDICAL MALPRACTICE ACTION WAS INITIATED AGAINST HIM CONCERNING HIS TREATMENT IN THIS CASE, HE SENT COPIES OF THIS PATIENT'S MEDICAL RECORDS TO HIS INSURANCE CARRIER THAT HE HAD ALTERED TO INCLUDE A TEST WHICH HE HAD NOT IN FACT ORDERED. DECREE OF CENSURE.

GOODMAN, HERBERT D MD, WAS DISCIPLINED BY NEVADA ON JANUARY 16, 1993
DISCIPLINARY ACTION: FINE; REPRIMAND
OFFENSE: NONCOMPLIANCE WITH A PROFESSIONAL RULE

NOTES: ON 12/16/92 COMPLAINT FILED WHERE HE WAS CHARGED WITH FAILURE TO REPORT TO THE BOARD A CLAIM OF NEGLIGENCE AGAINST HIM BY THE ARIZONA MEDICAL BOARD, AND THE SUBSEQUENT DISPOSITION THEREOF WITHIN 90 DAYS AFTER THE CLAIM WAS FILED OR THE DISPOSITION OF THE CLAIM. MUST PAY A $1,000 FINE.

GOODMAN, HERBERT D MD, DATE OF BIRTH FEBRUARY 2, 1940, LICENSE NUMBER 0028104 OF 6726 E. MONTECITO AVENUE, SCOTTSDALE, AZ, WAS DISCIPLINED BY NEW JERSEY ON FEBRUARY 1, 1994
DISCIPLINARY ACTION: REPRIMAND
OFFENSE: DISCIPLINARY ACTION BY ANOTHER STATE OR AGENCY

NOTES: DISCIPLINARY ACTION TAKEN IN THE STATE OF ARIZONA. PRIOR TO RESUMING PRACTICE, MUST APPEAR FOR A STATUS CONFERENCE BEFORE A COMMITTEE OF THE NEW JERSEY BOARD.

GOODMAN, MARGARET E MD, WAS DISCIPLINED BY NEVADA ON MARCH 18, 1997
OFFENSE: PROFESSIONAL MISCONDUCT

NOTES: ENGAGED IN CONDUCT INTENDED TO DECEIVE IN THAT SHE, ON NUMEROUS OCCASIONS, KNOWINGLY AND FALSELY MISREPRESENTED HERSELF AS A BOARD CERTIFIED NEUROLOGIST, WHEN IN FACT SHE WAS NOT. SHALL PAY $5,000 AS DISGORGEMENT OF PAYMENTS WHICH MAY HAVE BEEN RECEIVED BY HER HAVING ENGAGED IN SUCH CONDUCT.

GRAY, JOHN E MD, LICENSE NUMBER FE21668 OF LAS VEGAS, NV, WAS DISCIPLINED BY CALIFORNIA ON JUNE 17, 1998
DISCIPLINARY ACTION: SURRENDER OF LICENSE

NOTES: WHILE CHARGES PENDING.

GRAY, JOHN E MD, LICENSE NUMBER 165870 OF 9624 BEACH WATER CIRCLE, LAS VEGAS, NV, WAS DISCIPLINED BY NEW YORK ON NOVEMBER 9, 1998
DISCIPLINARY ACTION: SURRENDER OF LICENSE
OFFENSE: DISCIPLINARY ACTION BY ANOTHER STATE OR AGENCY

NOTES: DISCIPLINED BY THE CALIFORNIA BOARD FOR GROSS NEGLIGENCE AND REPEATED NEGLIGENCE DURING HIS TREATMENT OF A PATIENT.

GRAY, JOHN E MD, DATE OF BIRTH JULY 6, 1924 OF 9624 BEACH WATER CIRCLE, LAS VEGAS, NV, WAS DISCIPLINED BY MEDICARE ON JANUARY 20, 1999
DISCIPLINARY ACTION: EXCLUSION FROM THE MEDICARE AND/OR MEDICAID PROGRAM
OFFENSE: DISCIPLINARY ACTION BY ANOTHER STATE OR AGENCY

NOTES: LICENSE REVOKED, SUSPENDED, SURRENDERED OR OTHERWISE LOST FOR REASONS BEARING ON PROFESSIONAL PERFORMANCE, PROFESSIONAL COMPETENCE OR FINANCIAL INTEGRITY.

GREGORIO, ARTEMIO O MD, DATE OF BIRTH JANUARY 16, 1929 OF 33 JOYCE DRIVE, RIVERHEAD, NY, WAS DISCIPLINED BY MEDICARE ON AUGUST 10, 1994
DISCIPLINARY ACTION: EXCLUSION FROM THE MEDICARE AND/OR MEDICAID PROGRAM
OFFENSE: DISCIPLINARY ACTION BY ANOTHER STATE OR AGENCY

NOTES: LICENSE SURRENDERED FOR REASONS BEARING ON PROFESSIONAL COMPETENCE.

GREGORIO, ARTEMIO O MD, DATE OF BIRTH JANUARY 16, 1929, LICENSE NUMBER 031195L OF 5592 EDISTO CIRCLE, LAS VEGAS, NV, WAS DISCIPLINED BY PENNSYLVANIA ON MARCH 28, 1995
DISCIPLINARY ACTION: SURRENDER OF LICENSE
OFFENSE: DISCIPLINARY ACTION BY ANOTHER STATE OR AGENCY

NOTES: DISCIPLINARY ACTION TAKEN IN NEW YORK FOR MULTIPLE ACTS OF SEXUAL MISCONDUCT.

VOLUNTARY SURRENDER.

HADUONG, QUAN MD, LICENSE NUMBER G57891 OF HENDERSON, NV, WAS DISCIPLINED BY CALIFORNIA ON SEPTEMBER 6, 1999
DISCIPLINARY ACTION: 60-MONTH PROBATION
NOTES: SUSPENSION STAYED.

HANDSFIELD, RODNEY L MD, WAS DISCIPLINED BY NEVADA ON OCTOBER 6, 1999
DISCIPLINARY ACTION: LICENSE SUSPENSION
NOTES: INABILITY TO PRACTICE MEDICINE WITH REASONABLE SKILL AND SAFETY BECAUSE OF ILLNESS, A MENTAL OR PHYSICAL CONDITION OR THE USE OF ALCOHOL, DRUGS, NARCOTICS OR ANY OTHER SUBSTANCE. LICENSE SUBJECT TO FOLLOWING TERMS AND CONDITIONS: SHALL ENTER TALBOTT RECOVERY CAMPUS FOR AN OPEN-ENDED EVALUATION, RECOMMENDATION, AND TREATMENT IF RECOMMENDED; UPON RELEASE, SHALL ENTER INTO A FIVE YEAR CONTRACT WITH THE DIVERSION PROGRAM; REQUIRED TO PETITION THE BOARD FOR RESTORATION OF HIS LICENSE; SHALL PAY $2,000 IN COSTS.

HARRISON, WILLIAM O MD OF 2621 NORTH LOSEE ROAD, NORTH LAS VEGAS, NV, WAS DISCIPLINED BY DEA ON NOVEMBER 10, 1998
DISCIPLINARY ACTION: SURRENDER OF CONTROLLED SUBSTANCE LICENSE

HARRISON, WILLIAM O MD OF BUSTER STREET BLDG 650, MERCURY, NV, WAS DISCIPLINED BY DEA ON MARCH 11, 1999
DISCIPLINARY ACTION: SURRENDER OF CONTROLLED SUBSTANCE LICENSE

HARRISON, WILLIAM O MD, WAS DISCIPLINED BY NEVADA ON AUGUST 28, 1999
DISCIPLINARY ACTION: DENIAL OF NEW LICENSE
OFFENSE: DISCIPLINARY ACTION BY ANOTHER STATE OR AGENCY
NOTES: REVOCATION OF CALIFORNIA LICENSE; CRIMINAL CONVICTION IN NEVADA; IN 6/98 SURRENDERED HIS NEVADA LICENSE WHILE UNDER INVESTIGATION.

HARRISON, WILLIAM ORVILLE MD, LICENSE NUMBER G17944 OF LAS VEGAS, NV, WAS DISCIPLINED BY CALIFORNIA ON JULY 26, 1999
DISCIPLINARY ACTION: LICENSE REVOCATION
OFFENSE: DISCIPLINARY ACTION BY ANOTHER STATE OR AGENCY
NOTES: DISCIPLINED BY NEVADA FOR UNLAWFULLY SELLING PRESCRIPTIONS FOR SCHEDULE II AND III CONTROLLED SUBSTANCES AND CRIMINAL CONVICTION FOR POSSESSION OF CONTROLLED SUBSTANCES.

HIRSCH, NEIL R MD, DATE OF BIRTH JULY 16, 1948 OF 829 15TH STREET, MOLINE, IL, WAS DISCIPLINED BY MEDICARE ON OCTOBER 3, 1994
DISCIPLINARY ACTION: 60-MONTH EXCLUSION FROM THE MEDICARE AND/OR MEDICAID PROGRAM
OFFENSE: CRIMINAL CONVICTION OR PLEA OF GUILTY, NOLO CONTENDERE, OR NO CONTEST TO A CRIME
NOTES: CONVICTED OF A CRIME INVOLVING THE MEDICARE, MEDICAID, MATERNAL AND CHILD HEALTH SERVICES BLOCK GRANT OR BLOCK GRANTS TO STATES FOR SOCIAL SERVICES PROGRAMS.

HIRSCH, NEIL R MD OF MOLINE, IL, WAS DISCIPLINED BY ILLINOIS ON DECEMBER 1, 1995
DISCIPLINARY ACTION: 24-MONTH PROBATION
OFFENSE: CRIMINAL CONVICTION OR PLEA OF GUILTY, NOLO CONTENDERE, OR NO CONTEST TO A CRIME
NOTES: ENTERED INTO A PLEA AGREEMENT IN ARIZONA WHICH RESULTED IN A FELONY CONVICTION; TERMINATED FROM THE ILLINOIS DEPARTMENT OF PUBLIC AID MEDICAL ASSISTANCE PROGRAM BASED ON CONVICTION.

HIRSCH, NEIL R MD, LICENSE NUMBER 121240 OF 8433 PASEO VISTA DRIVE, LAS VEGAS, NV, WAS DISCIPLINED BY NEW YORK ON DECEMBER 17, 1997
DISCIPLINARY ACTION: 60-MONTH PROBATION
OFFENSE: DISCIPLINARY ACTION BY ANOTHER STATE OR AGENCY
NOTES: CONVICTED IN THE ARIZONA SUPERIOR COURT OF FRAUDULENT SCHEMES AND PRACTICES AND WILLFUL CONCEALMENT OF HIS FINANCIAL INTEREST IN TWO SUBCONTRACTS BETWEEN HEALTH CARE PROVIDERS OF ARIZONA, A STATE CONTRACTED PROVIDER OF HEALTH CARE SERVICES AND EYELITES INTERNATIONAL, A PROVIDER OF EYEGLASSES; DISCIPLINED BY THE ILLINOIS BOARD AND EXCLUDED FROM THE MEDICARE PROGRAM BASED UPON HIS CRIMINAL CONVICTION. FIVE YEAR SUSPENSION STAYED.

HIRSCH, NEIL RICHARD MD, LICENSE NUMBER G31451 OF LAS VEGAS, NV, WAS DISCIPLINED BY CALIFORNIA ON APRIL 3, 1998
DISCIPLINARY ACTION: 36-MONTH PROBATION
OFFENSE: DISCIPLINARY ACTION BY ANOTHER STATE OR AGENCY
NOTES: DISCIPLINED BY ILLINOIS BASED ON A FELONY CONVICTION IN ARIZONA FOR FRAUDULENT SCHEMES AND PRACTICES, WILLFUL CONCEALMENT, AND FACILITATION OF THEFT. REVOCATION STAYED.

HOFFMAN, JAMES F JR MD, DATE OF BIRTH FEBRUARY 12, 1938, LICENSE NUMBER 0014835 OF FT COLLINS, CO, WAS DISCIPLINED BY COLORADO ON MARCH 10, 1992
DISCIPLINARY ACTION: EMERGENCY SUSPENSION
OFFENSE: SUBSTANDARD CARE, INCOMPETENCE OR NEGLIGENCE
NOTES: AN ACT OR OMISSION CONSTITUTING GROSSLY NEGLIGENT PRACTICE, OR TWO OR MORE ACTS OF SUBSTANDARD CARE, AND FALSIFYING OR REPEATEDLY FAILING TO MAKE ESSENTIAL ENTRIES ON PATIENT RECORDS.

HOFFMAN, JAMES F JR MD, DATE OF BIRTH FEBRUARY 12, 1938, LICENSE NUMBER 0014835 OF FT COLLINS, CO, WAS DISCIPLINED BY COLORADO ON MAY 15, 1992
DISCIPLINARY ACTION: SURRENDER OF LICENSE
OFFENSE: SUBSTANDARD CARE, INCOMPETENCE OR NEGLIGENCE
NOTES: AN ACT OR OMISSION CONSTITUTING GROSSLY NEGLIGENT PRACTICE, OR TWO OR MORE ACTS OF SUBSTANDARD CARE, AND FALSIFYING OR REPEATEDLY FAILING TO MAKE ESSENTIAL ENTRIES ON PATIENT RECORDS. AGREES NEVER TO REAPPLY FOR LICENSURE IN COLORADO.

HOFFMAN, JAMES F JR MD, WAS DISCIPLINED BY NEVADA ON JANUARY 28, 1993
DISCIPLINARY ACTION: SURRENDER OF LICENSE
OFFENSE: NONCOMPLIANCE WITH A PROFESSIONAL RULE
NOTES: ON 12/04/92 COMPLAINT FILED WHERE HE WAS CHARGED WITH FAILURE TO REPORT WITHIN 30 DAYS, AND CONTINUAL FAILURE TO REPORT TO THE BOARD, THE SURRENDER OF HIS COLORADO LICENSE TO

PRACTICE MEDICINE.

HOFFMAN, JAMES F JR MD, DATE OF BIRTH FEBRUARY 12, 1938 OF 1845 KEDRON CIRCLE, FORT COLLINS, CO, WAS DISCIPLINED BY MEDICARE ON AUGUST 13, 1996
DISCIPLINARY ACTION: 180-MONTH EXCLUSION FROM THE MEDICARE AND/OR MEDICAID PROGRAM
OFFENSE: CRIMINAL CONVICTION OR PLEA OF GUILTY, NOLO CONTENDERE, OR NO CONTEST TO A CRIME

NOTES: CONVICTED OF A CRIME INVOLVING THE MEDICARE, MEDICAID, MATERNAL AND CHILD HEALTH SERVICES BLOCK GRANT OR BLOCK GRANTS TO STATES FOR SOCIAL SERVICES PROGRAMS.

HOSSAIN, MOHAMMAD MOAZZAM MD, DATE OF BIRTH DECEMBER 30, 1945 OF 627 BROOKSIDE AVENUE, REDLANDS, CA, WAS DISCIPLINED BY NEVADA ON DECEMBER 7, 1996
DISCIPLINARY ACTION: DENIAL OF NEW LICENSE
OFFENSE: DISCIPLINARY ACTION BY ANOTHER STATE OR AGENCY

NOTES: ACTION PENDING IN CALIFORNIA. ON 4/24/97 BOARD RECONSIDERED AND ACCEPTED HIS APPLICATION FOR LICENSURE AND HE WAS ISSUED A LICENSE TO PRACTICE IN NEVADA.

KATO, CHARLES K MD, LICENSE NUMBER 0010942 OF LOS ANGELES, CA, WAS DISCIPLINED BY CALIFORNIA ON JULY 7, 1990
DISCIPLINARY ACTION: LICENSE REVOCATION
OFFENSE: SUBSTANDARD CARE, INCOMPETENCE OR NEGLIGENCE

NOTES: EXCESSIVE PRESCRIBING OF CONTROLLED SUBSTANCES WITHOUT PRIOR EXAM AND MEDICAL INDICATION. GROSS NEGLIGENCE, INCOMPETENCE, REPEATED NEGLIGENCE, AND FALSE RECORDS IN HIS DIAGNOSES, RECORDS KEEPING, AND PRESCRIBING PRACTICES. NO APPEARANCE BY RESPONDENT. JUDICIAL REVIEW FILED - NO STAY ORDER ISSUED.

KATO, CHARLES K MD, DATE OF BIRTH OCTOBER 23, 1935 OF 5018 ALTA CANYADA ROAD, LA CANADA, CA, WAS DISCIPLINED BY MEDICARE ON JULY 24, 1991
DISCIPLINARY ACTION: EXCLUSION FROM THE MEDICARE AND/OR MEDICAID PROGRAM
OFFENSE: DISCIPLINARY ACTION BY ANOTHER STATE OR AGENCY

NOTES: LICENSE REVOCATION OR SUSPENSION.

KATO, CHARLES K MD, WAS DISCIPLINED BY NEVADA ON JUNE 10, 1994
DISCIPLINARY ACTION: DENIAL OF NEW LICENSE
OFFENSE: DISCIPLINARY ACTION BY ANOTHER STATE OR AGENCY

NOTES: CALIFORNIA LICENSE REVOKED.

KELLY, RONALD K MD, DATE OF BIRTH APRIL 15, 1953 OF DAVIS, CA, WAS DISCIPLINED BY CALIFORNIA ON MARCH 1, 1992
DISCIPLINARY ACTION: DENIAL OF NEW LICENSE

NOTES: DEFAULT DECISION.

KELLY, RONALD K MD, WAS DISCIPLINED BY NEVADA ON MARCH 20, 1996
DISCIPLINARY ACTION: EMERGENCY SUSPENSION

NOTES: COMPLAINT FILED ALLEGING THE CONTINUED PRACTICE OF MEDICINE WOULD ENDANGER THE HEALTH, SAFETY AND WELFARE OF HIS PATIENTS.

KELLY, RONALD K MD, WAS DISCIPLINED BY NEVADA ON JULY 2, 1996
DISCIPLINARY ACTION: LICENSE REVOCATION
OFFENSE: CRIMINAL CONVICTION OR PLEA OF GUILTY, NOLO CONTENDERE, OR NO CONTEST TO A CRIME

NOTES: FOUND GUILTY OF CONVICTION OF A FELONY; INABILITY TO PRACTICE MEDICINE WITH REASONABLE SKILL AND SAFETY BECAUSE OF ILLNESS, A MENTAL OR PHYSICAL CONDITION OR THE USE OF ALCOHOL, DRUGS, NARCOTICS, OR ANY OTHER SUBSTANCE; RENDERING PROFESSIONAL SERVICES TO A PATIENT WHILE THE PHYSICIAN IS UNDER THE INFLUENCE OF ALCOHOL OR ANY CONTROLLED SUBSTANCE. SHALL REIMBURSE THE BOARD FOR ALL EXPENSES INCURRED IN THE INVESTIGATION AND HEARING PROCESS.

KELLY, RONALD KAY MD, DATE OF BIRTH APRIL 15, 1953 OF 585 SAGE STREET, ELKO, NV, WAS DISCIPLINED BY MEDICARE ON JANUARY 12, 1997
DISCIPLINARY ACTION: EXCLUSION FROM THE MEDICARE AND/OR MEDICAID PROGRAM
OFFENSE: DISCIPLINARY ACTION BY ANOTHER STATE OR AGENCY

NOTES: LICENSE SUSPENDED FOR REASONS BEARING ON PROFESSIONAL PERFORMANCE.

KHALILI, ELI J MD, WAS DISCIPLINED BY NEVADA ON DECEMBER 24, 1991
DISCIPLINARY ACTION: LICENSE REVOCATION
OFFENSE: PROVIDING FALSE INFORMATION TO THE BOARD OR OTHER HEALTH AGENCY

NOTES: COMPLAINT FILED 8/5/91 STATED HE ENGAGED IN CONDUCT INTENDED TO DECEIVE THE BOARD, INTENTIONALLY MAKING A FALSE, MISLEADING, INACCURATE AND INCOMPLETE STATEMENT ON HIS APPLICATION FOR LICENSURE AS A RESIDENT PHYSICIAN IN NEVADA.

KHALILI, ELI J MD, DATE OF BIRTH JULY 24, 1962, LICENSE NUMBER 1059682 OF 100 MICHIGAN ST NE, GRAND RAPIDS, MI, WAS DISCIPLINED BY MICHIGAN ON APRIL 8, 1996
DISCIPLINARY ACTION: LICENSE REVOCATION; FINE
OFFENSE: CRIMINAL CONVICTION OR PLEA OF GUILTY, NOLO CONTENDERE, OR NO CONTEST TO A CRIME

NOTES: CRIMINAL CONVICTION; DIVERSION OR MISPRESCRIBING OF DRUGS. $1,000 FINE.

KHALILI, ELI J MD, DATE OF BIRTH JULY 24, 1962 OF 630 TEETOR ROAD, HAGERSTOWN, IN, WAS DISCIPLINED BY MEDICARE ON AUGUST 27, 1997
DISCIPLINARY ACTION: EXCLUSION FROM THE MEDICARE AND/OR MEDICAID PROGRAM
OFFENSE: DISCIPLINARY ACTION BY ANOTHER STATE OR AGENCY

NOTES: LICENSE REVOKED, SUSPENDED, SURRENDERED OR OTHERWISE LOST FOR REASONS BEARING ON PROFESSIONAL PERFORMANCE, PROFESSIONAL COMPETENCE OR FINANCIAL INTEGRITY.

KLEGON, NORMAN A DO, DATE OF BIRTH JANUARY 20, 1939 OF 18444 WEST TEN MILE, SOUTHFIELD, MI, WAS DISCIPLINED BY MEDICARE ON MARCH 19, 1990
DISCIPLINARY ACTION: 84-MONTH EXCLUSION FROM THE MEDICARE AND/OR MEDICAID PROGRAM
OFFENSE: CRIMINAL CONVICTION OR PLEA OF GUILTY, NOLO CONTENDERE, OR NO CONTEST TO A CRIME

NOTES: CONVICTION RELATING TO CONTROLLED SUBSTANCES. REINSTATED ON 4/1/96.

KLEGON, NORMAN A DO, DATE OF BIRTH JANUARY 20, 1939, LICENSE NUMBER 0005449 OF 18444 W TEN MILE, SOUTHFIELD, MI,

WAS DISCIPLINED BY MICHIGAN ON JUNE 20, 1992
DISCIPLINARY ACTION: RESTRICTION PLACED ON LICENSE

NOTES: REINSTATED WITH LIMITED LICENSE.

KLEGON, NORMAN A DO OF 1904 SOUTH MARYLAND PARKWAY, LAS VEGAS, NV, WAS DISCIPLINED BY DEA ON MAY 16, 1995
DISCIPLINARY ACTION: RESTRICTION PLACED ON CONTROLLED SUBSTANCE LICENSE
OFFENSE: PROFESSIONAL MISCONDUCT

NOTES: PLED GUILTY TO DRUG VIOLATION.

KLEGON, NORMAN A DO OF 1230 SOUTH MARLAND PARKWAY, LAS VEGAS, NV, WAS DISCIPLINED BY DEA ON APRIL 16, 1996
DISCIPLINARY ACTION: RESTRICTION PLACED ON CONTROLLED SUBSTANCE LICENSE
OFFENSE: PROFESSIONAL MISCONDUCT

NOTES: PLED GUILTY TO DRUG VIOLATION.

KRAUSE, ROBERT A MD, WAS DISCIPLINED BY NEW MEXICO ON JANUARY 1, 1997
DISCIPLINARY ACTION: LICENSE REVOCATION
OFFENSE: DISCIPLINARY ACTION BY ANOTHER STATE OR AGENCY

NOTES: MONTANA LICENSE REVOKED FOR UNPROFESSIONAL CONDUCT.

KRAUSE, ROBERT A MD, LICENSE NUMBER 21615, WAS DISCIPLINED BY MINNESOTA ON DECEMBER 21, 1998
DISCIPLINARY ACTION: LICENSE SUSPENSION

KRAUSE, ROBERT A MD, DATE OF BIRTH MAY 6, 1947 OF 6501 VEGAS DRIVE #1071, LAS VEGAS, NV, WAS DISCIPLINED BY MEDICARE ON JUNE 17, 1999
DISCIPLINARY ACTION: EXCLUSION FROM THE MEDICARE AND/OR MEDICAID PROGRAM
OFFENSE: DISCIPLINARY ACTION BY ANOTHER STATE OR AGENCY

NOTES: LICENSE REVOKED, SUSPENDED, SURRENDERED OR OTHERWISE LOST FOR REASONS BEARING ON PROFESSIONAL PERFORMANCE, PROFESSIONAL COMPETENCE OR FINANCIAL INTEGRITY.

KRAUSE, ROBERT ALAN MD, DATE OF BIRTH MAY 6, 1947, LICENSE NUMBER 0004514 OF 4504 BLACKTAIL LANE, BUTTE, MT, WAS DISCIPLINED BY MONTANA ON APRIL 11, 1996
DISCIPLINARY ACTION: EMERGENCY SUSPENSION
OFFENSE: SUBSTANCE ABUSE

NOTES: VIOLATED HIS MONTANA PROFESSIONAL ASSISTANCE PROGRAM AGREEMENT ENTERED INTO 1/24/96 FOR RECOVERY FROM ALCOHOL OR CHEMICAL DEPENDENCY; ON 3/13/96 INGESTED ALCOHOL AND DID NOT INFORM PROGRAM; IN 4/96 FAILED AND REFUSED TO REPORT FOR EVALUATION AND/OR TREATMENT AND FAILED TO REPORT TO A BOARD ORDERED EVALUATION; NOT IN RECOVERY OF HIS DISEASE OF ALCOHOLISM AND/OR CHEMICAL DEPENDENCY. SHALL SURRENDER LICENSE TO THE BOARD; AND SHALL CEASE AND DESIST FROM THE PRACTICE OF MEDICINE.

KRAUSE, ROBERT ALAN MD, DATE OF BIRTH MAY 6, 1947, LICENSE NUMBER 0004514 OF 4504 BLACKTAIL LANE, BUTTE, MT, WAS DISCIPLINED BY MONTANA ON JUNE 5, 1996
DISCIPLINARY ACTION: 60-MONTH PROBATION; MONITORING OF PHYSICIAN PERFORMANCE
OFFENSE: SUBSTANCE ABUSE

NOTES: VIOLATED AGREEMENT WITH PROFESSIONAL ASSISTANCE PROGRAM; ALCOHOL ABUSE. HAS NOW UNDERGONE A BOARD APPROVED EVALUATION RECEIVING A DIAGNOSIS OF ALCOHOL ABUSE, WITH POSSIBLE ALCOHOL DEPENDENCE. CONDITIONS OF PROBATION: SHALL ENTER INTO A REVISED AGREEMENT WITH THE MONTANA PROFESSIONAL ASSISTANCE PROGRAM; SHALL ABSTAIN FROM ANY USE OF ALCOHOL, MIND-ALTERING OR POTENTIALLY ADDICTING DRUGS OR MEDICATIONS, EXCEPT WHEN PRESCRIBED BY HIS PRIMARY CARE PHYSICIAN; SHALL NOTIFY THE BOARD IN ADVANCE OF TAKING ANY MEDICATION, EXCEPT IN THE CASE OF MEDICAL EMERGENCY; SHALL INFORM HIS PRIMARY CARE PHYSICIAN, DENTIST, AND ANY OTHER HEALTH CARE PROVIDER OF THIS ORDER; SHALL NOT WRITE PRESCRIPTIONS FOR ANY MOOD-ALTERING, ALCOHOL BASED OR POTENTIALLY ADDICTING DRUGS FOR HIMSELF OR ANY MEMBER OF HIS FAMILY; SHALL SUBMIT TO RANDOM BODY FLUID ANALYSIS FOR A MINIMUM OF ONE YEAR UPON BOARD REQUEST; AND SHALL RENEW HIS LICENSE IN A TIMELY FASHION FROM YEAR TO YEAR, DURING THE PROBATIONARY PERIOD.

KRAUSE, ROBERT ALAN MD, DATE OF BIRTH MAY 6, 1947, LICENSE NUMBER 0004514 OF 4504 BLACKTAIL LANE, BUTTE, MT, WAS DISCIPLINED BY MONTANA ON JUNE 27, 1996
DISCIPLINARY ACTION: EMERGENCY SUSPENSION; MONITORING OF PHYSICIAN PERFORMANCE
OFFENSE: FAILURE TO COMPLY WITH PREVIOUS BOARD ORDER

NOTES: VIOLATION OF PROBATION BY INGESTING ALCOHOL ON 6/13/96; PRESENTLY IN RELAPSE. SHALL SURRENDER LICENSE TO THE BOARD; SHALL CEASE AND DESIST ENTIRELY FROM THE PRACTICE OF MEDICINE; SHALL PRESENT HIMSELF FOR COMPLETE MENTAL, PHYSICAL AND CHEMICAL DEPENDENCY EVALUATION AND COOPERATE FULLY WITH THE EVALUATION PROCESS; SHALL FULFILL ANY RECOMMENDATIONS FOR TREATMENT AND OBTAIN A SATISFACTORY MEDICAL DISCHARGE PRIOR TO SEEKING REINSTATEMENT OF LICENSE; AND SHALL PROVIDE THE BOARD WITH RELEASES AND AUTHORIZATIONS TO OBTAIN FULL AND COMPLETE COPIES OF ALL RECORDS, REPORTS OR OTHER DOCUMENTS REGARDING THIS EVALUATION.

KRAUSE, ROBERT ALAN MD, DATE OF BIRTH MAY 6, 1947, LICENSE NUMBER 0004514 OF 4504 BLACKTAIL LANE, BUTTE, MT, WAS DISCIPLINED BY MONTANA ON SEPTEMBER 27, 1996
DISCIPLINARY ACTION: LICENSE REVOCATION
OFFENSE: FAILURE TO COMPLY WITH PREVIOUS BOARD ORDER

NOTES: BASED ON ALLEGATIONS OF PROBATION VIOLATION. DEFAULT ACTION.

KUGEL, HARVEY MD, LICENSE NUMBER 0031558 OF LAS VEGAS, NV, WAS DISCIPLINED BY FLORIDA ON FEBRUARY 9, 1993
DISCIPLINARY ACTION: FINE
OFFENSE: NONCOMPLIANCE WITH A PROFESSIONAL RULE

NOTES: CHARGED WITH FAILING TO TIMELY FURNISH THE PATIENT OR A LEGAL REPRESENTATIVE WITH COPIES OF THE PATIENT'S MEDICAL RECORDS; FAILING TO NOTIFY THE BOARD OF PRIMARY PLACE OF PRACTICE. $1,000 FINE; SHALL KEEP CURRENT RESIDENCE AND PRACTICE ADDRESSES ON FILE WITH THE BOARD AND NOTIFY THE BOARD OF CHANGE WITHIN 10 DAYS; SHALL MAINTAIN ADEQUATE OFFICE STAFF TO HANDLE REQUESTS FOR MEDICAL RECORDS AND FURNISH THEM WITHIN 20 WORKING DAYS INCLUDING X-RAYS AND INSURANCE INFORMATION OR THE ADDRESS OF THE PERSON WHO HAS THE MEDICAL RECORDS IF HE DOESN'T.

KUGEL, HARVEY L MD, WAS DISCIPLINED BY NEVADA ON JANUARY 22, 1994
DISCIPLINARY ACTION: FINE
OFFENSE: DISCIPLINARY ACTION BY ANOTHER STATE OR AGENCY

NOTES: ON 10/01/93 COMPLAINT FILED WHERE HE WAS CHARGED WITH ATTEMPTING TO RENEW NEVADA LICENSE TO PRACTICE MEDICINE BY A FALSE, MISLEADING, INACCURATE OR INCOMPLETE STATEMENT; ACTION TAKEN BY FLORIDA TO MODIFY LICENSE; FAILED TO ADVISE NEVADA OF THIS ON BIENNIAL FORM. MUST PAY A $100 FINE WITHIN 90 DAYS. ON 2/22/96 FOLLOWING COURT REMAND THE BOARD ORDERED HIM TO PAY THE FINE.

L'ARDENT, DENNIS R MD, LICENSE NUMBER 0151799 OF 301 EAST 38TH STREET, NEW YORK, NY, WAS DISCIPLINED BY NEW YORK ON MARCH 15, 1996
DISCIPLINARY ACTION: EMERGENCY SUSPENSION

NOTES: CONTINUED PRACTICE POSES AN IMMINENT DANGER TO PUBLIC HEALTH.

L'ARDENT, DENNIS R MD, LICENSE NUMBER 0151799 OF 6185 S PECOS #196, LAS VEGAS, NV, WAS DISCIPLINED BY NEW YORK ON APRIL 26, 1996
DISCIPLINARY ACTION: LICENSE REVOCATION
OFFENSE: DISCIPLINARY ACTION BY ANOTHER STATE OR AGENCY

NOTES: ACTION IN CALIFORNIA FOR GROSS NEGLIGENCE, INCOMPETENCE, AND SEXUAL MISCONDUCT INVOLVING HIS CARE AND TREATMENT OF THREE PATIENTS.

L'ARDENT, DENNIS R MD, DATE OF BIRTH AUGUST 18, 1946 OF 4632 S MARYLAND PKWY #71137, LAS VEGAS, NV, WAS DISCIPLINED BY MEDICARE ON JULY 18, 1996
DISCIPLINARY ACTION: EXCLUSION FROM THE MEDICARE AND/OR MEDICAID PROGRAM
OFFENSE: DISCIPLINARY ACTION BY ANOTHER STATE OR AGENCY

NOTES: LICENSE REVOKED FOR REASONS BEARING ON PROFESSIONAL PERFORMANCE.

L'ARDENT, DENNIS ROBERT MD, LICENSE NUMBER 0G31487 OF LAS VEGAS, NV, WAS DISCIPLINED BY CALIFORNIA ON AUGUST 31, 1995
DISCIPLINARY ACTION: LICENSE REVOCATION
OFFENSE: PROVIDING FALSE INFORMATION TO THE BOARD OR OTHER HEALTH AGENCY

NOTES: SEXUAL MISCONDUCT WITH FEMALE PATIENTS. GROSS NEGLIGENCE, REPEATED ACTS OF NEGLIGENCE, AND INCOMPETENCE. DISHONESTY IN FILING A FALSE DECLARATION ON HIS INTERIM SUSPENSION. DEFAULT ACTION.

LEVINGER, WILLIAM A MD, WAS DISCIPLINED BY NEVADA ON JUNE 20, 1997
DISCIPLINARY ACTION: MONITORING OF PHYSICIAN PERFORMANCE
OFFENSE: NONCOMPLIANCE WITH A PROFESSIONAL RULE

NOTES: FAILED TO REPORT, WITHIN 30 DAYS, THE REVOCATION, SUSPENSION OR SURRENDER OF HIS LICENSE IN IDAHO. MUST PAY $500 TO THE BOARD FOR INVESTIGATION COSTS; MUST ENTER INTO AGREEMENT WITH THE NEVADA HEALTH PROFESSIONALS ASSISTANCE FOUNDATION THAT THE IDAHO PHYSICIANS RECOVERY NETWORK WILL PROVIDE THEM WITH ALL REPORTS, CONCLUSIONS OR RECOMMENDATIONS CONCERNING HIS MONITORING.

LIES, BERT JR MD, WAS DISCIPLINED BY NEW MEXICO ON AUGUST 25, 1995
DISCIPLINARY ACTION: 36-MONTH PROBATION
OFFENSE: CRIMINAL CONVICTION OR PLEA OF GUILTY, NOLO CONTENDERE, OR NO CONTEST TO A CRIME

NOTES: CONVICTION OF FELONY. SAME TERMS AS COURT-ORDERED PROBATION. IN 8/98 BOARD REMOVED ALL STIPULATIONS FOR PROBATION FOR TAX EVASION, GIVING HIM AN UNRESTRICTED LICENSE.

LIES, BERT A JR MD, LICENSE NUMBER 0095843 OF 539 HARKLE ROAD, SANTA FE, NM, WAS DISCIPLINED BY NEW YORK ON SEPTEMBER 11, 1996
DISCIPLINARY ACTION: LICENSE SUSPENSION
OFFENSE: DISCIPLINARY ACTION BY ANOTHER STATE OR AGENCY

NOTES: DISCIPLINED BY THE NEW MEXICO BOARD FOR CONVICTION IN COURT OF FILING FALSE INCOME TAX STATEMENTS. SUSPENSION UNTIL HE COMPLETES ALL PROBATION TERMS IMPOSED BY THE NEW MEXICO BOARD AND AUTHORITIES.

LIES, BERT A JR MD, LICENSE NUMBER G14439 OF CRYSTAL BAY, NV, WAS DISCIPLINED BY CALIFORNIA ON JUNE 12, 1998
DISCIPLINARY ACTION: 60-MONTH PROBATION
OFFENSE: DISCIPLINARY ACTION BY ANOTHER STATE OR AGENCY

NOTES: DISCIPLINED BY NEW MEXICO BASED ON HIS FELONY CONVICTION FOR FILING FALSE INCOME TAX RETURNS. REVOCATION STAYED.

LIES, BERT A JR MD, LICENSE NUMBER G14439 OF CRYSTAL BAY, NV, WAS DISCIPLINED BY CALIFORNIA ON JUNE 24, 1998
DISCIPLINARY ACTION: SURRENDER OF LICENSE

NOTES: WHILE CHARGES PENDING.

LIM, RANULFO Y MD, LICENSE NUMBER A38719 OF SAN FRANCISCO, CA, WAS DISCIPLINED BY CALIFORNIA ON MARCH 28, 1997
DISCIPLINARY ACTION: 60-MONTH PROBATION
OFFENSE: SUBSTANDARD CARE, INCOMPETENCE OR NEGLIGENCE

NOTES: FAILED TO DIAGNOSE BOWEL CANCER RESULTING IN DELAYED TREATMENT AND METASTATIC SPREAD OF THE CANCER. REVOCATION STAYED.

LIM, RANULFO Y MD, WAS DISCIPLINED BY NEVADA ON DECEMBER 6, 1997
DISCIPLINARY ACTION: LICENSE REVOCATION
OFFENSE: DISCIPLINARY ACTION BY ANOTHER STATE OR AGENCY

NOTES: ACTION TAKEN BY CALIFORNIA AGAINST HIS LICENSE; FAILURE TO NOTIFY THE BOARD OF THIS CALIFORNIA ACTION; ATTEMPTING TO RENEW A LICENSE TO PRACTICE BY FRAUD, MISREPRESENTATION, OR FALSE, MISLEADING, INACCURATE OR INCOMPLETE STATEMENT; ENGAGING IN CONDUCT INTENDED TO DECEIVE THE BOARD.

LIM, RANULFO Y MD, DATE OF BIRTH MAY 28, 1927 OF 1096 SOUTHGATE AVENUE, DALY CITY, CA, WAS DISCIPLINED BY MEDICARE ON AUGUST 20, 1998
DISCIPLINARY ACTION: EXCLUSION FROM THE MEDICARE AND/OR MEDICAID PROGRAM
OFFENSE: DISCIPLINARY ACTION BY ANOTHER STATE OR AGENCY

NOTES: LICENSE REVOKED, SUSPENDED, SURRENDERED OR OTHERWISE LOST FOR REASONS BEARING ON PROFESSIONAL PERFORMANCE, PROFESSIONAL COMPETENCE OR FINANCIAL INTEGRITY.

LIMPIN, VIDAL C DR OF LINCOLNWOOD, IL, WAS DISCIPLINED BY ILLINOIS ON JULY 1, 1997
DISCIPLINARY ACTION: LICENSE SUSPENSION; SUSPENSION OF CONTROLLED SUBSTANCE LICENSE
OFFENSE: DISCIPLINARY ACTION BY ANOTHER STATE OR AGENCY

NOTES: VOLUNTARILY WITHDREW FROM THE MEDICAL ASSISTANCE PROGRAM OF THE ILLINOIS DEPARTMENT OF PUBLIC AID IN 1993, WHICH SUBSEQUENTLY DENIED HIS PETITIONS FOR REINSTATEMENT IN 1994 AND 1996.

LIMPIN, VIDAL C MD, WAS DISCIPLINED BY NEVADA ON DECEMBER 5, 1998
DISCIPLINARY ACTION: REPRIMAND; COMMUNITY SERVICE
OFFENSE: DISCIPLINARY ACTION BY ANOTHER STATE OR AGENCY

NOTES: LICENSE SUSPENDED IN ILLINOIS; FAILURE TO REPORT THE SUSPENSION TO NEVADA. MUST PERFORM 10 HOURS OF COMMUNITY SERVICE AT A BOARD APPROVED LOCATION WITHIN THREE MONTHS. $500 FOR ALL ADMINISTRATIVE EXPENSES INCURRED.

LIU, KUOCHIN MD, LICENSE NUMBER 107879 OF 1341 FOX ACRES, LAS VEGAS, NV, WAS DISCIPLINED BY NEW YORK ON JANUARY 11, 1999
DISCIPLINARY ACTION: SURRENDER OF LICENSE
OFFENSE: SUBSTANDARD CARE, INCOMPETENCE OR NEGLIGENCE

NOTES: NEGLIGENCE ON MORE THAN ONE OCCASION.

LODI, THOMAS LOUIS VIVANTE MD, DATE OF BIRTH JUNE 12, 1951, LICENSE NUMBER 0006666 OF 3535 LAS VEGAS BLVD, LAS VEGAS, NV, WAS DISCIPLINED BY NEVADA ON SEPTEMBER 21, 1996
DISCIPLINARY ACTION: SURRENDER OF LICENSE

NOTES: VOLUNTARY AND IRREVOCABLE SURRENDER.

LORANT, NIR Y MD, WAS DISCIPLINED BY NEVADA ON AUGUST 28, 1999
DISCIPLINARY ACTION: LICENSE REVOCATION
OFFENSE: PROFESSIONAL MISCONDUCT

NOTES: OBTAINING A LICENSE BY FRAUD OR MISREPRESENTATION, OR BY ANY FALSE, MISLEADING, INACCURATE OR INCOMPLETE STATEMENT; ENGAGING IN CONDUCT WHICH IS INTENDED TO DECEIVE.

LORANT, NIR YEHUDA MD, LICENSE NUMBER A49821 OF SAN LUIS OBISPO, CA, WAS DISCIPLINED BY CALIFORNIA ON MARCH 19, 1999
DISCIPLINARY ACTION: 60-MONTH PROBATION
OFFENSE: PROFESSIONAL MISCONDUCT

NOTES: COMMITTED ACTS OF UNPROFESSIONAL CONDUCT IN THAT HIS CONDUCT WHILE TREATING TWO FEMALE PATIENTS CROSSED THERAPEUTIC BOUNDARIES. REVOCATION STAYED.

MAHAKIAN, CHARLES G MD, LICENSE NUMBER G14144 OF WALNUT CREEK, CA, WAS DISCIPLINED BY CALIFORNIA ON JUNE 11, 1997
DISCIPLINARY ACTION: SURRENDER OF LICENSE

NOTES: WHILE CHARGES PENDING.

MAHAKIAN, CHARLES G MD, DATE OF BIRTH APRIL 20, 1940 OF 1808 DERBY SHIRE DRIVE, LAS VEGAS, NV, WAS DISCIPLINED BY MEDICARE ON JULY 20, 1998
DISCIPLINARY ACTION: EXCLUSION FROM THE MEDICARE AND/OR MEDICAID PROGRAM
OFFENSE: DISCIPLINARY ACTION BY ANOTHER STATE OR AGENCY

NOTES: LICENSE REVOKED, SUSPENDED, SURRENDERED OR OTHERWISE LOST FOR REASONS BEARING ON PROFESSIONAL PERFORMANCE, PROFESSIONAL COMPETENCE OR FINANCIAL INTEGRITY.

MANGIS, PHILLIP GEORGE MD, DATE OF BIRTH MARCH 3, 1935, LICENSE NUMBER 034894 OF 777 SOUTH VIRGINIA STREET, RENO, NV, WAS DISCIPLINED BY GEORGIA ON SEPTEMBER 8, 1995
DISCIPLINARY ACTION: LICENSE SUSPENSION
OFFENSE: DISCIPLINARY ACTION BY ANOTHER STATE OR AGENCY

NOTES: BASED ON ARIZONA REVOCATION; MAINTAINING INADEQUATE RECORDS; FALSIFICATION OF RECORDS AND INAPPROPRIATE PRESCRIBING. ON 5/8/98 LICENSE REINSTATED.

MANZUR, JUAN E MD, DATE OF BIRTH DECEMBER 17, 1958 OF 1621 E SAHARA AVENUE, LAS VEGAS, NV, WAS DISCIPLINED BY MEDICARE ON OCTOBER 20, 1998
DISCIPLINARY ACTION: EXCLUSION FROM THE MEDICARE AND/OR MEDICAID PROGRAM
OFFENSE: NONCOMPLIANCE WITH A PROFESSIONAL RULE

NOTES: DEFAULTED ON PUBLIC HEALTH SERVICE EDUCATION LOAN. REINSTATED ON 2/10/99.

MARLON, ANTHONY MD, WAS DISCIPLINED BY NEVADA ON SEPTEMBER 20, 1991
DISCIPLINARY ACTION: REPRIMAND
OFFENSE: CRIMINAL CONVICTION OR PLEA OF GUILTY, NOLO CONTENDERE, OR NO CONTEST TO A CRIME

NOTES: PLED GUILTY IN U.S. DISTRICT COURT FOR THE DISTRICT OF NEVADA TO A MISDEMEANOR FOR MAKING AND DELIVERING A CERTIFICATE TO THE FEDERAL GOVERNMENT CONTAINING A STATEMENT WHICH HE KNEW TO BE FALSE.

MARTELL, ALGIS MD, WAS DISCIPLINED BY NEVADA ON AUGUST 19, 1994
DISCIPLINARY ACTION: 60-MONTH PROBATION; FINE
OFFENSE: SUBSTANDARD CARE, INCOMPETENCE OR NEGLIGENCE

NOTES: COMPLAINT FILED ON 06/15/94 WHERE HE WAS CHARGED WITH GROSS MALPRACTICE IN TERMINATING A PREGNANCY WITHOUT ADEQUATELY DETERMINING UTERINE AGE OR GESTATIONAL SIZE AND IN FAILING TO COMPLETE THE TERMINATION. REVOCATION STAYED. CONDITIONS OF PROBATION AS FOLLOWS: MAY NOT PERFORM ANY PREGNANCY TERMINATION IN WHICH GESTATION HAS PROGRESSED BEYOND FOURTEEN WEEKS; MUST PERFORM AN ULTRASOUND EXAMINATION OF EVERY PREGNANCY TERMINATION PATIENT; MUST COMPLETE 20 HOURS OF CONTINUING MEDICAL EDUCATION IN OBSTETRICS AND/OR GYNECOLOGY, COVERING ASSESSMENT OF PREGNANCY AND PREGNANCY TERMINATIONS; MUST PROVIDE COMPLETE MEDICAL RECORDS FOR THE FIRST THIRTY PREGNANCY TERMINATIONS PERFORMED DURING PROBATION TO THE BOARD; MUST PAY $1,000 FOR REIMBURSEMENT OF INVESTIGATION COSTS; MUST RECEIVE A PUBLIC WRITTEN REPRIMAND TO BE PUBLISHED IN BOARD NEWSLETTER AND NEWSPAPERS IN 2 COUNTIES; MUST PAY A FINE OF $4,000.

MARTELL, ALGIS MD, LICENSE NUMBER 0C28968 OF RENO, NV, WAS DISCIPLINED BY CALIFORNIA ON OCTOBER 6, 1995
DISCIPLINARY ACTION: LICENSE REVOCATION
OFFENSE: DISCIPLINARY ACTION BY ANOTHER STATE OR AGENCY

NOTES: ACTION IN NEVADA FOR GROSS MALPRACTICE IN

OBSTETRICAL CARE. REVOCATION, STAYED. DEFAULT ACTION.

MARTELL, ALGIS MD, WAS DISCIPLINED BY NEVADA ON DECEMBER 2, 1995
DISCIPLINARY ACTION: RESTRICTION PLACED ON LICENSE
OFFENSE: FAILURE TO COMPLY WITH PREVIOUS BOARD ORDER

NOTES: CHARGED WITH VIOLATING BOARD ORDER OF 9/1/94; REPEATED MALPRACTICE; CONTINUAL FAILURE TO EXERCISE THE SKILL OR DILIGENCE OR USE THE METHODS ORDINARILY EXERCISED UNDER THE SAME CIRCUMSTANCES BY PHYSICIANS IN GOOD STANDING; DELEGATING RESPONSIBILITY FOR THE CARE OF A PATIENT TO A PERSON HE KNEW OR HAD REASON TO KNOW WAS NOT QUALIFIED TO UNDERTAKE THAT RESPONSIBILITY. HIS LICENSE IS RESTRICTED TO PROHIBIT HIS ENGAGING IN OR PERFORMING ANY PROCEDURE WHATSOEVER FOR TERMINATION OF PREGNANCY.

MARTELL, ALGIS MD, DATE OF BIRTH MARCH 12, 1933, LICENSE NUMBER 0002500 OF 2545 SOUTH BRUCE STREET #8, LAS VEGAS, NV, WAS DISCIPLINED BY NEVADA ON NOVEMBER 20, 1996
DISCIPLINARY ACTION: EMERGENCY SUSPENSION
OFFENSE: OVERPRESCRIBING OR MISPRESCRIBING DRUGS

NOTES: PRESCRIBED CONTROLLED SUBSTANCES, APPETITE SUPPRESSANTS, TO CONTROL THE WEIGHT OF APPROXIMATELY 41 PATIENTS WITHOUT DISPENSING AND/OR PRESCRIBING BEING PART OF A PROGRAM OF MEDICAL TREATMENT WHICH INCLUDES DIETARY RESTRICTIONS, MODIFICATION OF BEHAVIOR AND EXERCISE, WITHOUT DETERMINING IF THE PATIENTS' OBESITY REPRESENTED A THREAT TO THEIR HEALTH, AND WITHOUT OBTAINING A MEDICAL HISTORY AND PERFORMING A PHYSICAL EXAMINATION ON ANY OF THE PATIENTS AND/OR CONDUCTING APPROPRIATE STUDIES TO DETERMINE IF THERE WERE CONTRAINDICATIONS TO THE USE OF APPETITE SUPPRESSANT BY ANY OF THE PATIENTS; FAILED TO PROVIDE ADEQUATE SUPERVISION OF A MEDICAL ASSISTANT WHOM HE AIDED, ASSISTED, AND EMPLOYED DIRECTLY OR INDIRECTLY TO ENGAGE IN THE PRACTICE OF MEDICINE AND DELEGATED RESPONSIBILITY FOR THE CARE OF PATIENTS TO THIS PERSON WHO HE KNEW, OR HAD REASON TO KNOW WAS NOT QUALIFIED TO UNDERTAKE THAT RESPONSIBILITY.

MARTELL, ALGIS MD, DATE OF BIRTH MARCH 12, 1933, LICENSE NUMBER 0002500 OF 2545 SOUTH BRUCE ST SUITE #8, LAS VEGAS, NV, WAS DISCIPLINED BY NEVADA ON DECEMBER 7, 1996
DISCIPLINARY ACTION: SURRENDER OF LICENSE
OFFENSE: OVERPRESCRIBING OR MISPRESCRIBING DRUGS

NOTES: ALLEGATIONS THAT HE DISPENSED AND/OR PRESCRIBED CONTROLLED SUBSTANCES WHICH ARE APPETITE SUPPRESSANTS TO CONTROL THE WEIGHT OF A PATIENT WITHOUT BEING A PART OF A PROGRAM OF MEDICAL TREATMENT WHICH INCLUDES DIETARY RESTRICTIONS, MODIFICATION OF BEHAVIOR AND EXERCISE, WITHOUT A DETERMINATION THAT THE PATIENT'S OBESITY REPRESENTED A THREAT TO THE PATIENT'S HEALTH, WITHOUT OBTAINING A MEDICAL HISTORY AND PERFORMING A PHYSICAL EXAMINATION OF PATIENTS, AND WITHOUT CONDUCTING APPROPRIATE STUDIES TO DETERMINE IF THERE ARE ANY CONTRAINDICATIONS TO THE USE OF THE APPETITE SUPPRESSANTS BY THE PATIENTS; FAILED TO PROVIDE ADEQUATE SUPERVISION OF A MEDICAL ASSISTANT WHOM HE AIDED, ASSISTED, AND EMPLOYED, DIRECTLY OR INDIRECTLY TO ENGAGE IN THE PRACTICE OF MEDICINE; DELEGATED RESPONSIBILITY FOR THE CARE OF PATIENTS TO A PERSON, WHO HE KNEW WAS NOT QUALIFIED TO UNDERTAKE THAT RESPONSIBILITY. IRREVOCABLE VOLUNTARY SURRENDER.

MARTELL, ALGIS MD, DATE OF BIRTH MARCH 12, 1933 OF 129 WEST SIXTH STREET, #3, RENO, NV, WAS DISCIPLINED BY MEDICARE ON JULY 20, 1998
DISCIPLINARY ACTION: EXCLUSION FROM THE MEDICARE AND/OR MEDICAID PROGRAM
OFFENSE: DISCIPLINARY ACTION BY ANOTHER STATE OR AGENCY

NOTES: LICENSE REVOKED, SUSPENDED, SURRENDERED OR OTHERWISE LOST FOR REASONS BEARING ON PROFESSIONAL PERFORMANCE, PROFESSIONAL COMPETENCE OR FINANCIAL INTEGRITY.

MCCORMICK, THOMAS M MD, WAS DISCIPLINED BY NEVADA ON JULY 28, 1994
DISCIPLINARY ACTION: 36-MONTH PROBATION; FINE
OFFENSE: CRIMINAL CONVICTION OR PLEA OF GUILTY, NOLO CONTENDERE, OR NO CONTEST TO A CRIME

NOTES: CONVICTION OF 6 FELONIES INCLUDING FALSE STATEMENTS IN A PASSPORT APPLICATION AND CREDIT CARD APPLICATION; FRAUDULENT USE OF A SOCIAL SECURITY NUMBER AND POSSESSING FALSE IDENTIFICATION. REVOCATION STAYED. CONDITIONS OF PROBATION: MUST COMPLETE A COURSE IN MEDICAL ETHICS TO BE APPROVED IN ADVANCE BY THE BOARD; MUST PERFORM 40 HOURS OF MEDICALLY RELATED PUBLIC SERVICE APPROVED BY BOARD; MUST COMPLETE TERMS OF ANY PROBATION OR SENTENCE IMPOSED BY THE COURTS; MAY NOT PERSONALLY TAKE ANY SCHEDULES I THROUGH V CONTROLLED SUBSTANCES WITHOUT A WRITTEN PRESCRIPTION FROM A PHYSICIAN OR DENTIST RENDERING MEDICAL OR DENTAL CARE TO HIM; RANDOM URINE AND/OR BLOOD DRUG TESTING; MUST PAY $1500 FOR REIMBURSEMENT OF INVESTIGATION COSTS; ANY PERIOD OF TIME HE RESIDES OUTSIDE OF NEVADA DURING PERIOD OF PROBATION SHALL NOT BE CREDITED TO HIS PROBATION; MUST RECEIVE A PUBLIC WRITTEN REPRIMAND TO BE PUBLISHED IN BOARD NEWSLETTER AND FINED $500.

MCCORMICK, THOMAS MICHAEL MD, LICENSE NUMBER 0G23994 OF LAS VEGAS, NV, WAS DISCIPLINED BY CALIFORNIA ON JULY 3, 1996
DISCIPLINARY ACTION: 60-MONTH PROBATION
OFFENSE: DISCIPLINARY ACTION BY ANOTHER STATE OR AGENCY

NOTES: DISCIPLINARY ACTION IN NEVADA FOR CONVICTION IN FEDERAL DISTRICT COURT FOR SIX FELONY COUNTS INCLUDING: MAKING A FALSE STATEMENT ON A PASSPORT APPLICATION; FRAUDULENT USE OF A SOCIAL SECURITY NUMBER; POSSESSING A FALSE IDENTIFICATION DOCUMENT WITH INTENT TO DEFRAUD THE UNITED STATES; PRODUCTION OF ONE OR MORE COUNTERFEIT ACCESS DEVICES, A CITIBANK VISA CREDIT CARD; MAKING A MATERIALLY FALSE STATEMENT ON AN APPLICATION FOR A VISA CREDIT CARD TO CITIBANK; AND KNOWINGLY AND FRAUDULENTLY CONCEALING BANKRUPTCY ASSETS. REVOCATION, STAYED.

MCNAIR, KIMBLE II MD, LICENSE NUMBER 0037190 OF LAS VEGAS, NV, WAS DISCIPLINED BY FLORIDA ON MAY 7, 1991
DISCIPLINARY ACTION: LICENSE REVOCATION; FINE
OFFENSE: DISCIPLINARY ACTION BY ANOTHER STATE OR AGENCY

NOTES: $5,000 FINE.

MCNAIR, KIMBLE II MD, DATE OF BIRTH NOVEMBER 16, 1950 OF 3006 MARYLAND PKWY #675, LAS VEGAS, NV, WAS DISCIPLINED BY MEDICARE ON NOVEMBER 4, 1991
DISCIPLINARY ACTION: EXCLUSION FROM THE MEDICARE AND/OR MEDICAID PROGRAM
OFFENSE: DISCIPLINARY ACTION BY ANOTHER STATE OR AGENCY
NOTES: LICENSE REVOCATION OR SUSPENSION.

MCNAIR, KIMBLE II MD, WAS DISCIPLINED BY NEVADA ON MARCH 10, 1992
DISCIPLINARY ACTION: LICENSE REVOCATION
OFFENSE: CRIMINAL CONVICTION OR PLEA OF GUILTY, NOLO CONTENDERE, OR NO CONTEST TO A CRIME
NOTES: THE NEVADA SUPREME COURT HAS AFFIRMED HIS CONVICTION OF A FELONY.

MCQUILLAN, BERNARD P MD, WAS DISCIPLINED BY NEVADA ON DECEMBER 6, 1997
DISCIPLINARY ACTION: REPRIMAND
OFFENSE: PROFESSIONAL MISCONDUCT
NOTES: AIDING, ASSISTING, EMPLOYING OR ADVISING ANY UNLICENSED PERSON TO ENGAGE IN THE PRACTICE OF MEDICINE.

MCQUILLAN, BERNARD PATRICK MD, DATE OF BIRTH APRIL 19, 1935, LICENSE NUMBER 008960E OF 815 HARMONY ROAD, WINNEMUCCA, NV, WAS DISCIPLINED BY PENNSYLVANIA ON NOVEMBER 17, 1998
DISCIPLINARY ACTION: REPRIMAND
OFFENSE: DISCIPLINARY ACTION BY ANOTHER STATE OR AGENCY
NOTES: DISCIPLINARY ACTION TAKEN BY NEVADA.

MEISENHEIMER, KARL W MD, WAS DISCIPLINED BY NEVADA ON JULY 28, 1994
DISCIPLINARY ACTION: REQUIRED TO TAKE ADDITIONAL MEDICAL EDUCATION
OFFENSE: SUBSTANDARD CARE, INCOMPETENCE OR NEGLIGENCE
NOTES: ON 10/01/93 CHARGED WITH GROSS MALPRACTICE. MUST COMPLETE 20 HOURS OF CONTINUING MEDICAL EDUCATION APPROVED BY THE BOARD IN THE FIELD OF MEDICAL CARE OF THE ELDERLY, GERIATRICS OR GERONTOLOGY.

MEISENHEIMER, KARL WILLIAM MD, DATE OF BIRTH MARCH 11, 1948, LICENSE NUMBER 0003467, WAS DISCIPLINED BY NEVADA ON APRIL 4, 1996
DISCIPLINARY ACTION: 1-MONTH LICENSE SUSPENSION; FINE
OFFENSE: FAILURE TO COMPLY WITH PREVIOUS BOARD ORDER
NOTES: FAILURE TO COMPLY WITH AN ORDER OF THE BOARD IN THAT HE FAILED TO PAY A FINE AND PROVIDE REPORTS AS PER AN 11/95 ORDER. COMPLETION OF 40 HOURS UNCOMPENSATED COMMUNITY SERVICE. $2,000 FINE. $2,000 ADMINISTRATIVE COSTS.

MEISENHEIMER, KARL WILLIAM MD, DATE OF BIRTH MARCH 11, 1948, LICENSE NUMBER 0003467 OF 3121 SOUTH MARYLAND PKWY #101, LAS VEGAS, NV, WAS DISCIPLINED BY NEVADA ON SEPTEMBER 30, 1996
DISCIPLINARY ACTION: REPRIMAND; COMMUNITY SERVICE
OFFENSE: FAILURE TO COMPLY WITH PREVIOUS BOARD ORDER
NOTES: FAILURE TO COMPLY WITH AN ORDER OF THE BOARD IN THAT A $4,000 FINE IN 4/96 WAS NOT PAID IN 30 DAYS; IT WAS PAID ON 6/06/96. SHALL PERFORM 40 HOURS OF COMMUNITY SERVICE.

MILLER, ALBAN I MD, WAS DISCIPLINED BY NEVADA ON MARCH 15, 1999
DISCIPLINARY ACTION: 36-MONTH PROBATION; RESTRICTION PLACED ON LICENSE
OFFENSE: PROFESSIONAL MISCONDUCT
NOTES: CHARGED WITH ONE COUNT OF GROSS MALPRACTICE. REVOCATION STAYED WITH FOLLOWING TERMS AND CONDITIONS: REPRIMAND; WITHIN ONE YEAR SHALL OBTAIN 20 HOURS OF CONTINUING MEDICAL EDUCATION IN THE AREA OF CONSCIOUS AND DEEP CONSCIOUS SEDATION; SHALL PAY $3,177.00 IN COSTS; SHALL BE PRECLUDED FROM PERFORMING ANY SURGICAL PROCEDURE WHICH INVOLVES CONSCIOUS AND/OR DEEP CONSCIOUS SEDATION IN HIS OFFICE OR AT ANY LOCATION OTHER THAN A BOARD-APPROVED HOSPITAL SETTING, OR A CLINIC; ANY SUCH SURGICAL PROCEDURE MUST BE UNDER THE SUPERVISION OF AN ANESTHESIOLOGIST.

MILLER, JOHN J MD, WAS DISCIPLINED BY NEVADA ON OCTOBER 17, 1995
DISCIPLINARY ACTION: LICENSE REVOCATION
OFFENSE: DISCIPLINARY ACTION BY ANOTHER STATE OR AGENCY
NOTES: CONVICTION OF A FELONY; CHARGED WITH BEING FOUND GUILTY OF TWO FELONIES IN MONTANA; DISCIPLINARY ACTION AGAINST HIS LICENSE IN MONTANA; SUSPENSION OF LICENSE BY ANY OTHER JURISDICTION; FAILURE TO REPORT, WITHIN 30 DAYS, THE SUSPENSION OF HIS LICENSE TO PRACTICE MEDICINE IN ANOTHER JURISDICTION.

MILLER, JOHN J MD OF JACKSONVILLE, FL, WAS DISCIPLINED BY UTAH ON OCTOBER 28, 1995
DISCIPLINARY ACTION: LICENSE REVOCATION; REVOCATION OF CONTROLLED SUBSTANCE LICENSE
OFFENSE: PHYSICAL OR MENTAL ILLNESS INHIBITING THE ABILITY TO PRACTICE WITH SKILL AND SAFETY
NOTES: ADMISSION OF INABILITY TO SAFELY ENGAGE IN THE PRACTICE OF MEDICINE BECAUSE OF A MENTAL OR PHYSICAL CONDITION.

MILLER, JOHN J MD, LICENSE NUMBER 0D27191 OF HIDDEN LAKE DRIVE, JACKSONVILLE, FL, WAS DISCIPLINED BY MARYLAND ON NOVEMBER 7, 1995
DISCIPLINARY ACTION: PROBATION
OFFENSE: DISCIPLINARY ACTION BY ANOTHER STATE OR AGENCY
NOTES: ACTION BY MONTANA. REVOCATION STAYED.

MILLER, JOHN J MD, LICENSE NUMBER 0039841 OF DEER LODGE, MT, WAS DISCIPLINED BY FLORIDA ON MARCH 6, 1996
DISCIPLINARY ACTION: LICENSE REVOCATION
OFFENSE: DISCIPLINARY ACTION BY ANOTHER STATE OR AGENCY
NOTES: CONVICTED OF A CRIME DIRECTLY RELATING TO THE PRACTICE OF MEDICINE.

MILLER, JOHN JOSEPH MD, DATE OF BIRTH FEBRUARY 14, 1942, LICENSE NUMBER 0003980 OF 310 SUNNYVIEW LANE, KALISPELL, MT, WAS DISCIPLINED BY MONTANA ON AUGUST 23, 1994
DISCIPLINARY ACTION: EMERGENCY SUSPENSION
OFFENSE: SUBSTANCE ABUSE
NOTES: UNTREATED CHEMICAL DEPENDENCY. STIPULATION NOT TO SEEK REINSTATEMENT OF LICENSE UNTIL AFTER COMPLETION OF EVALUATION AND TREATMENT FOR ILLNESSES ON 8/31/94.

MILLER, JOHN JOSEPH MD, DATE OF BIRTH FEBRUARY 14, 1942, LICENSE NUMBER 00M5606, WAS DISCIPLINED BY IDAHO ON NOVEMBER 18, 1994

DISCIPLINARY ACTION: LICENSE SUSPENSION
OFFENSE: DISCIPLINARY ACTION BY ANOTHER STATE OR AGENCY

NOTES: ON 8/24/94 MONTANA ORDERED THAT LICENSE BE PLACED ON EMERGENCY SUSPENSION; ALSO REQUIRED HIM TO HAVE A COMPLETE MENTAL AND PHYSICAL EXAMINATION. THE IDAHO BOARD FOR THE PURPOSE OF THIS RECIPROCAL DISCIPLINE INCORPORATES THE TERMS AND CONDITIONS OF THIS ORDER AND ORDERS HIM TO FULLY COMPLY WITH THEM.

MILLER, JOHN JOSEPH MD, DATE OF BIRTH FEBRUARY 14, 1942, LICENSE NUMBER 0021472 OF JACKSONVILLE, FL, WAS DISCIPLINED BY TENNESSEE ON FEBRUARY 23, 1995
DISCIPLINARY ACTION: LICENSE REVOCATION
OFFENSE: DISCIPLINARY ACTION BY ANOTHER STATE OR AGENCY

NOTES: DISCIPLINARY ACTION TAKEN BY MONTANA BOARD. SUBSTANCE ABUSE. MUST APPEAR BEFORE BOARD IF REINSTATEMENT SOUGHT.

MILLER, JOHN JOSEPH MD, DATE OF BIRTH FEBRUARY 14, 1942, LICENSE NUMBER 00M5606, WAS DISCIPLINED BY IDAHO ON MAY 1, 1995
DISCIPLINARY ACTION: LICENSE REVOCATION
OFFENSE: DISCIPLINARY ACTION BY ANOTHER STATE OR AGENCY

NOTES: IN 8/94 ENGAGED IN THE EXCESSIVE USE OF ALCOHOL OR OTHER SUBSTANCES TO THE EXTENT THAT THE USE IMPAIRED HIM PHYSICALLY OR MENTALLY; AS A RESULT HE WAS IN AN AUTO ACCIDENT WHICH CAUSED THE DEATH OF TWO PERSONS; LICENSE IN TENNESSEE WAS REVOKED ON 2/23/95. THE IDAHO BOARD ADOPTS THE FINDING OF THE TENNESSEE ORDER AND INCORPORATES ALL OF THE TERMS AND CONDITIONS OF THE TENNESSEE ORDER.

MILLER, JOHN JOSEPH MD, DATE OF BIRTH FEBRUARY 14, 1942 OF 215 SUNNYVIEW LANE #7, KALISPELL, MT, WAS DISCIPLINED BY MEDICARE ON MAY 4, 1995
DISCIPLINARY ACTION: EXCLUSION FROM THE MEDICARE AND/OR MEDICAID PROGRAM
OFFENSE: DISCIPLINARY ACTION BY ANOTHER STATE OR AGENCY

NOTES: LICENSE SUSPENDED FOR REASONS BEARING ON PROFESSIONAL PERFORMANCE.

MILLER, JOHN JOSEPH MD, DATE OF BIRTH FEBRUARY 14, 1942, LICENSE NUMBER 0003980 OF 3459 HIDDEN LAKE DRIVE WEST, JACKSONVILLE, FL, WAS DISCIPLINED BY MONTANA ON MAY 19, 1995
DISCIPLINARY ACTION: PROBATION
OFFENSE: CRIMINAL CONVICTION OR PLEA OF GUILTY, NOLO CONTENDERE, OR NO CONTEST TO A CRIME

NOTES: CONVICTION OF FELONY; CHEMICAL DEPENDENCY. REVOCATION STAYED.

MILLER, JOHN JOSEPH MD, LICENSE NUMBER 0049431 OF JACKSONVILLE, FL, WAS DISCIPLINED BY VIRGINIA ON JUNE 13, 1995
DISCIPLINARY ACTION: LICENSE SUSPENSION
OFFENSE: DISCIPLINARY ACTION BY ANOTHER STATE OR AGENCY

NOTES: REVOCATION BY TENNESSEE AND SUSPENSION BY MONTANA AFTER HE ENGAGED IN THE EXCESSIVE USE OF ALCOHOL OR OTHER SUBSTANCES.

MILLER, JOHN JOSEPH MD, DATE OF BIRTH FEBRUARY 14, 1942, LICENSE NUMBER 0031991 OF 3459 HIDDEN LAKE DR W, JACKSONVILLE, FL, WAS DISCIPLINED BY GEORGIA ON AUGUST 3, 1995
DISCIPLINARY ACTION: LICENSE SUSPENSION
OFFENSE: CRIMINAL CONVICTION OR PLEA OF GUILTY, NOLO CONTENDERE, OR NO CONTEST TO A CRIME

NOTES: CONVICTION OF A CRIME. SUSPENDED INDEFINITELY.

MILLER, JOHN JOSEPH MD, DATE OF BIRTH FEBRUARY 14, 1942, LICENSE NUMBER 0009752 OF 3459 HIDDEN LAKE DRIVE WEST, JACKSONVILLE, FL, WAS DISCIPLINED BY WEST VIRGINIA ON NOVEMBER 20, 1995
DISCIPLINARY ACTION: LICENSE REVOCATION
OFFENSE: DISCIPLINARY ACTION BY ANOTHER STATE OR AGENCY

NOTES: FOUND GUILTY OF TWO FELONY COUNTS OF NEGLIGENT HOMICIDE IN 2/95 IN MONTANA; HIS EXCESSIVE USE OF ALCOHOL CAUSED HIM TO BE IMPAIRED AND TO CAUSE THE DEATHS OF TWO PERSONS IN A MOTOR VEHICLE ACCIDENT. IN 2/95 THE TENNESSEE BOARD REVOKED HIS LICENSE. IN 11/94 THE IDAHO BOARD SUSPENDED HIS LICENSE AND IN 5/95 REVOKED HIS LICENSE. IN 8/94 MONTANA SUSPENDED HIS LICENSE AND IN 4/95 REVOKED HIS LICENSE AND THEN STAYED THE REVOCATION AS PROBATION UNDER SEVERAL TERMS AND CONDITIONS.

MILLER, JOHN JOSEPH MD, DATE OF BIRTH FEBRUARY 14, 1942, LICENSE NUMBER 0030589, WAS DISCIPLINED BY COLORADO ON JANUARY 11, 1996
OFFENSE: CRIMINAL CONVICTION OR PLEA OF GUILTY, NOLO CONTENDERE, OR NO CONTEST TO A CRIME

NOTES: PLED GUILTY TO TWO FELONY CHARGES (NEGLIGENT HOMICIDE AS A RESULT OF A MOTOR VEHICLE ACCIDENT). ORDERED TO PERMANENTLY RELINQUISH HIS LICENSE TO PRACTICE MEDICINE IN COLORADO.

MILLER, JOHN JOSEPH MD, LICENSE NUMBER 0060453 OF DEER LODGE, MT, WAS DISCIPLINED BY OHIO ON FEBRUARY 14, 1996
DISCIPLINARY ACTION: LICENSE REVOCATION
OFFENSE: DISCIPLINARY ACTION BY ANOTHER STATE OR AGENCY

NOTES: PRIOR ACTION BY MONTANA MEDICAL BOARD WHICH WAS BASED ON HIS ADMISSIONS THAT HE HAD ENGAGED IN EXCESSIVE USE OF ALCOHOL SO THAT HE WAS MENTALLY AND PHYSICALLY IMPAIRED AND THAT WHILE HE WAS IMPAIRED, HE WAS INVOLVED IN A MOTOR VEHICLE ACCIDENT THAT CAUSED THE DEATH OF TWO PEOPLE. CONVICTION OF TWO FELONY COUNTS OF NEGLIGENT HOMICIDE. PERMANENT REVOCATION.

MINSKY, FRANCES MD, WAS DISCIPLINED BY NEVADA ON AUGUST 13, 1991
DISCIPLINARY ACTION: LICENSE REVOCATION; SURRENDER OF LICENSE
OFFENSE: DISCIPLINARY ACTION BY ANOTHER STATE OR AGENCY

NOTES: FAILED TO NOTIFY BOARD WITHIN 30 DAYS OF SUSPENSION OF LICENSE AND VOLUNTARY SURRENDER OF LICENSE IN ANOTHER STATE.

MINTON, GREGORY A MD, WAS DISCIPLINED BY NEVADA ON AUGUST 2, 1992
DISCIPLINARY ACTION: LICENSE REVOCATION
OFFENSE: SUBSTANDARD CARE, INCOMPETENCE OR NEGLIGENCE

NOTES: FOUND GUILTY OF 11 COUNTS OF INFLUENCING A PATIENT IN ORDER TO ENGAGE IN SEXUAL ACTIVITY WITH THE PATIENT; 9 COUNTS OF ENGAGING IN ANY CONDUCT WHICH IS INTENDED TO DECEIVE; 3 COUNTS OF GROSS MALPRACTICE.

MIRCHOU, RAFAEL MD, WAS DISCIPLINED BY NEVADA ON FEBRUARY 4, 1998
DISCIPLINARY ACTION: EMERGENCY SUSPENSION
OFFENSE: EXCEEDING PROFESSIONAL LIMITATIONS

NOTES: AIDING, ASSISTING, EMPLOYING OR ADVISING ANY UNLICENSED PERSON TO PRACTICE MEDICINE; PRACTICING OR OFFERING TO PRACTICE BEYOND THE SCOPE PERMITTED BY LAW OR PERFORMING SERVICES HE KNOWS OR HAS REASON TO KNOW HE IS NOT COMPETENT TO PERFORM.

MIRCHOU, RAFAEL MD, WAS DISCIPLINED BY NEVADA ON JUNE 15, 1998
DISCIPLINARY ACTION: PROBATION; REPRIMAND
OFFENSE: EXCEEDING PROFESSIONAL LIMITATIONS

NOTES: AIDING, ASSISTING, EMPLOYING OR ADVISING, DIRECTLY OR INDIRECTLY, ANY UNLICENSED PERSON TO ENGAGE IN THE PRACTICE OF MEDICINE; PRACTICING OR OFFERING TO PRACTICE BEYOND THE SCOPE PERMITTED BY LAW OR PERFORMING SERVICES WHICH HE KNOWS HE IS NOT COMPETENT TO PERFORM. REVOCATION STAYED. CONDITIONS OF PROBATION INCLUDE: MUST PAY $35,000 AS DISGORGEMENT OF INCOME WHICH MAY HAVE BEEN RECEIVED FROM PATIENTS WHO MAY HAVE BEEN SEEN BY PERSONS NOT LICENSED TO PRACTICE WHICH SHALL BE USED FOR FUTURE PUBLIC PROTECTION ENFORCEMENT AND PUBLIC AWARENESS EFFORTS. PLACED ON PROBATION FOR THE REMAINDER OF HIS TERM AS A RESIDENT PHYSICIAN; SHALL PAY $35,000 COSTS OF INVESTIGATION.

MOLDE, DONALD A MD, WAS DISCIPLINED BY NEVADA ON AUGUST 19, 1992
DISCIPLINARY ACTION: REPRIMAND
OFFENSE: SUBSTANDARD CARE, INCOMPETENCE OR NEGLIGENCE

NOTES: FOUND GUILTY OF 1 COUNT EACH OF ENGAGING IN CONDUCT WHICH THE BOARD HAS DETERMINED IS A VIOLATION OF THE STANDARDS OF PRACTICE ESTABLISHED BY REGULATION OF THE BOARD, ENGAGING IN THE PRACTICE OF WRITING PRESCRIPTIONS FOR CONTROLLED SUBSTANCES IN SUCH EXCESSIVE AMOUNTS AS TO CONSTITUTE A DEPARTURE FROM PREVAILING STANDARDS OF ACCEPTABLE MEDICAL PRACTICE, AND CONTINUAL FAILURE TO EXERCISE THE SKILL OR DILIGENCE OR USE THE METHODS ORDINARILY EXERCISED UNDER THE SAME CIRCUMSTANCES BY PHYSICIANS IN GOOD STANDING PRACTICING IN THE SAME SPECIALTY OR FIELD.

MOLDE, DONALD ALLEN MD, LICENSE NUMBER 0G17276 OF RENO, NV, WAS DISCIPLINED BY CALIFORNIA ON NOVEMBER 28, 1993
DISCIPLINARY ACTION: SURRENDER OF LICENSE

NOTES: VOLUNTARY SURRENDER OF LICENSE WHILE CHARGES PENDING.

MOLNAR, E MICHAEL MD, WAS DISCIPLINED BY NEVADA ON MARCH 15, 1991
DISCIPLINARY ACTION: REPRIMAND

NOTES: SECOND AMENDED ORDER; PUBLIC REPRIMAND AS PREVIOUSLY RENDERED, AND IF RETURNS TO NEVADA TO PRACTICE IS SUBJECT TO CONDITIONS TO RETURN TO ACTIVE LICENSURE STATUS.

MULLANNEY, PATRICK J MD, LICENSE NUMBER C26586 OF SAN DIEGO, CA, WAS DISCIPLINED BY CALIFORNIA ON NOVEMBER 1, 1997
DISCIPLINARY ACTION: SURRENDER OF LICENSE

NOTES: WHILE CHARGES PENDING.

MULLANNEY, PATRICK J MD, LICENSE NUMBER 26765 OF HENDERSON, NV, WAS DISCIPLINED BY OHIO ON MAY 3, 1999
DISCIPLINARY ACTION: SURRENDER OF LICENSE
OFFENSE: DISCIPLINARY ACTION BY ANOTHER STATE OR AGENCY

NOTES: PERMANENT SURRENDER OF MEDICAL LICENSE ACCEPTED BY THE BOARD IN LIEU OF FORMAL DISCIPLINARY PROCEEDINGS BASED ON HIS FAILING TO ADVISE THE OHIO BOARD ON LICENSE RENEWAL APPLICATION THAT ACTION HAD BEEN TAKEN AGAINST HIS CALIFORNIA LICENSE BY THAT STATE'S BOARD, AND THAT HE HAD SUBSEQUENTLY BEEN EXCLUDED FROM PARTICIPATION IN THE MEDICARE MEDICAID, AND ALL FEDERAL HEALTH PROGRAMS ON THE BASIS OF THE CALIFORNIA ACTION.

MULLANNEY, PATRICK JEROME MD OF 3405 KENYON #305, SAN DIEGO, CA, WAS DISCIPLINED BY DEA ON MARCH 23, 1998
DISCIPLINARY ACTION: SURRENDER OF CONTROLLED SUBSTANCE LICENSE

NOTES: IN LIEU OF PUBLIC INTEREST REVOCATION.

MURRAY, WILLIAM O MD OF VA, WAS DISCIPLINED BY NEVADA ON DECEMBER 4, 1999
DISCIPLINARY ACTION: LICENSE REVOCATION; FINE
OFFENSE: PROFESSIONAL MISCONDUCT

NOTES: FOUND GUILTY ON 59 DIFFERENT COUNTS, INCLUDING AIDING AND ASSISTING THE UNAUTHORIZED PRACTICE OF MEDICINE, IMPROPER DELEGATION OF MEDICAL CARE OF PATIENTS, IMPROPER FEE SPLITTING, FAILURE TO MAINTAIN MEDICAL RECORDS OF PATIENT, AND FAILURE TO DISCLOSE TO HIS PATIENTS FINANCIAL CONFLICTS OF INTEREST; FOUND GUILTY OF AIDING AND ASSISTING AN INDIVIDUAL WHO WAS NOT A PHYSICIAN IN PERFORMING CHELATION THERAPY, COLON THERAPY, LYMPHATIC DETOXIFICATION, OXYGENATION, AND MAGNETIC PULSE THERAPY. $5,000 FINE AND $19,637.10 IN COSTS; REPRIMAND.

MYERS, RONALD A MD, LICENSE NUMBER 0043456 OF PORT ANGELES, WA, WAS DISCIPLINED BY FLORIDA ON FEBRUARY 12, 1992
DISCIPLINARY ACTION: SURRENDER OF LICENSE

NOTES: AGREES NEVER AGAIN TO APPLY FOR LICENSURE AS A PHYSICIAN IN FLORIDA.

MYERS, RONALD A MD, LICENSE NUMBER 0019234, WAS DISCIPLINED BY ARIZONA ON OCTOBER 22, 1994
DISCIPLINARY ACTION: REQUIRED TO ENTER AN IMPAIRED PHYSICIAN PROGRAM OR SUBSTANCE ABUSE TREATMENT; MONITORING OF PHYSICIAN PERFORMANCE

NOTES: MUST IMMEDIATELY PARTICIPATE IN A BOARD-APPROVED MONITORED AFTERCARE TREATMENT PROGRAM, THE ONE SPONSORED BY ARIZONA BOARD IF HE IS IN ARIZONA OR, IF HE RESIDES IN ANOTHER STATE, A BOARD AFFILIATED PROGRAM IN THAT STATE; MUST PARTICIPATE IN A 12-STEP RECOVERY PROGRAM AND ATTEND AT LEAST THREE WEEKLY MEETINGS; SHALL OBTAIN A BOARD-APPROVED TREATING PHYSICIAN; SHALL ABSTAIN COMPLETELY FROM THE CONSUMPTION OF ALCOHOLIC BEVERAGES AND DRUGS EXCEPT WHEN PRESCRIBED BY HIS TREATING PHYSICIAN; MUST SUBMIT TO

WITNESSED RANDOM BIOLOGICAL FLUID COLLECTION; KEEP A LOG OF ANY AND ALL MEDICATIONS PRESCRIBED FOR HIM; SHALL SUBMIT TO ANY EXAMINATIONS OR THERAPY ORDERED BY BOARD; SHALL APPEAR BEFORE BOARD FOR INTERVIEWS UPON REQUEST; SHALL INFORM BOARD OF CHANGE OF ADDRESS OR IF AWAY FOR MORE THAN FIVE DAYS.

MYERS, RONALD A MD, WAS DISCIPLINED BY NEVADA ON MAY 5, 1995
DISCIPLINARY ACTION: SURRENDER OF LICENSE
OFFENSE: DISCIPLINARY ACTION BY ANOTHER STATE OR AGENCY

NOTES: CHARGED WITH DISCIPLINARY ACTION AGAINST HIS LICENSES IN FLORIDA AND CALIFORNIA; RENEWING AND ATTEMPTING TO RENEW A LICENSE BY FRAUD OR MISREPRESENTATION OR BY A FALSE, MISLEADING, INACCURATE OR INCOMPLETE STATEMENT; ENGAGING IN CONDUCT WHICH IS INTENDED TO DECEIVE; FAILING TO NOTIFY THE NEVADA BOARD OF THE DISCIPLINARY ACTIONS TAKEN AGAINST HIS LICENSE IN FLORIDA AND CALIFORNIA. VOLUNTARY SURRENDER OF LICENSE WHILE HE IS UNDER INVESTIGATION.

MYERS, RONALD A MD, LICENSE NUMBER 0019234, WAS DISCIPLINED BY ARIZONA ON AUGUST 5, 1996
DISCIPLINARY ACTION: REPRIMAND
OFFENSE: DISCIPLINARY ACTION BY ANOTHER STATE OR AGENCY

NOTES: IN 12/91, HE VOLUNTARILY RELINQUISHED HIS FLORIDA LICENSE AND AGREED NEVER AGAIN TO APPLY FOR LICENSURE IN FLORIDA IN ORDER TO AVOID ADMINISTRATIVE PROSECUTION FOR FAILING TO MAINTAIN AND SUBMIT DOCUMENTATION VERIFYING THE REQUIRED HOURS OF CONTINUING MEDICAL EDUCATION CREDITS FROM 1/1/88 THROUGH 12/31/89; HE RENEWED HIS FLORIDA LICENSE BY FRAUDULENT MISREPRESENTATION BY CERTIFYING HE HAD COMPLETED THESE CONTINUING MEDICAL EDUCATION REQUIREMENTS.

NOVAK, FREDDIE PATRICK DOUGLAS MD, LICENSE NUMBER 0015427 OF PORTLAND, OR, WAS DISCIPLINED BY OREGON ON AUGUST 23, 1991
DISCIPLINARY ACTION: EMERGENCY SUSPENSION

NOTES: NO LONGER SUSPENDED AS OF 1/28/92.

NOVAK, FREDDIE PATRICK MD, LICENSE NUMBER 0028055 OF 1848 N WINCHELL ST, PORTLAND, OR, WAS DISCIPLINED BY GEORGIA ON JULY 1, 1992
DISCIPLINARY ACTION: NONRENEWAL OF LICENSE
OFFENSE: DISCIPLINARY ACTION BY ANOTHER STATE OR AGENCY

NOTES: LICENSE SUSPENDED IN OREGON 1/9/92. REVOKED FOR NONRENEWAL.

NOVAK, FREDDIE PATRICK MD, LICENSE NUMBER 0025150 OF OR, WAS DISCIPLINED BY WASHINGTON ON DECEMBER 17, 1992
DISCIPLINARY ACTION: EMERGENCY SUSPENSION
OFFENSE: DISCIPLINARY ACTION BY ANOTHER STATE OR AGENCY

NOTES: SUSPENSION/REVOCATION AND OR RESTRICTION OF HIS LICENSE TO PRACTICE IN ANOTHER JURISDICTION AND BEING UNABLE TO PRACTICE WITH REASONABLE SKILL AND SAFETY.

NOVAK, FREDDIE PATRICK MD, LICENSE NUMBER 0025150, WAS DISCIPLINED BY WASHINGTON ON MARCH 19, 1993
DISCIPLINARY ACTION: PROBATION; FINE
OFFENSE: DISCIPLINARY ACTION BY ANOTHER STATE OR AGENCY

NOTES: ON 8/23/91 OREGON LICENSE SUSPENDED BASED ON EXCESSIVE USE OF CONTROLLED SUBSTANCES; URINE SAMPLE TESTED POSITIVE FOR COCAINE ON 11/29/91; SURRENDERED OREGON LICENSE IN LIEU OF FURTHER PROCEEDINGS IN 1/92. PROBATION SUBJECT TO TERMS AND CONDITIONS AS FOLLOWS: SHALL NOT PRACTICE MEDICINE IN WASHINGTON UNTIL HE UNDERGOES A PSYCHOLOGICAL AND PHYSICAL EXAMINATION; SHALL APPEAR BEFORE THE BOARD AND BE REQUIRED TO PRESENT EVIDENCE OF HIS RECOVERY FROM HIS ADDICTION TO DRUGS AND ALCOHOL, INCLUDING THE RESULTS OF THE PSYCHOLOGICAL AND PHYSICAL EXAMINATION; SHALL INFORM THE BOARD IN WRITING OF CHANGES IN PRACTICE AND/OR RESIDENCE ADDRESS; SHALL PAY A $250 FINE. ON 3/23/95 HIS REQUEST FOR MODIFICATION OF THIS ORDER WAS DENIED.

NOVAK, FREDDIE PATRICK MD, WAS DISCIPLINED BY NEVADA ON JUNE 30, 1993
DISCIPLINARY ACTION: LICENSE REVOCATION
OFFENSE: DISCIPLINARY ACTION BY ANOTHER STATE OR AGENCY

NOTES: ON 03/05/93 CHARGED WITH FAILING TO REPORT WITHIN 30 DAYS, AND CONTINUAL FAILURE TO REPORT TO THE BOARD, THE SUSPENSION AND SURRENDER OF HIS OREGON LICENSE TO PRACTICE MEDICINE.

NOVAK, FREDDIE PATRICK MD, LICENSE NUMBER 0G61059 OF PORTLAND, OR, WAS DISCIPLINED BY CALIFORNIA ON MAY 26, 1994
DISCIPLINARY ACTION: 60-MONTH PROBATION
OFFENSE: DISCIPLINARY ACTION BY ANOTHER STATE OR AGENCY

NOTES: DISCIPLINE BY OREGON BOARD FOR IMPAIRMENT DUE TO EXCESSIVE USE OF CONTROLLED DRUGS. REVOCATION STAYED.

NOVAK, FREDDIE PATRICK DOUGLAS MD, LICENSE NUMBER 0015427 OF PORTLAND, OR, WAS DISCIPLINED BY OREGON ON MAY 17, 1995
DISCIPLINARY ACTION: 120-MONTH PROBATION; RESTRICTION PLACED ON CONTROLLED SUBSTANCE LICENSE

NOTES: CANNOT PRESCRIBE SCHEDULE II CONTROLLED SUBSTANCES; MUST PROVIDE TRIPLICATE COPIES OF SCHEDULE III AND IV CONTROLLED SUBSTANCES PRESCRIPTIONS UNDER SUPERVISION OF HOSPITAL IN WHICH HE HAS PRIVILEGES.

NOVAK, FREDDIE PATRICK DOUGLAS MD, LICENSE NUMBER 0015427 OF PORTLAND, OR, WAS DISCIPLINED BY OREGON ON FEBRUARY 1, 1996
DISCIPLINARY ACTION: EMERGENCY SUSPENSION

NOVAK, FREDDIE PATRICK DOUGLAS MD, LICENSE NUMBER 15427 OF PORTLAND, OR, WAS DISCIPLINED BY OREGON ON JANUARY 24, 1997
DISCIPLINARY ACTION: LICENSE REVOCATION

NOVAK, FREDDIE PATRICK MD, LICENSE NUMBER 25150 OF PORTLAND, OR, WAS DISCIPLINED BY WASHINGTON ON MARCH 18, 1998
DISCIPLINARY ACTION: LICENSE REVOCATION
OFFENSE: PROFESSIONAL MISCONDUCT

NOVAK, FREDDIE PATRICK MD, DATE OF BIRTH OCTOBER 7, 1958 OF 1848 N WINCHELL STREET, PORTLAND, OR, WAS DISCIPLINED

BY MEDICARE ON OCTOBER 20, 1998
DISCIPLINARY ACTION: EXCLUSION FROM THE MEDICARE AND/OR MEDICAID PROGRAM
OFFENSE: DISCIPLINARY ACTION BY ANOTHER STATE OR AGENCY

NOTES: LICENSE REVOKED, SUSPENDED, SURRENDERED OR OTHERWISE LOST FOR REASONS BEARING ON PROFESSIONAL PERFORMANCE, PROFESSIONAL COMPETENCE OR FINANCIAL INTEGRITY.

NOVAK, FREDDIE PATRICK MD, LICENSE NUMBER FE61059 OF PORTLAND, OR, WAS DISCIPLINED BY CALIFORNIA ON JANUARY 27, 1999
DISCIPLINARY ACTION: SURRENDER OF LICENSE

NOTES: WHILE CHARGES PENDING.

NOVAK, FREDDIE PATRICK MD, DATE OF BIRTH OCTOBER 7, 1958 OF 1848 N WINCHELL STREET, PORTLAND, OR, WAS DISCIPLINED BY MEDICARE ON AUGUST 19, 1999
DISCIPLINARY ACTION: EXCLUSION FROM THE MEDICARE AND/OR MEDICAID PROGRAM
OFFENSE: CRIMINAL CONVICTION OR PLEA OF GUILTY, NOLO CONTENDERE, OR NO CONTEST TO A CRIME

NOTES: CONVICTED OF A FELONY INVOLVING CONTROLLED SUBSTANCES.

OKSENHOLT, LORRIE M DO, DATE OF BIRTH MAY 28, 1957 OF 75 PRINGLE, #301, RENO, NV, WAS DISCIPLINED BY MEDICARE ON APRIL 9, 1996
DISCIPLINARY ACTION: EXCLUSION FROM THE MEDICARE AND/OR MEDICAID PROGRAM
OFFENSE: NONCOMPLIANCE WITH A PROFESSIONAL RULE

NOTES: DEFAULTED ON PUBLIC HEALTH SERVICE EDUCATION LOAN. REINSTATED ON 4/24/96.

ONG, TENG C MD, WAS DISCIPLINED BY NEVADA ON MARCH 15, 1996
DISCIPLINARY ACTION: 48-MONTH PROBATION; 6-MONTH RESTRICTION PLACED ON CONTROLLED SUBSTANCE LICENSE
OFFENSE: OVERPRESCRIBING OR MISPRESCRIBING DRUGS

NOTES: CHARGED WITH REPEATED AND GROSS MALPRACTICE; WRITING PRESCRIPTIONS FOR CONTROLLED SUBSTANCES IN SUCH EXCESSIVE AMOUNTS AS TO CONSTITUTE A DEPARTURE FROM PREVAILING STANDARDS OF ACCEPTABLE PRACTICE. SUSPENSION STAYED. CONDITIONS OF PROBATION: SHALL NOT PRESCRIBE SCHEDULE II AND III CONTROLLED SUBSTANCES FOR A PERIOD OF 6 MONTHS; SHALL COMPLETE 60 HOURS OF CONTINUING MEDICAL EDUCATION IN PAIN MANAGEMENT AND 20 HOURS IN A COURSE DEALING WITH PRESCRIBING OF NARCOTIC MEDICATION AS DIRECTED BY BOARD; ON 5/1/96 DENIED 4/17/96 RECONSIDERATION MOTION. ON 7/9/97 THE BOARD SETTLED HIS NEVADA SUPREME COURT APPEAL OF THE DISTRICT COURT'S DECISION AFFIRMING THIS ORDER BY ORDERING THAT HIS LICENSE SHALL REMAIN SUSPENDED BUT THE SUSPENSION WILL BE STAYED AND THE PROBATION IS REDUCED FROM 4 TO 2 YEARS, COMMENCING ON 3/15/96. WHILE ON PROBATION, THE FOLLOWING CONDITIONS WILL APPLY: SHALL COMPLETE 30 HOURS OF CONTINUING MEDICAL EDUCATION IN PAIN MANAGEMENT AND 10 HOURS DEALING WITH PRESCRIBING OF NARCOTIC MEDICATION; HIS PROBATION SHALL NOT TERMINATE UNTIL SUCCESSFUL COMPLETION OF THE ADDED CONTINUING MEDICAL EDUCATION; HE SHALL REIMBURSE THE BOARD $5,000 FOR ITS EXPENSES.

PANICARI, MICHAEL R MD, WAS DISCIPLINED BY NEVADA ON JANUARY 22, 1999
DISCIPLINARY ACTION: FINE; REPRIMAND
OFFENSE: PROFESSIONAL MISCONDUCT

NOTES: FAILURE TO MAINTAIN MEDICAL RECORDS RELATING TO THE DIAGNOSIS, TREATMENT AND CARE OF A PATIENT; ENGAGING IN ANY CONDUCT WHICH IS INTENDED TO DECEIVE. MUST PERFORM 20 HOURS OF COMMUNITY SERVICE WITHIN THREE MONTHS; PAY $2,281.36 FOR ADMINISTRATIVE EXPENSES INCURRED; MUST PAY $1,000 FINE; MUST COMPLETE 20 HOURS OF CONTINUING MEDICAL EDUCATION IN MEDICAL RECORD KEEPING WITHIN SIX MONTHS.

PASTO, GEORGE N MD, WAS DISCIPLINED BY NEVADA ON DECEMBER 9, 1996
DISCIPLINARY ACTION: LICENSE REVOCATION
OFFENSE: DISCIPLINARY ACTION BY ANOTHER STATE OR AGENCY

NOTES: ARIZONA LICENSE SURRENDERED WHILE UNDER INVESTIGATION.

PASTO, GEORGE NICHOLAS MD, LICENSE NUMBER 06388 OF PORTLAND, OR, WAS DISCIPLINED BY OREGON ON MAY 4, 1998
DISCIPLINARY ACTION: LICENSE REVOCATION

PIMENTEL, HENRY T MD, DATE OF BIRTH FEBRUARY 3, 1937 OF CHICAGO, IL, WAS DISCIPLINED BY ILLINOIS ON APRIL 1, 1991
DISCIPLINARY ACTION: LICENSE SUSPENSION
OFFENSE: CRIMINAL CONVICTION OR PLEA OF GUILTY, NOLO CONTENDERE, OR NO CONTEST TO A CRIME

NOTES: PERFORMED SEVERAL OPERATIONS IN WHICH HE SIGNED ANOTHER DOCTOR'S NAME TO THE PUBLIC AID FORMS BECAUSE AT THE TIME HE WAS INELIGIBLE TO PARTICIPATE IN THE MEDICAL ASSISTANCE PROGRAM. ADDITIONALLY, FOR APPROXIMATELY SEVEN YEARS, HE WAS PRESCRIBING CONTROLLED SUBSTANCES WHILE HIS LICENSE WAS NONRENEWED. ALSO PLEADED GUILTY ON 05/11/90 TO VENDOR FRAUD IN THE CIRCUIT COURT OF COOK COUNTY. INDEFINITE SUSPENSION.

PIMENTEL, HENRY T MD, DATE OF BIRTH FEBRUARY 3, 1937 OF 6540 CHAUCER RD, WILLOWBROOK, IL, WAS DISCIPLINED BY MEDICARE ON JUNE 7, 1991
DISCIPLINARY ACTION: 84-MONTH EXCLUSION FROM THE MEDICARE AND/OR MEDICAID PROGRAM
OFFENSE: CRIMINAL CONVICTION OR PLEA OF GUILTY, NOLO CONTENDERE, OR NO CONTEST TO A CRIME

NOTES: PROGRAM-RELATED CONVICTION. REINSTATED ON 7/1/98.

PIMENTEL, HENRY T MD, DATE OF BIRTH FEBRUARY 3, 1937, LICENSE NUMBER 0055746 OF 1213 CEDAR AVENUE, IRON MOUNTAIN, MI, WAS DISCIPLINED BY MICHIGAN ON DECEMBER 6, 1993
DISCIPLINARY ACTION: 6-MONTH LICENSE SUSPENSION; 12-MONTH PROBATION
OFFENSE: CRIMINAL CONVICTION OR PLEA OF GUILTY, NOLO CONTENDERE, OR NO CONTEST TO A CRIME

NOTES: CONVICTION/INSURANCE FRAUD. $2,000 FINE.

PIMENTEL, HENRY T MD, DATE OF BIRTH FEBRUARY 3, 1937, WAS DISCIPLINED BY NEVADA ON JULY 8, 1994
DISCIPLINARY ACTION: LICENSE REVOCATION
OFFENSE: DISCIPLINARY ACTION BY ANOTHER STATE OR AGENCY

NOTES: ON 04/09/94 CHARGED WITH THE SUSPENSION, MODIFICATION AND LIMITATION OF HIS LICENSES TO

PRACTICE MEDICINE IN ILLINOIS AND MICHIGAN; CONVICTION OF VENDOR FRAUD FELONY INVOLVING THE PRACTICE OF MEDICINE IN ILLINOIS AND FAILURE TO NOTIFY THE NEVADA BOARD OF THE ACTIONS TAKEN AGAINST HIM IN ILLINOIS AND MICHIGAN.

PIMENTEL, HENRY T MD, DATE OF BIRTH FEBRUARY 3, 1937, LICENSE NUMBER 1038018 OF 1213 CEDAR AVENUE, IRON MOUNTAIN, MI, WAS DISCIPLINED BY INDIANA ON FEBRUARY 29, 1996
DISCIPLINARY ACTION: PROBATION; FINE
OFFENSE: DISCIPLINARY ACTION BY ANOTHER STATE OR AGENCY

NOTES: ON 5/11/90 CONVICTED OF VENDOR FRAUD IN ILLINOIS; ON 3/20/91 SIGNED A CONSENT ORDER WITH THE ILLINOIS BOARD; AND ON 3/04/94 THEY REINSTATED HIS MEDICAL LICENSE AND PLACED HIM ON PROBATION. ON 6/29/94 NEVADA REVOKED HIS LICENSE BASED ON THE ILLINOIS ORDER. ON 11/05/93 MICHIGAN PLACED HIS LICENSE ON A SIX MONTH SUSPENSION FOLLOWED BY PROBATION BASED ON THE ILLINOIS ORDER AND THAT HE WAS PRESCRIBING CONTROLLED SUBSTANCES WITHOUT A LICENSE. INDEFINITE PROBATION IN INDIANA UNDER TERMS AND CONDITIONS: MAY NOT PETITION FOR WITHDRAWAL FOR ONE YEAR; AND SHALL COMPLETE 50 HOURS OF CONTINUING MEDICAL EDUCATION EACH YEAR AND SHALL SUBMIT PROOF OF COMPLETION TO THE BOARD. $500 FINE. $50.00 ASSESSED COSTS.

POPE, FREDERICK E MD, DATE OF BIRTH NOVEMBER 19, 1928, LICENSE NUMBER 0028458 OF THE LAKES, NV, WAS DISCIPLINED BY KENTUCKY ON DECEMBER 1, 1992
DISCIPLINARY ACTION: FINE
OFFENSE: NONCOMPLIANCE WITH A PROFESSIONAL RULE

NOTES: FAILED TO COMPLETE REQUIRED CONTINUING MEDICAL EDUCATION IN THE AREA OF HIV/AIDS.

POPE, FREDERICK E MD, DATE OF BIRTH NOVEMBER 19, 1928, LICENSE NUMBER 1039832 OF 9501 W SAHARA, LAS VEGAS, NV, WAS DISCIPLINED BY INDIANA ON JUNE 29, 1995
DISCIPLINARY ACTION: LICENSE REVOCATION; FINE
OFFENSE: DISCIPLINARY ACTION BY ANOTHER STATE OR AGENCY

NOTES: ON 10/6/92, HIS KENTUCKY MEDICAL LICENSE WAS SUSPENDED AND HE WAS FINED FOR FAILURE TO COMPLETE REQUIRED AIDS EDUCATION COURSEWORK ON TIME; COURSEWORK COMPLETED ON 11/10/92; IN INDIANA RENEWAL APPLICATION OF 6/4/93, HE FAILED TO INFORM THE BOARD OF KENTUCKY DISCIPLINE. DEFAULT DECISION. $1,000 FINE; ASSESSED COSTS OF $327.29.

POPE, FREDERICK E MD, DATE OF BIRTH NOVEMBER 19, 1928, WAS DISCIPLINED BY NEVADA ON NOVEMBER 3, 1995
DISCIPLINARY ACTION: REPRIMAND
OFFENSE: DISCIPLINARY ACTION BY ANOTHER STATE OR AGENCY

NOTES: IN 10/92 KENTUCKY LICENSE WAS SUSPENDED FOR FAILING TO COMPLETE REQUIRED COURSEWORK; DID NOT NOTIFY NEVADA OF THIS ACTION; IN 8/95 INDIANA LICENSE WAS REVOKED WHICH HE ALSO FAILED TO INFORM NEVADA; LIED ABOUT THESE ACTIONS ON NEVADA REGISTRATION APPLICATION. SUSPENSION OF LICENSE; $300 ADMINISTRATIVE AND INVESTIGATIVE COSTS.

POPE, FREDERICK E MD, LICENSE NUMBER 0C37319 OF LAS VEGAS, NV, WAS DISCIPLINED BY CALIFORNIA ON FEBRUARY 22, 1996
DISCIPLINARY ACTION: REPRIMAND
OFFENSE: DISCIPLINARY ACTION BY ANOTHER STATE OR AGENCY

NOTES: ACTION IN INDIANA FOR FAILING TO DISCLOSE DISCIPLINE BY KENTUCKY FOR FAILURE TO COMPLETE AN AIDS COURSE IN A TIMELY MANNER.

POPE, FREDERICK E MD, LICENSE NUMBER 0001653 OF 9501 WEST SAHARA #2032, THE LAKES, NV, WAS DISCIPLINED BY HAWAII ON OCTOBER 30, 1996
DISCIPLINARY ACTION: FINE
OFFENSE: DISCIPLINARY ACTION BY ANOTHER STATE OR AGENCY

NOTES: ACTION IN KENTUCKY AND INDIANA. FAILED TO TIMELY NOTIFY THE HAWAII BOARD. $500.00 FINE.

RASMUSSEN, THOMAS W MD, WAS DISCIPLINED BY NEVADA ON MARCH 4, 1995
DISCIPLINARY ACTION: DENIAL OF NEW LICENSE
OFFENSE: DISCIPLINARY ACTION BY ANOTHER STATE OR AGENCY

NOTES: CALIFORNIA REVOKED HIS LICENSE.

RIDENOUR, GARY C MD, WAS DISCIPLINED BY NEVADA ON JUNE 10, 1994
DISCIPLINARY ACTION: 60-MONTH PROBATION; FINE
OFFENSE: CRIMINAL CONVICTION OR PLEA OF GUILTY, NOLO CONTENDERE, OR NO CONTEST TO A CRIME

NOTES: ON 04/25/94 CHARGED WITH CONVICTION OF A FELONY RELATING TO THE PRACTICE OF MEDICINE; ENGAGING IN ANY CONDUCT INTENDED TO DECEIVE THE BOARD; PRESCRIBING CONTROLLED SUBSTANCES TO OTHERS EXCEPT AS AUTHORIZED BY LAW; WRITING A PRESCRIPTION FOR CONTROLLED SUBSTANCES FOR ANY PERSON WITHOUT AN APPROPRIATE EXAMINATION WHICH CONFIRMS THE MEDICAL NECESSITY FOR THE CONTROLLED SUBSTANCES; FAILURE TO MAINTAIN MEDICAL RECORDS RELATING TO THE DIAGNOSIS, TREATMENT AND CARE OF A PATIENT. REVOCATION STAYED. TERMS AND CONDITIONS OF PROBATION AS FOLLOWS: MUST COMPLETE THE "APPROPRIATE PRESCRIBING WORKSHOP" CONDUCTED IN PORTLAND, OREGON; MUST COMPLETE A COURSE IN MEDICAL ETHICS TO BE APPROVED IN ADVANCE BY THE BOARD; MUST PERFORM 40 HOURS OF PUBLIC SERVICE, WITHOUT COMPENSATION IN THE AREA OF DRUG ABUSE PREVENTION OR DRUG EDUCATION TO BE APPROVED BY THE BOARD; MAY NOT POSSESS, DISPENSE OR PRESCRIBE SCHEDULES I THROUGH III CONTROLLED SUBSTANCES; MAY PRESCRIBE, DISPENSE OR POSSESS FOR PURPOSES OF DISPENSING TO PATIENTS, SCHEDULES IV AND V CONTROLLED SUBSTANCES AND PROVIDE THE BOARD WITH A LOG OF ALL OF THESE SUBSTANCES PRESCRIBED OR DISPENSED TO PATIENTS DURING THE PREVIOUS MONTH; MUST COMPLETE TERMS OF THE PROBATION IMPOSED UPON HIM BY COURT; MAY NOT PERSONALLY TAKE ANY SCHEDULES I THROUGH V CONTROLLED SUBSTANCES WITHOUT A WRITTEN PRESCRIPTION FROM A PHYSICIAN OR DENTIST RENDERING MEDICAL OR DENTAL CARE TO HIM; RANDOM URINE AND/OR BLOOD DRUG TESTING; MUST PAY $3,000 FOR REIMBURSEMENT OF INVESTIGATION COSTS; FINED $1,000; MUST RECEIVE A PUBLIC WRITTEN REPRIMAND TO BE PUBLISHED IN BOARD NEWSLETTER AND NEWSPAPER IN FALLON, NEVADA.

RIDENOUR, GARY C MD OF 625 WEST WILLIAMS, FALLON, NV, WAS DISCIPLINED BY DEA ON SEPTEMBER 27, 1994
DISCIPLINARY ACTION: RESTRICTION PLACED ON CONTROLLED SUBSTANCE LICENSE

OFFENSE: DISCIPLINARY ACTION BY ANOTHER STATE OR AGENCY

NOTES: STATE BOARD.

RIDENOUR, GARY C MD OF 1035 SOUTH TAYLOR, FALLON, NV, WAS DISCIPLINED BY DEA ON OCTOBER 20, 1995
DISCIPLINARY ACTION: RESTRICTION PLACED ON CONTROLLED SUBSTANCE LICENSE

NOTES: MEMO OF UNDERSTANDING.

ROBERTS, DONALD L MD, WAS DISCIPLINED BY NEVADA ON AUGUST 22, 1998
DISCIPLINARY ACTION: REPRIMAND; COMMUNITY SERVICE
OFFENSE: DISCIPLINARY ACTION BY ANOTHER STATE OR AGENCY

NOTES: SURRENDERED LICENSE IN CALIFORNIA. MUST PERFORM 10 HOURS OF COMMUNITY SERVICE AND PAY $500 FOR ALL INVESTIGATORY EXPENSES.

ROBERTS, DONALD LEE MD, LICENSE NUMBER G81739 OF SAN DIEGO, CA, WAS DISCIPLINED BY CALIFORNIA ON JULY 31, 1997
DISCIPLINARY ACTION: SURRENDER OF LICENSE

NOTES: WHILE CHARGES PENDING.

ROBERTS, DONALD LEE MD, DATE OF BIRTH MAY 10, 1961 OF 2040 W CHARLESTON #200, LAS VEGAS, NV, WAS DISCIPLINED BY MEDICARE ON JULY 20, 1999
DISCIPLINARY ACTION: EXCLUSION FROM THE MEDICARE AND/OR MEDICAID PROGRAM
OFFENSE: DISCIPLINARY ACTION BY ANOTHER STATE OR AGENCY

NOTES: LICENSE REVOKED, SUSPENDED, SURRENDERED OR OTHERWISE LOST FOR REASONS BEARING ON PROFESSIONAL PERFORMANCE, PROFESSIONAL COMPETENCE OR FINANCIAL INTEGRITY.

ROBERTSON, MACARTHUR M MD, WAS DISCIPLINED BY NEVADA ON DECEMBER 6, 1997
DISCIPLINARY ACTION: REPRIMAND
OFFENSE: DISCIPLINARY ACTION BY ANOTHER STATE OR AGENCY

NOTES: SURRENDERED HIS LICENSE IN CALIFORNIA WHILE UNDER INVESTIGATION. MUST PAY $1,440 IN INVESTIGATORY COSTS; MUST PASS A COMPETENCY EXAMINATION IN THE FIELD OF PRACTICE IN WHICH HE IS CURRENTLY ENGAGED.

ROBERTSON, MACARTHUR MICHAEL MD, LICENSE NUMBER G34725 OF LOS ANGELES, CA, WAS DISCIPLINED BY CALIFORNIA ON APRIL 4, 1997
DISCIPLINARY ACTION: SURRENDER OF LICENSE

NOTES: WHILE CHARGES PENDING.

ROCK, HERMAN H MD, LICENSE NUMBER G005460 OF CITRUS HEIGHTS, CA, WAS DISCIPLINED BY CALIFORNIA ON JULY 5, 1990
DISCIPLINARY ACTION: LICENSE REVOCATION
OFFENSE: DISCIPLINARY ACTION BY ANOTHER STATE OR AGENCY

NOTES: DISCIPLINARY ACTIONS BY NEVADA BOARD AND NEW MEXICO BOARD.

ROCK, HERMAN H MD, LICENSE NUMBER 0014843 OF RENO, NV, WAS DISCIPLINED BY WASHINGTON ON OCTOBER 18, 1991

NOTES: PERMANENTLY RETIRES FROM MEDICAL PRACTICE; STATEMENT OF CHARGES ISSUED AS RESULT OF BOARD INVESTIGATION WITHDRAWN. EFFECTIVE DATE OF RETIREMENT IS 10/28/91 OR UPON SERVICE TO THE PHYSICIAN, WHICHEVER IS SOONER.

ROLLER, FRANKLIN D MD OF 207 GOLDFIELD AVENUE, YERINGTON, NV, WAS DISCIPLINED BY DEA ON JANUARY 3, 1996
DISCIPLINARY ACTION: SURRENDER OF CONTROLLED SUBSTANCE LICENSE
OFFENSE: DISCIPLINARY ACTION BY ANOTHER STATE OR AGENCY

NOTES: STATE BOARD.

ROLLER, FRANKLIN DELANO MD, WAS DISCIPLINED BY WASHINGTON ON DECEMBER 14, 1990
DISCIPLINARY ACTION: PROBATION; MONITORING OF PHYSICIAN PERFORMANCE
OFFENSE: DISCIPLINARY ACTION BY ANOTHER STATE OR AGENCY

NOTES: NEVADA BOARD STAYED A REVOCATION AND PLACED HIS LICENSE ON PROBATION 4/3/87; CALIFORNIA BOARD STAYED A REVOCATION AND PLACED LICENSE ON PROBATION 6/8/87, AND THEN REVOKED LICENSE 12/12/88. WASHINGTON REVOCATION STAYED WITH THE FOLLOWING CONDITIONS OF PROBATION: SHALL COMPLY WITH ALL CONDITIONS OF NEVADA ORDER, AND WASHINGTON BOARD SHALL HAVE THE RIGHT TO MONITOR PRACTICE AS SET FORTH IN THE NEVADA ORDER; SHALL ALLOW BOARD TO OBTAIN INVESTIGATORY FILES FROM NEVADA; MAY PETITION FOR CHANGE IN TERMS OF ORDER ONLY AFTER NEVADA REINSTATES HIS LICENSE; SHALL INFORM BOARD IF HE MOVES OR LEAVES THE STATE.

ROSEN, BARUCH D MD, WAS DISCIPLINED BY NEVADA ON AUGUST 24, 1994
DISCIPLINARY ACTION: LICENSE REVOCATION
OFFENSE: DISCIPLINARY ACTION BY ANOTHER STATE OR AGENCY

NOTES: ACTION TAKEN BY THE ARIZONA MEDICAL BOARD AGAINST HIS ARIZONA MEDICAL LICENSE; FAILURE TO REPORT TO NEVADA BOARD WITHIN 30 DAYS OF THE ACTIONS TAKEN AGAINST HIS ARIZONA LICENSE.

ROSEN, BARUCH D MD OF 7555 EAST OSBORN #206, SCOTTSDALE, AZ, WAS DISCIPLINED BY DEA ON APRIL 20, 1995
DISCIPLINARY ACTION: RESTRICTION PLACED ON CONTROLLED SUBSTANCE LICENSE
OFFENSE: PROFESSIONAL MISCONDUCT

NOTES: PRIOR ALLEGED CONTROLLED SUBSTANCE VIOLATIONS.

ROSEN, BARUCH D MD, DATE OF BIRTH JULY 27, 1941 OF 5407 E ELMWOOD STREET, MESA, AZ, WAS DISCIPLINED BY MEDICARE ON DECEMBER 20, 1998
DISCIPLINARY ACTION: EXCLUSION FROM THE MEDICARE AND/OR MEDICAID PROGRAM
OFFENSE: DISCIPLINARY ACTION BY ANOTHER STATE OR AGENCY

NOTES: LICENSE REVOKED, SUSPENDED, SURRENDERED OR OTHERWISE LOST FOR REASONS BEARING ON PROFESSIONAL PERFORMANCE, PROFESSIONAL COMPETENCE OR FINANCIAL INTEGRITY.

ROSEN, BARUCH DANIEL MD, LICENSE NUMBER 0010880 OF 7555 EAST OSBORN RD #206, SCOTTSDALE, AZ, WAS DISCIPLINED BY ARIZONA ON APRIL 8, 1992
DISCIPLINARY ACTION: LICENSE REVOCATION
OFFENSE: PROVIDING FALSE INFORMATION TO THE BOARD OR OTHER HEALTH AGENCY

NOTES: HAD AT HIS PRACTICE A PHYSICIAN WHO WAS UNLICENSED IN ARIZONA, THEN FALSELY INFORMED THE BOARD THAT THIS DOCTOR WAS NOT PERFORMING PROCEDURES; MAINTAINED INADEQUATE AND/OR FALSE MEDICAL RECORDS SOME OF WHICH STATED HE HAD PERFORMED SURGERY WHICH HE HAD NOT PERFORMED; BILLED

PATIENT AND/OR HER INSURANCE CARRIER FOR A PROCEDURE ADVERTISED AS FREE; STATED ON 1988 LICENSE RENEWAL FORM AND IN 1990 BOARD INTERVIEW THAT HE WAS BOARD CERTIFIED WHEN IN FACT HIS CERTIFICATION EXPIRED 12/31/86; MADE FALSE CLAIMS ON HIS BUSINESS CARDS; ADMINISTERED CONTROLLED SUBSTANCES IN 1989 AFTER HAVING SURRENDERED IN MAY 1986 HIS DEA CONTROLLED SUBSTANCES REGISTRATION CERTIFICATE FOR SCHEDULES II AND IIN; THEN LIED TO BOARD ABOUT HIS ACTIONS; PERFORMED GROSSLY NEGLIGENT AND SUBSTANDARD COSMETIC SURGERIES WITHOUT PROPER CONSULTATION WITH PATIENTS. PERMANENT REVOCATION, NO OPPORTUNITY FOR REHEARING OR REVIEW. HE APPEALED THIS PERMANENT REVOCATION BY THE ARIZONA BOARD TO THE SUPERIOR COURT AND THE COURT GRANTED A PARTIAL STAY PENDING APPEAL. ON 5/6/93, SUPERIOR COURT AFFIRMED THE BOARD'S ORDER AND SUBSEQUENTLY GRANTED HIS REQUEST FOR STAY OF THE PERMANENT REVOCATION PENDING FURTHER APPEAL. THE STAY LIMITS HIM TO "PRACTICING TRADITIONAL FAMILY MEDICINE" ONLY. ON 1/24/94, THE BOARD REJECTED A SETTLEMENT PROPOSAL PRESENTED BY DR. ROSEN.

ROSEN, BARUCH DANIEL MD, LICENSE NUMBER 0010880, WAS DISCIPLINED BY ARIZONA ON FEBRUARY 23, 1994
DISCIPLINARY ACTION: 12-MONTH LICENSE SUSPENSION; 60-MONTH PROBATION
OFFENSE: PRACTICING WITHOUT A VALID CONTROLLED SUBSTANCE LICENSE

NOTES: DID NOT RECOMMEND OR SUGGEST THAT ONE OF HIS PATIENTS GO TO A HOSPITAL FOR EVALUATION OR TREATMENT FOR SYMPTOMS FOLLOWING A 7 FOOT FALL; PATIENT WENT INTO CARDIAC ARREST AND WAS TRANSPORTED TO A HOSPITAL EMERGENCY ROOM PRIOR TO DEATH; HAD NO RECORDS FOR THIS PATIENT; VIOLATED 10/15/93 ORDER BY REFUSING THE BOARD ACCESS TO HIS MEDICAL RECORDS FOR AN OFFICE PRACTICE SURVEY; PRESCRIBED SCHEDULE II SUBSTANCES TWICE IN 7/93 WITH NO DEA REGISTRATION. SHALL PROMPTLY TRANSFER PATIENT RECORDS TO OTHER HEALTH CARE PROVIDERS IN ORDER TO PROVIDE CONTINUITY OF PATIENT CARE. RECONSIDERATION WAS DENIED 4/15/94. COURT DISMISSED HIS APPEAL FOR LACK OF JURISDICTION; CASE PENDING IN COURT OF APPEALS. SUSPENSION ENDED IN 2/95. HIS MOTION TO CONSOLIDATE TWO CASES GRANTED 4/19/95; HIS MOTION FOR ORAL ARGUMENT DENIED BY COURTS.

ROSEN, BARUCH DANIEL MD OF 7555 E OSBORN SUITE 206, PHOENIX, AZ, WAS DISCIPLINED BY DEA ON JULY 18, 1994
DISCIPLINARY ACTION: SURRENDER OF CONTROLLED SUBSTANCE LICENSE
OFFENSE: DISCIPLINARY ACTION BY ANOTHER STATE OR AGENCY

NOTES: OTHER STATE.

ROSEN, BARUCH DANIEL MD, LICENSE NUMBER 0G22901 OF MESA, AZ, WAS DISCIPLINED BY CALIFORNIA ON DECEMBER 2, 1996
DISCIPLINARY ACTION: LICENSE REVOCATION
OFFENSE: DISCIPLINARY ACTION BY ANOTHER STATE OR AGENCY

NOTES: DISCIPLINED BY ARIZONA FOR MAKING FALSE AND FRAUDULENT STATEMENTS IN CONNECTION WITH HIS PRACTICE OF MEDICINE; ENGAGING IN CONDUCT DANGEROUS TO HIS PATIENTS; AND ASSISTING AN UNLICENSED PRACTITIONER.

ROSEN, ROBERT S MD, WAS DISCIPLINED BY NEVADA ON SEPTEMBER 24, 1997
DISCIPLINARY ACTION: FINE; REPRIMAND
OFFENSE: PROVIDING FALSE INFORMATION TO THE BOARD OR OTHER HEALTH AGENCY

NOTES: ANSWERED "NO" TO A QUESTION ON HIS RENEWAL APPLICATION WHEN THE CORRECT RESPONSE WAS "YES." MUST PAY AN INVESTIGATIVE COST OF $1,500; SHALL PAY A $500 FINE AND PERFORM 40 HOURS OF COMMUNITY SERVICE IN LAS VEGAS WITHOUT COMPENSATION WITHIN ONE YEAR.

ROSEN, RONALD C MD, WAS DISCIPLINED BY NEVADA ON AUGUST 28, 1999
DISCIPLINARY ACTION: REPRIMAND; COMMUNITY SERVICE
OFFENSE: DISCIPLINARY ACTION BY ANOTHER STATE OR AGENCY

NOTES: LIMITATION OF THE LICENSE TO PRACTICE MEDICINE IN CALIFORNIA. SHALL PERFORM 20 HOURS OF COMMUNITY SERVICE WITHIN THREE MONTHS; SHALL PAY $500 IN COSTS.

ROSEN, RONALD CARY MD, LICENSE NUMBER G40504 OF LAS VEGAS, NV, WAS DISCIPLINED BY CALIFORNIA ON MAY 14, 1999
DISCIPLINARY ACTION: 60-MONTH PROBATION
OFFENSE: PROFESSIONAL MISCONDUCT

NOTES: IMPROPERLY BILLED INSURANCE COMPANIES RELATED TOT HE TREATMENT RENDERED TO THREE PATIENTS. REVOCATION STAYED.

RUCKER, ELLESTON CRAIG MD, DATE OF BIRTH SEPTEMBER 20, 1956 OF 2200 SAPPHIRE VALLEY STREET, LAS VEGAS, NV, WAS DISCIPLINED BY MEDICARE ON JUNE 5, 1997
DISCIPLINARY ACTION: EXCLUSION FROM THE MEDICARE AND/OR MEDICAID PROGRAM
OFFENSE: NONCOMPLIANCE WITH A PROFESSIONAL RULE

NOTES: DEFAULTED ON PUBLIC HEALTH SERVICE EDUCATION LOAN. REINSTATED ON 8/22/97.

RUDELL, JEFFREY H MD, LICENSE NUMBER 0101320 OF 65 E 96TH ST, NEW YORK, NY, WAS DISCIPLINED BY NEW YORK ON AUGUST 17, 1992
DISCIPLINARY ACTION: LICENSE REVOCATION
OFFENSE: PROFESSIONAL MISCONDUCT

NOTES: THE HEARING COMMITTEE FOUND HIM GUILTY OF FRAUDULENT PRACTICE, MORAL UNFITNESS AND WILLFULLY ABUSING A PATIENT. THE BOARD SUSTAINED THE HEARING COMMITTEE'S DETERMINATION AND UPHELD THE PENALTY.

RUDELL, JEFFREY H MD, DATE OF BIRTH JULY 4, 1940, LICENSE NUMBER 0014835 OF POINT LOOKOUT, NY, WAS DISCIPLINED BY KENTUCKY ON NOVEMBER 18, 1993
DISCIPLINARY ACTION: LICENSE REVOCATION
OFFENSE: DISCIPLINARY ACTION BY ANOTHER STATE OR AGENCY

NOTES: ACTION TAKEN BY NEW YORK BOARD.

RUDELL, JEFFREY H MD, WAS DISCIPLINED BY NEVADA ON JANUARY 20, 1995
DISCIPLINARY ACTION: DENIAL OF NEW LICENSE
OFFENSE: DISCIPLINARY ACTION BY ANOTHER STATE OR AGENCY

NOTES: NEW YORK REVOKED HIS LICENSE.

RUDELL, JEFFREY H MD, LICENSE NUMBER 101320 OF 110 CEDARHURST AVENUE, POINT LOOKOUT, NY, WAS DISCIPLINED BY NEW YORK ON SEPTEMBER 7, 1999
DISCIPLINARY ACTION: DENIAL OF LICENSE REINSTATEMENT

RUECA, CARLOS N MD, WAS DISCIPLINED BY NEVADA ON JUNE 20, 1996
DISCIPLINARY ACTION: 36-MONTH PROBATION; 12-MONTH RESTRICTION PLACED ON CONTROLLED SUBSTANCE LICENSE
OFFENSE: OVERPRESCRIBING OR MISPRESCRIBING DRUGS

NOTES: PLED NO CONTEST TO 10 COUNTS OF OVERPRESCRIBING, ONE COUNT OF GROSS MALPRACTICE, 10 COUNTS OF PRESCRIBING THYROID SYNTHETICS FOR WEIGHT LOSS, AND ONE COUNT OF REPEATED MALPRACTICE. WRITTEN PUBLIC REPRIMAND. SUSPENSION, STAYED AS PROBATION UNDER THE FOLLOWING TERMS AND CONDITIONS: HIS AUTHORITY TO PRESCRIBE SCHEDULE II, III, AND IV CONTROLLED SUBSTANCES IS SUSPENDED FOR ONE YEAR; SHALL ATTEND 60 HOURS OF CONTINUING MEDICAL EDUCATION IN PAIN MANAGEMENT AND 20 HOURS IN APPROPRIATE PRESCRIBING OF NARCOTIC MEDICATION; FROM AND AFTER ONE YEAR DURING THE REMAINDER OF HIS THREE YEAR PROBATION, SHALL KEEP A LOG, BY MONTH, OF EACH INCIDENCE OF HIS PRESCRIBING OR DISPENSING A CONTROLLED SUBSTANCE TO A PATIENT. $7,500 FOR ALL ADMINISTRATIVE EXPENSES INCURRED IN THE INVESTIGATION AND HEARING PREPARATION PROCESS.

RUECA, CARLOS N MD, LICENSE NUMBER 131921 OF 3009 W CHARLESTON BLVD., LAS VEGAS, NV, WAS DISCIPLINED BY NEW YORK ON MARCH 12, 1997
DISCIPLINARY ACTION: LICENSE REVOCATION
OFFENSE: DISCIPLINARY ACTION BY ANOTHER STATE OR AGENCY

NOTES: DISCIPLINED BY THE NEVADA BOARD FOR WRITING PRESCRIPTIONS FOR EXCESSIVE AMOUNTS OF CONTROLLED SUBSTANCES AND INAPPROPRIATELY PRESCRIBING THYROID SYNTHETIC FOR WEIGHT LOSS.

RUECA, ROSALINDA PINEDA MD, DATE OF BIRTH NOVEMBER 18, 1942, LICENSE NUMBER 0003651 OF 3009 WEST CHARLESTON BOULEVARD, LAS VEGAS, NV, WAS DISCIPLINED BY NEVADA ON DECEMBER 7, 1996
DISCIPLINARY ACTION: 60-MONTH PROBATION; REPRIMAND
OFFENSE: FALSIFYING OR ALTERING PATIENT RECORDS

NOTES: WITH REGARD TO SIX HOSPITALIZED PATIENTS IN 3/95: CHARGED FOR NON-RENDERED SERVICES; ENGAGED IN CONDUCT INTENDED TO DECEIVE; ALTERED MEDICAL RECORDS OF PATIENTS; FALSIFIED RECORDS OF HEALTH CARE FOR PATIENTS; AND FALSIFIED THE MEDICAL RECORDS OF A HOSPITAL SO AS TO INDICATE HER PRESENCE AT A TIME WHEN SHE WAS NOT IN ATTENDANCE. LICENSE REVOKED, STAYED, PROBATION UNDER TERMS AND CONDITIONS: SHALL COMPLETE HER INPATIENT PRIMARY TREATMENT AND SHALL ONLY BE DISCHARGED THEREFROM AFTER COMPLETION OF THE PROGRAM AND RECOMMENDATION OF THE STAFF OF THE DIVERSION PROGRAM; SHALL ENTER INTO AN AGREEMENT WITH THE DIVERSION PROGRAM OF THE BOARD FOR A TERM OF FIVE YEARS; SHALL ABIDE BY ALL DIRECTIVES OF THE PROGRAM, AND PARTICIPATE IN ANY PROGRAM FOR REHABILITATION, INCLUDING PARTICIPATION IN THE PROGRAM'S SELECTED TREATMENT PROGRAMS; AND SHALL AUTHORIZE THE DIVERSION PROGRAM, AND ANY TREATMENT PROGRAM SHE PARTICIPATES IN, TO PROVIDE THE BOARD STATUS REPORTS OF HER PARTICIPATION AND PROGRESS, INCLUDING REPORTS ON ALL TESTS OF BODY FLUIDS TAKEN FROM HER, UPON BOARD REQUEST. $7,500 FINE AND COSTS.

RUECA, ROSALINDA PINEDA MD, DATE OF BIRTH NOVEMBER 18, 1942 OF 7145 TARA AVENUE, LAS VEGAS, NV, WAS DISCIPLINED BY MEDICARE ON SEPTEMBER 30, 1997
DISCIPLINARY ACTION: 60-MONTH EXCLUSION FROM THE MEDICARE AND/OR MEDICAID PROGRAM
OFFENSE: CRIMINAL CONVICTION OR PLEA OF GUILTY, NOLO CONTENDERE, OR NO CONTEST TO A CRIME

NOTES: CONVICTED OF A CRIME INVOLVING THE MEDICARE, MEDICAID, MATERNAL AND CHILD HEALTH SERVICES BLOCK GRANT OR BLOCK GRANTS TO STATES FOR SOCIAL SERVICES PROGRAMS.

SANDIDGE, ERNIE MD, WAS DISCIPLINED BY NEVADA ON JUNE 8, 1990
DISCIPLINARY ACTION: 60-MONTH PROBATION; FINE
OFFENSE: PROVIDING FALSE INFORMATION TO THE BOARD OR OTHER HEALTH AGENCY

NOTES: ON 2/22/88, CLINICAL PRIVILEGES AT THE GOODFELLOW CLINIC WERE REVOKED. LIED TO THE BOARD ON BIENNIAL REGISTRATION FORM OF 5/13/89 BY CLAIMING HE HAD NEVER HAD STAFF PRIVILEGES REVOKED. REPRIMAND AND COMMUNITY SERVICE.

SAVERY, FRANCOIS L MD, WAS DISCIPLINED BY NEVADA ON OCTOBER 6, 1999
DISCIPLINARY ACTION: SURRENDER OF LICENSE
OFFENSE: PROFESSIONAL MISCONDUCT

NOTES: CHARGED WITH AIDING, ASSISTING, EMPLOYING OR ADVISING, DIRECTLY OR INDIRECTLY, ANY UNLICENSED PERSON TO ENGAGE IN THE PRACTICE OF MEDICINE; DELEGATING RESPONSIBILITY FOR THE CARE OF A PATIENT TO A PERSON IF THE LICENSEE KNOWS, OR HAS REASON TO KNOW, THAT THE PERSON IS NOT QUALIFIED TO UNDERTAKE THAT RESPONSIBILITY. VOLUNTARY SURRENDER WHILE UNDER INVESTIGATION.

SCHIEVE, DONALD R MD, DATE OF BIRTH FEBRUARY 23, 1933 OF 1800 HWY 95, #4, BULLHEAD CITY, AZ, WAS DISCIPLINED BY MEDICARE ON JUNE 18, 1998
DISCIPLINARY ACTION: EXCLUSION FROM THE MEDICARE AND/OR MEDICAID PROGRAM
OFFENSE: DISCIPLINARY ACTION BY ANOTHER STATE OR AGENCY

NOTES: LICENSE REVOKED, SUSPENDED, SURRENDERED OR OTHERWISE LOST FOR REASONS BEARING ON PROFESSIONAL PERFORMANCE, PROFESSIONAL COMPETENCE OR FINANCIAL INTEGRITY.

SCHIEVE, DONALD R MD, LICENSE NUMBER C21402 OF BULLHEAD CITY, AZ, WAS DISCIPLINED BY CALIFORNIA ON DECEMBER 16, 1998
DISCIPLINARY ACTION: LICENSE REVOCATION
OFFENSE: DISCIPLINARY ACTION BY ANOTHER STATE OR AGENCY

NOTES: DISCIPLINED BY NEVADA FOR PERFORMING PHENOL FACE PEELS WITH AN UNLICENSED INDIVIDUAL.

SCHIEVE, DONALD REYNOLDS MD, DATE OF BIRTH FEBRUARY 23, 1933, LICENSE NUMBER 0002056 OF 1800 HIGHWAY 95 #4, BULLHEAD CITY, AZ, WAS DISCIPLINED BY NEVADA ON DECEMBER 7, 1996
DISCIPLINARY ACTION: 60-MONTH PROBATION; REPRIMAND
OFFENSE: PROFESSIONAL MISCONDUCT

NOTES: CHARGED WITH 4 COUNTS OF SIGNING A BLANK PRESCRIPTION FORM; 9 COUNTS OF ENGAGING IN ANY CONDUCT WHICH IS INTENDED TO DECEIVE; 2 COUNTS OF FAILURE TO MAINTAIN MEDICAL RECORDS RELATING TO THE DIAGNOSIS, TREATMENT AND CARE

OF A PATIENT; 7 COUNTS OF ALTERING MEDICAL RECORDS OF A PATIENT; 4 COUNTS OF ENGAGING IN ANY CONDUCT WHICH THE BOARD HAS DETERMINED IS A VIOLATION OF THE STANDARDS OF PRACTICE ESTABLISHED BY REGULATION OF THE BOARD; 2 COUNTS OF WRITING A PRESCRIPTION FOR CONTROLLED SUBSTANCES FOR ANY PERSON WITHOUT AN APPROPRIATE EXAMINATION WHICH CONFIRMS THE MEDICAL NECESSITY FOR THE CONTROLLED SUBSTANCES; 2 COUNTS OF ACQUIRING ANY CONTROLLED SUBSTANCES FROM ANY PHARMACY OR OTHER SOURCE BY MISREPRESENTATION, FRAUD, DECEPTION OR SUBTERFUGE; 9 COUNTS OF AIDING, ASSISTING, EMPLOYING OR ADVISING, DIRECTLY OR INDIRECTLY, ANY UNLICENSED PERSON TO ENGAGE IN THE PRACTICE OF MEDICINE CONTRARY TO THE PROVISION OR THE REGULATIONS OF THE BOARD; AND 1 COUNT OF PERFORMING SERVICES WHICH HE KNOWS OR HAS REASON TO KNOW THAT HE IS NOT COMPETENT TO PERFORM; ENGAGED IN THE MEDICAL PRACTICE OF PERFORMING "PHENOL FACE PEELS" TOGETHER WITH AN INDIVIDUAL NOT LICENSED TO PRACTICE MEDICINE IN NEVADA; ACTION HAD NO RELATIONSHIP TO HIS PRACTICE OF OPHTHALMOLOGY. LICENSE REVOCATION, STAYED, PROBATION UNDER TERMS AND CONDITIONS: SHALL NOT PRACTICE IN NEVADA DURING HIS PROBATIONARY PERIOD; SHALL, AT THE NEXT BI-ENNIAL LICENSING, ON 7/01/97, REQUEST TO BE PLACED ON INACTIVE STATUS IN NEVADA AND REMAIN ON INACTIVE STATUS DURING THE TERM OF HIS PROBATION. PUBLIC REPRIMAND. $7,500 FINE.

SCHIEVE, DONALD REYNOLDS MD, DATE OF BIRTH FEBRUARY 23, 1933, LICENSE NUMBER 028226E OF 1195 PINEVIEW DRIVE, MORGANTOWN, WV, WAS DISCIPLINED BY PENNSYLVANIA ON NOVEMBER 17, 1997
DISCIPLINARY ACTION: LICENSE REVOCATION
OFFENSE: DISCIPLINARY ACTION BY ANOTHER STATE OR AGENCY

NOTES: DISCIPLINARY ACTION TAKEN BY NEVADA.

SHALLENBERGER, FRANK A MD, LICENSE NUMBER 0G27254 OF GARDNERVILLE, NV, WAS DISCIPLINED BY CALIFORNIA ON APRIL 7, 1995
DISCIPLINARY ACTION: SURRENDER OF LICENSE

NOTES: VOLUNTARY SURRENDER WHILE CHARGES PENDING.

SHALLENBERGER, FRANK A MD, WAS DISCIPLINED BY NEVADA ON NOVEMBER 3, 1995
DISCIPLINARY ACTION: REPRIMAND
OFFENSE: DISCIPLINARY ACTION BY ANOTHER STATE OR AGENCY

NOTES: IN 3/95 SURRENDERED CALIFORNIA LICENSE AFTER BOARD FILED ALLEGATIONS REGARDING PATIENT CARE.

SHANKMAN, ANDREW S MD, DATE OF BIRTH FEBRUARY 11, 1954, LICENSE NUMBER 023876 OF PO BOX 30387, SEA ISLAND, GA, WAS DISCIPLINED BY GEORGIA ON FEBRUARY 27, 1997
DISCIPLINARY ACTION: EMERGENCY SUSPENSION
OFFENSE: SUBSTANDARD CARE, INCOMPETENCE OR NEGLIGENCE

NOTES: FAILURE TO COMPLY WITH THE MINIMAL STANDARDS OF ACCEPTABLE AND PREVAILING PRACTICE.

SHANKMAN, ANDREW S MD, DATE OF BIRTH FEBRUARY 11, 1954, LICENSE NUMBER 023876 OF PO BOX 30387, SEA ISLAND, GA, WAS DISCIPLINED BY GEORGIA ON NOVEMBER 7, 1997
DISCIPLINARY ACTION: SURRENDER OF LICENSE
OFFENSE: SUBSTANDARD CARE, INCOMPETENCE OR NEGLIGENCE

NOTES: PRACTICE BELOW MINIMUM ACCEPTABLE STANDARDS. VOLUNTARY SURRENDER; SAME AS REVOCATION.

SHANKMAN, ANDREW S MD, DATE OF BIRTH FEBRUARY 11, 1954 OF 868 NE 54TH TERRACE, COLEMAN, FL, WAS DISCIPLINED BY MEDICARE ON JANUARY 20, 1998
DISCIPLINARY ACTION: 240-MONTH EXCLUSION FROM THE MEDICARE AND/OR MEDICAID PROGRAM
OFFENSE: CRIMINAL CONVICTION OR PLEA OF GUILTY, NOLO CONTENDERE, OR NO CONTEST TO A CRIME

NOTES: CONVICTED OF A CRIME INVOLVING THE MEDICARE, MEDICAID, MATERNAL AND CHILD HEALTH SERVICES BLOCK GRANT OR BLOCK GRANTS TO STATES FOR SOCIAL SERVICES PROGRAMS.

SHANKMAN, ANDREW STUART MD, LICENSE NUMBER A40890 OF LAS VEGAS, NV, WAS DISCIPLINED BY CALIFORNIA ON DECEMBER 18, 1998
DISCIPLINARY ACTION: SURRENDER OF LICENSE

NOTES: WHILE CHARGES PENDING.

SKLAR, ALLEN L MD, LICENSE NUMBER 0026361 OF INCLINE VILLAGE, NV, WAS DISCIPLINED BY FLORIDA ON OCTOBER 12, 1994
DISCIPLINARY ACTION: FINE; REQUIRED TO TAKE ADDITIONAL MEDICAL EDUCATION
OFFENSE: NONCOMPLIANCE WITH A PROFESSIONAL RULE

NOTES: CHARGED WITH VIOLATING ANY RULE OR ORDER OF THE BOARD OR FAILING TO COMPLY WITH A SUBPOENA OF THE DEPARTMENT IN THAT HE FAILED TO DOCUMENT COMPLIANCE WITH THE CONTINUING EDUCATION REQUIREMENTS BY PROVIDING ADEQUATE VERIFICATION OF COMPLETION OF AT LEAST ONE HOUR OF CONTINUING EDUCATION IN THE AREA OF HIV/AIDS. $750 FINE; SHALL COMPLETE THE DEFICIENT CONTINUING MEDICAL EDUCATION CREDIT IN HIV/AIDS WITHIN ONE YEAR.

SOLI, DONALD E MD, WAS DISCIPLINED BY NEVADA ON AUGUST 22, 1998
DISCIPLINARY ACTION: 60-MONTH PROBATION; RESTRICTION PLACED ON LICENSE

NOTES: MALPRACTICE IN THE CASE OF TWO PATIENTS: ONE FOR WHOM HE FAILED TO PROPERLY TREAT OR APPROPRIATELY REFER TO WHOM HE GAVE CHELATION THERAPY FOR A DIAGNOSIS OF ARTERIOSCLEROTIC VASCULAR DISEASE AND LOWER EXTREMITY VASCULAR DISEASE; ANOTHER PATIENT HE TREATED IN 6/94 AND 8/94 PRESENTED WITH RECTAL BLEEDING AND OTHER GI SYMPTOMS; TOOK NO ACTION TO EVALUATE THE RECTAL BLEEDING; IN 3/95 THE PATIENT WAS TREATED BY ANOTHER PHYSICIAN WHEN A CARCINOMA WAS DETECTED. REVOCATION STAYED. CONDITIONS OF PROBATION ARE AS FOLLOWS: MUST COMPLETE 17 HOURS OF CONTINUING MEDICAL EDUCATION IN PROPER RECORD-KEEPING PRACTICES; MUST PAY $4,000 FOR ALL ADMINISTRATIVE EXPENSES INCURRED; MUST NOT USE THE EAV DERMATRON MACHINE OR ANY OTHER SIMILAR MACHINE AS THE SOLE SOURCE OF MEDICAL DIAGNOSIS OF PATIENTS; MUST NOT ENGAGE IN THE PRACTICE OF CHELATION THERAPY OR REFER PATIENTS TO OTHER HEALTH CARE PROFESSIONALS OR PHYSICIANS FOR THIS THERAPY; SHALL CONTACT THE AMERICAN COLLEGE FOR THE ADVANCEMENT OF MEDICINE AND REQUEST THAT IT REMOVE HIS NAME FROM THE LIST OF PHYSICIANS SPECIALIZING IN CHELATION THERAPY; MUST LIMIT

HIS PRACTICE TO ALLERGY AND GENERAL PRACTICE AND REQUIRE THAT ALL PATIENT RECORDS SHALL CONTAIN ALL TESTS, DIAGNOSTIC METHODS HISTORIES AND PHYSICAL EXAMINATIONS CONDUCTED ON PATIENTS TO ARRIVE AT A DIAGNOSIS AND TREATMENT; REPRIMAND.

SOMOSHEGYI-SZOKOL, ATTILA MD, WAS DISCIPLINED BY NEVADA ON JANUARY 20, 1995
DISCIPLINARY ACTION: DENIAL OF NEW LICENSE
OFFENSE: FAILURE TO COMPLY WITH PREVIOUS BOARD ORDER

NOTES: VIOLATED HIS STIPULATED AGREEMENT WITH THE INVESTIGATIVE COMMITTEE OF THE BOARD DURING HIS PERIOD OF TEMPORARY RESTRICTED LICENSURE FROM 1/31/94 - 1/30/95.

SPRINGER, MARTIN F MD, LICENSE NUMBER 0G57322 OF VACAVILLE, CA, WAS DISCIPLINED BY CALIFORNIA ON JUNE 16, 1995
DISCIPLINARY ACTION: 60-MONTH PROBATION
OFFENSE: CRIMINAL CONVICTION OR PLEA OF GUILTY, NOLO CONTENDERE, OR NO CONTEST TO A CRIME

NOTES: CONVICTION FOR SEXUAL BATTERY. REVOCATION STAYED.

SPRINGER, MARTIN F B MD, WAS DISCIPLINED BY NEVADA ON JUNE 29, 1995
DISCIPLINARY ACTION: NONRENEWAL OF LICENSE
OFFENSE: DISCIPLINARY ACTION BY ANOTHER STATE OR AGENCY

NOTES: DISCIPLINARY ACTION TAKEN IN CALIFORNIA.

STARK, ROY COSBY MD, DATE OF BIRTH JULY 13, 1959 OF 9404 VISTA RIDGE, LAS VEGAS, NV, WAS DISCIPLINED BY MEDICARE ON FEBRUARY 18, 1999
DISCIPLINARY ACTION: EXCLUSION FROM THE MEDICARE AND/OR MEDICAID PROGRAM
OFFENSE: DISCIPLINARY ACTION BY ANOTHER STATE OR AGENCY

NOTES: LICENSE REVOKED, SUSPENDED, SURRENDERED OR OTHERWISE LOST FOR REASONS BEARING ON PROFESSIONAL PERFORMANCE, PROFESSIONAL COMPETENCE OR FINANCIAL INTEGRITY.

STOERMER, DIETRICH A MD, WAS DISCIPLINED BY NEVADA ON MARCH 5, 1993
DISCIPLINARY ACTION: RESTRICTION PLACED ON CONTROLLED SUBSTANCE LICENSE; REPRIMAND
OFFENSE: OVERPRESCRIBING OR MISPRESCRIBING DRUGS

NOTES: FAILED TO MAKE MEDICAL RECORDS AVAILABLE TO PATIENTS AND EXCESSIVE PRESCRIBING OF CONTROLLED SUBSTANCES. CONDITIONS: SUSPENDED FROM PRESCRIBING SCHEDULE II DRUGS UNTIL FURTHER ORDER OF THE BOARD; MUST COMPLETE CONTINUING MEDICAL EDUCATION ON CHRONIC PAIN MANAGEMENT INCLUDING INAPPROPRIATE WRITING OF PRESCRIPTIONS FOR CONTROLLED SUBSTANCES AND A COURSE ON APPROPRIATE MEDICAL RECORD KEEPING/DOCUMENTATION.

STOERMER, DIETRICH A MD, LICENSE NUMBER 0C39091 OF LAS VEGAS, NV, WAS DISCIPLINED BY CALIFORNIA ON SEPTEMBER 1, 1994
DISCIPLINARY ACTION: LICENSE REVOCATION
OFFENSE: DISCIPLINARY ACTION BY ANOTHER STATE OR AGENCY

NOTES: DISCIPLINED BY NEVADA BOARD FOR FAILURE TO MAKE MEDICAL RECORDS AVAILABLE TO PATIENTS FOR INSPECTION AND COPYING, AS REQUIRED BY LAW. DEFAULT DECISION.

STOERMER, DIETRICH ALBERT MD, LICENSE NUMBER 00E5952 OF LAS VEGAS, NV, WAS DISCIPLINED BY TEXAS ON AUGUST 19, 1994
DISCIPLINARY ACTION: RESTRICTION PLACED ON CONTROLLED SUBSTANCE LICENSE; REQUIRED TO TAKE ADDITIONAL MEDICAL EDUCATION
OFFENSE: DISCIPLINARY ACTION BY ANOTHER STATE OR AGENCY

NOTES: LICENSE WAS DISCIPLINED BY ARIZONA BOARD ON 3/18/93. PRIOR TO PRACTICING IN TEXAS SHALL APPEAR BEFORE THE BOARD AND BE SUBJECT TO THE FOLLOWING RESTRICTIONS; SHALL NOT PRESCRIBE OR ADMINISTER SCHEDULE II CONTROLLED SUBSTANCES; SHALL ATTEND AT LEAST 50 HOURS PER YEAR OF CONTINUING MEDICAL EDUCATION INCLUDING AT LEAST 15 HOURS IN PAIN MANAGEMENT AND 6 HOURS IN RISK MANAGEMENT PER YEAR; SHALL GIVE A COPY OF THIS ORDER TO ANY HEALTH CARE ENTITY WHERE HE HAS PRIVILEGES; SHALL COOPERATE WITH THE BOARD IN VERIFYING COMPLIANCE; SHALL INFORM BOARD OF CHANGE OF ADDRESS WITHIN 10 DAYS. SHALL NOT SEEK MODIFICATION FOR ONE YEAR.

SUGARMAN, GERALD I MD, LICENSE NUMBER 00G8791 OF SHERMAN OAKS, CA, WAS DISCIPLINED BY CALIFORNIA ON JULY 23, 1996
DISCIPLINARY ACTION: 32-MONTH PROBATION
OFFENSE: CRIMINAL CONVICTION OR PLEA OF GUILTY, NOLO CONTENDERE, OR NO CONTEST TO A CRIME

NOTES: CONVICTED FOR MONEY LAUNDERING AND BANKRUPTCY FRAUD. REVOCATION, STAYED.

SUGARMAN, GERALD I MD, LICENSE NUMBER 016630 OF ARROYO GRANDE, CA, WAS DISCIPLINED BY VIRGINIA ON JANUARY 6, 1997
DISCIPLINARY ACTION: LICENSE SUSPENSION
OFFENSE: CRIMINAL CONVICTION OR PLEA OF GUILTY, NOLO CONTENDERE, OR NO CONTEST TO A CRIME

NOTES: BASED UPON FELONY CONVICTIONS FOR AIDING AND ABETTING BANKRUPTCY FRAUD AND MONEY LAUNDERING. LICENSE WAS SUBSEQUENTLY CONTINUED INDEFINITELY ON SUSPENSION 6/30/97, FOLLOWING HIS PETITION FOR REINSTATEMENT.

SUGARMAN, GERALD I MD, WAS DISCIPLINED BY NEVADA ON FEBRUARY 12, 1997
DISCIPLINARY ACTION: PROBATION
OFFENSE: DISCIPLINARY ACTION BY ANOTHER STATE OR AGENCY

NOTES: CONVICTION OF A FELONY; PROBATION BY CALIFORNIA BOARD. REVOCATION STAYED WITH FOLLOWING TERMS AND CONDITIONS: PROBATION SHALL RUN CONCURRENT WITH THE CALIFORNIA PROBATIONARY PERIOD; SHALL PAY $1,000 IN COSTS.

TARVER, ANGELO A MD OF 4727 WEST PARK DRIVE, ZACHARY, LA, WAS DISCIPLINED BY DEA ON AUGUST 3, 1993
DISCIPLINARY ACTION: SURRENDER OF CONTROLLED SUBSTANCE LICENSE
OFFENSE: SUBSTANCE ABUSE

NOTES: DUE TO SELF ABUSE OF CONTROLLED SUBSTANCES.

TARVER, ANGELO A MD, WAS DISCIPLINED BY NEVADA ON NOVEMBER 17, 1994
DISCIPLINARY ACTION: PROBATION
OFFENSE: DISCIPLINARY ACTION BY ANOTHER STATE OR AGENCY

NOTES: LICENSE TO PRACTICE MEDICINE IN LOUISIANA SUSPENDED AND REINSTATED ON A FIVE YEAR

PROBATION BY THE LOUISIANA BOARD OF MEDICAL EXAMINERS. CONDITIONS OF PROBATION INCLUDE: MUST COMPLY WITH ALL TERMS OF HIS PROBATION IN LOUISIANA, WILL DIRECT HIS TREATING AND MONITORING PHYSICIANS IN LOUISIANA TO SUBMIT TO THE NEVADA BOARD REPORTS ON HIS TREATMENT PROGRAM AND COMPLIANCE WITH HIS PROBATION IN LOUISIANA. HE WILL ALSO DIRECT LOUISIANA BOARD TO PROVIDE VERIFICATION TO THE NEVADA BOARD OF HIS COMPLIANCE WITH HIS PROBATION IN LOUISIANA; UPON SUCCESSFUL COMPLETION OF ALL PROBATIONARY TERMS IN LOUISIANA HIS LICENSE TO PRACTICE MEDICINE IN NEVADA WILL RETURN TO UNRESTRICTED STATUS.

TARVER, ANGELO ANTHONY MD OF ZACHARY, LA, WAS DISCIPLINED BY LOUISIANA ON MAY 26, 1993
DISCIPLINARY ACTION: REVOCATION OF CONTROLLED SUBSTANCE LICENSE; LICENSE SUSPENSION
OFFENSE: SUBSTANCE ABUSE

NOTES: HABITUAL OR RECURRING ABUSE OF DRUGS INCLUDING ALCOHOL; PRESCRIBING, DISPENSING OR ADMINISTERING CONTROLLED SUBSTANCES IN OTHER THAN A LEGAL OR LEGITIMATE MANNER. CONSENT ORDER ISSUED SUSPENDING LICENSE PENDING DISCHARGE FROM INPATIENT TREATMENT, AFTERCARE AND FAVORABLE OPINIONS OF TWO PHYSICIANS; SUBJECT TO REINSTATEMENT THEREAFTER ON PROBATION FOR FIVE YEARS, SUBJECT TO CONTINUING TREATMENT AND PERIODIC REPORTS TO THE BOARD, LIFETIME PROHIBITION ON PRESCRIPTION OF CONTROLLED SUBSTANCES, MAINTENANCE OF COMPLETE ABSTINENCE FROM USE OF MOOD-ALTERING SUBSTANCES, AND COMPLETION OF SPECIFIED CONTINUING MEDICAL EDUCATION.

THOMPSON, LARRY W MD, WAS DISCIPLINED BY NEVADA ON APRIL 9, 1992
DISCIPLINARY ACTION: LICENSE REVOCATION
OFFENSE: PROFESSIONAL MISCONDUCT

NOTES: CHARGED WITH LACK OF CARE OF A PATIENT TO THE POINT OF CONSCIOUS INDIFFERENCE TO THE SAFETY AND WELFARE OF SAID PATIENT CONSTITUTING GROSS MALPRACTICE.

THOMPSON, LARRY W MD, LICENSE NUMBER 0011653, WAS DISCIPLINED BY ARIZONA ON JULY 15, 1993
DISCIPLINARY ACTION: RESTRICTION PLACED ON LICENSE

NOTES: HE SHALL NOT PERFORM ANY PREGNANCY TERMINATION, SURGERY, OR INVASIVE PROCEDURE EXCEPT AT A LICENSED HEALTH CARE FACILITY. ON 1/25/94 BOARD ACCEPTED HIS REQUEST FOR INACTIVE STATUS.

THORP, THEODORE M MD, WAS DISCIPLINED BY NEVADA ON NOVEMBER 27, 1990
DISCIPLINARY ACTION: REPRIMAND; REQUIRED TO TAKE ADDITIONAL MEDICAL EDUCATION
OFFENSE: OVERPRESCRIBING OR MISPRESCRIBING DRUGS

NOTES: FROM 11/9/88 THROUGH 6/20/90 HE PRESCRIBED CONTROLLED SUBSTANCES TO A PATIENT IN EXCESSIVE AMOUNTS, AND FAILED TO MAINTAIN ADEQUATE MEDICAL RECORDS FOR THIS PATIENT. MUST COMPLETE APPROPRIATE PRESCRIBING WORKSHOP.

THURAIRATNAM, INDRAN RAJPAL MD, LICENSE NUMBER 0166118 OF 323 HAMPTON GREEN, STATEN ISLAND, NY, WAS DISCIPLINED BY NEW YORK ON MAY 12, 1994
DISCIPLINARY ACTION: DENIAL OF LICENSE REINSTATEMENT

THURAIRATNAM, INDRAN RAJPAL MD, LICENSE NUMBER 0166118 OF 323 HAMPTON GREEN, STATEN ISLAND, NY, WAS DISCIPLINED BY NEW YORK ON JUNE 14, 1994
DISCIPLINARY ACTION: LICENSE REVOCATION
OFFENSE: PRACTICING WITHOUT A VALID LICENSE

NOTES: PRACTICED WHILE LICENSE WAS INACTIVE; HAD A PSYCHIATRIC CONDITION WHICH IMPAIRED HIS ABILITY TO PRACTICE; PRACTICED WHILE IMPAIRED.

THURAIRATNAM, INDRAN RAJPAL MD, DATE OF BIRTH JANUARY 11, 1948 OF 323 HAMPTON GREEN, STATEN ISLAND, NY, WAS DISCIPLINED BY MEDICARE ON DECEMBER 18, 1995
DISCIPLINARY ACTION: EXCLUSION FROM THE MEDICARE AND/OR MEDICAID PROGRAM
OFFENSE: DISCIPLINARY ACTION BY ANOTHER STATE OR AGENCY

NOTES: LICENSE REVOKED FOR REASONS BEARING ON PROFESSIONAL COMPETENCE.

THURAIRATNAM, INDRAN RAJPAL MD, LICENSE NUMBER 166118 OF 4999 TOPAZ AVENUE APT 26, LAS VEGAS, NV, WAS DISCIPLINED BY NEW YORK ON APRIL 19, 1999
DISCIPLINARY ACTION: DENIAL OF LICENSE REINSTATEMENT

NOTES: ALSO KNOWN AS INDRAN RATNAM.

TIFFANY, FRANK J MD, WAS DISCIPLINED BY NEVADA ON JUNE 8, 1995
DISCIPLINARY ACTION: RESTRICTION PLACED ON LICENSE

NOTES: PROHIBITED FROM PRACTICING OR PERFORMING ANY SERVICES IN THE FIELD OF OBSTETRICS AND GYNECOLOGY UNTIL FURTHER ORDER OF THE BOARD

TYLER, PETER D MD, LICENSE NUMBER 0013460 OF INCLINE VILLA, NV, WAS DISCIPLINED BY FLORIDA ON FEBRUARY 25, 1993
DISCIPLINARY ACTION: FINE
OFFENSE: SUBSTANDARD CARE, INCOMPETENCE OR NEGLIGENCE

NOTES: FAILING TO PRACTICE MEDICINE WITH AN ACCEPTABLE LEVEL OF CARE AND SKILL. MUST PAY $3,000 FINE; ISSUED LETTER OF CONCERN.

TYLER, PETER D MD, LICENSE NUMBER 0013460 OF INCLINE VILLAGE, NV, WAS DISCIPLINED BY FLORIDA ON JUNE 27, 1994
DISCIPLINARY ACTION: LICENSE SUSPENSION; FINE
OFFENSE: FAILURE TO COMPLY WITH PREVIOUS BOARD ORDER

NOTES: VIOLATED PREVIOUS BOARD ORDER IN THAT HE FAILED TO PAY A FINE. $1000 FINE; SUSPENSION UNTIL HE PAYS FINE IMPOSED BY THIS ORDER AND THE $3,000 FINE IMPOSED BY PREVIOUS ORDER.

VANCE, ROBERT BLISS DO OF 801 SOUTH RANCHO DRIVE SUITE F2, LAS VEGAS, NV, WAS DISCIPLINED BY DEA ON SEPTEMBER 18, 1995
DISCIPLINARY ACTION: RESTRICTION PLACED ON CONTROLLED SUBSTANCE LICENSE

NOTES: VIOLATIVE CONTROLLED SUBSTANCE HISTORY.

VANETTI, CHARLES MD, WAS DISCIPLINED BY NEVADA ON MARCH 20, 1992
DISCIPLINARY ACTION: REQUIRED TO TAKE ADDITIONAL MEDICAL EDUCATION

NOTES: 1/21/92: ORDERED BY BOARD TO UNDERGO MEDICAL COMPETENCY EXAMINATIONS, INCLUDING SPEX.

SUBSEQUENTLY FAILED SPEX, CONSTITUTING FAILURE TO BE FOUND COMPETENT TO PRACTICE MEDICINE. 3/20/92: THE BOARD ORDERED HIM TO TAKE INTENSIVE REFRESHER COURSES IN HIS SPECIALTY AND TO RE-TAKE SPEX. SHOULD HE PASS SPEX, DISCIPLINARY ACTION WILL TERMINATE. SHOULD HE FAIL SPEX, HIS LICENSE WILL BE SUMMARILY SUSPENDED UNTIL SUCH TIME THAT HE PROVES HIS COMPETENCY TO THE BOARD, BY SUCH MEANS AS THE BOARD DEEMS APPROPRIATE.

VOLOSHIN, PETER J MD, LICENSE NUMBER 0A22795 OF NEWPORT BEACH, CA, WAS DISCIPLINED BY CALIFORNIA ON MARCH 16, 1995
DISCIPLINARY ACTION: 3-MONTH LICENSE SUSPENSION; 57-MONTH PROBATION
OFFENSE: INSURANCE, MEDICARE OR MEDICAID FRAUD

NOTES: PERFORMED PLASTIC SURGERIES FOR COSMETIC PURPOSES; MISREPRESENTED IN FALSE REPORTS AND BILLING TO INSURANCE THE SURGERIES WERE FOR PATHOLOGY OR FUNCTIONAL DISORDERS. FAILED TO MAINTAIN PROPER MEDICAL RECORDS AND CHARTS. PROCURED BUSINESS FROM VIETNAMESE SECTOR THROUGH A PAID RUNNER OR STEERER. REVOCATION STAYED.

VOLOSHIN, PETER J MD, WAS DISCIPLINED BY NEVADA ON JUNE 29, 1995
DISCIPLINARY ACTION: SURRENDER OF LICENSE
OFFENSE: DISCIPLINARY ACTION BY ANOTHER STATE OR AGENCY

NOTES: CHARGED WITH HAVING ACTION TAKEN AGAINST HIS LICENSE IN CALIFORNIA AND FAILING TO NOTIFY THE NEVADA BOARD OF THIS ACTION. VOLUNTARY SURRENDER OF LICENSE WHILE HE IS UNDER INVESTIGATION.

WARD, JOSEPH C MD, DATE OF BIRTH AUGUST 6, 1946, LICENSE NUMBER 0039761 OF 9717 CEDAR ISLAND ROAD, WHITE LAKE, MI, WAS DISCIPLINED BY MICHIGAN ON MAY 21, 1993
DISCIPLINARY ACTION: 36-MONTH PROBATION; RESTRICTION PLACED ON LICENSE
OFFENSE: SUBSTANCE ABUSE

NOTES: MENTAL/PHYSICAL INABILITY TO PRACTICE -- DRUG/ALCOHOL RELATED. ON 2/3/95 RECLASSIFIED WITH UNLIMITED LICENSE.

WARD, JOSEPH C MD, LICENSE NUMBER 0039507 OF 2799 W GRAND BOULEVARD, DETROIT, MI, WAS DISCIPLINED BY MASSACHUSETTS ON MARCH 23, 1994
DISCIPLINARY ACTION: NONRENEWAL OF LICENSE

NOTES: RESIGNATION OF INCHOATE RIGHT TO RENEW.

WARD, JOSEPH CHARLES MD, LICENSE NUMBER 0035155 OF RENO, NV, WAS DISCIPLINED BY OHIO ON APRIL 28, 1994
DISCIPLINARY ACTION: LICENSE SUSPENSION; PROBATION
OFFENSE: DISCIPLINARY ACTION BY ANOTHER STATE OR AGENCY

NOTES: MICHIGAN BOARD ACTION DUE TO HISTORY OF TREATMENT FOR MAJOR DEPRESSION, SUBSTANCE ABUSE, AND IMPAIRMENT OF ABILITY TO PRACTICE MEDICINE, AS WELL AS HIS PLEA OF GUILTY TO OPERATING A MOTOR VEHICLE WHILE UNDER THE INFLUENCE ON TWO SEPARATE OCCASIONS; FAILURE TO RESPOND TO QUESTIONS ON APPLICATION FOR RENEWAL OF OHIO MEDICAL LICENSE PERTAINING TO CRIMINAL ACTIVITIES AND SUBSTANCE ABUSE. PERMANENT REVOCATION STAYED; INDEFINITE SUSPENSION, MINIMUM 90 DAYS; CONDITIONS FOR REINSTATEMENT; SUBSEQUENT PROBATION FOR AT LEAST FIVE YEARS.

WILCOURT, ROBIN J MD OF RENO, NV, WAS DISCIPLINED BY NEVADA ON DECEMBER 4, 1999
DISCIPLINARY ACTION: COMMUNITY SERVICE
OFFENSE: CRIMINAL CONVICTION OR PLEA OF GUILTY, NOLO CONTENDERE, OR NO CONTEST TO A CRIME

NOTES: CONVICTED OF A CRIME INVOLVING MORAL TURPITUDE. SHALL PAY $4,055.35 IN COSTS; SHALL PERFORM 20 HOURS OF UNCOMPENSATED PUBLIC SERVICE, TO BE APPROVED IN ADVANCE BY THE BOARD.

WILLARD, RICHARD MD, WAS DISCIPLINED BY NEVADA ON FEBRUARY 1, 1990
DISCIPLINARY ACTION: 24-MONTH PROBATION; FINE
OFFENSE: FALSIFYING OR ALTERING PATIENT RECORDS

NOTES: ALTERED MEDICAL RECORDS OF A PATIENT. ALSO REPRIMAND. ON 8/14/92 COMPLETED AND RELEASED FROM 2-YEAR PROBATION. LICENSE IS UNRESTRICTED.

WYCKOFF, STUART M MD, WAS DISCIPLINED BY NEVADA ON JANUARY 19, 1991
DISCIPLINARY ACTION: RESTRICTION PLACED ON LICENSE; REPRIMAND
OFFENSE: SUBSTANDARD CARE, INCOMPETENCE OR NEGLIGENCE

NOTES: TREATED PATIENTS IN A MATTER NOT RECOGNIZED SCIENTIFICALLY AS BEING BENEFICIAL, FAILED TO EXERCISE SKILL OR DILIGENCE, SPECIFICALLY IN THE AREA OF ADOLESCENT PSYCHIATRY, REPEATED MALPRACTICE. CANNOT PROVIDE PSYCHIATRIC TREATMENT TO ANY PERSON UNDER 18; LICENSE STATUS INACTIVE FOR 3 YEARS SUBJECT TO CONDITIONS FOR REINSTATEMENT TO ACTIVE STATUS.

WYCKOFF, STUART M MD, LICENSE NUMBER 00E2955 OF FORT FAIRFIELD, ME, WAS DISCIPLINED BY TEXAS ON OCTOBER 5, 1991
DISCIPLINARY ACTION: 60-MONTH PROBATION; RESTRICTION PLACED ON LICENSE
OFFENSE: DISCIPLINARY ACTION BY ANOTHER STATE OR AGENCY

NOTES: MAINE BOARD FOUND THAT DURING HIS TREATMENT OF ADOLESCENT PATIENTS WHILE PRACTICING AS A PSYCHIATRIST IN THE STATE OF NEVADA, HE VIOLATED STANDARDS OF PROFESSIONAL BEHAVIOR IN THE PRACTICE OF PSYCHIATRY, INCLUDING THE INAPPROPRIATE USE OF PROFANITY, CONFRONTATIONAL STYLE, AND EXTREME AND INAPPROPRIATE DISCIPLINARY MEASURES; LICENSE RESTRICTED IN BOTH MAINE AND NEVADA. FIVE YEAR SUSPENSION STAYED, PROBATION ISSUED UNDER FOLLOWING CONDITIONS: SHALL TREAT NO INVOLUNTARY PATIENTS IN ANY PRACTICE SETTING; SHALL TREAT ONLY THOSE PATIENTS WHO SEEK HIS SERVICES INTENTIONALLY WITHOUT COERCION OF ANY KIND; SHALL NOT PROVIDE PROFESSIONAL TREATMENT TO ANY PERSON UNDER THE AGE OF 18 IN ANY PRACTICE SETTING EXCEPT UNDER CERTAIN CONDITIONS, INCLUDING GROUP OR FAMILY THERAPY; SUPERVISORY ROLE LIMITED TO ADMINISTRATIVE PERSONNEL; SHALL PROVIDE TEXAS WITH COPIES OF REPORTS SENT TO MAINE; MUST APPEAR BEFORE BOARD BEFORE PRACTICING; TIME SPENT OUTSIDE OF TEXAS OR MAINE DOES NOT COUNT TOWARD PROBATION; SHALL COOPERATE WITH BOARD IN VERIFYING COMPLIANCE; SHALL APPEAR BEFORE BOARD ONCE A YEAR; MAY FILE FOR TERMINATION OF ORDER AFTER 8/1/92.

WYCKOFF, STUART MORELY MD, DATE OF BIRTH OCTOBER 13, 1949, LICENSE NUMBER 0013113 OF PO BOX 612, FORT FAIRFIELD, ME, WAS DISCIPLINED BY MAINE ON MAY 31, 1991
DISCIPLINARY ACTION: RESTRICTION PLACED ON LICENSE
OFFENSE: PROFESSIONAL MISCONDUCT

NOTES: ISSUED MODIFIED, CONDITIONAL LICENSE BASED ON UNPROFESSIONAL CONDUCT ALLEGED TO HAVE OCCURRED IN NEVADA.

YBALLE, DANILO N MD OF 11 EAST PACIFIC, HENDERSON, NV, WAS DISCIPLINED BY DEA ON MAY 31, 1995
DISCIPLINARY ACTION: RESTRICTION PLACED ON CONTROLLED SUBSTANCE LICENSE
OFFENSE: PROFESSIONAL MISCONDUCT

NOTES: PRIOR ALLEGED CONTROLLED SUBSTANCE VIOLATIONS.

NEW MEXICO

1999 serious action rate: 3.14/1000
1999 ranking: 27th

The New Mexico Board of Medical Examiners provided a list of actions for 1990 through 1999. The list includes the physician's name, degree, the type of action taken, and sometimes a brief description of the reason for the action. The listing contains information on modifications and terminations of board actions but not on court decisions affecting board actions.Nebraska stated that court decisions would be included in the information we received. New Mexico stated that court decisions would be included in the information we received. In some cases, New Mexico did not list a date in their newsletters, in which case we used the first day of the year.

The New Mexico Board of Osteopathic Medical Examiners provided a list of actions from 1990 through 1999. The list includes the physician's name, degree, license number, the date and type of action taken and a brief description of the reason for the action. The listing contains information on modifications and terminations of board actions but not on court decisions affecting board actions. New Mexico stated that court decisions would be included in the information we received. The information provided covers disciplinary actions taken against allopathic physicians (MDs) and osteopathic physicians (DOs).

Besides disciplinary actions taken by the State Medical Boards, this listing also includes actions taken by the Medicare/Medicaid programs, the FDA, and the DEA against physicians located in this state. Actions taken by other states against physicians located in New Mexico or that match a physician disciplined by New Mexico (see Appendix 2 for an explanation of the matching protocol) are also included.

Although we have made every effort to match physicians' names correctly, some materials we received did not include complete information on middle names, license numbers, birth dates or addresses. Therefore, consumers should remember that non-disciplined physicians and physicians with different disciplinary actions may have similar names to those disciplined physicians listed in this state. Consumers should also remember that if they want the most current information on the status on a physician's license, they should contact the medical board of the state in which the physician practices or had practiced.

According to the Federation of State Medical Boards, New Mexico took 13 serious disciplinary actions against MDs in 1999. Compared to the 4,138 MDs licensed in the state, New Mexico had a serious disciplinary action rate of 3.14 serious actions per 1,000 MDs and a ranking of 27th on that list (see Table A, Findings, pg. 14).

The tables below summarize the data Public Citizen received from New Mexico.

Table 1. Disciplinary Actions Against MDs and DOs 1990 through 1999*

Action	Number	Percent**
Revocation	32	22.1%
Surrender	28	19.3%
Suspension	14	9.7%
Probation	14	9.7%
Practice Restriction	18	12.4%
Action Taken Against Controlled Substance License	4	2.8%
Other Actions	35	24.1%
Total Actions	**145**	**100.0%**

* This table lists only the two most serious disciplinary actions taken against a physician.
** Percentages may not total 100% due to rounding.

Table 2. Offenses for which MDs and DOs were Disciplined 1990 through 1999*

Offense	Number	Percent
Criminal Conviction	7	5.7%
Sexual Abuse of or Sexual Misconduct with a Patient	0	0.0%
Substandard Care, Incompetence or Negligence	4	3.3%
Misprescribing or Overprescribing Drugs	7	5.7%
Substance Abuse	44	35.8%
Disciplinary Action Taken Against License by Another State or Agency	15	12.2%
Other Offenses	46	37.4%
Total Records With Offense Listed	**123**	**100.0%**

* Includes only those actions for which an offense was listed and for which we had a corresponding term in our database.

Table 3. Disciplinary Actions Taken for Substance Abuse

Action	Number	Percent
Revocation	3	11.1%
Surrender	4	14.8%
Suspension	3	11.1%
Probation	3	11.1%
Restriction on Controlled Substance License	2	7.4%
Required to Enter an Impaired Physician Program or Substance Abuse Treatment	4	14.8%
Other Actions	8	29.6%
Total Actions	**27**	**100.0%**

If you feel that your doctor has not given you proper medical care or has mistreated you in any way--whether or not he or she is listed in this report--it is important that you let your state medical board know. Even if they do not immediately act on your complaint, it is important that the information be recorded in their files because it is possible that other people may have filed or will file complaints about the same doctor. Send a brief written description of what occurred to the addresses below or call the phone numbers listed for more information on how to file a complaint.

Addresses

New Mexico State Board of Medical Examiners
Kristen A. Hedrick, Executive Secretary
491 Old Santa Fe Trail
2nd Floor, Lamy Bldg.
Santa Fe, NM 87501
(505) 827-5022
Fax: (505) 827-7377

New Mexico Board of Osteopathic Medical Examiners
Michelle McGinnis, Executive Director
PO Box 25101
Santa Fe, NM 87504
(505) 476-7120/9632

Listing of Doctors Sanctioned by Offense

Substandard Care, Incompetence, or Negligence

DUNN, TERRY
HEDGES, DONALD W
PARADA, JOSEPH A

Criminal Conviction or Plea of Guilty, Nolo Contendere, or No Contest to a Crime

DABBS, THURMAN C
DAVIS, ROBERT C
GRAOR, ROBERT
JARAMILLO, JAMES D
LAMURE, DAVID S
LIES, BERT

Misprescribing or Overprescribing Drugs

BLEAKLY, JEFFREY W
FLOWERS, JEFFERSON
GRENKO, PETE J
MADDOX, A DANIEL
MAGLIOZZI, JOSEPH
NOVOSAD, CHARLES LOUIS
SEWELL, JAMES W

Substance Abuse

ALVORD, REX
BARBER, WAYNE S
BETTINGER, CARL
BIAZAK, ROBERT A
BORRA, HENRY
BUSSEY, WILLIAM J
BYRD, MARCIA
CLEMENTS, MICHAEL P
GARCIA, IGNACIO
GORDON, IRA J
GRAHAM, JACK L
GRAY, ROBERT H
HOLLAND, MARK
HOPPER, JAMES
JUTILA, CHARLOTTE K
LEIDICH, RAYMOND
LOMBARDO, MICHAEL
MCMILLAN, TERRY H
MOORHEAD, PETER
MORO, MICHELE
NEWVILLE, BETTY
OSSORIO, JULIO M
OSTERHOLTZ, ROGER L
ROY, JERRY
SHEFFIELD, JERRY
SHEFFIELD, JERRY W
SMITH, NEILSON
SMITH, PAUL R
SOKOLL, MARTIN D
SWOBODA, JAYE T
TALBOT, WILLIAM A
TRUJILLO, RONALD
VAN OSTEN, KATHLEEN
VAN WORMER, MARK E
WAGNER, JON D
WEBSTER, MICHELE
WHALEN, THOMAS J
YU, ELMER

Caution: This list is designed to be used only in conjunction with the rest of this book which includes additional information on each physician such as license number, date of action and more complete descriptions of the offenses.

ABUD-SANCHEZ, DANILO MD, WAS DISCIPLINED BY NEW MEXICO ON JUNE 12, 1992
DISCIPLINARY ACTION: SURRENDER OF LICENSE
NOTES: IN LIEU OF DISCIPLINARY HEARING.

AKERY, EARL MD, WAS DISCIPLINED BY NEW MEXICO ON APRIL 1, 1998
DISCIPLINARY ACTION: LICENSE REVOCATION
OFFENSE: NONCOMPLIANCE WITH A PROFESSIONAL RULE
NOTES: FAILURE TO RESPOND TO THE BOARD. MAY NEVER REAPPLY.

AKERY, EARL J MD, DATE OF BIRTH MAY 1, 1929 OF PO BOX 711, DEMING, NM, WAS DISCIPLINED BY MEDICARE ON FEBRUARY 13, 1996
DISCIPLINARY ACTION: EXCLUSION FROM THE MEDICARE AND/OR MEDICAID PROGRAM
OFFENSE: DISCIPLINARY ACTION BY ANOTHER STATE OR AGENCY
NOTES: SUSPENDED OR EXCLUDED BY A FEDERAL OR STATE HEALTH CARE PROGRAM FOR REASONS BEARING ON PROFESSIONAL PERFORMANCE.

AKES, LINDY K MD OF HWY 84-64 #17333, TIERRA AMARILLA, NM, WAS DISCIPLINED BY DEA ON DECEMBER 19, 1997
DISCIPLINARY ACTION: SURRENDER OF CONTROLLED SUBSTANCE LICENSE

AKES, LINDY K MD, WAS DISCIPLINED BY NEW MEXICO ON APRIL 1, 1998
DISCIPLINARY ACTION: 6-MONTH LICENSE SUSPENSION; PROBATION
NOTES: PERMANENT PROHIBITION TO PRESCRIBE SCHEDULE II AND III CONTROLLED SUBSTANCES.

ALLON, DAN ERNEST MD, LICENSE NUMBER 136054 OF 141 CAMINO DE LAS CRUCITAS, SANTA FE, NM, WAS DISCIPLINED BY NEW YORK ON SEPTEMBER 10, 1998
DISCIPLINARY ACTION: RESTRICTION PLACED ON LICENSE
OFFENSE: SUBSTANDARD CARE, INCOMPETENCE OR NEGLIGENCE
NOTES: NEGLIGENCE ON MORE THAN ONE OCCASION DURING HIS CARE AND TREATMENT OF THREE SURGICAL PATIENTS. LICENSE LIMITATION PROHIBITING THE PRACTICE OF SURGERY.

ALVORD, REX JR MD OF 407A IRONDALE DRIVE, EL PASO, TX, WAS DISCIPLINED BY NEW MEXICO ON OCTOBER 6, 1994
OFFENSE: SUBSTANCE ABUSE
NOTES: LICENSE PLACED UNDER UNSPECIFIED CONDITIONS. IN 5/98 ALL STIPULATIONS REMOVED; UNRESTRICTED LICENSE.

ANDREWS, MARK LEROY MD, LICENSE NUMBER 18103 OF SAN DIEGO, CA, WAS DISCIPLINED BY OREGON ON APRIL 15, 1999
DISCIPLINARY ACTION: REPRIMAND

ANDREWS, MARK LEROY MD, LICENSE NUMBER G82221 OF ALAMOGORDO, NM, WAS DISCIPLINED BY CALIFORNIA ON OCTOBER 25, 1999
DISCIPLINARY ACTION: REPRIMAND

ANGELES, JAIME MD OF 3616 RIO RANCHO BLVD NW, ALBUQUERQUE, NM, WAS DISCIPLINED BY NEW MEXICO ON DECEMBER 15, 1993
DISCIPLINARY ACTION: REPRIMAND
OFFENSE: PROVIDING FALSE INFORMATION TO THE BOARD OR OTHER HEALTH AGENCY
NOTES: MISINFORMATION ON APPLICATION.

ARMIJO, JOSE B MD, DATE OF BIRTH SEPTEMBER 4, 1953 OF 1331 SAN ANDRES AVENUE NW, ALBUQUERQUE, NM, WAS DISCIPLINED BY MEDICARE ON JULY 17, 1994
DISCIPLINARY ACTION: 36-MONTH EXCLUSION FROM THE MEDICARE AND/OR MEDICAID PROGRAM
OFFENSE: CRIMINAL CONVICTION OR PLEA OF GUILTY, NOLO CONTENDERE, OR NO CONTEST TO A CRIME
NOTES: CONVICTED OF A CRIME RELATED TO THE DELIVERY OF HEALTH CARE OR FINANCIAL MISCONDUCT INVOLVING A GOVERNMENT-OPERATED PROGRAM.

ARMIJO, JOSE BRUNO MD OF 1331 SAN ANDREAS AVENUE, ALBUQUERQUE, NM, WAS DISCIPLINED BY DEA ON SEPTEMBER 12, 1990
DISCIPLINARY ACTION: REVOCATION OF CONTROLLED SUBSTANCE LICENSE
OFFENSE: DISCIPLINARY ACTION BY ANOTHER STATE OR AGENCY
NOTES: NEW MEXICO SUSPENDED HIS LICENSE 8/11/88 BASED ON HIS INABILITY TO PRACTICE WITH REASONABLE SKILL DUE TO EXCESSIVE USE OF ALCOHOL OR DRUGS. HE ALSO OVERPRESCRIBED DILAUDID, A SCHEDULE II NARCOTIC. NEW MEXICO REVOKED HIS LICENSE 6/30/89 SINCE HE PRESCRIBED CONTROLLED SUBSTANCES 107 TIMES FOR NO LEGITIMATE MEDICAL PURPOSE.

ARONSON, KARON S MD, DATE OF BIRTH SEPTEMBER 14, 1948, LICENSE NUMBER 0019791, WAS DISCIPLINED BY COLORADO ON SEPTEMBER 26, 1995
DISCIPLINARY ACTION: EMERGENCY SUSPENSION

ARONSON, KARON S MD, DATE OF BIRTH SEPTEMBER 14, 1948, LICENSE NUMBER 0019791, WAS DISCIPLINED BY COLORADO ON APRIL 11, 1996
DISCIPLINARY ACTION: LICENSE REVOCATION
OFFENSE: PHYSICAL OR MENTAL ILLNESS INHIBITING THE ABILITY TO PRACTICE WITH SKILL AND SAFETY
NOTES: MENTAL DISABILITY.

ARONSON, KARON S MD, WAS DISCIPLINED BY IDAHO ON JUNE 24, 1996
DISCIPLINARY ACTION: LICENSE REVOCATION
NOTES: SUPPLEMENTAL ORDER FOR RECIPROCAL DISCIPLINE.

ARONSON, KARON S MD, WAS DISCIPLINED BY NEW MEXICO ON JANUARY 1, 1997
DISCIPLINARY ACTION: LICENSE REVOCATION
OFFENSE: NONCOMPLIANCE WITH A PROFESSIONAL RULE
NOTES: FAILURE TO NOTIFY THE BOARD OF LICENSE REVOCATION IN COLORADO.

ARONSON, KARON SZELWACH MD, LICENSE NUMBER 0G73845 OF DENVER, CO, WAS DISCIPLINED BY CALIFORNIA ON NOVEMBER 21, 1996
DISCIPLINARY ACTION: LICENSE REVOCATION
OFFENSE: DISCIPLINARY ACTION BY ANOTHER STATE OR AGENCY
NOTES: DISCIPLINED BY COLORADO FOR MENTAL IMPAIRMENT. DEFAULT ACTION.

AUGE, WAYNE K III MD, WAS DISCIPLINED BY NEW MEXICO ON JANUARY 1, 1997

DISCIPLINARY ACTION: RESTRICTION PLACED ON LICENSE
OFFENSE: DISCIPLINARY ACTION BY ANOTHER STATE OR AGENCY

NOTES: LICENSED WITH RESTRICTIONS BASED ON OHIO COURT AND BOARD ACTIONS REGARDING PRESCRIPTIONS. AS OF 2/98, STIPULATIONS REDUCED BY REMOVING REQUIREMENTS FOR THE MONITORED TREATMENT PROGRAM. ON 2/1/99 REDUCED TO BIANNUAL VISITS WITH THE BOARD. ON 8/1/99 GRANTED UNRESTRICTED LICENSE.

AUGE, WAYNE KENNETH II MD, LICENSE NUMBER 64142 OF SANTA FE, NM, WAS DISCIPLINED BY OHIO ON JANUARY 10, 1997
DISCIPLINARY ACTION: EMERGENCY SUSPENSION
OFFENSE: CRIMINAL CONVICTION OR PLEA OF GUILTY, NOLO CONTENDERE, OR NO CONTEST TO A CRIME

NOTES: FOUND GUILTY OF ONE FELONY COUNT OF ILLEGAL PROCESSING OF DRUG DOCUMENTS.

AUGE, WAYNE KENNETH II MD, LICENSE NUMBER 64142 OF SANTA FE, NM, WAS DISCIPLINED BY OHIO ON JULY 1, 1997
DISCIPLINARY ACTION: LICENSE SUSPENSION; PROBATION
OFFENSE: CRIMINAL CONVICTION OR PLEA OF GUILTY, NOLO CONTENDERE, OR NO CONTEST TO A CRIME

NOTES: FOUND GUILTY OF ONE FELONY COUNT OF ILLEGAL PROCESSING OF DRUG DOCUMENTS AND VIOLATION OF BOARD RULES PERTAINING TO UTILIZATION OF STEROIDS AND SPECIFIED HORMONES. MEDICAL LICENSE SUSPENDED FOR AT LEAST TWO YEARS; CONDITIONS FOR REINSTATEMENT AND SUBSEQUENT PROBATIONARY TERMS, CONDITIONS, AND LIMITATIONS FOR AT LEAST THREE YEARS ESTABLISHED. NOTICE OF APPEAL OF THIS ORDER FILED IN FRANKLIN COUNTY COURT OF COMMON PLEAS ON 7/15/97. BY DECISION FILED ON 1/6/98 THE COURT AFFIRMED BOARD'S ORDER. NOTICE OF APPEAL TO TENTH DISTRICT COURT OF APPEALS FILED ON 2/11/98. ON 11/17/98 THIS COURT AFFIRMED THE DECISION OF THE LOWER COURT WHICH HAD UPHELD THE BOARD'S ORDER.

AUGE, WAYNE KENNETH II MD, LICENSE NUMBER G80901 OF SANTA FE, NM, WAS DISCIPLINED BY CALIFORNIA ON AUGUST 24, 1998
DISCIPLINARY ACTION: 6-MONTH LICENSE SUSPENSION; 78-MONTH PROBATION
OFFENSE: DISCIPLINARY ACTION BY ANOTHER STATE OR AGENCY

NOTES: DISCIPLINED BY NEW MEXICO FOLLOWING HIS CRIMINAL CONVICTION FOR WRITING A PRESCRIPTION FOR WINSTROL, A SCHEDULE III STEROID, FOR A FICTITIOUS PATIENT. REVOCATION STAYED.

BAILLIE, JON-ERIC MD, WAS DISCIPLINED BY NEW MEXICO ON JANUARY 1, 1997
DISCIPLINARY ACTION: SURRENDER OF CONTROLLED SUBSTANCE LICENSE; RESTRICTION PLACED ON LICENSE
OFFENSE: PROFESSIONAL MISCONDUCT

NOTES: INAPPROPRIATE DRUG USAGE; LICENSE LIMITED INCLUDING THE SURRENDER OF HIS DEA PERMIT. AS OF 8/98, STIPULATIONS AMENDED TO ALLOW HIM TO APPLY FOR LIMITED DEA PERMIT; SCHEDULES III, IV, AND V ONLY. ON 5/1/99 BOARD AMENDED STIPULATIONS FOR SUBSTANCE ABUSE TO ALLOW HIM TO BE AN ACTIVE PARTICIPANT IN THE IDAHO PHYSICIAN RECOVERY NETWORK WITH PROGRESS REPORTS BEING SENT TO NEW MEXICO; SHALL BE REQUIRED TO APPEAR BEFORE THE BOARD ON AN ANNUAL BASIS; ALL OTHER STIPULATIONS REMAIN THE SAME.

BARBER, WAYNE S MD, WAS DISCIPLINED BY NEW MEXICO ON JANUARY 1, 1997
OFFENSE: SUBSTANCE ABUSE

NOTES: ISSUED NEW MEXICO LICENSE WITH STANDARD STIPULATIONS FOR SUBSTANCE ABUSE. AS OF 2/98, ALL STIPULATIONS REMOVED; UNRESTRICTED LICENSE.

BARRICKMAN, LES L DO, DATE OF BIRTH NOVEMBER 2, 1953, LICENSE NUMBER 0001988 OF 938 TALWRN COURT, IOWA CITY, IA, WAS DISCIPLINED BY IOWA ON JUNE 3, 1993
DISCIPLINARY ACTION: 48-MONTH PROBATION; FINE
OFFENSE: CRIMINAL CONVICTION OR PLEA OF GUILTY, NOLO CONTENDERE, OR NO CONTEST TO A CRIME

NOTES: ALLEGATIONS OF CRIMINAL CONVICTIONS RELATED TO ILLEGAL POSSESSION OF CONTROLLED DRUGS. $5,000 CIVIL PENALTY.

BARRICKMAN, LES L DO, DATE OF BIRTH NOVEMBER 2, 1953, LICENSE NUMBER 0099794, WAS DISCIPLINED BY NEW MEXICO ON FEBRUARY 12, 1994
DISCIPLINARY ACTION: PROBATION
OFFENSE: DISCIPLINARY ACTION BY ANOTHER STATE OR AGENCY

NOTES: ACTION IN ANOTHER STATE. ON 10/21/95 A PERMANENT LICENSE WITH FULL PRIVILEGES ISSUED.

BARRICKMAN, LES L DO, DATE OF BIRTH NOVEMBER 2, 1953, LICENSE NUMBER 0002676 OF 2316 CAMIO DE LOS ARTESANOS NW, ALBUQUERQUE, NM, WAS DISCIPLINED BY ARIZONA ON MAY 13, 1994
DISCIPLINARY ACTION: MONITORING OF PHYSICIAN PERFORMANCE
OFFENSE: DISCIPLINARY ACTION BY ANOTHER STATE OR AGENCY

NOTES: ACTION IN NEW MEXICO ON 2/12/94 BASED ON TWO GUILTY PLEAS TO POSSESSION OF A CONTROLLED SUBSTANCE ON 1/15/93 IN IOWA; ON 6/3/93 IOWA LICENSE PLACED ON PROBATION BASED ON THESE ACTIONS. AGREEMENT WITH ARIZONA: SHALL COMPLY WITH THE NEW MEXICO BOARD ORDER; SHALL MEET WITH THE BOARD UPON REQUEST; SHALL AUTHORIZE NEW MEXICO TO RELEASE TO THE BOARD UPON REQUEST A RECORD OF COMPLIANCE WITH THE TERMS AND CONDITIONS IN NEW MEXICO; IF HE CHOOSES TO PRACTICE IN ARIZONA BOARD RESERVES THE RIGHT TO REVIEW THE COMPLIANCE WITH THIS ORDER.

BARRICKMAN, LES L DO, DATE OF BIRTH NOVEMBER 2, 1953, LICENSE NUMBER 0025600 OF IOWA CITY, IA, WAS DISCIPLINED BY COLORADO ON MAY 20, 1994
DISCIPLINARY ACTION: SURRENDER OF LICENSE
OFFENSE: DISCIPLINARY ACTION BY ANOTHER STATE OR AGENCY

NOTES: BASED ON IOWA DISCIPLINE. NO UNPROFESSIONAL CONDUCT IDENTIFIED. PERMANENT LICENSE SURRENDER.

BARRICKMAN, LES L DO OF HI, WAS DISCIPLINED BY IOWA ON MAY 22, 1997
DISCIPLINARY ACTION: SURRENDER OF LICENSE
OFFENSE: DISCIPLINARY ACTION BY ANOTHER STATE OR AGENCY

NOTES: CHARGED WITH VIOLATING THE TERMS OF A PREVIOUS AGREEMENT WITH THE BOARD AS WELL AS IN CONNECTION WITH DISCIPLINE TAKEN BY ARIZONA.

BARRICKMAN, LES L DO, LICENSE NUMBER 782 OF 509 UNIVERSITY AVENUE, #104, HONOLULU, HI, WAS DISCIPLINED BY HAWAII ON

DECEMBER 11, 1998
DISCIPLINARY ACTION: FINE
OFFENSE: DISCIPLINARY ACTION BY ANOTHER STATE OR AGENCY

NOTES: FAILED TO TIMELY INFORM THE HAWAII BOARD OF DISCIPLINARY ACTIONS AGAINST HIS LICENSE IN ARIZONA AND IOWA; ACTION ALSO TAKEN IN NEW MEXICO. $500 FINE

BASHIR, NAIM MD, WAS DISCIPLINED BY NEW MEXICO ON FEBRUARY 1, 1999

NOTES: LICENSE ISSUED WITH STIPULATIONS FOR CONTINUED MEDICAL CARE.

BEALE, MARK MD OF LAS VEGAS MEDICAL CENTER, LAS VEGAS, NM, WAS DISCIPLINED BY NEW MEXICO ON JUNE 15, 1993
DISCIPLINARY ACTION: REQUIRED TO TAKE ADDITIONAL MEDICAL EDUCATION

NOTES: LICENSE ISSUED UNDER CONDITIONS: ADDITIONAL CONTINUING MEDICAL EDUCATION ORDERED. CONDITIONS FULFILLED 11/93.

BENNETT, JOHN II MD, WAS DISCIPLINED BY NEW MEXICO ON APRIL 1, 1998
DISCIPLINARY ACTION: SURRENDER OF LICENSE

NOTES: VOLUNTARY SURRENDER AND MAY NEVER REAPPLY.

BERGSRUD, ROBERT MD OF 5419 LOVINGTON HWY, HOBBS, NM, WAS DISCIPLINED BY NEW MEXICO ON DECEMBER 7, 1993

NOTES: LICENSE ISSUED UNDER CONDITIONS: THERAPY ORDERED. CONDITIONS FULFILLED 5/20/94.

BETTINGER, CARL MD, WAS DISCIPLINED BY NEW MEXICO ON JANUARY 1, 1997
DISCIPLINARY ACTION: RESTRICTION PLACED ON LICENSE
OFFENSE: SUBSTANCE ABUSE

NOTES: DRUG USE.

BIAZAK, ROBERT A MD, WAS DISCIPLINED BY NEW MEXICO ON JANUARY 1, 1997
DISCIPLINARY ACTION: SURRENDER OF LICENSE
OFFENSE: SUBSTANCE ABUSE

NOTES: VOLUNTARY SURRENDER OF LICENSE UNDER THE TERMS OF THE IMPAIRED PHYSICIAN HEALTH CARE PROVIDER ACT FOR SUBSTANCE ABUSE.

BIAZAK, ROBERT A MD, WAS DISCIPLINED BY NEW MEXICO ON FEBRUARY 1, 1998
DISCIPLINARY ACTION: LICENSE REINSTATEMENT
OFFENSE: SUBSTANCE ABUSE

NOTES: LICENSE RESTORED FROM VOLUNTARY SURRENDER UNDER THE TERMS OF THE IMPAIRED HEALTH CARE PROVIDERS ACT. LICENSE PLACED UNDER STANDARD STIPULATIONS FOR SUBSTANCE ABUSE.

BISLA, RANJIT MD, WAS DISCIPLINED BY NEW MEXICO ON MARCH 20, 1995
DISCIPLINARY ACTION: LICENSE REVOCATION
OFFENSE: DISCIPLINARY ACTION BY ANOTHER STATE OR AGENCY

NOTES: REVOCATION BY ANOTHER STATE; FAILURE TO RESPOND.

BLEAKLY, JEFFREY W MD OF 8800 MONTGOMERY NE, ALBUQUERQUE, NM, WAS DISCIPLINED BY NEW MEXICO ON DECEMBER 22, 1993
DISCIPLINARY ACTION: LICENSE REVOCATION
OFFENSE: OVERPRESCRIBING OR MISPRESCRIBING DRUGS

NOTES: UNPROFESSIONAL CONDUCT; INJUDICIOUS PRESCRIBING.

BORRA, HENRY MD, WAS DISCIPLINED BY NEW MEXICO ON AUGUST 1, 1996
OFFENSE: SUBSTANCE ABUSE

NOTES: SUBSTANCE ABUSE. ISSUED LICENSE WITH STANDARD STIPULATIONS.

BORRA, HENRY MD, WAS DISCIPLINED BY NEW MEXICO ON JANUARY 1, 1997
DISCIPLINARY ACTION: SURRENDER OF LICENSE
OFFENSE: SUBSTANCE ABUSE

NOTES: VOLUNTARY SURRENDER OF LICENSE UNDER THE TERMS OF THE IMPAIRED PHYSICIAN HEALTH CARE PROVIDER ACT FOR SUBSTANCE ABUSE.

BORRA, HENRY MD, WAS DISCIPLINED BY NEW MEXICO ON FEBRUARY 1, 1998
DISCIPLINARY ACTION: LICENSE REINSTATEMENT
OFFENSE: SUBSTANCE ABUSE

NOTES: LICENSE RESTORED FROM VOLUNTARY SURRENDER UNDER THE TERMS OF THE IMPAIRED HEALTH CARE PROVIDERS ACT. LICENSE PLACED UNDER STANDARD STIPULATIONS FOR SUBSTANCE ABUSE.

BROOKS, BANCROFT MD OF ALBUQUERQUE, NM, WAS DISCIPLINED BY MISSOURI ON NOVEMBER 2, 1992
DISCIPLINARY ACTION: LICENSE REVOCATION
OFFENSE: DISCIPLINARY ACTION BY ANOTHER STATE OR AGENCY

NOTES: NO REAPPLICATION FOR FIVE YEARS.

BROWN, DAVID M MD, WAS DISCIPLINED BY NEW MEXICO ON JUNE 12, 1992
DISCIPLINARY ACTION: FINE; REPRIMAND
OFFENSE: PROFESSIONAL MISCONDUCT

NOTES: IMPROPER SUPERVISION OF A PHYSICIANS ASSISTANT.

BROWN, DAVID MICHAEL MD, LICENSE NUMBER 17687 OF PUYALLUP, WA, WAS DISCIPLINED BY WASHINGTON ON JUNE 5, 1999
DISCIPLINARY ACTION: PROBATION; FINE
OFFENSE: SEXUAL ABUSE OF OR SEXUAL MISCONDUCT WITH A PATIENT

NOTES: SEXUAL CONTACT WITH A PATIENT. ON PROBATION UNTIL COMPLETION OF SEVEN CONTINUING MEDICAL EDUCATION HOURS AND PAYMENT OF A FINE. ON 9/9/99 REQUEST FOR RECONSIDERATION DENIED.

BRUDER, MURRAY MD, WAS DISCIPLINED BY NEW MEXICO ON MAY 1, 1999
DISCIPLINARY ACTION: RESTRICTION PLACED ON LICENSE

NOTES: MAY NOT PRACTICE OBSTETRICS AND DESIGNATED GYNECOLOGICAL PROCEDURES FOR AS LONG AS HE HOLDS A NEW MEXICO LICENSE.

BULL, KENNETH H MD, WAS DISCIPLINED BY NEW MEXICO ON FEBRUARY 1, 1996
DISCIPLINARY ACTION: REPRIMAND
OFFENSE: PROFESSIONAL MISCONDUCT

NOTES: UNPROFESSIONAL CONDUCT.

BURSTEIN, ERIC MD, DATE OF BIRTH DECEMBER 22, 1951, LICENSE NUMBER 0041396 OF 6409 TURNBERRY LANE, NE, ALBUQUERQUE, NM, WAS DISCIPLINED BY OHIO ON MAY 21, 1992
DISCIPLINARY ACTION: LICENSE REVOCATION
OFFENSE: SEXUAL ABUSE OF OR SEXUAL MISCONDUCT WITH A PATIENT

NOTES: FAILURE TO CONFORM TO MINIMAL STANDARDS OF CARE AND VIOLATION OF CODE OF PROFESSIONAL ETHICS BASED ON DOCTOR'S HAVING ENGAGED IN A SEXUAL RELATIONSHIP WITH PATIENT WHILE HE WAS HER TREATING PSYCHIATRIST. PERMANENT REVOCATION. APPEAL FILED IN FRANKLIN COUNTY COURT OF COMMON PLEAS ON 06/04/92; LIMITED STAY PROHIBITING HIM FROM PRACTICING IN OHIO GRANTED ON 7/6/92. 3/11/93 DECISION AFFIRMED 5/13/92 ORDER OF PERMANENT REVOCATION. REVOCATION EFFECTIVE 4/1/93.

BURSTEIN, ERIC MD OF 4724 HOMESTEAD NW, ALBUQUERQUE, NM, WAS DISCIPLINED BY NEW MEXICO ON AUGUST 16, 1993
DISCIPLINARY ACTION: LICENSE REVOCATION
OFFENSE: PROFESSIONAL MISCONDUCT

BURSTEIN, ERIC A MD, WAS DISCIPLINED BY NEW MEXICO ON SEPTEMBER 14, 1992
DISCIPLINARY ACTION: LICENSE REVOCATION

BURT, HUGH A MD, DATE OF BIRTH FEBRUARY 6, 1957 OF 405 CIRCLE DRIVE, CLOVIS, NM, WAS DISCIPLINED BY MEDICARE ON DECEMBER 30, 1996
DISCIPLINARY ACTION: EXCLUSION FROM THE MEDICARE AND/OR MEDICAID PROGRAM
OFFENSE: NONCOMPLIANCE WITH A PROFESSIONAL RULE

NOTES: DEFAULTED ON PUBLIC HEALTH SERVICE EDUCATION LOAN. INDEFINITE EXCLUSION. REINSTATED ON 2/24/97.

BUSSEY, WILLIAM J MD, DATE OF BIRTH DECEMBER 23, 1962, LICENSE NUMBER 0032929 OF FT. COLLINS, CO, WAS DISCIPLINED BY COLORADO ON JUNE 17, 1994
DISCIPLINARY ACTION: LICENSE REVOCATION
OFFENSE: FAILURE TO COMPLY WITH PREVIOUS BOARD ORDER

NOTES: VIOLATION OF BOARD ORDER.

BUSSEY, WILLIAM J MD, DATE OF BIRTH DECEMBER 23, 1962 OF 1306 ASH DRIVE, FT COLLINS, CO, WAS DISCIPLINED BY MEDICARE ON DECEMBER 5, 1994
DISCIPLINARY ACTION: EXCLUSION FROM THE MEDICARE AND/OR MEDICAID PROGRAM
OFFENSE: DISCIPLINARY ACTION BY ANOTHER STATE OR AGENCY

NOTES: LICENSE REVOKED FOR REASONS BEARING ON PROFESSIONAL COMPETENCE. REINSTATED ON 12/13/94.

BUSSEY, WILLIAM J MD OF 1306 ASH DRIVE, FT COLLINS, CO, WAS DISCIPLINED BY NEW MEXICO ON JANUARY 1, 1997
OFFENSE: SUBSTANCE ABUSE

NOTES: LICENSE ISSUED UNDER UNSPECIFIED CONDITIONS. IN 1997 STIPULATIONS FOR SUBSTANCE ABUSE REDUCED TO ANNUAL VISITS WITH THE BOARD. IN 11/98 REMOVED ALL STIPULATIONS FOR SUBSTANCE ABUSE; UNRESTRICTED LICENSE.

BUSSEY, WILLIAM J MD, DATE OF BIRTH DECEMBER 23, 1962, LICENSE NUMBER 36582, WAS DISCIPLINED BY COLORADO ON OCTOBER 9, 1997
DISCIPLINARY ACTION: 60-MONTH PROBATION; MONITORING OF PHYSICIAN PERFORMANCE

NOTES: NO UNPROFESSIONAL CONDUCT IDENTIFIED. PROBATIONARY TERMS INCLUDE: ABSTINENCE FROM ADDICTIVE SUBSTANCES, TREATMENT MONITORING AND PRACTICE MONITORING.

BUSSEY, WILLIAM J MD, WAS DISCIPLINED BY IOWA ON MARCH 12, 1998
DISCIPLINARY ACTION: REQUIRED TO ENTER AN IMPAIRED PHYSICIAN PROGRAM OR SUBSTANCE ABUSE TREATMENT; MONITORING OF PHYSICIAN PERFORMANCE

NOTES: RECEIVED AN IOWA MEDICAL LICENSE UNDER TERMS AND CONDITIONS: PROHIBITED FROM USING ALCOHOL OR OTHER CONTROLLED SUBSTANCES NOT PRESCRIBED BY A QUALIFIED HEALTH CARE PROVIDER; REQUIRED TO SEEK CONTINUING SUBSTANCE ABUSE TREATMENT, FILE REGULAR REPORTS ON HIS PROGRESS AND PROVIDE BLOOD OR URINE SAMPLES ON DEMAND.

BYRD, MARCIA MD, WAS DISCIPLINED BY NEW MEXICO ON JANUARY 1, 1997
OFFENSE: SUBSTANCE ABUSE

NOTES: ISSUED NEW MEXICO LICENSE WITH STANDARD STIPULATIONS FOR SUBSTANCE ABUSE.

CAMERO, ELAINE MD, WAS DISCIPLINED BY NEW MEXICO ON FEBRUARY 9, 1990

NOTES: LICENSE STIPULATED.

CANTU, ADEX H MD, WAS DISCIPLINED BY NEW MEXICO ON JANUARY 1, 1997
DISCIPLINARY ACTION: RESTRICTION PLACED ON LICENSE
OFFENSE: PROFESSIONAL MISCONDUCT

NOTES: FRAUDULENT TREATMENT. ENTERED INTO AN AGREEMENT THAT HE WOULD NO LONGER PERFORM INTRAVENOUS HYDROGEN PEROXIDE THERAPY. BOARD DISMISSED NOTICE OF CONTEMPLATED ACTION.

CARMODY, EUGENE MD, DATE OF BIRTH MARCH 30, 1940 OF 5021 SAN MATEO LANE, ALBUQUERQUE, NM, WAS DISCIPLINED BY MEDICARE ON JUNE 9, 1992
DISCIPLINARY ACTION: 60-MONTH EXCLUSION FROM THE MEDICARE AND/OR MEDICAID PROGRAM
OFFENSE: CRIMINAL CONVICTION OR PLEA OF GUILTY, NOLO CONTENDERE, OR NO CONTEST TO A CRIME

NOTES: PROGRAM-RELATED CONVICTION.

CARTER, H EUGENE MD, LICENSE NUMBER 0011460, WAS DISCIPLINED BY ARIZONA ON JULY 21, 1995
DISCIPLINARY ACTION: LICENSE REVOCATION
OFFENSE: SUBSTANDARD CARE, INCOMPETENCE OR NEGLIGENCE

NOTES: BETWEEN 10/89 AND 11/94, VIOLATIONS RELATING TO HIS PRACTICE OF PAIN MANAGEMENT AND OUTPATIENT ANESTHESIA IN SIX PATIENTS. ENGAGED IN MEDICAL RECORDS VIOLATIONS IN THAT HE CREATED AND MAINTAINED MEDICAL RECORDS WHICH HE DID NOT PREPARE CONTEMPORANEOUSLY; MECHANICALLY REPRODUCED SIGNATURES, CREATED RECORDS OF TREATMENT, WHICH WERE NOT ACCURATE AS TO THE INJECTION SITES FOR THE REGIONAL ANESTHETIC PROCEDURES AND THE DRUGS USED

ARE NOT RECORDED, MAINTAINED INCOMPLETE OFFICE RECORDS WITH THE EXPECTATION THAT SUPPLEMENTARY TREATMENT INFORMATION COULD BE OBTAINED; NO EVIDENCE THAT HE DID SO; MAINTAINED INCOMPLETE TREATMENT RECORDS, CONTAINING INSUFFICIENT INFORMATION FOR ANOTHER PRACTITIONER TO ASSUME CONTINUITY OF CARE; FAILURE TO RECORD A TREATMENT PLAN IN THE MEDICAL RECORDS WHEREBY THERE IS NO JUSTIFICATION FOR THE TREATMENTS PROVIDED; FAILURE TO UPDATE TREATMENT RECORDS; FAILURE TO DOCUMENT ADVICE AND CAUTIONARY WARNINGS TO PATIENTS; CHARGING VIOLATIONS FOR THESE SIX PATIENTS, FEES WERE UNREASONABLE OVER EXTENDED LENGTHS OF TIME AND NOT JUSTIFIED IN THE MEDICAL RECORDS. ENGAGED IN PRACTICE THAT IS OR MIGHT BE HARMFUL OR DANGEROUS TO THE HEALTH OF THE PATIENT IN THAT HE FAILED TO SEEK A PSYCHOLOGICAL EVALUATION OF THREE PATIENTS PRIOR TO IMPLANTING A DORSAL COLUMN STIMULATOR; FOR THREE PATIENTS, USED REGIONAL ANESTHETIC TECHNIQUES WHICH WERE NOT MEDICALLY NECESSARY AS SET FORTH IN MEDICARE GUIDELINES; AND PERFORMED A CAUDAL EPIDUREAL BLOCK ON A PATIENT WHICH LEFT PATIENT WEAK AND UNABLE TO WALK AND WHICH RESULTED IN HER HOSPITALIZATION. ENGAGED IN PRESCRIBING PRACTICES WHICH ARE OR MIGHT BE HARMFUL OR DANGEROUS TO THE HEALTH OF TWO PATIENTS IN THAT HE PRESCRIBED NUMEROUS NARCOTIC MEDICATIONS, INCLUDING ROXICET, HYDROCET, DEMEROL, LORCET AND DURAGESIC PATCHES FOR OTHER THAN ACCEPTED THERAPEUTIC PURPOSES. AS MEDICAL DIRECTOR OF PAIN GROUP, FAILED TO SUPERVISE THE MEDICAL TREATMENT PROVIDED TO TWO PATIENTS BY ANOTHER PHYSICIAN WHO WAS PERMITTED TO PERFORM A MYRIAD OF REGIONAL ANESTHETIC PROCEDURES WHICH WERE NOT MEDICALLY NECESSARY AND FAILED TO DIRECT PHYSICIAN'S CLINICAL ACTIONS. ON 9/23/98 ARIZONA SUPREME COURT DENIED HIS PETITION FOR REVIEW AND AFFIRMED BOARD'S REVOCATION ORDER.

CARTER, H EUGENE MD, WAS DISCIPLINED BY NEW MEXICO ON MAY 1, 1996
DISCIPLINARY ACTION: LICENSE REVOCATION
OFFENSE: NONCOMPLIANCE WITH A PROFESSIONAL RULE

NOTES: FAILED TO REPORT REVOCATION IN ANOTHER STATE.

CHALMERS, THOMAS MD, WAS DISCIPLINED BY NEW MEXICO ON NOVEMBER 1, 1996

NOTES: MUST NOTIFY THE BOARD IN WRITING 90 DAYS PRIOR TO PRACTICING UNDER NEW MEXICO LICENSE OR RETURNING TO NEW MEXICO.

CHESTER, ALVIN A MD, WAS DISCIPLINED BY NEW MEXICO ON DECEMBER 2, 1992
DISCIPLINARY ACTION: LICENSE REVOCATION

CHESTER, ALVIN A MD, LICENSE NUMBER 0102512 OF 1305 TIJERAS AVENUE NW, ALBUQUERQUE, NM, WAS DISCIPLINED BY NEW YORK ON NOVEMBER 30, 1993
DISCIPLINARY ACTION: LICENSE REVOCATION
OFFENSE: DISCIPLINARY ACTION BY ANOTHER STATE OR AGENCY

NOTES: LICENSE REVOKED BY THE NEW MEXICO BOARD.

CHESTER, ALVIN A MD, DATE OF BIRTH JANUARY 16, 1937 OF 6611 W PEORIA AVENUE #5, GLENDALE, AZ, WAS DISCIPLINED BY MEDICARE ON APRIL 5, 1995
DISCIPLINARY ACTION: EXCLUSION FROM THE MEDICARE AND/OR MEDICAID PROGRAM
OFFENSE: DISCIPLINARY ACTION BY ANOTHER STATE OR AGENCY

NOTES: LICENSE REVOKED FOR REASONS BEARING ON PROFESSIONAL PERFORMANCE.

CLEMENTS, MICHAEL P MD, WAS DISCIPLINED BY NEW MEXICO ON NOVEMBER 1, 1996
OFFENSE: SUBSTANCE ABUSE

NOTES: SUBSTANCE ABUSE. ISSUED LICENSE WITH STANDARD NEW MEXICO STIPULATIONS. IN 8/98 ORDER AMENDED; STIPULATIONS FOR SUBSTANCE ABUSE REDUCED TO BI-ANNUALLY.

COHN, FREDERICK MD OF ALBUQUERQUE, NM, WAS DISCIPLINED BY ILLINOIS ON AUGUST 1, 1992
DISCIPLINARY ACTION: PROBATION
OFFENSE: DISCIPLINARY ACTION BY ANOTHER STATE OR AGENCY

NOTES: DISCIPLINED BY NEW MEXICO FOR GROSS NEGLIGENCE IN PERFORMING AN ABORTION. LICENSE ISSUED AND PLACED ON INDEFINITE PROBATION.

COHN, FREDERICK MD, DATE OF BIRTH APRIL 11, 1932, LICENSE NUMBER 0030026 OF ALBUQUERQUE, NM, WAS DISCIPLINED BY KENTUCKY ON SEPTEMBER 30, 1993
DISCIPLINARY ACTION: 24-MONTH PROBATION; RESTRICTION PLACED ON LICENSE
OFFENSE: DISCIPLINARY ACTION BY ANOTHER STATE OR AGENCY

NOTES: ACTION TAKEN BY NEW MEXICO BOARD. CONDITIONS OF PROBATION: MAY NOT PRACTICE OBSTETRIC MEDICINE OR PERFORM/ASSIST ABORTIONS; NO GYNECOLOGIC SURGERY WITHOUT PRIOR CONSULTATION AND ASSISTANCE DURING SURGERY.

COHN, FREDERICK MD, LICENSE NUMBER 0065955 OF ALBUQUERQUE, NM, WAS DISCIPLINED BY OHIO ON OCTOBER 13, 1993
DISCIPLINARY ACTION: RESTRICTION PLACED ON LICENSE
OFFENSE: DISCIPLINARY ACTION BY ANOTHER STATE OR AGENCY

NOTES: PRIOR ACTIONS BY NEW MEXICO, CALIFORNIA AND ILLINOIS MEDICAL BOARDS DUE TO HIS PERFORMANCE OF AN ABORTION ON A 16-YEAR-OLD GIRL WITHOUT CONDUCTING AN ADEQUATE DIAGNOSTIC WORKUP, WHICH WOULD HAVE REVEALED THAT THE PATIENT WAS 28 WEEKS PREGNANT, RATHER THAN TWO MONTHS PREGNANT AS BOTH THE PATIENT AND HER MOTHER HAD PURPORTED. LICENSURE GRANTED, BUT LICENSE PERMANENTLY LIMITED TO PROHIBIT HIM FROM AIDING, ABETTING, ASSISTING OR PERFORMING ABORTIONS AND FROM ENGAGING IN THE PRACTICE OF OBSTETRICS AND GYNECOLOGY, EXCEPT IN THE EVENT OF LIFE THREATENING EMERGENCY.

COHN, FREDERICK MD OF ALBUQUERQUE, NM, WAS DISCIPLINED BY MISSOURI ON FEBRUARY 18, 1994
DISCIPLINARY ACTION: DENIAL OF NEW LICENSE
OFFENSE: DISCIPLINARY ACTION BY ANOTHER STATE OR AGENCY

COHN, FREDERICK MD, WAS DISCIPLINED BY NEW MEXICO ON JANUARY 1, 1997
DISCIPLINARY ACTION: RESTRICTION PLACED ON LICENSE

NOTES: STIPULATED AGREEMENT: AS LONG AS HE HOLDS A LICENSE TO PRACTICE IN NEW MEXICO, HE SHALL NOT PRACTICE OBSTETRIC MEDICINE, AND SHALL NOT AID, ABET, ASSIST OR PERFORM ABORTIONS. IN 1997 PROBATION COMPLETED; LIFETIME

RESTRICTIONS FROM PRACTICING OBSTETRICS FOR AS LONG AS HE HOLDS A NEW MEXICO LICENSE.

CONNELLY, CHRISTOPHER F DO, LICENSE NUMBER 0075983, WAS DISCIPLINED BY NEW MEXICO ON APRIL 8, 1991
DISCIPLINARY ACTION: SURRENDER OF LICENSE
OFFENSE: NONCOMPLIANCE WITH A PROFESSIONAL RULE

NOTES: FAILED TO APPEAR BEFORE THE BOARD. VOLUNTARY SURRENDER.

CONNELLY, CHRISTOPHER FOUST DO, DATE OF BIRTH MARCH 6, 1955 OF 3675 LAKEVIEW ROAD, CARSON CITY, NV, WAS DISCIPLINED BY MEDICARE ON FEBRUARY 19, 1998
DISCIPLINARY ACTION: EXCLUSION FROM THE MEDICARE AND/OR MEDICAID PROGRAM
OFFENSE: NONCOMPLIANCE WITH A PROFESSIONAL RULE

NOTES: DEFAULTED ON PUBLIC HEALTH SERVICE EDUCATION LOAN.

CORDON, RICARDO MD, WAS DISCIPLINED BY NEW MEXICO
DISCIPLINARY ACTION: LICENSE SUSPENSION

NOTES: LICENSE SUSPENDED UNTIL SPEX IS SUCCESSFULLY TAKEN. IN 1997 ALL STIPULATIONS REMOVED REGARDING LICENSE RE-QUALIFICATION AND SUSPENSION TERMINATED.

CORDON, RICARDO M MD, LICENSE NUMBER 0015499, WAS DISCIPLINED BY ARIZONA ON JULY 15, 1993
OFFENSE: DISCIPLINARY ACTION BY ANOTHER STATE OR AGENCY

NOTES: FAILURE TO REPORT RESTRICTION IN PRIVILEGES BY THE MILITARY IN 1989 ON HIS LICENSE RENEWAL FORM; FAILED THE SPEX EXAMINATION IN ARIZONA. SHALL NOT ENGAGE IN THE PRACTICE OF MEDICINE IN ARIZONA UNTIL HE HAS FIRST ADVISED THE BOARD OF HIS INTENTION TO DO SO. THE BOARD MAY REQUIRE ADDITIONAL EXAMS OR INVESTIGATION IN ORDER TO SATISFY ITSELF THAT HE IS MEDICALLY COMPETENT TO PRACTICE.

CORDON, RICARDO M MD OF 1211 E AZTEC, GALLUP, NM, WAS DISCIPLINED BY DEA ON MAY 17, 1995
DISCIPLINARY ACTION: SURRENDER OF CONTROLLED SUBSTANCE LICENSE
OFFENSE: DISCIPLINARY ACTION BY ANOTHER STATE OR AGENCY

NOTES: STATE BOARD.

CORDOVA, EDMUND S MD, WAS DISCIPLINED BY NEW MEXICO ON FEBRUARY 16, 1995
DISCIPLINARY ACTION: LICENSE REVOCATION
OFFENSE: PROFESSIONAL MISCONDUCT

NOTES: SEXUAL MISCONDUCT; UNPROFESSIONAL CONDUCT.

CORDOVA, EDMUND S MD, LICENSE NUMBER 0D25096 OF 4231 POSTAL COURT, STE 102, PASADENA, MD, WAS DISCIPLINED BY MARYLAND ON MARCH 22, 1995
DISCIPLINARY ACTION: EMERGENCY SUSPENSION
OFFENSE: DISCIPLINARY ACTION BY ANOTHER STATE OR AGENCY

NOTES: BASED ON REVOCATION OF LICENSE IN NEW MEXICO FOR SEXUAL MISCONDUCT WITH PATIENTS IN THAT STATE AND A 1984 REPRIMAND BY THE U.S. ARMY FOR "UNPROFESSIONAL AND INDECENT CONDUCT DURING HIS MEDICAL EXAMINATION OF SEVERAL WOMEN PATIENTS;" AND A 1986 REPRIMAND FROM THE ARMY FOR UNPROFESSIONAL CONDUCT IN THE PRACTICE OF MEDICINE.

CORDOVA, EDMUND S MD OF 4231 POSTAL COURT, PASADENA, MD, WAS DISCIPLINED BY DEA ON APRIL 24, 1995
DISCIPLINARY ACTION: SURRENDER OF CONTROLLED SUBSTANCE LICENSE
OFFENSE: DISCIPLINARY ACTION BY ANOTHER STATE OR AGENCY

NOTES: STATE BOARD.

CORDOVA, EDMUND S MD, LICENSE NUMBER 0D25096 OF 7669 RONA COURT, APT. J, GLEN BURNIE, MD, WAS DISCIPLINED BY MARYLAND ON AUGUST 1, 1995
DISCIPLINARY ACTION: SURRENDER OF LICENSE
OFFENSE: DISCIPLINARY ACTION BY ANOTHER STATE OR AGENCY

NOTES: INVESTIGATION CONDUCTED BASED ON ACTIONS THE UNITED STATES ARMY TOOK AGAINST HIM FOR UNPROFESSIONAL AND INDECENT CONDUCT DURING MEDICAL EXAMINATIONS OF WOMEN PATIENTS AT ARMY HOSPITALS IN ALASKA AND OKLAHOMA; ALSO HAD LICENSE REVOKED IN NEW MEXICO FOR SEXUAL ABUSE OF TWO WOMEN PATIENTS.

CORDOVA, EDMUND S MD, LICENSE NUMBER 0016849 OF PO BOX 1296, PASADENA, MD, WAS DISCIPLINED BY OKLAHOMA ON OCTOBER 2, 1995
DISCIPLINARY ACTION: LICENSE REVOCATION
OFFENSE: DISCIPLINARY ACTION BY ANOTHER STATE OR AGENCY

NOTES: ACTION IN NEW MEXICO ON 2/23/95 WHICH REVOKED HIS LICENSE FOR INAPPROPRIATE CONDUCT WITH TWO FEMALE PATIENTS. IN 1990 WHILE IN THE MILITARY FORCES OF THE UNITED STATES, THE MILITARY RECEIVED COMPLAINTS THAT HE HAD FONDLED WOMEN IN ALASKA AND OKLAHOMA AND THAT THE COMPLAINTS HAD ADDRESSED HIS USE OF A STETHOSCOPE WHEN EXAMINING FEMALE PATIENTS' HEARTS. THE MILITARY REQUIRED HIM TO HAVE CHAPERONES PRESENT FOR EXAMINATIONS UNLESS DURING EXTREME EMERGENCY. STAFF PRIVILEGES WERE SUSPENDED IN A HOSPITAL IN 10/93 BASED ON THIS TYPE OF COMPLAINT.

CORDOVA, EDMUND S MD, DATE OF BIRTH JANUARY 5, 1947 OF C/O 4231 POSTAL COURT, PASADENA, MD, WAS DISCIPLINED BY MEDICARE ON DECEMBER 20, 1995
DISCIPLINARY ACTION: EXCLUSION FROM THE MEDICARE AND/OR MEDICAID PROGRAM
OFFENSE: DISCIPLINARY ACTION BY ANOTHER STATE OR AGENCY

NOTES: LICENSE SUSPENDED FOR REASONS BEARING ON PROFESSIONAL PERFORMANCE.

CORTELYOU, MARIE MD, WAS DISCIPLINED BY NEW MEXICO ON NOVEMBER 1, 1996

NOTES: MUST NOTIFY THE BOARD IN WRITING 90 DAYS PRIOR TO PRACTICING UNDER NEW MEXICO LICENSE OR RETURNING TO NEW MEXICO.

CORTELYOU, MARIE MD, WAS DISCIPLINED BY NEW MEXICO ON AUGUST 1, 1999
DISCIPLINARY ACTION: LICENSE REVOCATION
OFFENSE: DISCIPLINARY ACTION BY ANOTHER STATE OR AGENCY

NOTES: FAILURE TO NOTIFY THE BOARD OF ACTION IN ANOTHER STATE AND REVOCATION OF PRIVILEGES ON MILITARY INSTALLATION.

DABBS, THURMAN C MD OF 810 WEST APACHE, FARMINGTON, NM, WAS DISCIPLINED BY NEW MEXICO ON SEPTEMBER 3, 1993
DISCIPLINARY ACTION: LICENSE SUSPENSION
OFFENSE: FAILURE TO COMPLY WITH PREVIOUS BOARD ORDER

NOTES: UNPROFESSIONAL CONDUCT.

DABBS, THURMAN C MD, WAS DISCIPLINED BY NEW MEXICO ON NOVEMBER 1, 1996
DISCIPLINARY ACTION: LICENSE REVOCATION
OFFENSE: CRIMINAL CONVICTION OR PLEA OF GUILTY, NOLO CONTENDERE, OR NO CONTEST TO A CRIME

NOTES: FELONY CONVICTION FOR CRIMINAL CONTACT WITH A MINOR. LICENSE REVOKED WITH CONDITION TO NEVER REAPPLY.

DAIL, ROBERT W MD OF CHATTANOOGA, TN, WAS DISCIPLINED BY TENNESSEE ON MARCH 1, 1995
DISCIPLINARY ACTION: 6-MONTH LICENSE SUSPENSION; 30-MONTH PROBATION
OFFENSE: DISCIPLINARY ACTION BY ANOTHER STATE OR AGENCY

NOTES: DISCIPLINARY ACTION TAKEN BY TEXAS. REMAINDER OF THREE YEAR SUSPENSION STAYED; MUST APPEAR BEFORE BOARD TWICE A YEAR DURING PROBATION; MUST EXECUTE A CONTRACT WITH THE IMPAIRED PHYSICIANS PROGRAM; A RANDOM SAMPLING OF HIS MEDICAL CHARTS AND BILLING RECORDS WILL BE REVIEWED SEMIANNUALLY BY THE MEDICAL DIRECTOR OF THE BOARD OF MEDICAL EXAMINERS.

DAIL, ROBERT W MD, WAS DISCIPLINED BY NEW MEXICO ON JULY 17, 1995
DISCIPLINARY ACTION: LICENSE REVOCATION
OFFENSE: NONCOMPLIANCE WITH A PROFESSIONAL RULE

NOTES: FAILURE TO REPORT ACTION BY ANOTHER BOARD.

DAIL, ROBERT WOOD MD, LICENSE NUMBER 00E3244 OF CHATTANOOGA, TN, WAS DISCIPLINED BY TEXAS ON APRIL 15, 1994
DISCIPLINARY ACTION: SURRENDER OF LICENSE
OFFENSE: PROFESSIONAL MISCONDUCT

NOTES: ALLEGATIONS CONCERNING ORDERING OF MULTIPLE MODALITIES FOR AUTO ACCIDENT PATIENTS; BOARD FINDS THAT VARIOUS PATIENTS RECEIVED UNNECESSARY TREATMENT; PRACTICES IN TENNESSEE AND DOES NOT PLAN ON PRACTICING IN TEXAS. SHALL NOT SEEK REINSTATEMENT OF LICENSE.

DAVIS, ROBERT C MD OF 1519 WEST 90TH SOUTH, WEST JORDAN, UT, WAS DISCIPLINED BY NEW MEXICO ON DECEMBER 15, 1993
DISCIPLINARY ACTION: LICENSE REVOCATION
OFFENSE: CRIMINAL CONVICTION OR PLEA OF GUILTY, NOLO CONTENDERE, OR NO CONTEST TO A CRIME

NOTES: CRIMINAL CONVICTION IN ANOTHER STATE.

DAVIS, ROBERT CHARLES MD, DATE OF BIRTH OCTOBER 25, 1953, LICENSE NUMBER 0005035 OF 1781 WEST 90TH S, WEST JORDAN, UT, WAS DISCIPLINED BY MONTANA ON JANUARY 24, 1991
DISCIPLINARY ACTION: SURRENDER OF LICENSE
OFFENSE: NONCOMPLIANCE WITH A PROFESSIONAL RULE

NOTES: FAILURE TO DISCLOSE UTAH DISCIPLINARY ACTION IN A TIMELY MANNER.

DAVIS, ROBERT CHARLES MD OF SANDY, UT, WAS DISCIPLINED BY UTAH ON JULY 19, 1993
DISCIPLINARY ACTION: LICENSE REVOCATION; REVOCATION OF CONTROLLED SUBSTANCE LICENSE
OFFENSE: CRIMINAL CONVICTION OR PLEA OF GUILTY, NOLO CONTENDERE, OR NO CONTEST TO A CRIME

NOTES: CONVICTION OF CRIMES OF MORAL TURPITUDE WHICH RELATE TO HIS PRACTICE OF MEDICINE AND DEMONSTRATE A THREAT TO THE PUBLIC HEALTH, SAFETY AND WELFARE. HE FILED A REQUEST FOR AGENCY REVIEW ON 07/08/93 AND THE REVOCATION WAS STAYED PENDING THE ISSUANCE OF AN ORDER ON THE REQUEST. ORDER WAS UPHELD IN ITS ENTIRETY.

DAVIS, ROBERT CHARLES MD, DATE OF BIRTH OCTOBER 25, 1953, LICENSE NUMBER 0023956 OF 1519 WEST 90TH STREET, WEST JORDAN, UT, WAS DISCIPLINED BY IOWA ON JUNE 6, 1994
DISCIPLINARY ACTION: LICENSE REVOCATION
OFFENSE: DISCIPLINARY ACTION BY ANOTHER STATE OR AGENCY

NOTES: CHARGES THAT UTAH TOOK ACTION FOR FRAUD.

DAVIS, ROBERT CHARLES MD, DATE OF BIRTH OCTOBER 25, 1953 OF RR 2 BOX 9000, SAFFORD, AZ, WAS DISCIPLINED BY MEDICARE ON OCTOBER 10, 1994
DISCIPLINARY ACTION: 300-MONTH EXCLUSION FROM THE MEDICARE AND/OR MEDICAID PROGRAM
OFFENSE: CRIMINAL CONVICTION OR PLEA OF GUILTY, NOLO CONTENDERE, OR NO CONTEST TO A CRIME

NOTES: CONVICTED OF A CRIME INVOLVING THE MEDICARE, MEDICAID, MATERNAL AND CHILD HEALTH SERVICES BLOCK GRANT OR BLOCK GRANTS TO STATES FOR SOCIAL SERVICES PROGRAMS.

DEBLANC, GEORGE BRUCE MD OF 2226B WYOMING NE #304, ALBUQUERQUE, NM, WAS DISCIPLINED BY DEA ON FEBRUARY 9, 1998
DISCIPLINARY ACTION: SURRENDER OF CONTROLLED SUBSTANCE LICENSE

NOTES: IN LIEU OF PUBLIC INTEREST REVOCATION.

DENAPLES, MARK MD, WAS DISCIPLINED BY NEW MEXICO ON MAY 1, 1996
DISCIPLINARY ACTION: SURRENDER OF LICENSE

NOTES: IN LIEU OF PROSECUTION.

DICIANNO, JULIE MD, WAS DISCIPLINED BY NEW MEXICO ON AUGUST 1, 1998
OFFENSE: DISCIPLINARY ACTION BY ANOTHER STATE OR AGENCY

NOTES: SHE REQUESTED REINSTATEMENT OF HER NEW MEXICO LICENSE FROM INACTIVE STATUS. BASED ON STIPULATED STATUS IN ARKANSAS, LICENSE WAS REINSTATED WITH STANDARD STIPULATIONS FOR SUBSTANCE ABUSE.

DILLON, VALERIE G MD, WAS DISCIPLINED BY NEW MEXICO ON JANUARY 1, 1997
DISCIPLINARY ACTION: RESTRICTION PLACED ON LICENSE
OFFENSE: PROFESSIONAL MISCONDUCT

NOTES: CONDUCT UNBECOMING, SELF-PRESCRIBING, AND PRACTICING VETERINARY MEDICINE WITHOUT A LICENSE. ON 2/1/99 ORDER AMENDED ALLOWING HER TO PRACTICE PATIENT CARE FOR DISABILITY EVALUATIONS UNDER THE DIRECT SUPERVISION OF PHYSICIAN APPROVED BY THE BOARD; ALL OTHER STIPULATIONS REMAIN THE SAME.

DITTEMORE, HAROLD E MD OF 3400 ANDREWS HIGHWAY, MIDLAND, TX, WAS DISCIPLINED BY NEW MEXICO ON DECEMBER 22, 1993
DISCIPLINARY ACTION: SURRENDER OF LICENSE

NOTES: IN LIEU OF ACTION.

DITTEMORE, HAROLD E MD, LICENSE NUMBER 00E3897 OF MIDLAND, TX, WAS DISCIPLINED BY TEXAS ON MARCH 2, 1996
DISCIPLINARY ACTION: SURRENDER OF LICENSE

NOTES: VOLUNTARY AND PERMANENT SURRENDER; SHALL IMMEDIATELY RETIRE FROM THE PRACTICE OF MEDICINE.

DITTEMORE, HAROLD E MD OF 3400 ANDREWS HIGHWAY, MIDLAND, TX, WAS DISCIPLINED BY DEA ON APRIL 29, 1996
DISCIPLINARY ACTION: SURRENDER OF CONTROLLED SUBSTANCE LICENSE

NOTES: IN LIEU OF ORDER TO SHOW CAUSE.

DITTEMORE, HAROLD EUGENE MD, LICENSE NUMBER C34845 OF MIDLAND, TX, WAS DISCIPLINED BY CALIFORNIA ON NOVEMBER 25, 1997
DISCIPLINARY ACTION: SURRENDER OF LICENSE

NOTES: WHILE CHARGES PENDING.

DUNCAN, MARILYN MD, WAS DISCIPLINED BY NEW MEXICO ON AUGUST 1, 1998
DISCIPLINARY ACTION: SURRENDER OF LICENSE

NOTES: VOLUNTARY SURRENDER IN LIEU OF FURTHER DISCIPLINARY ACTION, AND MAY NEVER REAPPLY.

DUNN, TERRY MD, WAS DISCIPLINED BY NEW MEXICO ON JULY 30, 1990
DISCIPLINARY ACTION: LICENSE SUSPENSION
OFFENSE: SUBSTANDARD CARE, INCOMPETENCE OR NEGLIGENCE

NOTES: INCOMPETENCE AND GROSS NEGLIGENCE. SUSPENSION STAYED AND LICENSE PLACED ON PROBATION 5/28/91.

DWYER, PATRICK JR MD, WAS DISCIPLINED BY NEW MEXICO ON MARCH 2, 1999
DISCIPLINARY ACTION: EMERGENCY SUSPENSION
OFFENSE: FAILURE TO COMPLY WITH PREVIOUS BOARD ORDER

NOTES: FAILURE TO COMPLY WITH STIPULATIONS.

DWYER, PATRICK JR MD, WAS DISCIPLINED BY NEW MEXICO ON MAY 1, 1999
DISCIPLINARY ACTION: SURRENDER OF LICENSE

NOTES: VOLUNTARY SURRENDER UNDER THE TERMS OF IMPAIRED HEALTH CARE PROVIDER ACT; SURRENDER RUNS CONCURRENTLY WITH EMERGENCY SUSPENSION OF 3/2/99 AND WILL BE ADDRESSED WHEN HE PETITIONS FOR REINSTATEMENT.

EASTON, KARL MD, WAS DISCIPLINED BY NEW MEXICO ON APRIL 1, 1998
DISCIPLINARY ACTION: SURRENDER OF LICENSE

NOTES: VOLUNTARY SURRENDER AND MAY NEVER REAPPLY.

ESCALANTE-SAUTO, GILBERTO MD, WAS DISCIPLINED BY NEW MEXICO ON NOVEMBER 1, 1998
DISCIPLINARY ACTION: LICENSE REVOCATION
OFFENSE: DISCIPLINARY ACTION BY ANOTHER STATE OR AGENCY

NOTES: DISCIPLINARY ACTION TAKEN IN FLORIDA (REVOKED FOR A FELONY CONVICTION) AND FOR FAILURE TO NOTIFY NEW MEXICO BOARD OF FLORIDA ACTION.

EVANS, STEPHEN D MD, WAS DISCIPLINED BY NEW MEXICO ON SEPTEMBER 6, 1995
DISCIPLINARY ACTION: PROBATION; FINE

NOTES: NO PHYSICIAN ASSISTANT SUPERVISION FOR THREE YEARS.

FARMER, GARY L MD, DATE OF BIRTH AUGUST 2, 1945, LICENSE NUMBER 1055170 OF PO BOX 23054, ALBUQUERQUE, NM, WAS DISCIPLINED BY MICHIGAN ON MAY 21, 1997
DISCIPLINARY ACTION: LICENSE SUSPENSION
OFFENSE: DISCIPLINARY ACTION BY ANOTHER STATE OR AGENCY

NOTES: LICENSE SUSPENDED FOR A MINIMUM OF ONE DAY. ON 1/29/98 REINSTATEMENT DENIED.

FLOWERS, JEFFERSON III MD, WAS DISCIPLINED BY NEW MEXICO ON NOVEMBER 1, 1998
DISCIPLINARY ACTION: LICENSE SUSPENSION
OFFENSE: OVERPRESCRIBING OR MISPRESCRIBING DRUGS

NOTES: LICENSE SUSPENDED FOR TEN DAYS FROM 12/3/98 TO 12/13/98 FOR INJUDICIOUS PRESCRIBING.

FOLLETT, WILLIAM III MD, WAS DISCIPLINED BY NEW MEXICO ON MAY 31, 1995
DISCIPLINARY ACTION: SURRENDER OF LICENSE
OFFENSE: PROFESSIONAL MISCONDUCT

NOTES: SEXUAL MISCONDUCT.

FOLLETT, WILLIAM WALLACE III MD, LICENSE NUMBER 00D4118 OF EL PASO, TX, WAS DISCIPLINED BY TEXAS ON MARCH 5, 1994
DISCIPLINARY ACTION: 84-MONTH PROBATION; REQUIRED TO TAKE ADDITIONAL MEDICAL EDUCATION
OFFENSE: PROFESSIONAL MISCONDUCT

NOTES: FROM 5/27/92 THROUGH 6/2/92 MAINTAINED AN INAPPROPRIATE SOCIAL RELATIONSHIP WITH A FEMALE PATIENT; FAILED TO RECOGNIZE THE OCCURRENCE OF TRANSFERENCE AND COUNTERTRANSFERENCE WHILE TREATING THE PATIENT AND THAT SHE WAS IN A VULNERABLE POSITION RELATING TO THE DEATH OF HER HUSBAND; PATIENT BELIEVES SHE WAS EXPLOITED BY DR. FOLLETT; HE DOES NOT HAVE A PAST DISCIPLINARY HISTORY. SUSPENSION STAYED. CONDITIONS OF PROBATION: SHALL ATTEND AT LEAST 50 HOURS OF CONTINUING MEDICAL EDUCATION AND AN ADDITIONAL SIX HOURS OF ETHICS COURSES PER YEAR; SHALL SUBMIT HIMSELF TO A BOARD-APPROVED PSYCHIATRIST FOR EVALUATION AND FOLLOW RECOMMENDATIONS FOR CARE AND TREATMENT IF ANY; SHALL GIVE THIS PSYCHIATRIST A COPY OF THE BOARD ORDER; SHALL APPEAR BEFORE THE BOARD ONCE A YEAR; SHALL NOT MAINTAIN A PERSONAL OR SOCIAL RELATIONSHIP WITH PATIENTS; WITHIN ONE YEAR SHALL SUBMIT A PUBLISHABLE PAPER REGARDING DOCTOR-PATIENT BOUNDARIES; SHALL COOPERATE WITH THE BOARD IN VERIFYING COMPLIANCE; SHALL INFORM BOARD OF CHANGE OF ADDRESS WITHIN 10 DAYS OR IF HE LEAVES THE STATE; TIME SPENT OUT OF TEXAS DOES NOT COUNT TOWARD PROBATION. SHALL NOT SEEK MODIFICATION FOR ONE YEAR. ON 4/4/98 ORDER TERMINATED.

FRANKLIN, JAMES E DO, LICENSE NUMBER 20A1931 OF ALBUQUERQUE, NM, WAS DISCIPLINED BY CALIFORNIA ON JUNE 22, 1990
DISCIPLINARY ACTION: LICENSE REVOCATION
OFFENSE: DISCIPLINARY ACTION BY ANOTHER STATE OR AGENCY

NOTES: ACTION TAKEN BY ANOTHER STATE.

FRANKLIN, JAMES E DO, LICENSE NUMBER 20A1931 OF

ALBUQUERQUE, NM, WAS DISCIPLINED BY CALIFORNIA ON DECEMBER 3, 1996
DISCIPLINARY ACTION: DENIAL OF LICENSE REINSTATEMENT

GALLAGHER, CHRISTOPHER MD, WAS DISCIPLINED BY NEW MEXICO ON MAY 22, 1992
DISCIPLINARY ACTION: RESTRICTION PLACED ON LICENSE

NOTES: LICENSE STIPULATED, UNSPECIFIED. IN 1996 ALL STIPULATIONS REMOVED.

GALLOWAY, ROBERT MD, WAS DISCIPLINED BY NEW MEXICO ON SEPTEMBER 5, 1995
DISCIPLINARY ACTION: REPRIMAND
OFFENSE: PROVIDING FALSE INFORMATION TO THE BOARD OR OTHER HEALTH AGENCY

NOTES: MISSTATEMENT OF CREDENTIALS.

GARCIA, IGNACIO MD OF 6004 MADRE CT NE, ALBUQUERQUE, NM, WAS DISCIPLINED BY NEW MEXICO ON MAY 19, 1994
OFFENSE: SUBSTANCE ABUSE

NOTES: LICENSE PLACED UNDER UNSPECIFIED CONDITIONS. IN 8/98 REMOVED ALL STIPULATIONS FOR SUBSTANCE ABUSE; UNRESTRICTED LICENSE.

GASIS, ALBERT J MD, DATE OF BIRTH FEBRUARY 16, 1931, LICENSE NUMBER 0017944 OF ALBUQUERQUE, NM, WAS DISCIPLINED BY COLORADO ON OCTOBER 15, 1993
DISCIPLINARY ACTION: 60-MONTH PROBATION; RESTRICTION PLACED ON LICENSE
OFFENSE: SUBSTANDARD CARE, INCOMPETENCE OR NEGLIGENCE

NOTES: ALLEGATIONS OF SUBSTANDARD PATIENT CARE. PROBATIONARY PERIOD INCLUDES PRACTICE MONITORING; ORDER PROHIBITS SURGICAL PRACTICE.

GEER, RICHARD MD OF 137 EAST TENTH STREET, DURANGO, CO, WAS DISCIPLINED BY NEW MEXICO ON JULY 28, 1993
OFFENSE: PROFESSIONAL MISCONDUCT

NOTES: LICENSE PLACED UNDER UNSPECIFIED CONDITIONS. PROBATION TERMINATED IN 1995; DONATED 1,000 FREE PATIENT VISITS.

GILMOUR, EDWARD E MD, LICENSE NUMBER 48980 OF P.O. BOX 10108, POJOAQUE VALLEY, NM, WAS DISCIPLINED BY MASSACHUSETTS ON JULY 28, 1999
DISCIPLINARY ACTION: NONRENEWAL OF LICENSE
OFFENSE: PROFESSIONAL MISCONDUCT

NOTES: FAILED TO MAINTAIN PROPER BOUNDARIES IN THAT HE ENGAGED IN A PERSONAL AND SOCIAL, AS WELL AS ECONOMIC, RELATIONSHIP WITH A PATIENT; HE ALSO DISCLOSED TO THE PATIENT THE DETAILS OF HIS PERSONAL AND FINANCIAL LIFE. REVOCATION OF RIGHT TO RENEW LICENSE.

GILMOUR, EDWARD E MD, LICENSE NUMBER 090115 OF 1040 DON DIEGO, SANTA FE, NM, WAS DISCIPLINED BY NEW YORK ON DECEMBER 3, 1999
DISCIPLINARY ACTION: SURRENDER OF LICENSE
OFFENSE: DISCIPLINARY ACTION BY ANOTHER STATE OR AGENCY

NOTES: DISCIPLINED BY THE MASSACHUSETTS BOARD FOR ENGAGING IN A PERSONAL, SOCIAL, AND ECONOMIC RELATIONSHIP WITH A PATIENT.

GOLDMAN, SIDNEY M MD, WAS DISCIPLINED BY NEW MEXICO ON JANUARY 1, 1997
DISCIPLINARY ACTION: SURRENDER OF LICENSE

NOTES: REFERRED TO AN IMPAIRED PHYSICIANS COMMITTEE REGARDING MENTAL COGNITIVE SKILLS; VOLUNTARY AND PERMANENT SURRENDER OF HIS LICENSE TO PRACTICE MEDICINE.

GORDON, IRA J MD, WAS DISCIPLINED BY NEW MEXICO ON FEBRUARY 1, 1998
DISCIPLINARY ACTION: RESTRICTION PLACED ON LICENSE
OFFENSE: SUBSTANCE ABUSE

NOTES: ISSUED NEW MEXICO LICENSE WITH STANDARD STIPULATIONS FOR SUBSTANCE ABUSE. AS OF 11/98 STIPULATIONS REDUCED TO BIANNUAL VISITS WITH THE BOARD.

GRAHAM, JACK L MD, LICENSE NUMBER 0007439, WAS DISCIPLINED BY NEW MEXICO ON JUNE 17, 1996
DISCIPLINARY ACTION: PROBATION; MONITORING OF PHYSICIAN PERFORMANCE
OFFENSE: SUBSTANCE ABUSE

NOTES: SUBSTANCE ABUSE. CONDITIONS OF PROBATION: SHALL ABSTAIN FROM THE USE OF MIND-ALTERING SUBSTANCES, CONTROLLED SUBSTANCES OR ALCOHOL EXCEPT AS LEGITIMATELY PRESCRIBED BY A LICENSED PHYSICIAN; SHALL BE AN ACTIVE PARTICIPANT IN THE NEW MEXICO MONITORED TREATMENT PROGRAM INCLUDING SUBMITTING TO RANDOM BIOLOGICAL FLUID TESTING. THE PROGRAM SHALL RELEASE THE RESULTS OF SUCH TEST TO THE BOARD; SHALL APPEAR BEFORE THE BOARD AND SUBMIT QUARTERLY REPORTS. IN 8/98 STIPULATIONS FOR SUBSTANCE ABUSE REDUCED TO BIANNUAL VISITS WITH THE BOARD. IN 8/99 REDUCED TO ANNUAL VISITS.

GRAHAM, JACK L MD, WAS DISCIPLINED BY ALASKA ON JULY 1, 1997
DISCIPLINARY ACTION: RESTRICTION PLACED ON LICENSE; MONITORING OF PHYSICIAN PERFORMANCE
OFFENSE: SUBSTANCE ABUSE

NOTES: HISTORY OF SUBSTANCE ABUSE. DURATION ON PRACTICE TO BE 7/1 97--7/20/97; MUST ENTER INTO AMERICAN STUDENTS MEDICAL ASSOCIATION PAC; MUST CONSUME NO CONTROLLED DRUG, ALCOHOL, OR LEGEND DRUG UNLESS PRESCRIBED BY HIS DOCTOR OR DENTIST; MUST PARTICIPATE IN HEALTH CARE PROVIDER SUPPORT GROUP; MUST HAVE URINE, BLOOD AND HAIR TESTS; WORK LOCATION RESTRICTION; AND EMPLOYER REPORTS; MUST NOTIFY HOSPITALS OF MEMORANDUM OF AGREEMENT.

GRAHAM, JACK L MD, LICENSE NUMBER 4076, WAS DISCIPLINED BY ALASKA ON JUNE 30, 1998
DISCIPLINARY ACTION: FINE; REPRIMAND
OFFENSE: FAILURE TO COMPLY WITH PREVIOUS BOARD ORDER

NOTES: VIOLATED CONDITIONS OF MEMORANDUM OF AGREEMENT DATED 7/1/98 FOR FAILURE TO CONTACT PAC PROGRAM. FINE OF $1,000; MEMORANDUM OF AGREEMENT FOR CHEMICAL DEPENDENCY.

GRAHAM, JACKIE LYNN MD OF 1600 S.E. MAIN STREET, ROSWELL, NM, WAS DISCIPLINED BY DEA ON DECEMBER 4, 1995
DISCIPLINARY ACTION: SURRENDER OF CONTROLLED SUBSTANCE LICENSE

NOTES: IN LIEU OF ORDER TO SHOW CAUSE.

GRAOR, ROBERT MD, WAS DISCIPLINED BY NEW MEXICO ON

FEBRUARY 1, 1998
OFFENSE: CRIMINAL CONVICTION OR PLEA OF GUILTY, NOLO CONTENDERE, OR NO CONTEST TO A CRIME

NOTES: ISSUED LICENSE WITH STIPULATION TO DISCLOSE FELONY CONVICTION TO ALL EMPLOYERS.

GRAY, ROBERT H MD, WAS DISCIPLINED BY NEW MEXICO ON NOVEMBER 17, 1995
DISCIPLINARY ACTION: PROBATION; REQUIRED TO ENTER AN IMPAIRED PHYSICIAN PROGRAM OR SUBSTANCE ABUSE TREATMENT
OFFENSE: SUBSTANCE ABUSE

NOTES: INFORMED THE BOARD OF HIS HISTORY OF SUBSTANCE ABUSE AND OF HIS SUBSEQUENT AND CONTINUING REHABILITATION. LICENSE LIMITED AS FOLLOWS: SHALL ABSTAIN FROM THE USE OF MIND-ALTERING SUBSTANCES, CONTROLLED SUBSTANCE OR ALCOHOLIC BEVERAGES EXCEPT AS PRESCRIBED BY A LICENSED PHYSICIAN; SHALL BE AN ACTIVE PARTICIPANT IN THE NEW MEXICO MONITORED TREATMENT PROGRAM; SHALL SUBMIT TO RANDOM FLUID TESTING; SHALL APPEAR BEFORE THE BOARD ON A QUARTERLY BASIS OR UPON REQUEST; SHALL SUBMIT QUARTERLY REPORTS TO THE BOARD ATTESTING TO HIS COMPLIANCE WITH THIS STIPULATION. IN 1996, HE WAS IN FULL COMPLIANCE WITH ALL CONDITIONS AND ALL STIPULATIONS WERE REMOVED.

GREELEY, PHILIP H MD OF 839 PASEO DE PERALTA, SANTA FE, NM, WAS DISCIPLINED BY NEW MEXICO
OFFENSE: PROFESSIONAL MISCONDUCT

NOTES: IMPAIRMENT. LICENSE PLACED UNDER UNSPECIFIED CONDITIONS. IN 1996 ORDER AMENDED ALLOWING FOR REAPPLICATION OF DEA LICENSE. IN 1997 REMOVED STIPULATION THAT REQUIRED HE BE PROCTORED WHILE PRACTICING MEDICINE. IN 8/98 REMOVED ALL STIPULATIONS FOR PHYSICAL HEALTH PROBLEMS, GIVING HIM AN UNRESTRICTED NEW MEXICO LICENSE.

GREEN, JAMES E MD, LICENSE NUMBER 83209, WAS DISCIPLINED BY NEW MEXICO
DISCIPLINARY ACTION: PROBATION; REQUIRED TO ENTER AN IMPAIRED PHYSICIAN PROGRAM OR SUBSTANCE ABUSE TREATMENT

NOTES: TERMS AND CONDITIONS: SHALL ABSTAIN FROM THE USE OF MIND-ALTERING SUBSTANCES, CONTROLLED SUBSTANCES OR ALCOHOLIC BEVERAGES EXCEPT AS PRESCRIBED BY A LICENSED PHYSICIAN; SHALL BE AN ACTIVE PARTICIPANT IN THE NEW MEXICO MONITORED TREATMENT PROGRAM; SHALL SUBMIT TO RANDOM BIOLOGICAL FLUID TESTING; SHALL APPEAR ANNUALLY BEFORE THE BOARD OR UPON REQUEST; SHALL SUBMIT QUARTERLY REPORTS TO THE BOARD ATTESTING TO HIS COMPLIANCE. IN 1997 ALL STIPULATIONS FOR SUBSTANCE ABUSE TERMINATED.

GRENKO, PETE J MD, WAS DISCIPLINED BY NEW MEXICO ON NOVEMBER 13, 1991
DISCIPLINARY ACTION: LICENSE REVOCATION
OFFENSE: OVERPRESCRIBING OR MISPRESCRIBING DRUGS

NOTES: INJUDICIOUS PRESCRIBING.

GREYEYES, ROGER MD OF SHIPROCK, NM, WAS DISCIPLINED BY UTAH ON MARCH 3, 1999
DISCIPLINARY ACTION: LICENSE REVOCATION; REVOCATION OF CONTROLLED SUBSTANCE LICENSE
OFFENSE: SUBSTANCE ABUSE

NOTES: HIS CONTINUED USE OF ALCOHOL MAY REASONABLY BE CONSIDERED TO HAVE IMPAIRED HIS ABILITY TO PRACTICE MEDICINE.

GUARDIA, DAVID K MD, WAS DISCIPLINED BY NEW MEXICO ON MAY 1, 1996
DISCIPLINARY ACTION: LICENSE REVOCATION
OFFENSE: FAILURE TO COMPLY WITH PREVIOUS BOARD ORDER

NOTES: NONCOMPLIANCE WITH STIPULATIONS.

GUARDIA, DAVID KING MD OF 2211 LOMAS BLVD N.E., ALBUQUERQUE, NM, WAS DISCIPLINED BY DEA ON MAY 14, 1996
DISCIPLINARY ACTION: SURRENDER OF CONTROLLED SUBSTANCE LICENSE
OFFENSE: DISCIPLINARY ACTION BY ANOTHER STATE OR AGENCY

NOTES: STATE BOARD.

GUNDZIK, JOHN MD OF 664 EAST BARCELONA, SANTA FE, NM, WAS DISCIPLINED BY NEW MEXICO ON FEBRUARY 18, 1993
DISCIPLINARY ACTION: SURRENDER OF LICENSE

NOTES: IN LIEU OF ACTION.

GUTTMAN, STUART T MD OF 860 POLARIS BLVD SE, RIO RANCHO, NM, WAS DISCIPLINED BY NEW MEXICO ON JUNE 15, 1993
OFFENSE: DISCIPLINARY ACTION BY ANOTHER STATE OR AGENCY

NOTES: LICENSE PLACED UNDER UNSPECIFIED CONDITIONS: THERAPY.

GUTTMAN, STUART THOMAS MD, DATE OF BIRTH JANUARY 30, 1945, LICENSE NUMBER 0011184 OF 17 MARKS RD, OCEAN SPRINGS, MS, WAS DISCIPLINED BY MISSISSIPPI ON MAY 21, 1992
DISCIPLINARY ACTION: LICENSE SUSPENSION
OFFENSE: LOSS OR RESTRICTION OF HOSPITAL PRIVILEGES

NOTES: DISCIPLINED BY THE MEDICAL STAFF OF A LICENSED HOSPITAL AND VOLUNTARILY SURRENDERED HIS HOSPITAL STAFF PRIVILEGES WHILE AN INVESTIGATION WAS BEING CONDUCTED BY A MEDICAL STAFF COMMITTEE. SUSPENSION WILL BE STAYED AT SUCH TIME AS HE COMPLIES WITH THE FOLLOWING: SUBMITS TO COMPREHENSIVE PSYCHIATRIC AND PSYCHOLOGICAL EVALUATION; WHEN PSYCHIATRIST INFORMS BOARD THAT HE IS CAPABLE OF PRACTICING WITH REASONABLE SKILL AND SAFETY HE MAY PETITION BOARD FOR RECONSIDERATION.

GUTTMAN, STUART THOMAS MD, DATE OF BIRTH JANUARY 30, 1945, LICENSE NUMBER 0011184 OF 210 COOK AVENUE, RATON, NM, WAS DISCIPLINED BY MISSISSIPPI ON OCTOBER 15, 1992
DISCIPLINARY ACTION: RESTRICTION PLACED ON LICENSE; MONITORING OF PHYSICIAN PERFORMANCE

NOTES: AUTHORIZED TO RETURN TO PRACTICE UNDER THE FOLLOWING CONDITIONS: SHALL RETURN TO BOARD-APPROVED PSYCHIATRIST FOR PSYCHOANALYTIC PSYCHOTHERAPY ON AN ONGOING BASIS WITH MONTHLY REPORTS TO BOARD; MAY THEN RETURN TO ACTIVE PRACTICE OF GENERAL INTERNAL MEDICINE, BUT SHALL BE PROHIBITED FROM PRACTICING PULMONARY MEDICINE OR PERFORMING ANY INVASIVE PROCEDURES; CAN PETITION IN 12 MONTHS FOR RECONSIDERATION, HOWEVER, BOARD NOT OBLIGATED TO RETURN PRIVILEGES IN THOSE AREAS UNTIL HE HAS BECOME BOARD CERTIFIED IN PULMONARY MEDICINE AND TAKEN ADDITIONAL

TRAINING IN THE PERFORMANCE OF INVASIVE PROCEDURES AS PERTAINS TO PULMONARY AND CRITICAL CARE MEDICINE WITH CERTIFICATION THEREOF. ON 11/19/92 PETITION FOR RECONSIDERATION OF THE BOARD'S DECISIONS DENIED. ON 4/21/94 ALL RESTRICTIONS REMOVED FROM LICENSE IN ORDER FOR HIM TO PURSUE PULMONARY DISEASE EXAMINATION ADMINISTERED BY THE AMERICAN BOARD OF INTERNAL MEDICINE. IF HE FAILS THIS EXAMINATION OR FAILS TO OBTAIN CERTIFICATION, THE BOARD RESERVES THE RIGHT TO INITIATE PROCEEDINGS TO PROHIBIT HIM FROM PRACTICING PULMONARY MEDICINE.

HARBIN, CHARLES C C MD OF SILVER CITY, NM, WAS DISCIPLINED BY NORTH DAKOTA ON NOVEMBER 22, 1991
DISCIPLINARY ACTION: SURRENDER OF LICENSE

NOTES: BOARD MAY FIND ALLEGATIONS OF COMPLAINT TRUE, LICENSE WILL NOT BE RENEWED OR REINSTATED AT ANY TIME.

HARMSTON, JOHN C MD, WAS DISCIPLINED BY NEW MEXICO ON AUGUST 1, 1996
DISCIPLINARY ACTION: REPRIMAND
OFFENSE: NONCOMPLIANCE WITH A PROFESSIONAL RULE

NOTES: FAILURE TO RESPOND TO BOARD INQUIRIES.

HART, ALRUNDUS MD, WAS DISCIPLINED BY NEW MEXICO ON FEBRUARY 16, 1995
DISCIPLINARY ACTION: LICENSE REVOCATION
OFFENSE: PROFESSIONAL MISCONDUCT

NOTES: FAILURE TO RESPOND TO BOARD; UNPROFESSIONAL CONDUCT.

HART, ALRUNDUS MD OF 2001 S BROADWAY PO BOX 1107, TRUTH OR CONSEQUENCE, NM, WAS DISCIPLINED BY DEA ON MARCH 16, 1995
DISCIPLINARY ACTION: SURRENDER OF CONTROLLED SUBSTANCE LICENSE

NOTES: IN LIEU OF ORDER TO SHOW CAUSE.

HART, ALRUNDUS MD, DATE OF BIRTH JULY 23, 1952 OF 2001 S BROADWAY, TRUTH OR CONSEQUENCES, NM, WAS DISCIPLINED BY MEDICARE ON AUGUST 10, 1995
DISCIPLINARY ACTION: EXCLUSION FROM THE MEDICARE AND/OR MEDICAID PROGRAM
OFFENSE: DISCIPLINARY ACTION BY ANOTHER STATE OR AGENCY

NOTES: LICENSE REVOKED FOR REASONS BEARING ON PROFESSIONAL PERFORMANCE.

HEDGES, DON W DO, DATE OF BIRTH OCTOBER 2, 1940 OF 6463 FOURTH STREET NW, ALBUQUERQUE, NM, WAS DISCIPLINED BY MEDICARE ON JUNE 14, 1991
DISCIPLINARY ACTION: 60-MONTH EXCLUSION FROM THE MEDICARE AND/OR MEDICAID PROGRAM
OFFENSE: CRIMINAL CONVICTION OR PLEA OF GUILTY, NOLO CONTENDERE, OR NO CONTEST TO A CRIME

NOTES: PROGRAM-RELATED CONVICTION. REINSTATED ON 11/22/96.

HEDGES, DON WALTER DO, LICENSE NUMBER 00E3303 OF ALBUQUERQUE, NM, WAS DISCIPLINED BY TEXAS ON MARCH 5, 1994
DISCIPLINARY ACTION: REPRIMAND
OFFENSE: INSURANCE, MEDICARE OR MEDICAID FRAUD

NOTES: WHILE PRACTICING IN NEW MEXICO HE INTENTIONALLY SUBMITTED INACCURATE DIAGNOSES TO MEDICARE FOR FIVE PATIENTS HE WAS TREATING WITH A DIET PLAN SO THAT HE WOULD RECEIVE REIMBURSEMENT SINCE THE DIET PLAN WAS NOT A COVERED BENEFIT.

HEDGES, DONALD W DO, LICENSE NUMBER A62474, WAS DISCIPLINED BY NEW MEXICO ON MAY 26, 1997
DISCIPLINARY ACTION: REPRIMAND
OFFENSE: SUBSTANDARD CARE, INCOMPETENCE OR NEGLIGENCE

NOTES: FAILURE TO MAINTAIN PROFESSIONAL STANDARDS.

HEMPSTEAD, RICHARD MD, WAS DISCIPLINED BY NEW MEXICO ON FEBRUARY 1, 1999
DISCIPLINARY ACTION: PROBATION

NOTES: ENTERED INTO ORDER OF PROBATION FOR CONTINUED MEDICAL CARE AND CONTINUED COMPLIANCE WITH STATE PROBATION.

HOCHMAN, JOEL MD OF 153 WEST ZIA ROAD, SANTA FE, NM, WAS DISCIPLINED BY NEW MEXICO ON MARCH 2, 1993
OFFENSE: PROFESSIONAL MISCONDUCT

NOTES: SUSPENSION STAYED. LICENSE PLACED UNDER UNSPECIFIED CONDITIONS.

HOCHMAN, JOEL S MD, WAS DISCIPLINED BY NEW MEXICO
DISCIPLINARY ACTION: RESTRICTION PLACED ON CONTROLLED SUBSTANCE LICENSE

NOTES: ORDER LIMITING USE OF CONTROLLED SUBSTANCES.

HOCHMAN, JOEL S MD, WAS DISCIPLINED BY NEW MEXICO ON JANUARY 1, 1997
DISCIPLINARY ACTION: SURRENDER OF LICENSE
OFFENSE: FAILURE TO COMPLY WITH PREVIOUS BOARD ORDER

NOTES: VIOLATED THE TERMS OF HIS PROBATION BY PRESCRIBING CONTROLLED SUBSTANCES WITHOUT AUTHORITY AS SET FORTH IN THE AUGUST 1996 ORDER; VOLUNTARY SURRENDER WITH CONDITION THAT HE MAY NEVER REAPPLY.

HOCHMAN, JOEL S MD, WAS DISCIPLINED BY NEW MEXICO ON JANUARY 1, 1997
DISCIPLINARY ACTION: EMERGENCY SUSPENSION
OFFENSE: FAILURE TO COMPLY WITH PREVIOUS BOARD ORDER

NOTES: VIOLATED 8/96 BOARD ORDER BY PRESCRIBING CONTROLLED SUBSTANCES WITHOUT AUTHORITY.

HOLLAND, MARK MD, WAS DISCIPLINED BY NEW MEXICO ON FEBRUARY 1, 1999
DISCIPLINARY ACTION: REQUIRED TO ENTER AN IMPAIRED PHYSICIAN PROGRAM OR SUBSTANCE ABUSE TREATMENT
OFFENSE: SUBSTANCE ABUSE

NOTES: LICENSE PLACED UNDER STANDARD STIPULATIONS FOR SUBSTANCE ABUSE. MUST ACTIVELY PARTICIPATE IN NEW MEXICO MONITORED TREATMENT PROGRAM.

HOPPER, JAMES MD OF 315 WEST WASHINGTON, ARTESIA, NM, WAS DISCIPLINED BY NEW MEXICO ON SEPTEMBER 19, 1994
OFFENSE: SUBSTANCE ABUSE

NOTES: SUSPENSION STAYED. LICENSE PLACED UNDER UNSPECIFIED CONDITIONS.

HOPPER, JAMES F MD, WAS DISCIPLINED BY NEW MEXICO ON

SEPTEMBER 25, 1992
DISCIPLINARY ACTION: RESTRICTION PLACED ON LICENSE

NOTES: LICENSE STIPULATED, UNSPECIFIED.

HOPPER, JAMES F MD, WAS DISCIPLINED BY NEW MEXICO ON JANUARY 1, 1997
DISCIPLINARY ACTION: SURRENDER OF LICENSE

NOTES: BOARD ACCEPTED HIS VOLUNTARY SURRENDER OF STIPULATED LICENSE.

HURLEY, LLOYD A MD, LICENSE NUMBER 12087 OF PO BOX 2374, CORRALES, NM, WAS DISCIPLINED BY KENTUCKY ON NOVEMBER 19, 1999
DISCIPLINARY ACTION: NONRENEWAL OF LICENSE
OFFENSE: CRIMINAL CONVICTION OR PLEA OF GUILTY, NOLO CONTENDERE, OR NO CONTEST TO A CRIME

NOTES: ADMITTED CONVICTION OF A MINOR MISDEMEANOR AND TWO PENDING MALPRACTICE ACTIONS IN HIS 1999 APPLICATION FOR REGISTRATION; WAS ABLE TO TERMINATE A PENDING NEW MEXICO DISCIPLINARY ACTION BY AGREEING TO STOP PRACTICING.

HURLEY, LLOYD A MD, LICENSE NUMBER 079071 OF PO BOX 2374, CORRALES, NM, WAS DISCIPLINED BY NEW YORK ON DECEMBER 27, 1999
DISCIPLINARY ACTION: SURRENDER OF LICENSE
OFFENSE: DISCIPLINARY ACTION BY ANOTHER STATE OR AGENCY

NOTES: VOLUNTARILY RETIRED HIS LICENSE IN NEW MEXICO WHEN FACED WITH ALLEGATIONS OF MAKING FALSE STATEMENTS ON HIS RENEWAL APPLICATIONS, HAVING A SEXUAL RELATIONSHIP WITH A PATIENT HAD HAVING BEEN CONVICTED OF LEWD ACTS.

JAMESON, JOHN MD, WAS DISCIPLINED BY NEW MEXICO ON APRIL 3, 1990
DISCIPLINARY ACTION: REPRIMAND

JARAMILLO, JAMES D C MD, DATE OF BIRTH JANUARY 30, 1946 OF PO BOX 640, LOS LUNAS, NM, WAS DISCIPLINED BY MEDICARE ON FEBRUARY 13, 1996
DISCIPLINARY ACTION: 120-MONTH EXCLUSION FROM THE MEDICARE AND/OR MEDICAID PROGRAM
OFFENSE: CRIMINAL CONVICTION OR PLEA OF GUILTY, NOLO CONTENDERE, OR NO CONTEST TO A CRIME

NOTES: CONVICTED OF A CRIME INVOLVING THE MEDICARE, MEDICAID, MATERNAL AND CHILD HEALTH SERVICES BLOCK GRANT OR BLOCK GRANTS TO STATES FOR SOCIAL SERVICES PROGRAMS.

JARAMILLO, JAMES D C MD, WAS DISCIPLINED BY NEW MEXICO ON JUNE 1, 1996
DISCIPLINARY ACTION: LICENSE SUSPENSION
OFFENSE: CRIMINAL CONVICTION OR PLEA OF GUILTY, NOLO CONTENDERE, OR NO CONTEST TO A CRIME

NOTES: FELONY CONVICTION: MEDICARE/MEDICAID FRAUD.

JARAMILLO, JAMES D C MD, WAS DISCIPLINED BY NEW MEXICO ON FEBRUARY 1, 1999

NOTES: MUST PASS SPEX WITH A MINIMUM SCORE OF 75 FOR CONSIDERATION OF REINSTATEMENT OF LICENSE.

JUTILA, CHARLOTTE K MD OF 10524 GRIFFITH PARK NE, ALBUQUERQUE, NM, WAS DISCIPLINED BY NEW MEXICO ON DECEMBER 13, 1994
DISCIPLINARY ACTION: LICENSE SUSPENSION
OFFENSE: SUBSTANCE ABUSE

NOTES: NOTICE OF CONTEMPLATED ACTION ISSUED.

JUTILA, CHARLOTTE K MD, WAS DISCIPLINED BY NEW MEXICO ON FEBRUARY 1, 1996
DISCIPLINARY ACTION: LICENSE REVOCATION
OFFENSE: SUBSTANCE ABUSE

NOTES: SUBSTANCE ABUSE.

JUTILA, CHARLOTTE K MD OF 10524 GRIFFITH PK DRIVE NE, ALBUQUERQUE, NM, WAS DISCIPLINED BY DEA ON MAY 16, 1996
DISCIPLINARY ACTION: SURRENDER OF CONTROLLED SUBSTANCE LICENSE
OFFENSE: DISCIPLINARY ACTION BY ANOTHER STATE OR AGENCY

NOTES: STATE BOARD.

KHALSA, DHARMA K MD, LICENSE NUMBER 7986, WAS DISCIPLINED BY NEW MEXICO ON JANUARY 1, 1997
OFFENSE: PROFESSIONAL MISCONDUCT

NOTES: UNPROFESSIONAL CONDUCT. SUSPENSION STAYED PENDING COURT REVIEW. IN THE INTERESTS OF SETTLING LITIGATION, ON 12/29/97 AGREEMENT REACHED AS FOLLOWS: WITHIN THIRTY DAYS SHALL MAIL A LETTER OF APOLOGY TO SPECIFIED DOCTOR IN A FORM FIRST APPROVED BY THE BOARD; WITHIN SIXTY DAYS SHALL SUBMIT TO THE BOARD A TWELVE PAGE ESSAY ON A TOPIC RELATING TO MEDICAL ETHICS; AFTER THESE CONDITIONS ARE MET REPRIMAND SHALL BE ISSUED.

KIM, DONGSUK MD, WAS DISCIPLINED BY NEW MEXICO
DISCIPLINARY ACTION: LICENSE REVOCATION
OFFENSE: PROFESSIONAL MISCONDUCT

NOTES: SEXUAL MISCONDUCT. UNPROFESSIONAL CONDUCT. TEMPORARY COURT STAY. IN 1997 REVOCATION OF LICENSE FOR INAPPROPRIATE SEXUAL BEHAVIOR REMANDED TO THE BOARD BY DISTRICT COURT FOR RECONSIDERATION; DECISION UPON REMAND BEING REVIEWED BY DISTRICT COURT. IN 5/98 SECOND REMAND HEARING; BOARD UPHELD PRIOR REVOCATION; DISTRICT COURT REVIEW PENDING. IN 8/98 DISTRICT COURT LIFTED THE STAY AND UPHELD THE BOARD'S REVOCATION FOR SEXUAL MISCONDUCT WITH A PATIENT.

KLEIN, ALFRED L MD, WAS DISCIPLINED BY NEW MEXICO ON MAY 1, 1996
DISCIPLINARY ACTION: SURRENDER OF LICENSE

NOTES: VOLUNTARY SURRENDER WITH AGREEMENT TO NEVER REAPPLY IN NEW MEXICO.

KLEIN, ALFRED L MD, DATE OF BIRTH SEPTEMBER 21, 1935 OF LA SALLE GENERAL DRIVE #2, JENA, LA, WAS DISCIPLINED BY MEDICARE ON FEBRUARY 20, 1997
DISCIPLINARY ACTION: 120-MONTH EXCLUSION FROM THE MEDICARE AND/OR MEDICAID PROGRAM
OFFENSE: NONCOMPLIANCE WITH A PROFESSIONAL RULE

NOTES: BASED ON A RECOMMENDATION FROM A PEER REVIEW ORGANIZATION THAT HE VIOLATED STATUTORY OBLIGATIONS.

KLEIN, ALFRED LEONARD MD OF JENA, LA, WAS DISCIPLINED BY LOUISIANA ON APRIL 28, 1997
DISCIPLINARY ACTION: LICENSE REVOCATION
OFFENSE: DISCIPLINARY ACTION BY ANOTHER STATE OR AGENCY

NOTES: ACTION AGAINST LICENSE BY NEW MEXICO; DECEIT IN OBTAINING A LICENSE; PROVIDING FALSE INFORMATION TO THE BOARD.

KLINGHARDT, DIETRICH MD OF 1468 ST FRANCIS DRIVE, SANTA FE, NM, WAS DISCIPLINED BY NEW MEXICO ON FEBRUARY 18, 1993
OFFENSE: PROFESSIONAL MISCONDUCT

NOTES: SUSPENSION STAYED; LICENSE PLACED UNDER UNSPECIFIED CONDITIONS. IN 1996 PROBATION TERMINATED.

KNOTT, RANDALL O MD, WAS DISCIPLINED BY NEW MEXICO ON DECEMBER 17, 1992
DISCIPLINARY ACTION: MONITORING OF PHYSICIAN PERFORMANCE

NOTES: AGREEMENT TO PRACTICE ONLY UNDER SUPERVISION.

KRAMER, RALPH LEWIS MD, LICENSE NUMBER 0039409 OF 7428 LEW WALLACE DRIVE, NE, ALBUQUERQUE, NM, WAS DISCIPLINED BY VIRGINIA ON MARCH 1, 1995
DISCIPLINARY ACTION: REPRIMAND
OFFENSE: SEXUAL ABUSE OF OR SEXUAL MISCONDUCT WITH A PATIENT

NOTES: FAILED TO ESTABLISH AND MAINTAIN BOUNDARIES APPROPRIATE TO THE PHYSICIAN/PATIENT RELATIONSHIP IN THAT HE ENGAGED IN HUGGING AND KISSING A PATIENT DURING THE PERIOD OF 4/90 THROUGH 9/90.

KRAUSE, ROBERT A MD, WAS DISCIPLINED BY NEW MEXICO ON JANUARY 1, 1997
DISCIPLINARY ACTION: LICENSE REVOCATION
OFFENSE: DISCIPLINARY ACTION BY ANOTHER STATE OR AGENCY

NOTES: MONTANA LICENSE REVOKED FOR UNPROFESSIONAL CONDUCT.

KRAUSE, ROBERT A MD, LICENSE NUMBER 21615, WAS DISCIPLINED BY MINNESOTA ON DECEMBER 21, 1998
DISCIPLINARY ACTION: LICENSE SUSPENSION

KRAUSE, ROBERT A MD, DATE OF BIRTH MAY 6, 1947 OF 6501 VEGAS DRIVE #1071, LAS VEGAS, NV, WAS DISCIPLINED BY MEDICARE ON JUNE 17, 1999
DISCIPLINARY ACTION: EXCLUSION FROM THE MEDICARE AND/OR MEDICAID PROGRAM
OFFENSE: DISCIPLINARY ACTION BY ANOTHER STATE OR AGENCY

NOTES: LICENSE REVOKED, SUSPENDED, SURRENDERED OR OTHERWISE LOST FOR REASONS BEARING ON PROFESSIONAL PERFORMANCE, PROFESSIONAL COMPETENCE OR FINANCIAL INTEGRITY.

KRAUSE, ROBERT ALAN MD, DATE OF BIRTH MAY 6, 1947, LICENSE NUMBER 0004514 OF 4504 BLACKTAIL LANE, BUTTE, MT, WAS DISCIPLINED BY MONTANA ON APRIL 11, 1996
DISCIPLINARY ACTION: EMERGENCY SUSPENSION
OFFENSE: SUBSTANCE ABUSE

NOTES: VIOLATED HIS MONTANA PROFESSIONAL ASSISTANCE PROGRAM AGREEMENT ENTERED INTO 1/24/96 FOR RECOVERY FROM ALCOHOL OR CHEMICAL DEPENDENCY; ON 3/13/96 INGESTED ALCOHOL AND DID NOT INFORM PROGRAM; IN 4/96 FAILED AND REFUSED TO REPORT FOR EVALUATION AND/OR TREATMENT AND FAILED TO REPORT TO A BOARD ORDERED EVALUATION; NOT IN RECOVERY OF HIS DISEASE OF ALCOHOLISM AND/OR CHEMICAL DEPENDENCY. SHALL SURRENDER LICENSE TO THE BOARD; AND SHALL CEASE AND DESIST FROM THE PRACTICE OF MEDICINE.

KRAUSE, ROBERT ALAN MD, DATE OF BIRTH MAY 6, 1947, LICENSE NUMBER 0004514 OF 4504 BLACKTAIL LANE, BUTTE, MT, WAS DISCIPLINED BY MONTANA ON JUNE 5, 1996
DISCIPLINARY ACTION: 60-MONTH PROBATION; MONITORING OF PHYSICIAN PERFORMANCE
OFFENSE: SUBSTANCE ABUSE

NOTES: VIOLATED AGREEMENT WITH PROFESSIONAL ASSISTANCE PROGRAM; ALCOHOL ABUSE. HAS NOW UNDERGONE A BOARD APPROVED EVALUATION RECEIVING A DIAGNOSIS OF ALCOHOL ABUSE, WITH POSSIBLE ALCOHOL DEPENDENCE. CONDITIONS OF PROBATION: SHALL ENTER INTO A REVISED AGREEMENT WITH THE MONTANA PROFESSIONAL ASSISTANCE PROGRAM; SHALL ABSTAIN FROM ANY USE OF ALCOHOL, MIND-ALTERING OR POTENTIALLY ADDICTING DRUGS OR MEDICATIONS, EXCEPT WHEN PRESCRIBED BY HIS PRIMARY CARE PHYSICIAN; SHALL NOTIFY THE BOARD IN ADVANCE OF TAKING ANY MEDICATION, EXCEPT IN THE CASE OF MEDICAL EMERGENCY; SHALL INFORM HIS PRIMARY CARE PHYSICIAN, DENTIST, AND ANY OTHER HEALTH CARE PROVIDER OF THIS ORDER; SHALL NOT WRITE PRESCRIPTIONS FOR ANY MOOD-ALTERING, ALCOHOL BASED OR POTENTIALLY ADDICTING DRUGS FOR HIMSELF OR ANY MEMBER OF HIS FAMILY; SHALL SUBMIT TO RANDOM BODY FLUID ANALYSIS FOR A MINIMUM OF ONE YEAR UPON BOARD REQUEST; AND SHALL RENEW HIS LICENSE IN A TIMELY FASHION FROM YEAR TO YEAR, DURING THE PROBATIONARY PERIOD.

KRAUSE, ROBERT ALAN MD, DATE OF BIRTH MAY 6, 1947, LICENSE NUMBER 0004514 OF 4504 BLACKTAIL LANE, BUTTE, MT, WAS DISCIPLINED BY MONTANA ON JUNE 27, 1996
DISCIPLINARY ACTION: EMERGENCY SUSPENSION; MONITORING OF PHYSICIAN PERFORMANCE
OFFENSE: FAILURE TO COMPLY WITH PREVIOUS BOARD ORDER

NOTES: VIOLATION OF PROBATION BY INGESTING ALCOHOL ON 6/13/96; PRESENTLY IN RELAPSE. SHALL SURRENDER LICENSE TO THE BOARD; SHALL CEASE AND DESIST ENTIRELY FROM THE PRACTICE OF MEDICINE; SHALL PRESENT HIMSELF FOR COMPLETE MENTAL, PHYSICAL AND CHEMICAL DEPENDENCY EVALUATION AND COOPERATE FULLY WITH THE EVALUATION PROCESS; SHALL FULFILL ANY RECOMMENDATIONS FOR TREATMENT AND OBTAIN A SATISFACTORY MEDICAL DISCHARGE PRIOR TO SEEKING REINSTATEMENT OF LICENSE; AND SHALL PROVIDE THE BOARD WITH RELEASES AND AUTHORIZATIONS TO OBTAIN FULL AND COMPLETE COPIES OF ALL RECORDS, REPORTS OR OTHER DOCUMENTS REGARDING THIS EVALUATION.

KRAUSE, ROBERT ALAN MD, DATE OF BIRTH MAY 6, 1947, LICENSE NUMBER 0004514 OF 4504 BLACKTAIL LANE, BUTTE, MT, WAS DISCIPLINED BY MONTANA ON SEPTEMBER 27, 1996
DISCIPLINARY ACTION: LICENSE REVOCATION
OFFENSE: FAILURE TO COMPLY WITH PREVIOUS BOARD ORDER

NOTES: BASED ON ALLEGATIONS OF PROBATION VIOLATION. DEFAULT ACTION.

LAMURE, DAVID S MD, WAS DISCIPLINED BY NEW MEXICO ON MAY 24, 1991
DISCIPLINARY ACTION: SURRENDER OF LICENSE
OFFENSE: CRIMINAL CONVICTION OR PLEA OF GUILTY, NOLO CONTENDERE, OR NO CONTEST TO A CRIME

NOTES: PENDING APPEAL ON CONVICTION.

LAMURE, DAVID S SR MD, LICENSE NUMBER 00D6695 OF DEXTER, NM, WAS DISCIPLINED BY TEXAS ON OCTOBER 9, 1992
DISCIPLINARY ACTION: LICENSE REVOCATION
OFFENSE: CRIMINAL CONVICTION OR PLEA OF GUILTY, NOLO CONTENDERE, OR NO CONTEST TO A CRIME

NOTES: CONVICTION OF A FELONY.

LAMURE, DAVID S MD OF DEXTER, NM, WAS DISCIPLINED BY NEW MEXICO ON JUNE 14, 1993
DISCIPLINARY ACTION: LICENSE REVOCATION
OFFENSE: CRIMINAL CONVICTION OR PLEA OF GUILTY, NOLO CONTENDERE, OR NO CONTEST TO A CRIME

NOTES: CRIMINAL CONVICTION.

LAMURE, DAVID S MD OF DEXTER, NM, WAS DISCIPLINED BY MISSOURI ON SEPTEMBER 20, 1993
DISCIPLINARY ACTION: LICENSE REVOCATION
OFFENSE: CRIMINAL CONVICTION OR PLEA OF GUILTY, NOLO CONTENDERE, OR NO CONTEST TO A CRIME

NOTES: FELONY CONVICTION. NO REAPPLICATION FOR SEVEN YEARS.

LAWYER, JAMES T MD OF 3248 NORTH MOUNTAIN LANE, BOISE, ID, WAS DISCIPLINED BY NEW MEXICO ON DECEMBER 21, 1994

NOTES: LICENSE PLACED UNDER UNSPECIFIED CONDITIONS. IN 5/99 BASED ON SIMILAR ACTION IN IDAHO, ALL STIPULATIONS FOR SUBSTANCE ABUSE ON HIS LICENSE WERE REMOVED; UNRESTRICTED LICENSE.

LEIDICH, RAYMOND MD, WAS DISCIPLINED BY NEW MEXICO ON APRIL 22, 1995
OFFENSE: SUBSTANCE ABUSE

NOTES: HISTORY OF ALCOHOL ABUSE. LICENSE WITH CONDITIONS.

LERNER, BERNARD MD, WAS DISCIPLINED BY NEW MEXICO ON FEBRUARY 27, 1992
DISCIPLINARY ACTION: RESTRICTION PLACED ON LICENSE

NOTES: LICENSE STIPULATED, UNSPECIFIED.

LEVEY, IRWIN L MD, WAS DISCIPLINED BY NEW MEXICO ON DECEMBER 17, 1992
DISCIPLINARY ACTION: SURRENDER OF LICENSE

NOTES: IN LIEU OF HEARING.

LIES, BERT JR MD, WAS DISCIPLINED BY NEW MEXICO ON AUGUST 25, 1995
DISCIPLINARY ACTION: 36-MONTH PROBATION
OFFENSE: CRIMINAL CONVICTION OR PLEA OF GUILTY, NOLO CONTENDERE, OR NO CONTEST TO A CRIME

NOTES: CONVICTION OF FELONY. SAME TERMS AS COURT-ORDERED PROBATION. IN 8/98 BOARD REMOVED ALL STIPULATIONS FOR PROBATION FOR TAX EVASION, GIVING HIM AN UNRESTRICTED LICENSE.

LIES, BERT A JR MD, LICENSE NUMBER 0095843 OF 539 HARKLE ROAD, SANTA FE, NM, WAS DISCIPLINED BY NEW YORK ON SEPTEMBER 11, 1996
DISCIPLINARY ACTION: LICENSE SUSPENSION
OFFENSE: DISCIPLINARY ACTION BY ANOTHER STATE OR AGENCY

NOTES: DISCIPLINED BY THE NEW MEXICO BOARD FOR CONVICTION IN COURT OF FILING FALSE INCOME TAX STATEMENTS. SUSPENSION UNTIL HE COMPLETES ALL PROBATION TERMS IMPOSED BY THE NEW MEXICO BOARD AND AUTHORITIES.

LIES, BERT A MD, LICENSE NUMBER 0029966 OF SANTA FE, NM, WAS DISCIPLINED BY WASHINGTON ON NOVEMBER 15, 1996
DISCIPLINARY ACTION: PROBATION

NOTES: PROBATION UNDER TERMS AND CONDITIONS.

LIES, BERT A MD, DATE OF BIRTH APRIL 22, 1939, LICENSE NUMBER 30316, WAS DISCIPLINED BY COLORADO ON AUGUST 13, 1997
DISCIPLINARY ACTION: LICENSE REVOCATION
OFFENSE: CRIMINAL CONVICTION OR PLEA OF GUILTY, NOLO CONTENDERE, OR NO CONTEST TO A CRIME

NOTES: FELONY CONVICTION.

LIES, BERT A JR MD, LICENSE NUMBER G14439 OF CRYSTAL BAY, NV, WAS DISCIPLINED BY CALIFORNIA ON JUNE 12, 1998
DISCIPLINARY ACTION: 60-MONTH PROBATION
OFFENSE: DISCIPLINARY ACTION BY ANOTHER STATE OR AGENCY

NOTES: DISCIPLINED BY NEW MEXICO BASED ON HIS FELONY CONVICTION FOR FILING FALSE INCOME TAX RETURNS. REVOCATION STAYED.

LIES, BERT A JR MD, LICENSE NUMBER G14439 OF CRYSTAL BAY, NV, WAS DISCIPLINED BY CALIFORNIA ON JUNE 24, 1998
DISCIPLINARY ACTION: SURRENDER OF LICENSE

NOTES: WHILE CHARGES PENDING.

LIND, JOHN MD, WAS DISCIPLINED BY NEW MEXICO ON AUGUST 17, 1990
DISCIPLINARY ACTION: DENIAL OF NEW LICENSE
OFFENSE: DISCIPLINARY ACTION BY ANOTHER STATE OR AGENCY

NOTES: FELONY CONVICTION AND ACTION IN ANOTHER STATE

LIPANA, OSCAR MD, WAS DISCIPLINED BY NEW MEXICO ON MAY 1, 1999
DISCIPLINARY ACTION: PROBATION; REQUIRED TO TAKE ADDITIONAL MEDICAL EDUCATION

NOTES: REQUIREMENTS FOR FURTHER TRAINING.

LOMBARDO, MICHAEL MD OF 3901 72ND STREET NW, ALBUQUERQUE, NM, WAS DISCIPLINED BY NEW MEXICO ON AUGUST 26, 1993
OFFENSE: SUBSTANCE ABUSE

NOTES: LICENSE PLACED UNDER UNSPECIFIED CONDITIONS.

LOMBARDO, MICHAEL J MD, WAS DISCIPLINED BY NEW MEXICO ON NOVEMBER 1, 1996
DISCIPLINARY ACTION: EMERGENCY SUSPENSION
OFFENSE: FAILURE TO COMPLY WITH PREVIOUS BOARD ORDER

NOTES: NOTICE OF CONTEMPLATED ACTION FOR VIOLATION OF STIPULATION.

MADDOX, A DANIEL MD, WAS DISCIPLINED BY NEW MEXICO ON FEBRUARY 1, 1996
DISCIPLINARY ACTION: LICENSE REVOCATION
OFFENSE: OVERPRESCRIBING OR MISPRESCRIBING DRUGS

NOTES: INJUDICIOUS PRESCRIBING.

MAGLIOZZI, JOSEPH MD, WAS DISCIPLINED BY NEW MEXICO ON JANUARY 1, 1997
DISCIPLINARY ACTION: SURRENDER OF LICENSE

OFFENSE: OVERPRESCRIBING OR MISPRESCRIBING DRUGS

NOTES: IN LIEU OF PROSECUTION FOR INJUDICIOUS PRESCRIBING, HE VOLUNTARILY SURRENDERED HIS LICENSE AND MAY NEVER REAPPLY.

MAGLIOZZI, JOSEPH R MD, LICENSE NUMBER G34335 OF PLACITAS, NM, WAS DISCIPLINED BY CALIFORNIA ON JANUARY 14, 1999
DISCIPLINARY ACTION: SURRENDER OF LICENSE

NOTES: WHILE CHARGES PENDING.

MARCUS, M BENNETT MD, LICENSE NUMBER 0A17220 OF WHITTIER, CA, WAS DISCIPLINED BY CALIFORNIA ON APRIL 14, 1995
DISCIPLINARY ACTION: LICENSE REVOCATION
OFFENSE: SUBSTANDARD CARE, INCOMPETENCE OR NEGLIGENCE

NOTES: GROSS NEGLIGENCE, INCOMPETENCE AND REPEATED NEGLIGENT ACTS IN OBSTETRICAL PRACTICE. DEFAULT DECISION.

MARCUS, M BENNETT MD, LICENSE NUMBER 0079192 OF 1300 VISTA MORADA, SANTE FE, NM, WAS DISCIPLINED BY NEW YORK ON AUGUST 5, 1996
DISCIPLINARY ACTION: LICENSE REVOCATION
OFFENSE: DISCIPLINARY ACTION BY ANOTHER STATE OR AGENCY

NOTES: ACTION IN CALIFORNIA FOR GROSS NEGLIGENCE AND NEGLIGENCE AND INCOMPETENCE ON MORE THAN ONE OCCASION FOR PERFORMING AN UNNECESSARY CESAREAN SECTION AND FOR CUTTING THE UMBILICAL CORD CAUSING THE INFANT TO LOSE BLOOD AND REQUIRE A TRANSFUSION.

MARON, BARRY R MD, DATE OF BIRTH NOVEMBER 30, 1938, LICENSE NUMBER 0020300 OF IA, WAS DISCIPLINED BY ARIZONA ON APRIL 15, 1993

NOTES: BOARD HAS INVESTIGATED INFORMATION THAT HE HAS BIPOLAR DISORDER AND SELF MEDICATES HIMSELF. CURRENTLY PRACTICING IN IOWA. SHALL NOT PRACTICE MEDICINE IN ARIZONA UNTIL HE HAS FIRST ADVISED THE BOARD OF HIS INTENTION TO DO SO AND RECEIVED AUTHORIZATION.

MARON, BARRY R MD, DATE OF BIRTH NOVEMBER 30, 1938, LICENSE NUMBER 0021140 OF BOX 1707, BORGER, TX, WAS DISCIPLINED BY NEW JERSEY ON NOVEMBER 2, 1994

NOTES: AGREES TO COMPLY WITH ALL REQUIREMENTS OF AN ORDER DATED 06/16/93 ISSUED BY THE BOARD OF MEDICAL EXAMINERS OF ARIZONA. SHALL PROVIDE NOTICE TO NEW JERSEY OF ANY CHANGE IN ANY OF THE TERMS OF THE ARIZONA AGREEMENT OR HIS MEDICAL CONDITION. PRIOR TO ENGAGING IN ACTIVE PRACTICE IN NEW JERSEY, SHALL APPEAR BEFORE THE BOARD OR A COMMITTEE OF THE BOARD TO RESPOND TO QUESTIONS CONCERNING HIS STATUS, HEALTH AND PLANS.

MARON, BARRY R MD, LICENSE NUMBER 0G16120 OF ALBUQUERQUE, NM, WAS DISCIPLINED BY CALIFORNIA ON MAY 19, 1995
DISCIPLINARY ACTION: 60-MONTH PROBATION
OFFENSE: DISCIPLINARY ACTION BY ANOTHER STATE OR AGENCY

NOTES: ARIZONA ORDER RESTRICTING RESUMPTION OF PRACTICE WITH PRECONDITIONS, SUCH AS PSYCHIATRIC EVALUATION FOR SAFE PRACTICE. REVOCATION STAYED.

MARON, BARRY R MD, DATE OF BIRTH NOVEMBER 30, 1938, LICENSE NUMBER 0028935 OF 408 NORTH MAIN STREET, WARSAW, NY, WAS DISCIPLINED BY IOWA ON AUGUST 8, 1996

NOTES: AGREED THAT HE WILL NOT RETURN TO PRACTICE IN IOWA UNLESS HE GIVES THE BOARD 30 DAYS NOTICE IN WRITING AND IF HE DOES RETURN SHALL ENTER INTO A CONSENT AGREEMENT PLACING ANY RESTRICTIONS ON HIS LICENSE THAT THE BOARD DEEMS NECESSARY.

MCMILLAN, TERRY H MD OF 2930 HILLRISE, LAS CRUCES, NM, WAS DISCIPLINED BY NEW MEXICO ON AUGUST 26, 1993
OFFENSE: SUBSTANCE ABUSE

NOTES: LICENSE PLACED UNDER UNSPECIFIED CONDITIONS. IN 8/98 REMOVED ALL STIPULATIONS FOR SUBSTANCE ABUSE; UNRESTRICTED LICENSE.

MONTOYA, DONALD H MD OF 1290 EAST 32ND STREET, SILVER CITY, NM, WAS DISCIPLINED BY NEW MEXICO ON JUNE 24, 1993
OFFENSE: PROFESSIONAL MISCONDUCT

NOTES: LICENSE PLACED UNDER UNSPECIFIED CONDITIONS. IN 1997 STIPULATION FOR CHAPERONED PRACTICE OF MEDICINE REDUCED TO ANNUAL VISITS WITH THE BOARD.

MOORHEAD, PETER MD OF 703 COBEAN DRIVE, ROSWELL, NM, WAS DISCIPLINED BY NEW MEXICO ON DECEMBER 17, 1993
DISCIPLINARY ACTION: LICENSE SUSPENSION
OFFENSE: SUBSTANCE ABUSE

MOORHEAD, PETER MD, WAS DISCIPLINED BY NEW MEXICO ON AUGUST 1, 1998
DISCIPLINARY ACTION: RESTRICTION PLACED ON CONTROLLED SUBSTANCE LICENSE
OFFENSE: SUBSTANCE ABUSE

NOTES: SUSPENSION IS LIFTED AND A STIPULATED LICENSE WITH STANDARD STIPULATIONS FOR SUBSTANCE ABUSE, AS WELL AS A LIFETIME RESTRICTION FROM HOLDING A DEA PERMIT IS ISSUED. ON 8/1/99 STIPULATIONS FOR SUBSTANCE ABUSE REDUCED TO BIANNUAL VISITS WITH THE BOARD; ALL OTHER STIPULATIONS REMAIN THE SAME.

MOORHEAD, PETER B MD, WAS DISCIPLINED BY NEW MEXICO ON DECEMBER 17, 1992
DISCIPLINARY ACTION: RESTRICTION PLACED ON LICENSE

NOTES: LICENSE STIPULATED, UNSPECIFIED.

MOORHEAD, PETER B MD, WAS DISCIPLINED BY NEW MEXICO ON JULY 1, 1997
DISCIPLINARY ACTION: 12-MONTH LICENSE SUSPENSION; REQUIRED TO TAKE ADDITIONAL MEDICAL EDUCATION
OFFENSE: FAILURE TO COMPLY WITH PREVIOUS BOARD ORDER

NOTES: VIOLATION OF STIPULATION AND CONTRACT; SUSPENDED BEGINNING IN 7/97 DURING WHICH TIME HE IS TO CONTINUE WITH THE MONITORED TREATMENT PROGRAM AND HIS CONTINUING MEDICAL EDUCATION REQUIREMENTS. BOARD WILL EVALUATE PHYSICIAN AT THE END OF THE SUSPENSION.

MOORHEAD, PETER BRIAN MD OF 1621 N WASHINGTON, ROSWELL, NM, WAS DISCIPLINED BY DEA ON DECEMBER 1, 1993
DISCIPLINARY ACTION: SURRENDER OF CONTROLLED SUBSTANCE LICENSE
OFFENSE: DISCIPLINARY ACTION BY ANOTHER STATE OR AGENCY

NOTES: BASED ON SUSPENSION OF MEDICAL LICENSE.

MORO, MICHELE MD, WAS DISCIPLINED BY NEW MEXICO ON AUGUST 1, 1998
OFFENSE: SUBSTANCE ABUSE

NOTES: STANDARD STIPULATIONS FOR VOLUNTARY TREATMENT OF SUBSTANCE ABUSE.

MOTE, PAUL S MD, DATE OF BIRTH AUGUST 28, 1947, LICENSE NUMBER 0029142, WAS DISCIPLINED BY COLORADO ON APRIL 18, 1996
DISCIPLINARY ACTION: 60-MONTH PROBATION; REQUIRED TO TAKE ADDITIONAL MEDICAL EDUCATION
OFFENSE: SUBSTANDARD CARE, INCOMPETENCE OR NEGLIGENCE

NOTES: SUBSTANDARD CARE. FIVE YEAR PROBATION WITH RE-EDUCATION ACTIVITIES AND PRACTICE MONITORING.

MOTE, PAUL S MD, DATE OF BIRTH AUGUST 28, 1947, LICENSE NUMBER 0029142, WAS DISCIPLINED BY COLORADO ON JUNE 20, 1996
DISCIPLINARY ACTION: SURRENDER OF LICENSE

NOTES: NO UNPROFESSIONAL CONDUCT IDENTIFIED.

MOTE, PAUL S MD, WAS DISCIPLINED BY NEW MEXICO ON JANUARY 1, 1997
DISCIPLINARY ACTION: SURRENDER OF LICENSE
OFFENSE: PROVIDING FALSE INFORMATION TO THE BOARD OR OTHER HEALTH AGENCY

NOTES: PROVIDED FALSE INFORMATION TO THE BOARD ON A LICENSE RENEWAL AND FAILURE TO NOTIFY THE BOARD; VOLUNTARY SURRENDER OF NEW MEXICO LICENSE WITH THE CONDITION THAT HE MAY NEVER REAPPLY.

MULDOON, THOMAS N MD, DATE OF BIRTH JUNE 3, 1936 OF FED CORR INST - PO BOX 1000, ANTHONY, NM, WAS DISCIPLINED BY MEDICARE ON FEBRUARY 10, 1992
DISCIPLINARY ACTION: EXCLUSION FROM THE MEDICARE AND/OR MEDICAID PROGRAM
OFFENSE: DISCIPLINARY ACTION BY ANOTHER STATE OR AGENCY

NOTES: LICENSE REVOCATION OR SUSPENSION.

NARAYAN, VENKAT MD, WAS DISCIPLINED BY NEW MEXICO ON AUGUST 1, 1998
DISCIPLINARY ACTION: RESTRICTION PLACED ON LICENSE

NOTES: MAY ONLY HOLD PRIVILEGES AT SPECIFIED HOSPITAL AND MUST FOLLOW HOSPITAL GUIDELINES FOR SURGICAL PROCEDURES.

NASH, ROBERT MD OF PO BOX 177, EVANSTON, WY, WAS DISCIPLINED BY NEW MEXICO ON MAY 20, 1994
OFFENSE: DISCIPLINARY ACTION BY ANOTHER STATE OR AGENCY

NOTES: LICENSE PLACED UNDER UNSPECIFIED CONDITIONS.

NEWVILLE, BETTY MD, WAS DISCIPLINED BY NEW MEXICO ON AUGUST 1, 1998
OFFENSE: SUBSTANCE ABUSE

NOTES: LICENSE PLACED UNDER STANDARD STIPULATIONS FOR SUBSTANCE ABUSE.

NOVOSAD, CHARLES L JR MD, DATE OF BIRTH DECEMBER 19, 1930 OF PO BOX 3498, POJOAQUE, NM, WAS DISCIPLINED BY MEDICARE ON SEPTEMBER 15, 1996
DISCIPLINARY ACTION: EXCLUSION FROM THE MEDICARE AND/OR MEDICAID PROGRAM
OFFENSE: DISCIPLINARY ACTION BY ANOTHER STATE OR AGENCY

NOTES: LICENSE REVOKED FOR REASONS BEARING ON PROFESSIONAL PERFORMANCE.

NOVOSAD, CHARLES LOUIS JR MD OF 210 NORTH HIGHWAY 285, POJOAQUE, NM, WAS DISCIPLINED BY NEW MEXICO ON MAY 20, 1994
DISCIPLINARY ACTION: LICENSE REVOCATION
OFFENSE: OVERPRESCRIBING OR MISPRESCRIBING DRUGS

NOTES: UNPROFESSIONAL CONDUCT; INJUDICIOUS PRESCRIBING.

NOVOSAD, CHARLES LOUIS JR MD, LICENSE NUMBER 0008996, WAS DISCIPLINED BY OKLAHOMA ON SEPTEMBER 9, 1994
DISCIPLINARY ACTION: LICENSE REVOCATION
OFFENSE: DISCIPLINARY ACTION BY ANOTHER STATE OR AGENCY

NOTES: ON 5/20/94 NEW MEXICO BOARD REVOKED HIS LICENSE BASED ON OVER-PRESCRIPTION AND IMPROPER PRESCRIPTION OF CONTROLLED DANGEROUS SUBSTANCES.

NOVOSAD, CHARLES LOUIS JR MD, LICENSE NUMBER 00C4483 OF POJOAQUE, NM, WAS DISCIPLINED BY TEXAS ON JANUARY 6, 1995
OFFENSE: DISCIPLINARY ACTION BY ANOTHER STATE OR AGENCY

NOTES: ON 5/20/94 NEW MEXICO BOARD REVOKED HIS LICENSE ON THE GROUNDS OF INJUDICIOUS PRESCRIBING TO SEVERAL PATIENTS; PRESENTLY SEEKING JUDICIAL REVIEW OF THIS ORDER. SHALL NOT PRACTICE IN TEXAS UNTIL HE REQUESTS PERMISSION IN WRITING FROM THE TEXAS BOARD TO RESUME PRACTICE, PERSONALLY APPEARS BEFORE THE BOARD AND PROVIDES SUFFICIENT EVIDENCE THAT HE IS PHYSICALLY, MENTALLY AND OTHERWISE COMPETENT TO PRACTICE INCLUDING AT A MINIMUM CERTIFICATION OF REVERSAL OF THE NEW MEXICO REVOCATION; SHALL COOPERATE WITH THE BOARD IN VERIFYING COMPLIANCE; SHALL INFORM BOARD OF CHANGE OF ADDRESS WITHIN 10 DAYS.

NOVOSAD, CHARLES LOUIS JR MD OF POJOAQUE, NM, WAS DISCIPLINED BY DEA ON OCTOBER 11, 1995
DISCIPLINARY ACTION: REVOCATION OF CONTROLLED SUBSTANCE LICENSE
OFFENSE: DISCIPLINARY ACTION BY ANOTHER STATE OR AGENCY

NOTES: ON 5/20/94 NEW MEXICO BOARD ORDERED THE REVOCATION OF HIS LICENSE; ON 9/15/94 THE NEW MEXICO PHARMACY BOARD REVOKED HIS STATE REGISTRATION TO HANDLE CONTROLLED SUBSTANCES.

OSSORIO, JULIO M MD, DATE OF BIRTH JULY 9, 1948, LICENSE NUMBER 0032219 OF CANON CITY, CO, WAS DISCIPLINED BY COLORADO ON DECEMBER 1, 1992
DISCIPLINARY ACTION: EMERGENCY SUSPENSION
OFFENSE: PROVIDING FALSE INFORMATION TO THE BOARD OR OTHER HEALTH AGENCY

NOTES: RESORTING TO FRAUD, MISREPRESENTATION, OR DECEPTION IN APPLYING FOR AND SECURING A MEDICAL LICENSE; HABITUAL INTEMPERANCE; PHYSICAL OR MENTAL DISABILITY WHICH RENDERS HIM UNABLE TO PRACTICE WITH SKILL AND SAFETY; FAILURE TO MEET GENERALLY ACCEPTED STANDARDS OF MEDICAL PRACTICE.

OSSORIO, JULIO M MD, DATE OF BIRTH JULY 9, 1948, LICENSE NUMBER 0032219 OF CANON CITY, CO, WAS DISCIPLINED BY COLORADO ON MARCH 19, 1993

DISCIPLINARY ACTION: SURRENDER OF LICENSE
OFFENSE: SUBSTANCE ABUSE

NOTES: HABITUAL INTEMPERANCE.

OSSORIO, JULIO M MD OF 3695 HOT SPRINGS BLVD, LAS VEGAS, NM, WAS DISCIPLINED BY NEW MEXICO ON AUGUST 26, 1993
OFFENSE: SUBSTANCE ABUSE

NOTES: LICENSE PLACED UNDER UNSPECIFIED CONDITIONS. IN 11/98 REMOVED ALL STIPULATIONS FOR SUBSTANCE ABUSE, GIVING HIM AN UNRESTRICTED LICENSE.

OSSORIO, JULIO M MD, LICENSE NUMBER 0117727 OF 1001 RUPPEL STREET APT 521, PUEBLO, CO, WAS DISCIPLINED BY NEW YORK ON NOVEMBER 15, 1993
DISCIPLINARY ACTION: LICENSE REVOCATION
OFFENSE: DISCIPLINARY ACTION BY ANOTHER STATE OR AGENCY

NOTES: SURRENDERED HIS LICENSE IN COLORADO.

OSTERHOLTZ, ROGER L MD, WAS DISCIPLINED BY NEW MEXICO ON MAY 17, 1995
OFFENSE: SUBSTANCE ABUSE

NOTES: HISTORY OF SUBSTANCE ABUSE. LICENSE WITH CONDITIONS. NO LONGER STIPULATED AS OF 8/22/95. IN 1996 ALL STIPULATIONS REMOVED.

PALMER, ROBERT C MD, WAS DISCIPLINED BY NEW MEXICO ON NOVEMBER 1, 1996
DISCIPLINARY ACTION: RESTRICTION PLACED ON LICENSE

NOTES: REQUESTED VOLUNTARY RESTRICTION OF LICENSE.

PALMER, ROBERT CLEMMER MD, LICENSE NUMBER 0G20990 OF ALBUQUERQUE, NM, WAS DISCIPLINED BY CALIFORNIA ON JANUARY 18, 1995
DISCIPLINARY ACTION: SURRENDER OF LICENSE

NOTES: VOLUNTARY SURRENDER OF LICENSE WHILE CHARGES PENDING.

PARADA, JOSEPH A MD, WAS DISCIPLINED BY NEW MEXICO ON JANUARY 1, 1997
DISCIPLINARY ACTION: SURRENDER OF LICENSE
OFFENSE: SUBSTANDARD CARE, INCOMPETENCE OR NEGLIGENCE

NOTES: NOTICE OF CONTEMPLATED ACTION FOR REPEATED SIMILAR NEGLIGENT ACTS WHILE PRACTICING MEDICINE. AGREED ORDER OF DISMISSAL WITH VOLUNTARY SURRENDER OF LICENSE. SURRENDERED LICENSE NOT TO AVOID INQUIRY BUT BECAUSE HE HAS NO INTENTION OF PRACTICING IN NEW MEXICO.

PARKER, WAYLON M MD OF MARRERO, LA, WAS DISCIPLINED BY LOUISIANA ON APRIL 29, 1996
DISCIPLINARY ACTION: 16-MONTH LICENSE SUSPENSION
OFFENSE: DISCIPLINARY ACTION BY ANOTHER STATE OR AGENCY

NOTES: ACTION IN MISSISSIPPI. SURRENDER OF LICENSE IN TEXAS WHILE UNDER INVESTIGATION. MISREPRESENTATION AND DECEIT IN OBTAINING RENEWAL OF LICENSURE. APPLICATION FOR LICENSURE UPON COMPLETION OF PROBATION IMPOSED IN MISSISSIPPI; SHALL PAY ALL COSTS OF PROCEEDINGS.

PARKER, WAYLON M MD, WAS DISCIPLINED BY NEW MEXICO ON JANUARY 1, 1997
DISCIPLINARY ACTION: LICENSE REVOCATION
OFFENSE: DISCIPLINARY ACTION BY ANOTHER STATE OR AGENCY

NOTES: FAILURE TO INFORM BOARD OF SUSPENSION AND REVOCATION OF OTHER STATE LICENSES, AND HE MAY NEVER REAPPLY. AS OF 5/98, THE BOARD ACCEPTED PROPOSED ORDER TO WITHDRAW REVOCATION AND ALLOW HIM TO VOLUNTARILY SURRENDER NEW MEXICO LICENSE WITH CONDITION THAT HE MAY NEVER REAPPLY.

PARKER, WAYLON MORRIS MD, DATE OF BIRTH MAY 18, 1956, LICENSE NUMBER 00G7301 OF GULFPORT, MS, WAS DISCIPLINED BY TEXAS ON AUGUST 19, 1994
DISCIPLINARY ACTION: SURRENDER OF LICENSE
OFFENSE: OVERPRESCRIBING OR MISPRESCRIBING DRUGS

NOTES: ALLEGATIONS OF NON-THERAPEUTIC PRESCRIBING; HE DOES NOT ADMIT THIS BUT WISHES TO AVOID EXPENSE OF LITIGATION. SURRENDER IN LIEU OF FURTHER INVESTIGATION. SHALL NOT PETITION FOR REINSTATEMENT OF LICENSE.

PARKER, WAYLON MORRIS MD, DATE OF BIRTH MAY 18, 1956, LICENSE NUMBER 0012804 OF 4700 WICHERS DRIVE, SUITE 101, MARRERO, LA, WAS DISCIPLINED BY MISSISSIPPI ON SEPTEMBER 21, 1995
OFFENSE: DISCIPLINARY ACTION BY ANOTHER STATE OR AGENCY

NOTES: ON 8/15/94 TEXAS LICENSE SURRENDERED WHILE UNDER INVESTIGATION FOR NON-THERAPEUTIC PRESCRIBING TO A PATIENT HE HAD PREVIOUSLY IDENTIFIED AS HIS WIFE AND LATER SAID HE WAS TRYING TO PROTECT FROM SPOUSAL ABUSE. FIVE YEAR SUSPENSION STAYED SUBJECT TO CERTAIN CONDITIONS. ORDER MODIFIED ON 5/14/96 REQUIRING HIM TO RECEIVE PSYCHIATRIC TREATMENT/THERAPY FOR TWO YEARS WITH QUARTERLY REPORTS TO THE BOARD; SHALL COMPLETE THE COURSE "CLINICAL, LEGAL, AND ETHICAL ISSUES IN PRESCRIBING ABUSABLE DRUGS" OR AN EQUIVALENT BOARD APPROVED COURSE; PRACTICE LIMITED TO A GROUP SETTING WITH MONITORING; SHALL LIMIT PRACTICE TO PEDIATRICS AND SHALL NOT TREAT ADULTS OR FAMILY MEMBERS OR ANY SEXUALLY AND/OR PHYSICALLY ABUSED PATIENTS; CONTROLLED SUBSTANCES REGISTRATION CERTIFICATE LIMITED TO SCHEDULE V DRUGS WITH EXCEPTION OF BUPRENEX; ALSO CANNOT PRESCRIBE, ADMINISTER, DISPENSE OR POSSESS STADOL, NUBAIN, DALGEN, SOMA OR BUTALBITAL PRODUCTS.

PIZARRO, CECILIO MD, WAS DISCIPLINED BY NEW MEXICO ON FEBRUARY 1, 1998
DISCIPLINARY ACTION: LICENSE REVOCATION
OFFENSE: NONCOMPLIANCE WITH A PROFESSIONAL RULE

NOTES: FAILURE TO KEEP THE BOARD INFORMED OF CURRENT ADDRESS; MAY NEVER REAPPLY.

PLATTER, DANIEL H MD, DATE OF BIRTH JULY 22, 1960 OF 14213 LA CUEVA AVENUE NE, ALBUQUERQUE, NM, WAS DISCIPLINED BY MEDICARE ON MARCH 6, 1994
DISCIPLINARY ACTION: EXCLUSION FROM THE MEDICARE AND/OR MEDICAID PROGRAM
OFFENSE: NONCOMPLIANCE WITH A PROFESSIONAL RULE

NOTES: DEFAULTED ON PUBLIC HEALTH SERVICE EDUCATION LOAN.

POE, BRYAN S DO, LICENSE NUMBER 0A83486, WAS DISCIPLINED BY NEW MEXICO ON JANUARY 31, 1995
OFFENSE: PROFESSIONAL MISCONDUCT

NOTES: UNPROFESSIONAL AND NEGLIGENT CONDUCT. UNSPECIFIED STIPULATION AND ORDER ISSUED. ON 2/18/97 RESTRICTION REMOVED FROM LICENSE.

POE, BRYAN S DO OF 406 POST OFFICE SQUARE, AZTEC, NM, WAS DISCIPLINED BY DEA ON MAY 8, 1995
DISCIPLINARY ACTION: RESTRICTION PLACED ON CONTROLLED SUBSTANCE LICENSE
OFFENSE: DISCIPLINARY ACTION BY ANOTHER STATE OR AGENCY

NOTES: STATE BOARD.

POE, BRYAN S DO, LICENSE NUMBER A83486, WAS DISCIPLINED BY NEW MEXICO ON MAY 1, 1998
DISCIPLINARY ACTION: 12-MONTH LICENSE SUSPENSION
OFFENSE: PROFESSIONAL MISCONDUCT

NOTES: IMMORAL, DISHONORABLE, AND UNPROFESSIONAL CONDUCT. ON 5/15/99 LICENSE REINSTATED AS HE HAD COMPLIED WITH CONDITIONS OF THE ORDER.

PRIOR, WILLIAM FRANKLIN MD OF 28 CAMINO DES ALTES #977, PLACITAS, NM, WAS DISCIPLINED BY DEA ON AUGUST 31, 1998
DISCIPLINARY ACTION: SURRENDER OF CONTROLLED SUBSTANCE LICENSE

QUARMBY, ROBERT MD, WAS DISCIPLINED BY NEW MEXICO ON AUGUST 1, 1998
DISCIPLINARY ACTION: RESTRICTION PLACED ON LICENSE; MONITORING OF PHYSICIAN PERFORMANCE

NOTES: PRACTICE LIMITED TO INCLUDE MONITORING OF SCHEDULE II AND III CONTROLLED SUBSTANCE PRESCRIPTIONS AND LIMITATIONS ON TRIGGER POINT INJECTIONS.

QUARMBY, ROBERT MD, WAS DISCIPLINED BY NEW MEXICO ON AUGUST 26, 1999
DISCIPLINARY ACTION: EMERGENCY SUSPENSION
OFFENSE: FAILURE TO COMPLY WITH PREVIOUS BOARD ORDER

NOTES: NONCOMPLIANCE WITH TERMS OF PROBATION.

QUARMBY, ROBERT MD, LICENSE NUMBER 156855 OF 2604 EAST MAIN STREET, FARMINGTON, NM, WAS DISCIPLINED BY NEW YORK ON NOVEMBER 18, 1999
DISCIPLINARY ACTION: EMERGENCY SUSPENSION
OFFENSE: DISCIPLINARY ACTION BY ANOTHER STATE OR AGENCY

NOTES: LICENSE SUSPENDED BY THE NEW MEXICO BOARD FOR BREACHING AN ORDER LIMITING HIS PRACTICE BY PRESCRIBING SCHEDULE II DRUGS WITHOUT THE APPROVAL OF AN EVALUATING PHYSICIAN.

REED, TERESA MD, WAS DISCIPLINED BY NEW MEXICO ON NOVEMBER 22, 1991

NOTES: LICENSE STIPULATED.

RICE, SCOTT W MD, WAS DISCIPLINED BY NEW MEXICO ON JANUARY 1, 1997
DISCIPLINARY ACTION: SURRENDER OF LICENSE

NOTES: REFERRED TO AN IMPAIRED PHYSICIANS COMMITTEE FOR EVALUATION OF HEALTH MATTERS; VOLUNTARY SURRENDER OF LICENSE UNDER THE TERMS OF THE IMPAIRED HEALTH CARE PROVIDER ACT.

ROGERS, CHERYL MD, WAS DISCIPLINED BY NEW MEXICO ON AUGUST 17, 1990

NOTES: LICENSE STIPULATED TO CONCUR WITH STIPULATIONS ON TEXAS LICENSE.

ROSEIN, IGOR MD, WAS DISCIPLINED BY NEW MEXICO ON AUGUST 29, 1990

NOTES: LICENSE STIPULATED.

ROSEN, BARUCH MD OF 7555 EAST OSBORN ROAD, SCOTTSDALE, AZ, WAS DISCIPLINED BY NEW MEXICO ON DECEMBER 16, 1994
DISCIPLINARY ACTION: LICENSE REVOCATION
OFFENSE: DISCIPLINARY ACTION BY ANOTHER STATE OR AGENCY

ROSS, RICHARD B MD, WAS DISCIPLINED BY NEW MEXICO ON AUGUST 1, 1996

NOTES: ENTERED INTO STIPULATED AGREEMENT WITH THE BOARD. IN 8/98 REMOVED ALL RESTRICTIONS FOR BEHAVIORAL THERAPY; UNRESTRICTED LICENSE.

ROTERMUND, KURT H DO, DATE OF BIRTH OCTOBER 2, 1939, LICENSE NUMBER 0020418 OF TAOS, NM, WAS DISCIPLINED BY KENTUCKY ON NOVEMBER 27, 1991
DISCIPLINARY ACTION: LICENSE REVOCATION
OFFENSE: DISCIPLINARY ACTION BY ANOTHER STATE OR AGENCY

NOTES: REVOCATION OF LICENSE IN NEW MEXICO; FELONY CONVICTIONS.

ROTERMUND, KURT H DO OF BRECKENRIDGE, MI, WAS DISCIPLINED BY MISSOURI ON SEPTEMBER 20, 1993
DISCIPLINARY ACTION: LICENSE REVOCATION
OFFENSE: DISCIPLINARY ACTION BY ANOTHER STATE OR AGENCY

NOTES: BASED ON REVOCATION IN ANOTHER STATE. NO REAPPLICATION FOR SEVEN YEARS.

ROY, JERRY MD, WAS DISCIPLINED BY NEW MEXICO ON NOVEMBER 16, 1995
DISCIPLINARY ACTION: PROBATION; REQUIRED TO ENTER AN IMPAIRED PHYSICIAN PROGRAM OR SUBSTANCE ABUSE TREATMENT
OFFENSE: SUBSTANCE ABUSE

NOTES: INFORMED THE BOARD OF HIS HISTORY OF SUBSTANCE ABUSE AND CONTINUING REHABILITATION. TERMS AND CONDITIONS: SHALL ABSTAIN FROM THE USE OF MIND-ALTERING SUBSTANCES, CONTROLLED SUBSTANCES OR ALCOHOLIC BEVERAGES EXCEPT AS PRESCRIBED BY A LICENSED PHYSICIAN; SHALL BE AN ACTIVE PARTICIPANT IN THE NEW MEXICO MONITORED TREATMENT PROGRAM; SHALL SUBMIT TO RANDOM FLUID TESTING; SHALL APPEAR BEFORE THE BOARD ON A QUARTERLY BASIS OR UPON REQUEST; SHALL SUBMIT QUARTERLY REPORTS TO THE BOARD ATTESTING TO HIS COMPLIANCE WITH THIS STIPULATION. IN 1997 MEETINGS WITH THE BOARD WERE REDUCED TO BIANNUALLY.

ROY, SAMIR MD, WAS DISCIPLINED BY NEW MEXICO ON FEBRUARY 1, 1996
DISCIPLINARY ACTION: LICENSE REVOCATION
OFFENSE: PROFESSIONAL MISCONDUCT

NOTES: SEXUAL MISCONDUCT AND UNPROFESSIONAL CONDUCT.

ROY, SAMIR MD, DATE OF BIRTH NOVEMBER 20, 1945, LICENSE NUMBER 27494 OF 705 SAGEBRUSH TRAIL S.E., ALBUQUERQUE, NM, WAS DISCIPLINED BY WISCONSIN ON JANUARY 23, 1997
DISCIPLINARY ACTION: SURRENDER OF LICENSE

OFFENSE: DISCIPLINARY ACTION BY ANOTHER STATE OR AGENCY

NOTES: ON 2/29/96 THE NEW MEXICO BOARD REVOKED HIS LICENSE DUE TO ENGAGING IN A SEXUAL RELATIONSHIP WITH A FEMALE PATIENT. STARTING IN 5/93 OR 6/93 BEGAN A SEXUAL RELATIONSHIP WITH HER INCLUDING INTERCOURSE AND ORAL SEX; HAD PREVIOUSLY COMMITTED NUMEROUS OTHER BOUNDARY VIOLATIONS WITH THE PATIENT, INCLUDING VISITING HER AT HER HOME, CONSUMING ALCOHOL WITH HER, AND GIVING HER GIFTS. A PSYCHIATRIST TESTIFIED THAT HE SUFFERED FROM RECURRENT MAJOR DEPRESSION. ALSO INDICATED ON A LICENSE RENEWAL FORM THAT HE WAS BOARD CERTIFIED IN PSYCHIATRY WHEN HE HAD NOT TAKEN THE ORAL EXAM REQUIRED FOR CERTIFICATION. HAS APPEALED NEW MEXICO DECISION TO STATE SUPREME COURT. VOLUNTARY SURRENDER.

ROY, SAMIR MD, DATE OF BIRTH NOVEMBER 20, 1945 OF 705 SAGEBRUSH TRAIL SE, ALBUQUERQUE, NM, WAS DISCIPLINED BY MEDICARE ON MAY 20, 1999
DISCIPLINARY ACTION: EXCLUSION FROM THE MEDICARE AND/OR MEDICAID PROGRAM
OFFENSE: DISCIPLINARY ACTION BY ANOTHER STATE OR AGENCY

NOTES: LICENSE REVOKED, SUSPENDED, SURRENDERED OR OTHERWISE LOST FOR REASONS BEARING ON PROFESSIONAL PERFORMANCE, PROFESSIONAL COMPETENCE OR FINANCIAL INTEGRITY.

ROY, SAMIR M MD OF 4263 MONTGOMERY BLVD. NE STE 120, ALBUQUERQUE, NM, WAS DISCIPLINED BY DEA ON MAY 14, 1996
DISCIPLINARY ACTION: SURRENDER OF CONTROLLED SUBSTANCE LICENSE
OFFENSE: DISCIPLINARY ACTION BY ANOTHER STATE OR AGENCY

NOTES: STATE BOARD.

SANCHEZ, ISHMAEL B MD, DATE OF BIRTH JULY 4, 1952 OF 47 SECTION ROAD, LALUZ, NM, WAS DISCIPLINED BY MEDICARE ON JANUARY 5, 1997
DISCIPLINARY ACTION: EXCLUSION FROM THE MEDICARE AND/OR MEDICAID PROGRAM
OFFENSE: NONCOMPLIANCE WITH A PROFESSIONAL RULE

NOTES: DEFAULTED ON PUBLIC HEALTH SERVICE EDUCATION LOAN.

SEWELL, JAMES W MD, WAS DISCIPLINED BY NEW MEXICO ON JULY 30, 1990
DISCIPLINARY ACTION: SURRENDER OF LICENSE
OFFENSE: OVERPRESCRIBING OR MISPRESCRIBING DRUGS

NOTES: INJUDICIOUS PRESCRIBING. SURRENDER IN LIEU OF BOARD ACTION.

SHEFFIELD, JERRY MD OF 12550 CENTRAL SW #240, ALBUQUERQUE, NM, WAS DISCIPLINED BY NEW MEXICO ON NOVEMBER 18, 1994
DISCIPLINARY ACTION: LICENSE SUSPENSION
OFFENSE: SUBSTANCE ABUSE

NOTES: NOTICE OF CONTEMPLATED ACTION ISSUED.

SHEFFIELD, JERRY W MD, WAS DISCIPLINED BY NEW MEXICO ON FEBRUARY 16, 1995
DISCIPLINARY ACTION: LICENSE REVOCATION
OFFENSE: SUBSTANCE ABUSE

SHEFFIELD, JERRY WAYNE MD, LICENSE NUMBER 0006587 OF BIRMINGHAM, AL, WAS DISCIPLINED BY ALABAMA ON JULY 10, 1995
DISCIPLINARY ACTION: RESTRICTION PLACED ON CONTROLLED SUBSTANCE LICENSE; MONITORING OF PHYSICIAN PERFORMANCE
OFFENSE: SUBSTANCE ABUSE

NOTES: VOLUNTARY RESTRICTION DUE TO HIS TREATMENT FOR SUBSTANCE ABUSE. SHALL PARTICIPATE IN THE PHYSICIANS RECOVERY NETWORK; SHALL UTILIZE SEQUENTIALLY NUMBERED TRIPLICATE PRESCRIPTIONS FOR ALL CONTROLLED SUBSTANCES PRESCRIBED BY HIM TO PATIENTS; PROHIBITED FROM REGISTERING AS A DISPENSING PHYSICIAN; PROHIBITED FROM MAINTAINING ANY SAMPLES OF ANY CONTROLLED SUBSTANCES IN HIS MEDICAL OFFICE. ON 11/4/98 APPLICATION FOR REINSTATEMENT DENIED.

SHEFFIELD, JERRY WAYNE MD, DATE OF BIRTH JANUARY 10, 1948, LICENSE NUMBER 0006775 OF 329 GREENLEAF DRIVE, BIRMINGHAM, AL, WAS DISCIPLINED BY MISSISSIPPI ON JULY 20, 1995
DISCIPLINARY ACTION: SURRENDER OF LICENSE

NOTES: VOLUNTARILY AND UNCONDITIONALLY SURRENDERED HIS LICENSE TO AVOID A DISCIPLINARY HEARING BEFORE THE BOARD.

SHEFFIELD, JERRY WAYNE MD, LICENSE NUMBER 6587, WAS DISCIPLINED BY ALABAMA ON OCTOBER 31, 1997
DISCIPLINARY ACTION: LICENSE REVOCATION
OFFENSE: DISCIPLINARY ACTION BY ANOTHER STATE OR AGENCY

NOTES: HAS A HISTORY OF DRUG DEPENDENCE SINCE 1981; RELAPSED IN 1988 AND LICENSE WAS UNDER VOLUNTARY RESTRICTION THROUGH 1993; NEW MEXICO LICENSE REVOKED 4/3/95 BASED ON RELAPSE ON HYDROCODONE IN 1994 AND SUBSEQUENT TREATMENT; ON 7/10/95 AGREED TO VOLUNTARY RESTRICTIONS ON ALABAMA LICENSE WHICH HE VIOLATED ON 10/29/96 WHEN URINE TESTED POSITIVE FOR ULTRAM; CONTINUED TO TEST POSITIVE THROUGH 4/97; ON 6/17/95 VOLUNTARILY SURRENDERED MISSISSIPPI LICENSE.

SHEFFIELD, JERRY WAYNE MD, WAS DISCIPLINED BY ALABAMA ON NOVEMBER 4, 1998
DISCIPLINARY ACTION: DENIAL OF LICENSE REINSTATEMENT

SHEFFIELD, JERRY WAYNE MD, DATE OF BIRTH JANUARY 10, 1948 OF 329 GREENLEAF DRIVE, BIRMINGHAM, AL, WAS DISCIPLINED BY MEDICARE ON DECEMBER 20, 1998
DISCIPLINARY ACTION: EXCLUSION FROM THE MEDICARE AND/OR MEDICAID PROGRAM
OFFENSE: DISCIPLINARY ACTION BY ANOTHER STATE OR AGENCY

NOTES: LICENSE REVOKED, SUSPENDED, SURRENDERED OR OTHERWISE LOST FOR REASONS BEARING ON PROFESSIONAL PERFORMANCE, PROFESSIONAL COMPETENCE OR FINANCIAL INTEGRITY.

SHOBIN, DAVID M MD OF 498 ROUTE 111, SMITHTOWN, NY, WAS DISCIPLINED BY DEA ON OCTOBER 6, 1995
DISCIPLINARY ACTION: SURRENDER OF CONTROLLED SUBSTANCE LICENSE

NOTES: IN LIEU OF ORDER TO SHOW CAUSE.

SHOBIN, DAVID M MD, WAS DISCIPLINED BY NEW MEXICO ON NOVEMBER 1, 1996

NOTES: MUST NOTIFY THE BOARD IN WRITING 90 DAYS PRIOR TO PRACTICING UNDER NEW MEXICO LICENSE OR RETURNING TO NEW MEXICO.

SHOBIN, DAVID MICHAEL MD OF 498 ROUTE 111, SMITHTOWN, NY, WAS DISCIPLINED BY DEA ON MAY 6, 1996
DISCIPLINARY ACTION: RESTRICTION PLACED ON CONTROLLED SUBSTANCE LICENSE
OFFENSE: SUBSTANCE ABUSE

NOTES: ALLEGED ABUSE OF CONTROLLED SUBSTANCES.

SHOLLENBERGER, JOHN C MD, DATE OF BIRTH MARCH 13, 1942, LICENSE NUMBER 0004002 OF 7045 S CHRISTOPHER, BELEN, NM, WAS DISCIPLINED BY MONTANA ON JUNE 19, 1990
DISCIPLINARY ACTION: SURRENDER OF LICENSE
OFFENSE: DISCIPLINARY ACTION BY ANOTHER STATE OR AGENCY

NOTES: SURRENDER PENDING DISCIPLINARY ACTION.

SHOLLENBERGER, JOHN C MD, WAS DISCIPLINED BY NEW MEXICO ON DECEMBER 22, 1992
DISCIPLINARY ACTION: LICENSE SUSPENSION
OFFENSE: FAILURE TO COMPLY WITH PREVIOUS BOARD ORDER

NOTES: VIOLATION OF STIPULATION.

SHOLLENBERGER, JOHN C MD OF ALBUQUERQUE, NM, WAS DISCIPLINED BY NEW MEXICO ON SEPTEMBER 24, 1993
DISCIPLINARY ACTION: LICENSE REVOCATION
OFFENSE: PROFESSIONAL MISCONDUCT

SIMPSON, GARY MD, WAS DISCIPLINED BY NEW MEXICO ON SEPTEMBER 7, 1990
DISCIPLINARY ACTION: LICENSE SUSPENSION
OFFENSE: FAILURE TO COMPLY WITH PREVIOUS BOARD ORDER

NOTES: VIOLATION OF LICENSE STIPULATION. INDEFINITE SUSPENSION.

SIMPSON, GARY F MD, WAS DISCIPLINED BY NEW MEXICO ON MARCH 13, 1992
DISCIPLINARY ACTION: PROBATION

NOTES: SUSPENSION, STAYED; INDEFINITE PROBATION.

SIMPSON, GARY L MD, WAS DISCIPLINED BY NEW MEXICO ON JANUARY 1, 1997
DISCIPLINARY ACTION: RESTRICTION PLACED ON LICENSE
OFFENSE: FAILURE TO COMPLY WITH PREVIOUS BOARD ORDER

NOTES: VIOLATION OF STIPULATION AND CONTRACT REGARDING SUBSTANCE ABUSE; AS OF 2/98, ALL STIPULATIONS REMOVED; UNRESTRICTED LICENSE.

SMITH, NEILSON MD, WAS DISCIPLINED BY NEW MEXICO ON MARCH 1, 1995
DISCIPLINARY ACTION: SURRENDER OF LICENSE
OFFENSE: SUBSTANCE ABUSE

SMITH, NEILSON A MD, WAS DISCIPLINED BY NEW MEXICO ON JUNE 15, 1992
DISCIPLINARY ACTION: PROBATION

NOTES: SUSPENSION, STAYED; INDEFINITE PROBATION.

SMITH, PAUL R MD, WAS DISCIPLINED BY NEW MEXICO ON JANUARY 1, 1997
OFFENSE: SUBSTANCE ABUSE

NOTES: ISSUED A NEW MEXICO LICENSE WITH STANDARD STIPULATIONS FOR SUBSTANCE ABUSE. AS OF 2/98, ALL STIPULATIONS REMOVED; UNRESTRICTED LICENSE.

SMITH, TAMARA L MD, WAS DISCIPLINED BY NEW MEXICO ON MAY 22, 1992
DISCIPLINARY ACTION: RESTRICTION PLACED ON LICENSE

NOTES: LICENSE STIPULATED, UNSPECIFIED.

SOKOLL, MARTIN D MD, DATE OF BIRTH OCTOBER 14, 1932, LICENSE NUMBER 0016762 OF UNIV IOWA - ANESTHESIA DEPT, IOWA CITY, IA, WAS DISCIPLINED BY IOWA ON JULY 13, 1994
DISCIPLINARY ACTION: 48-MONTH PROBATION
OFFENSE: SUBSTANCE ABUSE

NOTES: SETTLEMENT TO CHARGES OF EXCESSIVE DRUG USE, EXCESSIVE ALCOHOL USE, SUBSTANDARD MEDICINE BY PRESCRIBING SCHEDULE II &/OR III CONTROLLED DRUGS TO TWO PATIENTS WITHOUT EXAMINATION.

SOKOLL, MARTIN D MD, WAS DISCIPLINED BY NEW MEXICO ON OCTOBER 4, 1995
OFFENSE: SUBSTANCE ABUSE

NOTES: SAME TERMS AS OTHER STATE STIPULATION; LICENSE WITH CONDITIONS.

SOKOLL, MARTIN D MD OF U OF IA HOP DEPT OF ANESTHESIA, IOWA CITY, IA, WAS DISCIPLINED BY DEA ON JANUARY 5, 1996
DISCIPLINARY ACTION: RESTRICTION PLACED ON CONTROLLED SUBSTANCE LICENSE
OFFENSE: DISCIPLINARY ACTION BY ANOTHER STATE OR AGENCY

NOTES: STATE BOARD.

SOKOLL, MARTIN DAVID MD, DATE OF BIRTH OCTOBER 14, 1932, LICENSE NUMBER 0011331 OF UNIVERSITY OF IOWA, IOWA CITY, IA, WAS DISCIPLINED BY WEST VIRGINIA ON NOVEMBER 28, 1994
DISCIPLINARY ACTION: SURRENDER OF LICENSE

SOKOLL, MARTIN DAVID MD, DATE OF BIRTH OCTOBER 14, 1932, LICENSE NUMBER 026931L OF UNIVERSITY OF IOWA HOSP, IOWA CITY, IA, WAS DISCIPLINED BY PENNSYLVANIA ON JULY 25, 1995
DISCIPLINARY ACTION: 48-MONTH PROBATION
OFFENSE: DISCIPLINARY ACTION BY ANOTHER STATE OR AGENCY

NOTES: RECIPROCAL ACTION FROM IOWA.

SOKOLL, MARTIN DAVID MD, LICENSE NUMBER 0C41608 OF IOWA CITY, IA, WAS DISCIPLINED BY CALIFORNIA ON OCTOBER 20, 1995
DISCIPLINARY ACTION: 60-MONTH PROBATION
OFFENSE: DISCIPLINARY ACTION BY ANOTHER STATE OR AGENCY

NOTES: ACTION IN IOWA FOR PRESCRIBING CONTROLLED SUBSTANCES TO PATIENTS WITHOUT APPROPRIATE EXAMINATION AND MEDICAL NEED AND FOR EXCESSIVE SELF-USE OF DRUGS AND ALCOHOL. REVOCATION, STAYED.

SOKOLL, MARTIN DAVID MD, LICENSE NUMBER 0041448 OF IOWA CITY, IA, WAS DISCIPLINED BY OHIO ON OCTOBER 9, 1996
DISCIPLINARY ACTION: LICENSE SUSPENSION
OFFENSE: DISCIPLINARY ACTION BY ANOTHER STATE OR AGENCY

NOTES: ACTION IN WEST VIRGINIA. SURRENDERED HIS LICENSE IN LIEU OF FURTHER ACTION. ACTION IN IOWA. PLACED ON PROBATION FOR HIS EXCESSIVE USE OR ABUSE OF DRUGS, INCLUDING ALCOHOL. MINIMUM THREE YEAR SUSPENSION. CONDITIONS FOR RESTORATION ESTABLISHED; SUBSEQUENT PROBATIONARY TERMS, CONDITIONS, AND LIMITATIONS TO BE ESTABLISHED BY CONSENT AGREEMENT OR BOARD ORDER AS A CONDITION FOR RESTORATION. AGREEMENT TO REMAIN IN EFFECT

FOR A MINIMUM OF TWO YEARS PRIOR TO ANY REQUEST FOR TERMINATION.

STAGGENBORG, RICHARD MD, WAS DISCIPLINED BY NEW MEXICO ON NOVEMBER 8, 1995

NOTES: CONTINUATION OF THERAPY. LICENSE WITH CONDITIONS.

STIRMAN, JERRY A MD, DATE OF BIRTH OCTOBER 13, 1924, LICENSE NUMBER 0013957 OF 653 CANYON ROAD #6, SANTA FE, NM, WAS DISCIPLINED BY COLORADO ON JANUARY 24, 1994
OFFENSE: SUBSTANDARD CARE, INCOMPETENCE OR NEGLIGENCE

NOTES: ACTION BASED ON ALLEGATIONS OF SUBSTANDARD CARE--TWO OR MORE ACTS OR OMISSIONS WHICH FAIL TO MEET GENERALLY ACCEPTED STANDARDS OF MEDICAL PRACTICE IN PRACTICE HE PROVIDED TO PATIENTS IN THE EMERGENCY ROOM IN 4/91. HE DENIES SUBSTANDARD CARE. AGREES TO NO FURTHER MEDICAL PRACTICE IN COLORADO, TO ALLOW HIS LICENSE TO PERMANENTLY LAPSE.

STIRMAN, JERRY A MD, DATE OF BIRTH OCTOBER 13, 1924 OF 653 CANYON ROAD #6, SANTA FE, NM, WAS DISCIPLINED BY MEDICARE ON NOVEMBER 9, 1994
DISCIPLINARY ACTION: EXCLUSION FROM THE MEDICARE AND/OR MEDICAID PROGRAM
OFFENSE: DISCIPLINARY ACTION BY ANOTHER STATE OR AGENCY

NOTES: LICENSE REVOKED FOR REASONS BEARING ON PROFESSIONAL PERFORMANCE.

STIRMAN, JERRY A MD OF 653 CANYON ROAD, SANTA FE, NM, WAS DISCIPLINED BY NEW MEXICO ON DECEMBER 1, 1994
DISCIPLINARY ACTION: SURRENDER OF LICENSE

NOTES: IN LIEU OF ACTION.

STOOPS, DONALD DO, DATE OF BIRTH AUGUST 15, 1925 OF 800 E 9TH STREET, TRUTH OR CONSEQUENCES, NM, WAS DISCIPLINED BY MEDICARE ON SEPTEMBER 14, 1993
DISCIPLINARY ACTION: 120-MONTH EXCLUSION FROM THE MEDICARE AND/OR MEDICAID PROGRAM
OFFENSE: NONCOMPLIANCE WITH A PROFESSIONAL RULE

NOTES: VIOLATED THE SOCIAL SECURITY ACT.

STOOPS, DONALD E DO, LICENSE NUMBER 0001315, WAS DISCIPLINED BY OKLAHOMA ON MARCH 17, 1994
DISCIPLINARY ACTION: LICENSE SUSPENSION
OFFENSE: DISCIPLINARY ACTION BY ANOTHER STATE OR AGENCY

NOTES: ON 5/06/93 ON HIS APPLICATION FOR LICENSURE RENEWAL INDICATED THAT HE HAD NOT BEEN DISCIPLINED IN THE PAST YEAR. NEW MEXICO SUSPENDED HIS LICENSE FOR ONE YEAR EFFECTIVE 1993 AND HE IS EXCLUDED FROM PARTICIPATION IN MEDICARE FOR 10 YEARS. INDEFINITE SUSPENSION. $485.00 ADMINISTRATIVE COSTS.

STOOPS, DONALD E DO, LICENSE NUMBER 0051969, WAS DISCIPLINED BY NEW MEXICO ON NOVEMBER 19, 1994
DISCIPLINARY ACTION: LICENSE REVOCATION
OFFENSE: PROFESSIONAL MISCONDUCT

NOTES: UNPROFESSIONAL CONDUCT.

STOOPS, DONALD E DO OF TRUTH OR CONSEQUENCES, NM, WAS DISCIPLINED BY DEA ON SEPTEMBER 9, 1996
DISCIPLINARY ACTION: REVOCATION OF CONTROLLED SUBSTANCE LICENSE
OFFENSE: DISCIPLINARY ACTION BY ANOTHER STATE OR AGENCY

NOTES: ON 11/19/94 THE NEW MEXICO BOARD REVOKED HIS STATE LICENSE TO PRACTICE OSTEOPATHIC MEDICINE.

STOUGHTON, NED MD, WAS DISCIPLINED BY NEW MEXICO ON JANUARY 1, 1997
DISCIPLINARY ACTION: SURRENDER OF LICENSE; REPRIMAND
OFFENSE: NONCOMPLIANCE WITH A PROFESSIONAL RULE

NOTES: NONDISCLOSURE OF INFORMATION ON LICENSE APPLICATION. VOLUNTARILY SURRENDERED HIS NEW MEXICO LICENSE UNDER THE TERMS OF THE IMPAIRED HEALTH CARE PROVIDER ACT.

STOUGHTON, NED S MD, LICENSE NUMBER 4660 OF 9005 MONTROSE WAY, SAN DIEGO, CA, WAS DISCIPLINED BY HAWAII ON APRIL 9, 1999
OFFENSE: DISCIPLINARY ACTION BY ANOTHER STATE OR AGENCY

NOTES: DISCIPLINED BY NEW MEXICO FOR FAILURE TO REVEAL A HISTORY OF PSYCHIATRIC ILLNESS ON HIS 1995 APPLICATION. AGREES NOT TO PRACTICE IN HAWAII UNLESS AND UNTIL THE BOARD BELIEVES HE IS FIT TO DO SO. HE MUST NOTIFY THE BOARD 90 DAYS PRIOR TO RETURNING TO PRACTICE. HE MUST SUBMIT A LETTER FROM HIS TREATING PSYCHIATRIST INFORMING THE BOARD OF HIS PRESENT MENTAL CONDITION AND STATING THAT HE IS FIT TO PRACTICE MEDICINE AND POSES NO HARM TO THE PUBLIC.

STOUGHTON, NED STANLEY MD, LICENSE NUMBER G34753 OF ALBUQUERQUE, NM, WAS DISCIPLINED BY CALIFORNIA ON APRIL 7, 1998
DISCIPLINARY ACTION: REPRIMAND
OFFENSE: DISCIPLINARY ACTION BY ANOTHER STATE OR AGENCY

NOTES: DISCIPLINED BY NEW MEXICO FOR FAILING TO REVEAL HISTORY OF PSYCHIATRIC ILLNESS ON HIS APPLICATION FOR LICENSURE.

SWOBODA, JAYE T MD OF 1525 MORRIS ROAD, LOS LUNAS, NM, WAS DISCIPLINED BY NEW MEXICO
OFFENSE: SUBSTANCE ABUSE

NOTES: LICENSE PLACED UNDER UNSPECIFIED CONDITIONS. IN 1997 BOARD REMOVED ALL STIPULATIONS FOR SUBSTANCE ABUSE FROM LICENSE, GIVING HIM AN UNRESTRICTED LICENSE.

SZALANSKI, DAVID L MD, DATE OF BIRTH JUNE 29, 1960 OF 901 EAST SANGER STREET, HOBBS, NM, WAS DISCIPLINED BY MEDICARE ON JANUARY 5, 1997
DISCIPLINARY ACTION: EXCLUSION FROM THE MEDICARE AND/OR MEDICAID PROGRAM
OFFENSE: NONCOMPLIANCE WITH A PROFESSIONAL RULE

NOTES: DEFAULTED ON PUBLIC HEALTH SERVICE EDUCATION LOAN. REINSTATED ON 9/11/98.

TADIAN, JOELLA MD, WAS DISCIPLINED BY NEW MEXICO ON MAY 16, 1991
DISCIPLINARY ACTION: REPRIMAND

TALBOT, WILLIAM A MD, WAS DISCIPLINED BY NEW MEXICO ON JANUARY 1, 1997
OFFENSE: SUBSTANCE ABUSE

NOTES: LICENSE PLACED UNDER STANDARD STIPULATIONS FOR SUBSTANCE ABUSE. AS OF 8/98 STIPULATIONS REDUCED TO BIANNUAL VISITS WITH THE BOARD.

TARASZKA, STEVEN R MD, LICENSE NUMBER 0009157 OF ATLANTA, GA, WAS DISCIPLINED BY VERMONT ON FEBRUARY 8, 1996
DISCIPLINARY ACTION: SURRENDER OF LICENSE
OFFENSE: SUBSTANCE ABUSE

NOTES: ADMITTED HE SUFFERS FROM CHEMICAL ADDICTION. VOLUNTARY SURRENDER IN LIEU OF SUMMARY SUSPENSION HEARING; AGREED THAT HE SHALL NEVER SEEK LICENSURE IN VERMONT, AND THAT TERMS OF THE STIPULATION AND UNDERLYING FACTUAL BASIS CAN BE DISCLOSED TO OTHER LICENSING AUTHORITIES.

TARASZKA, STEVEN R MD, LICENSE NUMBER 00AAAA2, WAS DISCIPLINED BY RHODE ISLAND ON MARCH 13, 1996
DISCIPLINARY ACTION: DENIAL OF NEW LICENSE
OFFENSE: DISCIPLINARY ACTION BY ANOTHER STATE OR AGENCY

NOTES: ACTS IN ANOTHER JURISDICTION WHICH ARE GROUNDS FOR DISCIPLINE IN RHODE ISLAND.

TARASZKA, STEVEN R MD, WAS DISCIPLINED BY ALASKA ON MAY 2, 1996
OFFENSE: SUBSTANCE ABUSE

NOTES: SUBSTANCE ABUSE. CANNOT PRACTICE IN ALASKA UNTIL HE CAN PROVE HE CAN DO SO SAFELY. MUST COMPLY WITH RECOMMENDATIONS OF THE TREATMENT FACILITY AND BOARD PRIOR TO RESUMING HIS MEDICAL PRACTICE.

TARASZKA, STEVEN R MD, WAS DISCIPLINED BY KANSAS ON JULY 1, 1996
DISCIPLINARY ACTION: DENIAL OF NEW LICENSE
OFFENSE: DISCIPLINARY ACTION BY ANOTHER STATE OR AGENCY

NOTES: SURRENDERED HIS LICENSE IN VERMONT ON 2/8/96 BASED IN PART ON AN ADMISSION OF CHEMICAL ADDICTION.

TARASZKA, STEVEN R MD, WAS DISCIPLINED BY NEW MEXICO ON SEPTEMBER 1, 1996

NOTES: BOARD ACCEPTED WITHDRAWAL OF APPLICATION WITH AGREEMENT TO NEVER REAPPLY IN NEW MEXICO.

TARASZKA, STEVEN R MD, DATE OF BIRTH APRIL 22, 1965, LICENSE NUMBER 0063345 OF 4060 PEACHTREE RD NE SUITE D-252, ATLANTA, GA, WAS DISCIPLINED BY NEW JERSEY ON OCTOBER 21, 1996
DISCIPLINARY ACTION: SURRENDER OF LICENSE
OFFENSE: DISCIPLINARY ACTION BY ANOTHER STATE OR AGENCY

NOTES: ACTION IN VERMONT FOR SUBSTANCE ABUSE. MINIMUM THREE MONTH SURRENDER. SHALL APPEAR BEFORE THE BOARD TO DISCUSS HIS COMPLIANCE AND DEMONSTRATE HIS FITNESS TO REENTER ACTIVE PRACTICE PRIOR TO RESTORATION OF LICENSE.

TARASZKA, STEVEN R MD, WAS DISCIPLINED BY ALABAMA ON OCTOBER 30, 1996
DISCIPLINARY ACTION: LICENSE REVOCATION
OFFENSE: DISCIPLINARY ACTION BY ANOTHER STATE OR AGENCY

NOTES: VOLUNTARY SURRENDER OF HIS LICENSE IN VERMONT; AGREEMENT TO NEVER SEEK RELICENSURE THERE AND HIS ADMISSION THAT HE SUFFERS FROM THE DISEASE OF CHEMICAL ADDICTION.

TARASZKA, STEVEN R MD, DATE OF BIRTH APRIL 22, 1963, LICENSE NUMBER 0036885 OF 4060 PEACHTREE ROAD, SUITE D-252, ATLANTA, GA, WAS DISCIPLINED BY GEORGIA ON NOVEMBER 8, 1996
DISCIPLINARY ACTION: LICENSE SUSPENSION

NOTES: SHALL NOT PRACTICE AS A PHYSICIAN IN GEORGIA UNTIL FURTHER ORDER OF THE BOARD. INDEFINITE SUSPENSION.

TARASZKA, STEVEN R MD, LICENSE NUMBER 053145 OF ATLANTA, GA, WAS DISCIPLINED BY VIRGINIA ON JANUARY 7, 1997
DISCIPLINARY ACTION: LICENSE SUSPENSION
OFFENSE: DISCIPLINARY ACTION BY ANOTHER STATE OR AGENCY

NOTES: SUSPENSION OF LICENSE BY FLORIDA MEDICAL BOARD, DUE TO ACTION TAKEN BY VERMONT MEDICAL BOARD FOR CHEMICAL DEPENDENCY.

TARASZKA, STEVEN R MD, DATE OF BIRTH APRIL 22, 1963, LICENSE NUMBER 036885 OF 4060 PEACHTREE ROAD, SUITE D-252, ATLANTA, GA, WAS DISCIPLINED BY GEORGIA ON OCTOBER 2, 1997
DISCIPLINARY ACTION: 60-MONTH PROBATION
OFFENSE: DISCIPLINARY ACTION BY ANOTHER STATE OR AGENCY

NOTES: DISCIPLINARY ACTION IN VERMONT; IMPAIRMENT.

TARASZKA, STEVEN ROBERT MD, LICENSE NUMBER 0069664 OF ATLANTA, GA, WAS DISCIPLINED BY FLORIDA ON FEBRUARY 16, 1996
DISCIPLINARY ACTION: EMERGENCY SUSPENSION
OFFENSE: DISCIPLINARY ACTION BY ANOTHER STATE OR AGENCY

NOTES: BEING UNABLE TO PRACTICE MEDICINE WITH REASONABLE SKILL AND SAFETY TO PATIENTS BY REASON OF ILLNESS OR USE OF ALCOHOL, DRUGS, NARCOTICS, CHEMICALS, OR ANY OTHER TYPE OF MATERIAL OR AS A RESULT OF ANY MENTAL OR PHYSICAL CONDITION.

TARASZKA, STEVEN ROBERT MD, LICENSE NUMBER 0069664 OF ATLANTA, GA, WAS DISCIPLINED BY FLORIDA ON JULY 15, 1996
DISCIPLINARY ACTION: LICENSE SUSPENSION
OFFENSE: DISCIPLINARY ACTION BY ANOTHER STATE OR AGENCY

NOTES: CHARGED WITH HAVING LICENSE ACTED UPON BY ANOTHER JURISDICTION. BEING UNABLE TO PRACTICE MEDICINE WITH REASONABLE SKILL AND SAFETY TO PATIENTS BY REASON OF ILLNESS OR USE OF ALCOHOL, DRUGS, NARCOTICS, CHEMICALS OR ANY OTHER TYPE OF MATERIAL, OR AS A RESULT OF ANY MENTAL OR PHYSICAL CONDITION. SUSPENSION UNTIL HE APPEARS AND DEMONSTRATES TO THE BOARD THAT HE CAN PRACTICE MEDICINE WITH REASONABLE SKILL AND SAFETY.

TARASZKA, STEVEN ROBERT MD, DATE OF BIRTH APRIL 22, 1965, LICENSE NUMBER 0014396 OF 4060 PEACHTREE ROAD, SUITE D252, ATLANTA, GA, WAS DISCIPLINED BY MISSISSIPPI ON JULY 18, 1996
DISCIPLINARY ACTION: LICENSE REVOCATION

TARASZKA, STEVEN ROBERT MD OF ATLANTA, GA, WAS DISCIPLINED BY UTAH ON OCTOBER 4, 1996
DISCIPLINARY ACTION: LICENSE REVOCATION
OFFENSE: DISCIPLINARY ACTION BY ANOTHER STATE OR AGENCY

NOTES: ACTION IN VERMONT.

TARASZKA, STEVEN ROBERT MD, DATE OF BIRTH APRIL 22, 1965, LICENSE NUMBER 9600070 OF ATLANTA, GA, WAS DISCIPLINED BY NORTH CAROLINA ON OCTOBER 17, 1996

DISCIPLINARY ACTION: EMERGENCY SUSPENSION
OFFENSE: DISCIPLINARY ACTION BY ANOTHER STATE OR AGENCY

NOTES: SURRENDERED HIS LICENSE IN VERMONT DUE TO ALLEGATIONS OF NARCOTIC ADDICTION. MAY BE UNABLE TO PRACTICE MEDICINE WITH REASONABLE SKILL AND SAFETY BY REASON OF DRUNKENNESS, EXCESSIVE USE OF ALCOHOL, DRUGS, CHEMICALS, OR ANY OTHER TYPE OF MATERIAL. ON 3/18/98 SUMMARY SUSPENSION LIFTED AND DISMISSED WITHOUT PREJUDICE. LICENSE LIMITED AS FOLLOWS: SHALL NOT PRACTICE ANESTHESIA; MAY PRACTICE ONLY IN A BOARD-APPROVED STRUCTURED SETTING; UNLESS LAWFULLY PRESCRIBED BY SOMEONE ELSE, SHALL REFRAIN FROM THE USE OF MIND OR MOOD ALTERING SUBSTANCES AND FROM THE USE OF ALCOHOL; SHALL REPORT TO THE BOARD WITHIN TWO WEEKS ANY USE OF SUCH MEDICATION OR ALCOHOL, INCLUDING THE IDENTIFICATION OF THE PRESCRIBER AND THE PHARMACY FILLING THE PRESCRIPTION; SHALL UNDERGO DRUG AND ALCOHOL SCREENS AS REQUESTED BY THE BOARD; IF HE RESIDES IN NORTH CAROLINA, SHALL MAINTAIN AND ABIDE BY A CONTRACT WITH THE NORTH CAROLINA PHYSICIANS HEALTH PROGRAM; SHALL NOT PRESCRIBE ANY DRUG FOR HIS OWN USE; MUST COMPLY WITH OTHER CONDITIONS.

TARASZKA, STEVEN ROBERT MD, LICENSE NUMBER 1044378 OF 4060 PEACHTREE ROAD NE #D252, ATLANTA, GA, WAS DISCIPLINED BY INDIANA ON FEBRUARY 6, 1997
DISCIPLINARY ACTION: LICENSE SUSPENSION
OFFENSE: DISCIPLINARY ACTION BY ANOTHER STATE OR AGENCY

NOTES: ON 2/1/96 VERMONT FILED A PETITION FOR EMERGENCY SUSPENSION AGAINST HIS MEDICAL LICENSE ALLEGING THAT ON 11/7/95 THE BOARD HAD BEEN NOTIFIED BY THE SPRINGFIELD POLICE DEPARTMENT THAT DRUG PARAPHERNALIA HAD BEEN FOUND IN THE MOTEL ROOM VACATED BY HIM, A LICENSED PHYSICIAN SPECIALIZING IN ANESTHESIOLOGY. THE MATERIALS FOUND IN THE TOILET HAD CAUSED THE SEPTIC SYSTEM OF THE HOTEL TO BE SHUT DOWN ON TWO OCCASIONS. THE EMPTY GLASS VIALS THAT WERE FOUND THERE WERE LABELED VERSED AND STADOL AND MARKED WITH LOT NUMBERS THAT CORRESPONDED WITH THOSE DISPENSED TO THE SPRINGFIELD HOSPITAL. 21 SYRINGES WERE SUBSEQUENTLY FOUND IN THE BASE OF THE TOILET OF HIS HOTEL ROOM. SPRINGFIELD HOSPITAL OFFICIALS DISCOVERED AFTER AUDITING PHARMACY RECORDS THAT THE ANESTHESIOLOGY DEPARTMENT HAD ORDERED UNUSUALLY LARGE AMOUNTS OF CONTROLLED SUBSTANCES DURING THE MONTHS THAT HE WORKED AT THE FACILITY, AND POLICE DISCOVERED THAT HE HAD WRITTEN SOME UNUSUAL PRESCRIPTIONS. IN 11/95 HE WASTED A VIAL OF COCAINE WITHOUT A WITNESS TO CO-SIGN THE WASTAGE AS REQUIRED BY HOSPITAL POLICY. IN 1995 HE ALSO FORMED A RELATIONSHIP WITH A FEMALE PATIENT, FOR WHOM HE WROTE PRESCRIPTIONS AND HAD HER FILL THE PRESCRIPTIONS AND THEN DELIVER THE MEDICATION TO HIM. ON 2/7/96 HE ENTERED INTO AN AGREEMENT FOR VOLUNTARY SURRENDER OF LICENSE WITH THE VERMONT BOARD, CONTAINING HIS ADMISSIONS THAT HE SUFFERS FROM CHEMICAL ADDICTION AND THAT HIS DISEASE CONSTITUTES A THREAT TO THE HEALTH, SAFETY, AND WELFARE OF HIS PATIENTS. HE AGREED NEVER TO SEEK RELICENSURE IN VERMONT.

TARASZKA, STEVEN ROBERT MD, LICENSE NUMBER 19620 OF ATLANTA, OR, WAS DISCIPLINED BY OREGON ON MAY 1, 1997
DISCIPLINARY ACTION: LICENSE REVOCATION

NOTES:

TARASZKA, STEVEN ROBERT MD, DATE OF BIRTH APRIL 22, 1965 OF 4060 PEACHTREE ROAD, SUITE D252, ATLANTA, GA, WAS DISCIPLINED BY MEDICARE ON SEPTEMBER 7, 1997
DISCIPLINARY ACTION: EXCLUSION FROM THE MEDICARE AND/OR MEDICAID PROGRAM
OFFENSE: DISCIPLINARY ACTION BY ANOTHER STATE OR AGENCY

NOTES: LICENSE REVOKED, SUSPENDED, SURRENDERED OR OTHERWISE LOST FOR REASONS BEARING ON PROFESSIONAL PERFORMANCE, PROFESSIONAL COMPETENCE OR FINANCIAL INTEGRITY. REINSTATED ON 4/1/98.

TARASZKA, STEVEN ROBERT MD, DATE OF BIRTH APRIL 22, 1965, LICENSE NUMBER 056084L OF 7202 SLOAN SQUARE NE, ATLANTA, GA, WAS DISCIPLINED BY PENNSYLVANIA ON OCTOBER 21, 1997
DISCIPLINARY ACTION: LICENSE REVOCATION
OFFENSE: DISCIPLINARY ACTION BY ANOTHER STATE OR AGENCY

NOTES: DISCIPLINARY ACTION TAKEN AGAINST HIS LICENSE BY VERMONT, NORTH CAROLINA, RHODE ISLAND, KANSAS, FLORIDA, MISSISSIPPI, TENNESSEE, ILLINOIS, GEORGIA, AND VIRGINIA FOR PERSONAL USE/ADDICTION.

TARASZKA, STEVEN ROBERT MD, LICENSE NUMBER 69933 OF ATLANTA, GA, WAS DISCIPLINED BY OHIO ON DECEMBER 4, 1997
DISCIPLINARY ACTION: LICENSE REVOCATION
OFFENSE: SUBSTANCE ABUSE

NOTES: INABILITY TO PRACTICE ACCORDING TO ACCEPTABLE AND PREVAILING STANDARDS OF CARE DUE TO HABITUAL OR EXCESSIVE USE OF DRUGS, ALCOHOL, OR OTHER SUBSTANCES THAT IMPAIR ABILITY TO PRACTICE. PERMANENT REVOCATION AUTHORIZED BY DOCTOR IN LIEU OF FORMAL DISCIPLINARY PROCEEDINGS.

TODD, W DAVID MD, WAS DISCIPLINED BY NEW MEXICO ON MARCH 20, 1995
DISCIPLINARY ACTION: LICENSE REVOCATION
OFFENSE: DISCIPLINARY ACTION BY ANOTHER STATE OR AGENCY

NOTES: REVOCATION IN ANOTHER STATE; ALCOHOL ABUSE.

TONG, ROLANDO MD, WAS DISCIPLINED BY NEW MEXICO ON APRIL 1, 1998
DISCIPLINARY ACTION: SURRENDER OF LICENSE

NOTES: VOLUNTARY SURRENDER AND MAY ONLY REAPPLY IF WISCONSIN LICENSE IS REINSTATED.

TONG, ROLANDO MERCADO MD, DATE OF BIRTH MARCH 15, 1949, LICENSE NUMBER 020419E OF PO BOX 668, CHAMA, NM, WAS DISCIPLINED BY PENNSYLVANIA ON JANUARY 26, 1999
DISCIPLINARY ACTION: SURRENDER OF LICENSE
OFFENSE: DISCIPLINARY ACTION BY ANOTHER STATE OR AGENCY

NOTES: DISCIPLINARY ACTION TAKEN BY WISCONSIN AND NEW MEXICO. VOLUNTARY SURRENDER. MAY REAPPLY IN PENNSYLVANIA ONLY IF WISCONSIN REINSTATES HIS LICENSE

TONG, ROLONDO MERCADO MD, DATE OF BIRTH MARCH 15, 1949, LICENSE NUMBER 36529 OF 799 NORTH CEDAR, CHAMA, NM, WAS DISCIPLINED BY WISCONSIN ON OCTOBER 22, 1997
DISCIPLINARY ACTION: SURRENDER OF LICENSE
OFFENSE: SUBSTANDARD CARE, INCOMPETENCE OR NEGLIGENCE

NOTES: ALLEGATIONS, FROM THE CLARK COUNTY SHERIFF'S DEPARTMENT THAT A 26 YEAR OLD NURSE AND FORMER PATIENT OF HIS WAS GIVEN MIDAZOLAM, A CONTROLLED SUBSTANCE, FOR NON-MEDICAL PURPOSES IN 3/96, IN A FORM NOT APPROVED BY THE FDA; SHE AND THE DOCTOR WERE HAVING AN AFFAIR, AND THE PROVIDING OF THESE SUBSTANCES OCCURRED IN THE CONTEXT OF THEIR MEETING FOR THE PURPOSE OF SEXUAL ACTIVITY AND THE CONSUMPTION OF ALCOHOLIC BEVERAGES; HE AGAIN GAVE HER ORAL DOSAGE FORMS OF MIDAZOLAM AND ALPRAZOLAM (XANAX), OUTSIDE THE COURSE OF LEGITIMATE PRACTICE, IN 4/96; A SEARCH WARRANT OF HIS HOME FOUND QUANTITIES OF AN ORAL DOSAGE FORM OF MIDAZOLAM; IMPORTATION OF THIS FORM OF MIDAZOLAM IS NOT LAWFUL UNLESS PURSUANT TO LEGITIMATE RESEARCH OR FOR PERSONAL USE PURSUANT TO LEGITIMATE PRESCRIPTION, AND THERE IS NO REASON TO BELIEVE THAT HE IS PARTICIPATING IN ANY LEGITIMATE RESEARCH RELATING TO THIS SUBSTANCE OR THAT HE HAS A PRESCRIPTION FOR PERSONAL USE OF THIS MEDICATION; THE SEARCH WARRANT HAS BEEN FOUND TO BE INVALID BY A CIRCUIT JUDGE AND SUCH RULING IS PRESENTLY ON APPEAL IN THE WISCONSIN COURT OF APPEALS; ANOTHER STATEMENT FROM SHERIFF'S DEPARTMENT ALLEGES THAT AN 18 YEAR OLD FORMER PATIENT OF HIS WAS INVITED BY HIM ON A DATE ON 7/21/96; AT THAT TIME, HE DID NOT HAVE ANY KNOWLEDGE OF HER OTHER THAN AS A PATIENT AND ATTEMPTED TO ENGAGE HER IN SEXUAL ACTIVITY AND OFFERED HER ALCOHOLIC BEVERAGES; SHERIFF'S DETECTIVES FOUND HYDROCODONE SAMPLES AND MIDAZOLAM BLISTER-TYPE PACKAGES WITH SOME TABLETS REMOVED ALONG WITH A CAMERA BAG WITH A NAMETAG BEARING HIS NAME WHICH CONTAINED A BOX DESIGNED TO CONTAIN 10 AMPOULES OF VERSED (INJECTIBLE MIDAZOLAM) OF WHICH 5 WERE PRESENT AND 5 WERE MISSING; AND A BOX DESIGNED TO CONTAIN 10 AMPOULES OF FENTANYL, OF WHICH 8 WERE PRESENT AND 2 WERE MISSING; VERSED AND FENTANYL ARE CONTROLLED SUBSTANCES USED IN HOSPITALS, SURGICAL SUITES, AND RADIOLOGY FACILITIES FOR SURGICAL PATIENTS AND BY NURSES DOING CERTAIN PROCEDURES; THERE IS NO LEGITIMATE REASON FOR A SURGEON TO MAINTAIN OR STORE THEM AT A PRIVATE RESIDENCE; AT THAT TIME, HE WAS REGISTERED WITH THE DEA ONLY AT HIS OFFICE LOCATION AND THERE WAS NO RECORD OF NECESSARY FORMS FOR FENTANYL DELIVERED TO THAT ADDRESS; CONTROLLED SUBSTANCES PURCHASED MUST BE SHIPPED ONLY TO THE REGISTERED ADDRESS; ON 4/28/93 THE NEW MEXICO BOARD FOUND THAT THERE WAS SUBSTANTIAL EVIDENCE THAT HE WAS PROFESSIONALLY NEGLIGENT IN HIS TREATMENT OF A PATIENT HE HAD OPERATED ON TO REMOVE GALLSTONES BY WHICH, DURING THE COURSE OF SURGERY, HE SEVERED THE PATIENT'S COMMON BILE DUCT; ON 5/30/95 THE NEW MEXICO BOARD FOUND THAT THERE WAS SUBSTANTIAL EVIDENCE THAT HE WAS PROFESSIONALLY NEGLIGENT IN HIS TREATMENT OF ONE PATIENT WHO HAD CONSULTED HIM FOR THE PURPOSE OF HAVING HIM SET A BROKEN WRIST; CIVIL LITIGATION REGARDING THESE TWO MATTERS HAD YET TO BE RESOLVED AS OF THE DATE OF THIS ORDER; HE HAS RELOCATED TO NEW MEXICO WITH NO INTENTION OF RETURNING TO OR PRACTICING IN WISCONSIN AGAIN. SHALL PAY $300 IN COSTS.

TREW, GEORGE MD OF LOS ALAMOS, NM, WAS DISCIPLINED BY NEW MEXICO ON DECEMBER 15, 1993
DISCIPLINARY ACTION: DENIAL OF NEW LICENSE
OFFENSE: PROFESSIONAL MISCONDUCT

TRUJILLO, MARTIN MD, WAS DISCIPLINED BY NEW MEXICO
OFFENSE: DISCIPLINARY ACTION BY ANOTHER STATE OR AGENCY

NOTES: ACTION IN ANOTHER STATE; HISTORY OF SUBSTANCE ABUSE. INTERIM PERMIT WITH CONDITIONS. IN 1997 ORDER AMENDED DISCONTINUING URINE MONITORING REQUIREMENT. IN 5/98 ORDER AMENDED REDUCING VISITS TO THE BOARD FROM ANNUAL TO BIANNUAL. IN 5/99 REMOVED ALL STIPULATIONS FOR SUBSTANCE ABUSE, GIVING HIM AN UNRESTRICTED LICENSE.

TRUJILLO, RALPH E MD OF 33 MILL ROAD NW, ALBUQUERQUE, NM, WAS DISCIPLINED BY NEW MEXICO ON OCTOBER 25, 1993
OFFENSE: DISCIPLINARY ACTION BY ANOTHER STATE OR AGENCY

NOTES: LICENSE PLACED UNDER UNSPECIFIED CONDITIONS. IN 1996 ALL STIPULATIONS REMOVED.

TRUJILLO, RALPH EUSEBIO MD, DATE OF BIRTH SEPTEMBER 22, 1940, LICENSE NUMBER 0015931 OF 33 MILL ROAD, NW, ALBUQUERQUE, NM, WAS DISCIPLINED BY WEST VIRGINIA ON JUNE 1, 1993
DISCIPLINARY ACTION: SURRENDER OF LICENSE
OFFENSE: PROVIDING FALSE INFORMATION TO THE BOARD OR OTHER HEALTH AGENCY

NOTES: ON 7/7/89 APPLICATION FOR LICENSE TO PRACTICE MEDICINE, HE STATED THAT HE HAD NEVER BEEN DENIED A LICENSE TO PRACTICE MEDICINE WHEN IN FACT HE HAD BEEN DENIED A LICENSE BY THE STATE OF OKLAHOMA IN 1987. DENIES ANY VIOLATION. AGREES NOT TO APPLY FOR A LICENSE TO PRACTICE MEDICINE IN WEST VIRGINIA IN THE FUTURE.

TRUJILLO, RONALD MD, WAS DISCIPLINED BY NEW MEXICO ON MAY 1, 1999
DISCIPLINARY ACTION: REQUIRED TO ENTER AN IMPAIRED PHYSICIAN PROGRAM OR SUBSTANCE ABUSE TREATMENT
OFFENSE: SUBSTANCE ABUSE

NOTES: LICENSE PLACED UNDER STANDARD STIPULATIONS FOR SUBSTANCE ABUSE; MUST ACTIVELY PARTICIPATE IN NEW MEXICO MONITORED TREATMENT PROGRAM, MUST CONTINUE TO SEE PERSONAL PHYSICIANS FOR MANAGEMENT OF MEDICATIONS.

TWIEST, MELVIN MD, WAS DISCIPLINED BY NEW MEXICO ON FEBRUARY 15, 1995
DISCIPLINARY ACTION: REPRIMAND
OFFENSE: PROFESSIONAL MISCONDUCT

NOTES: UNPROFESSIONAL CONDUCT.

TYSON, JOHN T OF 701 SOLANO SE, ALBUQUERQUE, NM, WAS DISCIPLINED BY OKLAHOMA ON JULY 1, 1993
DISCIPLINARY ACTION: DENIAL OF NEW LICENSE

NOTES: EVIDENCE INDICATES THAT HE HAD BEEN PRESCRIBED VARIOUS ANTIDEPRESSANTS FOR THE PAST 10 YEARS AND ALSO HAD A MALPRACTICE LITIGATION HISTORY; THOSE ELEMENTS RAISED ISSUES AS TO HIS CLINICAL COMPETENCY. EVIDENCE DID NOT SHOW HE HAS THE MENTAL AND PSYCHIATRIC ABILITY TO PRACTICE.

VAN OSTEN, KATHLEEN MD, WAS DISCIPLINED BY NEW MEXICO

ON JANUARY 1, 1997
DISCIPLINARY ACTION: SURRENDER OF LICENSE
OFFENSE: SUBSTANCE ABUSE

NOTES: REFERRED TO AN IMPAIRED PHYSICIANS COMMITTEE FOR EVALUATION REGARDING SUBSTANCE ABUSE; VOLUNTARY SURRENDER OF LICENSE UNDER THE TERMS OF THE IMPAIRED HEALTH CARE PROVIDER ACT.

VAN OSTEN, KATHLEEN MD, WAS DISCIPLINED BY NEW MEXICO ON FEBRUARY 1, 1998
DISCIPLINARY ACTION: LICENSE REINSTATEMENT
OFFENSE: SUBSTANCE ABUSE

NOTES: LICENSE RESTORED FROM VOLUNTARY SURRENDER UNDER THE TERMS OF THE IMPAIRED HEALTH CARE PROVIDERS ACT. STANDARD STIPULATIONS FOR SUBSTANCE ABUSE REINSTATED. ON 8/1/99 STIPULATIONS FOR SUBSTANCE ABUSE REDUCED TO BIANNUAL VISITS WITH THE BOARD; ALL OTHER STIPULATIONS REMAIN THE SAME.

VAN WORMER, MARK E MD, WAS DISCIPLINED BY NEW MEXICO ON JUNE 1, 1996
OFFENSE: SUBSTANCE ABUSE

NOTES: SUBSTANCE ABUSE. STIPULATED LICENSE. IN 8/98 STIPULATIONS FOR SUBSTANCE ABUSE REDUCED TO BIANNUAL VISITS WITH THE BOARD. IN 8/99 REMOVED ALL STIPULATIONS FOR SUBSTANCE ABUSE; UNRESTRICTED LICENSE.

WAGNER, JON D MD, WAS DISCIPLINED BY NEW MEXICO ON NOVEMBER 1, 1996
DISCIPLINARY ACTION: REPRIMAND
OFFENSE: SUBSTANCE ABUSE

NOTES: SUBSTANCE ABUSE. LETTER OF REPRIMAND. IN 8/98 STIPULATIONS FOR SUBSTANCE ABUSE REDUCED TO BIANNUAL VISITS WITH THE BOARD.

WALLENFOTI, EVA MD, WAS DISCIPLINED BY NEW MEXICO ON FEBRUARY 20, 1992

NOTES: NOTICE OF CONTEMPLATED ACTION DISMISSED WHEN SHE VOLUNTARILY RETIRED.

WALSKY, PAUL MD, WAS DISCIPLINED BY NEW MEXICO ON FEBRUARY 1, 1998
DISCIPLINARY ACTION: RESTRICTION PLACED ON LICENSE

NOTES: LICENSE STIPULATED WITH CONDITIONS OF CONTINUING MEDICAL CARE.

WEBSTER, MICHELE MD OF UNM SCHOOL OF MEDICINE, ALBUQUERQUE, NM, WAS DISCIPLINED BY NEW MEXICO ON JULY 15, 1994
OFFENSE: SUBSTANCE ABUSE

NOTES: LICENSE PLACED UNDER UNSPECIFIED CONDITIONS. IN NOVEMBER 1999 BOARD REMOVED ALL SPECIFICATIONS FOR SUBSTANCE ABUSE GIVING HER AN UNRESTRICTED LICENSE.

WERNER, MARK MD, WAS DISCIPLINED BY NEW MEXICO ON FEBRUARY 22, 1991

NOTES: LICENSE STIPULATED.

WHALEN, THOMAS J MD, LICENSE NUMBER 0007442 OF MONTPELIER, VT, WAS DISCIPLINED BY VERMONT ON JUNE 19, 1995
DISCIPLINARY ACTION: RESTRICTION PLACED ON LICENSE; RESTRICTION PLACED ON CONTROLLED SUBSTANCE LICENSE

NOTES: LICENSE RESTRICTED AS FOLLOWS: PROHIBITED FROM BEING EMPLOYED OR PROVIDING SERVICES IN A HOSPITAL, HEALTH CARE FACILITY OR PHYSICIAN'S OFFICE; PROHIBITED FROM PROVIDING DIRECT OR INDIRECT MEDICAL CARE TO ANYONE; PROHIBITED FROM PROVIDING OR PRESCRIBING DRUGS TO ANYONE; SHALL ABSTAIN COMPLETELY FROM ALL MOOD ALTERING CHEMICALS INCLUDING ALCOHOL UNLESS THEY ARE PRESCRIBED BY A TREATING PHYSICIAN; RESTRICTIONS SHALL REMAIN IN EFFECT UNTIL PROCEEDINGS ARE CONCLUDED.

WHALEN, THOMAS J MD, LICENSE NUMBER 0007442, WAS DISCIPLINED BY VERMONT ON DECEMBER 5, 1996
DISCIPLINARY ACTION: LICENSE SUSPENSION; MONITORING OF PHYSICIAN PERFORMANCE
OFFENSE: SUBSTANCE ABUSE

NOTES: HAS SUFFERED FROM ADDICTION TO NARCOTICS. BETWEEN OCTOBER 15 AND 18, 1996 UNDERWENT A FOUR DAY EVALUATION AT THE WILLIAM J. FARLEY CENTER. MINIMUM SIX MONTH SUSPENSION: SHALL NOT CONSUME, INJECT, OR OTHERWISE SELF-MEDICATE WITH ANY CONTROLLED SUBSTANCE OR LEGAL DRUG WHICH HAS NOT BEEN PRESCRIBED BY ANOTHER DULY LICENSED PRACTITIONER FOR THERAPEUTIC OR MEDICALLY PROPER PURPOSES; SHALL NOT CONSUME ALCOHOLIC BEVERAGES; WITHIN 10 DAYS, SHALL ENTER INTO A CONTRACT WITH THE NEW MEXICO MONITORED TREATMENT PROGRAM TO DOCUMENT HIS RECOVERY AND ABSTINENCE; SHALL ACTIVELY ENGAGE IN A 12 STEP PROGRAM EITHER WITH AA OR NARCOTICS ANONYMOUS AT LEAST THREE TIMES PER WEEK AND PARTICIPATE IN A HEALTH CARE PROFESSIONAL SUPPORT GROUP AT LEAST ONCE A MONTH WITH QUARTERLY REPORTS; SHALL CONTINUE WITH INDIVIDUAL THERAPY AT LEAST ONCE EVERY TWO WEEKS WITH A BOARD APPROVED THERAPIST WITH QUARTERLY REPORTS; PRIOR TO THE TERMINATION OF HIS SUSPENSION THE THERAPIST SHALL ATTEST THAT IN HIS OR HER OPINION HE CAN SAFELY RETURN TO THE PRACTICE OF MEDICINE; SHALL CONSENT TO RANDOM TESTS OF BODY FLUID UPON BOARD REQUEST; SHALL NOTIFY THE BOARD OF ANY ARREST ON A DRUG OR ALCOHOL-RELATED OFFENSE WITHIN SEVEN DAYS; AND THE SUSPENSION SHALL BE LIFTED ONLY UPON COMPLIANCE WITH THE ABOVE CONDITIONS. AT THE END OF SUSPENSION: SHALL CONTINUE TO ABIDE BY THE ABOVE RESTRICTIONS FOR A PERIOD OF THREE YEARS; SHALL NOT WORK IN THE FIELD OF ANESTHESIOLOGY; IF HE SHOULD PRACTICE IN ANOTHER STATE SHALL INFORM THAT STATE OF THIS ORDER.

WHALEN, THOMAS J MD, WAS DISCIPLINED BY NEW MEXICO ON FEBRUARY 21, 1997
DISCIPLINARY ACTION: RESTRICTION PLACED ON CONTROLLED SUBSTANCE LICENSE; MONITORING OF PHYSICIAN PERFORMANCE
OFFENSE: SUBSTANCE ABUSE

NOTES: LICENSE PLACED UNDER THE FOLLOWING TERMS AND CONDITIONS: HE MAY NOT HOLD A DEA LICENSE; SHALL ABSTAIN FROM ALCOHOL AND ANY CONTROLLED SUBSTANCES UNLESS PRESCRIBED BY A LICENSED PHYSICIAN; SHALL BE AN ACTIVE PARTICIPANT IN THE NEW MEXICO MONITORED TREATMENT PROGRAM INCLUDING RANDOM BIOLOGICAL FLUID TESTING; SHALL APPEAR BEFORE THE BOARD UPON REQUEST; ON 10/27/97 BOARD REMOVED DEA RESTRICTION FROM HIS

STIPULATIONS ALLOWING HIM TO WRITE PRESCRIPTIONS ONLY AT A SPECIFIED CLINIC. ON 2/20/98 BOARD FURTHER AMENDED STIPULATION TO ALLOW HIM TO WRITE CONTROLLED SUBSTANCES FOR USE AS PRE-OPERATIVE MEDICATION ON HOSPITAL ORDERS ONLY; AS OF 5/29/98 AMENDED STIPULATION TO ALLOW HIM TO PRESCRIBE UNDER THE SAME RESTRICTIONS IN ANY BOARD APPROVED SETTING. AS OF 9/22/98 STIPULATIONS ARE REDUCED TO BIANNUAL VISITS WITH THE BOARD, AND HE MAY USE DEA PERMIT IN HIS INSTITUTIONAL PRACTICE. IN 2/99 BOARD REMOVED ALL STIPULATIONS FOR SUBSTANCE ABUSE GIVING HIM AN UNRESTRICTED LICENSE.

WILLOUGHBY, THOMAS M DO, DATE OF BIRTH OCTOBER 20, 1922 OF 10900 HAINES NE, ALBUQUERQUE, NM, WAS DISCIPLINED BY MEDICARE ON JULY 13, 1992
DISCIPLINARY ACTION: 84-MONTH EXCLUSION FROM THE MEDICARE AND/OR MEDICAID PROGRAM
OFFENSE: CRIMINAL CONVICTION OR PLEA OF GUILTY, NOLO CONTENDERE, OR NO CONTEST TO A CRIME

NOTES: PROGRAM-RELATED CONVICTION.

YU, ELMER MD, WAS DISCIPLINED BY NEW MEXICO ON DECEMBER 12, 1990
DISCIPLINARY ACTION: LICENSE REVOCATION
OFFENSE: SUBSTANCE ABUSE

NOTES: SUBSTANCE ABUSE.

UTAH

1999 serious action rate: 2.73/1000
1999 ranking: 33rd

The Utah Medical Board sent newsletters listing actions from 1990 through 1997. As of 1998, Utah requested that the same information be downloaded from their web site, which we did through 1999. The newsletters list the physician's name, city and state of residence, type of action taken, and reason for the action. The newsletters also contain information on modifications and terminations of board actions but not on court decisions affecting board actions. Utah informed us no such actions had taken place.

The information provided covers disciplinary actions taken against allopathic physicians (MDs) and osteopathic physicians (DOs).

Besides disciplinary actions taken by the State Medical Board, this listing also includes actions taken by the Medicare/Medicaid programs, the FDA, and the DEA against physicians located in this state. Disciplinary actions taken by other states against physicians located in Utah or that match a physician disciplined by Utah (see Appendix 2 for an explanation of the matching protocol) are also included.

Although we have made every effort to match physicians' names correctly, some materials we received did not include complete information on middle names, license numbers, birth dates or addresses. Therefore, consumers should remember that non-disciplined physicians and physicians with different disciplinary actions may have similar names to those disciplined physicians listed in this state. Consumers should also remember that if they want the most current information on the status on a physician's license, they should contact the medical board of the state in which the physician practices or had practiced. (See board address below.) Internet address: *http://www.commerce.state.ut.us/dopl/dopl1.htm.* This state has a web site which we have graded B on a scale of A (best) to X (worst). This is a measure of the completeness of the information on disciplined doctors. Those state licensing boards with web sites make independent choices about the type of information to be included on their site and how often it is updated.

According to the Federation of State Medical Boards, Utah took 13 serious disciplinary actions against MDs and DOs in 1999. Compared to the 4,770 MDs licensed in the state, Utah had a serious disciplinary action rate of 2.73 serious actions per 1,000 MDs and a ranking of 33rd on that list (see Table A, Findings, pg. 14).

The tables below summarize the data Public Citizen received from Utah.

Table 1. Disciplinary Actions Against MDs and DOs 1990 through 1999*

Action	Number	Percent**
Revocation	12	5.5%
Surrender	11	5.0%
Suspension	15	6.9%
Probation	62	28.4%
Practice Restriction	10	4.6%
Action Taken Against Controlled Substance License	89	40.8%
Other Actions	19	8.7%
Total Actions	**218**	**100.0%**

* This table lists only the two most serious disciplinary actions taken against a physician.

** Percentages may not total 100% due to rounding.

Table 2. Offenses for which MDs and DOs were Disciplined 1990 through 1999*

Offense	Number	Percent
Criminal Conviction	2	1.6%
Sexual Abuse of or Sexual Misconduct with a Patient	6	4.8%
Substandard Care, Incompetence or Negligence	3	2.4%
Misprescribing or Overprescribing Drugs	21	16.7%
Substance Abuse	8	6.3%
Disciplinary Action Taken Against License by Another State or Agency	29	23.0%
Other Offenses	57	45.2%
Total Records With Offense Listed	**126**	**100.0%**

* Includes only those actions for which an offense was listed and for which we had a corresponding term in our database.

Table 3. Disciplinary Actions Taken for Sexual Abuse of or Sexual Misconduct with a Patient

Action	Number	Percent
Revocation	1	8.3%
Suspension	2	16.7%
Probation	4	33.3%
Other Actions	5	41.7%
Total Actions	**12**	**100.0%**

Table 4. Disciplinary Actions Taken for Misprescribing or Overprescribing Drugs

Action	Number	Percent
Revocation	1	2.7%
Surrender	1	2.7%
Revocation, Surrender, or Suspension of Controlled Substance License	10	27.0%
Suspension	2	5.4%
Probation	12	32.4%
Restriction of Controlled Substance License	8	21.6%
Other Actions	3	8.1%
Total Actions	**37**	**100.0%**

Table 5. Disciplinary Actions Taken for Substance Abuse

Action	Number	Percent
Revocation	1	6.3%
Surrender	1	6.3%
Revocation, Surrender, or Suspension of Controlled Substance License	5	31.3%
Probation	6	37.5%
Restriction of Controlled Substance License	3	18.8%
Total Actions	**16**	**100.0%**

If you feel that your doctor has not given you proper medical care or has mistreated you in any way--whether or not he or she is listed in this report--it is important that you let your state medical board know. Even if they do not immediately act on your complaint, it is important that the information be recorded in their files because it is possible that other people may have filed or will file complaints about the same doctor. Send a brief written description of what occurred to the addresses below or call the phone numbers listed for more information on how to file a complaint.

Address

Utah Department of Commerce
Craig Jackson, Director
Director of Occupational and Professional Licensure
PO Box 146741
Salt Lake City, UT 84114-6741
(801) 530-6628/ 6733/ 6736
Fax: (801) 530-6511
E-mail: brdopl.klesh@email.state.ut.us

Listing of Doctors Sanctioned by Offense

Sexual Abuse of or Sexual Misconduct with a Patient

CULBERTSON, JOE C
KITSON, STEPHAN JAMES
PRATT, VON S
THOMASON, ISAAC RAY
TOPHAM, EARL BARRY
WILMOTH, JON DARRELL

Substandard Care, Incompetence, or Negligence

BROADBENT, DAVID H
BRUCE, STEPHEN J
DREZGA, GRMISLAV GREGORY

Criminal Conviction or Plea of Guilty, Nolo Contendere, or No Contest to a Crime

DAVIS, ROBERT CHARLES
JOHNSON, SHERMAN B

Misprescribing or Overprescribing Drugs

CLAYTON, DAVID N
DEFRIEZ, CURTIS B
DWYER, THOMAS D
ELDREDGE, STEPHEN J
FULLMER, MARK ALLEN
HAMMOND, SAMUEL JENSEN
HARLINE, WESLEY GRANT
HINES, WIRT A
HINTON, RAYMOND K
JENSEN, MICHAEL HENRIE
MATRAVERS, GARY W
OLSON, PAUL F
RIVERA-VELEZ, ABDIEL
STEWART, LAMAR H
STONE, STEVEN A
TIMPSON, DAVID G
WASHBURN, PHILIP
WERNER, SCOTT RULON
WHITE, GARY BANKS
WOLKOFF, KENNETH A

Substance Abuse

CALL, GREGORY K
CRAVEN, CATHERINE M
CROOKSTON, MICHAEL J
CURTIS, GLADE B
GREYEYES, ROGER
KAY, DENNIS L
PETERSON, DAVID A
STODDARD, LARRY D

Caution: This list is designed to be used only in conjunction with the rest of this book which includes additional information on each physician such as license number, date of action and more complete descriptions of the offenses.

AARON, JOSEPH MD, LICENSE NUMBER 072800 OF 2803 NORTH 700 EAST, PROVO, UT, WAS DISCIPLINED BY NEW YORK ON JANUARY 13, 1999
DISCIPLINARY ACTION: SURRENDER OF LICENSE

NOTES: MODIFIES THE PENALTY PREVIOUSLY IMPOSED. NOT A NEW DISCIPLINARY ACTION.

AARON, JOSEPH NORMAN MD OF PROVO, UT, WAS DISCIPLINED BY UTAH ON MAY 31, 1990
DISCIPLINARY ACTION: SURRENDER OF CONTROLLED SUBSTANCE LICENSE
OFFENSE: PROFESSIONAL MISCONDUCT

NOTES: UNLAWFULLY OBTAINED AND ADMINISTERED TO HIMSELF A CONTROLLED SUBSTANCE. SHALL CONTINUE WITH HIS VOLUNTARY RETIREMENT FROM THE ACTIVE PRACTICE OF MEDICINE.

AARON, JOSEPH NORMAN MD OF 2803 NORTH 700 EAST, PROVO, UT, WAS DISCIPLINED BY DEA ON SEPTEMBER 19, 1990
DISCIPLINARY ACTION: SURRENDER OF CONTROLLED SUBSTANCE LICENSE
OFFENSE: OVERPRESCRIBING OR MISPRESCRIBING DRUGS

NOTES: INVOLVED WITH FALSELY WRITING PRESCRIPTIONS FOR DEXTROAMPHETAMINE. VOLUNTARILY SURRENDERED STATE CONTROLLED SUBSTANCE LICENSE. NO AUTOMATIC RENEWAL OF REGISTRATION APPLIED 03/28/90.

AARON, JOSEPH NORMAN MD, LICENSE NUMBER 0072800 OF 2803 NORTH 700 EAST, PROVO, UT, WAS DISCIPLINED BY NEW YORK ON MARCH 31, 1993
DISCIPLINARY ACTION: 24-MONTH PROBATION
OFFENSE: DISCIPLINARY ACTION BY ANOTHER STATE OR AGENCY

NOTES: DISCIPLINED BY UTAH BOARD. IF HE INTENDS TO PRACTICE IN NEW YORK A 2 YEAR PROBATION WILL BE IMPOSED. ON 1/13/99, HE SURRENDERED HIS LICENSE.

ANDERSON, RICHARD EDWARD MD OF SALT LAKE CITY, UT, WAS DISCIPLINED BY UTAH ON JULY 1, 1997
DISCIPLINARY ACTION: 84-MONTH PROBATION; 84-MONTH CONTROLLED SUBSTANCE LICENSE PLACED ON PROBATION
OFFENSE: PROVIDING FALSE INFORMATION TO THE BOARD OR OTHER HEALTH AGENCY

NOTES: HE USED AND ABUSED CONTROLLED SUBSTANCES TO AN EXTENT THAT IT IMPAIRED HIS ABILITY TO SAFELY PRACTICE MEDICINE; FALSIFYING AN APPLICATION TO PRACTICE MEDICINE BY MAKING MISREPRESENTATIONS; ISSUING FALSE PRESCRIPTIONS FOR CONTROLLED SUBSTANCES TO PERSONS HE NEVER EXAMINED; VIOLATING PROFESSIONAL ETHICS BY FAILING TO PROVIDE COMPETENT MEDICAL SERVICES TO HIS PATIENTS, FAILING TO DEAL HONESTLY WITH PATIENTS AND COLLEAGUES AND DISOBEYING THE LAW; FAILURE TO MAINTAIN ADEQUATE RECORDS OF PRESCRIPTIONS OF CONTROLLED SUBSTANCES. LICENSES TO PRACTICE MEDICINE AND TO PRESCRIBE AND ADMINISTER CONTROLLED SUBSTANCES WERE REVOKED WITH A STAY OF ENFORCEMENT ON THE REVOCATIONS. PROBATIONS WITH CONDITIONS AND RESTRICTIONS: SHALL SUBMIT TO A CHEMICAL DEPENDENCY EVALUATION AND RECEIVE TREATMENT AND AFTERCARE AS RECOMMENDED WITH QUARTERLY REPORTS; SHALL SUBMIT A PROPOSED PRACTICE PLAN WHICH SHALL INCLUDE SUPERVISION AND PRESCRIPTIONS ONLY ON SERIALLY NUMBERED PRESCRIPTION FORMS; SHALL MEET QUARTERLY WITH THE BOARD; SHALL PARTICIPATE WITH AA OR NARCOTICS ANONYMOUS AT LEAST THREE TIMES A WEEK; SHALL SUBMIT A TREATMENT PLAN OF COUNSELING; SHALL ABSTAIN FROM ANY MOOD ALTERING SUBSTANCE INCLUDING ALCOHOL EXCEPT WHEN PRESCRIBED BY A LICENSED PHYSICIAN AND ALL SUCH PRESCRIPTIONS SHALL BE FILLED AT ONE PHARMACY; SHALL SUBMIT TO RANDOM TESTS OF BODILY FLUIDS; SHALL COMPLETE WITHIN ONE YEAR A COURSE ON PRESCRIBING; SHALL INFORM THE BOARD IF HE LEAVES THE STATE; TIME SPENT OUT OF UTAH DOES NOT COUNT TOWARD PROBATION.

APPLEBAUM, MICHAEL J MD, LICENSE NUMBER 00M5597, WAS DISCIPLINED BY IDAHO ON AUGUST 14, 1996
DISCIPLINARY ACTION: RESTRICTION PLACED ON CONTROLLED SUBSTANCE LICENSE; MONITORING OF PHYSICIAN PERFORMANCE
OFFENSE: CRIMINAL CONVICTION OR PLEA OF GUILTY, NOLO CONTENDERE, OR NO CONTEST TO A CRIME

NOTES: PLED GUILTY TO A FELONY COUNT OF ILLEGAL POSSESSION OF A CONTROLLED SUBSTANCE AND RECEIVED A WITHHELD JUDGMENT FOR FELONY; USED FALSE AND FRAUDULENT STATEMENTS IN CONNECTION WITH LICENSING IN THAT IN REQUESTING BOARD TO TERMINATE PREVIOUS STIPULATION, FALSELY STATED HE WAS IN FULL COMPLIANCE WITH THE ORDER; PRESCRIBED OR FURNISHED NARCOTIC OR HALLUCINOGENIC DRUGS TO HIMSELF, AN ADDICTED PERSON, TO MAINTAIN HIS ADDICTION AND LEVEL OF USAGE WITHOUT ATTEMPTING TO TREAT THE PRIMARY CONDITION REQUIRING THE USE OF NARCOTICS AND FOR OTHER THAN TREATMENT OF ANY DISEASE, INJURY OR MEDICAL CONDITION. LICENSE REVOCATION, STAYED UNDER THE FOLLOWING TERMS AND CONDITIONS FOR A MINIMUM OF EIGHT YEARS: SHALL EXECUTE A CONTRACT WITH THE IDAHO MEDICAL ASSOCIATION PHYSICIAN HEALTH PROGRAM AND SHALL COMPLY WITH THE TERMS AND CONDITIONS OF THAT CONTRACT WITH REGULAR STATUS REPORTS ON COMPLIANCE; SHALL BE INELIGIBLE TO HOLD, AND SHALL NOT APPLY FOR, REGISTRATION WITH DEA OR THE IDAHO STATE BOARD OF PHARMACY TO PRESCRIBE, DISPENSE, OR ADMINISTER CONTROLLED SUBSTANCES, EXCEPT PSYCHOTROPICS AND ANTI-DEPRESSANTS; SHALL NOT PRESCRIBE, ADMINISTER, DISPENSE, ORDER, WRITE ORDERS FOR, GIVE VERBAL ORDERS FOR, OR POSSESS ANY CONTROLLED SUBSTANCES, EXCEPT PSYCHOTROPICS AND ANTI-DEPRESSANTS; SHALL ABSTAIN COMPLETELY FROM THE PERSONAL USE OR POSSESSION OF DRUGS, EXCEPT THOSE PRESCRIBED, ADMINISTERED, OR DISPENSED TO HIM BY ANOTHER PHYSICIAN; SHALL ABSTAIN COMPLETELY FROM THE USE OF ALCOHOL; SHALL SUBMIT TO RANDOM URINE SCREENINGS FOR DRUGS OF A WEEKLY BASIS OR AS OTHERWISE DIRECTED BY THE IMA PHYSICIAN HEALTH PROGRAM OR UPON BOARD REQUEST WITHOUT PRIOR NOTICE AND WITH REPORTS MONTHLY; SHALL HAVE A BOARD APPROVED MONITORING PHYSICIAN WHO SHALL PROVIDE REPORTS ON A QUARTERLY BASIS; SHALL GIVE A COPY OF THIS ORDER TO ANY HEALTH CARE ENTITY WHERE HE HAS PRIVILEGES; SHALL SUBMIT QUARTERLY DECLARATIONS UNDER PENALTY OF PERJURY STATING WHETHER THERE HAS BEEN COMPLIANCE WITH ALL THE CONDITIONS OF THIS ORDER; SHALL APPEAR FOR INTERVIEWS BEFORE THE BOARD AT THREE MONTH INTERVALS OR AS OTHERWISE DIRECTED; IF HE LEAVES IDAHO FOR THREE CONTINUOUS MONTHS HE MUST NOTIFY THE BOARD IN WRITING; AND PERIODS OF TIME OUTSIDE IDAHO WILL NOT APPLY TO THE REDUCTION OF THIS

PERIOD.

APPLEBAUM, MICHAEL J MD OF 223 16TH AVENUE NORTH, NAMPA, ID, WAS DISCIPLINED BY DEA ON JANUARY 6, 1997
DISCIPLINARY ACTION: SURRENDER OF CONTROLLED SUBSTANCE LICENSE

NOTES: IN LIEU OF PUBLIC INTEREST REVOCATION.

APPLEBAUM, MICHAEL J MD OF NAMPA, ID, WAS DISCIPLINED BY UTAH ON MARCH 25, 1997
OFFENSE: DISCIPLINARY ACTION BY ANOTHER STATE OR AGENCY

NOTES: DISCIPLINARY ACTION TAKEN AGAINST HIS MEDICAL LICENSE IN IDAHO. UTAH SUSPENSION STAYED SO LONG AS HE REMAINS IN FULL COMPLIANCE WITH THE TERMS AND CONDITIONS OF THE IDAHO STIPULATION AND ORDER. ALSO HAS CONDITIONS TO BE MET IN UTAH.

BARRETT, ELMER L MD OF SALT LAKE CITY, UT, WAS DISCIPLINED BY MISSOURI ON MARCH 4, 1993
DISCIPLINARY ACTION: SURRENDER OF LICENSE
OFFENSE: DISCIPLINARY ACTION BY ANOTHER STATE OR AGENCY

NOTES: DISCIPLINARY ACTION TAKEN IN ANOTHER STATE. SUBSTANDARD CARE; PRESCRIPTION VIOLATION. NO REINSTATEMENT OF LICENSE FOR SEVEN YEARS.

BASINGER, GERALD T MD OF 923 DANA DRIVE SUITE 5, REDDING, CA, WAS DISCIPLINED BY DEA ON JUNE 15, 1995
DISCIPLINARY ACTION: SURRENDER OF CONTROLLED SUBSTANCE LICENSE
OFFENSE: DISCIPLINARY ACTION BY ANOTHER STATE OR AGENCY

NOTES: STATE BOARD.

BASINGER, GERALD T MD OF REDDING, CA, WAS DISCIPLINED BY UTAH ON JULY 12, 1996
DISCIPLINARY ACTION: LICENSE REVOCATION
OFFENSE: DISCIPLINARY ACTION BY ANOTHER STATE OR AGENCY

NOTES: DISCIPLINARY ACTION TAKEN AGAINST HIS LICENSE TO PRACTICE MEDICINE IN CALIFORNIA; HE DEMONSTRATED A LACK OF GOOD MORAL CHARACTER; SEXUALLY ABUSED A PATIENT IN THE PERFORMANCE OF HIS DUTIES AS A PHYSICIAN; SUFFERS FROM A MENTAL CONDITION WHICH DEMONSTRATES A THREAT TO THE PUBLIC HEALTH, SAFETY AND WELFARE.

BERGESON, PAUL S MD OF PHOENIX, AZ, WAS DISCIPLINED BY UTAH ON MAY 17, 1991
OFFENSE: DISCIPLINARY ACTION BY ANOTHER STATE OR AGENCY

NOTES: ABUSED ALCOHOL OR CONTROLLED SUBSTANCES IN ANOTHER JURISDICTION RESULTING IN SANCTIONS UPON HIS LICENSE IN THAT JURISDICTION. THE ORDER ENTERED INTO IN ARIZONA IS ADOPTED AS FULLY BINDING IN UTAH; IF HE WISHES TO PRACTICE IN UTAH, HE IS TO MEET WITH THE DIVISION TO DETERMINE IF ANY FURTHER CONDITIONS SHOULD APPLY TO HIS LICENSE. LICENSE REINSTATED WITH FULL PRIVILEGES EFFECTIVE 6/8/92.

BERNTSON, DALE RAMPTON MD OF SALT LAKE CITY, UT, WAS DISCIPLINED BY UTAH ON JUNE 14, 1990
DISCIPLINARY ACTION: 24-MONTH PROBATION
OFFENSE: PROFESSIONAL MISCONDUCT

NOTES: FOUND GUILTY OF UNPROFESSIONAL CONDUCT, AIDING AND ABETTING THE PRACTICE OF MEDICINE BY AN UNLICENSED PERSON, ENGAGING IN CONDUCT/PRACTICE WHICH MAY CONSTITUTE A DANGER TO THE HEALTH, WELFARE, OR SAFETY OF THE PATIENT OR THE PUBLIC, CONDUCT OR PRACTICE WHICH DOES OR MIGHT IMPAIR THE PHYSICIANS ABILITY TO PRACTICE MEDICINE SAFELY AND SKILLFULLY. 60 DAY SUSPENSION STAYED. PROBATION TERMINATED AND LICENSE REINSTATED WITH FULL PRIVILEGES ON 9/16/92.

BERNTSON, DALE RAMPTON MD OF SALT LAKE CITY, UT, WAS DISCIPLINED BY UTAH ON APRIL 19, 1994
DISCIPLINARY ACTION: SURRENDER OF CONTROLLED SUBSTANCE LICENSE

NOTES: SURRENDER OF LICENSE AS AN ALTERNATIVE TO THE DIVISION PROCEEDING WITH FORMAL DISCIPLINARY ACTION. AGREED TO VOLUNTARILY SURRENDER HIS LICENSE TO PRESCRIBE AND ADMINISTER CONTROLLED SUBSTANCES SCHEDULES II-V.

BERNTSON, DALE RAMPTON MD OF 2033 EAST 33RD SOUTH, SALT LAKE CITY, UT, WAS DISCIPLINED BY DEA ON JULY 8, 1994
DISCIPLINARY ACTION: SURRENDER OF CONTROLLED SUBSTANCE LICENSE

NOTES: IN LIEU OF PUBLIC INTEREST REVOCATION.

BLACKBURN, BRENT L MD OF OGDEN, UT, WAS DISCIPLINED BY UTAH ON SEPTEMBER 23, 1999
DISCIPLINARY ACTION: EMERGENCY SUSPENSION
OFFENSE: PROFESSIONAL MISCONDUCT

NOTES: ON 9/18/99 ARRESTED ON A CHARGE OF ATTEMPTED SODOMY OF A CHILD. AGREED TO IMMEDIATE SUSPENSION ON HIS LICENSES TO PRACTICE AND TO PRESCRIBE AND ADMINISTER CONTROLLED SUBSTANCES, AND TO CEASE AND DESIST IMMEDIATELY FROM THE PRACTICE OF MEDICINE AND FROM THE ADMINISTRATION AND PRESCRIPTION OF ALL CONTROLLED SUBSTANCES DURING THE PERIOD OF THE PENDENCY OF THE INVESTIGATION AND UNTIL FINAL DISPOSITION.

BOOR, SAMUEL V MD OF ROUNDUP, MT, WAS DISCIPLINED BY UTAH ON MAY 12, 1994
OFFENSE: DISCIPLINARY ACTION BY ANOTHER STATE OR AGENCY

NOTES: DISCIPLINARY ACTION IN ANOTHER STATE FOR ACTS AND PRACTICES WHICH ARE A BASIS FOR UTAH DISCIPLINE. LICENSE SUSPENDED FOR THREE YEARS WITH A STAY OF ENFORCEMENT ON THE SUSPENSION AS LONG AS HE REMAINS IN FULL COMPLIANCE WITH TERMS AND CONDITIONS OF HIS MONTANA PROBATION. ON 2/23/95 PROBATION TERMINATED AND LICENSE REINSTATED WITH FULL PRIVILEGES.

BOOR, SAMUEL VLADIMIR MD, DATE OF BIRTH OCTOBER 6, 1932, LICENSE NUMBER 0004717 OF P.O. BOX 97, ROUNDUP, MT, WAS DISCIPLINED BY MONTANA ON JANUARY 11, 1994
DISCIPLINARY ACTION: EMERGENCY SUSPENSION
OFFENSE: PROFESSIONAL MISCONDUCT

NOTES: PENDING FURTHER INVESTIGATION OF ALLEGATIONS OF UNPROFESSIONAL CONDUCT.

BOOR, SAMUEL VLADIMIR MD, DATE OF BIRTH OCTOBER 6, 1932, LICENSE NUMBER 0004717 OF PO BOX 97, ROUNDUP, MT, WAS DISCIPLINED BY MONTANA ON FEBRUARY 16, 1994
DISCIPLINARY ACTION: 36-MONTH PROBATION
OFFENSE: PHYSICAL OR MENTAL ILLNESS INHIBITING THE ABILITY TO PRACTICE WITH SKILL AND SAFETY

NOTES: DIAGNOSED AS HAVING BIPOLAR DISORDER. HE

CONTESTS THE DIAGNOSIS, HOWEVER, HE HAS FULLY COOPERATED WITH BOARD REQUIREMENTS FOR TREATMENT AND AFTERCARE. THE BOARD HAS NO CURRENT INFORMATION INDICATING THAT HE IS PRESENTLY UNABLE TO PRACTICE MEDICINE WITH REASONABLE SKILL AND SAFETY. ON 1/18/95 TERMINATION OF PROBATION; LACK OF CONTINUED NEED.

BOSTROM, PAUL D MD, DATE OF BIRTH JULY 20, 1940, LICENSE NUMBER 0017962, WAS DISCIPLINED BY COLORADO ON JUNE 15, 1995
DISCIPLINARY ACTION: 60-MONTH PROBATION

NOTES: TREATMENT MONITORING.

BOSTROM, PAUL D MD, DATE OF BIRTH JULY 20, 1940, LICENSE NUMBER 0017962, WAS DISCIPLINED BY COLORADO ON JANUARY 18, 1996

NOTES: INTERIM CESSATION OF PRACTICE RETROACTIVE TO 11/24/95.

BOSTROM, PAUL D MD, DATE OF BIRTH JULY 20, 1940, LICENSE NUMBER 17962, WAS DISCIPLINED BY COLORADO ON JUNE 19, 1997
DISCIPLINARY ACTION: SURRENDER OF LICENSE
OFFENSE: SEXUAL ABUSE OF OR SEXUAL MISCONDUCT WITH A PATIENT

NOTES: A SEXUAL ACT WITH A PATIENT; PHYSICAL OR MENTAL DISABILITY.

BOSTROM, PAUL DAVID MD OF CORTEZ, CO, WAS DISCIPLINED BY UTAH ON JANUARY 23, 1996
OFFENSE: DISCIPLINARY ACTION BY ANOTHER STATE OR AGENCY

NOTES: CURRENT DISCIPLINARY ACTION AGAINST HIS LICENSE TO PRACTICE MEDICINE IN COLORADO. UTAH SUSPENSION STAYED DURING THE FIVE YEAR COLORADO PROBATIONARY PERIOD SO LONG AS HE REMAINS IN FULL COMPLIANCE WITH THE TERMS AND CONDITIONS OF HIS COLORADO PROBATION.

BRILLIANT, LEE STEVEN MD OF ROOSEVELT, UT, WAS DISCIPLINED BY UTAH ON JULY 13, 1993
DISCIPLINARY ACTION: 50-MONTH PROBATION
OFFENSE: DISCIPLINARY ACTION BY ANOTHER STATE OR AGENCY

NOTES: DISCIPLINARY ACTION AGAINST CALIFORNIA LICENSE FOR ACTS AND PRACTICES WHICH CONSTITUTE UNPROFESSIONAL CONDUCT UNDER UTAH LAW.

BRILLIANT, LEE STEVEN MD OF ROOSEVELT, UT, WAS DISCIPLINED BY UTAH ON JULY 19, 1996
DISCIPLINARY ACTION: 32-MONTH PROBATION
OFFENSE: FAILURE TO COMPLY WITH PREVIOUS BOARD ORDER

NOTES: COMMITTED A PATTERN OF NEGLIGENT ACTS; UNPROFESSIONAL CONDUCT; VIOLATED PROVISIONS OF A PRIOR ORDER. DID NOT ADMIT TO OR DENY ANY OF THE ALLEGATIONS. PROBATIONARY PERIOD ON HIS LICENSE WAS EXTENDED ALONG WITH ADDITIONAL CONDITIONS IMPOSED. ON 6/11/98 PROBATION EXTENDED INDEFINITELY. ON 12/8/98 LICENSE REINSTATED.

BROADBENT, DAVID H MD OF PROVO, UT, WAS DISCIPLINED BY UTAH ON MARCH 22, 1990
DISCIPLINARY ACTION: 12-MONTH PROBATION
OFFENSE: SUBSTANDARD CARE, INCOMPETENCE OR NEGLIGENCE

NOTES: SECOND YEAR OF TWO YEAR PROBATION STAYED. LICENSE SHALL BE REINSTATED TO FULL PRIVILEGES AFTER ONE YEAR OF PROBATION UPON FULL COMPLIANCE WITH CONDITIONS. ON 10/9/91 PROBATION TERMINATED AND LICENSE REINSTATED WITH FULL PRIVILEGES.

BROADBENT, DAVID H MD, LICENSE NUMBER 0009129, WAS DISCIPLINED BY ARIZONA ON APRIL 10, 1992
DISCIPLINARY ACTION: RESTRICTION PLACED ON LICENSE
OFFENSE: DISCIPLINARY ACTION BY ANOTHER STATE OR AGENCY

NOTES: ON 3/22/90, DISCIPLINED BY UTAH BOARD FOR PERFORMING LIPOSUCTION PROCEDURES WHICH HE WAS NOT QUALIFIED TO DO. SHALL NOT PERFORM LIPOSUCTION PROCEDURES UNTIL FURTHER ORDER OF THE ARIZONA BOARD OF MEDICAL EXAMINERS, AND SHALL CONFINE HIS MEDICAL PRACTICE TO OBSTETRICS AND GYNECOLOGY.

BROADBENT, DAVID H MD, LICENSE NUMBER 0G29387 OF PROVO, UT, WAS DISCIPLINED BY CALIFORNIA ON APRIL 13, 1994
DISCIPLINARY ACTION: 24-MONTH PROBATION
OFFENSE: DISCIPLINARY ACTION BY ANOTHER STATE OR AGENCY

NOTES: DISCIPLINED BY UTAH DIVISION OF OCCUPATIONAL AND PROFESSIONAL LICENSING FOR POOR MEDICAL JUDGMENT, INADEQUATE MEDICAL HISTORY OBTAINED OR DOCUMENTED, ON 2 LIPOSUCTION PATIENTS. IN CALIFORNIA, SUSPENSION STAYED.

BROWN, IAN S MD, LICENSE NUMBER 126863 OF 5205 OCEAN FRONT WALK #101, MARINA DEL RAY, CA, WAS DISCIPLINED BY NEW YORK ON MAY 15, 1997
DISCIPLINARY ACTION: SURRENDER OF LICENSE
OFFENSE: DISCIPLINARY ACTION BY ANOTHER STATE OR AGENCY

NOTES: HAS NEITHER ADMITTED NOR DENIED THAT HE WAS DISCIPLINED BY THE CALIFORNIA BOARD FOR GROSS NEGLIGENCE; INCOMPETENCE AND NEGLIGENCE ON MORE THAN ONE OCCASION; PRACTICING THE PROFESSION FRAUDULENTLY; FAILING TO MAINTAIN ACCURATE PATIENT RECORDS.

BROWN, IAN STEVEN MD, LICENSE NUMBER 0G29640 OF BEVERLY HILLS, CA, WAS DISCIPLINED BY CALIFORNIA ON AUGUST 15, 1996
DISCIPLINARY ACTION: SURRENDER OF LICENSE

NOTES: WHILE CHARGES PENDING.

BROWN, IAN STEVEN MD OF BEVERLY HILLS, CA, WAS DISCIPLINED BY UTAH ON APRIL 22, 1997
DISCIPLINARY ACTION: LICENSE SUSPENSION; SUSPENSION OF CONTROLLED SUBSTANCE LICENSE
OFFENSE: DISCIPLINARY ACTION BY ANOTHER STATE OR AGENCY

NOTES: DISCIPLINARY ACTION TAKEN AGAINST HIS MEDICAL LICENSE IN CALIFORNIA.

BROWN, IAN STEVEN MD, DATE OF BIRTH AUGUST 17, 1948 OF 11608 CHAYOTE STREET SUITE 2, LOS ANGELES, CA, WAS DISCIPLINED BY MEDICARE ON NOVEMBER 20, 1997
DISCIPLINARY ACTION: EXCLUSION FROM THE MEDICARE AND/OR MEDICAID PROGRAM
OFFENSE: DISCIPLINARY ACTION BY ANOTHER STATE OR AGENCY

NOTES: LICENSE REVOKED, SUSPENDED, SURRENDERED OR OTHERWISE LOST FOR REASONS BEARING ON PROFESSIONAL PERFORMANCE, PROFESSIONAL COMPETENCE OR FINANCIAL INTEGRITY.

BRUCE, STEPHEN J MD OF OGDEN, UT, WAS DISCIPLINED BY UTAH ON OCTOBER 6, 1997
DISCIPLINARY ACTION: REQUIRED TO TAKE ADDITIONAL MEDICAL

EDUCATION
OFFENSE: SUBSTANDARD CARE, INCOMPETENCE OR NEGLIGENCE

NOTES: EMBARKED ON A COURSE OF TREATMENT OF A SERIOUS DISEASE BASED ON A PATIENT'S MISREPRESENTATIONS THAT HE HAD BEEN DIAGNOSED WITH A DISEASE; FAILED TO CONDUCT MEDICALLY RECOGNIZED TESTS TO CONFIRM THE EXISTENCE OF THE DISEASE AND THE PRESENCE OF OPPORTUNISTIC INFECTION; PRESCRIBED EXCESSIVE QUANTITIES OF NARCOTICS AND OTHER DRUGS BASED UPON THE PATIENT'S MISREPRESENTATIONS AND HIS FAILURE TO CONDUCT APPROPRIATE TESTS. HE SHALL ATTEND AND SUCCESSFULLY COMPLETE ONE OF THREE EDUCATIONAL PROGRAMS WITHIN ONE YEAR AND SHALL MEET WITH THE BOARD.

BURKETT, ROX C MD, DATE OF BIRTH APRIL 19, 1947 OF 819 17TH STREET, MODESTO, CA, WAS DISCIPLINED BY MEDICARE ON NOVEMBER 20, 1997
DISCIPLINARY ACTION: EXCLUSION FROM THE MEDICARE AND/OR MEDICAID PROGRAM
OFFENSE: DISCIPLINARY ACTION BY ANOTHER STATE OR AGENCY

NOTES: LICENSE REVOKED, SUSPENDED, SURRENDERED OR OTHERWISE LOST FOR REASONS BEARING ON PROFESSIONAL PERFORMANCE, PROFESSIONAL COMPETENCE OR FINANCIAL INTEGRITY.

BURKETT, ROX CHARLES MD, LICENSE NUMBER 0G29053 OF MODESTO, CA, WAS DISCIPLINED BY CALIFORNIA ON DECEMBER 6, 1992
DISCIPLINARY ACTION: 1-MONTH LICENSE SUSPENSION; 60-MONTH PROBATION

NOTES: REVOCATION STAYED.

BURKETT, ROX CHARLES MD, LICENSE NUMBER 00M5976 OF 10378 FAIRVIEW AVENUE, BOISE, ID, WAS DISCIPLINED BY IDAHO ON AUGUST 22, 1994

NOTES: SHALL NOT PRACTICE MEDICINE IN IDAHO PENDING HEARING.

BURKETT, ROX CHARLES MD, LICENSE NUMBER 0G29053 OF TIBURON, CA, WAS DISCIPLINED BY CALIFORNIA ON JANUARY 12, 1995
DISCIPLINARY ACTION: 2-MONTH LICENSE SUSPENSION; 58-MONTH PROBATION
OFFENSE: FAILURE TO COMPLY WITH PREVIOUS BOARD ORDER

NOTES: VIOLATED PROBATION OF PRIOR DISCIPLINE; LEFT CALIFORNIA TO PRACTICE IN IDAHO WITHOUT NOTIFYING THE BOARD. REVOCATION STAYED.

BURKETT, ROX CHARLES MD OF KETCHUM, ID, WAS DISCIPLINED BY UTAH ON AUGUST 22, 1995
DISCIPLINARY ACTION: 15-MONTH PROBATION
OFFENSE: DISCIPLINARY ACTION BY ANOTHER STATE OR AGENCY

NOTES: DISCIPLINARY ACTION BY ANOTHER STATE FOR GROSS AND REPEATED NEGLIGENCE. REVOCATION STAYED. ON 12/16/97 PROBATION TERMINATED; LICENSE REINSTATED.

BURKETT, ROX CHARLES MD, LICENSE NUMBER 00M5976 OF 10378 FAIRVIEW AVENUE, BOISE, ID, WAS DISCIPLINED BY IDAHO ON MAY 31, 1996
DISCIPLINARY ACTION: MONITORING OF PHYSICIAN PERFORMANCE
OFFENSE: DISCIPLINARY ACTION BY ANOTHER STATE OR AGENCY

NOTES: ON 4/91 LICENSE APPLICATION HE STATED HE HAD NOT BEEN SUBJECT TO PROCEEDINGS BY A BOARD OR CONVICTED OF A FELONY OR MISDEMEANOR WHEN IN FACT IN 9/92 HE SIGNED A STIPULATION WITH THE CALIFORNIA BOARD AND HE WAS CONVICTED OF DRIVING UNDER THE INFLUENCE OFFENSES IN 1985 AND 1991. LICENSE LAPSED AND HE SHALL NOT APPLY FOR A LICENSE TO PRACTICE MEDICINE IN IDAHO FOR A MINIMUM OF FIVE YEARS. SHALL SUBMIT QUARTERLY DECLARATIONS UNDER THE PENALTY OF PERJURY STATING WHETHER THERE HAS BEEN COMPLIANCE WITH ALL THE CONDITIONS OF THIS ORDER; SHALL REPORT TO THE BOARD, AT THREE MONTH INTERVALS; AND SHALL EXECUTE A RELEASE AUTHORIZING ANY PERSON OR ENTITY HAVING INFORMATION RELEVANT TO HIS COMPLIANCE WITH THE PROVISIONS OF THIS ORDER TO GIVE THE INFORMATION TO THE BOARD.

BURKETT, ROX CHARLES MD, LICENSE NUMBER G29053 OF MODESTO, CA, WAS DISCIPLINED BY CALIFORNIA ON MARCH 3, 1997
DISCIPLINARY ACTION: SURRENDER OF LICENSE

NOTES: WHILE CHARGES PENDING.

BUTLER, RONALD BAY MD OF OREM, UT, WAS DISCIPLINED BY UTAH ON JULY 21, 1997
DISCIPLINARY ACTION: SURRENDER OF CONTROLLED SUBSTANCE LICENSE
OFFENSE: NONCOMPLIANCE WITH A PROFESSIONAL RULE

NOTES: ALLEGATIONS THAT HE FAILED TO MAINTAIN RECORDS REGARDING HIS CONTROLLED SUBSTANCE STOCK. VOLUNTARY SURRENDER.

CALL, GREGORY K MD OF SALT LAKE CITY, UT, WAS DISCIPLINED BY UTAH ON JANUARY 20, 1998
DISCIPLINARY ACTION: 60-MONTH PROBATION; 60-MONTH CONTROLLED SUBSTANCE LICENSE PLACED ON PROBATION
OFFENSE: SUBSTANCE ABUSE

NOTES: SELF ABUSE OF ALCOHOL. ON 6/22/98 ONE PROBATIONARY CONDITION WAS ADDED REGARDING ATTENDANCE OF WEEKLY AFTERCARE MEETINGS AND ONE PROBATIONARY CONDITION REGARDING PARTICIPATION IN A SUPPORT GROUP WAS CHANGED TO ALLOW ATTENDANCE AT TWO NARCOTICS ANONYMOUS OR AA MEETINGS WEEKLY.

CALL, GREGORY K MD OF SALT LAKE CITY, UT, WAS DISCIPLINED BY UTAH ON OCTOBER 8, 1999
DISCIPLINARY ACTION: SURRENDER OF LICENSE; SURRENDER OF CONTROLLED SUBSTANCE LICENSE

NOTES: AN INVESTIGATION IS BEING CONDUCTED REGARDING RESTRICTIONS IMPOSED UPON HIM BY A PRIOR DIVISION ORDER TO REFRAIN FROM THE USE OF ALCOHOL. HE AGREED TO SURRENDER HIS LICENSES TO PRACTICE MEDICINE AND TO PRESCRIBE AND ADMINISTER CONTROLLED SUBSTANCES PENDING THE COMPLETION OF THE DIVISION'S INVESTIGATION AND ANY PROCEEDING THAT MAY ARISE FROM THAT INVESTIGATION.

CAMPBELL, STEVEN K MD, DATE OF BIRTH APRIL 15, 1949 OF 173-E CHICAGO, COLDWATER, MI, WAS DISCIPLINED BY MEDICARE ON MARCH 22, 1991
DISCIPLINARY ACTION: EXCLUSION FROM THE MEDICARE AND/OR MEDICAID PROGRAM
OFFENSE: DISCIPLINARY ACTION BY ANOTHER STATE OR AGENCY

NOTES: LICENSE REVOCATION OR SUSPENSION.

CAMPBELL, STEVEN K MD OF SALT LAKE CITY, UT, WAS DISCIPLINED BY UTAH ON NOVEMBER 24, 1991
DISCIPLINARY ACTION: LICENSE REVOCATION; REVOCATION OF CONTROLLED SUBSTANCE LICENSE
OFFENSE: DISCIPLINARY ACTION BY ANOTHER STATE OR AGENCY

NOTES: EMPLOYED FRAUD, DECEPTION, AND/OR MISREPRESENTATION IN SECURING LICENSE; REVOCATION OF LICENSE BY MICHIGAN, THE STATE FROM WHICH LICENSURE BY ENDORSEMENT IN UTAH WAS BASED.

CAMPBELL, STEVEN K MD OF 105 EAST CHICAGO ST, COLDWATER, MI, WAS DISCIPLINED BY DEA ON JANUARY 4, 1993
DISCIPLINARY ACTION: REVOCATION OF CONTROLLED SUBSTANCE LICENSE
OFFENSE: DISCIPLINARY ACTION BY ANOTHER STATE OR AGENCY

NOTES: ON 12/17/90, MEDICAL LICENSE IN MICHIGAN REVOKED UPON FINDING THAT HE HAD SUBMITTED DOCUMENTS THAT WERE FORGED AND FICTITIOUS TO HIS MEDICAL SCHOOL AND TO MICHIGAN TO ESTABLISH HIS ELIGIBILITY FOR LICENSURE. AS A RESULT, HE IS NOT AUTHORIZED TO HANDLE CONTROLLED SUBSTANCES IN MICHIGAN. RELOCATED TO UTAH IN 09/90. ON 10/24/91, UTAH REVOKED HIS LICENSES TO PRACTICE MEDICINE AND TO HANDLE CONTROLLED SUBSTANCES AFTER FINDING THAT HE HAD EMPLOYED AN ELABORATE SCHEME TO FALSIFY HIS QUALIFICATIONS FOR LICENSURE.

CANNON, MAX K MD OF 400 15TH AVENUE SOUTH, GREAT FALLS, MT, WAS DISCIPLINED BY DEA ON DECEMBER 8, 1994
DISCIPLINARY ACTION: SURRENDER OF CONTROLLED SUBSTANCE LICENSE

NOTES: IN LIEU OF PUBLIC INTEREST REVOCATION.

CANNON, MAX KENT MD, DATE OF BIRTH OCTOBER 28, 1958, LICENSE NUMBER 0007314 OF 400 15TH AVENUE, SUITE 105, GREAT FALLS, MT, WAS DISCIPLINED BY MONTANA ON MAY 24, 1994
DISCIPLINARY ACTION: EMERGENCY SUSPENSION
OFFENSE: PROFESSIONAL MISCONDUCT

NOTES: ALLEGATIONS OF SEXUAL MISCONDUCT RELATED TO PRACTICE OF MEDICINE; SUSPICION THAT HE MAY BE SUFFERING FROM A MENTAL OR PHYSICAL CONDITION WHICH MAKES HIM UNABLE TO SAFELY PRACTICE MEDICINE. SHALL IMMEDIATELY SURRENDER LICENSE AND ALL CERTIFICATES. ORDERED TO SUBMIT TO A COMPLETE MENTAL AND PHYSICAL EVALUATION, INCLUDING BUT NOT LIMITED TO A FULL CHEMICAL DEPENDENCY EVALUATION; SHALL PROVIDE BOARD WITH COPIES OF ALL RECORDS RELATING TO THIS EVALUATION. ON 9/6/94, SUSPENSION LIFTED FOR THREE WEEKS FOR THE SOLE PURPOSE OF ALLOWING HIM TO COMPLETE AND SIGN HOSPITAL CHARTS PENDING AT THE TIME OF SUSPENSION.

CANNON, MAX KENT MD, DATE OF BIRTH OCTOBER 28, 1958, LICENSE NUMBER 0007314 OF 1108 E PATTERSON SUITE 2, KINKSVILLE, MO, WAS DISCIPLINED BY MONTANA ON MARCH 10, 1995
DISCIPLINARY ACTION: PROBATION; RESTRICTION PLACED ON LICENSE
OFFENSE: PHYSICAL OR MENTAL ILLNESS INHIBITING THE ABILITY TO PRACTICE WITH SKILL AND SAFETY

NOTES: FROM 3/8/94 THROUGH 5/21/94 HE WAS TAKING CORTICOSTEROIDS PRESCRIBED BY HIS TREATING PHYSICIANS FOR A CERVICAL DISC CONDITION; HAS BEEN DIAGNOSED BY THREE PSYCHIATRISTS, WHOSE OPINIONS ARE ACCEPTED BY THE BOARD, AS HAVING HAD A RECOGNIZED SIDE EFFECT OF STEROIDS, I.E. A SUBSTANCE-INDUCED MOOD DISORDER WITH MANIC FEATURES, WHICH, DURING THAT PERIOD, RESULTED IN OFFENDING BEHAVIOR. SUSPENSION LIFTED. CONDITIONS OF PROBATION: SHALL ESTABLISH A MENTOR RELATIONSHIP WITH A BOARD APPROVED PHYSICIAN WHO HE SHALL CONSULT WITH ON A REGULAR BASIS; SHALL NOT WORK ANY MORE THAN 55 HOURS PER SEVEN DAY WEEK WITHOUT OBTAINING BOARD APPROVAL; SHALL KEEP A LOG OF HOURS WORKED; SHALL GET BOARD APPROVAL FOR PRACTICE LOCATION; SHALL ESTABLISH A RELATIONSHIP WITH A PRIMARY CARE PHYSICIAN WHO WILL ASSUME RESPONSIBILITY FOR HIS ONGOING CARE; SHALL CONTINUE HIS ONGOING RELATIONSHIP WITH PSYCHIATRIST; SHALL ABSTAIN COMPLETELY FROM THE USE OF ANY AND ALL POTENTIALLY MOOD-ALTERING SUBSTANCES EXCEPT WHEN PRESCRIBED BY A LICENSED PHYSICIAN; SHALL REPORT ANY SUCH PRESCRIPTIONS TO THE BOARD; SHALL NOT WRITE, PHONE IN OR OTHERWISE ORDER PRESCRIPTIONS FOR HIMSELF OR ANY MEMBER OF HIS FAMILY; SHALL ENTER INTO AN AGREEMENT WITH THE MONTANA PROFESSIONAL ASSISTANCE PROGRAM; SHALL EXECUTE ANY RELEASES NECESSARY FOR BOARD TO VERIFY COMPLIANCE WITH THIS AGREEMENT; SHALL MEET ANNUALLY WITH THE BOARD. ON 8/11/95 ORDER MODIFIED SUCH THAT RESTRICTIONS ON THE NUMBER OF HOURS PER WEEK HE MAY WORK ARE LEFT TO THE DISCRETION OF HIS TREATING PSYCHIATRIST. ON 1/29/99 PROBATION TERMINATED; LICENSE RESTORED.

CANNON, MAX KENT MD OF SALEM, UT, WAS DISCIPLINED BY UTAH ON SEPTEMBER 30, 1997
DISCIPLINARY ACTION: 12-MONTH PROBATION; 12-MONTH CONTROLLED SUBSTANCE LICENSE PLACED ON PROBATION
OFFENSE: DISCIPLINARY ACTION BY ANOTHER STATE OR AGENCY

NOTES: DISCIPLINARY ACTION TAKEN AGAINST HIS MEDICAL LICENSE IN MONTANA. ON 10/23/98 PROBATIONS TERMINATED AND LICENSES REINSTATED WITH FULL PRIVILEGES.

CHANDLER, SWITHIN JR MD, LICENSE NUMBER 019849L OF SALT LAKE CITY, UT, WAS DISCIPLINED BY PENNSYLVANIA ON APRIL 20, 1990
DISCIPLINARY ACTION: FINE; REPRIMAND
OFFENSE: DISCIPLINARY ACTION BY ANOTHER STATE OR AGENCY

NOTES: DID NOT ADVISE THE BOARD OF ACTION TAKEN AGAINST HIS LICENSE TO PRACTICE MEDICINE AND SURGERY BY THE STATE OF UTAH ON 10/26/86. $2,000 CIVIL PENALTY.

CHEIN, EDMUND MD OF BEVERLY HILLS, CA, WAS DISCIPLINED BY UTAH ON MAY 6, 1996
OFFENSE: DISCIPLINARY ACTION BY ANOTHER STATE OR AGENCY

NOTES: DISCIPLINARY ACTION TAKEN AGAINST HIS MEDICAL LICENSE IN CALIFORNIA. UTAH SUSPENSION STAYED SO LONG AS HE REMAINS IN FULL COMPLIANCE WITH THE TERMS AND CONDITIONS OF HIS CALIFORNIA PROBATION.

CHINGROS, WILLIAM N MD, LICENSE NUMBER 0165349 OF 843 FRANKLIN STREET, OGDEN, UT, WAS DISCIPLINED BY NEW YORK ON JULY 21, 1993
DISCIPLINARY ACTION: FINE; REPRIMAND
OFFENSE: CRIMINAL CONVICTION OR PLEA OF GUILTY, NOLO CONTENDERE, OR NO CONTEST TO A CRIME

NOTES: HAD BEEN FOUND GUILTY OF STUDENT LOAN FRAUD. $1,000 FINE.

CHINGROS, WILLIAM N MD, WAS DISCIPLINED BY NEVADA ON DECEMBER 3, 1993
DISCIPLINARY ACTION: REPRIMAND
OFFENSE: DISCIPLINARY ACTION BY ANOTHER STATE OR AGENCY

NOTES: ON 11/15/93, STATE BOARD IN NEW YORK IMPOSED A CENSURE AND REPRIMAND AND A $1,000 FINE UPON HIS LICENSE TO PRACTICE MEDICINE IN NEW YORK.

CLAYTON, DAVID N MD OF SANDY, UT, WAS DISCIPLINED BY UTAH ON AUGUST 8, 1994
DISCIPLINARY ACTION: SURRENDER OF CONTROLLED SUBSTANCE LICENSE; 60-MONTH PROBATION
OFFENSE: OVERPRESCRIBING OR MISPRESCRIBING DRUGS

NOTES: UNLAWFULLY AND UNPROFESSIONALLY OBTAINING AND ADMINISTERING CONTROLLED SUBSTANCES TO HIMSELF; PROCURING ADMINISTRATION OF CONTROLLED SUBSTANCES BY MISREPRESENTATION; ISSUING FALSE AND MISLEADING PRESCRIPTIONS. ON 12/11/95 PROBATIONARY CONDITION REQUIRING HIM TO MEET WITH THE PHYSICIANS LICENSING BOARD WAS CHANGED TO REQUIRE MEETINGS EVERY SIX MONTHS. ON 12/16/97 LICENSE TO PRESCRIBE AND ADMINISTER CONTROLLED SUBSTANCES SCHEDULES II-V WAS ISSUED AND PLACED ON PROBATION FOR THE DURATION OF THE PROBATION ON HIS LICENSE WITH ADDITIONAL CONDITIONS. ON 12/23/97 RESTRICTION REGARDING ACCESS TO CONTROLLED SUBSTANCES WAS TERMINATED. ON 8/10/99 PROBATIONS ON LICENSES TERMINATED.

CLAYTON, DAVID NAYLOR MD OF 5770 SOUTH 250 EAST SUITE 235, MURRAY, UT, WAS DISCIPLINED BY DEA ON JULY 14, 1995
DISCIPLINARY ACTION: SURRENDER OF CONTROLLED SUBSTANCE LICENSE

NOTES: IN LIEU OF ORDER TO SHOW CAUSE.

COHEN, NATHANIEL M MD, DATE OF BIRTH AUGUST 24, 1922, LICENSE NUMBER 0028463 OF SALT LAKE CITY, UT, WAS DISCIPLINED BY KENTUCKY ON DECEMBER 1, 1992
DISCIPLINARY ACTION: FINE
OFFENSE: NONCOMPLIANCE WITH A PROFESSIONAL RULE

NOTES: FAILED TO COMPLETE REQUIRED CONTINUING MEDICAL EDUCATION IN THE AREA OF HIV/AIDS.

COHEN, NATHANIEL M MD, DATE OF BIRTH AUGUST 24, 1922, LICENSE NUMBER 0021299 OF 258 HARVARD ST #323, BROOKLINE, MA, WAS DISCIPLINED BY MASSACHUSETTS ON JULY 26, 1995
DISCIPLINARY ACTION: RESTRICTION PLACED ON LICENSE
OFFENSE: LOSS OR RESTRICTION OF HOSPITAL PRIVILEGES

NOTES: LOSS OF HOSPITAL PRIVILEGES.

COHEN, NATHANIEL M MD, DATE OF BIRTH AUGUST 24, 1922, LICENSE NUMBER 1062523 OF 5655 EAST RIVER RD, STE 101-207, TUCSON, AZ, WAS DISCIPLINED BY MICHIGAN ON APRIL 17, 1996
DISCIPLINARY ACTION: RESTRICTION PLACED ON LICENSE
OFFENSE: DISCIPLINARY ACTION BY ANOTHER STATE OR AGENCY

NOTES: FAILURE TO REPORT/COMPLY.

COHEN, NATHANIEL M MD, DATE OF BIRTH AUGUST 24, 1922, LICENSE NUMBER 0028463 OF TUCSON, AZ, WAS DISCIPLINED BY KENTUCKY ON MAY 20, 1996
DISCIPLINARY ACTION: RESTRICTION PLACED ON LICENSE
OFFENSE: DISCIPLINARY ACTION BY ANOTHER STATE OR AGENCY

NOTES: DISCIPLINARY ACTION TAKEN BY THE MASSACHUSETTS BOARD. MAY NOT ATTEND DELIVERIES, PRACTICE IN AN EMERGENCY ROOM, NEONATAL OR PEDIATRIC INTENSIVE CARE UNIT OR ANY CRITICAL CARE SETTING; PROHIBITED FROM PRACTICING MEDICINE EXCEPT IN A GROUP PRACTICE OR INSTITUTIONAL SETTING WHERE SUPERVISION AND BACKUP ARE READILY AVAILABLE.

COHEN, NATHANIEL M MD, LICENSE NUMBER 0425680 OF 5655 EAST RIVER RD SUITE 101-207, TUCSON, AZ, WAS DISCIPLINED BY KANSAS ON JULY 23, 1996
DISCIPLINARY ACTION: RESTRICTION PLACED ON LICENSE
OFFENSE: DISCIPLINARY ACTION BY ANOTHER STATE OR AGENCY

NOTES: ACTION IN MASSACHUSETTS ON 7/26/95 LIMITING HIS KANSAS LICENSE FOR AN INDEFINITE PERIOD, BUT AT LEAST AS LONG AS THE MASSACHUSETTS BOARD MAINTAINS ITS LIMITATIONS. KANSAS PROHIBITS HIM FROM: ATTENDING DELIVERIES; PRACTICING IN AN EMERGENCY ROOM, NEONATAL OR PEDIATRIC INTENSIVE CARE UNIT, OR ANY CRITICAL CARE SETTING; AND PRACTICING MEDICINE EXCEPT IN A GROUP PRACTICE OR INSTITUTIONAL SETTING WHERE SUPERVISION AND BACK-UP ARE READILY AVAILABLE.

COHEN, NATHANIEL M MD, DATE OF BIRTH AUGUST 24, 1922, LICENSE NUMBER 0032717 OF 5655 EAST RIVER ROAD #107-207, TUCSON, AZ, WAS DISCIPLINED BY WISCONSIN ON AUGUST 22, 1996
DISCIPLINARY ACTION: RESTRICTION PLACED ON LICENSE; MONITORING OF PHYSICIAN PERFORMANCE
OFFENSE: DISCIPLINARY ACTION BY ANOTHER STATE OR AGENCY

NOTES: ON 7/25/95 THE MASSACHUSETTS BOARD IMPOSED DISCIPLINE UPON HIS LICENSE TO PRACTICE MEDICINE. HIS WISCONSIN LICENSE IS LIMITED AS FOLLOWS: SHALL REFRAIN FROM PRACTICING OBSTETRICS, EMERGENCY MEDICINE, NEONATAL MEDICINE, SURGERY, PEDIATRIC INTENSIVE CARE OR IN ANY OTHER CRITICAL CARE SETTING; SHALL REFRAIN FROM THE PRACTICE OF MEDICINE IN WISCONSIN OR THE PRACTICE OF MEDICINE ELSEWHERE UNDER THE USE OF HIS WISCONSIN LICENSE EXCEPT IN A GROUP PRACTICE OR INSTITUTIONAL SETTING AND UNDER SUPERVISION BY OTHER LICENSED PHYSICIANS; PRIOR TO ENGAGING IN THE PRACTICE OF MEDICINE IN WISCONSIN, SHALL SUBMIT AND OBTAIN APPROVAL BY THE BOARD OF A PLAN OF SUPERVISION FOR HIS PRACTICE; SHALL IMMEDIATELY SURRENDER ALL INDICIA OF WISCONSIN REGISTRATION TO THE DEPARTMENT MONITOR WHO SHALL REISSUE CREDENTIALS MARKED "LIMITED."

COHEN, NATHANIEL M MD, LICENSE NUMBER 00G1904 OF TUCSON, AZ, WAS DISCIPLINED BY CALIFORNIA ON AUGUST 30, 1996
DISCIPLINARY ACTION: SURRENDER OF LICENSE

NOTES: WHILE CHARGES PENDING.

COHEN, NATHANIEL M MD, DATE OF BIRTH AUGUST 24, 1922, LICENSE NUMBER J5730, WAS DISCIPLINED BY TEXAS ON MAY 10, 1997
OFFENSE: DISCIPLINARY ACTION BY ANOTHER STATE OR AGENCY

NOTES: ON 7/26/95 ENTERED INTO AN AGREED ORDER WITH THE MASSACHUSETTS BOARD RESTRICTING HIS LICENSE BASED ON SOME HOSPITAL PRIVILEGES BEING WITHDRAWN FOLLOWING TWO INCIDENTS IN WHICH HIS RESPONSE TO TWO CESAREAN SECTIONS WAS DEEMED TO BE INSUFFICIENTLY AGGRESSIVE;

FAILED TO REPORT RESTRICTION TO THE BOARD WITHIN 30 DAYS SHALL NOT PRACTICE MEDICINE IN TEXAS UNTIL HE REQUESTS PERMISSION IN WRITING TO RESUME THE PRACTICE OF MEDICINE THERE, AND PERSONALLY APPEARS BEFORE THE BOARD TO PROVIDE SUFFICIENT EVIDENCE THAT HE IS OTHERWISE COMPETENT TO PRACTICE MEDICINE SAFELY INCLUDING AT A MINIMUM: EVIDENCE THAT THE 7/26/95 ORDER'S TERMS AND CONDITIONS HAVE BEEN TERMINATED/LIFTED OR MODIFIED; AND EVIDENCE THAT HE IS NOT THE SUBJECT OF ANY OTHER STATE DISCIPLINARY ACTION, INVESTIGATION, OR PROCEEDINGS; SHALL COOPERATE WITH THE BOARD IN VERIFYING COMPLIANCE INCLUDING PROVIDING COPIES OF ANY DOCUMENTS SUBMITTED TO MASSACHUSETTS UPON REQUEST; SHALL GIVE A COPY OF THIS ORDER TO ANY HEALTH CARE ENTITY WHERE HE HAS PRIVILEGES; SHALL INFORM THE BOARD OF CHANGE OF ADDRESS WITHIN 10 DAYS; SHALL NOT SEEK MODIFICATION FOR ONE YEAR.

COHEN, NATHANIEL MAURICE MD, DATE OF BIRTH AUGUST 24, 1922, LICENSE NUMBER 0003379 OF 5655 EAST RIVER ROAD NO. 101-207, TUCSON, AZ, WAS DISCIPLINED BY HAWAII ON OCTOBER 30, 1996
DISCIPLINARY ACTION: RESTRICTION PLACED ON LICENSE; MONITORING OF PHYSICIAN PERFORMANCE
OFFENSE: DISCIPLINARY ACTION BY ANOTHER STATE OR AGENCY

NOTES: RESTRICTIONS ON LICENSES IN MICHIGAN (4/17/96), KANSAS (7/23/96), AND KENTUCKY (5/17/96). HAWAII ORDER FOR INDEFINITE LIMITED LICENSE. TERMS AND CONDITIONS: SHALL COMPLY WITH MICHIGAN, KANSAS, AND KENTUCKY TERMS AND CONDITIONS: PROHIBITED FROM ATTENDING DELIVERIES OR PRACTICING IN AN EMERGENCY ROOM, NEONATAL, OR PEDIATRIC INTENSIVE CARE UNIT, OR ANY CRITICAL CARE SETTING; SHALL ONLY PRACTICE MEDICINE IN A GROUP PRACTICE OR INSTITUTIONAL SETTING WHERE SUPERVISION AND BACK-UP ARE READILY AVAILABLE; RESTRICTIONS IN HAWAII FOR AT LEAST AS LONG AS MASSACHUSETTS MAINTAINS LIMITATIONS.

COLLETTE, DAVID J MD OF FLAGSTAFF, AZ, WAS DISCIPLINED BY UTAH ON DECEMBER 4, 1990
DISCIPLINARY ACTION: CONTROLLED SUBSTANCE LICENSE PLACED ON PROBATION

NOTES: LICENSE TO PRESCRIBE SCHEDULES II THROUGH V PLACED ON FIVE YEAR PROBATION WITH THE CONDITION THAT HE MAY ONLY PRESCRIBE CONTROLLED SUBSTANCES IN THE WORK CARE INDUSTRIAL CLINIC AND EMERGICARE CLINIC. ON 8/28/95 PROBATION TERMINATED IN FAVOR OF HIM AGREEING TO CERTAIN TERMS AND CONDITIONS REGARDING HIS RETURN TO MEDICINE IN UTAH.

COLLETTE, DAVID S MD OF SALT LAKE CITY, UT, WAS DISCIPLINED BY UTAH ON AUGUST 31, 1990
DISCIPLINARY ACTION: 60-MONTH PROBATION; 60-MONTH CONTROLLED SUBSTANCE LICENSE PLACED ON PROBATION
OFFENSE: PROFESSIONAL MISCONDUCT

NOTES: UNLAWFULLY OBTAINED A SCHEDULE II CONTROLLED SUBSTANCE AND ADMINISTERED IT TO HIMSELF. SUSPENSION OF MEDICAL AND CONTROLLED SUBSTANCE LICENSES STAYED. SHALL NOT PRACTICE ANESTHESIOLOGY FOR THE FIVE YEAR PROBATIONARY PERIOD.

CRAVEN, CATHERINE M MD OF SALT LAKE CITY, UT, WAS DISCIPLINED BY UTAH ON MARCH 8, 1994
DISCIPLINARY ACTION: 60-MONTH PROBATION; 60-MONTH CONTROLLED SUBSTANCE LICENSE PLACED ON PROBATION
OFFENSE: SUBSTANCE ABUSE

NOTES: PRESENCE OF MEDICAL CONDITION AND SUBSTANCE ABUSE TO THE EXTENT THAT HER ABILITY TO PRACTICE MEDICINE SAFELY AND SKILLFULLY MAY BE IMPAIRED. ORDER DATED 8/17/95 MODIFIED THIS ORDER BY ALLOWING HER TO PRACTICE ANATOMIC AND CLINICAL PATHOLOGY; ALL OTHER TERMS AND CONDITIONS REMAIN IN EFFECT. ON 3/5/99 PROBATION ON LICENSE TO PRACTICE MEDICINE TERMINATED AND LICENSE REINSTATED WITH FULL PRIVILEGES; LICENSE TO PRESCRIBE AND ADMINISTER CONTROLLED SUBSTANCES EXPIRED ON 12/31/94 WHEN SHE FAILED TO PAY RENEWAL FEES.

CROOKSTON, MICHAEL J MD OF SOUTH JORDAN, UT, WAS DISCIPLINED BY UTAH ON MAY 9, 1990
DISCIPLINARY ACTION: 60-MONTH PROBATION; 60-MONTH CONTROLLED SUBSTANCE LICENSE PLACED ON PROBATION
OFFENSE: SUBSTANCE ABUSE

NOTES: ENGAGED IN CONDUCT WHICH FAILED TO CONFORM TO THE ACCEPTED STANDARDS OF HIS OCCUPATION AND COULD JEOPARDIZE THE PUBLIC HEALTH, SAFETY, OR WELFARE. PRESCRIBED/ADMINISTERED TO HIMSELF NARCOTICS OR DANGEROUS CONTROLLED SUBSTANCES, IMPAIRING HIS ABILITY TO CONDUCT THE PRACTICE OF MEDICINE SAFELY. HAS VIOLATED FEDERAL OR STATE LAW RELATING TO CONTROLLED SUBSTANCES, AND ENGAGED IN FRAUDULENT BEHAVIOR TO ACQUIRE CONTROLLED SUBSTANCES. MEDICAL LICENSE AND CONTROLLED SUBSTANCE LICENSE REVOCATION STAYED. MAY NOT ENGAGE IN THE PRACTICE OF ANESTHESIOLOGY FOR THE FIVE YEAR PROBATIONARY PERIOD. ON 7/29/92 LICENSE TO PRESCRIBE SCHEDULE IV AND V CONTROLLED SUBSTANCES WAS REINSTATED. ON 2/9/93 LICENSE TO PRESCRIBE AND ADMINISTER SCHEDULE II AND III CONTROLLED SUBSTANCES WAS REINSTATED AND PLACED ON PROBATION CONSISTENT WITH CONDITIONS OF THIS ORDER. ON 5/9/95 PROBATIONS TERMINATED AND LICENSE REINSTATED WITH FULL PRIVILEGES.

CROSBY, W MICHAEL MD, LICENSE NUMBER 1026511 OF 1715 DARLING STREET, OGDEN, UT, WAS DISCIPLINED BY INDIANA ON JANUARY 10, 1990
DISCIPLINARY ACTION: PROBATION

NOTES: INDEFINITE PROBATION. PROBATION MODIFIED EFFECTIVE 3/28/91 TO ALLOW HIM TO HOLD A CONTROLLED SUBSTANCE REGISTRATION ONLY FOR THE PURPOSE OF PRESCRIBING OR ADMINISTERING IN OPERATING ROOM OR IN THE PRE- OR POST-OPERATIVE STAGE WITHIN A HOSPITAL.

CULBERTSON, JOE C MD OF SALT LAKE CITY, UT, WAS DISCIPLINED BY UTAH ON JUNE 6, 1997
DISCIPLINARY ACTION: 2-MONTH LICENSE SUSPENSION; 2-MONTH SUSPENSION OF CONTROLLED SUBSTANCE LICENSE
OFFENSE: SEXUAL ABUSE OF OR SEXUAL MISCONDUCT WITH A PATIENT

NOTES: ENGAGED IN AN INTIMATE AND SEXUAL RELATIONSHIP WITH A PATIENT. LICENSES TO PRACTICE MEDICINE AND TO PRESCRIBE AND ADMINISTER CONTROLLED SUBSTANCES WERE REVOKED WITH A STAY OF ENFORCEMENT ON THE REVOCATION. FOLLOWING THE PERIOD OF SUSPENSION, HIS LICENSES WILL BE PLACED ON PROBATION FOR FIVE YEARS WITH CONDITIONS. ON 9/6/97 HIS LICENSES WERE PLACED ON PROBATION.

CURTIS, GLADE B MD OF SANDY, UT, WAS DISCIPLINED BY UTAH ON APRIL 14, 1998
DISCIPLINARY ACTION: REVOCATION OF CONTROLLED SUBSTANCE LICENSE; 60-MONTH PROBATION
OFFENSE: SUBSTANCE ABUSE

NOTES: ENGAGED IN WRITING FICTITIOUS PRESCRIPTIONS IN ORDER TO OBTAIN CONTROLLED SUBSTANCES FOR HIS PERSONAL USE AND ABUSE. PROBATION WITH CONDITIONS AND RESTRICTIONS.

CURTIS, GLADE B MD OF 9600 SOUTH 1300 EAST #305, SANDY, UT, WAS DISCIPLINED BY DEA ON MARCH 2, 1999
DISCIPLINARY ACTION: SURRENDER OF CONTROLLED SUBSTANCE LICENSE

NOTES: IN LIEU OF PUBLIC INTEREST REVOCATION.

DAVIS, ROBERT C MD OF 1519 WEST 90TH SOUTH, WEST JORDAN, UT, WAS DISCIPLINED BY NEW MEXICO ON DECEMBER 15, 1993
DISCIPLINARY ACTION: LICENSE REVOCATION
OFFENSE: CRIMINAL CONVICTION OR PLEA OF GUILTY, NOLO CONTENDERE, OR NO CONTEST TO A CRIME

NOTES: CRIMINAL CONVICTION IN ANOTHER STATE.

DAVIS, ROBERT CHARLES MD, DATE OF BIRTH OCTOBER 25, 1953, LICENSE NUMBER 0005035 OF 1781 WEST 90TH S, WEST JORDAN, UT, WAS DISCIPLINED BY MONTANA ON JANUARY 24, 1991
DISCIPLINARY ACTION: SURRENDER OF LICENSE
OFFENSE: NONCOMPLIANCE WITH A PROFESSIONAL RULE

NOTES: FAILURE TO DISCLOSE UTAH DISCIPLINARY ACTION IN A TIMELY MANNER.

DAVIS, ROBERT CHARLES MD OF SANDY, UT, WAS DISCIPLINED BY UTAH ON JULY 19, 1993
DISCIPLINARY ACTION: LICENSE REVOCATION; REVOCATION OF CONTROLLED SUBSTANCE LICENSE
OFFENSE: CRIMINAL CONVICTION OR PLEA OF GUILTY, NOLO CONTENDERE, OR NO CONTEST TO A CRIME

NOTES: CONVICTION OF CRIMES OF MORAL TURPITUDE WHICH RELATE TO HIS PRACTICE OF MEDICINE AND DEMONSTRATE A THREAT TO THE PUBLIC HEALTH, SAFETY AND WELFARE. HE FILED A REQUEST FOR AGENCY REVIEW ON 07/08/93 AND THE REVOCATION WAS STAYED PENDING THE ISSUANCE OF AN ORDER ON THE REQUEST. ORDER WAS UPHELD IN ITS ENTIRETY.

DAVIS, ROBERT CHARLES MD, DATE OF BIRTH OCTOBER 25, 1953, LICENSE NUMBER 0023956 OF 1519 WEST 90TH STREET, WEST JORDAN, UT, WAS DISCIPLINED BY IOWA ON JUNE 6, 1994
DISCIPLINARY ACTION: LICENSE REVOCATION
OFFENSE: DISCIPLINARY ACTION BY ANOTHER STATE OR AGENCY

NOTES: CHARGES THAT UTAH TOOK ACTION FOR FRAUD.

DAVIS, ROBERT CHARLES MD, DATE OF BIRTH OCTOBER 25, 1953 OF RR 2 BOX 9000, SAFFORD, AZ, WAS DISCIPLINED BY MEDICARE ON OCTOBER 10, 1994
DISCIPLINARY ACTION: 300-MONTH EXCLUSION FROM THE MEDICARE AND/OR MEDICAID PROGRAM
OFFENSE: CRIMINAL CONVICTION OR PLEA OF GUILTY, NOLO CONTENDERE, OR NO CONTEST TO A CRIME

NOTES: CONVICTED OF A CRIME INVOLVING THE MEDICARE, MEDICAID, MATERNAL AND CHILD HEALTH SERVICES BLOCK GRANT OR BLOCK GRANTS TO STATES FOR SOCIAL SERVICES PROGRAMS.

DECKER, MARSHALL SMITH MD OF SALT LAKE CITY, UT, WAS DISCIPLINED BY UTAH ON APRIL 15, 1996
DISCIPLINARY ACTION: SURRENDER OF LICENSE
OFFENSE: PRACTICING WITHOUT A VALID CONTROLLED SUBSTANCE LICENSE

NOTES: ALLEGATIONS THAT HE ISSUED PRESCRIPTIONS FOR CONTROLLED SUBSTANCES AND OTHER PRESCRIPTION DRUGS FOR HIMSELF, WHEN SUCH DRUGS WERE INTENDED FOR AND USED BY HIS WIFE; HE PRESCRIBED CONTROLLED SUBSTANCES TO A PATIENT WITHOUT MAINTAINING ADEQUATE RECORDS OF SUCH PRESCRIPTIONS; HE PRESCRIBED CONTROLLED SUBSTANCES UNDER AN EXPIRED LICENSE. WITHOUT ADMITTING OR DENYING ANY OF THE ALLEGATIONS, HE AGREED TO VOLUNTARILY SURRENDER HIS LICENSE SINCE HE RETIRED FROM MEDICINE IN 1983. HE FURTHER AGREED THAT HE WILL NOT HEREAFTER REAPPLY FOR A LICENSE TO PRESCRIBE AND ADMINISTER CONTROLLED SUBSTANCES.

DEFRIEZ, CURTIS B MD OF SALT LAKE CITY, UT, WAS DISCIPLINED BY UTAH ON SEPTEMBER 27, 1994
DISCIPLINARY ACTION: SURRENDER OF CONTROLLED SUBSTANCE LICENSE

NOTES: VOLUNTARY SURRENDER WITHOUT ADMITTING OR DENYING ALLEGATIONS UNTIL SUCH TIME AS THE DIVISION'S DISCIPLINARY ACTION IS RESOLVED COMPLETELY.

DEFRIEZ, CURTIS B MD OF LOVELOCK, NV, WAS DISCIPLINED BY UTAH ON AUGUST 10, 1995
DISCIPLINARY ACTION: REVOCATION OF CONTROLLED SUBSTANCE LICENSE; LICENSE SUSPENSION
OFFENSE: OVERPRESCRIBING OR MISPRESCRIBING DRUGS

NOTES: POSSESSED AND USED CONTROLLED SUBSTANCES NOT OBTAINED UNDER A VALID PRESCRIPTION; ISSUED CONTROLLED SUBSTANCE PRESCRIPTIONS FOR OTHER THAN LEGITIMATE MEDICAL PURPOSES; PRESCRIBED CONTROLLED SUBSTANCES IN QUANTITIES IN EXCESS OF THAT MEDICALLY NECESSARY; MADE FALSE PRESCRIPTIONS AND GAVE FALSE INFORMATION TO OBTAIN PRESCRIPTIONS FOR CONTROLLED SUBSTANCES. MEDICAL LICENSE INDEFINITELY SUSPENDED WITH CONDITIONS TO BE MET DURING PERIOD OF SUSPENSION.

DEFRIEZ, CURTIS B MD, LICENSE NUMBER 0G59725 OF SALT LAKE CITY, UT, WAS DISCIPLINED BY CALIFORNIA ON OCTOBER 7, 1996
DISCIPLINARY ACTION: LICENSE REVOCATION

DREZGA, GRMISLAV G MD, DATE OF BIRTH AUGUST 14, 1936, LICENSE NUMBER 1059477 OF 1456 HUDSON ROAD, HILLSDALE, MI, WAS DISCIPLINED BY MICHIGAN ON FEBRUARY 28, 1999
DISCIPLINARY ACTION: LICENSE REVOCATION
OFFENSE: DISCIPLINARY ACTION BY ANOTHER STATE OR AGENCY

NOTES: FAILURE TO REPORT/COMPLY.

DREZGA, GRMISLAV GREGORY MD OF NEW YORK, NY, WAS DISCIPLINED BY UTAH ON MARCH 4, 1998
DISCIPLINARY ACTION: LICENSE REVOCATION; REVOCATION OF CONTROLLED SUBSTANCE LICENSE
OFFENSE: SUBSTANDARD CARE, INCOMPETENCE OR NEGLIGENCE

NOTES: BEHAVIOR REFLECTS A PATTERN OF INCOMPETENCY OR NEGLIGENCE; VERBALLY ABUSED AND EXPLOITED PATIENTS AND MEDICAL STAFF.

DREZGA, GRMISLAV GREGORY MD, DATE OF BIRTH AUGUST 14, 1936 OF 540 W BOSTON POST ROAD, MAMARONECK, NY, WAS DISCIPLINED BY MEDICARE ON FEBRUARY 18, 1999
DISCIPLINARY ACTION: EXCLUSION FROM THE MEDICARE AND/OR MEDICAID PROGRAM
OFFENSE: DISCIPLINARY ACTION BY ANOTHER STATE OR AGENCY

NOTES: LICENSE REVOKED, SUSPENDED, SURRENDERED OR OTHERWISE LOST FOR REASONS BEARING ON PROFESSIONAL PERFORMANCE, PROFESSIONAL COMPETENCE OR FINANCIAL INTEGRITY.

DWYER, THOMAS D MD OF WAIALUA, HI, WAS DISCIPLINED BY UTAH ON JANUARY 16, 1990
DISCIPLINARY ACTION: REVOCATION OF CONTROLLED SUBSTANCE LICENSE; 3-MONTH LICENSE SUSPENSION
OFFENSE: OVERPRESCRIBING OR MISPRESCRIBING DRUGS

NOTES: CHARGES FOUND GUILTY OF INCLUDE USING FALSE/FRAUDULENT STATEMENTS IN CONNECTION WITH THE PRACTICE OF MEDICINE, UNETHICAL PROFESSIONAL CONDUCT, UNSAFE/DANGEROUS CONDUCT OR MEDICAL PRACTICE, CONDUCT WHICH MAY IMPAIR HIS ABILITY TO PRACTICE MEDICINE SAFELY AND SKILLFULLY. ISSUANCE OF FALSE OR FORGED PRESCRIPTION OR WRITTEN ORDER FOR CONTROLLED SUBSTANCE; ALTERATION OF PRESCRIPTION OR WRITTEN ORDER, AND INAPPROPRIATE USE OF SCHEDULE II OR III CONTROLLED SUBSTANCES. VIOLATION OF FEDERAL OR STATE LAW RELATING TO CONTROLLED SUBSTANCES. SUSPENSION RETROACTIVE TO 12/01/89. AFTER SUSPENSION, LICENSE PLACED ON PROBATION FOR FIVE YEARS. SHALL SUBMIT A PRACTICE PLAN TO BOARD FOR APPROVAL PRIOR TO RESUMING PRACTICE. SHALL NOT REAPPLY FOR CONTROLLED SUBSTANCE LICENSE UNTIL 12/1/91. PROBATION TERMINATED ON 4/3/95; HOWEVER BOARD NOTED AT THAT TIME THAT LICENSE TO PRACTICE MEDICINE IN UTAH HAD PREVIOUSLY EXPIRED ON 12/31/90 FOR NONPAYMENT OF RENEWAL FEES. HIS LICENSE TO PRESCRIBE AND ADMINISTER CONTROLLED SUBSTANCES WILL REMAIN REVOKED.

DWYER, THOMAS D MD OF 9600 S 1300E, SANDY, UT, WAS DISCIPLINED BY DEA ON FEBRUARY 20, 1990
DISCIPLINARY ACTION: SURRENDER OF CONTROLLED SUBSTANCE LICENSE
OFFENSE: PROFESSIONAL MISCONDUCT

NOTES: FOR PERSONAL ABUSE.

DWYER, THOMAS D MD, WAS DISCIPLINED BY HAWAII ON JULY 18, 1990
DISCIPLINARY ACTION: 24-MONTH MONITORING OF PHYSICIAN PERFORMANCE

DWYER, THOMAS DANIEL DR OF WAIALUA, HI, WAS DISCIPLINED BY ILLINOIS ON AUGUST 1, 1991
DISCIPLINARY ACTION: REVOCATION OF CONTROLLED SUBSTANCE LICENSE; PROBATION
OFFENSE: DISCIPLINARY ACTION BY ANOTHER STATE OR AGENCY

NOTES: DISCIPLINED BY UTAH; PHYSICIAN AND SURGEON LICENSE ON PROBATION UNTIL 1995.

EGLI, DAVID LAMBERT MD OF SALT LAKE CITY, UT, WAS DISCIPLINED BY UTAH ON MARCH 3, 1992
DISCIPLINARY ACTION: 60-MONTH PROBATION

NOTES: CONDUCT OR PRACTICE CONTRARY TO THE RECOGNIZED STANDARDS OF ETHICS OF THE MEDICAL PROFESSION. PROBATION WITH CONDITIONS.

ELDREDGE, STEPHEN J MD OF SALT LAKE CITY, UT, WAS DISCIPLINED BY UTAH ON MARCH 30, 1995
DISCIPLINARY ACTION: 60-MONTH PROBATION; 60-MONTH RESTRICTION PLACED ON CONTROLLED SUBSTANCE LICENSE
OFFENSE: OVERPRESCRIBING OR MISPRESCRIBING DRUGS

NOTES: PRESCRIBING CONTROLLED SUBSTANCES FOR OTHER THAN LEGITIMATE MEDICAL PURPOSE AND IN EXCESSIVE QUANTITIES; MAKING FALSE PRESCRIPTIONS AND GIVING FALSE INFORMATION TO OBTAIN PRESCRIPTIONS; FAILURE TO PROVIDE COMPETENT MEDICAL SERVICES; FAILURE TO DEAL HONESTLY WITH A PATIENT. REVOCATION OF LICENSE AND CONTROLLED SUBSTANCES LICENSE STAYED. PROBATIONS WITH RESTRICTIONS AND CONDITIONS. SCHEDULES II-V RESTRICTED. HE MAY NOT PRESCRIBE TO TREAT ANY MEDICAL CONDITION. MAY ADMINISTER MORPHINE FOR MANAGEMENT OF A MYOCARDIAL INFARCT, CONSISTENT WITH TERMS OF HIS PRACTICE PLAN. MAY NOT ADMINISTER ANY OTHER CONTROLLED SUBSTANCES IN THE COURSE OF HIS EMPLOYMENT AT HILL AIR FORCE BASE EMERGENCY ROOM. ON 11/28/95 HIS PRACTICE PLAN WAS AMENDED TO ALLOW HIM TO PRACTICE MEDICINE AS AN EMPLOYEE OF WESTSIDE MEDICAL SERVICES. HIS PRACTICE IS LIMITED TO THE LAYTON AND CLINTON SITES. MAY ALSO CONTINUE TO PRACTICE AT THE HILL AIR FORCE BASE EMERGENCY ROOM CONSISTENT WITH THE TERMS AND RESTRICTIONS IDENTIFIED IN THIS PRACTICE PLAN. RESTRICTIONS ON HIS LICENSE TO PRESCRIBE AND ADMINISTER CONTROLLED SUBSTANCES REMAIN UNCHANGED.

ELDREDGE, STEPHEN J MD OF SALT LAKE CITY, UT, WAS DISCIPLINED BY UTAH ON JANUARY 27, 1997
DISCIPLINARY ACTION: 84-MONTH PROBATION; 84-MONTH CONTROLLED SUBSTANCE LICENSE PLACED ON PROBATION
OFFENSE: FAILURE TO COMPLY WITH PREVIOUS BOARD ORDER

NOTES: VIOLATION OF PROBATIONARY CONDITION BY PRESCRIBING AND ADMINISTERING SUFENTANIL TO A PATIENT. LICENSES TO PRACTICE MEDICINE AND TO PRESCRIBE AND ADMINISTER CONTROLLED SUBSTANCES WERE REVOKED WITH A STAY OF ENFORCEMENT ON THE REVOCATION. SAID LICENSES SUBJECT TO EXISTING CONDITIONS AND RESTRICTIONS. $2,500 FINE. ON 5/15/97 ORDER WAS AMENDED.

ELDREDGE, STEPHEN J MD OF SALT LAKE CITY, UT, WAS DISCIPLINED BY UTAH ON MAY 3, 1999
DISCIPLINARY ACTION: LICENSE REVOCATION; REVOCATION OF CONTROLLED SUBSTANCE LICENSE
OFFENSE: FAILURE TO COMPLY WITH PREVIOUS BOARD ORDER

NOTES: PRACTICED MEDICINE AT A LOCATION OTHER THAN AS AUTHORIZED BY THE PROBATIONARY TERMS AND CONDITIONS GOVERNING HIS LICENSES AND AVOIDED THE REQUIRED SUPERVISION OF HIS MEDICAL PRACTICE. VIOLATED PROBATIONARY CONDITIONS WHEN HE HANDLED CONTROLLED SUBSTANCES AND ADMINISTERED CONTROLLED SUBSTANCES TO A PATIENT. USED ALCOHOL TO AN EXTENT WHICH MAY HAVE CREATED THE POTENTIAL FOR INJURY TO ANY GIVEN PATIENT.

ELIASON, RICHARD JAMES MD OF SALT LAKE CITY, UT, WAS DISCIPLINED BY UTAH ON MAY 16, 1991
DISCIPLINARY ACTION: 60-MONTH PROBATION
OFFENSE: PROFESSIONAL MISCONDUCT

NOTES: ALLEGATION OF UNPROFESSIONAL PERSONAL CONDUCT IN A PHYSICIAN/PATIENT RELATIONSHIP; HE DOES NOT ADMIT TO THE ALLEGATIONS IN AMENDED ORDER, BUT ENTERS INTO THIS STIPULATION TO AVOID LITIGATION, AND TO PROVIDE REASONABLE ASSURANCE OF PUBLIC SAFETY IN HIS PRACTICE. PROBATION WITH CONDITIONS.

ENGEN, JUDY J MD OF SALT LAKE CITY, UT, WAS DISCIPLINED BY UTAH ON AUGUST 12, 1992
DISCIPLINARY ACTION: SUSPENSION OF CONTROLLED SUBSTANCE LICENSE; EMERGENCY SUSPENSION

NOTES: SUSPENSIONS SHALL REMAIN IN EFFECT UNTIL A WRITTEN STIPULATION HAS BEEN FINALIZED REGARDING THE SPECIFIC DISPOSITION OF HER LICENSURE.

ENGEN, JUDY J MD OF SALT LAKE CITY, UT, WAS DISCIPLINED BY UTAH ON SEPTEMBER 27, 1993
DISCIPLINARY ACTION: 60-MONTH PROBATION

NOTES: SUSPENSION TERMINATED IN FAVOR OF A RESTRICTED PRACTICE; LICENSE TO PRESCRIBE AND ADMINISTER CONTROLLED SUBSTANCES REMAINS SUSPENDED. ON 12/16/97 SUSPENSION ON LICENSE TO PRESCRIBE AND ADMINISTER CONTROLLED SUBSTANCES SCHEDULES II-V WAS TERMINATED; AND THIS LICENSE PLACED ON PROBATION FOR DURATION OF THE PROBATION ON HER LICENSE WITH ADDITIONAL CONDITIONS. ON 9/28/98 PROBATION TERMINATED; LICENSES REINSTATED WITH FULL PRIVILEGES.

ENGEN, JUDY JACOBSON MD OF 1950 EAST 7000 SOUTH, SALT LAKE CITY, UT, WAS DISCIPLINED BY DEA ON AUGUST 19, 1993
DISCIPLINARY ACTION: SURRENDER OF CONTROLLED SUBSTANCE LICENSE
OFFENSE: DISCIPLINARY ACTION BY ANOTHER STATE OR AGENCY

NOTES: STATE LICENSE REVOCATION. ARRESTED 08/06/91 AND 10/14/92 IN SALT LAKE COUNTY UTAH FOR PRESCRIPTION FRAUD. LICENSE SUSPENDED AROUND 8/18/92. CONVICTED 02/12/93. SENTENCED 02/12/93 TO PROBATION AND FINE.

FEINAUER, LYMAN R JR MD, LICENSE NUMBER 0A24710 OF SALT LAKE CITY, UT, WAS DISCIPLINED BY CALIFORNIA ON SEPTEMBER 7, 1991
DISCIPLINARY ACTION: LICENSE REVOCATION
OFFENSE: DISCIPLINARY ACTION BY ANOTHER STATE OR AGENCY

NOTES: DISCIPLINED BY UTAH BOARD FOR UNAUTHORIZED AND EXCESSIVE USE OF TYLENOL #4 AND FAILURE TO MAINTAIN DRUG RECORDS. DEFAULT DECISION.

FILSTEIN, MARK M MD OF BOUNTIFUL, UT, WAS DISCIPLINED BY UTAH ON JUNE 27, 1997
DISCIPLINARY ACTION: FINE; REPRIMAND
OFFENSE: PROFESSIONAL MISCONDUCT

NOTES: HE ENTERED INTO A PARTNERSHIP WITH A PERSON NOT LICENSED TO PRACTICE MEDICINE AND ALLOWED THAT PERSON TO PRACTICE MEDICINE UNDER HIS AUTHORITY. $2,000 FINE.

FLOYD, CHARLES P DR, LICENSE NUMBER 0021104, WAS DISCIPLINED BY MINNESOTA ON JANUARY 6, 1996
DISCIPLINARY ACTION: RESTRICTION PLACED ON LICENSE

NOTES: ON 7/11/98 UNCONDITIONAL LICENSE.

FLOYD, CHARLES PATRICK MD OF MARSHALL, MN, WAS DISCIPLINED BY UTAH ON JULY 30, 1996
DISCIPLINARY ACTION: PROBATION
OFFENSE: DISCIPLINARY ACTION BY ANOTHER STATE OR AGENCY

NOTES: ACTION IN MINNESOTA. PLACED ON PROBATION DURING THE MINNESOTA RESTRICTION PERIOD UNDER TERMS AND CONDITIONS. ON 8/10/98 LICENSE REINSTATED.

FREEMAN, TERRY M MD, LICENSE NUMBER A38863 OF REDONDO BEACH, CA, WAS DISCIPLINED BY CALIFORNIA ON JUNE 15, 1995
DISCIPLINARY ACTION: 60-MONTH PROBATION
OFFENSE: PHYSICAL OR MENTAL ILLNESS INHIBITING THE ABILITY TO PRACTICE WITH SKILL AND SAFETY

NOTES: SEVERE INJURIES FROM HEAD-ON AUTO COLLISION. IMPAIRMENT AFFECTING SAFE MEDICAL PRACTICE. REVOCATION STAYED.

FREEMAN, TERRY M MD, LICENSE NUMBER A38863 OF LOS ANGELES, CA, WAS DISCIPLINED BY CALIFORNIA ON MAY 14, 1997
DISCIPLINARY ACTION: SURRENDER OF LICENSE

NOTES: WHILE CHARGES PENDING.

FREEMAN, TERRY MITCHELL MD OF LOS ANGELES, CA, WAS DISCIPLINED BY UTAH ON AUGUST 7, 1996
OFFENSE: DISCIPLINARY ACTION BY ANOTHER STATE OR AGENCY

NOTES: ACTION IN CALIFORNIA. UTAH SUSPENSION STAYED SO LONG AS HE REMAINS IN FULL COMPLIANCE WITH THE TERMS AND CONDITIONS OF HIS CALIFORNIA PROBATION.

FREEMAN, TERRY MITCHELL MD, DATE OF BIRTH MARCH 17, 1947 OF 2262 S BEVERLY DRIVE, LOS ANGELES, CA, WAS DISCIPLINED BY MEDICARE ON NOVEMBER 20, 1997
DISCIPLINARY ACTION: EXCLUSION FROM THE MEDICARE AND/OR MEDICAID PROGRAM
OFFENSE: DISCIPLINARY ACTION BY ANOTHER STATE OR AGENCY

NOTES: LICENSE REVOKED, SUSPENDED, SURRENDERED OR OTHERWISE LOST FOR REASONS BEARING ON PROFESSIONAL PERFORMANCE, PROFESSIONAL COMPETENCE OR FINANCIAL INTEGRITY.

FULLMER, MARK ALLEN MD OF PROVO, UT, WAS DISCIPLINED BY UTAH ON OCTOBER 17, 1997
DISCIPLINARY ACTION: 60-MONTH PROBATION; 60-MONTH CONTROLLED SUBSTANCE LICENSE PLACED ON PROBATION
OFFENSE: OVERPRESCRIBING OR MISPRESCRIBING DRUGS

NOTES: OBTAINED CONTROLLED SUBSTANCES WITHOUT A VALID PRESCRIPTION OR APPROPRIATE ORDER FORM; FAILED TO KEEP APPROPRIATE CONTROLLED SUBSTANCE RECORDS; ISSUED A FICTITIOUS PRESCRIPTION TO OBTAIN CONTROLLED SUBSTANCES; TOOK SCHEDULE II CONTROLLED SUBSTANCES FROM HOSPITAL INVENTORY; AND PRESCRIBED CONTROLLED SUBSTANCES IN QUANTITIES IN EXCESS OF THAT NECESSARY TO TREAT HIS PATIENTS' CONDITIONS. PROBATION WITH CONDITIONS AND RESTRICTIONS

GARNER, FRANK A MD OF 1561 S.W. BIRDIE DRIVE, CORVALLIS, OR, WAS DISCIPLINED BY DEA ON OCTOBER 31, 1994
DISCIPLINARY ACTION: RESTRICTION PLACED ON CONTROLLED SUBSTANCE LICENSE
OFFENSE: OVERPRESCRIBING OR MISPRESCRIBING DRUGS

NOTES: QUESTIONABLE PRESCRIBING PRACTICES.

GARNER, FRANK A MD OF SANDY, UT, WAS DISCIPLINED BY UTAH ON AUGUST 1, 1996
OFFENSE: DISCIPLINARY ACTION BY ANOTHER STATE OR AGENCY

NOTES: ACTION IN OREGON. UTAH SUSPENSION STAYED AS LONG AS HE REMAINS IN FULL COMPLIANCE WITH THE TERMS AND CONDITIONS OF HIS OREGON PROBATION.

GARNER, FRANK ALFRED MD, LICENSE NUMBER 0014325 OF CORVALLIS, OR, WAS DISCIPLINED BY OREGON ON JULY 19, 1990
DISCIPLINARY ACTION: RESTRICTION PLACED ON CONTROLLED SUBSTANCE LICENSE

NOTES: VOLUNTARY LIMITATION. NO SCHEDULE II OR III PRESCRIBING EXCEPT INSTITUTIONAL PATIENTS.

GARNER, FRANK ALFRED MD, LICENSE NUMBER MD14325 OF CORVALLIS, OR, WAS DISCIPLINED BY OREGON ON APRIL 15, 1994
DISCIPLINARY ACTION: 120-MONTH PROBATION; RESTRICTION PLACED ON LICENSE

NOTES: LIMITED TO PSYCHIATRY IN APPROVED SETTING; 50 HOURS OF CONTINUING MEDICAL EDUCATION; NO PSYCHOPHARMACOLOGICAL DRUGS WITHOUT APPROVAL.

GIBBONS, DE LAMAR J MD OF KELLOGG, ID, WAS DISCIPLINED BY IDAHO ON SEPTEMBER 30, 1991
DISCIPLINARY ACTION: REQUIRED TO TAKE ADDITIONAL MEDICAL EDUCATION
OFFENSE: OVERPRESCRIBING OR MISPRESCRIBING DRUGS

NOTES: INAPPROPRIATE PRESCRIBING OF CONTROLLED SUBSTANCES. AGREED TO CONTINUING MEDICAL EDUCATION STUDY AND EXAMINATION. STIPULATION EXPIRED ON 10/15/92.

GIBBONS, DE LAMAR J MD, LICENSE NUMBER 00M5298 OF 204 OREGON STREET, KELLOGG, ID, WAS DISCIPLINED BY IDAHO ON DECEMBER 3, 1993
DISCIPLINARY ACTION: LICENSE REVOCATION
OFFENSE: OVERPRESCRIBING OR MISPRESCRIBING DRUGS

NOTES: PRESCRIBED OR FURNISHED NARCOTICS TO ADDICTED PERSONS TO MAINTAIN THEIR ADDICTIONS AND LEVEL OF USAGE WITHOUT ATTEMPTING TO TREAT THE PRIMARY CONDITION REQUIRING USE OF NARCOTICS IN 18 CASES; THIS PRACTICE OF EXCESSIVE, UNWARRANTED AND INAPPROPRIATE PRESCRIBING IS A PATTERN OF INTENTIONAL AND DELIBERATE MEDICAL PRACTICE THAT ENDANGERS THE HEALTH AND SAFETY OF HIS PATIENTS. ON 12/22/93 A REQUEST FOR RECONSIDERATION WAS DENIED.

GIBBONS, DE LAMAR J MD, DATE OF BIRTH FEBRUARY 16, 1929 OF PO BOX 521152, SALT LAKE CITY, UT, WAS DISCIPLINED BY MEDICARE ON MARCH 19, 1996
DISCIPLINARY ACTION: EXCLUSION FROM THE MEDICARE AND/OR MEDICAID PROGRAM
OFFENSE: DISCIPLINARY ACTION BY ANOTHER STATE OR AGENCY

NOTES: LICENSE REVOKED FOR REASONS BEARING ON PROFESSIONAL PERFORMANCE.

GIBBONS, DE LAMAR JOHNSON MD OF 204 OREGON STREET, KELLOGG, ID, WAS DISCIPLINED BY DEA ON DECEMBER 28, 1993
DISCIPLINARY ACTION: SURRENDER OF CONTROLLED SUBSTANCE LICENSE
OFFENSE: DISCIPLINARY ACTION BY ANOTHER STATE OR AGENCY

NOTES: IDAHO MEDICAL LICENSE REVOKED. LOST FEDERAL CONTROLLED SUBSTANCE PRIVILEGES.

GOATES, MICHAEL G MD OF SALEM, UT, WAS DISCIPLINED BY UTAH ON JULY 14, 1992
DISCIPLINARY ACTION: 24-MONTH PROBATION
OFFENSE: DISCIPLINARY ACTION BY ANOTHER STATE OR AGENCY

NOTES: IS UNDER CONSENT AGREEMENT WITH CONNECTICUT AND APPLIED FOR LICENSURE IN UTAH. LICENSE ISSUED AND PLACED ON PROBATION WITH CONDITIONS OR UNTIL CONNECTICUT CONSENT AGREEMENT IS TERMINATED. ON 7/19/94 PROBATION ON LICENSE TO PRACTICE MEDICINE WAS TERMINATED AND LICENSE REINSTATED WITH FULL PRIVILEGES.

GREGORY, BUFORD LORTAIN DO OF 193 SOUTH MAIN, LEWISTON, UT, WAS DISCIPLINED BY DEA ON JUNE 21, 1994
DISCIPLINARY ACTION: SURRENDER OF CONTROLLED SUBSTANCE LICENSE

NOTES: IN LIEU OF PUBLIC INTEREST REVOCATION.

GREYEYES, ROGER MD OF SHIPROCK, NM, WAS DISCIPLINED BY UTAH ON MARCH 3, 1999
DISCIPLINARY ACTION: LICENSE REVOCATION; REVOCATION OF CONTROLLED SUBSTANCE LICENSE
OFFENSE: SUBSTANCE ABUSE

NOTES: HIS CONTINUED USE OF ALCOHOL MAY REASONABLY BE CONSIDERED TO HAVE IMPAIRED HIS ABILITY TO PRACTICE MEDICINE.

GRIGSBY, JAMES LEE MD OF OMAHA, NE, WAS DISCIPLINED BY UTAH ON NOVEMBER 27, 1995
OFFENSE: PROFESSIONAL MISCONDUCT

NOTES: ALLEGED SEXUAL MISCONDUCT IN THE PRACTICE OF MEDICINE. WITHOUT ADMITTING ANY OF THE ALLEGATIONS CONTAINED IN THE PETITION, HE AGREES THAT HE WILL NOT FILE APPLICATIONS TO RENEW OR REINSTATE HIS LICENSE GIVEN THAT HE NO LONGER RESIDES IN UTAH AND HAS NO INTENT TO RETURN TO UTAH TO PRACTICE MEDICINE.

HALE, BOYD J MD OF PROVO, UT, WAS DISCIPLINED BY UTAH ON JANUARY 15, 1998
DISCIPLINARY ACTION: 60-MONTH PROBATION; 60-MONTH CONTROLLED SUBSTANCE LICENSE PLACED ON PROBATION
OFFENSE: PROFESSIONAL MISCONDUCT

NOTES: ALLEGATIONS THAT HE ENGAGED IN UNPROFESSIONAL CONDUCT AS A PHYSICIAN/SURGEON.

HAMMOND, SAMUEL JENSEN MD OF OREM, UT, WAS DISCIPLINED BY UTAH ON JULY 30, 1998
DISCIPLINARY ACTION: 12-MONTH PROBATION; 12-MONTH CONTROLLED SUBSTANCE LICENSE PLACED ON PROBATION
OFFENSE: OVERPRESCRIBING OR MISPRESCRIBING DRUGS

NOTES: OVERPRESCRIBED PAIN MEDICATION TO HIS PATIENTS. ON 8/6/99 PROBATIONS TERMINATED AND LICENSES REINSTATED WITH FULL PRIVILEGES.

HANSON, JOEL WALLACE MD OF CENTERVILLE, UT, WAS DISCIPLINED BY UTAH ON NOVEMBER 2, 1999
DISCIPLINARY ACTION: RESTRICTION PLACED ON LICENSE
OFFENSE: PROFESSIONAL MISCONDUCT

NOTES: FROM THE EARLY 1980S TO THE PRESENT, HE HAS ENGAGED IN VOYEURISTIC CONDUCT; IN 7/99, HE WAS CHARGED WITH TWO COUNTS OF WITNESS TAMPERING, BOTH THIRD DEGREE FELONIES, AND

ONE COUNT OF PRIVACY VIOLATION, A CLASS B MISDEMEANOR. REVOCATION STAYED AS LONG AS HE COMPLIES WITH CONDITIONS; SHALL NOT PERFORM PHYSICAL EXAMS OR MEET PRIVATELY WITH ANY PATIENT OR CLIENT UNTIL THE MATTER IS RESOLVED EITHER BY STIPULATION BY THE PARTIES OR FORMAL PROCEEDINGS; INDIVIDUAL COUNSELING MAY BE PERFORMED AS LONG AS HE HAS A THIRD PERSON ADULT PRESENT IN THE OFFICE.

HARBRECHT, DAVID J MD OF BOUNTIFUL, UT, WAS DISCIPLINED BY UTAH ON AUGUST 16, 1996
DISCIPLINARY ACTION: 24-MONTH PROBATION; 24-MONTH CONTROLLED SUBSTANCE LICENSE PLACED ON PROBATION
OFFENSE: PROFESSIONAL MISCONDUCT

NOTES: INAPPROPRIATELY OBTAINED DEMEROL AND FAILED TO KEEP ADEQUATE CONTROLLED SUBSTANCE AND PATIENT RECORDS. PROHIBITED FROM PRESCRIBING SCHEDULE II CONTROLLED SUBSTANCES UNTIL SUCH TIME AS THE DRUG ENFORCEMENT ADMINISTRATION ISSUES A NEW REGISTRATION UNDER A MEMORANDUM AGREEMENT BETWEEN HIMSELF AND THE DEA. ON 8/11/98 LICENSES REINSTATED.

HARBRECHT, DAVID J MD, LICENSE NUMBER 4309A, WAS DISCIPLINED BY WYOMING ON MARCH 24, 1997
DISCIPLINARY ACTION: PROBATION; RESTRICTION PLACED ON CONTROLLED SUBSTANCE LICENSE
OFFENSE: DISCIPLINARY ACTION BY ANOTHER STATE OR AGENCY

NOTES: ENTERED INTO A STIPULATION AND ORDER WITH THE UTAH BOARD ON 8/15/96 WHICH IMPOSED CONDITIONS UPON HIS UTAH LICENSE TO PRACTICE MEDICINE, HIS PRESCRIBING PRIVILEGES, AND IMPOSED A PERIOD OF PROBATION. PROBATION WITH THE FOLLOWING TERMS AND CONDITIONS: RESTRICTED FROM PRESCRIBING SCHEDULE II CONTROLLED SUBSTANCES UNTIL THE DEA ISSUES A NEW REGISTRATION UNDER A MEMORANDUM OF AGREEMENT; AND SHALL SUBMIT COPIES TO THE BOARD OF ALL REPORTS PREPARED IN CONJUNCTION WITH FULFILLMENT OF ALL CONDITIONS OF AGREEMENT WITH THE DEA.

HARLINE, WESLEY GRANT MD OF OGDEN, UT, WAS DISCIPLINED BY UTAH ON JUNE 18, 1992
DISCIPLINARY ACTION: RESTRICTION PLACED ON LICENSE

NOTES: RESTRICTED PENDING RESOLUTION OF RELATED PROCEEDINGS. ORDER DEALS WITH INFORMED CONSENT, CEASE AND DESIST FROM USING INJECTABLE LIQUID SILICONE, EMPLOYMENT OF QUALIFIED PERSONNEL, PROPER ADMINISTRATION OF ANESTHESIA AND FACILITY CONDITIONS AND INSPECTION. SOME RESTRICTIONS ORIGINALLY IMPOSED BY EMERGENCY ORDER JUNE 5, 1992. DR. HARLINE'S COUNSEL AGREED TO ACCEPT TERMS AND CONDITIONS OF THE ORDER ON 6/17/92 DURING AN APPEARANCE BEFORE THE THIRD DISTRICT COURT.

HARLINE, WESLEY GRANT MD OF OGDEN, UT, WAS DISCIPLINED BY UTAH ON DECEMBER 12, 1996
DISCIPLINARY ACTION: 60-MONTH PROBATION; RESTRICTION PLACED ON LICENSE
OFFENSE: OVERPRESCRIBING OR MISPRESCRIBING DRUGS

NOTES: FAILED TO PROVIDE INFORMED CONSENT TO PATIENTS PRIOR TO PERFORMING SURGICAL PROCEDURES; PERFORMED A NONMEDICALLY RECOGNIZED SURGERY; SUBSTITUTED SILICONE FOR SALINE DURING BREAST AUGMENTATION SURGERY CONTRARY TO THE PATIENT'S EXPRESS DIRECTIVE PRIOR TO SURGERY; USED AND OFFERED TO USE SILICONE INJECTIONS, A NON-FDA APPROVED MEDICAL DEVICE; ENGAGED IN UNLAWFUL DISPENSING OF CONTROLLED SUBSTANCES TO PATIENTS WITHOUT MEDICAL NEED OR PROPER CHARTING; AND IMPROPER OVER-PRESCRIPTION OF CONTROLLED SUBSTANCE STIMULANTS FOR DIET PURPOSES. HE DENIED ALL OF THE ABOVE ALLEGATIONS, BUT AGREED TO THE FOLLOWING RESTRICTIONS. THREE MONTH SUSPENSION, STAYED AS PROBATION WITH CONDITIONS AND RESTRICTIONS

HERZER, FRED E MD OF SANDY, UT, WAS DISCIPLINED BY UTAH ON AUGUST 22, 1994
DISCIPLINARY ACTION: 60-MONTH PROBATION; 60-MONTH RESTRICTION PLACED ON CONTROLLED SUBSTANCE LICENSE
OFFENSE: PRACTICING WITHOUT A VALID CONTROLLED SUBSTANCE LICENSE

NOTES: ALLEGATIONS OF ABUSE OF ALCOHOL AND DRUGS; PRESCRIBED CONTROLLED SUBSTANCES WHEN NOT LICENSED; ISSUED CONTROLLED SUBSTANCE PRESCRIPTIONS FOR OTHER THAN A LEGITIMATE MEDICAL PURPOSE; PRESCRIBED EXCESSIVE QUANTITIES OF CONTROLLED SUBSTANCES BEYOND MEDICAL NECESSITY; MADE FALSE PRESCRIPTIONS; GAVE FALSE INFORMATION TO OBTAIN CONTROLLED SUBSTANCES; FAILURE TO PROVIDE COMPETENT MEDICAL SERVICES AND OTHERWISE ACTING OUTSIDE THE STANDARDS AND ETHICS OF THE PROFESSION; ISSUING CONTROLLED SUBSTANCES PRESCRIPTIONS TO A DRUG DEPENDENT PERSON. NEITHER ADMITS NOR DENIES ALLEGATIONS. SHALL ONLY BE PERMITTED TO PRESCRIBE STIMULANTS IN SCHEDULE II AND III CONTROLLED SUBSTANCES; SHALL NOT BE PERMITTED TO PRESCRIBE ANY SCHEDULE V CONTROLLED SUBSTANCES, MAY PRESCRIBE SCHEDULE IV SUBSTANCES. ON 9/9/99 PROBATIONS ON LICENSES TERMINATED AND REINSTATED WITH FULL PRIVILEGES.

HERZER, FRED E III MD OF 5899 WEST RIVENDELL DRIVE, WEST JORDAN, UT, WAS DISCIPLINED BY DEA ON DECEMBER 20, 1994
DISCIPLINARY ACTION: RESTRICTION PLACED ON CONTROLLED SUBSTANCE LICENSE
OFFENSE: DISCIPLINARY ACTION BY ANOTHER STATE OR AGENCY

NOTES: STATE BOARD.

HEWETT, DAVID E MD OF OREM, UT, WAS DISCIPLINED BY UTAH ON OCTOBER 10, 1990
DISCIPLINARY ACTION: EMERGENCY SUSPENSION

NOTES: SUSPENSION PENDING HEARING SCHEDULED FOR 11/14/90 TO DETERMINE WHETHER HIS LICENSE SHOULD BE PERMANENTLY REVOKED.

HEWETT, DAVID E MD OF OREM, UT, WAS DISCIPLINED BY UTAH ON NOVEMBER 20, 1990
DISCIPLINARY ACTION: LICENSE SUSPENSION
OFFENSE: FAILURE TO COMPLY WITH PREVIOUS BOARD ORDER

NOTES: FAILED TO SUBMIT TO PHYSICAL AND/OR MENTAL EXAMINATION AS DIRECTED BY PREVIOUS BOARD ORDER, AND FINDING OF REASONABLE CAUSE TO BELIEVE HE IS UNABLE TO PRACTICE MEDICINE WITH REASONABLE SKILL AND SAFETY TO PATIENTS. LICENSE SHALL REMAIN SUSPENDED UNTIL HE SUBMITS TO SUCH AN EXAMINATION.

HEWETT, DAVID E MD, DATE OF BIRTH MARCH 1, 1939 OF PO BOX 1122, OREM, UT, WAS DISCIPLINED BY MEDICARE ON JULY 23, 1991

DISCIPLINARY ACTION: EXCLUSION FROM THE MEDICARE AND/OR MEDICAID PROGRAM
OFFENSE: DISCIPLINARY ACTION BY ANOTHER STATE OR AGENCY

NOTES: LICENSE REVOCATION OR SUSPENSION.

HIGGINBOTHAM, ROBERT WRIGHT MD OF SAN LUIS OBISPO, CA, WAS DISCIPLINED BY UTAH ON OCTOBER 3, 1996
OFFENSE: DISCIPLINARY ACTION BY ANOTHER STATE OR AGENCY

NOTES: ACTION IN CALIFORNIA. STAYED SUSPENSION AS LONG AS HE REMAINS IN FULL COMPLIANCE WITH THE CALIFORNIA PROBATION. CONDITIONS TO BE MET IN UTAH DURING THE CALIFORNIA PROBATIONARY PERIOD. ON 12/6/99 PROBATION TERMINATED AND LICENSE REINSTATED WITH FULL PRIVILEGES.

HINES, WIRT A JR MD OF SALT LAKE CITY, UT, WAS DISCIPLINED BY UTAH ON FEBRUARY 7, 1990
DISCIPLINARY ACTION: 1-MONTH SURRENDER OF LICENSE; REVOCATION OF CONTROLLED SUBSTANCE LICENSE
OFFENSE: OVERPRESCRIBING OR MISPRESCRIBING DRUGS

NOTES: CHARGES FOUND GUILTY OF INCLUDE FURNISHING DRUGS TO A DRUG-DEPENDENT PERSON, UNETHICAL PROFESSIONAL CONDUCT, UNSAFE/DANGEROUS CONDUCT OR MEDICAL PRACTICE, PRESCRIPTION VIOLATIONS AND INADEQUATE RECORD-KEEPING AND INVENTORY PROCEDURES IN CONNECTION WITH ADMINISTERING CONTROLLED SUBSTANCES. REVOCATION STAYED; 3 MONTH SUSPENSION RETROACTIVE TO 12/1/89. SURRENDERED LICENSE ON 2/7/90; DURING WEEK OF 2/1-2/7/90, PRACTICE LIMITED TO AFTERCARE OF PATIENTS WHO RECEIVED SERVICES PRIOR TO 2/1/90. MUST SUBMIT PRACTICE PLAN; IF APPROVED, MAY RESUME PRACTICE 2/28/90. AFTER SUSPENSION PERIOD, LICENSE WILL BE ON PROBATION FOR 5 YEARS. MAY APPLY FOR REVOKED CONTROLLED SUBSTANCE LICENSE ON 1/1/92. AFTER TWO YEAR PERIOD OF REVOCATION, CONTROLLED SUBSTANCE LICENSE WILL BE ON 3 YEAR PROBATION.

HINES, WIRT A JR MD OF SALT LAKE CITY, UT, WAS DISCIPLINED BY UTAH ON FEBRUARY 5, 1992
DISCIPLINARY ACTION: 36-MONTH CONTROLLED SUBSTANCE LICENSE PLACED ON PROBATION

NOTES: REVOCATION ON LICENSE TO PRESCRIBE AND ADMINISTER CONTROLLED SUBSTANCES WAS TERMINATED. THIS LICENSE ISSUED ON PROBATION CONSISTENT WITH THE TERMS AND CONDITIONS IDENTIFIED IN THE FEBRUARY 7, 1990 ORDER. ON 1/25/94 THE PROBATION ON HIS LICENSE TO PRACTICE MEDICINE AND PRESCRIBE AND ADMINISTER CONTROLLED SUBSTANCES WAS TERMINATED AND LICENSE REINSTATED WITH FULL PRIVILEGES.

HINES, WIRT A MD, LICENSE NUMBER 14488 OF SALT LAKE CITY, UT, WAS DISCIPLINED BY FLORIDA ON DECEMBER 30, 1997
DISCIPLINARY ACTION: SURRENDER OF LICENSE
OFFENSE: DISCIPLINARY ACTION BY ANOTHER STATE OR AGENCY

NOTES: CHARGED WITH HAVING A DISCIPLINARY ACTION IN ANOTHER JURISDICTION AND FAILING TO REPORT THIS WITHIN 30 DAYS. VOLUNTARY SURRENDER WITH AGREEMENT NEVER TO REAPPLY FOR A FLORIDA LICENSE.

HINES, WIRT ANDERSON MD, LICENSE NUMBER 0G20362 OF SALT LAKE CITY, UT, WAS DISCIPLINED BY CALIFORNIA ON FEBRUARY 14, 1994
DISCIPLINARY ACTION: LICENSE REVOCATION
OFFENSE: DISCIPLINARY ACTION BY ANOTHER STATE OR AGENCY

NOTES: DISCIPLINED BY THE UTAH BOARD FOR UNPROFESSIONAL CONDUCT. VIOLATED PROBATION OF PRIOR DISCIPLINE. DEFAULT DECISION.

HINTON, RAYMOND K MD OF WASHINGTON, UT, WAS DISCIPLINED BY UTAH ON JANUARY 19, 1996
DISCIPLINARY ACTION: 12-MONTH PROBATION; 12-MONTH CONTROLLED SUBSTANCE LICENSE PLACED ON PROBATION
OFFENSE: OVERPRESCRIBING OR MISPRESCRIBING DRUGS

NOTES: PRESCRIBING CONTROLLED SUBSTANCES IN EXCESS OF WHAT WAS MEDICALLY NECESSARY TO TREAT HIS PATIENTS' MEDICAL CONDITIONS. ON 3/6/97 LICENSES TO PRACTICE MEDICINE AND HANDLE CONTROLLED SUBSTANCES REINSTATED WITH FULL PRIVILEGES.

HOENES, DOUGLAS RADFORD MD OF KAYSVILLE, UT, WAS DISCIPLINED BY UTAH ON JANUARY 4, 1993
DISCIPLINARY ACTION: LICENSE REINSTATEMENT; PROBATION
OFFENSE: PHYSICAL OR MENTAL ILLNESS INHIBITING THE ABILITY TO PRACTICE WITH SKILL AND SAFETY

NOTES: MEDICAL DISABILITY. ON 7/13/93 CONDITIONS REQUIRING QUARTERLY PSYCHIATRIC REPORTS AND QUARTERLY MEETINGS WERE CHANGED TO ONCE EVERY SIX MONTHS. ON 1/3/95 THE PROBATIONARY CONDITIONS REQUIRING SEMIANNUAL PSYCHIATRIC REPORTS AND SEMIANNUAL MEETINGS WITH THE BOARD WERE PLACED ON HOLD UNLESS AND UNTIL HE IS ENGAGED IN THE PRACTICE OF MEDICINE INCLUDING AN ADMINISTRATIVE POSITION HELD BASED ON THE FACT THAT HE IS A PHYSICIAN.

HOLT, DEAN MD, DATE OF BIRTH FEBRUARY 8, 1927 OF 281 EAST 200 NORTH, LOGAN, UT, WAS DISCIPLINED BY MEDICARE ON MARCH 16, 1995
DISCIPLINARY ACTION: 60-MONTH EXCLUSION FROM THE MEDICARE AND/OR MEDICAID PROGRAM
OFFENSE: NONCOMPLIANCE WITH A PROFESSIONAL RULE

NOTES: EXCLUDED BASED ON A RECOMMENDATION FROM A PEER REVIEW ORGANIZATION THAT HE VIOLATED STATUTORY OBLIGATIONS.

HOLT, DEAN A MD OF LOGAN, UT, WAS DISCIPLINED BY UTAH ON FEBRUARY 23, 1995
DISCIPLINARY ACTION: SURRENDER OF LICENSE; SURRENDER OF CONTROLLED SUBSTANCE LICENSE
OFFENSE: PRACTICING WITHOUT A VALID CONTROLLED SUBSTANCE LICENSE

NOTES: ALLEGATIONS OF A PATTERN OF NEGLIGENT ACTS AND PRACTICES IN MEDICINE; ISSUED PRESCRIPTIONS FOR CONTROLLED SUBSTANCES WHEN NOT LICENSED TO DO SO. DOES NOT ADMIT OR DENY ANY DEFICIENCIES IN HIS PAST MEDICAL PRACTICE. VOLUNTARY SURRENDER.

HOPKINS, JAMES L MD, LICENSE NUMBER 0127538 OF SALT LAKE CITY, UT, WAS DISCIPLINED BY NEW YORK ON FEBRUARY 21, 1990
DISCIPLINARY ACTION: 12-MONTH PROBATION

NOTES: 1 YEAR SUSPENSION STAYED

HOPKINS, JAMES L MD OF 40 NORTH STATE STREET #7B, SALT LAKE CITY, UT, WAS DISCIPLINED BY DEA ON FEBRUARY 5, 1997
DISCIPLINARY ACTION: SURRENDER OF CONTROLLED SUBSTANCE LICENSE

NOTES: IN LIEU OF PUBLIC INTEREST REVOCATION.

HOPKINS, JAMES L MD, LICENSE NUMBER 127538 OF 150 SOUTH

800 EAST #E1, SALT LAKE CITY, UT, WAS DISCIPLINED BY NEW YORK ON MARCH 7, 1997
DISCIPLINARY ACTION: SURRENDER OF LICENSE
OFFENSE: DISCIPLINARY ACTION BY ANOTHER STATE OR AGENCY

NOTES: DISCIPLINED BY THE UTAH BOARD FOR BEING A HABITUAL USER OF DRUGS OR FOR HAVING A PSYCHIATRIC CONDITION WHICH IMPAIRS HIS ABILITY TO PRACTICE.

HOPKINS, JAMES L MD OF SALT LAKE CITY, UT, WAS DISCIPLINED BY IOWA ON OCTOBER 8, 1998
DISCIPLINARY ACTION: LICENSE SUSPENSION
OFFENSE: DISCIPLINARY ACTION BY ANOTHER STATE OR AGENCY

NOTES: BASED ON DISCIPLINARY ACTION TAKEN IN UTAH, WHERE HE WAS CHARGED WITH ABUSING CONTROLLED SUBSTANCES.

HOPKINS, JAMES LEWIS MD OF SALT LAKE CITY, UT, WAS DISCIPLINED BY UTAH ON OCTOBER 23, 1995

NOTES: DURING THE PENDENCY OF A DISCIPLINARY HEARING HE AGREED TO CEASE AND DESIST FROM THE PRACTICE OF MEDICINE AND THE ADMINISTRATION AND PRESCRIPTION OF ALL MEDICATIONS.

HOPKINS, JAMES LEWIS MD OF SALT LAKE CITY, UT, WAS DISCIPLINED BY UTAH ON SEPTEMBER 9, 1996
DISCIPLINARY ACTION: REVOCATION OF CONTROLLED SUBSTANCE LICENSE; 60-MONTH PROBATION

NOTES: UNABLE TO PRACTICE MEDICINE WITH REASONABLE SKILL AND SAFETY. PROBATION WITH CONDITIONS AND RESTRICTIONS.

HOPKINS, JAMES LEWIS MD OF SALT LAKE CITY, UT, WAS DISCIPLINED BY UTAH ON JULY 1, 1998
DISCIPLINARY ACTION: PROBATION; RESTRICTION PLACED ON LICENSE
OFFENSE: FAILURE TO COMPLY WITH PREVIOUS BOARD ORDER

NOTES: HE FAILED TO COMPLY WITH SOME OF THE PROBATIONARY CONDITIONS IMPOSED ON HIS LICENSE TO PRACTICE MEDICINE. ADDITIONAL RESTRICTIONS IMPOSED.

HUNTER, WILLARD S MD, LICENSE NUMBER 0002933 OF PHOENIX, AZ, WAS DISCIPLINED BY ARIZONA ON FEBRUARY 23, 1992
DISCIPLINARY ACTION: 36-MONTH PROBATION; RESTRICTION PLACED ON CONTROLLED SUBSTANCE LICENSE
OFFENSE: OVERPRESCRIBING OR MISPRESCRIBING DRUGS

NOTES: FAILING OR REFUSING TO MAINTAIN ADEQUATE RECORDS; PRESCRIBING, DISPENSING OR ADMINISTERING CONTROLLED SUBSTANCES FOR OTHER THAN ACCEPTED THERAPEUTIC PURPOSES AND IN EXCESSIVE AMOUNTS TO NUMEROUS PATIENTS; SUCH SUBSTANCES INCLUDED VALIUM, TYLENOL #4, SOMA, DEMEROL AND PERCOCET. DURING TERM OF PROBATION: SHALL NOT PRESCRIBE, ADMINISTER OR DISPENSE SCHEDULE II OR III CONTROLLED SUBSTANCES EXCEPT FOR HOSPITALIZED OR POSTOPERATIVE PATIENTS FOR UP TO TWO MONTHS AFTER SURGERY; SHALL OBTAIN 80 HOURS CONTINUING MEDICAL EDUCATION IN THE PRESCRIBING OF CONTROLLED SUBSTANCES. EFFECTIVE 1/26/94 BOARD ORDER TERMINATED AND IN SIX AND EIGHTEEN MONTHS AFTER TERMINATION, STAFF SHALL CONDUCT AN OFFICE AND PHARMACY SURVEY TO REVIEW HIS PRESCRIBING OF CONTROLLED SUBSTANCES.

HUNTER, WILLARD S MD OF PHOENIX, AZ, WAS DISCIPLINED BY UTAH ON DECEMBER 7, 1992
DISCIPLINARY ACTION: PROBATION; RESTRICTION PLACED ON CONTROLLED SUBSTANCE LICENSE
OFFENSE: DISCIPLINARY ACTION BY ANOTHER STATE OR AGENCY

NOTES: ARIZONA MEDICAL BOARD TOOK ACTION UPON FINDING THAT HE PRESCRIBED, DISPENSED OR ADMINISTERED CONTROLLED SUBSTANCES IN AMOUNTS AND IN A MANNER INCONSISTENT WITH THERAPEUTIC PURPOSES. SCHEDULE II AND III CONTROLLED SUBSTANCE LICENSE IS RESTRICTED. ON 9/2/94 PROBATION ON LICENSE TO PRACTICE MEDICINE AND PRESCRIBE AND ADMINISTER CONTROLLED SUBSTANCES WAS TERMINATED AND LICENSE WAS REINSTATED WITH FULL PRIVILEGES.

HUNTER, WILLARD S MD, LICENSE NUMBER 0C23614 OF PHOENIX, AZ, WAS DISCIPLINED BY CALIFORNIA ON FEBRUARY 20, 1995
DISCIPLINARY ACTION: REPRIMAND
OFFENSE: DISCIPLINARY ACTION BY ANOTHER STATE OR AGENCY

NOTES: DISCIPLINE BY ARIZONA BOARD FOR FAILING TO MAINTAIN ADEQUATE RECORDS REGARDING DRUGS TO PATIENTS, AND FOR DISPENSING DRUGS FOR OTHER THAN THERAPEUTIC PURPOSES. ALSO, DISCIPLINED BY UTAH BOARD BASED ON ARIZONA ACTION. BOTH BOARDS REINSTATED FULL PRIVILEGES.

HUNTER, WILLARD SMITH MD OF TEMPE, AZ, WAS DISCIPLINED BY UTAH ON JULY 11, 1996
OFFENSE: DISCIPLINARY ACTION BY ANOTHER STATE OR AGENCY

NOTES: ACTION IN ARIZONA. SUSPENSION WITH A STAY OF ENFORCEMENT ON THE SUSPENSION DURING THE ARIZONA PERIOD OF PROBATION SO LONG AS HE REMAINS IN FULL COMPLIANCE WITH THE TERMS AND CONDITIONS OF HIS ARIZONA PROBATION. HE HAS CONDITIONS TO BE MET DURING THIS PERIOD OF TIME.

JACOBSON, CECIL B MD, DATE OF BIRTH OCTOBER 2, 1936, LICENSE NUMBER 0027401 OF 461 W 4150 N, PROVO, UT, WAS DISCIPLINED BY VIRGINIA ON JUNE 3, 1992
DISCIPLINARY ACTION: LICENSE REVOCATION
OFFENSE: CRIMINAL CONVICTION OR PLEA OF GUILTY, NOLO CONTENDERE, OR NO CONTEST TO A CRIME

NOTES: ON 5/8/92 CONVICTED IN US DISTRICT COURT FOR THE EASTERN DISTRICT OF VIRGINIA, ALEXANDRIA DIVISION, OF 32 COUNTS OF MAIL FRAUD, 9 COUNTS OF WIRE FRAUD, 3 COUNTS OF TRAVEL FRAUD, AND 5 COUNTS OF PERJURY. SENTENCED TO 60 MONTHS IMPRISONMENT; ORDERED TO PAY SPECIAL ASSESSMENT OF $2600; SHALL BE ON SUPERVISED RELEASE FOR THREE YEARS AFTER RELEASE FROM PRISON; ORDERED TO MAKE RESTITUTION IN THE AMOUNT OF $39,205 TO THE VICTIMS INVOLVED IN THE DONOR FRAUD WHO WERE NOT COMPENSATED IN THE CIVIL SUITS; ORDERED TO PAY FINE OF $75,000.

JACOBSON, CECIL B MD, DATE OF BIRTH OCTOBER 2, 1936 OF 461 WEST 4150 NORTH, PROVO, UT, WAS DISCIPLINED BY MEDICARE ON NOVEMBER 16, 1992
DISCIPLINARY ACTION: EXCLUSION FROM THE MEDICARE AND/OR MEDICAID PROGRAM
OFFENSE: CRIMINAL CONVICTION OR PLEA OF GUILTY, NOLO CONTENDERE, OR NO CONTEST TO A CRIME

NOTES: CONVICTION RELATING TO FRAUD.

JENSEN, CLEL L MD OF SANDY, UT, WAS DISCIPLINED BY UTAH ON

OCTOBER 24, 1991
DISCIPLINARY ACTION: REVOCATION OF CONTROLLED SUBSTANCE LICENSE; 60-MONTH PROBATION
OFFENSE: FAILURE TO COMPLY WITH PREVIOUS BOARD ORDER

NOTES: USE OF A CONTROLLED SUBSTANCE WITHOUT PRESCRIPTION BY A PRACTITIONER; FAILURE TO SUBMIT TO RANDOM DRUG SCREENING AS REQUIRED UNDER A PROBATIONARY ORDER. REVOCATION OF CONTROLLED SUBSTANCES AUTHORITY TO BECOME EFFECTIVE 30 DAYS FROM ORDER. ON 10/6/94 PROBATION SHALL BE TERMINATED UPON RECEIPT OF AN INACTIVE LICENSURE APPLICATION AND APPROPRIATE FEE; IF AT ANY TIME IN THE FUTURE HE WISHED TO REACTIVATE HIS LICENSE TO PRACTICE MEDICINE, HE MUST FIRST MEET WITH THE BOARD.

JENSEN, MICHAEL HENRIE MD OF PROVO, UT, WAS DISCIPLINED BY UTAH ON OCTOBER 31, 1996
DISCIPLINARY ACTION: REPRIMAND
OFFENSE: OVERPRESCRIBING OR MISPRESCRIBING DRUGS

NOTES: ALLEGED THAT HE PRESCRIBED SCHEDULE IV CONTROLLED SUBSTANCES FOR THE PURPOSE OF WEIGHT REDUCTION WITHOUT COMPLYING WITH THE REQUIREMENTS; AND ADVISED A PATIENT HOW TO MISUSE A CONTROLLED SUBSTANCE AND OFFERED TO MAKE AN UNSUBSTANTIATED DIAGNOSIS TO SUPPORT A PRESCRIPTION. ADMITS THAT HE FAILED TO COMPLY WITH SOME OF THE REQUIREMENTS. AGREED TO ABIDE BY CONDITIONS FOR ONE YEAR.

JEPPSON, ROBERT L DO OF KAYSVILLE, UT, WAS DISCIPLINED BY UTAH ON OCTOBER 12, 1993
DISCIPLINARY ACTION: RESTRICTION PLACED ON LICENSE; RESTRICTION PLACED ON CONTROLLED SUBSTANCE LICENSE
OFFENSE: PHYSICAL OR MENTAL ILLNESS INHIBITING THE ABILITY TO PRACTICE WITH SKILL AND SAFETY

NOTES: UNABLE TO PRACTICE UNRESTRICTED MEDICINE DUE TO ILLNESS. ON 2/18/94 RESTRICTIONS LIFTED AND LICENSE REINSTATED WITH FULL PRIVILEGES.

JOHNSON, SHERMAN B MD OF OGDEN, UT, WAS DISCIPLINED BY UTAH ON JUNE 1, 1992
DISCIPLINARY ACTION: REVOCATION OF CONTROLLED SUBSTANCE LICENSE; LICENSE SUSPENSION
OFFENSE: CRIMINAL CONVICTION OR PLEA OF GUILTY, NOLO CONTENDERE, OR NO CONTEST TO A CRIME

NOTES: PRESCRIBING AND/OR ADMINISTERING CONTROLLED SUBSTANCES IN EXCESS OF RECOGNIZED APPROPRIATE QUANTITIES; FAILURE TO KEEP APPROPRIATE RECORDS OF CONTROLLED SUBSTANCES; AND CONVICTION OF A SECOND DEGREE FELONY RELATED TO THE PRACTICE OF MEDICINE. REVOCATION, STAYED. INDEFINITE SUSPENSION, NOT TO EXCEED FIVE YEARS. ON 8/31/99 SUSPENSION ON LICENSE TO PRACTICE MEDICINE TERMINATED AND REINSTATED WITH FULL PRIVILEGES EFFECTIVE 11/19/97; LICENSE TO PRESCRIBE AND ADMINISTER CONTROLLED SUBSTANCES SCHEDULES IV-V ONLY WAS REINSTATED EFFECTIVE 4/13/98.

JOHNSON, SHERMAN B MD, DATE OF BIRTH SEPTEMBER 5, 1939 OF 3905 HARRISON BLVD, OGDEN, UT, WAS DISCIPLINED BY MEDICARE ON APRIL 12, 1993
DISCIPLINARY ACTION: 120-MONTH EXCLUSION FROM THE MEDICARE AND/OR MEDICAID PROGRAM
OFFENSE: CRIMINAL CONVICTION OR PLEA OF GUILTY, NOLO CONTENDERE, OR NO CONTEST TO A CRIME

NOTES: CONVICTED OF MANSLAUGHTER OF A PATIENT.

JOHNSON, VAUGHN A MD, DATE OF BIRTH JULY 12, 1939, LICENSE NUMBER 0014849, WAS DISCIPLINED BY COLORADO ON AUGUST 14, 1996
DISCIPLINARY ACTION: 60-MONTH PROBATION; REQUIRED TO TAKE ADDITIONAL MEDICAL EDUCATION
OFFENSE: SUBSTANDARD CARE, INCOMPETENCE OR NEGLIGENCE

NOTES: SUBSTANDARD CARE (PRIMA FACIE TYPE ADMISSION ONLY. RE-EDUCATION ACTIVITIES AND PRACTICE MONITORING.

JOHNSON, VAUGHN A MD OF DURANGO, CO, WAS DISCIPLINED BY UTAH ON JUNE 12, 1997
DISCIPLINARY ACTION: PROBATION
OFFENSE: DISCIPLINARY ACTION BY ANOTHER STATE OR AGENCY

NOTES: DISCIPLINARY ACTION TAKEN AGAINST HIS MEDICAL LICENSE IN COLORADO. CONDITIONS ON LICENSE FOR THE DURATION OF HIS COLORADO PROBATION. AS OF 1/29/98, THE PROBATION WAS TERMINATED AND HIS MEDICAL LICENSE WAS REINSTATED WITH FULL PRIVILEGES.

KAY, DENNIS L MD OF SALT LAKE CITY, UT, WAS DISCIPLINED BY UTAH ON OCTOBER 1, 1995
DISCIPLINARY ACTION: SURRENDER OF LICENSE; SURRENDER OF CONTROLLED SUBSTANCE LICENSE
OFFENSE: SUBSTANCE ABUSE

NOTES: USE OF ALCOHOL IN A MANNER WHICH MAY HAVE IMPAIRED HIS ABILITY TO SAFELY PRACTICE MEDICINE

KITSON, STEPHAN JAMES MD OF PARK CITY, UT, WAS DISCIPLINED BY UTAH ON DECEMBER 29, 1997
DISCIPLINARY ACTION: LICENSE REVOCATION; REVOCATION OF CONTROLLED SUBSTANCE LICENSE
OFFENSE: SEXUAL ABUSE OF OR SEXUAL MISCONDUCT WITH A PATIENT

NOTES: HE ENGAGED IN MULTIPLE INSTANCES OF INAPPROPRIATE SEXUAL CONDUCT WITH TWO PATIENTS.

KOERPEL, BARRY J MD, LICENSE NUMBER 0008981, WAS DISCIPLINED BY ARIZONA ON OCTOBER 17, 1995
DISCIPLINARY ACTION: RESTRICTION PLACED ON LICENSE; REQUIRED TO TAKE ADDITIONAL MEDICAL EDUCATION
OFFENSE: DISCIPLINARY ACTION BY ANOTHER STATE OR AGENCY

NOTES: KNOWINGLY MADE FALSE OR FRAUDULENT STATEMENTS IN CONNECTION WITH APPLICATION FOR HOSPITAL PRIVILEGES IN THAT WHEN APPLYING FOR PRIVILEGES AT AN ARIZONA HOSPITAL IN 10/93. HE FAILED TO REPORT ACTION BY THE BOARD OF A UTAH HOSPITAL INITIATED IN 10/83 THAT INCLUDED A LETTER SENT IN 12/84 FOR INADEQUATE RESPONSE TIME, PROVIDING INADEQUATE CALL COVERAGE, POOR COMMUNICATION WITH COLLEAGUES AND FAILURE TO MAKE ROUNDS ON SIGNIFICANTLY ILL PATIENTS; ANOTHER SUSPENSION IN 4/86 FOR POOR RECORDKEEPING; AND ANOTHER LETTER IN 11/86 REGARDING INADEQUATE RESPONSE TIMES TO CRITICALLY ILL PATIENTS; DENIED THAT HIS LICENSE HAD EVER BEEN SUSPENDED, MODIFIED OR TERMINATED DESPITE 6/84 PROBATION BY UTAH BOARD FOR UNPROFESSIONAL CONDUCT INCLUDING THAT IN 1981 AND 1982, CONTINUED TO TREAT FOUR PATIENTS ON CHRONIC DIALYSIS TREATMENT WHEN SUCH TREATMENT WAS CONTRARY TO MEDICAL STANDARDS; PERMITTED SEVEN PATIENTS TO CONTINUE DIALYSIS TREATMENTS AFTER THEY WERE NO LONGER MEDICALLY NECESSARY; INITIATED

UNNECESSARY DIALYSIS TREATMENT ON ONE PATIENT; AND ALLOWED 10 PATIENTS TO RECEIVE INADEQUATE AND SUBSTANDARD DIALYSIS TREATMENTS; UTAH PROBATION TERMINATED ON 5/26/87. IN 4/85, HE WAS EXCLUDED FROM THE MEDICARE PROGRAM FOR 10 YEARS BY THE DEPARTMENT OF HEALTH AND HUMAN SERVICES FOR FURNISHING SERVICES FOUND TO BE IN EXCESS OF THE NEEDS OF HIS PATIENTS AND FURNISHING CARE WHICH DOES NOT MEET PROFESSIONALLY RECOGNIZED STANDARDS OF HEALTH CARE; TWO YEARS AFTER AN UNSUCCESSFUL APPEAL, REQUESTED REINSTATEMENT AS A MEDICARE PROVIDER WHICH WAS APPROVED ON 4/25/89; HAS NOT PRACTICED CLINICAL MEDICINE SINCE 1989. SHALL NOT PRACTICE CLINICAL MEDICINE IN ARIZONA UNTIL HE SUCCESSFULLY COMPLETES A BOARD-APPROVED ONE YEAR TRAINING EXPERIENCE; CENSURED.

KOERPEL, BARRY JON MD OF HAYWARD, WI, WAS DISCIPLINED BY UTAH ON JUNE 18, 1996
DISCIPLINARY ACTION: LICENSE SUSPENSION
OFFENSE: DISCIPLINARY ACTION BY ANOTHER STATE OR AGENCY

NOTES: DISCIPLINARY ACTION TAKEN AGAINST HIS LICENSE TO PRACTICE MEDICINE IN ARIZONA. UTAH MEDICAL LICENSE SUSPENDED DURING ARIZONA RESTRICTION PERIOD. HE HAS CONDITIONS TO BE MET DURING THE PERIOD OF SUSPENSION.

KORNMAYER, KARLA MD OF SALT LAKE CITY, UT, WAS DISCIPLINED BY UTAH ON OCTOBER 8, 1992
DISCIPLINARY ACTION: LICENSE SUSPENSION; SUSPENSION OF CONTROLLED SUBSTANCE LICENSE

NOTES: PERSONAL CONDITIONS WHICH HAVE RAISED CONCERNS REGARDING HER ABILITY TO SAFELY AND COMPETENTLY PRACTICE MEDICINE.

KORNMAYER, KARLA MD OF SALT LAKE CITY, UT, WAS DISCIPLINED BY UTAH ON FEBRUARY 22, 1993
DISCIPLINARY ACTION: LICENSE SUSPENSION; SUSPENSION OF CONTROLLED SUBSTANCE LICENSE
OFFENSE: PHYSICAL OR MENTAL ILLNESS INHIBITING THE ABILITY TO PRACTICE WITH SKILL AND SAFETY

NOTES: PHYSICAL AND PSYCHIATRIC CONDITIONS DIRECTLY AFFECTING HER ABILITY TO SAFELY AND COMPETENTLY PRACTICE MEDICINE. SUSPENSIONS TO LAST A MINIMUM OF ONE YEAR WITH CONDITIONS.

KORNMAYER, KARLA MD OF MIDVALE, UT, WAS DISCIPLINED BY UTAH ON DECEMBER 12, 1997
DISCIPLINARY ACTION: 12-MONTH PROBATION

NOTES: ON 1/21/99 PROBATION TERMINATED AND LICENSE REINSTATED WITH FULL PRIVILEGES. NO LICENSE TO PRESCRIBE AND ADMINISTER CONTROLLED SUBSTANCES WAS ISSUED AT THIS TIME.

LEDLIE, WILLIAM BOYER MD, DATE OF BIRTH JANUARY 4, 1950, LICENSE NUMBER 00E4475 OF 9218 MONTFORD, HOUSTON, TX, WAS DISCIPLINED BY TEXAS ON AUGUST 24, 1991
DISCIPLINARY ACTION: SURRENDER OF CONTROLLED SUBSTANCE LICENSE; 36-MONTH PROBATION
OFFENSE: SUBSTANCE ABUSE

NOTES: LICENSE SUSPENDED, STAYED; PROBATION TERMS ARE AS FOLLOWS: SHALL APPEAR BEFORE THE BOARD TWICE A YEAR; SHALL SURRENDER DEA AND DPS CONTROLLED SUBSTANCES REGISTRATION CERTIFICATES AND NOT ATTEMPT TO REREGISTER WITHOUT BOARD APPROVAL; SHALL SURRENDER ALL UNUSED TRIPLICATE PRESCRIPTION FORMS AND NOT ATTEMPT TO ORDER MORE WITHOUT BOARD APPROVAL; SHALL SURRENDER ALL CONTROLLED SUBSTANCES, INCLUDING SAMPLES; SHALL NOT TREAT OR OTHERWISE SERVE AS THE PHYSICIAN, PRESCRIBE, DISPENSE, OR ADMINISTER CONTROLLED SUBSTANCES, OR ANY OTHER DRUGS THAT MAY BE SUBJECT TO ABUSE, FOR SELF OR ANY MEMBER OF IMMEDIATE FAMILY; MAY ADMINISTER TO SELF OR IMMEDIATE FAMILY ONLY SUCH DRUGS AS ARE PRESCRIBED BY OTHER PHYSICIANS; SHALL ABSTAIN FROM CONSUMPTION OF ALCOHOL, CONTROLLED SUBSTANCES, DANGEROUS DRUGS, OR PRESCRIPTION DRUGS IN ANY FORM; SHALL PARTICIPATE WITH IMPAIRED PHYSICIANS PROGRAM; SHALL SUBMIT FOR ALCOHOL OR DRUG SCREENING; SHALL CONTINUE TREATMENT FROM TALBOTT-MARSH RECOVERY PROGRAM; SHALL FURNISH WRITTEN REPORTS WHEN REQUESTED; SHALL PARTICIPATE IN AA. ON 1/29/93 MODIFICATION OF ORDER GIVING HIM PERMISSION TO REAPPLY TO THE DRUG ENFORCEMENT ADMINISTRATION AND THE TEXAS DEPARTMENT OF PUBLIC SAFETY FOR SCHEDULES II, IIN, III, IIIN, IV OR V CONTROLLED SUBSTANCE AUTHORITY. ALL OTHER TERMS AND CONDITIONS REMAIN IN EFFECT.

LEDLIE, WILLIAM BOYER MD OF HOUSTON, TX, WAS DISCIPLINED BY UTAH ON MAY 7, 1992
DISCIPLINARY ACTION: SURRENDER OF LICENSE; SURRENDER OF CONTROLLED SUBSTANCE LICENSE
OFFENSE: DISCIPLINARY ACTION BY ANOTHER STATE OR AGENCY

NOTES: ENGAGING IN THE INTEMPERATE USE OF A CONTROLLED SUBSTANCE RESULTING IN DISCIPLINARY ACTION AGAINST HIS LICENSE IN TEXAS. AGREED NOT TO REAPPLY FOR LICENSURE FOR 2 1/2 YEARS.

LUDLOW, LESTER A MD, LICENSE NUMBER G8762 OF SANTA ANA, CA, WAS DISCIPLINED BY CALIFORNIA ON JULY 17, 1998
DISCIPLINARY ACTION: SURRENDER OF LICENSE

NOTES: WHILE CHARGES PENDING.

LUDLOW, LESTER ANDRUS MD OF OLD HICKORY, TN, WAS DISCIPLINED BY UTAH ON NOVEMBER 1, 1999
DISCIPLINARY ACTION: SURRENDER OF LICENSE
OFFENSE: DISCIPLINARY ACTION BY ANOTHER STATE OR AGENCY

NOTES: SURRENDERED LICENSE IN CALIFORNIA AFTER HE WAS CHARGED WITH ENGAGING IN GROSS NEGLIGENCE IN THE PRACTICE OF MEDICINE AND SUFFERED FROM MENTAL AND PHYSICAL IMPAIRMENT AFFECTING HIS COMPETENCY. VOLUNTARY SURRENDER AS HE IS RETIRED AND DOES NOT INTEND TO PRACTICE MEDICINE IN UTAH.

MACNEILL, MARTIN J MD, DATE OF BIRTH FEBRUARY 1, 1956 OF 10 NORTH MAIN, SALEM, UT, WAS DISCIPLINED BY MEDICARE ON JULY 26, 1990
DISCIPLINARY ACTION: 60-MONTH EXCLUSION FROM THE MEDICARE AND/OR MEDICAID PROGRAM
OFFENSE: CRIMINAL CONVICTION OR PLEA OF GUILTY, NOLO CONTENDERE, OR NO CONTEST TO A CRIME

NOTES: PROGRAM-RELATED CONVICTION.

MACNEILL, MARTIN J DO, WAS DISCIPLINED BY WASHINGTON ON MARCH 25, 1998
DISCIPLINARY ACTION: FINE; RESTRICTION PLACED ON LICENSE

OFFENSE: DISCIPLINARY ACTION BY ANOTHER STATE OR AGENCY

NOTES: FAILED TO SUBMIT MATERIAL FACTS ON 1997 LICENSE APPLICATION REGARDING HIS 1990 PLEA OF NOLO CONTENDERE TO A CRIMINAL OFFENSE RELATED TO THE DELIVERY OF AN ITEM OR SERVICE UNDER THE MEDICAID PROGRAM; WAS EXCLUDED FROM MEDICARE AND STATE HEALTH CARE PROGRAMS FOR FIVE YEARS. CONDITIONED LICENSE SUBJECT TO THE FOLLOWING TERMS AND CONDITIONS: SHALL SUBMIT QUARTERLY DECLARATIONS ATTESTING TO COMPLIANCE WITH ALL TERMS AND CONDITIONS; SHALL ABIDE BY TERMS OF MEDICARE AND HEALTH CARE PROGRAMS EXCLUSIONS; SHALL BE FINED $1,000; AN INVESTIGATOR OF THE BOARD SHALL AUDIT RECORDS AND REVIEW PRACTICE ON AN UNANNOUNCED BASIS UP TO TWICE A YEAR; IN THE EVENT THAT HE SHOULD LEAVE WASHINGTON TO RESIDE OR TO PRACTICE, HE MUST NOTIFY THE BOARD, IN WRITING, WITHIN 60 DAYS OF THE DEPARTURE DATE AND RETURN; SHALL INFORM THE BOARD OF ANY CHANGE IN ADDRESS.

MATRAVERS, GARY W MD OF TOOELE, UT, WAS DISCIPLINED BY UTAH ON FEBRUARY 4, 1997
DISCIPLINARY ACTION: 12-MONTH RESTRICTION PLACED ON LICENSE
OFFENSE: OVERPRESCRIBING OR MISPRESCRIBING DRUGS

NOTES: PRESCRIBED RITALIN IN EXCESS OF WHAT WAS MEDICALLY NECESSARY TO TREAT TWO PATIENTS' ALLEGED MEDICAL CONDITIONS, AND FAILED TO KEEP RECORDS OF SUCH PRESCRIPTIONS. LICENSE TO PRESCRIBE AND ADMINISTER CONTROLLED SUBSTANCES WAS SUSPENDED FOR 90 DAYS WITH A STAY OF ENFORCEMENT ON THE SUSPENSION. ON 4/27/98 THE CONDITIONS AND RESTRICTIONS ON HIS LICENSE TO PRESCRIBE AND ADMINISTER CONTROLLED SUBSTANCES WERE EXTENDED UNTIL 2/4/99. CONDITIONS AND RESTRICTIONS ON LICENSES TO PRACTICE MEDICINE AND TO PRESCRIBE AND ADMINISTER CONTROLLED SUBSTANCES WERE TERMINATED AND LICENSES WERE REINSTATED WITH FULL PRIVILEGES ON 3/5/99.

MCCLELLAN, MONTY MD OF WEST JORDAN, UT, WAS DISCIPLINED BY ILLINOIS ON APRIL 1, 1990
DISCIPLINARY ACTION: 60-MONTH LICENSE SUSPENSION
OFFENSE: CRIMINAL CONVICTION OR PLEA OF GUILTY, NOLO CONTENDERE, OR NO CONTEST TO A CRIME

NOTES: HE WAS CONVICTED OF 2 COUNTS OF BANKRUPTCY FRAUD IN U.S. DISTRICT COURT, CENTRAL DISTRICT OF ILLINOIS. MEDICAL LICENSE INDEFINITELY SUSPENDED, MINIMUM FIVE YEARS.

MCCLELLAN, MONTY P MD OF WEST JORDAN, UT, WAS DISCIPLINED BY UTAH ON FEBRUARY 27, 1990
DISCIPLINARY ACTION: RESTRICTION PLACED ON CONTROLLED SUBSTANCE LICENSE

NOTES: VOLUNTARILY SURRENDERED LICENSE TO PRESCRIBE CONTROLLED SUBSTANCES SCHEDULES II-V.

MCCLELLAN, MONTY P MD, WAS DISCIPLINED BY WISCONSIN ON NOVEMBER 26, 1994
DISCIPLINARY ACTION: DENIAL OF NEW LICENSE
OFFENSE: DISCIPLINARY ACTION BY ANOTHER STATE OR AGENCY

NOTES: DOCUMENTATION ON HIS APPLICATION OF DISCIPLINARY ACTIONS BY UTAH, KANSAS, ILLINOIS, DEA, AND THE MEDICARE PROGRAM; THESE ACTIONS STEMMED FROM HIS CONVICTION IN U.S. DISTRICT COURT OF FOUR COUNTS OF BANKRUPTCY FRAUD AND ONE COUNT OF MAIL FRAUD.

MCCLELLAN, MONTY PHILLIP MD OF 1715 WEST 7888 S P.O. BOX 457, WEST JORDAN, UT, WAS DISCIPLINED BY DEA ON APRIL 19, 1990
DISCIPLINARY ACTION: SURRENDER OF CONTROLLED SUBSTANCE LICENSE
OFFENSE: CRIMINAL CONVICTION OR PLEA OF GUILTY, NOLO CONTENDERE, OR NO CONTEST TO A CRIME

NOTES: SURRENDER DUE TO FEDERAL FRAUD CONVICTIONS IN ILLINOIS.

MCDERMOTT, ROBERT WILLIAM JR MD, DATE OF BIRTH APRIL 13, 1944, LICENSE NUMBER 6728 OF 3124 BEN HOGAN, BILLINGS, MT, WAS DISCIPLINED BY MONTANA ON DECEMBER 8, 1997
DISCIPLINARY ACTION: PROBATION
OFFENSE: SUBSTANCE ABUSE

NOTES: CHEMICAL DEPENDENCY AND BIPOLAR DISORDER RESULTING IN DRUG DIVERSION. ON 7/28/99 PROBATION AMENDED TO PERMIT REQUEST FOR DEA REGISTRATION AND PRESCRIBING OF SCHEDULE IV AND V DRUGS.

MCDERMOTT, ROBERT WILLIAM JR MD, DATE OF BIRTH APRIL 13, 1944, LICENSE NUMBER 0028882 OF BILLINGS, MT, WAS DISCIPLINED BY NORTH CAROLINA ON OCTOBER 27, 1998
DISCIPLINARY ACTION: RESTRICTION PLACED ON CONTROLLED SUBSTANCE LICENSE; REQUIRED TO TAKE ADDITIONAL MEDICAL EDUCATION
OFFENSE: DISCIPLINARY ACTION BY ANOTHER STATE OR AGENCY

NOTES: ON OR ABOUT 11/26/97, HE ENTERED INTO A PROBATIONARY AGREEMENT WITH THE MONTANA BOARD ADMITTING THAT HE HAS THE ILLNESSES OF BIPOLAR DISORDER AND CHEMICAL DEPENDENCY AND ADDICTION, AND THAT HE USED HIS MONTANA LICENSE AND DEA REGISTRATION TO WRITE THIRD-PARTY PRESCRIPTIONS FOR CONTROLLED SUBSTANCES THAT HE DIVERTED TO HIS OWN USE. HE SHALL COMPLY WITH THE TERMS AND CONDITIONS SET FORTH IN THE MONTANA ORDER; IF HE RETURNS TO NORTH CAROLINA, HE MUST REFRAIN FROM THE USE OF ALL MIND OR MOOD ALTERING SUBSTANCES, ALCOHOL, AND ALL CONTROLLED SUBSTANCES UNLESS LAWFULLY PRESCRIBED TO HIM BY SOMEONE ELSE; HE SHALL SUPPLY BODILY FLUIDS AND TISSUE SAMPLES AS REQUESTED BY THE BOARD FOR SCREENING PURPOSES; HE SHALL MAINTAIN AND ABIDE BY A CONTRACT WITH THE NORTH CAROLINA PHYSICIAN'S HEALTH PROGRAM; HE SHALL NOT REGISTER WITH THE DEA AND SHALL NOT PURCHASE, ADMINISTER, PRESCRIBE, DISPENSE, OR ORDER ANY CONTROLLED SUBSTANCES; HE SHALL APPEAR BEFORE THE BOARD BEFORE PRACTICING IN NORTH CAROLINA; HE SHALL OBTAIN AND DOCUMENT 50 HOURS OF RELEVANT CONTINUING MEDICAL EDUCATION PER YEAR; MUST COMPLY WITH OTHER CONDITIONS.

MCDERMOTT, ROBERT WILLIAM JR MD OF BILLINGS, MT, WAS DISCIPLINED BY UTAH ON AUGUST 20, 1999
DISCIPLINARY ACTION: PROBATION
OFFENSE: DISCIPLINARY ACTION BY ANOTHER STATE OR AGENCY

NOTES: DISCIPLINARY ACTION TAKEN AGAINST LICENSE IN MONTANA. REVOCATION STAYED; PROBATION FOR THE DURATION OF THE MONTANA PROBATION.

MERRITT, EDWARD G MD, DATE OF BIRTH OCTOBER 13, 1921,

LICENSE NUMBER 0011315 OF DELORES, CO, WAS DISCIPLINED BY COLORADO ON SEPTEMBER 17, 1993
DISCIPLINARY ACTION: SURRENDER OF LICENSE

NOTES: NO UNPROFESSIONAL CONDUCT IDENTIFIED. ACCORDING TO ORDER, AGREES TO PERMANENTLY RETIRE FROM THE PRACTICE OF MEDICINE EFFECTIVE 03/31/94.

MERRITT, EDWARD GEORGE MD OF CORTEZ, CO, WAS DISCIPLINED BY UTAH ON MARCH 10, 1994
DISCIPLINARY ACTION: SURRENDER OF LICENSE
OFFENSE: DISCIPLINARY ACTION BY ANOTHER STATE OR AGENCY

NOTES: SURRENDER OF LICENSE ON OFFER TO RETIRE PENDING INQUIRY INTO BASIS FOR CAUSE FOR DISCIPLINARY ACTION IN COLORADO. AGREED TO PERMANENTLY RETIRE FROM PRACTICE OF MEDICINE IN UTAH EFFECTIVE 03/31/94 AND AGREES HE WILL NOT REAPPLY FOR LICENSURE TO PRACTICE MEDICINE IN UTAH.

MICHAUD, ROBERT MERRILL DO OF JUNEAU, AK, WAS DISCIPLINED BY UTAH ON JANUARY 23, 1998
DISCIPLINARY ACTION: 60-MONTH PROBATION; 60-MONTH CONTROLLED SUBSTANCE LICENSE PLACED ON PROBATION
OFFENSE: EXCEEDING PROFESSIONAL LIMITATIONS

NOTES: SOLD SAMPLE DRUGS WHICH HAD BEEN LABELED AS NOT INTENDED FOR RESALE; DISPENSED DRUGS IN THE UNLICENSED PRACTICE OF PHARMACY; AND NEGLIGENTLY RETURNED EXCESS INJECTABLE MEDICATION TO SOURCE VIALS, REPEATEDLY UTILIZED A SINGLE SYRINGE TO ADMINISTER MEDICATIONS TO NUMEROUS PATIENTS AND REUSED EXCESS AND PURPORTEDLY STERILIZED SUTURE MATERIAL. ORDERED TO CEASE AND DESIST FROM THE UNLAWFUL SALE OF PRESCRIPTIVE SAMPLE MEDICATIONS OR OVER THE COUNTER MEDICATIONS AND FROM THE UNAUTHORIZED PRACTICE OF PHARMACY. ON 6/22/98 THE PROBATIONARY CONDITIONS REQUIRING HIM TO PARTICIPATE IN AND SUCCESSFULLY COMPLETE TRAINING THROUGH AN OSHA APPROVED COURSE ON STERILIZATION AND TO COMPLETE FIVE HOURS IN CONTINUING EDUCATION REGARDING PEDIATRIC PRESCRIPTIVE PRACTICE WERE CHANGED TO ALLOW HIM TO HAVE THOSE CONDITIONS MET VIA PERSONAL INSTRUCTION. ON 12/21/98 PROBATIONS TERMINATED AND LICENSES REINSTATED WITH FULL PRIVILEGES.

MICHAUD, ROBERT MERRILL DO, LICENSE NUMBER 3638, WAS DISCIPLINED BY ALASKA ON JUNE 16, 1999
DISCIPLINARY ACTION: SURRENDER OF LICENSE
OFFENSE: NONCOMPLIANCE WITH A PROFESSIONAL RULE

NOTES: LICENSE UNDER INVESTIGATION FOR QUESTIONS REGARDING THE VALIDITY OF ANSWERS TO QUESTIONS IN INITIAL APPLICATION; ALSO UNDER INVESTIGATION FOR ALLEGATIONS REGARDING PATIENT TREATMENT MATTERS. VOLUNTARY SURRENDER.

MICHAUD, ROBERT MERRILL DO, LICENSE NUMBER 2045 OF 3319 E. UNIVERSITY #341, MESA, AZ, WAS DISCIPLINED BY ARIZONA ON JULY 9, 1999
DISCIPLINARY ACTION: LICENSE SUSPENSION; 12-MONTH PROBATION
OFFENSE: DISCIPLINARY ACTION BY ANOTHER STATE OR AGENCY

NOTES: ON 1/23/98 UTAH PLACED HIS LICENSE ON PROBATION FOR THE FOLLOWING: BETWEEN 1992-1995 PERIODICALLY SOLD ROGAINE SAMPLES MARKED NOT FOR RESALE TO VARIOUS PATIENTS; DURING 2/95 PERIODICALLY SOLD CLEOCIN T & RETIN-A PRESCRIPTIVE MEDICATIONS TO CERTAIN PATIENTS; HE OBTAINED THE LATTER DRUG FROM MEXICO; ALSO DURING 2/95 SOLD CERTAIN OVER THE COUNTER MEDICATIONS TO PATIENTS; HE SUBSEQUENTLY CEASED THAT PRACTICE WHEN IT BECAME TOO TIME-CONSUMING AND HE DECIDED IT WAS NO LONGER COST EFFECTIVE; BETWEEN 1992-1995 PERIODICALLY RETURNED EXCESS CORTISONE SOLUTION TO SOURCE VIALS AFTER HE ADMINISTERED INJECTIONS TO VARIOUS PATIENTS; HE RETURNED THE UNUSED MEDICATION TO AVOID THE NEED TO SUBSEQUENTLY REMIX THE SOLUTION FOR LATER USE AT THE GIVEN CONCENTRATION; HE OCCASIONALLY DIRECTED HIS MEDICAL ASSISTANTS TO ALSO RETURN EXCESS CORTISONE SOLUTION TO THE SOURCE VIALS; DURING VARIOUS SURGICAL PROCEDURES, BETWEEN 1992-1995, HE USED A SINGLE SYRINGE FILLED WITH EPINEPHRINE AND XYLOCAINE FOR MULTIPLE PATIENTS; HE DID USE A SEPARATE NEEDLE FOR EACH INJECTION ON EVERY PATIENT, BUT BASED ON CREDIBLE TESTIMONY FROM HIS MEDICAL ASSISTANTS, HE OFTEN ASPIRATED THOSE INJECTIONS AND THUS COULD HAVE CONTAMINATED THE MEDICATION WITH A GIVEN PATIENT'S BLOOD PRIOR TO RETURNING THE UNUSED PORTION OF THE MEDICATION TO THE SOURCE VIAL; HE PERIODICALLY INSTRUCTED HIS MEDICAL ASSISTANTS TO ALSO RETAIN SUCH EXCESS MEDICATION FOR SUBSEQUENT USE; DURING THE SAME TIME PERIOD, HE REUSED EXCESS SUTURE MATERIAL WHICH HAD BEEN PULLED THROUGH THE TISSUE OF A PREVIOUS PATIENT; ON 8/5/95 WHEN A THREE YEAR OLD PATIENT BECAME AGITATED, HE OVER-PRESCRIBED AN ADULT DOSE OF VALIUM AND INSTRUCTED THE MOTHER TO ADMINISTER THAT MEDICATION ONE-HALF HOUR PRIOR TO THE NEXT SCHEDULED PROCEDURE; ON 8/10/95 THE PATIENT HAD AN ADVERSE REACTION TO VALIUM; HE THEN INSTRUCTED THE PATIENT'S MOTHER TO DOUBLE THE VALIUM DOSAGE PRIOR TO THE NEXT SCHEDULED PROCEDURE WHICH SHE DID NOT DO; THE MOTHER ALSO DID NOT INFORM HIM OF THE PREVIOUS ADVERSE REACTION NOR DID HE ASK; WHEN HE APPEARED BEFORE THE BOARD HE TESTIFIED HE HAD DONE NOTHING WRONG AND HIS UTAH PROBATION HAD BEEN TERMINATED. LICENSE PLACED ON PROBATION WITH THE FOLLOWING TERMS AND CONDITIONS: SUSPENSION NOT TO EXCEED SIX MONTHS AND SUSPENSION WILL BE TERMINATED AFTER HE COMPLETES 15 HOURS OF CONTINUING MEDICAL EDUCATION WITH 10 HOURS IN THE AREA OF MEDICAL ETHICS AND FIVE HOURS IN THE APPLICATION OF STERILE TECHNIQUES AND INFECTIOUS DISEASES; SHALL PROVIDE A COPY OF THIS ORDER TO ANY HEALTH CARE ENTITY WHERE HE HAS PRIVILEGES; SHALL INFORM THE BOARD IF HE CEASES TO PRACTICE IN ARIZONA; TIME SPENT OUT OF ARIZONA DOES NOT COUNT TOWARD PROBATION.

MICHAUD, ROBERT MERRILL DO, LICENSE NUMBER 3638, WAS DISCIPLINED BY ALASKA ON AUGUST 5, 1999
DISCIPLINARY ACTION: DENIAL OF LICENSE REINSTATEMENT
OFFENSE: DISCIPLINARY ACTION BY ANOTHER STATE OR AGENCY

NOTES: REQUEST FOR REINSTATEMENT DENIED BASED ON LICENSE SUSPENSION IN ARIZONA.

MILES, WILLIAM D DO, DATE OF BIRTH JUNE 7, 1947, LICENSE NUMBER 0002265 OF PULASKI COUNTY, KY, WAS DISCIPLINED BY KENTUCKY ON DECEMBER 28, 1990
DISCIPLINARY ACTION: 60-MONTH PROBATION; MONITORING OF PHYSICIAN PERFORMANCE

NOTES: LICENSE GRANTED ON CONDITIONS INCLUDING URINE SCREENS AND COOPERATION WITH IMPAIRED PHYSICIANS COMMITTEE.

MILES, WILLIAM D MD, LICENSE NUMBER 0035131 OF HAMPTON, VA, WAS DISCIPLINED BY VIRGINIA ON APRIL 26, 1993
DISCIPLINARY ACTION: LICENSE REVOCATION
OFFENSE: CRIMINAL CONVICTION OR PLEA OF GUILTY, NOLO CONTENDERE, OR NO CONTEST TO A CRIME

NOTES: FELONY CONVICTION FOR MAIL FRAUD.

MILES, WILLIAM D MD, LICENSE NUMBER 0035131 OF BOX 12237, ALEXANDRIA, LA, WAS DISCIPLINED BY VIRGINIA ON OCTOBER 25, 1993
DISCIPLINARY ACTION: MONITORING OF PHYSICIAN PERFORMANCE; COMMUNITY SERVICE
OFFENSE: CRIMINAL CONVICTION OR PLEA OF GUILTY, NOLO CONTENDERE, OR NO CONTEST TO A CRIME

NOTES: ON 1/22/93 CONVICTED OF ONE COUNT OF MAIL FRAUD; LIED TO LOUISIANA BOARD ABOUT 13 FELONY INDICTMENTS. REVOCATION STAYED WITH CONDITIONS: SHALL REMAIN IN COMPLIANCE WITH ALL CONDITIONS OF CRIMINAL PROBATION; SHALL PROVIDE AT LEAST 10 HOURS PER MONTH OF COMMUNITY SERVICE; SHALL APPEAR BEFORE AN INFORMAL COMMITTEE IN ONE YEAR WHICH SHALL PROVIDE ONGOING MONITORING.

MILES, WILLIAM D MD, DATE OF BIRTH JUNE 26, 1935 OF PO BOX 12237, ALEXANDRIA, LA, WAS DISCIPLINED BY MEDICARE ON APRIL 3, 1994
DISCIPLINARY ACTION: 60-MONTH EXCLUSION FROM THE MEDICARE AND/OR MEDICAID PROGRAM
OFFENSE: CRIMINAL CONVICTION OR PLEA OF GUILTY, NOLO CONTENDERE, OR NO CONTEST TO A CRIME

NOTES: CONVICTED OF A CRIME RELATED TO FINANCIAL MISCONDUCT.

MILES, WILLIAM D MD, LICENSE NUMBER 0035131 OF PO BOX 12237, ALEXANDRIA, LA, WAS DISCIPLINED BY VIRGINIA ON MAY 27, 1994
DISCIPLINARY ACTION: LICENSE SUSPENSION
OFFENSE: DISCIPLINARY ACTION BY ANOTHER STATE OR AGENCY

NOTES: ON 12/28/93 THE LOUISIANA BOARD SUSPENDED HIS LICENSE FOR ONE YEAR.

MILES, WILLIAM D MD, LICENSE NUMBER 0020725 OF ALEXANDRIA, LA, WAS DISCIPLINED BY TENNESSEE ON JUNE 27, 1995
DISCIPLINARY ACTION: 12-MONTH LICENSE SUSPENSION
OFFENSE: DISCIPLINARY ACTION BY ANOTHER STATE OR AGENCY

NOTES: DISCIPLINARY ACTION IN VIRGINIA AND LOUISIANA FOR FELONY CONVICTION; UNPROFESSIONAL CONDUCT. AFTER ONE YEAR, MUST PERSONALLY APPEAR BEFORE BOARD TO REQUEST REINSTATEMENT. LICENSE TO BE PLACED ON AN ADDITIONAL FIVE YEARS PROBATION IF REINSTATED.

MILES, WILLIAM D MD, DATE OF BIRTH JUNE 26, 1935, LICENSE NUMBER 0025234 OF BOX 12237, ALEXANDRIA, LA, WAS DISCIPLINED BY GEORGIA ON JULY 7, 1995
DISCIPLINARY ACTION: PROBATION
OFFENSE: DISCIPLINARY ACTION BY ANOTHER STATE OR AGENCY

NOTES: DISCIPLINARY ACTION IN VIRGINIA. CRIMINAL CONVICTION. PROBATION INDEFINITE. ON 5/13/99 ORDER TERMINATED.

MILES, WILLIAM D DO OF 9561 VILLA WAY, MIAMISBURG, OH, WAS DISCIPLINED BY DEA ON SEPTEMBER 20, 1995
DISCIPLINARY ACTION: SURRENDER OF CONTROLLED SUBSTANCE LICENSE

NOTES: IN LIEU OF PUBLIC INTEREST REVOCATION.

MILES, WILLIAM D DO, LICENSE NUMBER 006687E OF 9561 VILLA WAY, MIAMISBURG, OH, WAS DISCIPLINED BY PENNSYLVANIA ON JUNE 11, 1997
DISCIPLINARY ACTION: PROBATION; MONITORING OF PHYSICIAN PERFORMANCE
OFFENSE: DISCIPLINARY ACTION BY ANOTHER STATE OR AGENCY

NOTES: ON 11/8/95 THE OHIO BOARD PUT HIS LICENSE ON FIVE YEARS PROBATION SUBJECT TO CONDITIONS INCLUDING SUCCESSFUL PARTICIPATION IN A DRUG AND ALCOHOL REHAB PROGRAM. SUSPENSION UNTIL ALL TERMS PLACED ON HIS OHIO LICENSE ARE REMOVED; SUSPENSION STAYED FOR PROBATION UNDER THE FOLLOWING CONDITIONS: THE PROBATION WILL LAST UNTIL ALL TERMS ON HIS OHIO LICENSE ARE REMOVED; HE WILL ENSURE THAT DUPLICATES OF ALL MATERIALS SUBMITTED TO THE OHIO BOARD SHALL BE PROVIDED; HE MAY PRACTICE IN PENNSYLVANIA UNDER THE FOLLOWING CONDITIONS: HE WILL IMMEDIATELY NOTIFY THE BOARD OF HIS INTENTION TO PRACTICE IN PENNSYLVANIA; HE WILL ENTER INTO A CONTRACT WITH THE PROFESSIONAL HEALTH MONITORING PROGRAM (PHMP) UNTIL HIS OHIO AGREEMENT EXPIRES BUT FOR A MINIMUM OF ONE YEAR. HIS SUSPENSION IS ACTIVE FROM THE DATE OF HIS RETURN TO PENNSYLVANIA UNTIL HE ENTERS INTO A CONTRACT WITH PHMP. UPON EXPIRATION OF THE PHMP CONTRACT HIS SUSPENSION BECOMES ACTIVE UNTIL FURTHER NOTICE BY THE BOARD.

MILES, WILLIAM D DO, LICENSE NUMBER 02214 OF MIAMISBURG, OH, WAS DISCIPLINED BY IOWA ON MAY 27, 1999
DISCIPLINARY ACTION: SURRENDER OF LICENSE
OFFENSE: DISCIPLINARY ACTION BY ANOTHER STATE OR AGENCY

NOTES: ON 6/19/95 LICENSE SUSPENDED BY OHIO, AND SUBSEQUENTLY DISCIPLINED BY UTAH AND PENNSYLVANIA FOR SUBSTANCE ABUSE. VOLUNTARY SURRENDER.

MILES, WILLIAM DOUGLAS DO, LICENSE NUMBER 0004296 OF MIAMISBURG, OH, WAS DISCIPLINED BY OHIO ON JUNE 19, 1995
DISCIPLINARY ACTION: LICENSE SUSPENSION
OFFENSE: SUBSTANCE ABUSE

NOTES: ADMITTED IMPAIRMENT OF ABILITY TO PRACTICE BECAUSE OF HABITUAL OR EXCESSIVE USE OR ABUSE OF DRUGS, ALCOHOL OR OTHER SUBSTANCES; PUBLISHING A FALSE, FRAUDULENT, DECEPTIVE OR MISLEADING STATEMENT. INDEFINITE SUSPENSION FOR A MINIMUM OF THREE MONTHS. REINSTATEMENT REQUIREMENTS INCLUDE PREPARATION OF NEW CONSENT AGREEMENT WHICH WILL SET PROBATIONARY TERMS AND CONDITIONS.

MILES, WILLIAM DOUGLAS DO, LICENSE NUMBER 0004296 OF MIAMISBURG, OH, WAS DISCIPLINED BY OHIO ON NOVEMBER 8, 1995
DISCIPLINARY ACTION: PROBATION; RESTRICTION PLACED ON LICENSE
OFFENSE: SUBSTANCE ABUSE

NOTES: HISTORY OF CHEMICAL DEPENDENCE AND DEPRESSION FOR WHICH HE RECEIVED TREATMENT FROM AN APPROVED PROVIDER; FAILURE TO ADVISE BOARD OF IMPAIRMENT ON APPLICATION FOR LICENSURE. REINSTATED FROM SUSPENSION.

PROBATIONARY TERMS AND CONDITIONS FOR A MINIMUM OF FIVE YEARS. ON 2/12/97 REQUEST TO REDUCE REQUIRED PSYCHIATRIC TREATMENT TO ONCE PER MONTH GRANTED. ON 11/13/97 REQUEST TO REDUCE AA ATTENDANCE FROM FOUR TO THREE TIMES A WEEK AND REDUCE REQUIRED DRUG SCREENS FROM WEEKLY TO BIWEEKLY GRANTED. ON 5/13/98 REQUEST TO REDUCE REQUIRED PERSONAL APPEARANCES TO ONCE EVERY SIX MONTHS GRANTED. ON 12/10/98 REQUESTS TO REDUCE REQUIRED DRUG SCREENS TO MONTHLY AND PSYCHIATRIC TREATMENT TO ONCE EVERY THREE MONTHS GRANTED.

MILES, WILLIAM DOUGLAS DO OF MIAMISBURG, OH, WAS DISCIPLINED BY UTAH ON MAY 17, 1996
OFFENSE: DISCIPLINARY ACTION BY ANOTHER STATE OR AGENCY
NOTES: DISCIPLINARY ACTION TAKEN IN OHIO. FIVE YEAR SUSPENSION STAYED SO LONG AS HE REMAINS IN FULL COMPLIANCE WITH HIS OHIO PROBATION. HE ALSO HAS CONDITIONS TO BE MET DURING THE STAYED SUSPENSION PERIOD.

MILLER, JOHN J MD, WAS DISCIPLINED BY NEVADA ON OCTOBER 17, 1995
DISCIPLINARY ACTION: LICENSE REVOCATION
OFFENSE: DISCIPLINARY ACTION BY ANOTHER STATE OR AGENCY
NOTES: CONVICTION OF A FELONY; CHARGED WITH BEING FOUND GUILTY OF TWO FELONIES IN MONTANA; DISCIPLINARY ACTION AGAINST HIS LICENSE IN MONTANA; SUSPENSION OF LICENSE BY ANY OTHER JURISDICTION; FAILURE TO REPORT, WITHIN 30 DAYS, THE SUSPENSION OF HIS LICENSE TO PRACTICE MEDICINE IN ANOTHER JURISDICTION.

MILLER, JOHN J MD OF JACKSONVILLE, FL, WAS DISCIPLINED BY UTAH ON OCTOBER 28, 1995
DISCIPLINARY ACTION: LICENSE REVOCATION; REVOCATION OF CONTROLLED SUBSTANCE LICENSE
OFFENSE: PHYSICAL OR MENTAL ILLNESS INHIBITING THE ABILITY TO PRACTICE WITH SKILL AND SAFETY
NOTES: ADMISSION OF INABILITY TO SAFELY ENGAGE IN THE PRACTICE OF MEDICINE BECAUSE OF A MENTAL OR PHYSICAL CONDITION.

MILLER, JOHN J MD, LICENSE NUMBER 0D27191 OF HIDDEN LAKE DRIVE, JACKSONVILLE, FL, WAS DISCIPLINED BY MARYLAND ON NOVEMBER 7, 1995
DISCIPLINARY ACTION: PROBATION
OFFENSE: DISCIPLINARY ACTION BY ANOTHER STATE OR AGENCY
NOTES: ACTION BY MONTANA. REVOCATION STAYED.

MILLER, JOHN J MD, LICENSE NUMBER 0039841 OF DEER LODGE, MT, WAS DISCIPLINED BY FLORIDA ON MARCH 6, 1996
DISCIPLINARY ACTION: LICENSE REVOCATION
OFFENSE: DISCIPLINARY ACTION BY ANOTHER STATE OR AGENCY
NOTES: CONVICTED OF A CRIME DIRECTLY RELATING TO THE PRACTICE OF MEDICINE.

MILLER, JOHN JOSEPH MD, DATE OF BIRTH FEBRUARY 14, 1942, LICENSE NUMBER 0003980 OF 310 SUNNYVIEW LANE, KALISPELL, MT, WAS DISCIPLINED BY MONTANA ON AUGUST 23, 1994
DISCIPLINARY ACTION: EMERGENCY SUSPENSION
OFFENSE: SUBSTANCE ABUSE
NOTES: UNTREATED CHEMICAL DEPENDENCY. STIPULATION NOT TO SEEK REINSTATEMENT OF LICENSE UNTIL AFTER COMPLETION OF EVALUATION AND TREATMENT FOR ILLNESSES ON 8/31/94.

MILLER, JOHN JOSEPH MD, DATE OF BIRTH FEBRUARY 14, 1942, LICENSE NUMBER 00M5606, WAS DISCIPLINED BY IDAHO ON NOVEMBER 18, 1994
DISCIPLINARY ACTION: LICENSE SUSPENSION
OFFENSE: DISCIPLINARY ACTION BY ANOTHER STATE OR AGENCY
NOTES: ON 8/24/94 MONTANA ORDERED THAT LICENSE BE PLACED ON EMERGENCY SUSPENSION; ALSO REQUIRED HIM TO HAVE A COMPLETE MENTAL AND PHYSICAL EXAMINATION. THE IDAHO BOARD FOR THE PURPOSE OF THIS RECIPROCAL DISCIPLINE INCORPORATES THE TERMS AND CONDITIONS OF THIS ORDER AND ORDERS HIM TO FULLY COMPLY WITH THEM.

MILLER, JOHN JOSEPH MD, DATE OF BIRTH FEBRUARY 14, 1942, LICENSE NUMBER 0021472 OF JACKSONVILLE, FL, WAS DISCIPLINED BY TENNESSEE ON FEBRUARY 23, 1995
DISCIPLINARY ACTION: LICENSE REVOCATION
OFFENSE: DISCIPLINARY ACTION BY ANOTHER STATE OR AGENCY
NOTES: DISCIPLINARY ACTION TAKEN BY MONTANA BOARD. SUBSTANCE ABUSE. MUST APPEAR BEFORE BOARD IF REINSTATEMENT SOUGHT.

MILLER, JOHN JOSEPH MD, DATE OF BIRTH FEBRUARY 14, 1942, LICENSE NUMBER 00M5606, WAS DISCIPLINED BY IDAHO ON MAY 1, 1995
DISCIPLINARY ACTION: LICENSE REVOCATION
OFFENSE: DISCIPLINARY ACTION BY ANOTHER STATE OR AGENCY
NOTES: IN 8/94 ENGAGED IN THE EXCESSIVE USE OF ALCOHOL OR OTHER SUBSTANCES TO THE EXTENT THAT THE USE IMPAIRED HIM PHYSICALLY OR MENTALLY; AS A RESULT HE WAS IN AN AUTO ACCIDENT WHICH CAUSED THE DEATH OF TWO PERSONS; LICENSE IN TENNESSEE WAS REVOKED ON 2/23/95. THE IDAHO BOARD ADOPTS THE FINDING OF THE TENNESSEE ORDER AND INCORPORATES ALL OF THE TERMS AND CONDITIONS OF THE TENNESSEE ORDER.

MILLER, JOHN JOSEPH MD, DATE OF BIRTH FEBRUARY 14, 1942 OF 215 SUNNYVIEW LANE #7, KALISPELL, MT, WAS DISCIPLINED BY MEDICARE ON MAY 4, 1995
DISCIPLINARY ACTION: EXCLUSION FROM THE MEDICARE AND/OR MEDICAID PROGRAM
OFFENSE: DISCIPLINARY ACTION BY ANOTHER STATE OR AGENCY
NOTES: LICENSE SUSPENDED FOR REASONS BEARING ON PROFESSIONAL PERFORMANCE.

MILLER, JOHN JOSEPH MD, DATE OF BIRTH FEBRUARY 14, 1942, LICENSE NUMBER 0003980 OF 3459 HIDDEN LAKE DRIVE WEST, JACKSONVILLE, FL, WAS DISCIPLINED BY MONTANA ON MAY 19, 1995
DISCIPLINARY ACTION: PROBATION
OFFENSE: CRIMINAL CONVICTION OR PLEA OF GUILTY, NOLO CONTENDERE, OR NO CONTEST TO A CRIME
NOTES: CONVICTION OF FELONY; CHEMICAL DEPENDENCY. REVOCATION STAYED.

MILLER, JOHN JOSEPH MD, LICENSE NUMBER 0049431 OF JACKSONVILLE, FL, WAS DISCIPLINED BY VIRGINIA ON JUNE 13, 1995
DISCIPLINARY ACTION: LICENSE SUSPENSION
OFFENSE: DISCIPLINARY ACTION BY ANOTHER STATE OR AGENCY
NOTES: REVOCATION BY TENNESSEE AND SUSPENSION BY MONTANA AFTER HE ENGAGED IN THE EXCESSIVE USE OF ALCOHOL OR OTHER SUBSTANCES.

MILLER, JOHN JOSEPH MD, DATE OF BIRTH FEBRUARY 14, 1942, LICENSE NUMBER 0031991 OF 3459 HIDDEN LAKE DR W, JACKSONVILLE, FL, WAS DISCIPLINED BY GEORGIA ON AUGUST 3, 1995
DISCIPLINARY ACTION: LICENSE SUSPENSION
OFFENSE: CRIMINAL CONVICTION OR PLEA OF GUILTY, NOLO CONTENDERE, OR NO CONTEST TO A CRIME

NOTES: CONVICTION OF A CRIME. SUSPENDED INDEFINITELY.

MILLER, JOHN JOSEPH MD, DATE OF BIRTH FEBRUARY 14, 1942, LICENSE NUMBER 0009752 OF 3459 HIDDEN LAKE DRIVE WEST, JACKSONVILLE, FL, WAS DISCIPLINED BY WEST VIRGINIA ON NOVEMBER 20, 1995
DISCIPLINARY ACTION: LICENSE REVOCATION
OFFENSE: DISCIPLINARY ACTION BY ANOTHER STATE OR AGENCY

NOTES: FOUND GUILTY OF TWO FELONY COUNTS OF NEGLIGENT HOMICIDE IN 2/95 IN MONTANA; HIS EXCESSIVE USE OF ALCOHOL CAUSED HIM TO BE IMPAIRED AND TO CAUSE THE DEATHS OF TWO PERSONS IN A MOTOR VEHICLE ACCIDENT. IN 2/95 THE TENNESSEE BOARD REVOKED HIS LICENSE. IN 11/94 THE IDAHO BOARD SUSPENDED HIS LICENSE AND IN 5/95 REVOKED HIS LICENSE. IN 8/94 MONTANA SUSPENDED HIS LICENSE AND IN 4/95 REVOKED HIS LICENSE AND THEN STAYED THE REVOCATION AS PROBATION UNDER SEVERAL TERMS AND CONDITIONS.

MILLER, JOHN JOSEPH MD, DATE OF BIRTH FEBRUARY 14, 1942, LICENSE NUMBER 0030589, WAS DISCIPLINED BY COLORADO ON JANUARY 11, 1996
OFFENSE: CRIMINAL CONVICTION OR PLEA OF GUILTY, NOLO CONTENDERE, OR NO CONTEST TO A CRIME

NOTES: PLED GUILTY TO TWO FELONY CHARGES (NEGLIGENT HOMICIDE AS A RESULT OF A MOTOR VEHICLE ACCIDENT). ORDERED TO PERMANENTLY RELINQUISH HIS LICENSE TO PRACTICE MEDICINE IN COLORADO.

MILLER, JOHN JOSEPH MD, LICENSE NUMBER 0060453 OF DEER LODGE, MT, WAS DISCIPLINED BY OHIO ON FEBRUARY 14, 1996
DISCIPLINARY ACTION: LICENSE REVOCATION
OFFENSE: DISCIPLINARY ACTION BY ANOTHER STATE OR AGENCY

NOTES: PRIOR ACTION BY MONTANA MEDICAL BOARD WHICH WAS BASED ON HIS ADMISSIONS THAT HE HAD ENGAGED IN EXCESSIVE USE OF ALCOHOL SO THAT HE WAS MENTALLY AND PHYSICALLY IMPAIRED AND THAT WHILE HE WAS IMPAIRED, HE WAS INVOLVED IN A MOTOR VEHICLE ACCIDENT THAT CAUSED THE DEATH OF TWO PEOPLE. CONVICTION OF TWO FELONY COUNTS OF NEGLIGENT HOMICIDE. PERMANENT REVOCATION.

MOHR, ROBERT C MD OF 945 EAST 1ST SOUTH, SALT LAKE CITY, UT, WAS DISCIPLINED BY DEA ON APRIL 15, 1994
DISCIPLINARY ACTION: SURRENDER OF CONTROLLED SUBSTANCE LICENSE
OFFENSE: DISCIPLINARY ACTION BY ANOTHER STATE OR AGENCY

NOTES: STATE BOARD.

MOHR, ROBERT CARL MD, DATE OF BIRTH JUNE 5, 1929 OF 1965 BROWNING AVENUE, SALT LAKE CITY, UT, WAS DISCIPLINED BY MEDICARE ON MARCH 15, 1993
DISCIPLINARY ACTION: 60-MONTH EXCLUSION FROM THE MEDICARE AND/OR MEDICAID PROGRAM
OFFENSE: CRIMINAL CONVICTION OR PLEA OF GUILTY, NOLO CONTENDERE, OR NO CONTEST TO A CRIME

NOTES: CONVICTED OF A CRIME RELATED TO THE MEDICAID PROGRAM.

MOHR, ROBERT CARL MD, DATE OF BIRTH JUNE 5, 1929, LICENSE NUMBER 0014617 OF SALT LAKE CITY, UT, WAS DISCIPLINED BY UTAH ON APRIL 7, 1994
DISCIPLINARY ACTION: SURRENDER OF LICENSE
OFFENSE: PROVIDING FALSE INFORMATION TO THE BOARD OR OTHER HEALTH AGENCY

NOTES: 5555ALLEGATIONS INCLUDE: FROM ABOUT 10/87 THROUGH 9/89 HE PURSUED A PATIENT FOR SEXUAL RELATIONS, EXPLOITING THE KNOWLEDGE THAT SHE WAS DEPENDENT ON CONTROLLED SUBSTANCES BY PRESCRIBING THESE DRUGS TO HER IN EXCHANGE FOR SEXUAL RELATIONS; ENCOURAGED ONE PATIENT WHOM HE SAW FROM ABOUT 10/84 TO 7/86 TO HAVE TWO AFFAIRS WITH MARRIED MEN AS PART OF HER THERAPY; AFTER ONE SESSION WHERE THEY DISCUSSED SEXUAL RELATIONS AND ENGAGED IN TOUCHING HE TOLD HER HE WAS TERMINATING HER AS A PATIENT THAT DAY AND THEY BEGAN TO HAVE SEXUAL RELATIONS THAT EVENING WHICH CONTINUED FOR APPROXIMATELY FIVE YEARS; BEGINNING IN 3/91 PURSUED A PATIENT WHO TOLD HIM SHE WANTED TO DISCONTINUE THERAPY; SHE LATER MARRIED HIM; ON 12/16/91 APPLICATION FOR REAPPOINTMENT FOR STAFF PRIVILEGES TURNED DOWN BECAUSE HE FALSIFIED APPLICATION CONCERNING HIS TREATMENT FOR ALCOHOL ABUSE, FAILURE TO MAINTAIN MALPRACTICE INSURANCE, AND EXHIBITED UNPROFESSIONAL RELATIONS AND DISRUPTIVE CONDUCT WITH HIS PEERS AND STAFF; ALCOHOL WAS DETECTED ON HIS BREATH ON DIFFERENT OCCASIONS BY HIS PATIENTS AND OFFICE STAFF FROM 10/91 THROUGH 1/93 DURING NORMAL BUSINESS HOURS; ONE PATIENT SAW HIM DRINK ALCOHOL FROM A BOTTLE IN THE CLINIC PARKING LOT; OBTAINED PERSONAL LOANS FROM AT LEAST THREE PATIENTS FROM 1989 THROUGH 3/92; PROVIDED PSYCHIATRIC TREATMENT TO TWO PATIENTS BETWEEN 1980 AND 1990 WITHOUT MAKING ANY SIGNIFICANT PROGRESS NOTES OR PROVIDING THEM WITH AN ADEQUATE DIAGNOSIS OR PROGNOSIS OF THEIR CONDITION; BETWEEN 6/88 AND 12/92 ENGAGED IN AT LEAST FIVE INSTANCES OF BILLING FRAUD CAUSING FALSE CLAIMS TO BE SUBMITTED TO BLUE CROSS/BLUE SHIELD, UTAH WORKER'S COMPENSATION FUND AND OTHER INSURERS; URINATED IN HIS TROUSERS IN THE PRESENCE OF A PATIENT DURING TREATMENT SESSION ON AT LEAST TWO OCCASIONS; FAILED TO RESPOND TO PATIENT THREATENING SUICIDE ON 3/29/91 WHO COMMITTED SUICIDE TWO DAYS LATER. HE NEITHER ADMITTED NOR DENIED ANY OF THESE ALLEGATIONS. FURTHER AGREED NOT TO REAPPLY FOR LICENSURE TO PRACTICE MEDICINE IN UTAH.

MORGAN, ARTHUR J MD, LICENSE NUMBER 025231L OF SPRINGVILLE, UT, WAS DISCIPLINED BY PENNSYLVANIA ON NOVEMBER 26, 1991
DISCIPLINARY ACTION: 6-MONTH LICENSE SUSPENSION; 30-MONTH PROBATION
OFFENSE: CRIMINAL CONVICTION OR PLEA OF GUILTY, NOLO CONTENDERE, OR NO CONTEST TO A CRIME

NOTES: CONVICTION OF 40 COUNTS OF MEDICAID FRAUD IN HAWAII. REMAINDER OF 3 YEAR SUSPENSION STAYED.

MORROW, ROBERT E MD, DATE OF BIRTH DECEMBER 18, 1952, LICENSE NUMBER 032014E OF 243 E. BROWN STREET, EAST STROUDSBURG, PA, WAS DISCIPLINED BY PENNSYLVANIA ON SEPTEMBER 26, 1995

DISCIPLINARY ACTION: 1-MONTH LICENSE SUSPENSION; 36-MONTH PROBATION
OFFENSE: NONCOMPLIANCE WITH A PROFESSIONAL RULE

NOTES: NONCOMPLIANCE WITH MALPRACTICE INSURANCE REQUIREMENT, NON-PAYMENT OF MEDICAL PROFESSIONAL LIABILITY CATASTROPHIC LOSS FUND SURCHARGE FOR TWO YEARS. REMAINDER OF THREE YEAR SUSPENSION STAYED. CIVIL PENALTY OF $15,000. ON 9/26/98 PROBATION TERMINATED.

MORROW, ROBERT E MD OF SALT LAKE CITY, UT, WAS DISCIPLINED BY UTAH ON FEBRUARY 22, 1999
DISCIPLINARY ACTION: FINE; RESTRICTION PLACED ON CONTROLLED SUBSTANCE LICENSE
OFFENSE: PRACTICING WITHOUT A VALID CONTROLLED SUBSTANCE LICENSE

NOTES: ALLEGATIONS THAT HE PRESCRIBED CONTROLLED SUBSTANCES WITHOUT BEING REGISTERED WITH THE DEA; IMPROPERLY PRESCRIBED CONTROLLED SUBSTANCES; FAILED TO HAVE REQUIRED INFORMATION IN PATIENT CHARTS. HIS LICENSE TO PRACTICE MEDICINE WAS REVOKED WITH A STAY OF ENFORCEMENT ON THE REVOCATION, AND HIS LICENSE TO PRESCRIBE AND ADMINISTER CONTROLLED SUBSTANCES SCHEDULES II-V WAS SURRENDERED TO THE DIVISION. $1,000 FINE.

MURDOCK, KENNETH JOE MD OF AMERICAN FORK, UT, WAS DISCIPLINED BY UTAH ON AUGUST 28, 1997
DISCIPLINARY ACTION: REQUIRED TO TAKE ADDITIONAL MEDICAL EDUCATION
OFFENSE: NONCOMPLIANCE WITH A PROFESSIONAL RULE

NOTES: HE PRESCRIBED CONTROLLED SUBSTANCES TO A PATIENT WITHOUT MAINTAINING ADEQUATE RECORDS OF THE PRESCRIPTIONS AND PRESCRIBED NARCOTIC CONTROLLED SUBSTANCES FOR DETOXIFICATION CONTRARY TO FEDERAL LAW. VOLUNTARILY ATTENDED AN EDUCATIONAL PROGRAM ON PRESCRIBING PRACTICES IN 11/95.

MUSE, DEREK D MD OF SALT LAKE CITY, UT, WAS DISCIPLINED BY UTAH ON AUGUST 11, 1998
DISCIPLINARY ACTION: FINE
OFFENSE: PROFESSIONAL MISCONDUCT

NOTES: PRIOR TO 8/97, HE OCCASIONALLY PRE-SIGNED BLANK PRESCRIPTION FORMS THAT HE GAVE TO A PHYSICIAN ASSISTANT. THE PRE-SIGNED PRESCRIPTION FORMS WERE GIVEN TO THE PHYSICIAN ASSISTANT SO THAT HE COULD WRITE PRESCRIPTIONS TO TREAT WEIGHT LOSS PATIENTS. ANOTHER EMPLOYEE USED SOME OF THE PRE-SIGNED BLANK PRESCRIPTION FORMS TO OBTAIN CONTROLLED SUBSTANCES FOR HERSELF AND HER HUSBAND. $2,000 FINE.

NELSON, JOEL STEPHEN MD OF SOUTH JORDAN, UT, WAS DISCIPLINED BY UTAH ON SEPTEMBER 24, 1998
DISCIPLINARY ACTION: LICENSE SUSPENSION; SUSPENSION OF CONTROLLED SUBSTANCE LICENSE
OFFENSE: FAILURE TO COMPLY WITH PREVIOUS BOARD ORDER

NOTES: FAILED TO SUBMIT TO A PSYCHOLOGICAL EVALUATION AS ORDERED BY THE BOARD.

OGLESBY, RICHARD J MD, LICENSE NUMBER 003712A, WAS DISCIPLINED BY WYOMING ON JUNE 24, 1992
DISCIPLINARY ACTION: REQUIRED TO ENTER AN IMPAIRED PHYSICIAN PROGRAM OR SUBSTANCE ABUSE TREATMENT; MONITORING OF PHYSICIAN PERFORMANCE
OFFENSE: SUBSTANCE ABUSE

NOTES: ALLEGED THAT HE HAS ENGAGED IN REPEATED USE OF DRUGS AND/OR INTOXICANTS TO SUCH A DEGREE AS TO RENDER HIM UNABLE TO PRACTICE MEDICINE WITH REASONABLE SKILL AND SAFETY TO PATIENTS. CONDITIONS OF CONSENT ORDER ARE AS FOLLOWS: SHALL START AND CONTINUE REGULAR INVOLVEMENT IN A SUBSTANCE ABUSE AFTERCARE AND COUNSELING PROGRAM; SHALL SUBMIT TO RANDOM URINALYSIS UNDER SPECIFIED CONDITIONS WITH FAILURE CONSTITUTING GROUNDS FOR DISCIPLINE; SHALL APPEAR BEFORE THE BOARD FOR A PERSONAL INTERVIEW ON 6/93 TO DETERMINE WHETHER CONDITIONS SHOULD BE CONTINUED, MODIFIED OR TERMINATED. ON 6/15/93 NUMBER OF URINALYSIS SCREENS WERE REDUCED.

OGLESBY, RICHARD JAMES MD OF RAWLINS, WY, WAS DISCIPLINED BY UTAH ON JULY 3, 1995
OFFENSE: DISCIPLINARY ACTION BY ANOTHER STATE OR AGENCY

NOTES: DISCIPLINARY ACTION BY WYOMING FOR AN ACCUSATION OF ALCOHOL ABUSE; HOSPITAL STAFF PRIVILEGES JEOPARDIZED ON ALLEGATIONS OF SEXUAL HARASSMENT AND PRACTICING BELOW STANDARD OF CARE. LICENSE ISSUED SUBJECT TO CERTAIN TERMS AND CONDITIONS WHICH SHALL BE IN EFFECT UNTIL JUNE 1997. ON 6/19/97 LICENSE REINSTATED WITH FULL PRIVILEGES.

OLSON, PAUL F MD OF PROVO, UT, WAS DISCIPLINED BY UTAH ON MAY 31, 1991
DISCIPLINARY ACTION: REVOCATION OF CONTROLLED SUBSTANCE LICENSE; 60-MONTH PROBATION
OFFENSE: OVERPRESCRIBING OR MISPRESCRIBING DRUGS

NOTES: UNLAWFULLY OBTAINING AND USING A SCHEDULED CONTROLLED DRUG; ALSO UNLAWFUL AND/OR UNPROFESSIONAL ISSUANCE OF PRESCRIPTIONS FOR CONTROLLED SUBSTANCES. ON 3/8/93 HIS LICENSE TO PRESCRIBE AND ADMINISTER CONTROLLED SUBSTANCES SCHEDULES IV AND V WAS REINSTATED ON PROBATION CONSISTENT WITH TERMS AND CONDITIONS OF THIS ORDER. ON 1/8/96 PROBATIONS ON LICENSES TO PRACTICE MEDICINE AND TO PRESCRIBE AND ADMINISTER CONTROLLED SUBSTANCES SCHEDULES IV-V ONLY TERMINATED; LICENSES REINSTATED WITH FULL PRIVILEGES.

OWENS, WILLIAM SELD MD OF OREM, UT, WAS DISCIPLINED BY UTAH ON JULY 9, 1990
DISCIPLINARY ACTION: 60-MONTH PROBATION; 24-MONTH RESTRICTION PLACED ON CONTROLLED SUBSTANCE LICENSE
OFFENSE: FAILURE TO COMPLY WITH PREVIOUS BOARD ORDER

NOTES: ACTED UNPROFESSIONALLY IN PRESCRIBING MEDICATIONS OUTSIDE OF THE RECOGNIZED STANDARDS OF THE PROFESSION, VIOLATED PROVISIONS OF A PRIOR ORDER ISSUED BY THE DIVISION, AND AIDED THE UNLAWFUL USE OF PRESCRIPTION DRUGS BY A KNOWN HABITUATE. OWENS AGREED TO STIPULATION WITHOUT ADMISSION OF GUILT. LICENSE REVOCATION STAYED. PHYSICIAN AGREED THAT CONTROLLED SUBSTANCE LICENSE HAD LAPSED AND HE WOULD NOT ATTEMPT TO RENEW IT. HE MAY NOT PRESCRIBE ANY PRESCRIPTION DRUGS OR MEDICATIONS EXCEPT FOR A SPECIFIC LIST WHICH IS PROVIDED IN THE STIPULATION.

PETERSON, DAVID A MD OF SALT LAKE CITY, UT, WAS DISCIPLINED BY UTAH ON MARCH 25, 1997

DISCIPLINARY ACTION: SURRENDER OF CONTROLLED SUBSTANCE LICENSE; 60-MONTH PROBATION
OFFENSE: SUBSTANCE ABUSE

NOTES: ALLEGATIONS THAT HE ENGAGED IN WRITING FICTITIOUS PRESCRIPTIONS IN ORDER TO OBTAIN CONTROLLED SUBSTANCES FOR HIS PERSONAL USE AND ABUSE. VOLUNTARY SURRENDER. ON 3/10/98 REQUIREMENT OF COURSES HE NEEDED TO TAKE WAS MODIFIED. ON 12/4/98 PROBATIONARY CONDITION REQUIRING HIM TO PARTICIPATE IN GROUP COUNSELING SESSIONS WAS TERMINATED.

PICKENS, JAMES E MD OF SALT LAKE CITY, UT, WAS DISCIPLINED BY UTAH ON NOVEMBER 18, 1993
DISCIPLINARY ACTION: PROBATION; CONTROLLED SUBSTANCE LICENSE PLACED ON PROBATION
OFFENSE: PROFESSIONAL MISCONDUCT

NOTES: ALLEGATION, NOT ADMITTED OR DENIED BY HIM THAT HE FAILED TO MAINTAIN SUFFICIENT RECORDS REGARDING CONTROLLED SUBSTANCES AND ADMINISTERED CONTROLLED SUBSTANCES TO HIMSELF WITHOUT A PRESCRIPTION FROM AN AUTHORIZED PRACTITIONER. AGREED TO VARIOUS TERMS AND CONDITIONS TO BE MET FOR A PERIOD OF TWO YEARS. WITH RESPECT TO HIS LICENSE TO PRESCRIBE AND ADMINISTER CONTROLLED SUBSTANCES, SHALL BE PROHIBITED FROM PRESCRIBING COCAINE, INCLUDING MAINTAINING IT IN HIS OFFICE INVENTORY. PROBATIONS ON LICENSES TO PRACTICE MEDICINE AND TO PRESCRIBE AND ADMINISTER CONTROLLED SUBSTANCES WERE TERMINATED AND LICENSES REINSTATED WITH FULL PRIVILEGES ON 12/4/95.

PICKENS, JAMES E MD, LICENSE NUMBER 0013747 OF MURRAY, UT, WAS DISCIPLINED BY FLORIDA ON APRIL 11, 1995
DISCIPLINARY ACTION: LICENSE SUSPENSION; FINE
OFFENSE: DISCIPLINARY ACTION BY ANOTHER STATE OR AGENCY

NOTES: CHARGED WITH HAVING A LICENSE TO PRACTICE MEDICINE ACTED AGAINST BY THE UTAH LICENSING AUTHORITY AND FAILING TO NOTIFY BOARD OF THIS WITHIN 30 DAYS. $500 FINE; SUSPENSION UNTIL UTAH LICENSE IS FREE AND CLEAR OF ALL ENCUMBRANCES; SHALL APPEAR BEFORE BOARD PRIOR TO REINSTATEMENT AND DEMONSTRATE THAT HE CAN PRACTICE WITH REASONABLE SKILL AND SAFETY TO PATIENTS; DEMONSTRATION SHALL INCLUDE, BUT NOT BE LIMITED TO AN EVALUATION BY THE PHYSICIAN'S RECOVERY NETWORK; UPON REINSTATEMENT, BOARD MAY IMPOSE A PERIOD OF PROBATION.

POTTER, LEE H MD OF OGDEN, UT, WAS DISCIPLINED BY UTAH ON MARCH 2, 1993
DISCIPLINARY ACTION: 36-MONTH PROBATION; RESTRICTION PLACED ON CONTROLLED SUBSTANCE LICENSE
OFFENSE: PROFESSIONAL MISCONDUCT

NOTES: UNLAWFUL AND UNPROFESSIONAL OBTAINING AND USE OF CONTROLLED SUBSTANCES; FAILURE TO MAINTAIN PROPER CONTROLLED SUBSTANCE RECORDS; ENDANGERING PATIENT WELFARE BY SUBSTITUTING FOREIGN SUBSTANCE FOR CONTROLLED SUBSTANCE. LICENSE TO PRESCRIBE AND ADMINISTER CONTROLLED SUBSTANCES SCHEDULES 2-5 WAS REVOKED; HOWEVER, THERE WAS A STAY OF ENFORCEMENT WITH RESPECT TO SCHEDULES III THROUGH V AND THAT LICENSE WAS PLACED ON PROBATION FOR THREE YEARS WITH CONDITIONS. SHALL NOT POSSESS, ADMINISTER OR PRESCRIBE STADOL OR ANY GENERIC FORM OF THAT DRUG. ON 7/31/96 PROBATIONS ON LICENSES TO PRACTICE MEDICINE AND TO PRESCRIBE AND ADMINISTER CONTROLLED SUBSTANCES SCHEDULES III-V TERMINATED; LICENSES REINSTATED WITH FULL PRIVILEGES.

POTTS, ROBERT E MD OF SALINA, UT, WAS DISCIPLINED BY UTAH ON SEPTEMBER 24, 1990
DISCIPLINARY ACTION: PROBATION

NOTES: THIS LICENSE WAS PLACED ON PROBATION CONSISTENT WITH THE PROVISIONS OF THE 7/28/89 ORDER. ON 7/19/94 PROBATION TERMINATED AND LICENSE REINSTATED WITH FULL PRIVILEGES.

POTTS, ROBERT E MD OF SALINA, UT, WAS DISCIPLINED BY UTAH ON NOVEMBER 24, 1999
DISCIPLINARY ACTION: SURRENDER OF CONTROLLED SUBSTANCE LICENSE

NOTES: AN INVESTIGATION WAS BEING CONDUCTED REGARDING HIS CONDUCT WITH CONTROLLED SUBSTANCES. AGREED TO VOLUNTARILY SURRENDER HIS LICENSE TO PRESCRIBE AND ADMINISTER CONTROLLED SUBSTANCES.

PRATLEY, BRENT M MD OF 16661 VENTURA BLVD #710, ENCINO, CA, WAS DISCIPLINED BY DEA ON FEBRUARY 14, 1990
DISCIPLINARY ACTION: SURRENDER OF CONTROLLED SUBSTANCE LICENSE
OFFENSE: PROVIDING FALSE INFORMATION TO THE BOARD OR OTHER HEALTH AGENCY

NOTES: MATERIAL FALSIFICATION OF DEA APPLICATION.

PRATLEY, BRENT M MD OF 1055 NORTH WEST #501, PROVO, UT, WAS DISCIPLINED BY DEA ON SEPTEMBER 25, 1992
DISCIPLINARY ACTION: RESTRICTION PLACED ON CONTROLLED SUBSTANCE LICENSE
OFFENSE: PROVIDING FALSE INFORMATION TO THE BOARD OR OTHER HEALTH AGENCY

NOTES: VOLUNTARILY SURRENDERED DEA REGISTRATION 02/02/90 DUE TO FALSIFYING DEA APPLICATION FOR REGISTRATION. APPLICATION FOR REGISTRATION FOR SCHEDULES III-V APPROVED 10/30/90 IN SALT LAKE CITY, UTAH.

PRATLEY, BRENT M MD OF 1055 NORTH 300 WEST #501, PROVO, UT, WAS DISCIPLINED BY DEA ON JUNE 5, 1996
DISCIPLINARY ACTION: RESTRICTION PLACED ON CONTROLLED SUBSTANCE LICENSE
OFFENSE: PROFESSIONAL MISCONDUCT

NOTES: PRIOR ALLEGED CONTROLLED SUBSTANCE VIOLATIONS.

PRATT, VON S MD OF GUNNISON, UT, WAS DISCIPLINED BY UTAH ON JULY 31, 1995
DISCIPLINARY ACTION: 60-MONTH PROBATION; 60-MONTH CONTROLLED SUBSTANCE LICENSE PLACED ON PROBATION
OFFENSE: SEXUAL ABUSE OF OR SEXUAL MISCONDUCT WITH A PATIENT

NOTES: FAILING TO MAINTAIN PROPER RECORDS; PRESCRIBING CONTROLLED SUBSTANCES FOR OTHER THAN A RECOGNIZED MEDICAL PURPOSE; AND ENGAGING IN INTIMATE SEXUAL RELATIONSHIP WITH A PATIENT. LICENSE REVOCATION STAYED. ON 3/10/98 CONDITION REQUIRING HIM TO MEET WITH THE BOARD REDUCED FROM QUARTERLY TO EVERY SIX MONTHS. ON 5/27/99 PROBATIONS TERMINATED; LICENSES REINSTATED WITH FULL PRIVILEGES.

PURSER, DANNY C MD, DATE OF BIRTH AUGUST 31, 1959 OF 3200 NAVAJO LANE, PROVO, UT, WAS DISCIPLINED BY MEDICARE ON JUNE 17, 1999
DISCIPLINARY ACTION: EXCLUSION FROM THE MEDICARE AND/OR MEDICAID PROGRAM
OFFENSE: CRIMINAL CONVICTION OR PLEA OF GUILTY, NOLO CONTENDERE, OR NO CONTEST TO A CRIME

NOTES: CONVICTED OF A CRIME INVOLVING THE MEDICARE, MEDICAID, MATERNAL AND CHILD HEALTH SERVICES BLOCK GRANT OR BLOCK GRANTS TO STATES FOR SOCIAL SERVICES PROGRAMS.

PURVIN, JONATHAN MARK MD OF MIAMI BEACH, FL, WAS DISCIPLINED BY UTAH ON AUGUST 17, 1992
DISCIPLINARY ACTION: 60-MONTH PROBATION
OFFENSE: PROVIDING FALSE INFORMATION TO THE BOARD OR OTHER HEALTH AGENCY

NOTES: ACTS OR PRACTICES CONTRARY TO THE RECOGNIZED STANDARDS AND ETHICS OF THE PROFESSION; MAKING FALSE STATEMENTS IN AN APPLICATION FOR MEDICAL STAFF PRIVILEGES AT A HOSPITAL AND IN APPLYING FOR LICENSURE AS A PHYSICIAN IN ANOTHER STATE. THREE-MONTH SUSPENSION, STAYED. PROBATION WITH CONDITIONS. ON 9/18/97 LICENSE REINSTATED WITH FULL PRIVILEGES.

RADWIN, MARTIN MD OF OGDEN, UT, WAS DISCIPLINED BY UTAH ON JULY 28, 1999
DISCIPLINARY ACTION: 60-MONTH PROBATION; 60-MONTH CONTROLLED SUBSTANCE LICENSE PLACED ON PROBATION

RADWIN, MARTIN IRA MD OF OGDEN, UT, WAS DISCIPLINED BY UTAH ON SEPTEMBER 28, 1998
DISCIPLINARY ACTION: FINE
OFFENSE: PROFESSIONAL MISCONDUCT

NOTES: HAS TAKEN CONTROLLED SUBSTANCES WHICH HAD NOT BEEN PRESCRIBED TO HIM BY A PRACTITIONER; ASKED A COWORKER TO GIVE HIM CONTROLLED SUBSTANCES FROM THEIR PRESCRIPTIONS; ISSUED PRESCRIPTIONS TO COWORKERS WITH THE REQUEST THEY RETURN THE CONTROLLED SUBSTANCES TO HIM; PRESCRIBED MEDICATIONS TO PATIENTS WITHOUT MAINTAINING MEDICAL RECORDS. HE WAS ORDERED TO COMPLETE A SUBSTANCE ABUSE EVALUATION AND A MENTAL HEALTH EVALUATION. UPON SUCCESSFUL COMPLETION OF EITHER AN INPATIENT OR OUTPATIENT DRUG TREATMENT PROGRAM, IF REQUIRED BY THE BOARD, HIS LICENSES TO PRACTICE MEDICINE AND TO PRESCRIBE AND ADMINISTER CONTROLLED SUBSTANCES WILL BE PLACED ON PROBATION FOR FIVE YEARS WITH CONDITIONS AND RESTRICTIONS. $1,000 FINE.

RAVENSCROFT, WILLIAM III DO OF SALT LAKE CITY, UT, WAS DISCIPLINED BY MISSOURI ON MARCH 4, 1993
DISCIPLINARY ACTION: SURRENDER OF LICENSE
OFFENSE: DISCIPLINARY ACTION BY ANOTHER STATE OR AGENCY

NOTES: PRESCRIPTION VIOLATIONS AND SUBSTANDARD CARE. NO REINSTATEMENT OF LICENSE FOR SEVEN YEARS.

REDD, JAMES D MD, DATE OF BIRTH SEPTEMBER 15, 1948 OF 358 HILLSIDE DR, MOAB, UT, WAS DISCIPLINED BY MEDICARE ON JANUARY 15, 1992
DISCIPLINARY ACTION: 60-MONTH EXCLUSION FROM THE MEDICARE AND/OR MEDICAID PROGRAM
OFFENSE: CRIMINAL CONVICTION OR PLEA OF GUILTY, NOLO CONTENDERE, OR NO CONTEST TO A CRIME

NOTES: PROGRAM-RELATED CONVICTION.

REES, JOSEPH RICHARD MD OF OGDEN, UT, WAS DISCIPLINED BY UTAH ON NOVEMBER 25, 1991
DISCIPLINARY ACTION: 60-MONTH PROBATION; 60-MONTH CONTROLLED SUBSTANCE LICENSE PLACED ON PROBATION
OFFENSE: NONCOMPLIANCE WITH A PROFESSIONAL RULE

NOTES: SELF-ADMINISTRATION OF CONTROLLED SUBSTANCES WITHOUT AUTHORIZATION; FAILURE TO MAINTAIN REQUIRED RECORDS OF CONTROLLED SUBSTANCES PURCHASED AND ADMINISTERED. CONTROLLED SUBSTANCES LICENSE REVOCATION STAYED, AS WAS SUSPENSION ON MEDICAL LICENSE. ON 12/2/96 PROBATIONS ON LICENSES TO PRACTICE MEDICINE AND TO PRESCRIBE AND ADMINISTER CONTROLLED SUBSTANCES WERE TERMINATED AND LICENSES WERE REINSTATED WITH FULL PRIVILEGES.

REES, JOSEPH RICHARD MD OF 924 24TH STREET #4, OGDEN, UT, WAS DISCIPLINED BY WYOMING ON JUNE 23, 1993
DISCIPLINARY ACTION: 36-MONTH MONITORING OF PHYSICIAN PERFORMANCE
OFFENSE: SUBSTANCE ABUSE

NOTES: REVEALED IN HIS APPLICATION FOR LICENSURE THAT HE HAD A PRIOR HISTORY OF ALCOHOL DEPENDENCY. LICENSE ISSUED ON FOLLOWING CONDITIONS: SHALL PARTICIPATE IN A SUBSTANCE ABUSE AFTERCARE PROGRAM; SHALL SUBMIT SEMIANNUAL REPORTS OF HIS PARTICIPATION IN COUNSELING AND MEDICATION MONITORING; IF HE INTENDS TO PRACTICE IN WYOMING HE WILL INFORM THE BOARD 30 DAYS IN ADVANCE AND SHALL SUBMIT COPIES OF URINE SCREENS RECEIVED IN COMPLIANCE WITH AGREEMENT WITH UTAH. FOLLOWING COMPLIANCE WITH TERMS AND CONDITIONS OF THIS ORDER, ON 6/16/96 CONDITIONS EXPIRED AND LICENSE WAS UNRESTRICTED AND WITHOUT CONDITIONS.

REES, JOSEPH RICHARD MD, LICENSE NUMBER 0091549 OF 425 EAST 5350 SOUTH SUITE 120, OGDEN, UT, WAS DISCIPLINED BY NEW YORK ON JULY 19, 1994
DISCIPLINARY ACTION: 24-MONTH PROBATION
OFFENSE: DISCIPLINARY ACTION BY ANOTHER STATE OR AGENCY

NOTES: FOUND GUILTY OF PROFESSIONAL MISCONDUCT BY THE UTAH BOARD. 1 YEAR SUSPENSION STAYED.

REES, JOSEPH RICHARD MD, LICENSE NUMBER 0G15150 OF OGDEN, UT, WAS DISCIPLINED BY CALIFORNIA ON SEPTEMBER 25, 1995
DISCIPLINARY ACTION: 60-MONTH PROBATION
OFFENSE: DISCIPLINARY ACTION BY ANOTHER STATE OR AGENCY

NOTES: DISCIPLINARY ACTION IN UTAH ON 11/25/91 FOR SELF-USE OF DRUGS. ACTION IN WYOMING ON 6/23/93 FOR ALCOHOL ABUSE. ACTION BY THE U.S. AIR FORCE ON 1/29/93 FOR MEDICAL MISMANAGEMENT AND INADEQUATE DOCUMENTATION. REVOCATION, STAYED.

REES, JOSEPH RICHARD MD OF OGDEN, UT, WAS DISCIPLINED BY UTAH ON NOVEMBER 9, 1995
DISCIPLINARY ACTION: RESTRICTION PLACED ON CONTROLLED SUBSTANCE LICENSE
OFFENSE: FAILURE TO COMPLY WITH PREVIOUS BOARD ORDER

NOTES: PRESCRIBED HYDROCODONE OR OTHER

MEDICATIONS CONTAINING THAT CONTROLLED SUBSTANCE CONTRARY TO CURRENT RESTRICTIONS ON HIS LICENSE. HE MUST SUBMIT A COMPREHENSIVE LIST TO THE DIVISION WHICH SETS FORTH THE GENERIC NAMES OF ALL CONTROLLED SUBSTANCES HE BELIEVES ARE NECESSARY TO MAINTAIN HIS SURGICAL PRACTICE. THIS LIST IS TO BE REVIEWED AND APPROVED BY THE PHYSICIANS LICENSING BOARD. HE SHALL NOT PRESCRIBE OR ADMINISTER ANY CONTROLLED SUBSTANCES NOT SPECIFICALLY IDENTIFIED ON THIS LIST. ON 1/29/96 RESTRICTIONS TO PRESCRIBE AND ADMINISTER CONTROLLED SUBSTANCES SCHEDULES II-V WERE TERMINATED. ON 12/2/96 PROBATION ON HIS LICENSE TO PRACTICE MEDICINE AND TO PRESCRIBED AND ADMINISTER CONTROLLED SUBSTANCES WAS TERMINATED AND SAID LICENSES WERE REINSTATED WITH FULL PRIVILEGES.

RIDDLE, BRIAN T MD OF 175 NORTH 100 WEST #103, VERNAL, UT, WAS DISCIPLINED BY IDAHO ON APRIL 29, 1996
DISCIPLINARY ACTION: DENIAL OF NEW LICENSE
OFFENSE: DISCIPLINARY ACTION BY ANOTHER STATE OR AGENCY

NOTES: CONVICTED OF THREE CRIMES INVOLVING MORAL TURPITUDE, INCLUDING PETIT THEFT IN APRIL 1980; SOLICITING SEX ACTS ON OR AROUND JUNE 21, 1985, AND SOLICITING PROSTITUTION ON OR AROUND 4/10/86; PROVIDED INCORRECT INFORMATION ON HIS APPLICATION IN SAYING HE HAD NEVER BEEN SUBJECT TO PROCEEDINGS WHEN IN FACT THE ARMY FOUND PROBLEMS WITH HIS STANDARD OF CARE, AND REQUIRED 100% SUPERVISION FOR THREE MONTHS; DID NOT DISCLOSE THAT HALSTEAD HOSPITAL, KANSAS, DENIED HIS APPLICATION FOR PRIVILEGES; BASED ON THE PEER REVIEW PROCEEDINGS BY THE ARMY, HIS APPLICATION IS INCOMPLETE AND DOES NOT PROVIDE THE BOARD WITH SUFFICIENT INFORMATION TO ESTABLISH QUALIFICATION; FAILED TO APPEAR BEFORE THE BOARD ON THREE SEPARATE OCCASIONS.

RIVERA, ABDIEL MD OF 2400 WEST 7800 SOUTH, WEST JORDAN, UT, WAS DISCIPLINED BY DEA ON FEBRUARY 8, 1994
DISCIPLINARY ACTION: SURRENDER OF CONTROLLED SUBSTANCE LICENSE
OFFENSE: OVERPRESCRIBING OR MISPRESCRIBING DRUGS

NOTES: ARRESTED ON 10/13/93 IN UTAH FOR ISSUING PRESCRIPTIONS FOR SCHEDULE II, III AND IV CONTROLLED DRUGS FOR NO VALID MEDICAL REASON. ALIAS AL RIVERA, ABDIEL RIVERA-VELEZ.

RIVERA-VELEZ, ABDIEL MD OF LAYTON, UT, WAS DISCIPLINED BY UTAH ON OCTOBER 25, 1993
DISCIPLINARY ACTION: SUSPENSION OF CONTROLLED SUBSTANCE LICENSE

NOTES: LICENSE TO PRESCRIBE AND ADMINISTER CONTROLLED SUBSTANCE IS SUSPENDED UNTIL SUCH TIME AS A FINAL ORDER IS ENTERED.

RIVERA-VELEZ, ABDIEL MD OF LAYTON, UT, WAS DISCIPLINED BY UTAH ON JULY 1, 1994
DISCIPLINARY ACTION: LICENSE REVOCATION; REVOCATION OF CONTROLLED SUBSTANCE LICENSE
OFFENSE: OVERPRESCRIBING OR MISPRESCRIBING DRUGS

NOTES: ISSUING PRESCRIPTIONS FOR CONTROLLED SUBSTANCES FOR OTHER THAN LEGITIMATE MEDICAL PURPOSE; PRESCRIBING CONTROLLED SUBSTANCES IN EXCESSIVE QUANTITIES; MAKING FALSE PRESCRIPTIONS; ISSUING PRESCRIPTIONS TO PERSONS KNOWING INFORMATION PROVIDED HIM WAS FALSE; VIOLATION OF THE STANDARDS AND ETHICS OF THE PROFESSION AND ISSUED PRESCRIPTIONS FOR CONTROLLED SUBSTANCES TO KNOWN ADDICTS. HE NEITHER ADMITS TO NOR DENIES THESE ALLEGATIONS.

RODRIGUEZ, FRANCISCO E MD OF SALT LAKE CITY, UT, WAS DISCIPLINED BY ILLINOIS ON MAY 1, 1990
DISCIPLINARY ACTION: 60-MONTH PROBATION
OFFENSE: DISCIPLINARY ACTION BY ANOTHER STATE OR AGENCY

NOTES: LICENSE REVOKED BY LOUISIANA.

RODRIGUEZ, FRANCISCO EDGARDO MD, DATE OF BIRTH APRIL 4, 1950 OF 6832 W NORTH AVENUE, CHICAGO, IL, WAS DISCIPLINED BY MEDICARE ON AUGUST 8, 1990
DISCIPLINARY ACTION: EXCLUSION FROM THE MEDICARE AND/OR MEDICAID PROGRAM
OFFENSE: DISCIPLINARY ACTION BY ANOTHER STATE OR AGENCY

NOTES: LICENSE REVOCATION OR SUSPENSION. REINSTATED ON 4/23/96.

ROGERS, RANDY L MD OF OREM, UT, WAS DISCIPLINED BY UTAH ON SEPTEMBER 2, 1997
DISCIPLINARY ACTION: FINE
OFFENSE: PROFESSIONAL MISCONDUCT

NOTES: HE PRE-SIGNED BLANK PRESCRIPTION FORMS THAT HE GAVE TO A NURSE PRACTITIONER SO THAT SHE COULD WRITE PRESCRIPTIONS TO PATIENTS. THE NURSE PRACTITIONER USED FOUR OF THE PRE-SIGNED BLANK PRESCRIPTION FORMS TO OBTAIN CONTROLLED SUBSTANCES FOR HERSELF OR HER HUSBAND. $2,000 FINE.

ROHLFING, JEFFREY W MD OF FRESNO, CA, WAS DISCIPLINED BY UTAH ON DECEMBER 11, 1997

NOTES: DISCIPLINARY ACTION TAKEN AGAINST HIS MEDICAL LICENSE IN CALIFORNIA. HE AGREED NOT TO PRACTICE MEDICINE IN UTAH BEFORE OR AFTER THE EXPIRATION DATE OF HIS LICENSES TO PRACTICE MEDICINE AND TO PRESCRIBE AND ADMINISTER CONTROLLED SUBSTANCES (WHICH IS 1/31/98). HE AGREED NOT TO RENEW HIS LICENSES. HE FURTHER AGREED THAT NO APPLICATION TO REAPPLY FOR LICENSURE WOULD BE CONSIDERED FOR AT LEAST FIVE YEARS FROM THE DATE OF THE ORDER.

ROHLFING, JEFFREY WILLIAM MD, LICENSE NUMBER C37481 OF FRESNO, CA, WAS DISCIPLINED BY CALIFORNIA ON FEBRUARY 17, 1997
DISCIPLINARY ACTION: 60-MONTH PROBATION
OFFENSE: SUBSTANCE ABUSE

NOTES: IMPAIRMENT DUE TO MENTAL ILLNESS, USE OF ALCOHOLIC BEVERAGES TO AN EXTENT THAT HIS ABILITY TO PRACTICE MEDICINE SAFELY WAS IMPAIRED; FAILURE TO COMPLY WITH THE BOARD'S DIVERSION PROGRAM. REVOCATION STAYED.

ROHLFING, JEFFREY WILLIAM MD, LICENSE NUMBER D9640 OF FRESNO, CA, WAS DISCIPLINED BY TEXAS ON APRIL 4, 1998
OFFENSE: DISCIPLINARY ACTION BY ANOTHER STATE OR AGENCY

NOTES: IN 12/96 THE CALIFORNIA BOARD PLACED HIS LICENSE ON PROBATION FOR EXHIBITING BIZARRE, IRRATIONAL, AND DELUSIONAL BEHAVIOR AND COMMUNICATIONS. LICENSE LIMITED AS FOLLOWS: SHALL NOT PRACTICE MEDICINE IN TEXAS UNTIL HE REQUESTS TO RESUME PRACTICING, APPEARS

BEFORE THE BOARD WITH EVIDENCE THAT HE IS PHYSICALLY, MENTALLY AND OTHERWISE COMPETENT TO SAFELY PRACTICE; SHALL COMPLY WITH THE CALIFORNIA BOARD ORDER; SHALL SHOW THAT HE IS NOT THE SUBJECT OF ANY OTHER CIVIL, CRIMINAL OR ADMINISTRATIVE ACTION.

ROWLAND, GERALD KIM MD OF SALT LAKE CITY, UT, WAS DISCIPLINED BY UTAH ON OCTOBER 29, 1991
DISCIPLINARY ACTION: REPRIMAND
OFFENSE: PROFESSIONAL MISCONDUCT

NOTES: PARTICIPATION IN PREPARATION OF FALSE DOCUMENTS CONCERNING THE MEDICAL TRAINING OF ANOTHER. LETTER OF CENSURE ISSUED.

SANZENBACHER, ERIC D MD OF SALT LAKE CITY, UT, WAS DISCIPLINED BY UTAH ON MARCH 9, 1999
DISCIPLINARY ACTION: REVOCATION OF CONTROLLED SUBSTANCE LICENSE; LICENSE SUSPENSION
OFFENSE: PROVIDING FALSE INFORMATION TO THE BOARD OR OTHER HEALTH AGENCY

NOTES: HE PRESCRIBED CONTROLLED SUBSTANCES TO A NUMBER OF PERSONS WHEN THERE WAS NOT SUFFICIENT MEDICAL NEED FOR SUCH PRESCRIBING; PROVIDED FALSE INFORMATION ON FORMS REQUIRED BY THE UTAH CONTROLLED SUBSTANCE ACT; HAS A SUBSTANCE ABUSE PROBLEM THAT, IF LEFT UNTREATED, COULD IMPAIR HIS ABILITY TO PRACTICE MEDICINE SAFELY. HE MAY NOT REAPPLY FOR LICENSE TO PRESCRIBE AND ADMINISTER CONTROLLED SUBSTANCES FOR FIVE YEARS. LICENSE TO PRACTICE MEDICINE WAS REVOKED WITH A STAY OF ENFORCEMENT ON THE REVOCATION. LICENSE IS SUSPENDED UNTIL HE SUCCESSFULLY COMPLETES A DRUG TREATMENT PROGRAM AND PROVIDES DOCUMENTATION TO THE DIVISION. FOLLOWING THE SUSPENSION, LICENSE WILL BE PLACED ON PROBATION FOR FIVE YEARS WITH CONDITIONS AND RESTRICTIONS. $2,000 FINE.

SANZENBACHER, ERIC D MD OF SALT LAKE CITY, UT, WAS DISCIPLINED BY UTAH ON SEPTEMBER 14, 1999
DISCIPLINARY ACTION: LICENSE SUSPENSION
OFFENSE: NONCOMPLIANCE WITH A PROFESSIONAL RULE

NOTES: FAILED TO APPEAR FOR SCHEDULED DRUG TESTING; FAILED TO ATTEND ALL REQUIRED AFTERCARE MEETINGS; CONSUMED ALCOHOL; AND FAILED TO NOTIFY THE DIVISION OF CRIMINAL CHARGES FILED AGAINST HIM. REVOCATION STAYED; SUSPENSION FOR NOT LESS THAN SIX MONTHS WITH CONDITIONS TO BE MET DURING THE SUSPENSION.

SEEMAN, EUGENE F DO OF SALT LAKE CITY, UT, WAS DISCIPLINED BY UTAH ON DECEMBER 7, 1995
DISCIPLINARY ACTION: SURRENDER OF LICENSE
OFFENSE: PHYSICAL OR MENTAL ILLNESS INHIBITING THE ABILITY TO PRACTICE WITH SKILL AND SAFETY

NOTES: VOLUNTARILY SURRENDERED HIS MEDICAL LICENSE DUE TO HEALTH REASONS.

SHAFER, LELAND W DO OF SALT LAKE CITY, UT, WAS DISCIPLINED BY UTAH ON MAY 9, 1994
DISCIPLINARY ACTION: SURRENDER OF CONTROLLED SUBSTANCE LICENSE

NOTES: VOLUNTARY SURRENDER WITHOUT ADMITTING OR DENYING WRONGDOING, KNOWING OF AN ONGOING INVESTIGATION.

SHAFER, LELAND WILLIAM DO OF 3865 SO WASATCH BLVD #205, SALT LAKE CITY, UT, WAS DISCIPLINED BY DEA ON JUNE 8, 1994
DISCIPLINARY ACTION: SURRENDER OF CONTROLLED SUBSTANCE LICENSE
OFFENSE: DISCIPLINARY ACTION BY ANOTHER STATE OR AGENCY

NOTES: STATE BOARD.

SHARP, JEFFREY A MD, LICENSE NUMBER 0008664, WAS DISCIPLINED BY ARIZONA ON JANUARY 23, 1992
DISCIPLINARY ACTION: 60-MONTH PROBATION; RESTRICTION PLACED ON LICENSE
OFFENSE: SEXUAL ABUSE OF OR SEXUAL MISCONDUCT WITH A PATIENT

NOTES: SEXUAL RELATIONSHIPS WITH A NUMBER OF PATIENTS OVER A TEN YEAR PERIOD; HAS BEEN TREATED FOR DEPRESSION AND PSYCHOSEXUAL DISORDER. MAY PETITION FOR MODIFICATION OR TERMINATION OF PROBATION AFTER THREE YEARS. TERMS AND CONDITIONS: SHALL IMMEDIATELY ENTER INTO OUTPATIENT THERAPY WITH BOARD-APPROVED THERAPIST WHO SHALL RELEASE RECORDS TO BOARD AND SUBMIT QUARTERLY REPORTS; SHALL SUBMIT TO MENTAL OR PHYSICAL EXAMS REQUESTED BY BOARD; SHALL LIMIT PRACTICE TO ADULT MALES, AND WOMEN OVER AGE 55; SHALL APPEAR BEFORE THE BOARD FOR INTERVIEWS UPON REQUEST; SHALL INFORM BOARD OF CHANGE OF ADDRESS OR IF AWAY FOR MORE THAN FIVE DAYS. ISSUED A DECREE OF CENSURE. ON 8/8/98 PROBATION TERMINATED.

SHARP, JEFFREY ALAN MD OF SEDONA, AZ, WAS DISCIPLINED BY UTAH ON FEBRUARY 8, 1993
DISCIPLINARY ACTION: PROBATION; REPRIMAND
OFFENSE: DISCIPLINARY ACTION BY ANOTHER STATE OR AGENCY

NOTES: INAPPROPRIATE CONDUCT WITH A FEMALE PATIENT RESULTING IN DISCIPLINARY ACTION AGAINST HIS MEDICAL LICENSE IN ARIZONA. PROBATION CONSISTENT WITH TERMS OF THE ARIZONA ORDER.

SHUMAKER, SCOTT D MD, LICENSE NUMBER 12581 OF DUNCANSVILLE, PA, WAS DISCIPLINED BY WEST VIRGINIA ON AUGUST 27, 1998
DISCIPLINARY ACTION: SURRENDER OF LICENSE

SHUMAKER, SCOTT D MD, DATE OF BIRTH APRIL 3, 1952 OF 1838 N 2550 EAST, LAYTON, UT, WAS DISCIPLINED BY MEDICARE ON DECEMBER 20, 1998
DISCIPLINARY ACTION: EXCLUSION FROM THE MEDICARE AND/OR MEDICAID PROGRAM
OFFENSE: DISCIPLINARY ACTION BY ANOTHER STATE OR AGENCY

NOTES: LICENSE REVOKED, SUSPENDED, SURRENDERED OR OTHERWISE LOST FOR REASONS BEARING ON PROFESSIONAL PERFORMANCE, PROFESSIONAL COMPETENCE OR FINANCIAL INTEGRITY.

SHUMAKER, SCOTT DANIEL MD, LICENSE NUMBER FE43821 OF LAYTON, UT, WAS DISCIPLINED BY CALIFORNIA ON DECEMBER 26, 1997
DISCIPLINARY ACTION: LICENSE REVOCATION
OFFENSE: DISCIPLINARY ACTION BY ANOTHER STATE OR AGENCY

NOTES: DISCIPLINED BY THE U.S. AIR FORCE DUE TO DEFICIENCIES IN HIS ABILITY TO RECOGNIZE AND TREAT SERIOUS, LIFE-THREATENING ILLNESSES AND TO PROCESS DIAGNOSTIC DATA.

SMITH, TIMOTHY SCOTT DO, LICENSE NUMBER 20A5660 OF KAYSVILLE, UT, WAS DISCIPLINED BY CALIFORNIA ON FEBRUARY

23, 1992
DISCIPLINARY ACTION: LICENSE REVOCATION

NOTES: SELF-USE OF CONTROLLED SUBSTANCES.

SMITH, TIMOTHY SCOTT DO, LICENSE NUMBER 20A5660 OF FULLERTON, CA, WAS DISCIPLINED BY CALIFORNIA ON NOVEMBER 23, 1993
DISCIPLINARY ACTION: LICENSE REINSTATEMENT

NOTES: LICENSE REINSTATED WITH TERMS AND CONDITIONS.

SPAULDING, BRADLEY B MD, LICENSE NUMBER 00M4664, WAS DISCIPLINED BY IDAHO ON FEBRUARY 18, 1994
DISCIPLINARY ACTION: SURRENDER OF LICENSE
OFFENSE: SUBSTANDARD CARE, INCOMPETENCE OR NEGLIGENCE

NOTES: ALLEGATIONS THAT HE PROVIDED HEALTH CARE WHICH FAILS TO MEET COMMUNITY STANDARDS OF CARE WHICH HE DENIES. ON TWO SEPARATE OCCASIONS IN 1992 AND 1993, WAS APPARENTLY UNDER THE INFLUENCE OF DRUGS, ALCOHOL, OR OTHER SUBSTANCES WHILE TREATING THREE PATIENTS. HE SHALL NOT REAPPLY FOR AN IDAHO LICENSE FOR THREE YEARS FROM 6/25/93.

SPAULDING, BRADLEY B MD OF MILFORD, UT, WAS DISCIPLINED BY UTAH ON OCTOBER 18, 1994
DISCIPLINARY ACTION: 60-MONTH PROBATION; 60-MONTH CONTROLLED SUBSTANCE LICENSE PLACED ON PROBATION
OFFENSE: PROFESSIONAL MISCONDUCT

NOTES: UNLAWFULLY OBTAINING AND SELF-ADMINISTERING A SCHEDULE II CONTROLLED SUBSTANCE. REVOCATION STAYED TO PROBATION WITH CONDITIONS.

SPAULDING, BRADLEY B MD OF MILFORD, UT, WAS DISCIPLINED BY UTAH ON OCTOBER 21, 1995
DISCIPLINARY ACTION: 1-MONTH RESTRICTION PLACED ON CONTROLLED SUBSTANCE LICENSE; CONTROLLED SUBSTANCE LICENSE PLACED ON PROBATION
OFFENSE: FAILURE TO COMPLY WITH PREVIOUS BOARD ORDER

NOTES: FAILURE TO COMPLY WITH RESTRICTIONS IMPOSED ON HIS CONTROLLED SUBSTANCE LICENSE. REVOCATION STAYED SUBJECT TO RESTRICTIONS AND CONDITIONS. SCHEDULES II-V SUSPENDED FOR 30 DAYS. CAN ONLY PRESCRIBE AND ADMINISTER IN A HOSPITAL SETTING FOR INPATIENT OR EMERGENCY CARE PATIENTS DURING SUSPENSION. NO OUTPATIENT CARE PRESCRIPTIONS DURING SUSPENSION. FOLLOWING THE SUSPENSION PERIOD, HIS CONTROLLED SUBSTANCE LICENSE WILL REVERT TO ITS PRIOR PROBATIONARY STATUS. ON 11/30/95 SUSPENSION TERMINATED AND LICENSE PUT ON PROBATION CONSISTENT WITH PRIOR TERMS AND CONDITIONS.

SPAULDING, BRADLEY B MD OF MILFORD, UT, WAS DISCIPLINED BY UTAH ON MAY 21, 1997
DISCIPLINARY ACTION: LICENSE REVOCATION; REVOCATION OF CONTROLLED SUBSTANCE LICENSE
OFFENSE: FAILURE TO COMPLY WITH PREVIOUS BOARD ORDER

NOTES: VIOLATED PRIOR PROBATIONARY CONDITIONS; UNLAWFULLY OBTAINED AND USED CONTROLLED SUBSTANCES TO THE EXTENT THAT IT IMPAIRED HIS ABILITY TO SAFELY PRACTICE MEDICINE; ISSUED PRESCRIPTIONS OF CONTROLLED SUBSTANCES FOR OTHER THAN LEGITIMATE MEDICAL PURPOSES; MADE FALSE PRESCRIPTIONS AND GAVE FALSE INFORMATION TO OBTAIN CONTROLLED SUBSTANCES; FAILED TO KEEP RECORDS WITH REGARDS TO CONTROLLED SUBSTANCES.

SPENCER, MAITLAND G MD OF SALT LAKE CITY, UT, WAS DISCIPLINED BY UTAH ON NOVEMBER 25, 1998
DISCIPLINARY ACTION: SURRENDER OF CONTROLLED SUBSTANCE LICENSE; 4-MONTH RESTRICTION PLACED ON CONTROLLED SUBSTANCE LICENSE

NOTES: ENGAGED IN CONDUCT JUSTIFYING THE IMPOSITION OF SANCTIONS. LICENSE RESTRICTED TO SCHEDULES IV AND V, FOLLOWED BY SURRENDER OF LICENSE TO DIVISION.

STANZEL, CSILLA MARIA MD, DATE OF BIRTH APRIL 24, 1943, LICENSE NUMBER 035260L OF 1065 W 400 SOUTH, SALT LAKE CITY, UT, WAS DISCIPLINED BY PENNSYLVANIA ON DECEMBER 6, 1995
DISCIPLINARY ACTION: LICENSE REVOCATION
OFFENSE: DISCIPLINARY ACTION BY ANOTHER STATE OR AGENCY

NOTES: RECIPROCAL ACTION FROM CALIFORNIA.

STEWART, JOHN R MD, DATE OF BIRTH MAY 30, 1942 OF 6408 S. CANYON COVE DRIVE, HOLLADAY, UT, WAS DISCIPLINED BY MEDICARE ON APRIL 12, 1993
DISCIPLINARY ACTION: 60-MONTH EXCLUSION FROM THE MEDICARE AND/OR MEDICAID PROGRAM
OFFENSE: CRIMINAL CONVICTION OR PLEA OF GUILTY, NOLO CONTENDERE, OR NO CONTEST TO A CRIME

NOTES: CONVICTED OF FILING FALSE MEDICAID CLAIMS FOR SERVICES NOT RENDERED.

STEWART, LAMAR H MD OF GUNNISON, UT, WAS DISCIPLINED BY UTAH ON DECEMBER 2, 1996
DISCIPLINARY ACTION: 12-MONTH PROBATION; 12-MONTH CONTROLLED SUBSTANCE LICENSE PLACED ON PROBATION
OFFENSE: OVERPRESCRIBING OR MISPRESCRIBING DRUGS

NOTES: PRESCRIBED CONTROLLED SUBSTANCES IN EXCESS OF WHAT WAS MEDICALLY NECESSARY TO TREAT A PATIENT'S MEDICAL CONDITION. ON 12/23/97 PROBATION ON LICENSES TERMINATED; LICENSES REINSTATED WITH FULL PRIVILEGES.

STEWART, TERESA C MD, DATE OF BIRTH OCTOBER 23, 1953 OF 1062 GATES DRIVE, ROOSEVELT, UT, WAS DISCIPLINED BY MEDICARE ON NOVEMBER 5, 1990
DISCIPLINARY ACTION: 60-MONTH EXCLUSION FROM THE MEDICARE AND/OR MEDICAID PROGRAM
OFFENSE: CRIMINAL CONVICTION OR PLEA OF GUILTY, NOLO CONTENDERE, OR NO CONTEST TO A CRIME

NOTES: PROGRAM-RELATED CONVICTION.

STEWART, TERESA C MD, DATE OF BIRTH OCTOBER 23, 1953, LICENSE NUMBER 0043121 OF 1062 GATES DR, ROOSEVELT, UT, WAS DISCIPLINED BY NEW JERSEY ON APRIL 7, 1992
OFFENSE: DISCIPLINARY ACTION BY ANOTHER STATE OR AGENCY

NOTES: PROHIBITED FROM RESUMING NEW JERSEY PRACTICE UNTIL APPEARING BEFORE THE BOARD TO DISCUSS HER EXCLUSION FROM THE FEDERAL MEDICARE/MEDICAID PROGRAMS. AGREES TO REFRAIN FROM RESUMPTION OF PRACTICE UNTIL THE BOARD DETERMINES HER PRACTICE IS COMPATIBLE WITH THE PUBLIC HEALTH, SAFETY AND WELFARE.

STODDARD, LARRY MD OF 425 EAST 5350 SOUTH #255, OGDEN, UT, WAS DISCIPLINED BY DEA ON JULY 30, 1999
DISCIPLINARY ACTION: SURRENDER OF CONTROLLED SUBSTANCE LICENSE
OFFENSE: DISCIPLINARY ACTION BY ANOTHER STATE OR AGENCY

NOTES: STATE BOARD.

STODDARD, LARRY D MD OF LAYTON, UT, WAS DISCIPLINED BY UTAH ON DECEMBER 22, 1999
DISCIPLINARY ACTION: REVOCATION OF CONTROLLED SUBSTANCE LICENSE; 60-MONTH PROBATION
OFFENSE: SUBSTANCE ABUSE

NOTES: HISTORY OR DRUG ABUSE. FAILED TO MAINTAIN RECORDS WITH REGARDS TO RECEIPT AND DISPOSITION OF THE CONTROLLED SUBSTANCES HE PURCHASED FOR USE IN HIS MEDICAL PRACTICE. REVOCATION STAYED. PROBATION WITH RESTRICTIONS.

STODDARD, LARRY DOUGLAS MD OF LAYTON, UT, WAS DISCIPLINED BY UTAH ON JULY 26, 1999
DISCIPLINARY ACTION: EMERGENCY SUSPENSION

STONE, STEVEN A MD OF SALT LAKE CITY, UT, WAS DISCIPLINED BY UTAH ON MAY 12, 1994
DISCIPLINARY ACTION: SURRENDER OF CONTROLLED SUBSTANCE LICENSE
OFFENSE: OVERPRESCRIBING OR MISPRESCRIBING DRUGS

NOTES: ALLEGATIONS HE ISSUED PRESCRIPTIONS FOR CONTROLLED SUBSTANCES WITHOUT EXAMINING THE PATIENT AND FOR PURPOSE OF SPLITTING OR SHARING THE CONTROLLED SUBSTANCES OBTAINED USING SUCH PRESCRIPTIONS. DID NOT ADMIT OR DENY ANY OF THESE ALLEGATIONS.

STONE, STEVEN A MD OF 5770 SOUTH 250 EAST SUITE 330, MURRY, UT, WAS DISCIPLINED BY DEA ON MAY 13, 1994
DISCIPLINARY ACTION: SURRENDER OF CONTROLLED SUBSTANCE LICENSE

NOTES: IN LIEU OF ORDER TO SHOW CAUSE.

STONE, STEVEN A MD OF SANDY, UT, WAS DISCIPLINED BY UTAH ON APRIL 16, 1996
DISCIPLINARY ACTION: REVOCATION OF CONTROLLED SUBSTANCE LICENSE; PROBATION
OFFENSE: OVERPRESCRIBING OR MISPRESCRIBING DRUGS

NOTES: HE KNOWINGLY AND INTENTIONALLY: ISSUED PRESCRIPTION OF CONTROLLED SUBSTANCES FOR OTHER THAN LEGITIMATE MEDICAL PURPOSES; PRESCRIBED CONTROLLED SUBSTANCES FOR QUANTITIES IN EXCESS OF WHAT WAS MEDICALLY NECESSARY TO TREAT A PATIENT'S CONDITION; OMITTED ENTRIES IN PATIENT RECORDS FOR PRESCRIPTIONS OF CONTROLLED SUBSTANCES; PRESCRIBED CONTROLLED SUBSTANCES FOR PERSONS OTHER THAN HIS PATIENTS. OVER AN EXTENDED PERIOD HE: PRESCRIBED CONTROLLED SUBSTANCES TO HIS PATIENTS WITHOUT FIRST ESTABLISHING ANY MEDICAL NEED; MADE FALSE AND MISLEADING ENTRIES OR OMISSIONS IN PATIENT RECORDS; USED CONTROLLED SUBSTANCES OR ADMINISTERED THEM TO HIMSELF IN A MANNER DANGEROUS AND INJURIOUS TO HIMSELF; AND PRESCRIBED CONTROLLED SUBSTANCES TO A PATIENT HE KNEW TO BE AN ADDICT. LICENSE REVOKED AND STAYED TO PROBATION WITH RESTRICTIONS; NO FUTURE APPLICATION FOR A LICENSE TO PRESCRIBE AND ADMINISTER CONTROLLED SUBSTANCES WILL BE CONSIDERED FOR AT LEAST FIVE YEARS.

STONE, STEVEN A MD OF SANDY, UT, WAS DISCIPLINED BY UTAH ON DECEMBER 17, 1999
DISCIPLINARY ACTION: LICENSE REVOCATION
OFFENSE: FAILURE TO COMPLY WITH PREVIOUS BOARD ORDER

NOTES: FAILED TO COMPLY WITH PROBATIONARY CONDITIONS IMPOSED ON HIS LICENSE BY A PRIOR ORDER WHEN HE FAILED TO INFORM THE BOARD OF A PRIMARY CARE PHYSICIAN WHO WOULD BE RESPONSIBLE TO PRESCRIBE ANY DRUGS OR CONTROLLED SUBSTANCES FOR HIM; FAILED TO PROVIDE A COPY OF EACH CONTROLLED SUBSTANCE PRESCRIPTION WRITTEN FOR HIM TO THE BOARD WITHIN 48 HOURS; ENGAGED IN UNPROFESSIONAL CONDUCT WHEN HE PRACTICED MEDICINE ON THREE OCCASIONS AFTER CONSUMING ALCOHOL TO THE EXTENT IT MIGHT REASONABLY BE CONSIDERED TO HAVE IMPAIRED HIS ABILITY TO SAFELY PRACTICE MEDICINE; PRESCRIBED FIORICET, A CONTROLLED SUBSTANCE, AT TIMES THAT HIS LICENSE TO PRESCRIBE AND ADMINISTER CONTROLLED SUBSTANCES WAS REVOKED; ALSO PRACTICED WITHOUT AN APPROVED PRACTICE PLAN AND BEYOND THE SUPERVISION OF ANY DULY APPROVED PHYSICIAN.

SULLIVAN, WESLEY K MD OF TOOELE, UT, WAS DISCIPLINED BY UTAH ON MAY 31, 1991
DISCIPLINARY ACTION: 1-MONTH SUSPENSION OF CONTROLLED SUBSTANCE LICENSE; 60-MONTH PROBATION
OFFENSE: PROFESSIONAL MISCONDUCT

NOTES: UNLAWFULLY OBTAINING AND USING A SCHEDULED CONTROLLED DRUG. AFTER THE SUSPENSION PERIOD, MAY ORDER CONTROLLED SUBSTANCES IN A HOSPITAL SETTING, BUT SHALL HAVE NO DIRECT ACCESS TO OR ADMINISTER SUCH SUBSTANCES; SHALL HAVE NO ABILITY TO PRESCRIBE OR ADMINISTER CONTROLLED SUBSTANCES IN HIS PRIVATE PRACTICE OF MEDICINE FOR TWO YEARS. ORDER UPHELD IN ITS ENTIRETY 8/27/91. ON 12/16/97 PROBATION ON LICENSES TERMINATED; REINSTATED WITH FULL PRIVILEGES.

SULLIVAN, WESLEY K MD OF TOOELE, UT, WAS DISCIPLINED BY UTAH ON FEBRUARY 12, 1993
DISCIPLINARY ACTION: REPRIMAND; RESTRICTION PLACED ON CONTROLLED SUBSTANCE LICENSE
OFFENSE: PROFESSIONAL MISCONDUCT

NOTES: EXERCISE OF POOR JUDGMENT IN A PERSONAL RELATIONSHIP WITH A FEMALE PATIENT.

SULLIVAN, WESLEY KIM MD, LICENSE NUMBER 0024765 OF 170 E ALTAMIRA DR, CEDAR CITY, UT, WAS DISCIPLINED BY GEORGIA ON SEPTEMBER 26, 1991
DISCIPLINARY ACTION: NONRENEWAL OF LICENSE
OFFENSE: DISCIPLINARY ACTION BY ANOTHER STATE OR AGENCY

NOTES: DISCIPLINARY ACTION IN UTAH. ADMINISTRATIVE REVOCATION FOR FAILURE TO RENEW.

SULLIVAN, WESLEY KIM MD, DATE OF BIRTH NOVEMBER 18, 1954, LICENSE NUMBER 0066246 OF SHELBY, OH, WAS DISCIPLINED BY OHIO ON JANUARY 12, 1994
DISCIPLINARY ACTION: PROBATION; RESTRICTION PLACED ON LICENSE
OFFENSE: DISCIPLINARY ACTION BY ANOTHER STATE OR AGENCY

NOTES: PRIOR ACTION BY UTAH BOARD WHICH HAD BEEN BASED ON A HISTORY OF IMPAIRMENT; FAILURE TO PROVIDE OHIO MEDICAL BOARD WITH COMPLETE INFORMATION ABOUT DENIAL OF APPLICATION FOR MEDICAL LICENSURE IN CALIFORNIA AND ABOUT PETITION FILED BY UTAH BOARD ALLEGING THAT HE HAD ENGAGED IN A SEXUAL RELATIONSHIP WITH A PATIENT WHO HAD A HISTORY OF MANIC-

DEPRESSION. LICENSE GRANTED SUBJECT TO STAYED PERMANENT REVOCATION AND REPRIMAND. AGREEMENT TO REMAIN IN EFFECT FOR A MINIMUM OF THREE YEARS PRIOR TO ANY REQUEST FOR TERMINATION. PROBATION MODIFIED ON 5/11/94 TO REDUCE NUMBER OF REQUIRED AA MEETINGS TO TWO MEETINGS PER WEEK. PROBATION MODIFIED ON 11/10/94 GRANTING HIS REQUESTS TO SUBMIT TRIPLICATE PRESCRIPTION FORMS IN LIEU OF A LOG OF PRESCRIPTIONS, SUBMIT A COPY OF THE HOSPITAL PHARMACY LOG WITH HIS SIGNATURE ATTACHED IN PLACE OF HIS OWN LOG OF MEDICATIONS ORDERED BY HIM IN THE HOSPITAL FOR A TRIAL PERIOD OF SIX MONTHS, AND WAIVE THE COUNTERSIGNATURE REQUIREMENT. ON 5/11/95 THE BOARD GRANTED HIS REQUEST TO CHANGE HIS DRUG SCREENS FROM ONE RANDOM WEEKLY TO ONE RANDOM MONTHLY; HIS REQUEST FOR A CHANGE IN HIS APPEARANCE SCHEDULE FROM ONCE EVERY THREE MONTHS TO ONCE EVERY SIX MONTHS; AND TO CHANGE THE AA LOG REQUIREMENT TO ONE SIGNATURE PER WEEK.

TARASZKA, STEVEN R MD, LICENSE NUMBER 0009157 OF ATLANTA, GA, WAS DISCIPLINED BY VERMONT ON FEBRUARY 8, 1996
DISCIPLINARY ACTION: SURRENDER OF LICENSE
OFFENSE: SUBSTANCE ABUSE

NOTES: ADMITTED HE SUFFERS FROM CHEMICAL ADDICTION. VOLUNTARY SURRENDER IN LIEU OF SUMMARY SUSPENSION HEARING; AGREED THAT HE SHALL NEVER SEEK LICENSURE IN VERMONT, AND THAT TERMS OF THE STIPULATION AND UNDERLYING FACTUAL BASIS CAN BE DISCLOSED TO OTHER LICENSING AUTHORITIES.

TARASZKA, STEVEN R MD, LICENSE NUMBER 00AAAA2, WAS DISCIPLINED BY RHODE ISLAND ON MARCH 13, 1996
DISCIPLINARY ACTION: DENIAL OF NEW LICENSE
OFFENSE: DISCIPLINARY ACTION BY ANOTHER STATE OR AGENCY

NOTES: ACTS IN ANOTHER JURISDICTION WHICH ARE GROUNDS FOR DISCIPLINE IN RHODE ISLAND.

TARASZKA, STEVEN R MD, WAS DISCIPLINED BY ALASKA ON MAY 2, 1996
OFFENSE: SUBSTANCE ABUSE

NOTES: SUBSTANCE ABUSE. CANNOT PRACTICE IN ALASKA UNTIL HE CAN PROVE HE CAN DO SO SAFELY. MUST COMPLY WITH RECOMMENDATIONS OF THE TREATMENT FACILITY AND BOARD PRIOR TO RESUMING HIS MEDICAL PRACTICE.

TARASZKA, STEVEN R MD, WAS DISCIPLINED BY KANSAS ON JULY 1, 1996
DISCIPLINARY ACTION: DENIAL OF NEW LICENSE
OFFENSE: DISCIPLINARY ACTION BY ANOTHER STATE OR AGENCY

NOTES: SURRENDERED HIS LICENSE IN VERMONT ON 2/8/96 BASED IN PART ON AN ADMISSION OF CHEMICAL ADDICTION.

TARASZKA, STEVEN R MD, WAS DISCIPLINED BY NEW MEXICO ON SEPTEMBER 1, 1996

NOTES: BOARD ACCEPTED WITHDRAWAL OF APPLICATION WITH AGREEMENT TO NEVER REAPPLY IN NEW MEXICO.

TARASZKA, STEVEN R MD, DATE OF BIRTH APRIL 22, 1965, LICENSE NUMBER 0063345 OF 4060 PEACHTREE RD NE SUITE D-252, ATLANTA, GA, WAS DISCIPLINED BY NEW JERSEY ON OCTOBER 21, 1996
DISCIPLINARY ACTION: SURRENDER OF LICENSE
OFFENSE: DISCIPLINARY ACTION BY ANOTHER STATE OR AGENCY

NOTES: ACTION IN VERMONT FOR SUBSTANCE ABUSE. MINIMUM THREE MONTH SURRENDER. SHALL APPEAR BEFORE THE BOARD TO DISCUSS HIS COMPLIANCE AND DEMONSTRATE HIS FITNESS TO REENTER ACTIVE PRACTICE PRIOR TO RESTORATION OF LICENSE.

TARASZKA, STEVEN R MD, WAS DISCIPLINED BY ALABAMA ON OCTOBER 30, 1996
DISCIPLINARY ACTION: LICENSE REVOCATION
OFFENSE: DISCIPLINARY ACTION BY ANOTHER STATE OR AGENCY

NOTES: VOLUNTARY SURRENDER OF HIS LICENSE IN VERMONT; AGREEMENT TO NEVER SEEK RELICENSURE THERE AND HIS ADMISSION THAT HE SUFFERS FROM THE DISEASE OF CHEMICAL ADDICTION.

TARASZKA, STEVEN R MD, DATE OF BIRTH APRIL 22, 1963, LICENSE NUMBER 0036885 OF 4060 PEACHTREE ROAD, SUITE D-252, ATLANTA, GA, WAS DISCIPLINED BY GEORGIA ON NOVEMBER 8, 1996
DISCIPLINARY ACTION: LICENSE SUSPENSION

NOTES: SHALL NOT PRACTICE AS A PHYSICIAN IN GEORGIA UNTIL FURTHER ORDER OF THE BOARD. INDEFINITE SUSPENSION.

TARASZKA, STEVEN R MD, LICENSE NUMBER 053145 OF ATLANTA, GA, WAS DISCIPLINED BY VIRGINIA ON JANUARY 7, 1997
DISCIPLINARY ACTION: LICENSE SUSPENSION
OFFENSE: DISCIPLINARY ACTION BY ANOTHER STATE OR AGENCY

NOTES: SUSPENSION OF LICENSE BY FLORIDA MEDICAL BOARD, DUE TO ACTION TAKEN BY VERMONT MEDICAL BOARD FOR CHEMICAL DEPENDENCY.

TARASZKA, STEVEN R MD, DATE OF BIRTH APRIL 22, 1963, LICENSE NUMBER 036885 OF 4060 PEACHTREE ROAD, SUITE D-252, ATLANTA, GA, WAS DISCIPLINED BY GEORGIA ON OCTOBER 2, 1997
DISCIPLINARY ACTION: 60-MONTH PROBATION
OFFENSE: DISCIPLINARY ACTION BY ANOTHER STATE OR AGENCY

NOTES: DISCIPLINARY ACTION IN VERMONT; IMPAIRMENT.

TARASZKA, STEVEN ROBERT MD, LICENSE NUMBER 0069664 OF ATLANTA, GA, WAS DISCIPLINED BY FLORIDA ON FEBRUARY 16, 1996
DISCIPLINARY ACTION: EMERGENCY SUSPENSION
OFFENSE: DISCIPLINARY ACTION BY ANOTHER STATE OR AGENCY

NOTES: BEING UNABLE TO PRACTICE MEDICINE WITH REASONABLE SKILL AND SAFETY TO PATIENTS BY REASON OF ILLNESS OR USE OF ALCOHOL, DRUGS, NARCOTICS, CHEMICALS, OR ANY OTHER TYPE OF MATERIAL OR AS A RESULT OF ANY MENTAL OR PHYSICAL CONDITION.

TARASZKA, STEVEN ROBERT MD, LICENSE NUMBER 0069664 OF ATLANTA, GA, WAS DISCIPLINED BY FLORIDA ON JULY 15, 1996
DISCIPLINARY ACTION: LICENSE SUSPENSION
OFFENSE: DISCIPLINARY ACTION BY ANOTHER STATE OR AGENCY

NOTES: CHARGED WITH HAVING LICENSE ACTED UPON BY ANOTHER JURISDICTION. BEING UNABLE TO PRACTICE MEDICINE WITH REASONABLE SKILL AND SAFETY TO PATIENTS BY REASON OF ILLNESS OR USE OF ALCOHOL, DRUGS, NARCOTICS, CHEMICALS OR

ANY OTHER TYPE OF MATERIAL, OR AS A RESULT OF ANY MENTAL OR PHYSICAL CONDITION. SUSPENSION UNTIL HE APPEARS AND DEMONSTRATES TO THE BOARD THAT HE CAN PRACTICE MEDICINE WITH REASONABLE SKILL AND SAFETY.

TARASZKA, STEVEN ROBERT MD, DATE OF BIRTH APRIL 22, 1965, LICENSE NUMBER 0014396 OF 4060 PEACHTREE ROAD, SUITE D252, ATLANTA, GA, WAS DISCIPLINED BY MISSISSIPPI ON JULY 18, 1996
DISCIPLINARY ACTION: LICENSE REVOCATION

TARASZKA, STEVEN ROBERT MD OF ATLANTA, GA, WAS DISCIPLINED BY UTAH ON OCTOBER 4, 1996
DISCIPLINARY ACTION: LICENSE REVOCATION
OFFENSE: DISCIPLINARY ACTION BY ANOTHER STATE OR AGENCY
NOTES: ACTION IN VERMONT.

TARASZKA, STEVEN ROBERT MD, DATE OF BIRTH APRIL 22, 1965, LICENSE NUMBER 9600070 OF ATLANTA, GA, WAS DISCIPLINED BY NORTH CAROLINA ON OCTOBER 17, 1996
DISCIPLINARY ACTION: EMERGENCY SUSPENSION
OFFENSE: DISCIPLINARY ACTION BY ANOTHER STATE OR AGENCY
NOTES: SURRENDERED HIS LICENSE IN VERMONT DUE TO ALLEGATIONS OF NARCOTIC ADDICTION. MAY BE UNABLE TO PRACTICE MEDICINE WITH REASONABLE SKILL AND SAFETY BY REASON OF DRUNKENNESS, EXCESSIVE USE OF ALCOHOL, DRUGS, CHEMICALS, OR ANY OTHER TYPE OF MATERIAL. ON 3/18/98 SUMMARY SUSPENSION LIFTED AND DISMISSED WITHOUT PREJUDICE. LICENSE LIMITED AS FOLLOWS: SHALL NOT PRACTICE ANESTHESIA; MAY PRACTICE ONLY IN A BOARD-APPROVED STRUCTURED SETTING; UNLESS LAWFULLY PRESCRIBED BY SOMEONE ELSE, SHALL REFRAIN FROM THE USE OF MIND OR MOOD ALTERING SUBSTANCES AND FROM THE USE OF ALCOHOL; SHALL REPORT TO THE BOARD WITHIN TWO WEEKS ANY USE OF SUCH MEDICATION OR ALCOHOL, INCLUDING THE IDENTIFICATION OF THE PRESCRIBER AND THE PHARMACY FILLING THE PRESCRIPTION; SHALL UNDERGO DRUG AND ALCOHOL SCREENS AS REQUESTED BY THE BOARD; IF HE RESIDES IN NORTH CAROLINA, SHALL MAINTAIN AND ABIDE BY A CONTRACT WITH THE NORTH CAROLINA PHYSICIANS HEALTH PROGRAM; SHALL NOT PRESCRIBE ANY DRUG FOR HIS OWN USE; MUST COMPLY WITH OTHER CONDITIONS.

TARASZKA, STEVEN ROBERT MD, LICENSE NUMBER 1044378 OF 4060 PEACHTREE ROAD NE #D252, ATLANTA, GA, WAS DISCIPLINED BY INDIANA ON FEBRUARY 6, 1997
DISCIPLINARY ACTION: LICENSE SUSPENSION
OFFENSE: DISCIPLINARY ACTION BY ANOTHER STATE OR AGENCY
NOTES: ON 2/1/96 VERMONT FILED A PETITION FOR EMERGENCY SUSPENSION AGAINST HIS MEDICAL LICENSE ALLEGING THAT ON 11/7/95 THE BOARD HAD BEEN NOTIFIED BY THE SPRINGFIELD POLICE DEPARTMENT THAT DRUG PARAPHERNALIA HAD BEEN FOUND IN THE MOTEL ROOM VACATED BY HIM, A LICENSED PHYSICIAN SPECIALIZING IN ANESTHESIOLOGY. THE MATERIALS FOUND IN THE TOILET HAD CAUSED THE SEPTIC SYSTEM OF THE HOTEL TO BE SHUT DOWN ON TWO OCCASIONS. THE EMPTY GLASS VIALS THAT WERE FOUND THERE WERE LABELED VERSED AND STADOL AND MARKED WITH LOT NUMBERS THAT CORRESPONDED WITH THOSE DISPENSED TO THE SPRINGFIELD HOSPITAL. 21 SYRINGES WERE SUBSEQUENTLY FOUND IN THE BASE OF THE TOILET OF HIS HOTEL ROOM. SPRINGFIELD HOSPITAL OFFICIALS DISCOVERED AFTER AUDITING PHARMACY RECORDS THAT THE ANESTHESIOLOGY DEPARTMENT HAD ORDERED UNUSUALLY LARGE AMOUNTS OF CONTROLLED SUBSTANCES DURING THE MONTHS THAT HE WORKED AT THE FACILITY, AND POLICE DISCOVERED THAT HE HAD WRITTEN SOME UNUSUAL PRESCRIPTIONS. IN 11/95 HE WASTED A VIAL OF COCAINE WITHOUT A WITNESS TO CO-SIGN THE WASTAGE AS REQUIRED BY HOSPITAL POLICY. IN 1995 HE ALSO FORMED A RELATIONSHIP WITH A FEMALE PATIENT, FOR WHOM HE WROTE PRESCRIPTIONS AND HAD HER FILL THE PRESCRIPTIONS AND THEN DELIVER THE MEDICATION TO HIM. ON 2/7/96 HE ENTERED INTO AN AGREEMENT FOR VOLUNTARY SURRENDER OF LICENSE WITH THE VERMONT BOARD, CONTAINING HIS ADMISSIONS THAT HE SUFFERS FROM CHEMICAL ADDICTION AND THAT HIS DISEASE CONSTITUTES A THREAT TO THE HEALTH, SAFETY, AND WELFARE OF HIS PATIENTS. HE AGREED NEVER TO SEEK RELICENSURE IN VERMONT.

TARASZKA, STEVEN ROBERT MD, LICENSE NUMBER 19620 OF ATLANTA, OR, WAS DISCIPLINED BY OREGON ON MAY 1, 1997
DISCIPLINARY ACTION: LICENSE REVOCATION
NOTES:

TARASZKA, STEVEN ROBERT MD, DATE OF BIRTH APRIL 22, 1965 OF 4060 PEACHTREE ROAD, SUITE D252, ATLANTA, GA, WAS DISCIPLINED BY MEDICARE ON SEPTEMBER 7, 1997
DISCIPLINARY ACTION: EXCLUSION FROM THE MEDICARE AND/OR MEDICAID PROGRAM
OFFENSE: DISCIPLINARY ACTION BY ANOTHER STATE OR AGENCY
NOTES: LICENSE REVOKED, SUSPENDED, SURRENDERED OR OTHERWISE LOST FOR REASONS BEARING ON PROFESSIONAL PERFORMANCE, PROFESSIONAL COMPETENCE OR FINANCIAL INTEGRITY. REINSTATED ON 4/1/98.

TARASZKA, STEVEN ROBERT MD, DATE OF BIRTH APRIL 22, 1965, LICENSE NUMBER 056084L OF 7202 SLOAN SQUARE NE, ATLANTA, GA, WAS DISCIPLINED BY PENNSYLVANIA ON OCTOBER 21, 1997
DISCIPLINARY ACTION: LICENSE REVOCATION
OFFENSE: DISCIPLINARY ACTION BY ANOTHER STATE OR AGENCY
NOTES: DISCIPLINARY ACTION TAKEN AGAINST HIS LICENSE BY VERMONT, NORTH CAROLINA, RHODE ISLAND, KANSAS, FLORIDA, MISSISSIPPI, TENNESSEE, ILLINOIS, GEORGIA, AND VIRGINIA FOR PERSONAL USE/ADDICTION.

TARASZKA, STEVEN ROBERT MD, LICENSE NUMBER 69933 OF ATLANTA, GA, WAS DISCIPLINED BY OHIO ON DECEMBER 4, 1997
DISCIPLINARY ACTION: LICENSE REVOCATION
OFFENSE: SUBSTANCE ABUSE
NOTES: INABILITY TO PRACTICE ACCORDING TO ACCEPTABLE AND PREVAILING STANDARDS OF CARE DUE TO HABITUAL OR EXCESSIVE USE OF DRUGS, ALCOHOL, OR OTHER SUBSTANCES THAT IMPAIR ABILITY TO PRACTICE. PERMANENT REVOCATION AUTHORIZED BY DOCTOR IN LIEU OF FORMAL DISCIPLINARY PROCEEDINGS.

THOMASON, ISAAC RAY MD OF BOUNTIFUL, UT, WAS DISCIPLINED BY UTAH ON JULY 30, 1996
DISCIPLINARY ACTION: 60-MONTH PROBATION; 60-MONTH CONTROLLED SUBSTANCE LICENSE PLACED ON PROBATION
OFFENSE: SEXUAL ABUSE OF OR SEXUAL MISCONDUCT WITH A PATIENT

NOTES: ENGAGED IN INTIMATE PHYSICAL RELATIONS WITH A FEMALE PATIENT IN VIOLATION OF MEDICAL ETHICAL STANDARDS; FAILED TO KEEP ADEQUATE RECORDS OF PRESCRIPTIONS FOR CONTROLLED SUBSTANCES; FALSIFIED A PRESCRIPTION FOR A CONTROLLED SUBSTANCE. REVOCATION, STAYED. PROBATION WITH CONDITIONS.

THOMASON, ISAAC RAY MD OF BOUNTIFUL, UT, WAS DISCIPLINED BY UTAH ON APRIL 29, 1997
DISCIPLINARY ACTION: RESTRICTION PLACED ON LICENSE; RESTRICTION PLACED ON CONTROLLED SUBSTANCE LICENSE

NOTES: ADDITIONAL CONDITIONS AND RESTRICTIONS IMPOSED.

TIMPSON, DAVID G MD OF PROVO, UT, WAS DISCIPLINED BY UTAH ON NOVEMBER 9, 1994
DISCIPLINARY ACTION: 24-MONTH PROBATION; 24-MONTH CONTROLLED SUBSTANCE LICENSE PLACED ON PROBATION
OFFENSE: OVERPRESCRIBING OR MISPRESCRIBING DRUGS

NOTES: FAILURE TO MAINTAIN RECORDS OF CONTROLLED SUBSTANCES PRESCRIBED; PRESCRIBING CONTROLLED SUBSTANCES TO A DRUG DEPENDENT PATIENT FOR OTHER THAN LEGITIMATE MEDICAL PURPOSES. DID NOT ADMIT OR DENY ALLEGATIONS. ON 12/02/96 PROBATION TERMINATED AND REINSTATED WITH FULL PRIVILEGES.

TOPHAM, EARL BARRY MD, DATE OF BIRTH JANUARY 4, 1942, LICENSE NUMBER 0156285 OF SALT LAKE CITY, UT, WAS DISCIPLINED BY UTAH ON APRIL 15, 1991
DISCIPLINARY ACTION: 6-MONTH LICENSE SUSPENSION; 36-MONTH PROBATION
OFFENSE: SEXUAL ABUSE OF OR SEXUAL MISCONDUCT WITH A PATIENT

NOTES: ON OR ABOUT 5/24/89 A PATIENT HE WAS SEEING FOR ACNE TREATMENT ATTEMPTED SUICIDE; THE NEXT DAY THIS PATIENT SAW HIM FOR TREATMENT AND THEY DISCUSSED THE SUICIDE ATTEMPT; SHORTLY THEREAFTER HE ENGAGED THE PATIENT IN SEXUAL RELATIONS IN THE EXAMINATION ROOM; HAD BEEN FORMALLY CENSURED BY THE MEDICAL SOCIETY FOR THIS CONDUCT IN 10/90; ALSO, WAS PLACED ON PROBATION WITH CONDITIONS BY MEDICAL SOCIETY ON OR ABOUT 10/18/90; REMAINDER OF TWO YEAR SUSPENSION STAYED. CONDITIONS OF PROBATION: SHALL MEET WITH THE BOARD UPON REQUEST; SHALL CONTINUE IN TREATMENT WITH PERIODIC PROGRESS REPORTS TO THE BOARD; SHALL HAVE AN ADULT STAFF PERSON WITH HIM AT ALL TIMES WHEN TREATING AN UNACCOMPANIED FEMALE PATIENT. ON 10/17/91 SUSPENSION TERMINATED AND HE SHALL PRACTICE ON PROBATION UNDER THE TERMS OF THIS ORDER. ON 11/2/93 PROBATION TERMINATED AND LICENSE REINSTATED WITH FULL PRIVILEGES.

TOPHAM, EARL BARRY MD, LICENSE NUMBER 0156285 OF SALT LAKE CITY, UT, WAS DISCIPLINED BY UTAH ON DECEMBER 12, 1996
DISCIPLINARY ACTION: 60-MONTH RESTRICTION PLACED ON LICENSE; MONITORING OF PHYSICIAN PERFORMANCE
OFFENSE: PROFESSIONAL MISCONDUCT

NOTES: IN 3/94 ALLEGEDLY ENGAGED IN UNPROFESSIONAL CONDUCT WHILE TREATING A FEMALE PATIENT WHICH INVOLVED INAPPROPRIATE TOUCHING AND COMMENTS; HE THEN OFFERED HER $500 TO AVOID A LAWSUIT. HE DENIES ANY WRONGDOING BUT AGREES TO CONDITIONS AS FOLLOWS: WITHIN 90 DAYS MUST BE EVALUATED BY QUALIFIED HEALTH CARE PROVIDERS APPROVED BY THE BOARD; DURING A PERIOD NOT TO EXCEED FIVE YEARS, HE SHALL MEET WITH THE BOARD ON A QUARTERLY BASIS AND SUBMIT DOCUMENTATION THAT DEMONSTRATES HIS COMPLIANCE WITH THESE OR ANY SUBSEQUENT CONDITIONS; DURING THE ABOVE FIVE YEAR PERIOD, HE SHALL HAVE AN ADULT ASSISTANT PRESENT WHEN HE EXAMINES OR TREATS UNACCOMPANIED FEMALE PATIENTS WHO SHALL SIGN THE MEDICAL CHART ATTESTING TO THEIR ATTENDANCE DURING THE EXAMINATION OR TREATMENT; IF HE DECIDES TO LEAVE UTAH TO RESIDE OR PRACTICE MEDICINE IN ANOTHER STATE, HE SHALL NOTIFY THE BOARD IN WRITING WITHIN 14 DAYS PRIOR TO HIS DEPARTURE AND ANY SUCH PERIOD OF RESIDENCY OUTSIDE UTAH SHALL NOT COUNT TOWARDS THE ABOVE CONDITIONS UNLESS HE CONTINUES TO SHOW COMPLIANCE.

TOPHAM, EARL BARRY MD OF SALT LAKE CITY, UT, WAS DISCIPLINED BY UTAH ON JUNE 3, 1997
DISCIPLINARY ACTION: RESTRICTION PLACED ON LICENSE; RESTRICTION PLACED ON CONTROLLED SUBSTANCE LICENSE

NOTES: ADDITIONAL CONDITIONS AND RESTRICTIONS IMPOSED.

UDALL, MARC RICHARD MD OF OREM, UT, WAS DISCIPLINED BY UTAH ON SEPTEMBER 2, 1997
DISCIPLINARY ACTION: FINE
OFFENSE: PROFESSIONAL MISCONDUCT

NOTES: HE PRE-SIGNED BLANK PRESCRIPTION FORMS THAT HE GAVE TO A NURSE PRACTITIONER SO THAT SHE COULD WRITE PRESCRIPTIONS TO PATIENTS. THE NURSE PRACTITIONER USED FOUR OF THE PRE-SIGNED BLANK PRESCRIPTION FORMS TO OBTAIN CONTROLLED SUBSTANCES FOR HERSELF OR HER HUSBAND. $2,000 FINE.

VINCENT, PAMELA MD, DATE OF BIRTH NOVEMBER 15, 1952, LICENSE NUMBER 29118 OF 1055 NORTH 399TH WEST, PROVO, UT, WAS DISCIPLINED BY WISCONSIN ON NOVEMBER 20, 1997
DISCIPLINARY ACTION: NONRENEWAL OF LICENSE
OFFENSE: SUBSTANDARD CARE, INCOMPETENCE OR NEGLIGENCE

NOTES: INVESTIGATION INVOLVING ALLEGATIONS OF THE APPROPRIATENESS OF HER READING OF A PATIENT'S EKGS AT AN URGENT CARE CENTER AND THE TIMELINESS OF THE TRANSFER OF THAT PATIENT TO THE EMERGENCY ROOM; SHE HAS NOT PRACTICED MEDICINE AND SURGERY IN WISCONSIN SINCE 1993 AND IS CURRENTLY ENGAGED IN THE PRACTICE OF NEUROLOGY IN PROVO, UTAH. INVESTIGATION CLOSED WITHOUT FURTHER PROCEEDINGS. SHALL NOT REREGISTER AT ANY TIME IN THE FUTURE.

WADDINGHAM, RAND E MD, LICENSE NUMBER H5214 OF CRANE, TX, WAS DISCIPLINED BY TEXAS ON AUGUST 9, 1997
DISCIPLINARY ACTION: FINE; REQUIRED TO TAKE ADDITIONAL MEDICAL EDUCATION
OFFENSE: PROFESSIONAL MISCONDUCT

NOTES: HE TREATED A FAMILY MEMBER WHO HAD PREVIOUSLY ABUSED CONTROLLED SUBSTANCES, INSTEAD OF CONTACTING ANOTHER PHYSICIAN; HE FAILED TO KEEP ADEQUATE RECORDS CONCERNING HIS PRESCRIBING TO THIS PATIENT; HE PRESCRIBED AND ADMINISTERED CONTROLLED SUBSTANCES TO ANOTHER PATIENT WITH A POSSIBLE CHEMICAL DEPENDENCY; HE FAILED TO ADEQUATELY SUPERVISE A NURSE PRACTITIONER WHO IMPROPERLY ADMINISTERED PRESCRIPTION DRUGS TO ONE OF THESE TWO PATIENTS. SHALL ADHERE

TO THE FOLLOWING CONDITIONS FOR TWO YEARS: SHALL OBTAIN AT LEAST 50 HOURS PER YEAR OF CONTINUING MEDICAL EDUCATION INCLUDING ONE COURSE IN RISK MANAGEMENT AND ONE COURSE IN PAIN MANAGEMENT; SHALL TAKE AND PASS THE MEDICAL JURISPRUDENCE EXAM WITHIN ONE YEAR; $2,500 FINE TO BE PAID; SHALL GIVE A COPY OF THIS ORDER TO ANY HEALTH CARE ENTITY WHERE HE HAS PRIVILEGES; SHALL PROVIDE A COPY OF THIS ORDER TO ANYONE REQUESTING IT WITHIN 10 DAYS; TIME SPENT OUT OF TEXAS DOES NOT COUNT TOWARD RESTRICTION; SHALL INFORM THE BOARD OF CHANGE OF ADDRESS WITHIN 10 DAYS OR IF HE LEAVES THE STATE; SHALL NOT SEEK MODIFICATION FOR ONE YEAR. ON 8/22/98 THE ORDER WAS TERMINATED.

WADDINGHAM, RAND EDWARD MD OF ANDREWS, TX, WAS DISCIPLINED BY UTAH ON JULY 1, 1998
DISCIPLINARY ACTION: PROBATION; CONTROLLED SUBSTANCE LICENSE PLACED ON PROBATION
OFFENSE: DISCIPLINARY ACTION BY ANOTHER STATE OR AGENCY

NOTES: DISCIPLINARY ACTION TAKEN AGAINST HIS MEDICAL LICENSE IN TEXAS. LICENSE TO PRACTICE MEDICINE IN UTAH CONDITIONED CONSISTENT WITH THE TERMS AND CONDITIONS PLACED ON HIS TEXAS LICENSE. ON 10/23/98 PROBATION ON LICENSES TO PRACTICE MEDICINE AND TO PRESCRIBE AND ADMINISTER CONTROLLED SUBSTANCES WAS TERMINATED AND SAID LICENSES WERE REINSTATED WITH FULL PRIVILEGES.

WALLACE, SCOTT PYPER MD OF 1275 NORTH UNIVERSITY AVE, PROVO, UT, WAS DISCIPLINED BY DEA ON JUNE 6, 1991
DISCIPLINARY ACTION: RESTRICTION PLACED ON CONTROLLED SUBSTANCE LICENSE
OFFENSE: OVERPRESCRIBING OR MISPRESCRIBING DRUGS

NOTES: PRESCRIBED CONTROLLED SUBSTANCES WHILE POSSESSING SUSPENDED LICENSE 08/22/85 THROUGH 01/31/86. LICENSE SUSPENDED 08/05/85 FOR PRESCRIBING EXCESSIVE AMOUNTS OF CONTROLLED SUBSTANCES. SURRENDER OF PARTIAL REGISTRATION.

WALLACE, SCOTT PYPER MD OF PROVO, UT, WAS DISCIPLINED BY UTAH ON SEPTEMBER 27, 1999
DISCIPLINARY ACTION: SURRENDER OF LICENSE
OFFENSE: PRACTICING WITHOUT A VALID CONTROLLED SUBSTANCE LICENSE

NOTES: WROTE TEN PRESCRIPTIONS FOR SCHEDULES III-V CONTROLLED SUBSTANCES WITHOUT A VALID CONTROLLED SUBSTANCE LICENSE. VOLUNTARY SURRENDER.

WARBURTON, ROBERT L MD OF SALT LAKE CITY, UT, WAS DISCIPLINED BY UTAH ON NOVEMBER 2, 1999
DISCIPLINARY ACTION: LICENSE SUSPENSION
OFFENSE: FAILURE TO COMPLY WITH PREVIOUS BOARD ORDER

NOTES: FAILED TO SUBMIT TO A MENTAL AND PHYSICAL EVALUATION AS ORDERED.

WARDEN, DAVID R MD, DATE OF BIRTH JANUARY 6, 1938 OF 625 SOUTH GRAND OAKS, FRUIT HEIGHTS, UT, WAS DISCIPLINED BY MEDICARE ON NOVEMBER 4, 1991
DISCIPLINARY ACTION: 48-MONTH EXCLUSION FROM THE MEDICARE AND/OR MEDICAID PROGRAM
OFFENSE: CRIMINAL CONVICTION OR PLEA OF GUILTY, NOLO CONTENDERE, OR NO CONTEST TO A CRIME

NOTES: CONVICTION FOR PATIENT ABUSE OR NEGLECT.

REINSTATED ON 1/24/96.

WARREN, STEVEN E MD OF MONTICELLO, UT, WAS DISCIPLINED BY UTAH ON MAY 5, 1993
DISCIPLINARY ACTION: 60-MONTH PROBATION
OFFENSE: PROFESSIONAL MISCONDUCT

NOTES: UNLAWFULLY USING AND OBTAINING CONTROLLED SUBSTANCES; CONTAMINATION OF MULTI-DOSE CONTROLLED SUBSTANCE; FAILURE TO MAINTAIN ADEQUATE CONTROLLED SUBSTANCE RECORDS; FALSIFYING PRESCRIPTIONS FOR CONTROLLED SUBSTANCES. DEA REGISTRATION REVOKED. LICENSE REVOKED WITH A STAY OF ENFORCEMENT ON HIS REVOCATION. LICENSE TO PRESCRIBE AND ADMINISTER CONTROLLED SUBSTANCES HAD BEEN VOLUNTARILY SURRENDERED IN 10/92. SHALL NOT APPLY FOR REINSTATEMENT OF THAT LICENSE FOR AT LEAST TWO YEARS. ON 6/5/95 HIS LICENSE TO PRESCRIBE AND ADMINISTER CONTROLLED SUBSTANCES SCHEDULES II-V WAS REINSTATED AND ISSUED WITH FULL PRIVILEGES. ON 8/28/95 LICENSE TO PRESCRIBE AND ADMINISTER CONTROLLED SUBSTANCES CHANGED TO SCHEDULES III-V ONLY TO COMPLY WITH FEDERAL RULES AND THE ASSESSMENT MADE BY DEA. ON 6/19/97 ORDER AMENDED ADDING SCHEDULE II TO HIS LICENSE TO PRESCRIBE AND ADMINISTER CONTROLLED SUBSTANCES.

WARREN, STEVEN E MD, DATE OF BIRTH APRIL 7, 1952, LICENSE NUMBER 0026991 OF MONTICELLO, UT, WAS DISCIPLINED BY COLORADO ON DECEMBER 17, 1993
DISCIPLINARY ACTION: 36-MONTH RESTRICTION PLACED ON LICENSE; MONITORING OF PHYSICIAN PERFORMANCE
OFFENSE: CRIMINAL CONVICTION OR PLEA OF GUILTY, NOLO CONTENDERE, OR NO CONTEST TO A CRIME

NOTES: CONVICTION OF A FELONY; CONVICTION OF A VIOLATION OF FEDERAL LAW REGULATING THE POSSESSION, DISTRIBUTION, OR USE OF ANY CONTROLLED SUBSTANCE; ADMINISTERING, DISPENSING OR PRESCRIBING OR A CONTROLLED SUBSTANCE OTHER THAN IN THE COURSE OF LEGITIMATE PROFESSIONAL PRACTICE; EXCESSIVE USE OF A CONTROLLED SUBSTANCE; SELF-PRESCRIBING OF A CONTROLLED SUBSTANCE. REVOCATION STAYED FOR FIVE YEARS, PENDING COMPLIANCE WITH ALL TERMS OF THE STIPULATION, INCLUDING A PROHIBITION OF ANY MEDICAL PRACTICE IN COLORADO FOR THREE YEARS AND PRACTICE AND TREATMENT MONITORING UPON RESUMPTION OF ANY PRACTICE IN THIS STATE.

WARREN, STEVEN E MD OF 2075 NORTH 1200 WEST, LAYTON, UT, WAS DISCIPLINED BY DEA ON MAY 23, 1996
DISCIPLINARY ACTION: RESTRICTION PLACED ON CONTROLLED SUBSTANCE LICENSE
OFFENSE: CRIMINAL CONVICTION OR PLEA OF GUILTY, NOLO CONTENDERE, OR NO CONTEST TO A CRIME

NOTES: CONTROLLED SUBSTANCES.

WARREN, STEVEN E MD OF OGDEN, UT, WAS DISCIPLINED BY UTAH ON MARCH 11, 1999
DISCIPLINARY ACTION: 12-MONTH PROBATION; 12-MONTH CONTROLLED SUBSTANCE LICENSE PLACED ON PROBATION
OFFENSE: PROFESSIONAL MISCONDUCT

NOTES: HE PRESCRIBED THE MEDICATION STADOL TO FAMILY MEMBERS AND HE FAILED TO MAINTAIN PATIENT RECORDS. PROBATION WITH CONDITIONS AND RESTRICTIONS.

WASHBURN, PHILIP MD OF SPRINGVILLE, UT, WAS DISCIPLINED BY UTAH ON JUNE 18, 1996
DISCIPLINARY ACTION: SURRENDER OF CONTROLLED SUBSTANCE LICENSE
OFFENSE: OVERPRESCRIBING OR MISPRESCRIBING DRUGS

NOTES: THERE WAS A DIVISION INVESTIGATION INTO ISSUES RELATING TO HIS PRESCRIBING OF CONTROLLED SUBSTANCES. VOLUNTARY SURRENDER.

WEITZEL, ROBERT MD, LICENSE NUMBER H2895 OF SALT LAKE CITY, UT, WAS DISCIPLINED BY TEXAS ON OCTOBER 24, 1998
DISCIPLINARY ACTION: FINE; REPRIMAND
OFFENSE: DISCIPLINARY ACTION BY ANOTHER STATE OR AGENCY

NOTES: IN 1992 AFTER COMPLETING A PSYCHIATRY RESIDENCY IN CALIFORNIA AND TERMINATING HIS PHYSICIAN-PATIENT RELATIONSHIPS WITH ALL PATIENTS, HE RECEIVED A TELEPHONE CALL FROM A FORMER PATIENT WHOM HE HAD TREATED FOR DEPRESSION WHO WISHED TO BECOME INVOLVED IN A PERSONAL RELATIONSHIP WITH HIM; HE ENGAGED IN AN INTIMATE PERSONAL RELATIONSHIP WITHOUT ALLOWING SUFFICIENT TIME TO ELAPSE FROM THE DATE OF THE TERMINATION OF THE PHYSICIAN-PATIENT RELATIONSHIP TO THE ESTABLISHMENT OF THE PERSONAL RELATIONSHIP WHICH LASTED TWO YEARS; THE FORMER PATIENT FILED A LAWSUIT IN CALIFORNIA AGAINST HIM ALLEGING BOUNDARY VIOLATIONS IN THE CONTEXT OF THE PRIOR PHYSICIAN-PATIENT RELATIONSHIP WHICH HE HAS STEADFASTLY DENIED; LAWSUIT RESOLVED FOR WHAT HE CONSIDERED NUISANCE VALUE; HE SUBSEQUENTLY FAILED TO DISCLOSE THE MALPRACTICE SETTLEMENT AS WELL AS CALIFORNIA LICENSURE SURRENDER TO THE TEXAS BOARD, AND SUBMITTED AN INCORRECT RESPONSE TO A RELEVANT QUESTION ON HIS LICENSURE RENEWAL FORM FOR 1997; HAS ADMITTED THAT SUCH CONDUCT WAS IMPROPER; SINCE THE EVENTS WHICH LED TO HIS VOLUNTARY SURRENDER OF HIS CALIFORNIA LICENSE, HE HAS CEASED ENGAGING IN PSYCHOTHERAPY AND PRACTICES PSYCHIATRY WITH A PRIMARY FOCUS ON MEDICATION THERAPY. $3,500 FINE.

WEITZEL, ROBERT A MD OF SALT LAKE CITY, UT, WAS DISCIPLINED BY UTAH ON AUGUST 24, 1999
DISCIPLINARY ACTION: LICENSE SUSPENSION
OFFENSE: FAILURE TO COMPLY WITH PREVIOUS BOARD ORDER

NOTES: ON 8/13/99 FAILED TO SUBMIT TO AN EXAM AS ORDERED BY THE DIVISION.

WEITZEL, ROBERT ALLAN MD, LICENSE NUMBER A48888 OF SAN DIEGO, CA, WAS DISCIPLINED BY CALIFORNIA ON MARCH 27, 1997
DISCIPLINARY ACTION: SURRENDER OF LICENSE

NOTES: WHILE CHARGES PENDING.

WERNER, SCOTT RULON MD OF CEDAR CITY, UT, WAS DISCIPLINED BY UTAH ON FEBRUARY 24, 1998
DISCIPLINARY ACTION: 12-MONTH PROBATION; 12-MONTH CONTROLLED SUBSTANCE LICENSE PLACED ON PROBATION
OFFENSE: OVERPRESCRIBING OR MISPRESCRIBING DRUGS

NOTES: ALLEGATIONS THAT HE PRESCRIBED CONTROLLED SUBSTANCES IN EXCESS OF WHAT WAS MEDICALLY NECESSARY TO TREAT HIS PATIENT'S MEDICAL CONDITIONS. PROBATION WITH CONDITIONS AND ONE RESTRICTION. ON 4/8/98 THE PROBATIONARY CONDITION REQUIRING HIM TO PRACTICE MEDICINE UNDER THE SUPERVISION OF ANOTHER PHYSICIAN WAS DELETED AND REPLACED WITH A CONDITION THAT REQUIRED HIM TO WRITE ALL CONTROLLED SUBSTANCE PRESCRIPTIONS IN TRIPLICATE FORM AND PROVIDE THE BOARD WITH A COPY OF EACH SCRIPT WRITTEN. PROBATIONS TERMINATED AND LICENSES REINSTATED WITH FULL PRIVILEGES ON 2/25/99.

WHITE, GARY BANKS MD OF ROOSEVELT, UT, WAS DISCIPLINED BY UTAH ON AUGUST 12, 1990
DISCIPLINARY ACTION: 6-MONTH SUSPENSION OF CONTROLLED SUBSTANCE LICENSE; 60-MONTH PROBATION
OFFENSE: OVERPRESCRIBING OR MISPRESCRIBING DRUGS

NOTES: PRESCRIBED CONTROLLED SUBSTANCES TO A DRUG DEPENDENT PERSON, PRESCRIBED CONTROLLED SUBSTANCES IN EXCESSIVE QUANTITIES, AND FAILED TO DOCUMENT PATIENT RECORDS WITH RESPECT TO PRESCRIBING OF CONTROLLED SUBSTANCES. AFTER 6 MONTH SUSPENSION, CONTROLLED SUBSTANCE LICENSE SHALL BE PLACED ON FIVE YEAR PROBATION.

WHITE, GARY BANKS MD OF 210 WEST 300 NORTH 75-3, ROOSEVELT, UT, WAS DISCIPLINED BY DEA ON SEPTEMBER 28, 1990
DISCIPLINARY ACTION: SURRENDER OF CONTROLLED SUBSTANCE LICENSE
OFFENSE: DISCIPLINARY ACTION BY ANOTHER STATE OR AGENCY

NOTES: DISCIPLINED BY UTAH FOR PRESCRIBING TO ADDICTS IN 08/85. PRESCRIBED EXCESSIVE CONTROLLED SUBSTANCE TO ADDICTS.

WHITE, GARY BANKS MD OF ROOSEVELT, UT, WAS DISCIPLINED BY UTAH ON FEBRUARY 21, 1991
DISCIPLINARY ACTION: CONTROLLED SUBSTANCE LICENSE PLACED ON PROBATION

NOTES: SUSPENSION ON LICENSE TO PRESCRIBE AND ADMINISTER CONTROLLED SUBSTANCES WAS TERMINATED. THIS LICENSE PLACED ON PROBATION CONSISTENT WITH THE TERMS AND CONDITIONS OF 8/12/90 ORDER. ON 12/23/96 PROBATIONS ON LICENSES TO PRACTICE MEDICINE AND TO PRESCRIBE AND ADMINISTER CONTROLLED SUBSTANCES TERMINATED AND LICENSES WERE REINSTATED WITH FULL PRIVILEGES.

WILLIAMS, RYMAL G MD OF CEDAR CITY CLINIC, CEDAR CITY, UT, WAS DISCIPLINED BY DEA ON MAY 2, 1994
DISCIPLINARY ACTION: SURRENDER OF CONTROLLED SUBSTANCE LICENSE

NOTES: IN LIEU OF ORDER TO SHOW CAUSE.

WILLIAMS, RYMAL GRAFF MD OF CEDAR CITY, UT, WAS DISCIPLINED BY UTAH ON MARCH 22, 1994
DISCIPLINARY ACTION: SURRENDER OF CONTROLLED SUBSTANCE LICENSE

NOTES: VOLUNTARILY SURRENDERED LICENSE TO PRESCRIBE AND ADMINISTER CONTROLLED SUBSTANCES SCHEDULES II-V ACKNOWLEDGING THERE IS A PENDING INVESTIGATION WITH RESPECT TO THAT LICENSE.

WILMOTH, JON DARRELL MD OF BONNERS FERRY, ID, WAS DISCIPLINED BY UTAH ON MARCH 30, 1999
DISCIPLINARY ACTION: 24-MONTH PROBATION; RESTRICTION PLACED ON LICENSE
OFFENSE: SEXUAL ABUSE OF OR SEXUAL MISCONDUCT WITH A

PATIENT

NOTES: ENGAGED IN INTIMATE AND SEXUALLY-RELATED CONTACT WITH A PATIENT AND FAILED TO TIMELY TRANSFER MEDICAL RECORDS OF FORMER PATIENTS WHEN REQUESTED TO DO SO. LICENSE TO PRACTICE MEDICINE WAS REVOKED WITH A STAY OF ENFORCEMENT ON THE REVOCATION.

WOLKOFF, KENNETH A MD OF PALM BEACH GARDENS, FL, WAS DISCIPLINED BY UTAH ON APRIL 10, 1991
DISCIPLINARY ACTION: 36-MONTH CONTROLLED SUBSTANCE LICENSE PLACED ON PROBATION
OFFENSE: OVERPRESCRIBING OR MISPRESCRIBING DRUGS

NOTES: UNPROFESSIONAL PRESCRIBING PRACTICES AND/OR PRESCRIBING CONTROLLED SUBSTANCES IN EXCESSIVE QUANTITIES. ON 5/24/94 PROBATION ON HIS LICENSE TO PRESCRIBE AND ADMINISTER CONTROLLED SUBSTANCES WAS TERMINATED AND HIS LICENSE WAS REINSTATED WITH FULL PRIVILEGES.

WOLKOFF, KENNETH A MD, LICENSE NUMBER 0G27484 OF PALM BEACH GARDENS, FL, WAS DISCIPLINED BY CALIFORNIA ON JUNE 10, 1993
DISCIPLINARY ACTION: LICENSE REVOCATION

WOLKOFF, KENNETH A MD, LICENSE NUMBER 0G27484 OF PALM BEACH GARDENS, FL, WAS DISCIPLINED BY CALIFORNIA ON AUGUST 15, 1994
DISCIPLINARY ACTION: 60-MONTH PROBATION
OFFENSE: DISCIPLINARY ACTION BY ANOTHER STATE OR AGENCY

NOTES: DISCIPLINED BY UTAH BOARD FOR EXCESSIVE PRESCRIBING OF OXYCODONE OR HYDROCODONE TO THREE PATIENTS. REVOCATION STAYED.

WOLKOFF, KENNETH A MD, LICENSE NUMBER 0130957 OF PO BOX 358, OCEAN CITY, NY, WAS DISCIPLINED BY NEW YORK ON AUGUST 24, 1994
DISCIPLINARY ACTION: LICENSE REVOCATION
OFFENSE: DISCIPLINARY ACTION BY ANOTHER STATE OR AGENCY

NOTES: DISCIPLINARY ACTION TAKEN BY UTAH AND CALIFORNIA BOARDS.

WOLKOFF, KENNETH A MD, LICENSE NUMBER 0004277 OF 13768 SAND CRANE DRIVE, PALM BEACH GARDENS, FL, WAS DISCIPLINED BY HAWAII ON DECEMBER 14, 1994
DISCIPLINARY ACTION: 24-MONTH PROBATION; RESTRICTION PLACED ON CONTROLLED SUBSTANCE LICENSE
OFFENSE: DISCIPLINARY ACTION BY ANOTHER STATE OR AGENCY

NOTES: ENTERED INTO A SETTLEMENT AGREEMENT WITH THE UTAH BOARD ON 4/5/91 WHICH INCLUDED A 3 YEAR PROBATION ON HIS LICENSE TO PRESCRIBE CONTROLLED SUBSTANCES; THE ORDER WAS BASED ON PRESCRIPTION VIOLATIONS; LICENSE REINSTATED WITH FULL PRIVILEGES ON 5/24/94. BASED ON THE UTAH ACTION CALIFORNIA LICENSE WAS PLACED ON PROBATION FOR FIVE YEARS ON 8/15/94. NEITHER OF THESE ACTIONS WAS REPORTED TO HAWAII. DR. WOLKOFF REPRESENTS THAT ALTHOUGH HE SIGNED UTAH AGREEMENT CERTAIN FACTS WERE INACCURATE AND HE BELIEVED HE WOULD HAVE THE OPPORTUNITY TO SUBMIT FURTHER FACTS AND THAT HE WAS UNAWARE OF THE REPORTING PROVISIONS IN HAWAII. CONDITIONS OF THE HAWAII ORDER: SHALL INFORM THE BOARD IF HE MOVES TO HAWAII AND INTENDS TO PRACTICE; TERMS OF PROBATION WILL BE ESTABLISHED BY THE BOARD; IF HE TREATS PATIENTS DURING SHORT TRIPS TO HAWAII SHALL NOT PRESCRIBE ANY SCHEDULE I THROUGH III CONTROLLED SUBSTANCES; SHALL PAY $250 TO THE COMPLIANCE RESOLUTION FUND.

WOLKOFF, KENNETH A MD, DATE OF BIRTH MAY 14, 1948 OF 13768 SAND CRANE DRIVE, PALM BEACH GARDEN, FL, WAS DISCIPLINED BY MEDICARE ON FEBRUARY 13, 1996
DISCIPLINARY ACTION: EXCLUSION FROM THE MEDICARE AND/OR MEDICAID PROGRAM
OFFENSE: DISCIPLINARY ACTION BY ANOTHER STATE OR AGENCY

NOTES: LICENSE REVOKED FOR REASONS BEARING ON PROFESSIONAL COMPETENCE.

WOOD, JOHN R MD, DATE OF BIRTH DECEMBER 17, 1947 OF 1845 WEST 4400 SOUTH, ROY, UT, WAS DISCIPLINED BY MEDICARE ON JULY 23, 1991
DISCIPLINARY ACTION: 60-MONTH EXCLUSION FROM THE MEDICARE AND/OR MEDICAID PROGRAM
OFFENSE: CRIMINAL CONVICTION OR PLEA OF GUILTY, NOLO CONTENDERE, OR NO CONTEST TO A CRIME

NOTES: PROGRAM-RELATED CONVICTION. REINSTATED ON 8/21/96.

WOOD, JOHN RUSSELL MD OF OGDEN, UT, WAS DISCIPLINED BY UTAH ON NOVEMBER 18, 1991
DISCIPLINARY ACTION: 12-MONTH PROBATION
OFFENSE: INSURANCE, MEDICARE OR MEDICAID FRAUD

NOTES: MAKING FALSE STATEMENTS IN REPORTS OR CLAIM FORMS FOR REIMBURSEMENT FOR PROFESSIONAL SERVICES. FOUR OF FIVE YEARS OF PROBATION ARE CONDITIONALLY SUSPENDED UPON COMPLETION OF CONDITIONS. PROBATION TERMINATED AND LICENSE REINSTATED TO FULL PRIVILEGES ON 2/4/93.

WORKMAN, DAVID HENRY MD OF KAYSVILLE, UT, WAS DISCIPLINED BY UTAH ON OCTOBER 8, 1998
DISCIPLINARY ACTION: SURRENDER OF CONTROLLED SUBSTANCE LICENSE

NOTES: PENDING THE COMPLETION OF AN INVESTIGATION INTO HIS CONDUCT WITH CONTROLLED SUBSTANCES, HE AGREED TO VOLUNTARILY SURRENDER HIS LICENSE.

WORKMAN, DAVID HENRY MD, DATE OF BIRTH SEPTEMBER 22, 1957 OF 667 EAST 1250 SOUTH, KAYSVILLE, UT, WAS DISCIPLINED BY MEDICARE ON SEPTEMBER 20, 1999
DISCIPLINARY ACTION: EXCLUSION FROM THE MEDICARE AND/OR MEDICAID PROGRAM
OFFENSE: CRIMINAL CONVICTION OR PLEA OF GUILTY, NOLO CONTENDERE, OR NO CONTEST TO A CRIME

NOTES: CONVICTED OF A CRIME INVOLVING THE MEDICARE, MEDICAID, MATERNAL AND CHILD HEALTH SERVICES BLOCK GRANT OR BLOCK GRANTS TO STATES FOR SOCIAL SERVICES PROGRAMS.

YURTH, DANIEL A MD, DATE OF BIRTH APRIL 9, 1948 OF 3835 ADAMS, OGDEN, UT, WAS DISCIPLINED BY MEDICARE ON JANUARY 23, 1990
DISCIPLINARY ACTION: EXCLUSION FROM THE MEDICARE AND/OR MEDICAID PROGRAM
OFFENSE: DISCIPLINARY ACTION BY ANOTHER STATE OR AGENCY

NOTES: LICENSE REVOCATION OR SUSPENSION.

Public Citizen

Buyers Up • Congress Watch • Critical Mass • Global Trade Watch • Health Research Group • Litigation Group
Joan Claybrook, President

30+ Years of Consumer Activism

Dear Friend,

The year 2001 marks 30 years since a hardy group of enterprising young people came to the nation's capital to start an experiment in citizenship. The first "Nader's Raiders" showed special grit, integrity, and idealism that still serve us. You hold in your hands a book that is an example of the important work we do every day. Public Citizen is the only organization with the courage to write *Questionable Doctors*, because we are a completely independent organization representing citizens and consumers. I am writing to ask all buyers of *Questionable Doctors* to please help us continue this work by joining *Public Citizen* today.

When you join Public Citizen with a gift of $35 or more you'll get our monthly *Health Letter,* which will update you with new information important to your health and safety. You'll also receive our bi-monthly member publication *Public Citizen News*, which will keep you abreast of issues affecting citizens across the country.

We've helped purge cancer-producing additives from dozens of food products. We've pushed OSHA so that workplaces have fewer safety and health hazards. Many ineffective, unsafe drugs and medical devices have been forced from the market as a result of our tireless efforts. We have helped force government decision-making out of the smoke-filled back rooms. Still there is so much left to do.

We need to remove the flood of soft money polluting our political system, stop federal give-aways to corporate fat cats, rewrite unfair trade legislation that hurts American workers and weakens our environmental laws, pass new and improved laws to protect our health and safety, and compel federal agencies to enforce the laws we already have. *But we can't do it without you.*

To retain its independence, Public Citizen does not accept government or corporate funds. Our support comes from individual members who believe there should be full-time advocates of democratic principles working on their behalf and from foundation grants and publication sales. To remain effective, Public Citizen needs you. Please join us. As Ralph Nader reminds us, "together we *can* make a difference."

Sincerely,

Joan Claybrook
President

Ralph Nader, Founder

1600 20th Street NW • Washington, DC 20009-1001 • (202) 588-1000
www.citizen.org

Public Citizen

Corporations, trade associations and other special interest groups send lobbyists to Washington, D.C., to advance their very particular agendas. Most speak for business or industry.

Public Citizen speaks for you—
before Congress
in the courts,
in the hallways and offices of
federal regulatory agencies

Ralph Nader founded Public Citizen to empower ordinary citizens with a voice in the halls of power and to protect the rights of consumers.

Public Citizen exposes threats to health and safety and presses for freedom of information and public disclosure. We've won important victories for citizens and consumers on issues concerning health care, injury prevention, campaign finance reform, cutting corporate subsidies, and fair trade.

Join together with thousands of other like-minded citizens, and you can help transform many issues at the national level.

"There can be no daily democracy without daily citizenship."

—Ralph Nader, founder of Public Citizen

1971

■ Public Citizen founded by Ralph Nader as an organization dedicated to protecting health, safety and democracy.

1972

■ Public Citizen files lawsuit resulting in new compensation system for airline passengers on overbooked flights.

■ Public Citizen plays key role in creation of Consumer Product Safety Commission.

1973

■ In response to Public Citizen's suit, President Nixon's firing of Watergate prosecutor Archibald Cox is ruled illegal.

1974

■ Public Citizen persuades Congress to override President Ford's veto and pass major improvements to Freedom of Information Act.

1975

■ Public Citizen wins Supreme Court ruling forbidding lawyers and other professionals from price fixing.

■ Public Citizen successfully lobbies Congress for energy conservation legislation, including fuel economy requirements for cars.

1976

■ FDA bans Red Dye No. 2 after Public Citizen's four-year campaign against the carcinogenic food dye.

■ Public Citizen petition leads to FDA ban on use of cancer-causing chloroform in cough medicines and toothpaste.

1977

■ Public Citizen mobilizes citizens who persuade President Carter to halt construction of Clinch River breeder reactor.

■ Public Citizen challenges airline industry's failure to provide adequate seating for nonsmokers.

1978

■ Congress passes Public Citizen's National Consumer Cooperative Bill authorizing $300 million in seed money for consumer cooperatives.

■ Public Citizen is instrumental in stopping the spraying of DDT in airline passenger cabins to control Japanese beetles on California-bound flights.

1979

■ Public Citizen petition leads to an Environmental Protection Agency ban on use of DBCP, a pesticide proven to cause sterility in men.

■ Public Citizen helps defeat legislation raising sugar price supports, thereby saving consumers $300 million a year.

1980

■ Public Citizen publishes best-selling *Pills That Don't Work*, a consumer guide to ineffective drugs.

■ Public Citizen plays critical role in passage of Superfund law, which requires cleanup of toxic waste sites.

■ Public Citizen lawsuit forces government to keep records of closed-door proceedings of Chrysler bailout.

1981

■ Public Citizen helps thwart President Reagan's attempts to dismantle Clean Air Act and to diminish authority of Consumer Product Safety Commission.

1982

■ The arthritis drug Oraflex is withdrawn from the market after Public Citizen exposes deaths and injuries caused by the drug.

■ After an extensive campaign, cancer-causing urea formaldehyde is banned in home insulation.

1983

■ Public Citizen wins historic separation of powers case; Supreme Court strikes down legislative veto.

■ *Over the Counter Pills That Don't Work* is published and becomes a national best-seller.

■ Public Citizen participates in landmark Supreme Court decision overturning President Reagan's revocation of auto safety standards for automatic restraints such as air bags.

1984

■ Following AT&T's divestiture, Public Citizen mounts nationwide "Campaign for Affordable Phones" to oppose rate hikes for residential customers.

■ Public Citizen wins court order forcing EPA to recall 700,000 GM cars with faulty emission controls.

1985

■ FDA requires a Reye's Syndrome warning for children on aspirin labels following three-year campaign by Public Citizen.

■ Public Citizen reveals the locations of more than 250 work sites nationwide where workers have been exposed to hazardous chemicals.

1986

■ Congress requires health warning labels on chewing tobacco and snuff, capping Public Citizen's two-year campaign.

■ Public Citizen wins court order forbidding President from stopping expenditure of appropriated funds without express authorization from Congress.

1987

■ Public Citizen helps persuade Congress to pass legislation restricting the time banks can hold checks.

1988

■ After seven years of litigation by Public Citizen, the Occupational Safety and Health Administration (OSHA) imposes standards for exposure to cancer-causing ethylene oxide.

■ Public Citizen sells 400,000 copies of *Worst Pills/Best Pills*, a consumer guide to dangerous and ineffective drugs and their preferable alternatives.

1989

■ Public Citizen and Ralph Nader stop the $45,500 congressional pay raise, forcing Congress to take a smaller raise and ban honoraria.

■ Public Citizen helps persuade California voters to shut down Rancho Seco nuclear plant.

■ Public Citizen obtains court order forcing the FDA to require labels warning women that high-absorbency tampons are more likely to cause Toxic Shock Syndrome.

1990

■ Public Citizen court victory forces the Nuclear Regulatory Commission to issue mandatory training requirements for nuclear plant workers.

■ Public Citizen publishes *Who Robbed America?*, a citizen's guide to the savings and loan scandal that cost taxpayers billions of dollars.

1991

■ Public Citizen plays key role in passage of new auto and truck safety law requiring air bags and head injury protections, and limiting the expansion of big rigs.

■ Public Citizen publishes *They Love To Fly ...And It Shows,* exposing House members who took nearly 4,000 privately-funded trips in 1989-90.

1992

■ Public Citizen's four-year campaign leads the FDA to severely restrict use of silicone gel breast implants.

■ OSHA imposes standard to protect workers from cadmium, linked to lung cancer and kidney damage, after Public Citizen wins court order.

1993

■ Public Citizen wins landmark court victory that prevents destruction of electronic records of the White House under Presidents Reagan, Bush and Clinton.

■ Public Citizen plays a leading role in opposing the North American Free Trade Agreement (NAFTA), launching a new citizens' trade movement.

1994

■ Public Citizen helps to enlist nearly 100 cosponsors for single-payer health care reform bill modeled after the Canadian system.

■ Public Citizen helps win legislation protecting consumers from home equity scams.

1995

■ Congressional gift ban and lobbying registration reform enacted after major Public Citizen campaign.

■ Public Citizen successfully defends tobacco industry whistle-blower who released key documents to Congress and the FDA, against civil damages and criminal contempt charges.

1996

■ Public Citizen wins Supreme Court decision upholding the right of people injured by defective medical devices to sue for compensation.

■ Public Citizen forges historic settlement to secure release of Nixon's White House tapes after 15 years of litigation.

■ Public Citizen successfully opposes legislation mandating temporary transport of nuclear waste to Nevada for storage.

1997

■ Public Citizen leads multi-year campaign that results in defeat of damaging Fast Track trade authority.

1998

■ Public Citizen protests and helps force redesign of unethical AIDS research in Africa, which would have denied known effective treatment to HIV-positive pregnant women.

■ Public Citizen helps lead a global citizens' campaign that results in the scuttling of the Multilateral Agreement on Investments, a proposed global investment treaty.

■ Public Citizen wins passage of legislation mandating safer air bags to protect women and children.

■ Public Citizen releases latest compilation of *16,638 Questionable Doctors*, the only publicly available, national compendium of disciplined doctors.

1999

■ Public Citizen publishes third edition of its best-selling *Worst Pills, Best Pills*, a consumer's guide to avoiding drug-induced death or illness.

■ Public Citizen wins release of historic grand jury records relating to the 1948 indictment of alleged Soviet agent Alger Hiss.

■ Public Citizen publishes *Whose Trade Organization? Corporate Globalization and the Erosion of Democracy*, a book exposing the WTO's five-year record of weakening health, safety, environmental and labor standards.

■ Public Citizen works successfully to pass major truck safety legislation, which creates the new Federal Motor Carrier Safety Administration.

■ Public Citizen leads global coalition to organize massive demonstrations in Seattle against the unaccountable, undemocratic World Trade Organization.

2000

■ Public Citizen petition leads to ban on diabetes drug Rezulin after 63 deaths from liver toxicity.

■ Public Citizen releases latest compilation of *Questionable Doctors*, a national compendium of disciplined doctors.

Cut here to order or pass along to a friend.

ORDER FORM

Public Citizen

1600 20th Street, NW, Washington, DC 20009-1001
www.citizen.org

Publications from Public Citizen

Qty.	Item Description	Price	Subtotal
	F6672 *Worst Pills/Best Pills* 1999 ed.	$16	
	FQON *Questionable Doctors* 4-volume National Edition	$407.50	
	2000 Edition Questionable Doctors Regional Editions		
	FQ001 Arkansas, Louisiana, Mississippi	$23.50	
	FQ002 Alaska, Idaho, Montana, Oregon, Washington, Wyoming	$23.50	
	FQ003 Arizona, Colorado, Nevada, New Mexico, Utah	$23.50	
	FQ004 California, Hawaii	$23.50	
	FQ005 Connecticut, Maine, Massachusetts, New Hampshire, Rhode Island, Vermont	$23.50	
	FQ006 Delaware, New Jersey	$23.50	
	FQ007 District of Columbia, Maryland, Virginia	$23.50	
	FQ008 Florida	$23.50	
	FQ009 Alabama, Georgia	$23.50	
	FQ010 Illinois, Indiana	$23.50	
	FQ011 Iowa, Missouri	$23.50	
	FQ012 New York	$23.50	
	FQ013 Kentucky, North Carolina, South Carolina, Tennessee	$23.50	
	FQ014 Kansas, Nebraska, North Dakota, South Dakota	$23.50	
	FQ015 Oklahoma, Texas	$23.50	
	FQ016 Minnesota, Wisconsin	$23.50	
	FQ017 Michigan, Ohio	$23.50	
	FQ018 Pennsylvania, West Virginia	$23.50	
Subtotal (1)			

Public Citizen Membership/Newsletter Subscriptio

	Price	Subtotal
Basic Membership (includes *PC News*)	$20	
Combination Membership with *Health Letter*	$35	
Special Introductory subscription to *Worst Pills, Best Pills News* for 12 months	$10	
I want to help even more with an additional contribution		
Subtotal (2)		
Add (1) and (2)	TOTAL	

Ordered By:

Name ____________________

Address (National Edition can only be shipped to a street address)

____

____

City ____________ State ______ Zip ________

E-mail ____________________

Phone number (___) ____________________

Please use an additional sheet of paper for gift orders.

❑ Payment enclosed (check or money order payable to "Public Citizen")

❑ Charge to credit card ❑ VISA ❑ MC ❑ AMEX ❑ Discover

Credit Card # ____________________

Exp. Date ____________________

Signature ____________________

U.S. orders only. Please allow 6-8 weeks for delivery.

BOQDBK

Public Citizen

Health Research Group Publications

Questionable Doctors

www.questionabledoctors.org

This is the only state-by-state listing of doctors who have been disciplined by state and federal agencies—doctors who may be continuing to treat unsuspecting patients. Order for friends and family.

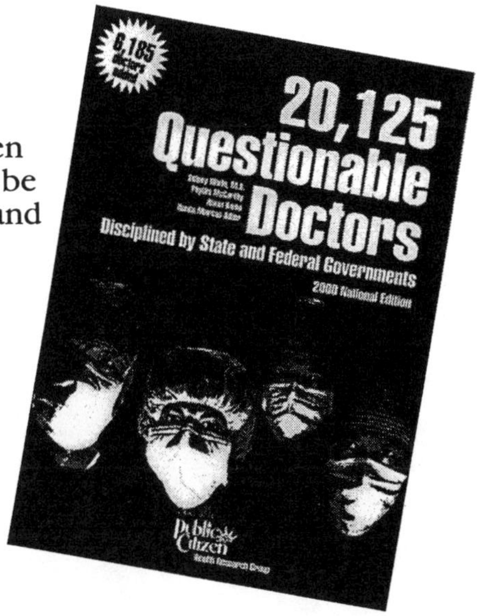

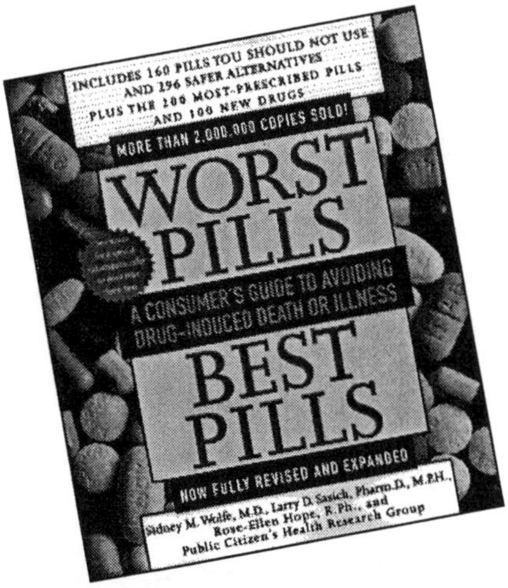

Worst Pills, Best Pills, 1999 edition

www.worstpills.org

What you can do to protect yourself and your loved ones from dangerous pharmaceuticals.

Pharmaceutical companies have gotten legislation passed to weaken FDA oversight of drug approvals. You can no longer be sure that just because a drug is on the market that it will be safe to use. *Worst Pills, Best Pills* is an excellent reference for you to find out which drugs are really safe, how to prevent adverse drug reactions, and which drugs should not be taken together. Every year, more and more drugs come onto the market. To stay up to date with the latest drugs, subscribe to *Worst Pills, Best Pills News.*

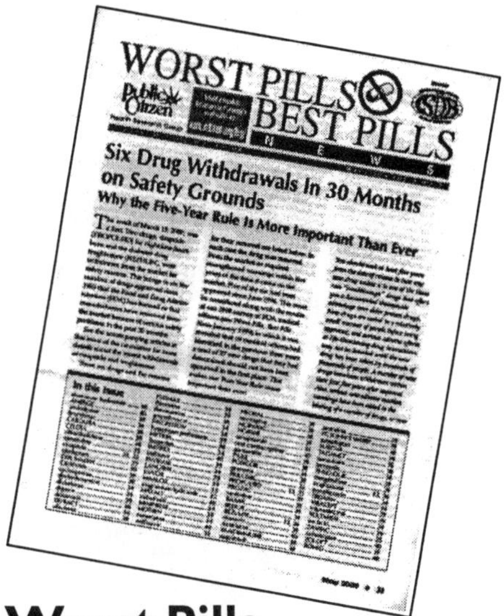

Worst Pills, Best Pills News

Get answers to your questions about the medical advice and care you receive—and how to ask your doctor important questions about the drugs prescribed for you. We are offering *Worst Pills, Best Pills News* at half price for new subscribers.

Order these publications by calling 1-877-747-1616 or use the form on the next page.